Williams' Basic Nutrition and Diet Therapy

15
EDITION

Williams' Basic Nutrition and Diet Therapy

Staci Nix, MS, RD, CD
Assistant Professor, Lecturer
Department of Nutrition and Integrative Physiology
Adjunct Faculty, School Of Medicine
University of Utah
Salt Lake City, Utah

ELSEVIER

ELSEVIER

3251 Riverport Lane
St. Louis, Missouri 63043

Library of Congress Cataloging-in-Publication Data

Names: Nix, Staci, author.
Title: Williams' basic nutrition and diet therapy / Staci Nix.
Other titles: Basic nutrition and diet therapy
Description: 15th edition. | St. Louis, Missouri : Elsevier/Mosby, [2017] | Includes bibliographical references and index.
Identifiers: LCCN 2016006019 | ISBN 9780323377317 (pbk. : alk. paper)
Subjects: | MESH: Diet Therapy | Nutritional Physiological Phenomena | Nutritional Requirements | Food Habits
Classification: LCC RM216 | NLM WB 400 | DDC 615.8/54—dc23 LC record available at http://lccn.loc.gov/2016006019

Director, Traditional Education: Kristin Geen
Content Development Manager: Laurie Gower
Senior Content Development Specialist: Lisa P. Newton
Publishing Services Manager: Jeff Patterson
Senior Project Manager: Tracey Schriefer
Design Direction: Renee Duenow

Printed in China

Last digit is the print number: 9 8 7 6 5 4 3 2

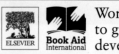

Working together
to grow libraries in
developing countries

www.elsevier.com • www.bookaid.org

Contributors and Reviewers

CONTRIBUTORS

Kelli Boi, MS, RD
Adjunct Nutrition Instructor
Weber State University
Ogden, Utah

Caiti Christensen, BS
Technician, Memorial Clinic
Sunset, Utah

Theresa Dvorak, MS, RDN, CSSD, ATC
Associate Instructor
Department of Nutrition and Integrative Physiology
University of Utah
Salt Lake City, Utah

Sara O. Harcourt, MPH, MS, RD
Clinical Dietitian
Salt Lake Regional Medical Center
Salt Lake City, Utah

Jennifer Schmidt, MS, RD
Clinical Nutrition Supervisor
University of Utah Healthcare
Salt Lake City, Utah

Kary Woodruff, MS, RD, CSSD
Associate Instructor
Department of Nutrition and Integrative Physiology
University of Utah
Salt Lake City, Utah

REVIEWERS

Penny Fauber, RN, BSN, MS, PhD
Program Head/Associate Professor
Director Practical Nursing Program
Dabney S. Lancaster Community College
Clifton Forge, Virginia

Janelle Hennes, MSN, RN
Clinical Instructor
Lead Instructor, On Campus and Off Campus BSN
    Program
College of Nursing and Health Innovation
University of Texas at Arlington
Arlington, Texas

Elizabeth A. Summers, MSN, RN, CNE
Coordinator of Practical Nursing Program
Cass Career Center
Harrisonville, Missouri

Nancy York, MSN, RN-BC
District 1199c Training & Upgrading Fund
Health & Technology Institute
Philadelphia, Pennsylvania

Preface to the Instructor

The field of nutrition is a dynamic human endeavor that is continuously expanding and evolving. Three main factors continue to change the modern face of nutrition. First, the science of nutrition continues to grow rapidly with exciting research. New knowledge in any science challenges some traditional ideas and lends to the development of new ones. Instead of primarily focusing on nutrition in the treatment of disease, we are expanding the search for disease prevention and general enhancement of life through nutrition and healthy lifestyles. Thus was the spirit during the establishment of the current Dietary Reference Intakes. Second, the rapidly increasing multiethnic diversity of the United States population enriches our food patterns and presents a variety of health care opportunities and needs. Third, the public is more aware and concerned about health promotion and the role of nutrition, largely because of the media's increasing attention. Clients and patients seek more self-directed involvement in their health care, and an integral part of that care is nutrition.

This new edition continues to reflect upon the evolving face of nutrition science. Its guiding principle is our own commitment, along with that of our publisher, to the integrity of the material. Our basic goal is to produce a new book for today's needs, with updated content, and to meet the expectations and changing needs of students, faculty, and practitioners of basic health care.

AUDIENCE

This text is primarily designed for students in licensed practical or vocational nursing (LPN/LVN) programs and associate degree programs (ADN/RN), as well as for diet technicians or aides. It is also appropriate for programs in various professions related to health care.

CONCEPTUAL APPROACH

The general purpose of this text is to introduce the basic scientific principles of nutrition and their applications in person-centered care. As in previous editions, basic concepts are carefully explained when introduced. In addition, our personal concerns are ever present, as follows: (1) that this introduction to the science and practice we love will continue to lead students and readers to enjoy learning about nutrition in the lives of people and stimulate further reading in areas of personal interest; (2) that caretakers will be alert to nutrition news and questions raised by their increasingly diverse clients and patients; and (3) that contact and communication with professionals in the field of nutrition will help build a strong team approach to clinical nutrition problems in all patient care.

ORGANIZATION

In keeping with the previous format, we have updated content areas to meet the needs of a rapidly developing science and society.

In **Part 1**, *Introduction to Basic Principles of Nutritional Science,* Chapter 1 focuses on the directions of health care and health promotion, risk reduction for disease prevention, and community health care delivery systems, with emphasis on team care and the active role of clients in self-care. Descriptions and illustrations accompany the new *Healthy People 2020* objectives, the *2015–2020 Dietary Guidelines for Americans,* and MyPlate guidelines. The Dietary Reference Intakes (DRIs) are incorporated throughout chapter discussions in Part 1 as well as throughout the rest of the text. New and improved illustrations for the visual learner are in this edition of the text for complicated metabolic pathways. Current research updates all of the basic nutrient and energy chapters in the remainder of Part 1.

In **Part 2**, *Nutrition throughout the Life Cycle,* Chapters 10, 11, and 12 reflect current material on human growth and development needs in different parts of the life cycle. Current National Academy of Science guidelines for positive weight gain to meet the metabolic demands of pregnancy and lactation are reinforced. Positive growth support for infancy, childhood, and adolescence is emphasized. The expanding health maintenance needs of a growing adult population through the aging process focus on building a healthy lifestyle to reduce disease risks. In all cases, statistics represent the most recent publications available at the time of print.

In **Part 3**, *Community Nutrition and Health Care,* a strong focus on community nutrition is coordinated with an emphasis on weight management and physical fitness as they pertain to health care benefits and risk reduction. The Nutrition Labeling and Education Act is discussed in terms of its current regulations and helpful label format as well as its effects on food marketing. Issues of malnutrition and the cycle of despair are discussed and illustrated in Chapter 13. Highlights of food-borne diseases reinforce concerns about food safety in a changing marketplace. Chapter 14 highlights information on America's multiethnic cultural food patterns and various religious dietary practices. New information on the topics of obesity and genetics, along with the use of alternative weight-loss methods, is included in Chapter 15 by a contributing author who is a certified specialist in weight management. Chapter 16 was written by a certified sports dietitian and discusses aspects of athletics, the proliferation of sports drinks, and the performance benefits of a well-hydrated and nourished athlete.

In **Part 4**, *Clinical Nutrition,* chapters are updated to reflect current medical nutrition therapy and approaches to nutrition education and management. As with previous editions, Drug-Nutrient Interaction boxes in this section address specific concerns with nutrition and medication interactions. Special areas include developments in gastrointestinal disease, heart disease, diabetes mellitus, renal disease, surgery, cancer, and HIV.

CONTENT AND FEATURES

- **Book format and design.** The chapter format and use of color continue to enhance the book's appeal. Basic chapter concepts and overview, illustrations, tables, boxes, definitions, headings, and subheadings make the content easier and more interesting to read.
- **Learning supplements.** Educational aids have been developed to assist both students and instructors in the teaching and learning process. Please see the *Ancillaries* section on the next page for more detailed information.
- **Illustrations.** Color illustrations, including artwork, graphs, charts, and photographs, help students and practitioners better understand the concepts and clinical practices presented.
- **Content threads.** This book shares a number of features—reading level; Key Concepts; Key Terms; Critical Thinking Questions; Chapter Challenge Questions; References; Further Reading and Resources; Glossary; and Cultural Considerations, For Further Focus, Drug-Nutrient Interactions, and Clinical Applications boxes—with other Elsevier books intended for students in demanding and fast-paced nursing curricula. These common threads help promote and hone the skills these students must master. (See the Content Threads page after this preface for more detailed information on these learning features.)

LEARNING AIDS

As indicated, this new edition is especially significant because of its use of many learning aids throughout the text.
- **Part openers.** To provide the "big picture" of the book's overall focus on nutrition and health, the

four main sections are introduced as successive developing parts of that unifying theme.
- **Chapter openers.** To immediately draw students into the topic for study, each chapter opens with a short list of the basic concepts involved and a brief chapter overview leading into the topic to "set the stage."
- **Chapter headings.** Throughout each chapter, the major headings and subheadings in special type or color indicate the organization of the chapter material, providing easy reading and understanding of the key ideas. Main concepts and terms also are highlighted with color or bold type and italics.
- **Special boxes.** The inclusion of For Further Focus, Cultural Considerations, Drug-Nutrient Interactions, and Clinical Applications boxes leads students a step further on a given topic or presents a case study for analysis. These boxes enhance understanding of concepts through further exploration or application.
- **Case studies.** In clinical care chapters, case studies are provided in **Clinical Applications** boxes to focus students' attention on related patient care problems. Each case is accompanied by questions for case analysis. Students can use these examples for similar patient care needs in their own clinical assignments.
- **Diet therapy guides.** In clinical chapters, medical nutrition therapy guides provide practical help in patient care and education.
- **Definitions of terms.** Key terms important to students' understanding and application of the material in patient care are presented in two ways. They are identified in the body of the text and are listed in a glossary at the back of the book for quick reference.
- **Summaries.** A brief summary in bulleted format reviews chapter highlights and helps students see how the chapter contributes to the book's "big picture." Students then can return to any part of the material for repeated study and clarification of details as needed.
- New **Chapter Review Questions.** In addition, self-test questions in multiple choice format are provided at the end of each chapter to allow students to test their basic knowledge of the chapter's contents.
- **References.** Background references throughout the text provide resources used in each chapter for students who may want to probe a particular topic of interest.
- **Further Reading and Resources.** To encourage further reading of useful materials, expand students' knowledge of key concepts, and help students apply material in practical ways for patient care and education, a brief list of annotated resources—including books, journals, and websites—is provided at the end of the book.

ANCILLARIES

TEACHING AND LEARNING RESOURCES FOR THE INSTRUCTORS

Instructor Resources on Evolve: available at www .evolve.elsevier.com/Williams/basic/—provides a wealth of material to help you make your nutrition instruction a success. In addition to all of the Student Resources, the following are provided for faculty:

- **TEACH Lesson Plans:** Based on textbook chapter Learning Objectives, serve as ready-made, modifiable lesson plans and a complete roadmap to link all parts of the educational package. These concise and straightforward lesson plans can be modified or combined to meet your particular scheduling and teaching needs.
- **Examview Test Bank:** Contains approximately 700 multiple-choice and alternate-format questions for the NCLEX Examination. Each question is coded for correct answer, rationale, page reference, Nursing Process Step, NCLEX Client Needs Category, and Cognitive Level.
- **Image Collection:** These images can be used in a unique presentation or as visual aids.
- **PowerPoint Presentations** with incorporated **Audience Response Questions** and unfolding **Case Study** to accompany each chapter guide classroom lectures.

FOR STUDENTS

- *Nutritrac Nutrition Analysis Program, Version 5.0 (Online):* The new edition of this popular tool is designed to allow the user to calculate and analyze food intake and energy expenditure, taking the guesswork out of nutrition planning. The new version features comprehensive databases containing more than 5000 foods organized into 18 different categories and more than 175 common/daily recreational, sporting, and occupational activities. The *Personal Profile* feature allows users to enter and edit the intake and output of an unlimited number of individuals, and the *Weight Management Planner* helps outline healthy lifestyles tailored to various personal profiles. In addition to foods and activities, new program features include an ideal body weight (IBW) calculator, a Harris-Benedict calculator to estimate total daily energy needs, and the complete *Exchange Lists for Meal Planning*.
- **Evolve Resources**
  - **Answers to Textbook Case Studies**—Answers to detailed case studies are found in specific chapters of the textbook.
  - **Case Studies** engage students with the opportunity to apply the knowledge they have learned in real-life situations.
- **Food Composition Tables** allow you to search the nutrient values of more than 5000 foods contained in *Nutritrac Nutrition Analysis Program, Version 5.0 (Online).* It is separated and alphabetized into 18 different food categories.
- **Infant and Child Growth Charts, United States** are available as useful handouts to encourage use of these valuable resources inside and outside of the classroom.
- **Self-Test Questions:** More than 350 self-assessment questions that provide students with practice questions and immediate feedback to help them prepare for exams.
- **Nutrition Resource Center website:** This informative website is available at http://nutrition .elsevier.com to provide the reader access to information about all Elsevier nutrition texts in one convenient location.

ACKNOWLEDGMENTS

Throughout this process, various staff members from Elsevier have kindly provided guidance and assistance, and I am grateful to all of them. I would like to especially acknowledge the professionalism, fortitude, and diligence of Kristin Geen, Director, Traditional Education; Laurie Gower, Content Development Manager; Lisa P. Newton, Senior Content Development Specialist; Tracey Schriefer, Senior Project Manager; and Beth Welch, Copyeditor. Your vision for this text is the true power behind the print.

I would like to acknowledge the hard work and dedication of Elsevier's Nursing Marketing Department for supporting this book through its many editions. Their ability to bridge the gap between a product and the end point—students who will hopefully learn from and enjoy this text—is integral to the success of this project. The contributions from content experts for Weight Management and Sports Nutrition by Theresa Dvorak and Kary Woodruff are cherished and lends an element of expertise to those chapters that will increase the value of the text overall. In addition, I am grateful to the reviewers who have provided constructive feedback on this edition. Your involvement provides the strength and thoroughness that no author can accomplish alone.

Finally, I want to thank my husband, family, and friends who have compassionately dealt with me and "the book." Your abundant support sustains me.

Staci Nix

Content Threads

The fifteenth edition of *Williams' Basic Nutrition and Diet Therapy* shares a number of learning features with other Elsevier titles used in nursing programs. These user-friendly Content Threads are designed to streamline the learning process among the variety of books and content areas included in this fast-paced and demanding curriculum.

Shared elements included in *Williams' Basic Nutrition and Diet Therapy,* fifteenth edition, include the following:

- **Reading level:** The easy-to-read and user-friendly format, as well as the often personal writing style, engage the reader and help unfold the information simply and effectively.
- **Cover design:** Graphic similarities help readers to instantly recognize the book as containing content and features relevant to today's nursing curricula.
- Bulleted lists of **Key Concepts** on each chapter opening page help focus the student on the "big picture" content presented.

- **Key Terms** presented in color are readily apparent throughout the book. In addition, key terms boxes presented on the book pages in which the terms are discussed provide complete definitions to help with memory association.
- New **Chapter Review Questions** presented in multiple-choice format help students test their comprehension of various content areas. Answers are provided in Appendix A at the end of this textbook.
- A complete list of **References** is accompanied by **Further Reading and Resources,** a section that includes a wealth of resources—books, journal articles, and websites—that supplement the information provided in the textbook.
- Four types of boxes—**Cultural Considerations, For Further Focus, Clinical Applications, and Drug-Nutrient Interaction**—explore current hot topics in nutrition today and provide insight beyond the information presented in the chapter text.

Preface to the Student

Williams' Basic Nutrition and Diet Therapy is a market leader in nutrition textbooks for support personnel in health care. It provides careful explanations of the basic principles of scientific nutrition and presents their applications in person-centered care in health and disease.

The author, Staci Nix, provides this important information in an easy-to-read, user-friendly format by including helpful learning tools throughout the text. Check out the following features to familiarize yourself with the book and help you get the most value out of this text.

A short list of **Key Concepts** and a brief **Chapter Overview** begin each chapter to immediately draw you into the subject at hand.

Key Terms Boxes throughout the text identify and define key terms important to your understanding and application of the material.

---

chapter

15

Weight Management

Theresa Dvorak, MS, RDN, CSSD, ATC

Key Concepts

- Underlying causes of obesity include a host of various genetic, environmental, and psychologic factors.
- Short-term food patterns or fads often stem from food misinformation that appeals to some human psychologic need; however, these fads do not necessarily meet physiologic needs.
- Realistic weight management focuses on individual needs and health promotion, including meal pattern planning and regular physical activity.
- Severe underweight carries physiologic and psychologic risk to the body.

Currently 68.5% of adults in the United States are overweight, of which 35% are obese and 6.4% are extremely obese. This epidemic—which results in large part from poor diet, physical inactivity, and genetics—is not limited to adults.[1] The National Center for Health Statistics reported that 17% of children and adolescents between the ages of 2 and 19 years are also obese.[1] Weight-loss diets are abundant and do not lack in variety with regard to the philosophy of the methods used to shed unwanted pounds. This variety also leads to greater confusion about weight-loss methods and expectations. Despite an apparent obsession with weight and the multibillion dollar industry of weight-loss diets and products, Americans continue to grow in undesirable directions (Figure 15-1). This chapter examines the problem of weight management and seeks a more positive and realistic health model that recognizes personal needs and sound weight goals.

OBESITY AND WEIGHT CONTROL

BODY WEIGHT VERSUS BODY FAT

Obesity develops from many interwoven factors—including personal, physical, psychologic, and genetic—and is difficult to pinpoint. As used in the traditional medical sense, *obesity* is a clinical term for excess body fat, and it is generally used to describe people who are at least 20% above a desired weight for height. The terms *overweight* and *obesity* are often used interchangeably, but they technically have different meanings. *Overweight* denotes a body weight that is above a population weight-for-height standard. Meanwhile, the word *obesity* is a more specific term that refers to the degree of fatness (i.e., the relative excess amount of fat in the total body composition). Over the past 5 decades, the percentage of obese adults (i.e., those with a body mass index [BMI] of 30 or greater) 20 years of age and older has increased from 13.4% of the

population to 35.3%.[2] Although the relative prevalence of overweight and obesity among adults in America has not increased in the past decade, it still remains at epidemic proportions.

Box 15-1 provides the classifications of BMI and the BMI chart is located on the inside back cover of the text. BMI can be tracked from childhood to adulthood with the Centers for Disease Control and Prevention growth charts (see Chapter 11). BMI is a reliable method of predicting the relative risk of becoming an overweight adult on the basis of the presence or absence of excess weight at various times throughout childhood. Children and adolescents who are overweight or obese are significantly more likely to continue to suffer from obesity as they age.[3]

Every person is different, and normal weight ranges vary in healthy people. Until recently, the important factor of age for setting a reasonable body weight for adults had been overlooked. With advancing age, body weight usually increases until approximately the age of 50 years for men and the age of 70 years for women, after which it declines.

The exclusive use of BMI to define obesity has undergone criticism because it does not measure body fat per se but rather total body weight relative to height. This method classifies some individuals as obese when they do not have excess body fat. For example, a football player in peak condition can be extremely "overweight" according to standard height/weight charts. In other words, he can weigh

body composition the relative sizes of the four body compartments that make up the total body: lean body mass (muscle mass), fat, water, and bone.
body mass index (BMI) the body weight in kilograms divided by the square of the height in meters (i.e., kg/m²).

245

x

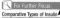
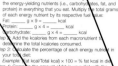
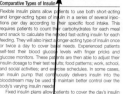
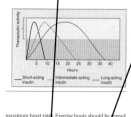
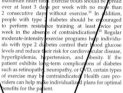

For Further Focus, Cultural Considerations, Clinical Applications, and **Drug-Nutrient Interaction boxes** take you one step further in the discussion of a given topic, enhancing your understanding of concepts through further exploration or application.

A bulleted **Summary** is included at the end of every chapter to review content highlights and help you see how particular chapters contribute to the book's overall focus.

New Chapter Review Questions are presented after each chapter summary for review and analysis and allow you to apply key concepts to patient care problems.

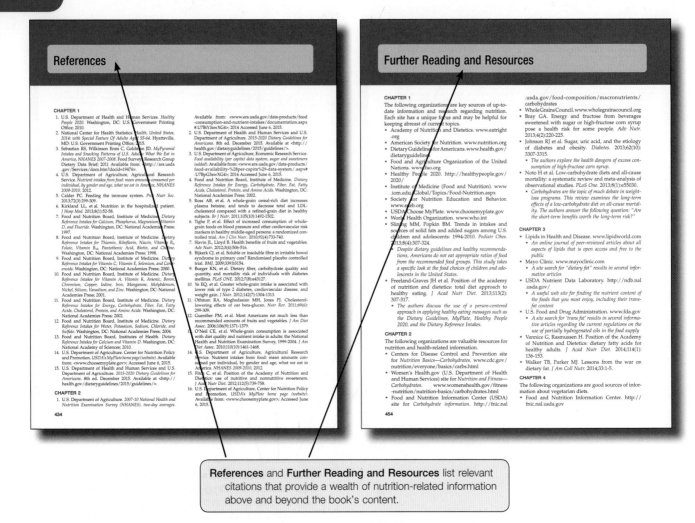

References and **Further Reading and Resources** list relevant citations that provide a wealth of nutrition-related information above and beyond the book's content.

Nutritrac Nutrition Analysis Program, Version 5.0 **(Online):** This popular tool is designed to allow the user to calculate and analyze food intake and energy expenditure, taking the guesswork out of nutrition planning. The new version features comprehensive databases containing more than 5000 foods organized into 18 different categories and more than 175 common/daily recreational, sporting, and occupational activities. The *Personal Profile* feature allows users to enter and edit the intake and output of an unlimited number of individuals, and the *Weight Management Planner* helps outline healthy lifestyles tailored to various personal profiles. In addition to foods and activities, new program features include an ideal body weight (IBW) calculator, a Harris-Benedict calculator to estimate total daily energy needs, and the complete *Exchange Lists for Meal Planning*.

Be sure to visit our two websites of interest.

1. An **Evolve** website has been created specifically for this book at http://evolve.elsevier.com/Williams/basic/. (See the Evolve page at the beginning of this text for more information.) The following exciting features are available:

- **Answers to Textbook Case Studies**—Answers to detailed case studies are found in specific chapters of the textbook.
- **Case Studies** are an integral tool to reinforce your understanding of key concepts and provide real-life examples.
- **Self-Test Questions** give you a chance to practice for your exams and receive immediate feedback.
- **Infant and Child Growth Charts, United States** are available as useful handouts to encourage use of these valuable resources inside and outside of the classroom.

2. A **Nutrition Resource Center** website is available at http://nutrition.elsevier.com to provide you access to all the Elsevier nutrition texts in one convenient location.

We are pleased that you have included *Williams' Basic Nutrition and Diet Therapy* as a part of your nutrition education. Be sure to check out our website at www.elsevierhealth.com for all your health science educational needs!

Contents

PART I   INTRODUCTION TO BASIC
          PRINCIPLES OF NUTRITION
          SCIENCE, 1

1 Food, Nutrition, and Health, 1

Health Promotion, 1
    Basic Definitions, 1
    Importance of a Balanced Diet, 2
Functions of Nutrients in Food, 3
    Energy Sources, 3
    Tissue Building, 4
    Regulation and Control, 4
Nutritional States, 5
    Optimal Nutrition, 5
    Malnutrition, 5
Nutrient and Food Guides for Health Promotion, 5
    Nutrient Standards, 5
    Food Guides and Recommendations, 7
    Individual Needs, 10

2 Carbohydrates, 12

Nature of Carbohydrates, 12
    Relation to Energy, 12
    Classes of Carbohydrates, 13
Functions of Carbohydrates, 20
    Basic Fuel Supply, 20
    Reserve Fuel Supply, 20
    Special Tissue Functions, 21
Food Sources of Carbohydrates, 21
    Starches, 21
    Sugars, 21
Digestion of Carbohydrates, 22
    Mouth, 22
    Stomach, 23
    Small Intestine, 23
Recommendations for Dietary Carbohydrate, 23
    Dietary Reference Intakes, 23
    Dietary Guidelines for Americans, 24
    MyPlate, 25

3 Fats, 27

The Nature of Fats, 27
    Dietary Importance, 27
    Structure and Classes of Fats, 27
    Classification of Fatty Acids, 27
Functions of Fat, 31
    Fat in Foods, 31
    Fat in the Body, 32

Food Sources of Fat, 32
    Variety of Sources, 32
    Characteristics of Food Fat Sources, 33
Food Label Information, 33
Digestion of Fats, 34
    Mouth, 34
    Stomach, 34
    Small Intestine, 34
    Digestibility of Food Fats, 37
Recommendations for Dietary Fat, 37
    Dietary Fat and Health, 37
    Dietary Reference Intakes, 39

4 Proteins, 41

The Nature of Proteins, 41
    Amino Acids, 41
    Classes of Amino Acids, 41
    Balance, 42
Functions of Protein, 44
    Primary Tissue Building, 44
    Additional Body Functions, 44
Food Sources of Protein, 44
    Types of Dietary Proteins, 44
    Vegetarian Diets, 45
Digestion of Proteins, 47
    Mouth, 47
    Stomach, 47
    Small Intestine, 48
Recommendations for Dietary Protein, 49
    Influential Factors of Protein Needs, 49
    Dietary Deficiency or Excess, 51
    Dietary Guides, 52

5 Digestion, Absorption, and Metabolism, 56

Digestion, 56
    Basic Principles, 56
    Mechanical and Chemical Digestion, 56
    Digestion in the Mouth and Esophagus, 58
    Digestion in the Stomach, 58
    Digestion in the Small Intestine, 59
Absorption and Transport, 60
    Absorption in the Small Intestine, 63
    Absorption in the Large Intestine, 65
    Transport, 65
Metabolism, 66
    Catabolism and Anabolism, 66
    Energy Density, 67
    Storing Extra Energy, 67

Errors in Digestion and Metabolism, 68
   The Genetic Defect, 68
   Other Intolerances or Allergies, 69

6 Energy Balance, 71

Human Energy System, 71
   Energy Needs, 71
   Measurement of Energy, 71
   Food as Fuel for Energy, 71
Energy Balance, 72
   Energy Intake, 72
   Energy Output, 73
Recommendations for Dietary Energy
   Intake, 80
   General Life Cycle, 80
   Dietary Reference Intakes, 80
   Dietary Guidelines for Americans, 80
   MyPlate, 80

7 Vitamins, 83

The Nature of Vitamins, 83
   Discovery, 83
   Definition, 84
   Functions of Vitamins, 84
   Vitamin Metabolism, 85
   Dietary Reference Intakes, 85
SECTION 1   FAT-SOLUBLE VITAMINS, 85
Vitamin A (Retinol), 85
   Functions, 85
   Requirements, 86
   Deficiency, 86
   Toxicity, 86
   Food Sources and Stability, 87
Vitamin D (Calciferol), 87
   Functions, 88
   Requirements, 88
   Deficiency, 89
   Toxicity, 89
   Food Sources and Stability, 89
Vitamin E (Tocopherol), 89
   Functions, 90
   Requirements, 90
   Deficiency, 90
   Toxicity, 90
   Food Sources and Stability, 90
Vitamin K, 91
   Functions, 91
   Requirements, 92
   Deficiency, 92
   Toxicity, 92
   Food Sources and Stability, 92
SECTION 2   WATER-SOLUBLE
VITAMINS, 93
Vitamin C (Ascorbic Acid), 93
   Functions, 93
   Requirements, 94
   Deficiency, 94
   Toxicity, 94
   Food Sources and Stability, 94

Thiamin (Vitamin B$_1$), 95
   Functions, 95
   Requirements, 95
   Deficiency, 95
   Toxicity, 96
   Food Sources and Stability, 96
Riboflavin (Vitamin B$_2$), 96
   Functions, 96
   Requirements, 96
   Deficiency, 96
   Toxicity, 96
   Food Sources and Stability, 96
Niacin (Vitamin B$_3$), 97
   Functions, 97
   Requirements, 97
   Deficiency, 97
   Toxicity, 97
   Food Sources and Stability, 98
Vitamin B$_6$, 98
   Functions, 98
   Requirements, 98
   Deficiency, 99
   Toxicity, 99
   Food Sources and Stability, 99
Folate, 99
   Functions, 99
   Requirements, 99
   Deficiency, 100
   Toxicity, 100
   Food Sources and Stability, 100
Cobalamin (Vitamin B$_{12}$), 101
   Functions, 101
   Requirements, 101
   Deficiency, 101
   Toxicity, 102
   Food Sources and Stability, 102
Pantothenic Acid, 102
   Functions, 102
   Requirements, 102
   Deficiency, 102
   Toxicity, 102
   Food Sources and Stability, 102
Biotin, 102
   Functions, 102
   Requirements, 103
   Deficiency, 103
   Toxicity, 103
   Food Sources and Stability, 103
Choline, 103
   Functions, 103
   Requirements, 103
   Deficiency, 103
   Toxicity, 105
   Food Sources and Stability, 105
SECTION 3   PLANT NUTRIENTS, 105
Phytochemicals, 105
   Function, 105
   Recommended Intake, 105
   Food Sources, 105

SECTION 4   NUTRIENT SUPPLEMENTATION, 106
Recommendations for Nutrient
    Supplementation, 106
    Life Cycle Needs, 107
    Lifestyle and Health Status, 107
Supplementation Principles, 107
    Basic Principles, 107
    Megadoses, 108
Functional Foods, 108

8 Minerals, 110

Nature of Minerals in Human Nutrition, 110
    Classes of Minerals, 110
    Functions of Minerals, 110
    Mineral Metabolism, 111
Major Minerals, 111
    Calcium, 111
    Phosphorus, 114
    Sodium, 116
    Potassium, 117
    Chloride, 118
    Magnesium, 119
    Sulfur, 119
Trace Minerals, 120
    Iron, 120
    Iodine, 123
    Zinc, 126
    Selenium, 127
    Fluoride, 128
    Copper, 128
    Manganese, 129
    Molybdenum, 129
    Chromium, 129
    Other Essential Trace Minerals, 129
Mineral Supplementation, 131
    Life Cycle Needs, 131
    Clinical Needs, 131

9 Water and Electrolyte Balance, 133

Body Water Functions and Requirements, 133
    Water: the Fundamental Nutrient, 133
    Body Water Functions, 133
    Body Water Requirements, 134
    Dehydration, 135
    Water Intoxication, 136
Water Balance, 136
    Body Water: the Solvent, 136
    Solute Particles in Solution, 138
    Separating Membranes, 139
    *Forces Moving Water and Solutes Across
        Membranes, 140*
    Capillary Fluid Shift Mechanism, 141
    Organ System Circulation, 141
    Hormonal Controls, 143
Acid-Base Balance, 144
    Acids and Bases, 144
    Buffer Systems, 145

PART 2 NUTRITION THROUGHOUT THE LIFE CYCLE, 147

10 Nutrition during Pregnancy and Lactation, 147

Nutritional Demands of Pregnancy, 147
    Energy Needs, 147
    Protein Needs, 148
    Key Mineral and Vitamin Needs, 149
    Weight Gain during Pregnancy, 151
    Daily Food Plan, 152
General Concerns, 152
    Gastrointestinal Problems, 152
    High-Risk Pregnancies, 153
    Complications of Pregnancy, 157
Lactation, 158
    Trends, 158
    The Baby-Friendly Hospital Initiative, 159
    Physiologic Process of Lactation, 159
    Nutrition and Lifestyle Needs, 163
    Long-Term Impacts of Feeding Methods, 163
    Additional Resources, 164

11 Nutrition during Infancy, Childhood, and Adolescence, 166

Growth and Development, 166
    Life Cycle Growth Pattern, 166
    Measuring Childhood Growth, 166
Nutritional Requirements for Growth, 167
    Energy Needs, 167
    Protein Needs, 171
    Water Requirements, 171
    Mineral and Vitamin Needs, 171
Nutrition Requirements during Infancy, 173
    Infant Classifications, 173
    *Considerations Regarding Feeding Premature
        Infants, 173*
    *What, How, and When to Feed the Mature
        Infant, 174*
Nutrition Requirements during
    Childhood, 178
    Toddlers (1 to 3 Years Old), 178
    Preschool-Aged Children (3 to 5 Years Old), 178
    School-Aged Children (5 to 12 Years Old), 178
    Nutrition Problems during Childhood, 180
Nutrition Requirements during Adolescence
    (12 to 18 Years Old), 183
    Physical Growth, 183
    Eating Patterns, 184
    Eating Disorders, 184

12 Nutrition for Adults: The Early, Middle, and Later Years, 186

Adulthood: Continuing Human Growth and
    Development, 186
    Coming of Age in America, 186
    *Shaping Influences on Adult Growth and
        Development, 187*

The Aging Process and Nutrition Needs, 190
   General Physiologic Changes, 190
   Nutrition Needs, 191
Clinical Needs of the Elderly, 193
   Health Promotion and Disease Prevention, 193
   Chronic Diseases of Aging, 197
Community Resources, 198
   Government Programs for Older Americans, 198
   Professional Organizations and Resources, 199
Alternative Living Arrangements, 200
   Congregate Care Arrangements, 200
   Continuing Care Retirement Communities, 200
   Assisted Living Facilities, 200
   Nursing Homes, 200

PART 3   COMMUNITY NUTRITION AND HEALTH CARE, 202

13   Community Food Supply and Health, 202

Food Safety and Health Promotion, 202
   The U.S. Food and Drug Administration, 202
   Food Labels, 203
Food Technology, 207
   Agricultural Pesticides, 207
   Food Additives, 210
Food-Borne Disease, 212
   Prevalence, 212
   Food Safety, 212
   Food Contamination, 215
Food Needs and Costs, 223
   Hunger and Malnutrition, 223
   Food Assistance Programs, 224
   Food Buying and Handling Practices, 225

14   Food Habits and Cultural Patterns, 228

Social, Psychologic, and Economic Influences on Food Habits, 228
   Social Impact, 228
   Factors That Influence Personal Food Choices, 228
Cultural Development of Food Habits, 229
   Strength of Personal Culture, 229
   Traditional Culture-Specific Food Patterns, 229
   Religious Dietary Laws, 238
Changing American Food Patterns, 241
   Household Dynamics, 241
   With Whom and Where We Eat, 243
   How Often and How Much We Eat, 243
   Economical Buying, 244

15   Weight Management, 245

Obesity and Weight Control, 245
   Body Weight versus Body Fat, 245
   Body Composition, 246
   Measures of Weight Maintenance Goals, 248
   Obesity and Health, 250
   Causes of Obesity, 250
   Individual Differences and Extreme Practices, 252

A Sound Weight-Management Program, 258
   Essential Characteristics, 258
   Behavior Modification, 258
   Dietary Modification, 258
Food Misinformation and Fads, 264
   Food Fads, 264
   What is the Answer?, 265
Underweight, 266
   General Causes and Treatment, 266
   Disordered Eating, 268

16   Nutrition and Physical Fitness, 272

Physical Activity Recommendations and Benefits, 272
   Guidelines and Recommendations, 272
   Health Benefits, 273
   Types of Physical Activity, 277
   Meeting Personal Needs, 278
Dietary Needs during Exercise, 279
   Muscle Action and Fuel, 279
   Fluid and Energy Needs, 280
   Macronutrient and Micronutrient Recommendations, 281
Athletic Performance, 282
   General Training Diet, 282
   Competition, 284
   Ergogenic Aids and Misinformation, 285

PART 4   CLINICAL NUTRITION, 288

17   Nutrition Care, 288

The Therapeutic Process, 288
   Setting and Focus of Care, 288
   Health Care Team, 288
Phases of the Care Process, 291
   Nutrition Assessment, 291
   Nutrition Diagnosis, 297
   Nutrition Intervention, 298
   Nutrition Monitoring and Evaluation, 299
Diet-Drug Interactions, 300
   Drug-Food Interactions, 300
   Drug-Nutrient Interactions, 301
   Drug-Herb Interactions, 301

18   Gastrointestinal and Accessory Organ Problems, 304

The Upper Gastrointestinal Tract, 304
   Mouth, 304
   Esophagus, 307
   Stomach and Duodenum: Peptic Ulcer Disease, 308
Lower Gastrointestinal Tract, 312
   Small Intestine Diseases, 312
   Large Intestine Diseases, 317
Food Intolerances and Allergies, 318
   Food Intolerances, 319
   Food Allergies, 319

Gastrointestinal Accessory Organs, 320
    Liver Disease, 321
    Gallbladder Disease, 324
    Pancreatic Disease, 325

19 Coronary Heart Disease and Hypertension, 327

Coronary Heart Disease, 327
    Atherosclerosis, 327
    Acute Cardiovascular Disease, 334
    Heart Failure, 336
Essential Hypertension, 338
    Incidence and Nature, 338
    Hypertensive Blood Pressure Levels, 339
    Principles of Medical Nutrition Therapy, 340
    Additional Lifestyle Factors, 343
Education and Prevention, 343
    Practical Food Guides, 343
    Education Principles, 344

20 Diabetes Mellitus, 347

The Nature of Diabetes, 347
    Defining Factor, 347
    Classification of Diabetes Mellitus and Glucose
        Intolerance, 347
    Symptoms of Diabetes, 352
The Metabolic Pattern of Diabetes, 352
    Energy Supply and Control of Blood
        Glucose, 352
    Abnormal Metabolism in Uncontrolled
        Diabetes, 355
    Long-Term Complications, 355
General Management of Diabetes, 357
    Early Detection and Monitoring, 357
    Basic Goals of Care, 357
Medical Nutrition Therapy for Individuals with
    Diabetes, 361
    Medical Nutrition Therapy, 361
    Total Energy Balance, 362
    Nutrient Balance, 362
    Food Distribution, 364
    Diet Management, 365

21 Kidney Disease, 371

Basic Structure and Function of the Kidney, 371
    Structures, 371
    Function, 373
Disease Process and Dietary Considerations, 373
    General Causes of Kidney Disease, 373
    Medical Nutrition Therapy in Kidney
        Disease, 375
Nephron Diseases, 375
    Acute Glomerulonephritis or Nephritic
        Syndrome, 375
    Nephrotic Syndrome, 375
Kidney Failure, 376
    Acute Kidney Injury, 376
    Chronic Kidney Disease, 378
    End-Stage Renal Disease, 380

Kidney Stone Disease, 386
    Disease Process, 387
    Medical Nutrition Therapy, 388

22 Surgery and Nutrition Support, 390

Nutrition Needs of General Surgery
    Patients, 390
    Preoperative Nutrition Care: Nutrient
        Reserves, 390
    Postoperative Nutrition Care: Nutrient Needs for
        Healing, 392
General Dietary Management, 394
    Initial Intravenous Fluid and
        Electrolytes, 394
    Methods of Nutrition Support, 395
Special Nutrition Needs after Gastrointestinal
    Surgery, 404
    Mouth, Throat, and Neck Surgery, 404
    Gastric Surgery, 405
    Bariatric Surgery, 405
    Gallbladder Surgery, 407
    Intestinal Surgery, 407
    Rectal Surgery, 408
Special Nutrition Needs for Patients with
    Burns, 408
    Type and Extent of Burns, 408
    Stages of Nutrition Care, 408

23 Nutrition Support in Cancer and HIV, 411

SECTION I   CANCER, 411
Process of Cancer Development, 411
    The Nature of Cancer, 411
    Causes of Cancer Cell Development, 411
    The Body's Defense System, 412
Nutrition Complications of Cancer
    Treatment, 413
    Surgery, 413
    Radiation, 413
    Chemotherapy, 414
    Drug-Nutrient Interactions, 414
Medical Nutrition Therapy in the Patient with
    Cancer, 414
    Nutrition Problems Related to the Disease
        Process, 414
    Basic Objectives of the Nutrition Plan, 415
    Medical Nutrition Therapy, 416
    Nutrition Management, 418
Cancer Prevention, 420
    American Cancer Society, World Cancer
        Research Fund, and the American Institute
        for Cancer Research: Guidelines for Cancer
        Prevention, 420
    Diets and Supplements Promoted as "Cancer
        Cures", 422
SECTION 2   HUMAN IMMUNODEFICIENCY
VIRUS, 422
Progression of Human Immunodeficiency
    Virus, 422

*Evolution of Human Immunodeficiency
    Virus, 422*
Parasitic Nature of the Virus, 423
Medical Management of the Patient with
    HIV/AIDS, 425
Initial Evaluation and Goals, 425
Drug Therapy, 426
Medical Nutrition Therapy, 430
Assessment, 430
Intervention, 430
*Wasting Effects of HIV on Nutritional
    Status, 430*

*Nutrition Counseling, Education, and Supportive
    Care, 431*
Personal Food Management Skills, 432

References, 434

Further Reading and Resources, 454

Glossary, 460

Appendix A, 470

Appendix B, 471

Appendix C, 480

Food, Nutrition, and Health

Key Concepts

- Optimal personal and community nutrition are major components of health promotion and disease prevention.
- Nutrients in food are essential to our health and well-being.

- Food and nutrient guides help us to plan a balanced diet that is in accordance with our individual needs and goals.

We live in a world of rapidly changing elements, including our environment, food supply, population, and scientific knowledge. Within different environments, our bodies, emotional responses, needs, and goals change. To be realistic within the concepts of change and balance, the study of food, nutrition, and health care must focus on **health promotion**. Although we may define health and disease in a variety of ways, the primary basis for promoting health and preventing disease must start with a balanced diet and the nutrition it provides. The study of nutrition is of primary importance in the following two ways: it is fundamental for our own health, and it is essential for the health and well-being of our patients and clients.

HEALTH PROMOTION

BASIC DEFINITIONS

Nutrition and Dietetics

Nutrition is the food people eat and how their bodies use it. **Nutrition science** comprises the body of scientific knowledge that governs nutrient requirements for all aspects of life such as growth, activity, reproduction, and maintenance. **Dietetics** is the health profession responsible for applying nutrition science to promote human health and treat disease. The **registered dietitian (RD),** who is also referred to as a *clinical nutrition specialist, a registered dietitian nutritionist,* or a *public health nutritionist,* is the nutrition authority on the health care team; this health care professional carries the major responsibility of nutrition care for patients and clients.

Health and Wellness

High-quality nutrition is essential for good health throughout life, beginning with prenatal life and continuing through old age. In its simplest terms, the word **health** is defined as the absence of disease.

However, life experience shows that the definition of health is much more complex. It must include extensive attention to the roots of health for the meeting of basic needs (e.g., physical, mental, psychologic, and social well-being). This approach recognizes the individual as a whole and relates health to both internal and external environments. The concept of *wellness* broadens this approach one step further. Wellness seeks the full development of potential for all people within their given environments. It implies a balance between activities and goals: work and leisure,

health promotion the active engagement in behaviors or programs that advance positive well-being.

nutrition the sum of the processes involved with the intake of nutrients as well as assimilating and using them to maintain body tissue and provide energy; a foundation for life and health.

nutrition science the body of science, developed through controlled research, that relates to the processes involved in nutrition internationally, clinically, and in the community.

dietetics the management of the diet and the use of food; the science concerned with nutrition planning and the preparation of foods.

registered dietitian (RD) a professional dietitian accredited with an academic degree from an undergraduate or graduate study program who has passed required registration examinations administered by the Commission on Dietetic Registration (CDR). The RD and RDN (registered dietitian nutritionist) credentials are legally protected titles that may only be used by authorized practitioners and by the CDR. The term *nutritionist* alone is not a legally protected title in most states and may be used by virtually anyone. See *www.eatright.org* for more details.

health a state of optimal physical, mental, and social well-being; relative freedom from disease or disability.

lifestyle choices and health risks, and personal needs versus others' expectations. The term *wellness* implies a positive dynamic state that motivates a person to seek a higher level of functioning.

National Health Goals

The wellness movement continues to be a fundamental response to the health care system's burden of illness and disease treatment and the rising costs of medical care. Since the 1970s, holistic health and health promotion have focused on lifestyle and personal choice when it comes to helping individuals and families develop plans for maintaining health and wellness. The U.S. national health goals continue to reflect this wellness philosophy. The most recent report in the *Healthy People* series published by the U.S. Department of Health and Human Services, *Healthy People 2020*, continues to focus on the nation's main objective of positive health promotion and disease prevention[1] (Figure 1-1). The guidelines encompass four overarching goals with the ultimate vision of a "society in which all people live long, healthy lives."[1]

A major theme throughout the report is the encouragement of healthy choices in diet, promotion of weight control, and education about other risk factors for disease, especially in the report's specific nutrition objectives. The *Healthy People 2020* topics, objectives, interventions, resources, and national data are all available on their website (www.healthypeople.gov). Some of the specific national goals under *Nutrition and Weight Status* include the following: promoting healthier food access, improving the presence of nutrition in the health care and worksite settings, improving the overall healthy weight status of the nation's population, reducing food insecurity, improving overall food and nutrient consumption, and reducing iron deficiency. Other objectives involving nutrition may be found under the topics *Adolescent Health, Diabetes, Education and Community-Based Programs, Food Safety,* and *Heart Disease and Stroke.*

Traditional and Preventive Approaches to Health

The preventive health care approach involves identifying risk factors in advance that increase a person's chances of developing a particular health problem. Knowing these factors, people can choose dietary and lifestyle behaviors that will prevent or minimize their risks for disease. Alternatively, the traditional health care approach only attempts change when symptoms of illness or disease already exist, at which point those who are ill seek a physician to diagnose, treat, and "cure" the condition (see the Drug-Nutrient Interaction box, "Introduction to Drug-Nutrient Interactions"). The traditional health care approach has much less value for lifelong positive health. Major chronic problems (e.g., heart disease, cancer, diabetes) may develop long before signs become apparent.

IMPORTANCE OF A BALANCED DIET

Signs of Good Nutrition

A lifetime of good nutrition is evidenced by a well-developed body, the ideal weight for height and body composition (i.e., the ratio of muscle mass to fat mass), and good muscle development. In addition, a healthy person's skin is smooth and clear, the hair is glossy, and the eyes are clear and bright. Appetite, digestion, and elimination are normal. Well-nourished people are more likely to be mentally and physically alert and to have a positive outlook on life. They are also more able to resist infectious diseases as compared with undernourished people. This is particularly important with our current trends of population growth and

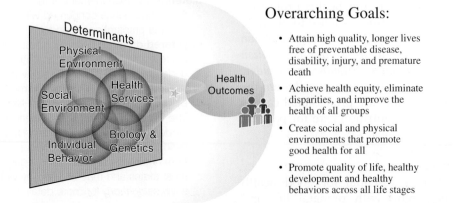

Healthy People 2020

A society in which all people live long, healthy lives

Overarching Goals:

- Attain high quality, longer lives free of preventable disease, disability, injury, and premature death

- Achieve health equity, eliminate disparities, and improve the health of all groups

- Create social and physical environments that promote good health for all

- Promote quality of life, healthy development and healthy behaviors across all life stages

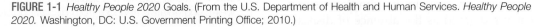

FIGURE 1-1 *Healthy People 2020* Goals. (From the U.S. Department of Health and Human Services. *Healthy People 2020.* Washington, DC: U.S. Government Printing Office; 2010.)

Drug-Nutrient Interaction

Introduction to Drug-Nutrient Interactions

SARA HARCOURT

Part of the traditional approach to medicine is "curing" the condition or disease. This often includes medications, surgery, or other interventions to alleviate symptoms or to treat the condition. For the purpose of the Drug-Nutrient Interaction boxes in this text, we will focus on the potential for interactions with nutrients in the diet and both over-the-counter and prescribed medications.

Drug regimens should be strictly followed. Many medications have potentially dangerous side effects, such as heart arrhythmias, hypertension, dizziness, and tingling in the hands and feet, when they are consumed inappropriately. Furthermore, some medications may interact with nutrients in food or dietary supplements, thereby creating a drug-nutrient interaction. The presence of food in the stomach may increase or decrease drug absorption, thus potentially enhancing or diminishing the effects of the intended medication. Dietary supplements that contain vitamins and minerals can be especially dangerous if they are consumed at the same time as a drug. Knowing which drugs are influenced by nutrients and how to work with a patient's diet is essential to the development of a complete medical plan.

In the following chapters of this book, look for the Drug-Nutrient Interaction boxes to learn about some of the more common interactions that may be encountered in the health care setting.

ever-increasing life expectancy. The national vital statistics report published in 2015 stated that life expectancy in the United States reached a high of 76.4 years for men and 81.2 years for women.[2]

Food and Health

Food is a necessity of life. However, many people are only concerned with food insofar as it relieves their hunger or satisfies their appetite and not with whether it supplies their bodies with all of the components of proper nutrition. Nutrients provided by the diet are further divided into the categories of essential, nonessential, and energy-yielding nutrients.

The six essential nutrients in human nutrition are the following:
1. Carbohydrates
2. Proteins
3. Fats
4. Vitamins
5. Minerals
6. Water

The core practitioners of the health care team (e.g., physician, dietitian, nurse) are all aware of the important part that food plays in maintaining good health and recovering from illness. Therefore, assessing a patient's nutritional status and identifying his or her nutrition needs are primary activities in the development of a health care plan.

FUNCTIONS OF NUTRIENTS IN FOOD

To sustain life, the nutrients in foods must perform the following three basic functions within the body:
1. Provide energy
2. Build tissue
3. Regulate metabolic processes

Metabolism refers to the sum of all body processes that accomplish the basic life-sustaining tasks. Close metabolic relations exist among all nutrients and their metabolic products. This is the fundamental principle of *nutrient interaction,* which involves two concepts. First, the individual nutrients have many specific metabolic functions, including primary and supporting roles. Second, no nutrient ever works alone; this key principle of nutrient interaction is demonstrated more clearly in the following chapters. Although the nutrients may be separated for study purposes, remember that they do not exist that way in the human body or in the food that we eat. They always interact as a dynamic whole to produce and maintain the body.

ENERGY SOURCES

Human energy is measured in heat units called **kilocalories,** which is abbreviated as *kcalories* or *kcal* (see Chapter 6). Of the six essential nutrients, there are three energy-yielding nutrients. These include carbohydrates, fat, and protein. The only other energy-yielding substance in the diet comes from alcohol. Because alcohol has no essential function in the body, it is not a *nutrient.* Although not a nutrient, alcohol does provide energy. There are 7 kcal/gram of alcohol.

---

essential nutrient nutrients a person must obtain from food because the body cannot make them for itself in sufficient quantity to meet physiologic needs.

nonessential nutrient a nutrient that can be manufactured in the body by means of other nutrients. Thus, it is not essential to consume this nutrient regularly in the diet.

energy-yielding nutrient nutrients that break down to yield energy within the body, including carbohydrates, fat, and protein.

metabolism the sum of all chemical changes that take place in the body by which it maintains itself and produces energy for its functioning; products of the various reactions are called *metabolites.*

kilocalorie the general term *calorie* refers to a unit of heat measure, and it is used alone to designate the small calorie; the calorie that is used in nutrition science and the study of metabolism is the large Calorie or kilocalorie, which avoids the use of large numbers in calculations; a kilocalorie, which is composed of 1000 calories, is the measure of heat that is necessary to raise the temperature of 1000 g (1 L) of water by 1° C.

Carbohydrates

Dietary carbohydrates (e.g., starches, sugars) provide the body's primary and preferred source of fuel for energy. Carbohydrates also maintain the body's reserve store of quick energy as **glycogen** (see Chapter 2). Each gram of carbohydrate consumed yields 4 kcal of body energy. In a well-balanced diet, carbohydrates from all sources should provide approximately 45% to 65% of the total kilocalories.

Fats

Dietary fats from both animal and plant sources provide the body's secondary or storage form of energy. This form is more concentrated, yielding 9 kcal for each gram consumed. In a well-balanced diet, fats should provide about 20% to 35% of the total kilocalories. Approximately two thirds of this amount should be from plant sources, which provide monounsaturated and polyunsaturated fats, and no more than 10% of kilocalories should come from saturated fat (see Chapter 3).

Proteins

Ideally protein would not be used for energy by the body. Rather, it should be preserved for other critical functions, such as structure, enzyme and hormone production, fluid balance, and so on. However, in the event that necessary energy from carbohydrates and fat is insufficient, the body may draw from dietary or tissue protein to obtain required energy. When protein is used for energy it yields 4 kcal/g. In a well-balanced diet, protein should provide approximately 10% to 35% of the total kilocalories (see Chapter 4).

Thus, the recommended intake of each energy-yielding nutrient, as a percent of total kilocalories, is as follows:
- Carbohydrate: 45% to 65%
- Fat: 20% to 35%
- Protein: 10% to 35%

Figure 1-2 illustrates the acceptable ranges of caloric intake for each macronutrient as part of the whole diet. Because individual needs vary, there are no exact recommendations for any macronutrient. If the diet is on the lower end of kilocalories from one of the macronutrients, then a necessary increase in percentage of total kilocalories will come from one or both of the other macronutrients.

TISSUE BUILDING

Proteins

The primary function of protein is tissue building. **Amino acids** are the building blocks of protein that are necessary for constructing and repairing body tissues (e.g., organs, muscles, cells, blood proteins). Tissue building is a constant process that ensures the growth and maintenance of a strong body structure as well as the creation of vital substances for cellular functions.

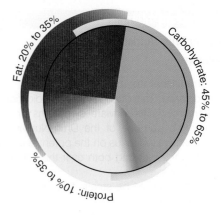

FIGURE 1-2 The recommended intake of each energy-yielding nutrient as a percentage of total energy intake.

Other Nutrients

Several other nutrients contribute to the building and maintenance of tissues. Some examples are provided here.

Vitamins and minerals. Vitamins and minerals are essential nutrients that help to regulate many body processes. An example of the use of a vitamin in tissue building is that of vitamin C in developing collagen. Collagen is the protein found in fibrous tissues such as cartilage, bone matrix, skin, and tendons. Two major minerals, calcium and phosphorus, participate in building and maintaining bone tissue. Another example is the mineral iron, which contributes to building the oxygen carrier protein hemoglobin in red blood cells. Several other vitamins and minerals are respectively discussed in greater detail in Chapters 7 and 8 with regard to their functions, which include tissue building.

Fatty acids. Fatty acids, the building blocks of lipids, help to build the central fat substance that is necessary in all cell membranes, and they promote the transport of fat-soluble nutrients throughout the body.

REGULATION AND CONTROL

The multiple chemical processes in the body that are necessary for providing energy and building tissue are carefully regulated and controlled to maintain a constant dynamic balance among all body parts and processes. Several of these regulatory functions involve essential nutrients. Some examples are provided here.

---

glycogen a polysaccharide; the main storage form of carbohydrate in the body, which is stored primarily in the liver and to a lesser extent in muscle tissue.

amino acids the nitrogen-bearing compounds that form the structural units of protein; after digestion, amino acids are available for the synthesis of required proteins.

Vitamins

Many vitamins function as coenzyme factors, which are components of cell enzymes, in the governing of chemical reactions during metabolism. This is true for most of the B-complex vitamins. In other words, the body must have an adequate supply of the B vitamins in order to yield energy (in the form of adenosine triphosphate [ATP]) from the metabolism of the energy-yielding nutrients (see Chapter 7).

Minerals

Many minerals also serve as coenzyme factors with enzymes in cell metabolism. For example, cobalt, which is a central constituent of vitamin B_{12} (cobalamin), functions with this vitamin in the synthesis of heme for hemoglobin formation.

Water and Fiber

Water and fiber also function as regulatory agents. In fact, water is the fundamental agent for life itself, providing the essential base for all metabolic processes. The adult body is approximately 50% to 70% water. Dietary fiber helps to regulate the passage of food material through the gastrointestinal tract, and it influences the absorption of nutrients.

NUTRITIONAL STATES

OPTIMAL NUTRITION

Optimal nutrition means that a person receives and uses adequate nutrients obtained from a varied and balanced diet of carbohydrates, fats, proteins, minerals, vitamins, and water. The desired amount of each essential nutrient should be balanced to cover variations in health and disease and to provide reserve supplies without unnecessary excesses.

MALNUTRITION

Malnutrition refers to a condition that is caused by an improper or insufficient diet. Both *undernutrition* and *overnutrition* are forms of malnutrition. Dietary surveys have shown that the average American diet is suboptimal. Intakes of fruits, vegetables, and dairy foods or dairy substitutes are lower than the recommended intake levels. Meanwhile, the average American intake of foods containing undesirable components such as saturated fat, alcohol, and added sugar is considerably higher than recommended.[3,4] That does not necessarily mean that all of these individuals are undernourished. But it does indicate poor dietary choices and suboptimal nutritional intake. Some people can maintain health on somewhat less than the optimal amounts of various nutrients in a state of borderline nutrition. However, on average, someone who is receiving less than the desired amounts of essential nutrients has a greater risk for physical illness and compromised immunity as compared with someone who is receiving optimal nutrition.[5] Such nutritionally deficient people

are limited with regard to their physical work capacity, immune system function, and mental activity. They lack the nutritional reserves to meet any added physiologic or metabolic demands from injury or illness or to sustain fetal development during pregnancy or proper growth during childhood. This state may result from many situations including poor eating habits, a continuously stressful environment with little or no available food, or a disease state.

Undernutrition

Undernutrition, a subcategory of malnutrition, appears when nutritional reserves are depleted and nutrient and energy intakes are not sufficient to meet daily needs or added metabolic stress. Many undernourished people live in conditions of poverty or illness. Such conditions influence the health of all involved but especially that of the most vulnerable populations: pregnant women, infants, children, and elderly adults. In the United States, which is one of the wealthiest countries in the world, widespread hunger and undernutrition among the poor still exist, which indicates that food security problems involve urban development issues, economic policies, and more general poverty issues (see the Cultural Considerations box, "Food Insecurity").

Undernutrition sometimes occurs in hospitalized patients as well. For example, acute trauma or chronic illness places added stress on the body, and the daily nutrient and energy intake may be insufficient to meet the needs of these patients. This is common despite the supply of nutritionally balanced meals and nutrition support provided by the hospital. Think about a patient you have seen before in a hospital—were they eager to eat? People are hospitalized because their health is in a state of serious distress. Illness and pain are often the cause for anorexia and decreased appetite. Thus, this form of malnutrition may result in patients that had a good nutritional standing before illness required hospitalization.[6]

Overnutrition

Some people are in a state of overnutrition, which results from excess nutrient and/or energy intake over time. Overnutrition is another form of malnutrition, especially when excess caloric intake produces harmful body weight (i.e., morbid obesity; see Chapter 15). Harmful overnutrition can also occur among people who consistently use excessive amounts of dietary supplements, which can result in vitamin or mineral toxicities (see Chapters 7 and 8).

NUTRIENT AND FOOD GUIDES FOR HEALTH PROMOTION

NUTRIENT STANDARDS

Most of the developed countries of the world have established nutrient standard recommendations. These

Cultural Considerations

Food Insecurity

Food insecurity is defined by the U.S. Department of Agriculture as the limited or uncertain availability of nutritious and adequate food. Using this definition, the Food Assistance and Nutrition Research Program of the U.S. Department of Agriculture reported that 17.6 million households (i.e., 14.5% of all U.S. households) qualify as having food insecurity. Furthermore, homes with children report almost double the rate of food insecurity as compared to homes without children (20% and 11.9%, respectively).[1] There is widespread hunger and malnutrition among the poor, especially among the growing number of homeless, including mothers with young children. Such problems may manifest as physical, psychologic, and sociofamilial disturbances in all age groups, with a significant negative impact on health status (including mental health) and the risk of chronic disease.

Individuals suffering from chronic illness are also at increased risk of suffering from food insecurity independent of their sociodemographic status.[2] In other words, individuals otherwise *food secure* may find themselves in a situation where disease complications create an environment in which food is not readily available, thus exacerbating their overall decline in health. In addition, food insecure patients with chronic disease are often faced with the choice between purchasing necessary medications or food. Many of these individuals are unable to take medications as prescribed because of inadequate funds and the overriding need for food instead of medications.[3,4]

Feeding America, which is the nation's largest organization of emergency food providers, estimated that 14 million children in the United States receive emergency food services each year.[5] Malnourished children are at an increased risk for stunted growth and episodes of infection and disease, which often have lasting effects on their intellectual development. Hunger is a chronic issue (i.e., persisting 8 months or more per year) among most households that report food insecurity. The prevalence of food insecurity is substantially higher among households that are headed by single mothers and in African-American and Hispanic households.[1] A variety of federal and nonfederal programs are available to address hunger issues in all cultural and age groups. The U.S. Department of Agriculture's Food and Nutrition Service provides detailed information about such programs on its website at www.fns.usda.gov.

REFERENCES

1. Coleman-Jensen A, Nord M, Singh A. *Household Food Security in the United States in 2012*. Washington, DC: Economic Research Service, U.S. Department of Agriculture; 2013.
2. Tarasuk V, et al. Chronic physical and mental health conditions among adults may increase vulnerability to household food insecurity. *J Nutr*. 2013;143(11):1785-1793.
3. Berkowitz SA, Seligman HK, Choudhry NK. Treat or eat: food insecurity, cost-related medication underuse, and unmet needs. *Am J Med*. 2014;127(4):303-310, e3.
4. Sattler EL, Lee JS. Persistent food insecurity is associated with higher levels of cost-related medication nonadherence in low-income older adults. *J Nutr Gerontol Geriatr*. 2013;32(1):41-58.
5. Mabli J, Potter F, Zhao Z. *Hunger in America 2010; National Report Prepared for Feeding America*. Chicago: Feeding America; 2010.

standards serve as a reference for intake levels of the essential nutrients to meet the known nutrition needs of most healthy population groups. Although these standards are similar in most countries, they vary according to the philosophies of the scientists and practitioners with regard to the purpose and use of such standards. In the United States, these standards are referred to as the **Dietary Reference Intakes (DRIs).**

U.S Standards: Dietary Reference Intakes

Since 1941, the **Recommended Dietary Allowances (RDAs),** which are published by the National Academy of Sciences, have been the authoritative source for setting standards for the minimum amounts of nutrients necessary to protect almost all people against the risk for nutrient deficiency. The U.S. RDA standards were first published during World War II as a guide for planning and obtaining food supplies for national defense and for providing population standards as a goal for good nutrition. These standards are revised and expanded every 5 to 10 years to reflect increasing scientific knowledge.

Public awareness and research attention have shifted from the original goal of *preventing deficiency disease* to reflect an increasing emphasis on nutrient requirements for *maintaining optimal health*. Following World War II, nutrient deficiencies were a major concern to the health of the nation. However, that is not the case today for the majority of the population. With food fortification and enrichment, few overt nutrient deficiencies exist in an otherwise balanced diet. This change of emphasis resulted in the DRIs project. This project was established to examine how much of a nutrient should be consumed to produce optimal health. For example, the original goal was to find out how much vitamin C had to be consumed in order to prevent the disease scurvy. The current DRIs represent an ideal amount of each nutrient that will maximize the health benefits of each nutrient (i.e., the optimal amount of vitamin C one should consume in order to receive all of the health benefits of that nutrient). For some nutrients, this shift in focus made a significant difference in the recommendations. And for others, the ideal intakes did not change.

The creation of the DRIs involved distinguished U.S. and Canadian scientists, who were divided into six functional panels (Box 1-1) and who have examined thousands of nutrition studies addressing the health

Dietary Reference Intakes (DRIs) reference values for the nutrient intake needs of healthy individuals for each gender and age group.

Recommended Dietary Allowances (RDAs) the average daily dietary intake level that is sufficient to meet the nutrient requirement of nearly all healthy individuals in a group.

Box 1-1	Dietary Reference Intake Panels of the Institute of Medicine of the National Academy of Sciences

1. Calcium, vitamin D, phosphorus, magnesium, and fluoride
2. Folate and other B vitamins
3. Antioxidants
4. Macronutrients
5. Trace elements
6. Electrolytes and water

benefits of nutrients and the hazards of consuming too much of a nutrient. The working group of nutrition scientists responsible for these standards forms the Food and Nutrition Board of the Institute of Medicine. The original DRI recommendations were published over several years in a series of six volumes.[7-12] They are continually updated as science indicates.[13]

The DRIs include recommendations for each gender and age group as well as recommendations for pregnancy and lactation (see Appendix B). For the first time, excessive amounts of nutrients were identified as tolerable upper intakes. The DRIs encompass the following four interconnected categories of nutrient recommendations:

1. *RDA.* This is the daily intake of a nutrient that meets the needs of almost all (i.e., 97.5%) healthy individuals of a specific age and gender. Individuals should use the RDA as a guide to achieve optimal nutrient intake. RDAs are established only when enough scientific evidence exists about a specific nutrient.
2. *Estimated Average Requirement.* This is the intake level that meets the needs of half of the individuals in a specific group. This quantity is used as the basis for the development of the RDA.
3. *Adequate Intake.* The Adequate Intake is used as a guide when insufficient scientific evidence is available to establish the RDA. Both the RDA and the Adequate Intake may be used as goals for individual intake.
4. *Tolerable Upper Intake Level.* This indicator is not a recommended intake. Rather, it sets the maximal intake that is unlikely to pose adverse health risks in almost all healthy individuals. For most nutrients, the Tolerable Upper Intake Level refers to the daily intake from food, fortified food, and nutrient supplements combined.

Other Standards

Historically, Canadian and European standards have been similar to the U.S. standards. In less developed countries, where factors such as the quality of available food must be considered, individuals refer to standards such as those set by the Food and Agriculture Organization and World Health Organization. Nonetheless, all standards provide a guideline to help health care workers who work with a variety of population groups to promote good health and prevent disease through sound nutrition.

FOOD GUIDES AND RECOMMENDATIONS

To interpret and apply nutrient standards, health care workers need practical food guides to use for nutrition education and food planning with individuals and families. Such tools include the U.S. Department of Agriculture's MyPlate system and the *Dietary Guidelines for Americans.*

MyPlate

The **MyPlate** food guidance system (Figure 1-3), which was released in June 2011 by the U.S. Department of Agriculture, provides the public with a valuable nutrition education tool. The goal of this food guide is to promote variety, proportionality, moderation, gradual improvements, and physical activity.[14] Participants are encouraged to personalize their own plans via the public website www.choosemyplate.gov by creating a profile and entering their age, gender, weight, height, and activity level. The system will create a plan with individualized calorie levels and specific recommendations for serving amounts from each food group. In addition, the MyPlate site provides participants with worksheets, resources, and individualized tools such as the Food Tracker, Physical Activity Tracker, and Weight Manager. Other helpful information can be found on the plan's website, including the following:

* Tips for consuming more whole grains, fruits, and vegetables
* Serving size information
* Health benefits and nutrients associated with each food group
* Sample menus

Dietary Guidelines for Americans

The *Dietary Guidelines for Americans* were issued as a result of growing public concern that began in the 1960s and the subsequent Senate investigations studying hunger and nutrition in the United States. These guidelines are based on developing alarm about chronic health problems in an aging population and a changing food environment. An updated statement is issued every 5 years. This publication encompasses a comprehensive evaluation of the scientific evidence regarding diet and health in a report jointly issued by the U.S. Department of Agriculture and the U.S. Department of Health and Human Services.[15]

Figure 1-4 shows the five key recommendations of the *Dietary Guidelines for Americans 2015-2020.* The

---

MyPlate a visual pattern of the current basic five food groups—grains, vegetables, fruits, dairy, and protein—arranged on a plate to indicate proportionate amounts of daily food choices.

10 tips
Nutrition Education Series

choose MyPlate
10 tips to a great plate

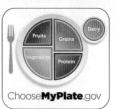
ChooseMyPlate.gov

Making food choices for a healthy lifestyle can be as simple as using these 10 Tips.
Use the ideas in this list to *balance your calories*, to choose foods to *eat more often*, and to cut back on foods to *eat less often*.

1 balance calories
Find out how many calories YOU need for a day as a first step in managing your weight. Go to www.ChooseMyPlate.gov to find your calorie level. Being physically active also helps you balance calories.

2 enjoy your food, but eat less
Take the time to fully enjoy your food as you eat it. Eating too fast or when your attention is elsewhere may lead to eating too many calories. Pay attention to hunger and fullness cues before, during, and after meals. Use them to recognize when to eat and when you've had enough.

3 avoid oversized portions
Use a smaller plate, bowl, and glass. Portion out foods before you eat. When eating out, choose a smaller size option, share a dish, or take home part of your meal.

4 foods to eat more often
Eat more vegetables, fruits, whole grains, and fat-free or 1% milk and dairy products. These foods have the nutrients you need for health—including potassium, calcium, vitamin D, and fiber. Make them the basis for meals and snacks.

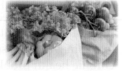

5 make half your plate fruits and vegetables
Choose red, orange, and dark-green vegetables like tomatoes, sweet potatoes, and broccoli, along with other vegetables for your meals. Add fruit to meals as part of main or side dishes or as dessert.

6 switch to fat-free or low-fat (1%) milk
They have the same amount of calcium and other essential nutrients as whole milk, but fewer calories and less saturated fat.

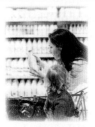

7 make half your grains whole grains
To eat more whole grains, substitute a whole-grain product for a refined product—such as eating whole-wheat bread instead of white bread or brown rice instead of white rice.

8 foods to eat less often
Cut back on foods high in solid fats, added sugars, and salt. They include cakes, cookies, ice cream, candies, sweetened drinks, pizza, and fatty meats like ribs, sausages, bacon, and hot dogs. Use these foods as occasional treats, not everyday foods.

9 compare sodium in foods
Use the Nutrition Facts label to choose lower sodium versions of foods like soup, bread, and frozen meals. Select canned foods labeled "low sodium," "reduced sodium," or "no salt added."

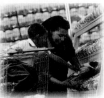

10 drink water instead of sugary drinks
Cut calories by drinking water or unsweetened beverages. Soda, energy drinks, and sports drinks are a major source of added sugar, and calories, in American diets.

Center for Nutrition Policy and Promotion

Go to www.ChooseMyPlate.gov for more information.

DG TipSheet No. 1
June 2011
USDA is an equal opportunity provider and employer.

FIGURE 1-3 MyPlate food guidance system recommendations. (From the U.S. Department of Agriculture, Center for Nutrition Policy and Promotion. *Choose MyPlate mini-poster* (website): <www.choosemyplate.gov>; Accessed June 16, 2014.)

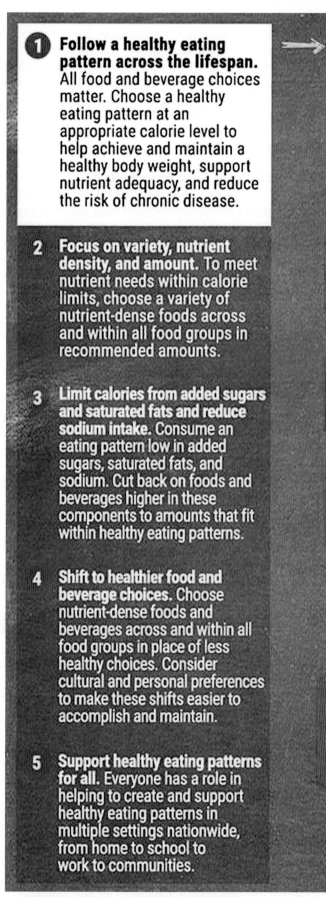

① **Follow a healthy eating pattern across the lifespan.** All food and beverage choices matter. Choose a healthy eating pattern at an appropriate calorie level to help achieve and maintain a healthy body weight, support nutrient adequacy, and reduce the risk of chronic disease.

2 **Focus on variety, nutrient density, and amount.** To meet nutrient needs within calorie limits, choose a variety of nutrient-dense foods across and within all food groups in recommended amounts.

3 **Limit calories from added sugars and saturated fats and reduce sodium intake.** Consume an eating pattern low in added sugars, saturated fats, and sodium. Cut back on foods and beverages higher in these components to amounts that fit within healthy eating patterns.

4 **Shift to healthier food and beverage choices.** Choose nutrient-dense foods and beverages across and within all food groups in place of less healthy choices. Consider cultural and personal preferences to make these shifts easier to accomplish and maintain.

5 **Support healthy eating patterns for all.** Everyone has a role in helping to create and support healthy eating patterns in multiple settings nationwide, from home to school to work to communities.

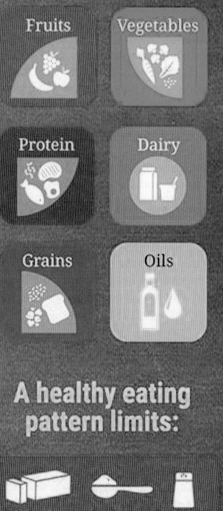

Follow a healthy eating pattern over time to help support a healthy body weight and reduce the risk of chronic disease.

A healthy eating pattern includes:

Fruits

Vegetables

Protein

Dairy

Grains

Oils

A healthy eating pattern limits:

Saturated fats and *trans* fats

Added sugars

Sodium

FIGURE 1-4 Summary of the *Dietary Guidelines for Americans, 2015-2020*. (From the U.S. Department of Health and Human Services and U.S. Department of Agriculture. *2015-2020 Dietary Guidelines for Americans. 8th Edition. December 2015.* Available at http://health.gov/dietaryguidelines/2015/guidelines/.)

current guidelines continue to serve as a useful overall guide for promoting dietary and lifestyle choices that reduce the risk for chronic disease. Although no guidelines can guarantee health or well-being and although people differ widely with regard to their food needs and preferences, these statements are meant to help evaluate food habits and move toward general improvements. Good food habits that are based on moderation and variety can help to build healthy bodies.

The current DRIs, MyPlate guidelines, and *Dietary Guidelines for Americans* are in sync with one another and supported by scientific literature. They reflect sound, although broad, guidelines for a healthy diet.

Other Recommendations

Organizations such as the American Cancer Society, the American Heart Association, and the American Diabetes Association also have their own independent dietary guidelines. In most cases, the guidelines set by various national organizations are modeled after the *Dietary Guidelines for Americans*. This may seem a bit repetitive, but the difference is the added emphasis on the prevention of specific chronic diseases, such as heart disease, cancer, and diabetes.

INDIVIDUAL NEEDS

Person-Centered Care

Regardless of the type of food guide or recommendations used, health care professionals must remember that food patterns vary with individual needs, tastes, habits, living situations, economic status, and energy demands. Cookie-cutter meal plans without regard to the individual's preferences are not useful. Food is a basic enjoyment of life and this should always be considered when implementing dietary changes for oneself or for a patient. Use the food guides to identify healthy food groups to choose from and then use a person-centered approach to more specifically select suitable foods within those food groups to meet the patient's needs.

Changing Food Environment

Our food environment has been rapidly changing in recent decades. American food habits appear to have deteriorated in some ways, with a heightened reliance on fast, processed, and prepackaged foods. However, Americans do recognize the relationship between food and overall health. More than ever, Americans are being selective about what they eat. Regardless of how much the food environment changes, the one thing that never goes out of style is the invention of food fads and popular diets. Health care professionals can address such concerns with a person-centered approach and ensure that the general dietary needs are still being met in accordance with the DRIs. Following a fad diet is a personal preference. If health care professionals dismiss such preferences in favor of a cookie-cutter meal plan, they are more likely to garner resistance from the patient instead of making any potential improvements. Most fad diets can provide an overall balanced diet with good judgment, guidance, and perhaps a few judgment.

Putting It All Together

Summary

- Good food and key nutrients are essential to life and health.
- In our changing world, an emphasis on health promotion and disease prevention by reducing health risks has become a primary health goal.
- The importance of a balanced diet for meeting this goal via the functioning of its nutrients is fundamental. Functions of nutrients include providing energy, building tissue, and regulating metabolic processes.
- Malnutrition exists in the United States in both overnutrition and undernutrition states.
- Food guides that help with the planning of an individualized healthy diet include the DRIs, MyPlate, and *Dietary Guidelines for Americans*.
- A person-centered approach is best when developing individual dietary recommendations that take personal factors into account.

Chapter Review Questions

See answers in Appendix A.

1. *Healthy People 2020* focuses on the ultimate vision of:
   a. A society in which all people live long, healthy lives.
   b. A society where there is zero tolerance for disease.
   c. A society where food in the United States is supplied by local plant sources.
   d. A society consuming a primarily plant-based diet.

2. Nutrient interactions involve the following two concepts:
   a. Nutrients have specific metabolic functions and work together to maintain the body.
   b. Nutrients have specific metabolic functions and work independently to maintain the body.
   c. Nutrients generally have independent functions in a healthy body but interact to promote healing during illness.
   d. Specific nutrients have similar metabolic functions and may be substituted for one another.

3. The most important and unique role of dietary protein is to:
   a. Provide energy.
   b. Build tissue.
   c. Provide essential fatty acids.
   d. Function as a coenzyme.

4. Forms of malnutrition include:
   a. Overnutrition only.
   b. Undernutrition only.
   c. Conditions associated with poverty only.
   d. Overnutrition and undernutrition.

5. The DRIs serve as a useful overall guide for promoting dietary and lifestyle choices for all people throughout life by recommending:
   a. Ideal intakes for each nutrient according to age and gender.
   b. Minimum intakes of each nutrient regardless of age and gender.
   c. Optimal intakes of each nutrient regardless of age and gender.
   d. Minimum intakes of each nutrient to prevent deficiency diseases.

Additional Learning Resources

evolve http://evolve.elsevier.com/Williams/basic/

References and **Further Reading and Resources** in the back of the book provide additional resources for enhancing knowledge.

2

Carbohydrates

Key Concepts

- Carbohydrate foods provide practical energy sources because of their wide availability, relatively low cost, and excellent storage capabilities.
- Carbohydrate structures vary from simple to complex, thus providing both quick and extended energy for the body.

- Dietary fiber, which is an indigestible carbohydrate, serves other functions within the gastrointestinal tract.

As discussed in Chapter 1, key nutrients in food sustain life and promote health. The unique functions of each nutrient provide the body with three essential elements for life: (1) energy to do work; (2) building materials to maintain form and functions; and (3) control agents to regulate these processes efficiently. These three basic functions of nutrients are closely related, and it is important to remember that no nutrient ever works alone.

This chapter looks specifically at the body's primary fuel source: carbohydrates. Carbohydrates are plentiful in the food supply, and they are an important contribution to a well-balanced diet. Controversy over the past decade surrounding the use, abuse, and misunderstanding of this critical macronutrient should be better interpreted after evaluating its functions within the body.

NATURE OF CARBOHYDRATES

RELATION TO ENERGY

Basic Fuel Source

Energy is required for organisms to live. All energy systems must have a basic fuel supply. In the Earth's energy system, vast energy resources from the sun enable plants, through **photosynthesis,** to transform solar energy into carbohydrate, which is the stored fuel form in plants. The human body can rapidly break down plant sources of carbohydrates through digestion and metabolism to yield our major source of energy, glucose.

Throughout this text, the term *energy* is used interchangeably with the terms *calorie, kilocalorie,* and *kcal* (see the definition of *kilocalorie* in Chapter 1). Our bodies need energy to survive. Both involuntary (e.g., heart and lung function) and voluntary actions (e.g., walking, talking) require energy, and that energy is derived from the digestion and metabolism of food.

Energy-Production System

A successful energy system, whether a living organism or a machine, must be able to do the following three things to produce energy from a fuel source:

1. Change the basic fuel to a refined fuel that the machine is designed to use.
2. Carry this refined fuel to the places that need it.
3. Burn this refined fuel in the special equipment set up at these places.

The body easily does these three things more efficiently than any manmade machine. It digests its basic fuel, carbohydrate, thereby releasing glucose. The body then absorbs and, through blood circulation, carries this refined fuel to cells that need it. Glucose is metabolized in the specific and intricate equipment in these cells. Ultimately energy in the form of adenosine triphosphate (ATP) is released through the process of cellular metabolism. Because the human body can rapidly digest the starches and sugars that are eaten to yield energy, carbohydrates are considered quick-energy foods.

Dietary Importance

Practical reasons also exist for the large quantities of carbohydrates found in diets all over the world. First, carbohydrates are widely available and easily grown (e.g., grains, legumes, vegetables, fruits). In some countries, carbohydrate foods make up almost the entire diet. Second, carbohydrates are relatively low in cost as compared with many other food items. Third, carbohydrate foods are easily stored. They can

photosynthesis the process by which plants that contain chlorophyll are able to manufacture carbohydrate by combining carbon dioxide and water; sunlight is used as energy, and chlorophyll is a catalyst.

be kept in dry storage for relatively long periods without spoilage, and modern processing and packaging can extend the shelf life of carbohydrate products for years.

The U.S. Department of Agriculture regularly surveys food intake. These reports indicate that Americans consume 6.5 oz of grain products per day, on average.[1] The *Dietary Guidelines for Americans* encourage people to make at least half of all grains consumed whole grains.[2] However, the average American consumes 88% of their grain products in the form of refined grains and only 12% as whole grains. Additionally, the average American continues to consume an excess of added sugar daily.[1]

CLASSES OF CARBOHYDRATES

The word *carbohydrate* is derived from the chemical nature of the substance. A carbohydrate is composed of carbon (C), hydrogen (H), and oxygen (O). Its abbreviated name, *CHO,* is the combination of the chemical symbols of its three components. The term **saccharide** is used as a carbohydrate class name, and it comes from the Latin word *saccharum,* which means "sugar." Carbohydrates are classified according to the number of saccharide units that make up their structure: *mono*saccharides have one unit; *di*saccharides have two units; and *poly*saccharides have many units. Monosaccharides and disaccharides are small, simple structures of respectively only one and two saccharide units; thus they are referred to as **simple carbohydrates.** However, polysaccharides are large, complex compounds

of many saccharide units in long chains; thus they are called **complex carbohydrates.** For example, starch, which is the most significant polysaccharide in human nutrition, is composed of many coiled and branching chains in a treelike structure. Each of the multiple branching chains is composed of 24 to 30 units of glucose, which are gradually released during digestion to supply a steady source of energy over time. Table 2-1 summarizes these classes of carbohydrates and demonstrates their basic structure.

Monosaccharides

The three single saccharides are glucose, fructose, and galactose. Monosaccharides, which are the building

---

saccharide the chemical name for sugar molecules; may occur as single molecules in monosaccharides (glucose, fructose, galactose), two molecules in disaccharides (sucrose, lactose, maltose), or multiple molecules in polysaccharides (starch, dietary fiber, glycogen).
simple carbohydrates sugars with a simple structure of one or two single-sugar (saccharide) units; a monosaccharide is composed of one sugar unit, and a disaccharide is composed of two sugar units.
complex carbohydrates large complex molecules of carbohydrates composed of many sugar units (polysaccharides); the complex forms of dietary carbohydrates are starch and dietary fiber.

Table **2-1** Summary of Carbohydrate Classes

CHEMICAL CLASS NAME	CLASS MEMBERS	SOURCES
Monosaccharides (simple carbohydrates)	Glucose (dextrose)	Corn syrup (commonly used in processed foods)
	Fructose	Fruits, honey
	Galactose	Lactose (milk, milk products)
Disaccharides (simple carbohydrates)	Sucrose	Table sugar (sugar cane, sugar beets)
	Lactose	Milk, milk products
	Maltose	Molasses
		Starch digestion, intermediate
		Sweetener in food products
Polysaccharides (complex carbohydrates)	Starch	Grains and grain products (cereal, bread, crackers, baked goods)
		Rice, corn, bulgur
		Legumes
		Potatoes and other vegetables
	Glycogen	Storage form of carbohydrate in animal tissue (not a dietary source)

blocks for all carbohydrates, require no digestion. They are quickly absorbed from the intestine into the bloodstream and transported to the liver. Energy demands will determine if the monosaccharides are then used for immediate energy or stored as **glycogen** for later use.

Glucose. The basic single sugar in human metabolism is glucose, which is the form of sugar circulating in the blood. It is the primary fuel for cells. Glucose, a moderately sweet sugar, usually is not found as such in the diet, except in corn syrup or processed food items. The body's supply of glucose mainly comes from the digestion of starch. Glucose is also called *dextrose* to denote the structure of the molecule (i.e., six carbons).

Fructose. Fructose is primarily found in fruits (from which it gets its name) and in honey. Although honey is sometimes thought of as a sugar substitute, it is a sugar itself; therefore, it cannot be considered a substitute. The amount of fructose found in fruits depends on the degree of ripeness. As a fruit ripens, some of its stored starch turns to sugar. Fructose is the sweetest of the simple sugars.

High-fructose corn syrups, which are manufactured by changing the glucose in cornstarch into fructose, are heavily used in processed food products, canned and frozen fruits, and soft drinks. These syrups are inexpensive sweeteners, and contribute to increased sugar intake in the United States. The per-capita consumption of high-fructose corn syrup increased from zero in 1967 to a height of 19.7 teaspoons (tsp) per day in 1999 and was most recently estimated to be down to 14.4 tsp per day.[3] While the change in high-fructose corn syrup intake has fluctuated significantly over the past 50 years, the overall intake of all caloric sweeteners has remained high. Figure 2-1 demonstrates the total added sugar in the American diet and that which comes from high-fructose corn syrup. Note that high-fructose corn syrup is only one of the sweeteners regularly used in the typical American diet.

Galactose. Galactose is not usually found as a free monosaccharide in the diet; rather, it is a product of lactose (milk sugar) digestion.

Disaccharides

Disaccharides are simple double sugars that are composed of two single-sugar units linked together. The three disaccharides that are important in human nutrition are sucrose, lactose, and maltose.

$$Sucrose = Glucose + Fructose$$
$$Lactose = Glucose + Galactose$$
$$Maltose = Glucose + Glucose$$

Sucrose. Sucrose is common table sugar. Its two single-sugar units are glucose and fructose. Sucrose is

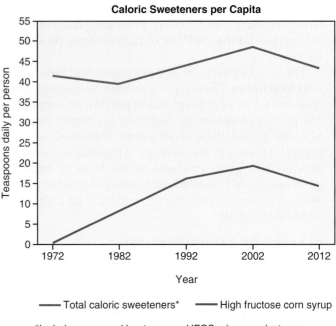

Caloric Sweeteners per Capita

*Includes cane and beet sugars, HFCS, glucose, dextrose, edible syrups, and honey.

FIGURE 2-1 Daily intake of caloric sweeteners in the United States per person. (Data from U.S. Department of Agriculture, Economic Research Service. *Food availability (per capita) data system, sugar and sweeteners (added).* Available from: <www.ers.usda.gov/data-products/food-availability-%28per-capita%29-data-system/.aspx#.U7BpG3awXG4>; Accessed June 6, 2015.)

used in the form of granulated, powdered, or brown sugar, and it is made from sugar cane or sugar beets. Molasses, which is a by-product of sugar production, is also a form of sucrose. When people speak of sugar in the diet, they usually mean sucrose.

Lactose. The sugar in milk, which is formed in mammary glands, is lactose. Its two single-sugar units are glucose and galactose. Lactose is the only common sugar that is not found in plants. It is less soluble and less sweet than sucrose. Lactose remains in the intestine longer than other sugars, and it encourages the growth of certain useful bacteria. Cow's milk contains 4.8% lactose, and human milk contains 7% lactose. Because lactose promotes the absorption of calcium and phosphorus, the presence of all three nutrients in milk is advantageous for absorption.

Maltose. Maltose is not usually found as such in food form. It is derived within the body from the intermediate digestive breakdown of starch. Starch is made up entirely of glucose units. Therefore, during the breakdown of starch, many disaccharide units of maltose are released. Synthetically derived maltose is used in various processed foods.

> **glycogen** a complex carbohydrate found in animal tissue that is composed of many glucose units linked together.

Polysaccharides

Polysaccharides are complex carbohydrates that are composed of many sugar units. The important polysaccharides in human nutrition include starch, glycogen, and dietary fiber.

Starch. Starches are by far the most significant polysaccharides in the diet. They are found in grains, legumes, and other vegetables and in some fruits in small amounts. Starches are more complex in structure than simple sugars, so they break down more slowly and supply energy over a longer period of time. Cooking starch improves its flavor and also softens and ruptures the starch cells, thereby making digestion easier and faster. Starch mixtures thicken when cooked, because the portion that encases the starch granules has a gel-like quality that thickens the starch mixture in the same way that pectin causes jelly to set.

The Dietary Reference Intakes (DRIs; see Chapter 1) recommend that 45% to 65% of total kilocalories consumed come from carbohydrates, with a greater portion of that intake coming from complex carbohydrates.[4] For countries in which starch is the staple food, carbohydrates make up an even higher proportion of the diet. The major food sources of starch (Figure 2-2) include grains in the form of cereal, pasta, crackers, bread, and other baked goods; legumes in the form of beans and peas; potatoes, rice, corn, and bulgur; and other vegetables, especially of the root variety.

The term *whole grain* is used for food products such as flours, breads, or cereals that are produced from unrefined grain. Unrefined grains retain the outer bran layers, the inner germ, and the endosperm (Figure 2-3) and thus the nutrients found within (i.e., dietary fiber, vitamins, and minerals). *Enriched grains* are refined grain products to which some (but not all) vitamins and minerals that were removed during the refining process—for example, riboflavin, niacin, thiamin, folate, iron—have been added back to some extent. *Fortified* foods are those that have nutrients added to them that would not naturally occur in that food regardless of how it was processed (e.g., calcium-fortified orange juice). Many enriched grains, such as ready-to-eat breakfast cereals, are also fortified with additional vitamins and minerals.

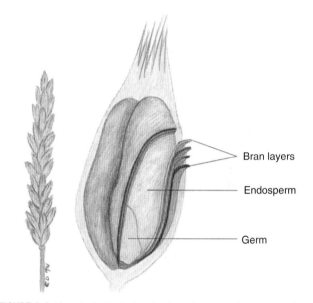

FIGURE 2-3 Kernel of wheat showing bran layers, endosperm, and germ. (Courtesy Eileen Draper.)

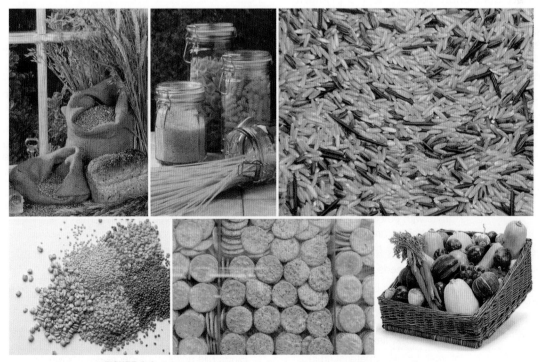

FIGURE 2-2 Complex carbohydrate foods. (Copyright JupiterImages Corp.)

Glycogen. Glycogen is not a dietary carbohydrate. Rather, it is a carbohydrate that is formed within the body's tissues, and it is crucial to the body's metabolism and energy balance. Glycogen is found in the liver and muscles, where it is constantly recycled (i.e., broken down to form glucose for immediate energy needs and synthesized for storage). These small stores of glycogen help to sustain normal blood glucose levels during short-term fasting periods (e.g., sleep), and they provide immediate fuel for muscle action. These reserves also protect cells from depressed metabolic function and injury. The process of blood glucose regulation with regard to glycogen breakdown is discussed in greater detail in Chapter 20.

Dietary fiber. Humans lack the necessary enzymes to digest dietary fiber; therefore, these polysaccharides do not have a direct energy value like other carbohydrates. However, their inability to be digested makes them an important dietary asset. The beneficial relationship between a diet high in fiber and disease prevention and/or management (e.g., cardiovascular disease, gastrointestinal problems, diabetes) is well established.[5-10]

Dietary fiber is divided into two groups on the basis of solubility. Cellulose, lignin, and most hemicelluloses are not soluble in water. The rest of the dietary fibers (i.e., most pectins, β-glucans, gums, mucilages) are water soluble. These two classes of dietary fiber are listed in Table 2-2. The looser physical structure and greater water-holding capacity of gums, mucilages, pectins, and algal polysaccharides partly account for their greater water solubility. Recommendations for specific types of fiber to consume often are based on the water-solubility distinction. Soluble fiber is primarily noted for its ability to bind bile acids and ultimately lower blood cholesterol levels.[11] Alternatively, insoluble fiber is particularly helpful for the prevention of constipation. However, you will notice from Table 2-2 that many of these functions overlap the soluble/insoluble categories and many high-fiber foods will contain both types of fiber. It is more important to include a variety of high-fiber foods in the diet than to be overly concerned with the specific form of fiber found in your grains, fruits, and vegetables.

Cellulose. Cellulose is the chief component of cell walls in plants. It remains undigested in the gastrointestinal tract of humans, and it adds important bulk to the diet. This bulk helps to move the food mass along, it stimulates normal muscle action in the intestine, and it forms soft feces for the elimination of waste products. The main sources of cellulose are the stems and leaves of vegetables and the coverings of seeds and grains. Within the same area of the plant, phosphorus is stored in the form of phytic acid; this compound is undigested in humans because of the lack of a necessary enzyme (phytase). Phytic acid is a strong **chelator** of important minerals (see the Drug-Nutrient Interaction box, "Phytic Acid and Mineral Absorption").

Lignin. Lignin, which is the only noncarbohydrate type of dietary fiber, is a large compound that forms the woody part of certain plants. It binds the cellulose fibers in plants, thereby giving added strength and

chelator a ligand that binds to a metal to form a metal complex.

Table 2-2 Summary of Dietary Fiber Classes

DIETARY FIBER CLASS	SOURCE	FUNCTION
Insoluble Fiber		
Cellulose	Main cell wall constituent of plants (stalks and leaves of vegetables; outer coverings of seeds, such as are found in whole grains)	Holds water; reduces elevated colonic intraluminal pressure
Hemicellulose	Cell wall plant material (bran, whole grains)	Holds water and increases stool bulk; reduces elevated colonic pressure; binds bile acids, thus decreasing serum cholesterol level
Lignin	Woody part of plants (broccoli stems; fruits with edible seeds, such as strawberries and flaxseeds)	Antioxidant; binds bile acids, thus decreasing serum cholesterol level; binds minerals
Soluble Fiber		
Algal polysaccharides	Algae, seaweeds	Used as thickener in food products
β-Glucans	Oats and barley bran	Binds bile acids, thus decreasing serum cholesterol level
Gums	Oats, legumes, guar, barley	Decreases gastric emptying; slows digestion, gut transit time, and glucose absorption
Mucilages	Psyllium husk, flaxseed	Holds water
Pectins	Intercellular plant material (fruit)	Binds bile acids, thus decreasing serum cholesterol level; binds minerals

Drug-Nutrient Interaction

Phytic Acid and Mineral Absorption

SARA HARCOURT

Some compounds that are naturally found in food bind minerals, thereby making them unavailable for absorption. Phytic acid is one such compound, and it is found in legumes, wheat bran, and seeds. Iron also is naturally found in these foods, but, because of the phytic acid interference, as little as 2% of the available iron may be absorbed.

A diet that consists of high-fiber foods containing phytic acid coupled with a low intake of iron-rich foods (e.g., meat, poultry) may intensify iron deficiency. This can especially be a problem in the developing world where grains and legumes are a staple in the diet. The World Health Organization classifies iron deficiency anemia as one of the top 10 most serious health problems in the world today.[1]

Although iron deficiency anemia is not nearly as common in the United States as other developing countries, it is a concern among pregnant and premenopausal women. If the anemia is severe enough, a physician may prescribe an iron supplement. The consumption of foods that contain high amounts of phytic acid along with the supplement would inhibit iron absorption just as it would if the iron were part of the food.

Phytic acid binds to other minerals that have a similar charge as iron, including calcium, magnesium, and zinc. Calcium supplements are often prescribed for those who may be losing bone mass (e.g., postmenopausal women) or for those who do not get enough calcium in the diet (e.g., teens, the elderly). Food sources of phytic acid that are eaten with calcium supplements may inhibit absorption. When recommending that patients take an iron or calcium supplement, also advise them to take the supplement with foods that do not contain phytate in order to maximize the bioavailability of the minerals and minimize the drug-nutrient interaction.

REFERENCE

1. World Health Organization; Centers for Disease Control and Prevention, de Benoist B, McLean E, Egli I, Cogswell M, eds. *Worldwide prevalence of anaemia 1993-2005: WHO Global Database on Anaemia* (website): <http://whqlibdoc.who.int/publications/2008/9789241596657_eng.pdf>; Accessed July 14, 2014.

stiffness to plant cell walls. Although it is an insoluble fiber, it also combines with bile acids and cholesterol in the human intestine to prevent their absorption.

Noncellulose polysaccharides. Hemicellulose, pectins, gums, mucilages, and algal substances are noncellulose polysaccharides. They absorb water and swell to a larger bulk, thus slowing the emptying of the food mass from the stomach (aiding satiety), binding bile acids in the intestine, and preventing spastic colon pressure by providing bulk for normal muscle action. Noncellulose polysaccharides also provide fermentation material on which colon bacteria can work.

Table 2-2 provides a summary of these dietary fiber classes along with some sources and functions of each. Table 2-3 provides the grams of carbohydrate and dietary fiber per serving of commonly used foods.

In general, the food groups that provide needed dietary fiber include whole grains, legumes, vegeta-

Clinical Applications

Case Study: Identifying Carbohydrates and Fiber

A patient comes to you for dietary analysis. He is trying to eat a diet that is consistent with the dietary guidelines of 45% to 65% carbohydrate and 38 g of dietary fiber per day. On the basis of the 1-day diet record that he provides you, answer the questions that follow regarding his dietary analysis.

BREAKFAST
- 2 cups of Cheerios
- 1¼ cups of skim milk
- 1 medium banana
- 16 oz of coffee with 1 Tbsp of sugar and 2 Tbsp of whole-milk creamer

LUNCH
- Turkey sandwich (2 slices of whole-wheat bread, 3 oz of lean turkey, 1 oz of cheddar cheese, 1 slice of tomato, 2 lettuce leaves, 2 tsp of yellow mustard, and ½ Tbsp of mayonnaise)
- 1 oz of pretzels
- 1½ cups of mixed green salad with 2 Tbsp of crushed pecans and 2 Tbsp of fat-free Italian dressing
- 20 oz of water

SNACK
- 1 medium apple
- 1 package of peanut-butter crackers (6 crackers)

DINNER
- 4 oz of grilled chicken breast
- ½ cup of green beans
- ¾ cup of mashed potatoes made with skim milk and butter
- ½ cup of roasted red peppers
- 1 whole-wheat roll
- 16 oz of sweet tea

QUESTIONS FOR ANALYSIS
1. Identify all of the foods that contain carbohydrates.
2. With the use of the dietary analysis on Evolve or the Choose MyPlate Food Tracker available at www.choosemyplate.gov, analyze this 1-day diet to determine the following:
   a. How many total grams of carbohydrate did this individual consume?
   b. How many grams of sugar did he consume?
   c. How many grams of soluble and total fiber did he consume?
   d. What was the percentage of total calories from carbohydrates?
3. Did this individual meet the dietary guidelines for the percentage of calories from carbohydrates and grams of fiber on this day?
4. What additional recommendations would you make for improvement?

bles, and fruits with as much of their skin remaining as possible. Whole grains provide a special natural "package" of both the complex carbohydrate starch and the fiber in its coating. In addition, whole grains contain an abundance of vitamins and minerals (see the Clinical Applications box, "Case Study: Identifying Carbohydrates and Fiber").

Table 2-3 Carbohydrate Content, Dietary Fiber, and Caloric Value for Selected Foods

FOOD SOURCE	SERVING SIZE	CARBOHYDRATE (g)	DIETARY FIBER (g)	TOTAL KILOCALORIES
Concentrated Sweets				
Sugar				
Granulated	1 tsp	4.2	0	16
Powdered	1 tsp	2.49	0	10
Maple	1 tsp	2.73	0	11
Honey	1 Tbsp	17.3	0	64
Syrup				
High-fructose corn	1 Tbsp	14.44	0	53
Maple	1 Tbsp	13.42	0	52
Jam and preserves	1 Tbsp	13.77	0.2	56
Carbonated beverage, cola	12 oz	35.18	0	136
Candy				
Skittles	1 package (1.8 oz)	46.42	0	205
Starburst fruit chews	1 package (2.07 oz)	48.72	0	241
Twizzlers	4 pieces from an 8-oz package	35.88	0	158
Baked Goods				
Brownie	1 square (1 oz)	18.12	0.6	115
Butter cookie	1 medium (1 oz)	19.53	0.2	132
Doughnut, glazed	1 medium (3-inch diameter)	22.86	0.7	192
Fruit				
Apple, raw with skin	1 medium (3-inch diameter)	25.13	4.4	95
Apricots, dried, no sugar added	½ cup	27.69	3.2	106
Banana	1 medium (7.5 to 7⅞ inches long)	26.95	3.1	105
Cherries, sweet, raw	15 cherries	19.69	2.6	77
Orange	1 medium (2⅞-inch diameter)	17.56	3.1	69
Pineapple	1 slice (3½-inch diameter × ¾-inch thick)	11.02	1.2	42
Strawberries	10 medium (1¼-inch diameter)	9.22	2.4	38
Vegetables				
Asparagus, cooked	½ cup	3.7	1.8	20
Beans, kidney, cooked	½ cup	20.18	5.7	112
Broccoli, cooked	½ cup	5.6	2.6	27
Carrots, raw	½ cup chopped, raw	6.13	1.8	26
Corn, sweet, yellow, cooked	½ cup, cut	15.63	1.8	72
Green beans (snap beans, cooked)	½ cup	4.92	2	22
Lettuce, green leaf, raw	1 cup shredded	1	0.5	5
Potato, with skin, baked	1 medium (2¼ to 3¼ inches in diameter)	36.59	3.8	161
Potato, sweet, baked	1 medium (2-inch diameter, 5 inches long)	23.61	3.8	103
Squash, summer	½ cup cooked slices	3.41	1	17
Tomatoes, red, raw	½ medium (2¾-inch diameter)	2.39	0.7	11

Table 2-3	Carbohydrate Content, Dietary Fiber, and Caloric Value for Selected Foods—cont'd			
FOOD SOURCE	SERVING SIZE	CARBOHYDRATE (g)	DIETARY FIBER (g)	TOTAL KILOCALORIES
Dairy Products				
Milk				
Skim	1 cup	12.15	0	83
2%	1 cup	13.5	0	138
Whole	1 cup	11.03	0	146
Cheese				
Cheddar	½ cup, shredded	0.72	0	228
Cottage, 2% milk fat	½ cup	4.14	0	97
Grain Products				
Bread				
Wheat	1 slice	14.34	1.2	78
White	1 slice	12.6	0.7	66
Rye	1 slice	15.46	1.9	83
Cereal (Dry)				
Corn flakes	1 cup	22.20	0.3	101
Rice, puffed	1 cup	12.57	0.2	56
Wheat, shredded	1 cup	39.89	6.1	172
Cereal (Cooked)				
Grits, corn, cooked with water	1 cup	37.93	2.1	182
Oatmeal, cooked with water	1 cup	28.08	4.0	166
Wheat, cooked with water	1 cup	33.15	3.9	150
Crackers, saltines	5	11.03	0.4	62
Pasta, cooked	1 cup	39.07	6.7	176
Rice				
Brown	½ cup, cooked	22.39	1.8	108
White	½ cup, cooked	26.59	0.3	121

Data from the U.S. Department of Agriculture, Agricultural Research Service, Nutrient Data Laboratory. *USDA national nutrient database for standard reference* (website): <http://ndb.nal.usda.gov/>; Accessed July 12, 2014.

Many health organizations have recommended increasing the intake of complex carbohydrates in general and dietary fiber in particular (see the For Further Focus box, "Fiber: What's All the Fuss About?").[2,4] The Food and Nutrition Board of the Institute of Medicine has always indicated that a desirable fiber intake should not be exclusively achieved by adding concentrated fiber supplements to the diet. Instead, the recommendations are to eat a high-fiber diet that is rich in whole foods. The recommended daily intake of fiber for women and men aged 19 to 50 years old is 25 and 38 g/day, respectively. The DRIs are reduced to 21 and 30 g/day for women and men who are older than 50 years of age.[4] This intake requires the consistent use of whole grains, legumes, vegetables, fruits, seeds, and nuts in the daily diet. Unfortunately, the average American does not consume the recommended servings of these food groups on a daily basis. In fact, results from the National Health and Nutrition Examination Survey (NHANES) revealed that only 40% of Americans meet the recommended servings

of fruits and vegetables per day.[12] Also, less than 5% of the U.S. adult population (ages 19 to 50) and 6.6% of adults older than age 51 consume the recommended three servings per day of whole grains.[13] In other words, the average American diet is very low in foods that provide necessary fiber. Subsequently, the mean fiber intake for women and men in the United States is 15.5 and 18.7 grams per day, respectively.[14] These averages are remarkably lower than the recommended fiber intake and contribute to health problems.

As with many things in nutrition, too much of a good thing also can be problematic. Sudden increases in fiber intake can result in uncomfortable gas, bloating, and constipation. Fiber intake should be gradually increased (along with water intake) to an appropriate amount for the individual. In addition, excessive amounts of dietary fiber can trap (by chelation) small amounts of minerals and prevent their absorption in the gastrointestinal tract. This function of fiber is beneficial when trapping or binding bile acids, but it may compromise nutritional status if fiber intake greatly

🔍 **For Further Focus**

Fiber: What's All the Fuss About?

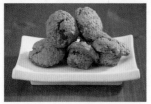

The National Institutes of Health and the World Health Organization—along with most other health-related agencies in the world—have been promoting the intake of fiber for years. The benefits have been defined in several clinical trials related to a variety of chronic illnesses (see references 5-11 in the Reference section in the back of the book).

However, the average fiber intake in a typical American diet remains substantially lower than the current recommendations. Scientists are confident that consuming a well-balanced diet high in whole grains, fruits, and vegetables providing ample fiber imparts the following health benefits:

- It lowers blood cholesterol levels.
- It promotes normal bowel function and prevents constipation.
- It increases satiety, which helps with the prevention of obesity.
- It protects against disorders of the small and large intestines (e.g., irritable bowel syndrome, diverticulosis).
- It slows glucose absorption, thereby reducing blood glucose spikes and insulin secretion.

Health professionals can assist members of the public with evaluating their fiber intake by educating and encouraging the use of food labels. Food labels list the total dietary fiber found in each serving of food. Manufacturers may also voluntarily list the specific type of fiber (i.e., soluble or insoluble).

Increases in dietary fiber intake should be made gradually. A sudden boost in dietary fiber can lead to uncomfortable bloating, gas, and cramping; this can be avoided by making small changes over time and by including an appropriate fluid intake of 8 glasses of water per day.

exceeds the recommendations to the point of reducing mineral absorption.

Other Sweeteners

Sugar alcohols and alternative sweeteners often are used as sugar replacements. Sweeteners that contribute to total calorie intake (e.g., sugar alcohols) are considered *nutritive* sweeteners. *Nonnutritive sweeteners* or *alternative sweeteners* are sugar substitutes that do not have a notable caloric value.

Nutritive sweeteners. The sugar alcohols **sorbitol**, mannitol, and xylitol are the alcohol forms of sucrose, mannose, and xylose, respectively. Sugar alcohols provide 2 to 3 kcal/g as compared with other carbohydrates, which provide 4 kcal/g. The most well-known sugar alcohol is sorbitol, which has been widely used as a sucrose substitute in various foods, candies, chewing gum, and beverages. Both glucose and sugar alcohols are absorbed in the small intestine. However,

the sugar alcohols are absorbed more slowly and do not increase the blood sugar level as rapidly as glucose. Therefore, sugar alcohols are often used in products that are intended for individuals who cannot tolerate a high blood sugar level (e.g., those with diabetes). Another advantage of using a sugar alcohol to replace sugar is a lowered risk of dental caries, because oral bacteria cannot use the alcohol for fuel. The downside of using excessive amounts of sugar alcohols in food products is that the slowed digestion may result in osmotic diarrhea.

Nonnutritive sweeteners. Nonnutritive sweeteners are specifically manufactured to be used as alternative or artificial sweeteners in food products. Because nonnutritive sweeteners do not provide kilocalories, they provide the sweet taste without contributing to an individual's total energy intake. People typically associate these sweeteners with "diet foods." The artificial sweeteners that are most commonly used in the United States are acesulfame-K, aspartame, luohan guo (monk fruit extract), neotame, saccharin, stevia, and sucralose.[15] Nonnutritive sweeteners are much sweeter than sucrose; therefore, extremely small quantities can be used to produce the same sweet taste. Table 2-4 provides a summary of nutritive and nonnutritive sweeteners and their relative sweetness value as compared with table sugar.

FUNCTIONS OF CARBOHYDRATES

BASIC FUEL SUPPLY

The main function of carbohydrates is to provide fuel for the body. Carbohydrates burn in the body at the rate of 4 kcal/g; thus, the fuel factor of carbohydrates is 4. Carbohydrates furnish readily available energy that is needed for physical activities as well as for the work of body cells. Fat also serves as a source of fuel for the body, but the body only needs a small amount of dietary fat to supply the essential fatty acids (see Chapter 3).

RESERVE FUEL SUPPLY

The total amount of carbohydrate in the body, including both stored glycogen and blood sugar, is

---

sugar alcohols nutritive sweeteners that provide 2 to 3 kcal/g; examples include sorbitol, mannitol, and xylitol; these are produced in food-industry laboratories for use as sweeteners in candies, chewing gum, beverages, and other foods.

sorbitol a sugar alcohol that is often used as a nutritive sugar substitute; it is named for where it was discovered in nature, in ripe berries of the *Sorbus aucuparia* tree; it also occurs naturally in small quantities in various other berries, cherries, plums, and pears.

Table 2-4 Sweetness of Sugars and Artificial Sweeteners

SUBSTANCE	SWEETNESS VALUE RELATIVE TO SUCROSE
Nutritive Sweeteners	
D-Tagatose	75 to 92
Glucose	74
Erythritol	60 to 80
Isomalt	45 to 65
Isomaltulose	50
Lactitol	30 to 40
Maltitol	90
Mannitol	50 to 70
Sorbitol	50 to 70
Sucrose	100
Trehalose	45
Xylitol	100
Nonnutritive Sweeteners (Approved for Use in the U.S.)*	
Acesulfame-K (Sunette and Sweet One)	200
Aspartame (NutraSweet and Equal)	160 to 220
Luohan guo extract (*Siraitia grosvenorii*, monk fruit)	150 to 300
Neotame (NutraSweet)	7000 to 13000
Saccharin (Sweet'N Low and Sugar Twin)	300
Stevia (*Stevia rebaudiana*)	250
Sucralose (Splenda)	600

Adapted from Fitch C, et al. Position of the Academy of Nutrition and Dietetics: use of nutritive and nonnutritive sweeteners. *J Acad Nutr Diet.* 2012;112(5):739-758.
*Some artificial sweeteners provide a small amount of calories. Example: 1 packet of Splenda provides 3 kcal, and 1 packet of Equal provides 4 kcal. Because the relative sweetness compared to sucrose is so great, very little of the artificial sweeteners is used to achieve the same level of sweetness as sugar and thus the kilocalories provided are minimal.

relatively small. Healthy, well-nourished adults store approximately 100 g of glycogen in the liver, which is about 8% of the liver mass weight. On average, 300 to 400 g of glycogen can be stored in the skeletal muscle, which is about 1% to 2% of the muscle mass weight. Glycogen in the liver is primarily earmarked to maintain blood glucose levels and to ensure brain function. Without refueling, the total amount of available glucose in the muscle only provides enough energy for 1 to 2 hours of aerobic activity at 66% maximum capacity. Therefore, to maintain a normal blood glucose level and to prevent the breakdown of fat and protein in tissue, individuals must eat carbohydrate foods regularly to meet energy demands.

SPECIAL TISSUE FUNCTIONS

Carbohydrates also serve special functions in many body tissues and organs.

Liver

Glycogen stores in the liver provide a reservoir of available energy to ensure the whole body's energy needs are met. These reserves protect cells from depressed metabolic function and resulting injury.

Central Nervous System

Constant carbohydrate intake and reserves are necessary for the proper functioning of the central nervous system. The brain has no stored supply of glucose; therefore, it is especially dependent on a minute-to-minute supply of glucose from the blood. Sustained and profound shock from low blood sugar may cause brain damage and can result in coma or death.

Protein and Fat Sparing

Carbohydrates help to regulate both protein and fat metabolism. If dietary carbohydrate is sufficient to meet energy needs, protein does not have to be sacrificed to supply energy. This protein-sparing action of carbohydrate protects protein for its major roles in tissue growth and maintenance; these are crucial functions for which the other macronutrients cannot serve as a substitute. Likewise, with sufficient carbohydrate for energy, fat is not needed to supply large amounts of energy. This is significant, because a rapid breakdown of fat may result in the production of ketones, which are products of incomplete fat oxidation in the cells. Ketones are strong acids. The condition of acidosis or ketosis upsets the normal acid-base balance of the body and could result in cellular damage in severe cases. This protective action of carbohydrate is called its *antiketogenic effect.*

FOOD SOURCES OF CARBOHYDRATES

STARCHES

Starch is the most important carbohydrate in a balanced diet. Whole-grain starches such as rice, wheat, corn, and potatoes provide important sources of fiber and other essential nutrients (see Table 2-3).

SUGARS

Sugar per se is not necessarily a villain. After all, the form of carbohydrate that is found in fruit is a disaccharide (a simple sugar). The difference between this type of sugar and the sugar in candy is that fruit also provides fiber, water, and vitamins. The problem with excess added sugar in the diet (e.g., sweets, desserts, candy, soda) is the large quantities of "empty calories" that many people consume, often to the exclusion of other important foods. The per capita availability of caloric sweeteners in the United States is 43.1 tsp daily.[3] That is a total of 690 kcal of "empty calories" every day. As with most things, moderation is the key.

See the For Further Focus box, "Carbohydrate Complications," for a brief discussion of two controversial hot topics in mass-media coverage of nutrition: the glycemic index and "net carbs."

For Further Focus

Carbohydrate Complications

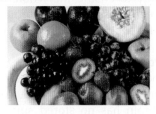

GLYCEMIC INDEX

The glycemic index (GI), which was developed by researchers at the University of Toronto in 1987, was thought to be an ideal tool for controlling blood glucose levels, specifically for individuals with diabetes. However, the use of this tool has been controversial.

How it Works

The GI ranks foods according to how fast blood glucose levels rise after consuming a specific amount (50 g) as compared with a reference food such as white bread or pure glucose. Foods that produce a higher peak in blood sugar within 2 hours of eating them are given a higher GI ranking. Thus, low GI foods do not produce high blood glucose spikes and are favorable. In addition, low GI foods are generally high in fiber.

Complications of Use

The primary reason why this tool is controversial is because of its high variability. The GI of a food can vary significantly in the following ways:

- From person to person
- With the quantity of food eaten
- From one time of day to another
- When a food is eaten alone versus when it is eaten with other foods
- Depending on the ripeness, variety, cooking method used, degree of processing, and site of origin

In addition, the GI of a food does not indicate the nutritious quality of the food. For example, ice cream has a lower GI value than pineapple.

Potential Benefits of Consistent Use

One recently published meta-analysis concluded that individuals who were consuming a low-GI diet had reduced risks for obesity-associated health disease.[1] Other studies evaluating the long-term benefits of a low-GI diet on risks for developing type 2 diabetes and cardiovascular risk factors have not been consistent.

NET CARBS

Food manufacturers invented a category of carbohydrates called "net carbs" as a marketing tactic to capitalize on the low-carbohydrate diet craze. The U.S. Food and Drug Administration regulates all information provided in the Nutrition Facts label, including total carbohydrates, dietary fiber, and sugars, and it does not acknowledge or approve of the "net carb" category.

The concept was developed during the height of carbohydrate-phobic diets. Food manufacturers reasoned that, because dietary fiber and sugar alcohols have lower GI values, these carbohydrates can simply be subtracted from the total carbohydrates in a food serving. For example, a food may have 30 g of total carbohydrates with 18 g of sugar alcohols and 3 g of fiber, thereby leaving 9 g of "net carbs"; these were sometimes referred to as "impact carbs" or "active carbs."

Problems with the "Net Carb" Theory

- Sugar alcohols do have calories and can raise blood sugar levels.
- The excessive use of sugar alcohols in foods has not been studied, but this type of labeling encourages manufacturers to increase the use of products such as sorbitol to lower their "net carb" claim.
- Excess intake of sugar alcohols can cause diarrhea.
- The idea of zero "net carbs" does not explain the fact that the food still has calories.

The bottom line is that the U.S. Food and Drug Administration maintains that, for weight management, no substitute exists for the formula of "calories in must equal calories out." Total calories count more than the quantity—or lack thereof—of high-GI carbohydrates, low-GI carbohydrates, or "net carbs."

REFERENCE

1. Schwingshackl L, Hoffmann G. Long-term effects of low glycemic index/load vs. high glycemic index/load diets on parameters of obesity and obesity-associated risks: a systematic review and meta-analysis. *Nutr Metab Cardiovasc Dis*. 2013;23(8):699-706.

DIGESTION OF CARBOHYDRATES

MOUTH

The digestion of carbohydrate foods, starches, and sugars begins in the mouth and progresses through the successive parts of the gastrointestinal tract. It is accomplished by two types of actions: (1) muscle actions that mechanically break the food mass into smaller particles; and (2) chemical processes in which specific **enzymes** break down the nutrients into still smaller usable metabolic products. The chewing of food, which is called *mastication,* breaks food into fine particles and mixes it with saliva. During this process, the enzyme salivary amylase (also called *ptyalin*) is

enzymes the proteins produced in the body that digest or change nutrients in specific chemical reactions without being changed themselves during the process; thus their action is that of a catalyst; digestive enzymes in gastrointestinal secretions act on food substances to break them down into simpler compounds. (An enzyme usually is named after the substance [i.e., substrate] on which it acts, with the common word ending of *-ase;* for example, sucrase is the specific enzyme for sucrose, which it breaks down into glucose and fructose.)

secreted by the parotid glands, which lie under each ear at the back of the jaw. Salivary amylase acts on starch to begin its breakdown into dextrins (i.e., intermediate starch breakdown products) and disaccharides (primarily maltose). Monosaccharides do not require further digestion; thus they travel unchanged to the stomach and small intestines for absorption.

STOMACH

Wavelike contractions of the stomach muscles continue the mechanical digestive process. This action, called *peristalsis,* further mixes food particles with gastric secretions to facilitate chemical digestion. The gastric secretions contain no specific enzymes for the breakdown of carbohydrates. Gastric secretions include hydrochloric acid, which inhibits the action of salivary amylase. However, before the food completely mixes with the acidic stomach secretions, up to 20% to 30% of the starch may have been changed to maltose. Muscle action continues to mix the food mass and then moves the food to the lower part of the stomach. Here, the food mass is a thick and creamy chyme, ready for its controlled emptying through the pyloric valve and into the duodenum, which is the first portion of the small intestine.

SMALL INTESTINE

Peristalsis continues to help with digestion in the small intestine by mixing and moving chyme along the length of the organ. The chemical digestion of carbohydrate is completed in the small intestine by specific enzymes from both the pancreas and the intestine.

Pancreatic Secretions

Secretions from the pancreas enter the duodenum through the common bile duct. These secretions contain the starch-splitting enzyme *pancreatic amylase* for the continued breakdown of starch into disaccharides and monosaccharides.

Intestinal Secretions

Enzymes from the **brush border** (i.e., microvilli) of the intestinal tract contain three disaccharidases: *sucrase, lactase,* and *maltase.* These specific enzymes act on their respective disaccharides to render the monosaccharides—glucose, galactose, and fructose—ready for absorption directly into the **portal** blood circulation.

Lactose intolerance, which is the inability to break lactose down into its monosaccharide units, results from a deficiency of the enzyme lactase. Symptoms include bloating, gas, abdominal pain, and diarrhea. Lactose intolerance affects 65% to 75% of adults worldwide, with a much higher prevalence in certain countries and ethnic groups (see the Cultural Considerations box, "Ethnicity and Lactose Intolerance").

A summary of the major aspects of carbohydrate digestion through the successive parts of the gastrointestinal tract is shown in Figure 2-4. The overall process

of the absorption and metabolism of all energy-yielding nutrients (i.e., carbohydrate, fat, and protein) is discussed in Chapter 5.

RECOMMENDATIONS FOR DIETARY CARBOHYDRATE

DIETARY REFERENCE INTAKES

Energy needs are listed as total kilocalories, and these amounts include caloric intake from fat and protein as well as carbohydrate. According to the most recent DRIs, 45% to 65% of an adult's total caloric intake should come from carbohydrate foods.[4] This translates

brush border the cells that are located on the microvilli within the lining of the intestinal tract; the microvilli are tiny hair-like projections that protrude from the mucosal cells that help to increase surface area for the digestion and absorption of nutrients.
portal an entrance or gateway; for example, the portal blood circulation designates the entry of blood vessels from the intestines into the liver; it carries nutrients for liver metabolism, and it then drains into the body's main systemic circulation to deliver metabolic products to body cells.

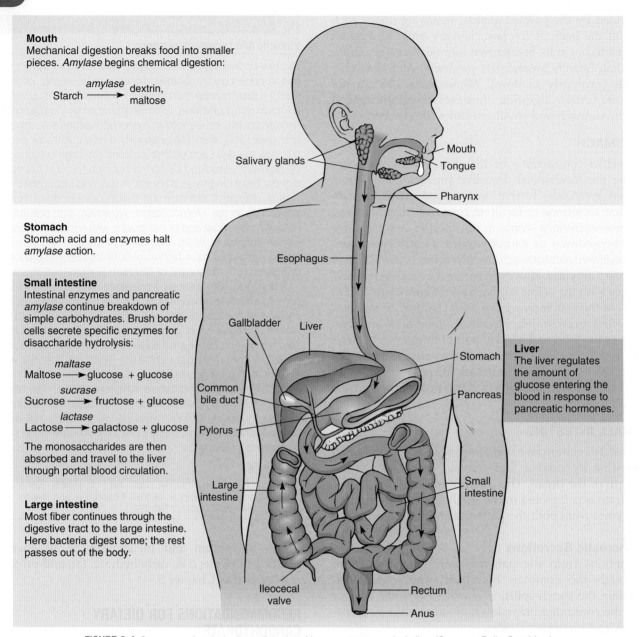

Mouth
Mechanical digestion breaks food into smaller pieces. *Amylase* begins chemical digestion:

Starch $\xrightarrow{\text{amylase}}$ dextrin, maltose

Stomach
Stomach acid and enzymes halt *amylase* action.

Small intestine
Intestinal enzymes and pancreatic *amylase* continue breakdown of simple carbohydrates. Brush border cells secrete specific enzymes for disaccharide hydrolysis:

Maltose $\xrightarrow{\text{maltase}}$ glucose + glucose

Sucrose $\xrightarrow{\text{sucrase}}$ fructose + glucose

Lactose $\xrightarrow{\text{lactase}}$ galactose + glucose

The monosaccharides are then absorbed and travel to the liver through portal blood circulation.

Large intestine
Most fiber continues through the digestive tract to the large intestine. Here bacteria digest some; the rest passes out of the body.

Liver
The liver regulates the amount of glucose entering the blood in response to pancreatic hormones.

Mouth
Tongue
Pharynx
Salivary glands
Esophagus
Gallbladder
Liver
Common bile duct
Pylorus
Stomach
Pancreas
Large intestine
Small intestine
Ileocecal valve
Rectum
Anus

FIGURE 2-4 Summary of carbohydrate digestion. Note: enzymes are in *italics*. (Courtesy Rolin Graphics.)

to 225 to 325 g of carbohydrates for a 2000 kcal/day diet. The recommended fiber intake can be achieved by choosing carbohydrate foods such as whole grains, legumes, vegetables, and fruits. In addition, the DRIs recommend limiting added sugar to no more than 25% of the total calories consumed. See the Clinical Applications box entitled "What Is Your Dietary Reference Intake for Carbohydrates?" to calculate your specific carbohydrate recommendation.

DIETARY GUIDELINES FOR AMERICANS

The *Dietary Guidelines for Americans* are general guidelines for the promotion of health (see Figure 1-4). The

2015-2020 *Guidelines* advise individuals to do the following with regard to carbohydrate-rich foods[2]:
- Consume at least half of all grains as whole grains. Increase whole-grain intake by replacing refined grains with whole grains.
- Increase vegetable and whole fruit intake. Eat a variety of vegetables from all subgroups—dark-green, red, and orange vegetables, legumes (beans and peas), and starchy vegetables.
- Choose more nutrient-dense foods and less foods and beverages with added sugar.
- Reduce the intake of calories from added sugars to less than 10% of total calories in the diet.

Clinical Applications

What Is Your Dietary Reference Intake for Carbohydrates?

On the basis of the current Dietary Reference Intakes (DRIs), calculate the amount of calories and grams of carbohydrates that you are recommended to consume daily. This requires you to know how many total calories you consume on a daily basis.

Step 1: Keep track of everything you eat for 1 day. You can use Nutritrac that is included on Evolve to calculate your daily food intake. This is your *total energy intake.* (Chapter 6 discusses the evaluation of total energy intake relative to body weight and activity needs.)

Total energy intake = _____ kcal

Step 2: Multiply your total energy intake by 45% (0.45) and 65% (0.65) to get the recommended number of *kilocalories from carbohydrates (CHO).*

_____ total kcal × 0.45 = _____ kcal
_____ total kcal × 0.65 = _____ kcal

Example:
2200 total kcal × 0.45 = 990 kcal
2200 total kcal × 0.65 = 1430 kcal

Thus, the recommended range of total kilocalories from CHO for this example is 990 to 1430 kcal/day.

Step 3: Determine how many *grams of CHO* you need on the basis of these recommendations.

Each gram of CHO has 4 kcal; therefore, divide your recommended range of kilocalories from CHO (as determined previously) by 4.

_____ kcal/day from CHO ÷ 4 = _____ g of CHO/day

Example:
990 to 1430 kcal/day from CHO ÷ 4 = 247.5 to 357.5 g of CHO/day

Thus, after rounding the nearest whole number, the recommended range of total grams of CHO for this example is 248 to 358 g of CHO/day.

Step 4: What is the maximum amount of total kilocalorie consumption that can come from *added sugars,* according to the DRIs? Added sugars are added to food and beverages during production. The majority of added sugars in American diets come from candy, soft drinks, fruit drinks, pastries, and other sweets. The DRIs recommend limiting added sugar intake to no more than 25% of the total kilocalories consumed.

Multiply your total energy intake by 25% (0.25) to get the maximum number of *kilocalories from added sugars.*

_____ total kcal × 0.25 = _____ kcal

Example:
2200 total kcal × 0.25 = 550 kcal

Thus, the maximum amount of total kilocalories from added sugar for this example is 550 kcal/day.

Step 5: Determine the number of grams of added sugar by dividing the maximum kcal/day of added sugar by 4.

_____ kcal/day from added sugar ÷ 4 = _____ g of added sugar/day

Example:
550 kcal/day from added sugar ÷ 4 = 137.5 g of added sugar/day

Therefore, the 137.5 g of added sugar is the recommended *limit* per day for this example.

NOTE: There is no dietary need for added sugar in the diet. This is only a reference for a *maximum* consumption.

MYPLATE

The MyPlate food guidance system provides recommendations that are specific to age, gender, height, weight, and physical activity when reported as part of the MyPlate plan (see Chapter 1).[16]

The MyPlate Tracker is an assessment tool available to MyPlate participants that allows the user to enter his or her own menu for an evaluation of diet quality. This is a great resource for feedback about dietary sources of carbohydrate, including the consumption of fiber, whole grains, fruits, vegetables, and added sugars.

Putting It All Together

Summary

- The primary source of energy for most of the world's population is carbohydrate foods. These foods are from widely distributed plant sources. For the most part, these food products can be stored easily and are relatively low in cost.
- Two basic types of carbohydrates supply energy: simple and complex. Simple carbohydrates are single- and double-sugar units (i.e., monosaccharides and disaccharides, respectively). Because simple carbohydrates are easy to digest and absorb, they provide quick energy. Complex carbohydrates (i.e., polysaccharides) are composed of many sugar units linked together. They break down more slowly and thus provide sustained energy over a longer period.
- Dietary fiber is a complex carbohydrate that is not digestible by humans. It mainly occurs as the structural parts of plants, and it provides important bulk in the diet, affects nutrient absorption, and benefits health.
- Carbohydrate digestion starts briefly in the mouth with the initial action of salivary amylase to begin digesting

starch into smaller units. No enzyme for starch digestion is present in the stomach, but muscle action continues to mix the food mass and move it to the small intestine, where pancreatic amylase continues the chemical digestion. Final starch and disaccharide digestion occurs in the small intestine with the action of sucrase, lactase, and maltase to produce single-sugar units of glucose, fructose, and galactose. These monosaccharides are then absorbed into the portal blood circulation to the liver.

Chapter Review Questions

See answers in Appendix A.

1. John is trying to increase dietary fiber in his diet. A good food choice to recommend is:
   a. Whole-grain toast with apple slices.
   b. Toaster pastry with blueberry filling.
   c. Hot dog on plain white bun.
   d. Milkshake with low-fat potato chips.

2. A patient asks the nurse for examples of refined grains. The nurse may give the following examples of refined grains:
   a. Popcorn and steel cut oats
   b. Carrots and celery
   c. Chocolate chip cookies and saltine crackers
   d. Parmesan cheese and cantaloupe

3. A patient has been recently diagnosed with lactose intolerance and comes into the clinic with complaints of gas and bloating. After reviewing foods eaten, the most likely cause would be:
   a. Roasted chicken with parsley.
   b. Chocolate pudding.
   c. Baked potato with butter.
   d. Dried fruit mix.

4. Anna requires 1700 calories per day. An appropriate amount of carbohydrate calories per day for her would be:
   a. 255 to 425 calories.
   b. 425 to 935 calories.
   c. 765 to 1105 calories.
   d. 825 to 1225 calories.

5. Which of the following food items would provide the quickest source of energy?
   a. Oat bran muffin
   b. Orange juice
   c. Pretzels
   d. 2% milk

Additional Learning Resources

evolve Please refer to this text's Evolve website for answers to the Case Study questions. http://evolve.elsevier.com/Williams/basic/

References and **Further Reading and Resources** in the back of the book provide additional resources for enhancing knowledge.

Fats

Key Concepts

- Dietary fat is essential to the body as both an energy fuel and a structural material.
- Foods from animal and plant sources supply distinct forms of fat that affect health in different ways.
- Excess dietary fat, especially in an otherwise unbalanced diet, is a risk factor for poor health.

General awareness regarding health concerns and the risk of chronic disease from poor food selections has influenced dietary choices for decades. More knowledge of "heart-healthy" fats is helpful for the public to identify beneficial sources of dietary fat and to create a well-rounded diet.

This chapter examines the various aspects of fat as an essential nutrient, a concentrated storage form of energy, and a savory food component. In addition, we will review the types of fat and the health implications when dietary fat intake or body fat are unchecked.

THE NATURE OF FATS

DIETARY IMPORTANCE

Fats are a concentrated fuel source for the human energy system. A large amount of energy can be stored in a relatively small space within adipose tissue as compared with carbohydrates that are stored as glycogen. As such, fats supplement carbohydrates (the primary fuel) as an additional energy source. In food, fats occur in the form of either solid fat or liquid oil. Fats are not soluble in water, and they have a greasy texture.

STRUCTURE AND CLASSES OF FATS

The overall name of the chemical group of fats and fat-related compounds is **lipids**, which comes from the Greek word *lipos*, meaning "fat." The word *lipid* appears in combination words that are used for fat-related health conditions. For example, an elevated level of fat in the blood is called *hyperlipidemia*.

All lipids are composed of the same basic chemical elements as carbohydrates: carbon, hydrogen, and oxygen. The majority of dietary fats are **glycerides**, which are composed of **fatty acids** attached to glycerol. Most natural fats, whether in animal or plant sources, have three fatty acids attached to their glycerol base, thus the chemical name of **triglyceride** (Figure 3-1).

CLASSIFICATION OF FATTY ACIDS

Fatty acids, which are the building blocks of triglycerides, can be classified by their length as short-, medium-, or long-chain fatty acids. The chains contain carbon atoms with a methyl group (CH_3) on one end (also known as the *omega end*) and an acid carboxyl group (COOH) on the other end. Short-chain fatty acids have 2 to 4 carbons, medium-chain fatty acids have 6 to 10 carbons, and long-chain fatty acids have more than 12 carbons. Fatty acids can also be classified according to their saturation or essentiality, both of which are significant characteristics.

Saturated Fatty Acid

When a substance is described as **saturated**, it contains all of the material that it is capable of holding (Figure 3-2, *A*). For example, a sponge is saturated with water when it holds all of the water that it can contain. Similarly, fatty acids are saturated or unsaturated according to whether each carbon is filled with hydrogen. Thus, a saturated fatty acid is heavy and dense

---

lipids the chemical group name for organic substances of a fatty nature; the lipids include fats, oils, waxes, and other fat-related compounds such as cholesterol.

glycerides the chemical group name for fats; fats are formed from a glycerol base with one, two, or three fatty acids attached to make monoglycerides, diglycerides, and triglycerides, respectively; glycerides are the principal constituents of adipose tissue, and they are found in animal and vegetable fats and oils.

fatty acids the major structural components of fats.

triglycerides the chemical name for fats in the body or in food; three fatty acids attached to a glycerol base.

saturated the state of being filled; the state of fatty acid components being filled in all their available carbon bonds with hydrogen, thus making the fat harder and more solid at room temperature; such solid food fats are generally from animal sources.

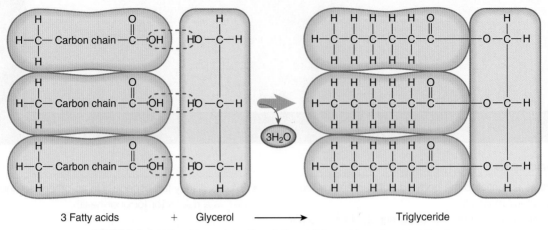

3 Fatty acids   +   Glycerol   ⟶   Triglyceride

FIGURE 3-1 A triglyceride contains three fatty acids bound to a glycerol molecule.

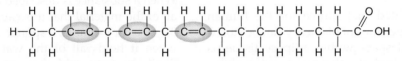

Methyl or omega end   **Acid groups**

A   Saturated fatty acid: palmitic acid

B   Monounsaturated fatty acid: oleic acid (omega-9)

C   Polyunsaturated fatty acid: linoleic acid (omega-6)

D   Polyunsaturated fatty acid: alpha-linolenic acid (omega-3)

FIGURE 3-2 Types of fatty acids. **A,** Saturated palmitic acid. **B,** Monounsaturated oleic acid (omega-9). **C,** Polyunsaturated linoleic acid (omega-6). **D,** Polyunsaturated alpha-linolenic acid (omega-3). (Adapted from Grodner M, Escott-Stump S, Dorner S. *Nutritional Foundations and Clinical Applications: A Nursing Approach*, 6th ed. St. Louis: Mosby; 2016.)

(i.e., solid at room temperature). If most of the fatty acids in a triglyceride are saturated, that fat is said to be a *saturated fat.* Most saturated fats are of animal origin. Figure 3-3 shows a variety of foods with saturated fat, including meat, dairy, and eggs.

Unsaturated Fatty Acid

A fatty acid that is not completely filled with all of the hydrogen that it can hold is unsaturated; as a result, it is less heavy and less dense (i.e., liquid at room temperature). If most of the fatty acids in a triglyceride are unsaturated, that fat is said to be an *unsaturated fat.* If the fatty acids have one unfilled spot (i.e., one double bond between the carbon atoms), the fat is called a *monounsaturated fat* (see Figure 3-2, *B*). Examples of foods that contain monounsaturated fats include the vegetable oils: olive, canola (rapeseed), peanut; nuts

such as macadamia, hazelnuts, almonds, and pecans; and avocados. If the fatty acids have two or more unfilled spots (i.e., more than one double bond between the carbon atoms), the fat is called a *polyunsaturated fat* (see Figure 3-2, *C* and *D*). Examples of foods that contain polyunsaturated fats are the vegetable oils: safflower, sunflower, corn, and soybean. Fats from plant and fish sources are mostly unsaturated (Figure 3-4). However, notable exceptions are the tropical oils (palm and coconut oils), which are predominantly saturated.

Nomenclature of unsaturated fatty acids. Unsaturated fatty acids are further classified according to the location of the first double bond from the omega end (i.e., the methyl group end). For example, when the first double bond starts on the third carbon from the

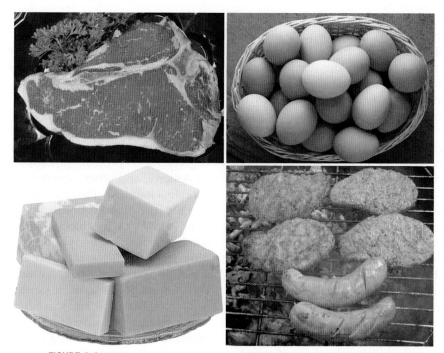

FIGURE 3-3 Dietary sources of saturated fats. (Copyright JupiterImages Corp.)

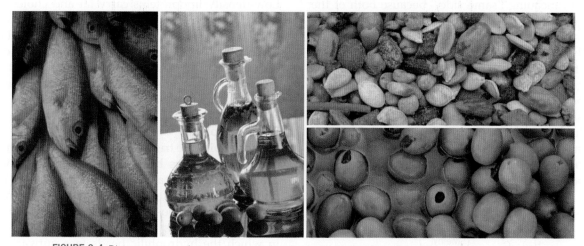

FIGURE 3-4 Dietary sources of monounsaturated and polyunsaturated fats. (Copyright JupiterImages Corp.)

methyl end, it is known as an *omega-3 fatty acid* (see Figure 3-2, *D*). When the first double bond starts on the sixth carbon from the methyl end, it is known as an *omega-6 fatty acid* (see Figure 3-2, *C*).

Essential fatty acids. The term *essential* or *nonessential* is applied to a nutrient according to its necessity in the diet. A nutrient is essential if either of the following is true: (1) its absence will create a specific deficiency disease; or (2) the body cannot manufacture it in sufficient amounts and must obtain it from the diet. A diet with 10% or less of its total kilocalories from fat cannot supply adequate amounts of essential fatty acids. The only fatty acids known to be essential for complete human nutrition are the polyunsaturated fatty acids **linoleic acid** and **alpha-linolenic acid.** Both essential fatty acids serve important functions related to tissue strength, **cholesterol** metabolism, muscle tone, blood

linoleic acid an essential fatty acid that consists of 18 carbon atoms and 2 double bonds. The first double bond is located at the sixth carbon from the omega end, making it an omega-6 fatty acid. Found in vegetable oils.

alpha-linolenic acid an essential fatty acid with 18 carbon atoms and 3 double bonds. The first double bond is located at the third carbon from the omega end, making it an omega-3 fatty acid. Found in soybean, canola, and flaxseed oil.

cholesterol a fat-related compound called a sterol that is synthesized only in animal tissues; a normal constituent of bile and a principal constituent of gallstones; in the body, cholesterol is primarily synthesized in the liver; in the diet, cholesterol is found in animal food sources.

clotting, and heart action. Essential fatty acids must come from the foods we eat. With an adequate dietary supply of the essential fatty acids, the body is capable of manufacturing saturated, monounsaturated, and other polyunsaturated fatty acids, as well as cholesterol. Therefore, no Dietary Reference Intake (DRI) exists for fat compounds other than the two essential fatty acids.

The terms omega-3 fatty acid and alpha-linolenic acid are often erroneously used interchangeably. This is also a point of confusion for omega-6 fatty acid and linoleic acid. There are several omega-3 and omega-6 fatty acids, of which alpha-linolenic and linoleic are two examples. Other examples of omega-3 fatty acids are eicosapentaenoic acid and docosahexaenoic acid. Thus, it is not accurate to use the term omega-3 when meaning to indicate the essential fatty acid alpha-linolenic acid. The same is true for omega-6 and linoleic acid—the terms are not synonymous.

Trans-fatty acids. Naturally occurring unsaturated fatty acid molecules have a bend in the chain of atoms at the point of the carbon double bond. This form is called *cis*, meaning "same side," because both of the hydrogen atoms around the carbon double bond are on the same side of the bond. When vegetable oils are partially hydrogenated to produce a more solid, shelf-stable fat, the normal bend is changed so that the hydrogen atoms around the carbon double bond are on opposite sides. This form is called *trans*, meaning "opposite side," and the process is called *hydrogenation.* The following illustration shows the *cis* form and the *trans* form of a molecule of oleic acid, which is a common monounsaturated fatty acid with a chain of 18 carbon atoms.

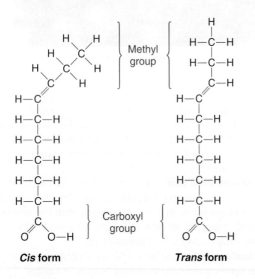

Cis form   **Trans form**

Commercially hydrogenated fats in margarine, snack items, fast food, and many other food products used to be high in trans fat. Trans fats are unnecessary in human nutrition and pose a great number of negative health consequences related to cardiovascular disease.[1-3] The current dietary recommendations by the American Heart Association, the Academy of Nutrition and Dietetics, the Institute of Medicine, and the *Dietary Guidelines for Americans* are to avoid trans fat in the diet as much as possible.

Lipoproteins

Lipoproteins, which are the major vehicles for lipid transport in the bloodstream, are combinations of triglycerides, protein (apoprotein), phospholipids, cholesterol, and other fat-soluble substances (e.g., fat-soluble vitamins). Because fat is insoluble in water and because blood is predominantly water, fat cannot freely travel in the bloodstream; it needs a water-soluble carrier. The body solves this problem by wrapping small particles of fat in a covering of protein, which is hydrophilic (i.e., "water loving"). The blood then transports these packages of fat to and from the cells throughout the body to supply needed nutrients. A lipoprotein's relative load of fat and protein determines its density. The higher the protein load, the higher the lipoprotein's density. The lower the protein load, the lower the lipoprotein's density (Figure 3-5). Low-density lipoproteins carry fat and cholesterol to cells. High-density lipoproteins carry free cholesterol from body tissues back to the liver for metabolism. Circulating levels of lipoproteins are indicative of lipid disorder risks and with the underlying blood vessel disease atherosclerosis. These relationships are discussed in greater detail in Chapter 19.

Phospholipids

Phospholipids are triglyceride derivatives in which the one fatty acid has been replaced with a phosphate group. The result is a molecule that is partially hydrophobic (i.e., "water fearing") and partially hydrophilic (because of the phosphate group). This combination results in what is called an *amphiphilic molecule,* in which the hydrophilic heads face outward to the aqueous environment and the hydrophobic heads bind fats and oils and face each other (Figure 3-6). Phospholipids are major constituents in cell membranes and allow for membrane fluidity.

Lecithin. Lecithin, which is a lipid substance produced by the liver, is a key building block of cell membranes. It is a combination of **glycolipids**, triglycerides,

lipoproteins chemical complexes of fat and protein that serve as the major carriers of lipids in the plasma; they vary in density according to the size of the fat load being carried (i.e., the lower the density, the higher the fat load); the combination package with water-soluble protein makes possible the transport of non–water-soluble fatty substances in the water-based blood circulation.

glycolipid a lipid with a carbohydrate attached.

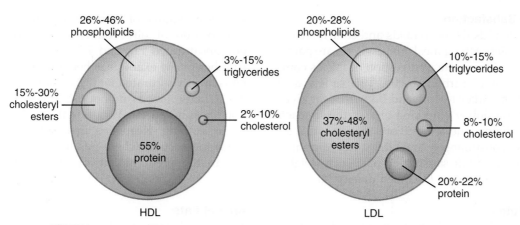

FIGURE 3-5 Composition of high-density lipoproteins (HDL) and low-density lipoproteins (LDL).

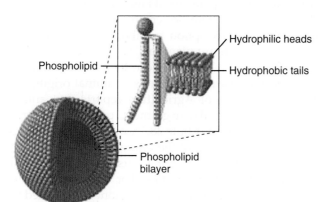

FIGURE 3-6 Phospholipid bilayer. (Reprinted from the NASA Astrobiology Institute. *Project 4. Prebiotic molecular selection and organization (website):* <http://nai.nasa.gov>; Accessed July 6, 2007.)

and phospholipids. The amphiphilic quality in lecithin makes it ideal for transporting fats and cholesterol.

Eicosanoids. Eicosanoids are signaling hormones that exert control over multiple functions in the body (e.g., the inflammatory response, immunity), and they are messengers for the central nervous system. Eicosanoids are divided into four classes: (1) prostaglandins; (2) prostacyclins; (3) thromboxanes; and (4) leukotrienes. Eicosanoids are derived from the essential fatty acids.

Sterols

Sterols are a subgroup of steroids, and they are amphipathic in nature. Sterols made by plants are called *phytosterols*, and sterols produced by animals are called *zoosterols*. Sterols play a variety of important roles, including membrane fluidity and cellular signaling. Cholesterol is the most significant zoosterol.

Cholesterol. Cholesterol is vital to membranes; it is a precursor for some hormones, and it plays other important roles in human metabolism. It occurs

naturally in foods of animal origin. The main food sources of cholesterol are egg yolks, organ meats (e.g., liver, kidney), and other meats. To ensure that it always has the relatively small amount of cholesterol necessary for sustaining life, the human body synthesizes endogenous cholesterol in many body tissues, particularly in the liver as well as in small amounts in the adrenal cortex, the skin, the intestines, the testes, and the ovaries. Consequently, no biologic requirement for dietary cholesterol exists, and no DRI has been set for cholesterol consumption. The *Dietary Guidelines for Americans* and the DRIs recommend consuming a diet that is low in cholesterol.[4,5] Although epidemiologic studies have found strong correlations between the dietary intake of trans fats with coronary heart disease,[1,3] the association with such risk factors and dietary cholesterol is less well-defined. Subsequently, the current recommendations to limit dietary cholesterol intake to <300 mg/day are being challenged by lack of scientific support.[6]

FUNCTIONS OF FAT

FAT IN FOODS

Energy

In addition to carbohydrates, fats serve as a fuel for energy production. Excess caloric intake from any macronutrient source is converted into stored fat throughout the body. Fat is a much more concentrated form of fuel, yielding 9 kcal/g when burned by the body as compared with carbohydrate's yield of 4 kcal/g.

Essential Nutrients

Dietary fat supplies the body with the essential fatty acids (linoleic and alpha-linolenic acid). As long as adequate amounts of essential fatty acids are consumed, the body is capable of endogenously producing other fats and cholesterol as needed. Also, foods high in fat are generally a good source of fat-soluble vitamins (see Chapter 7), and fat aids in the absorption of those vitamins.

Flavor and Satisfaction

Fat in the diet adds flavor to foods and contributes to a feeling of satiety after a meal. These effects are partly caused by the slower rate of digestion of fats as compared with that of carbohydrates. This satiety also results from the fuller texture and body that fat gives to food and the slower emptying time of the stomach that it necessitates. The absence of satiation while an individual is consuming a low-fat/fat-free diet may contribute to overall dissatisfaction with such weight-loss attempts that remove too much dietary fat.

Fat Substitutes

Several fat substitutes, which are compounds that are not absorbed and thus contribute little or no kilocalories, are available to provide improved flavor and physical texture to low-fat/fat-free foods and to help reduce total dietary fat intake. Fat substitutes that are currently on the market are considered safe by the U.S. Food and Drug Administration (FDA). However, the risks and benefits of long-term use of fat substitutes are not well established. There are many different types of fat substitutes. Two of the more common examples are Simplesse (CP Kelco, Atlanta, Ga), which is made by reshaping the protein of milk whey or egg whites, and Olean (Olestra, Procter & Gamble, Cincinnati, Ohio), which is an indigestible form of sucrose.

FAT IN THE BODY

Adipose Tissue

Fat that is stored in various parts of the body is called **adipose** *tissue*, from the Latin word *adiposus*, meaning "fatty." A weblike padding of fat tissue supports and protects vital organs, and a layer of fat directly under the skin is important for the regulation of body temperature.

Cell Membrane Structure

Fat forms the fatty center of cell membranes, thereby creating the selectively permeable lipid bilayer. Proteins are embedded within this layer and allow for the transport of various nutrients in and out of the cells. In addition, the protective myelin sheath that surrounds neurons is largely composed of fat.

FOOD SOURCES OF FAT

VARIETY OF SOURCES

It is common that foods are classified as being a source of one type of fat or another. In reality, most foods contain a combination of different types of fats. For example, we generally think of olive oil as a "heart-healthy" monounsaturated fat. Although it is a

---

significant source of monounsaturated fat, the actual composition of olive oil is 14% saturated fat, 9% polyunsaturated fat, and 77% monounsaturated fat. Another prime example is beef fat. It is true that beef fat is mostly saturated fat (52% of the fat is saturated), but a hefty 44% is monounsaturated fat and 4% is polyunsaturated fat. Very few things in nutrition are all or nothing. Keep this in mind as you read the following section where fats are categorized according to the predominant, but not exclusive, source of fat.

Animal Fats

The chief dietary supply of saturated fat and cholesterol comes from animal sources, the most concentrated of which include meat fats (e.g., bacon, sausage), dairy fats (e.g., cream, ice cream, butter, cheese), and egg yolks. The exception to this rule is coconut and palm oils, which are plant fats and also contain saturated fatty acids. The American diet has traditionally featured meats and other foods of animal origin. The U.S. Department of Agriculture reports that animal products in particular (e.g., meat, poultry, fish, eggs, dairy products) contribute 38.1% of the total fat to U.S. diets as well as 53.8% of the saturated fat and 95.3% of the cholesterol.[7] Some animal fats also contain small amounts of unsaturated fats. For example, 6 oz of sockeye salmon provides 4.2 g of monounsaturated fat and 3 g of polyunsaturated fat, in addition to 2.5 g of saturated fat.

Although animal products supply saturated fat and cholesterol to the diet, all types of animal-derived foods are not created equal. One study found that, regardless of the protein source, when consuming lean beef, lean fish, and poultry without skin in a well-balanced diet that also includes a high ratio of polyunsaturated fat to saturated fat and ample fiber, similar benefits for blood cholesterol levels are found.[8] In other words, although animal products are higher in cholesterol and saturated fat than plant foods, lean portions do not have the same hypercholesterolemic effects as their full-fat counterparts when they are consumed with diets that are high in fiber.[9]

Some studies show that cholesterol-lowering effects can be achieved from a diet that is low in trans-fatty acids and that involves the regular moderate use of unsaturated fat in the place of saturated fat.[10,11] However, other scientists argue that there is not enough definitive evidence to support the recommendation of substituting animal fats (high in cholesterol and saturated fat) with *unspecified* polyunsaturated fats.[12-15] The basis for this argument is that there are many dietary factors that affect the overall lipid profile of an individual. Making the singular recommendation that people reduce animal foods may or may not make improvements in their cardiovascular disease risk. This is particularly problematic if omega-6 fatty acids (inflammatory when consumed in excess of omega-3

---

adipose fat stored in the cells of adipose (fatty) tissue.

fatty acids) are used in place of saturated fats.[15] The whole diet and lifestyle must be taken into consideration.

Plant Fats

Plant foods supply mostly monounsaturated and polyunsaturated fats, including the essential fatty acids. Food sources for unsaturated fats include vegetable oils (e.g., safflower, corn, cottonseed, soybean, peanut, olive; see Figure 3-4). However, as indicated previously, coconut and palm oils are exceptions; these plants provide saturated fats and are widely used in commercially processed food items.

CHARACTERISTICS OF FOOD FAT SOURCES

For practical purposes, food fats can be classified as visible or invisible fats.

Visible Fat

The obvious fats are easy to see and include butter, margarine, separate cream, salad oils and dressings, lard, shortening, fatty meats (e.g., bacon, sausage, salt pork), and the visible fat of any meat. Visible fats are easier to control in the diet than those that are less apparent.

Invisible Fat

Some dietary fats are less visible, so individuals who want to control dietary fat must be aware of these food sources. Invisible fats include cheese, the cream portion of homogenized milk, nuts, seeds, olives, avocados, and lean meat. Basically, invisible fats are those that you cannot cut out of the food. Even when all of the visible fat has been removed from meat (e.g., the skin on poultry and the obvious fat on the lean portions), approximately 6% of the total fat surrounding the muscle fibers remains.

Table 3-1 provides a list of commonly eaten foods and their fat content.

FOOD LABEL INFORMATION

The FDA food-labeling regulations for nutrition facts panel content provide the following mandatory and voluntary (italicized below) information relating to dietary fat in food products (Figure 3-7):

- Total fat
- Saturated fat
- Trans fat
- *Polyunsaturated fat*
- *Monounsaturated fat*
- Cholesterol

The FDA has approved a series of health claims that link one or more dietary components to the reduced risk of a specific disease.[16] Approved health claims that involve dietary fat include the following:

- A diet that is low in total fat may reduce the risk of some cancers.

Table 3-1 Fat in Food Servings

FOOD	SERVING SIZE	FAT CONTENT (g)
Fats		
Butter or margarine	1 Tbsp	11
Cream cheese	1 Tbsp	10
Mayonnaise	1 Tbsp	11
Salad dressing	1 Tbsp	7
Vegetables		
Broccoli	½ cup	Trace
Carrots	½ cup	Trace
Potato, baked	1	Trace
Fruit		
Apple	1	Trace
Banana	1	Trace
Fruit juice	1 cup	Trace
Orange	1	Trace
Bread and Grains		
Bagel	1	Trace
Muffin	1 medium	6
Rice or pasta	½ cup	Trace
Dairy		
American cheese	2 oz	18
Cheddar cheese	1½ oz	14
Frozen yogurt	½ cup	2
Ice cream	⅓ cup	7
Low-fat milk	1 cup	5
Skim milk	1 cup	Trace
Whole milk	1 cup	8
Eggs, Fish, Meat, and Nuts		
Bologna (2 slices)	1 oz	16
Egg	1	5
Fish	3 oz	6
Ground beef	3 oz	16
Lean beef	3 oz	6
Poultry	3 oz	6
Nuts (⅓ cup)	1 oz	22
Other		
Danish pastry	1 medium	13
French fries	1 cup	8

Adapted from Grodner M, Escott-Stump S, Dorner S. *Nutritional Foundations and Clinical Applications: A Nursing Approach*, 6th ed. St. Louis: Mosby; 2016.

- Diets that are low in saturated fat and cholesterol may reduce the risk of coronary heart disease.

See the label claim information published by the FDA at www.fda.gov (search "Health Claims") for more information about FDA-approved health claims. This website provides updates regarding approved health claims, pending claims, and the appropriate use

Nutrition Facts

8 servings per container

Serving size	2/3 cup (55g)

Amount per 2/3 cup

Calories 230

% DV*

12%	**Total Fat** 8g	
5%	Saturated Fat 1g	
	Trans Fat 0g	
0%	**Cholesterol** 0mg	
7%	**Sodium** 160mg	
12%	**Total Carbs** 37g	
14%	Dietary Fiber 4g	
	Sugars 1g	
	Added Sugars 0g	
	Protein 3g	

10%	Vitamin D 2mcg	
20%	Calcium 260mg	
45%	Iron 8mg	
5%	Potassium 235mg	

* Footnote on Daily Values (DV) and calories reference to be inserted here.

FIGURE 3-7 Example of nutrition facts panel listing the trans-fat content. (From the U.S. Food and Drug Administration, U.S. Department of Health and Human Services. *Proposed Changes to the Nutrition Facts Label* (website): http://www.fda.gov/Food/GuidanceRegulation/GuidanceDocumentsRegulatoryInformation/LabelingNutrition/ucm385663.htm#images; Accessed January 27, 2016.)

of the claims on food products. Food labels and health claims are discussed further in Chapter 13.

DIGESTION OF FATS

MOUTH

As with other macronutrients (i.e., carbohydrates and proteins), fats are broken down into their basic building blocks, fatty acids, through the process of digestion (summarized in Figure 3-8). When foods are eaten, some initial fat breakdown may begin in the mouth by the action of lingual lipase, an enzyme that is secreted by the Ebner's glands at the back of the tongue. Lingual lipase is only important for digestion during infancy. For adults, the primary digestive action that occurs in the mouth is mechanical. Foods are broken into smaller particles through chewing and moistened for passage into the stomach.

STOMACH

Little if any chemical digestion of fat occurs in the stomach. General muscle action continues to mix the fat with the stomach contents. No significant amounts

of fat enzymes are present in the gastric secretions except gastric lipase (tributyrinase), which acts on emulsified butterfat. Although the primary gastric enzymes act on other protein in the food mix, fat is isolated and prepared for its major, enzyme-specific breakdown in the small intestine.

SMALL INTESTINE

Fat digestion largely occurs in the small intestine, where the major enzymes that are necessary for the chemical changes are present. These digestive agents come from three major sources: an emulsification agent from the gallbladder and two specific enzymes from the pancreas and the small intestine itself.

Bile from the Gallbladder

The **bile** is first produced in large dilute amounts in the liver, and the liver then sends the bile to the gallbladder for concentration and storage so that it is ready for use during fat digestion as needed. The fat that comes into the duodenum, which is the first section of the small intestine, stimulates the secretion of cholecystokinin, a hormone that is released from glands in the intestinal walls. In turn, cholecystokinin causes the gallbladder to contract, relax its opening, and subsequently secrete bile into the intestine by way of the common bile duct. Bile is not an enzyme that acts in the chemical digestive process; rather, it functions as an **emulsifier.** This emulsification process accomplishes the following two important tasks: (1) it breaks the fat into small particles, thereby greatly increasing the total surface area available for enzymatic action; and (2) it lowers the surface tension of the finely dispersed and suspended fat particles, thus allowing the enzymes to penetrate more easily. The bile also provides an alkaline medium that is necessary for the action of pancreatic lipase, which is the chief lipid enzyme.

Enzymes from the Pancreas

Pancreatic juice flowing into the small intestine contains one enzyme for triglycerides and another for cholesterol. First, pancreatic lipase breaks off one fatty acid at a time from the glycerol base of triglycerides. One free fatty acid plus a diglyceride and then another fatty acid plus a monoglyceride are produced in turn (Figure 3-9). Each succeeding step of this breakdown

---

bile an emulsifying agent produced by the liver and transported to the gallbladder for concentration and storage; it is released into the duodenum with the entry of fat to facilitate enzymatic fat digestion by acting as an emulsifier.

emulsifier an agent that breaks down large fat globules into smaller, uniformly distributed particles; the action is chiefly accomplished in the intestine by bile acids, which lower the surface tension of the fat particles, thereby breaking the fat into many smaller droplets and facilitating contact with the fat-digesting enzymes.

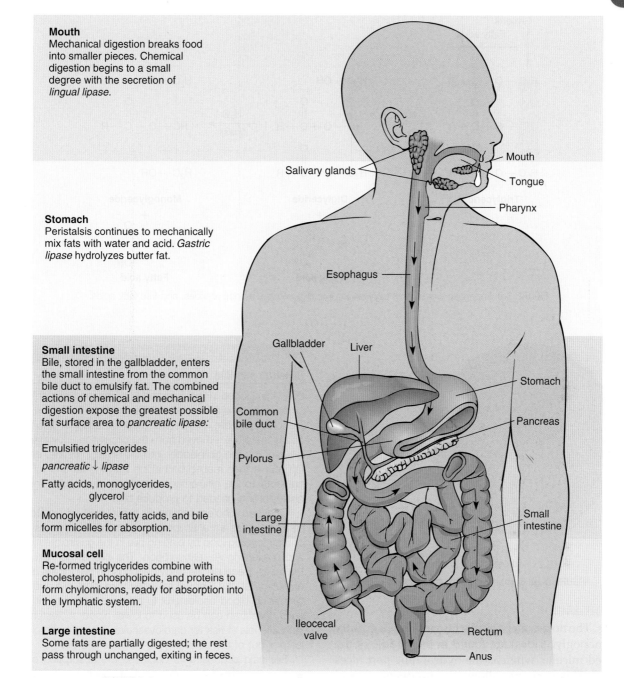

Mouth
Mechanical digestion breaks food into smaller pieces. Chemical digestion begins to a small degree with the secretion of *lingual lipase.*

Stomach
Peristalsis continues to mechanically mix fats with water and acid. *Gastric lipase* hydrolyzes butter fat.

Small intestine
Bile, stored in the gallbladder, enters the small intestine from the common bile duct to emulsify fat. The combined actions of chemical and mechanical digestion expose the greatest possible fat surface area to *pancreatic lipase:*

Emulsified triglycerides

pancreatic ↓ lipase

Fatty acids, monoglycerides,
　　　　glycerol

Monoglycerides, fatty acids, and bile form micelles for absorption.

Mucosal cell
Re-formed triglycerides combine with cholesterol, phospholipids, and proteins to form chylomicrons, ready for absorption into the lymphatic system.

Large intestine
Some fats are partially digested; the rest pass through unchanged, exiting in feces.

Salivary glands — Mouth
Tongue
Pharynx
Esophagus
Gallbladder — Liver — Stomach
Common bile duct — Pancreas
Pylorus
Large intestine — Small intestine
Ileocecal valve — Rectum
Anus

FIGURE 3-8 Summary of lipid digestion. NOTE: Enzymes are in *italics.* (Courtesy Rolin Graphics.)

occurs with increasing difficulty. In fact, the separation of the final fatty acid from the remaining monoglyceride is such a slow process that less than one third of the total fat present reaches complete breakdown. The final products of fat digestion to be absorbed are fatty acids, monoglycerides, and glycerol. Some small amounts of remaining fat may pass into the large intestine for fecal elimination. The enzyme *cholesterol esterase* acts on cholesterol esters (not free cholesterol) to form a combination of free cholesterol and fatty acids in preparation for absorption into the lacteals (lymph vessels) and finally into the bloodstream (see Chapter 5).

Enzyme from the Small Intestine

The small intestine secretes an enzyme in the intestinal juice called *lecithinase*, which breaks down lecithin for absorption. Figure 3-8 summarizes fat digestion in the successive parts of the gastrointestinal tract.

Absorption

Fat absorption into the gastrointestinal cells and bloodstream is more involved than the absorption of other macronutrients. Triglycerides are not soluble in water and thus cannot directly enter the bloodstream, which is mostly water. Within the small intestines, bile salts surround the monoglycerides and fatty acids to form

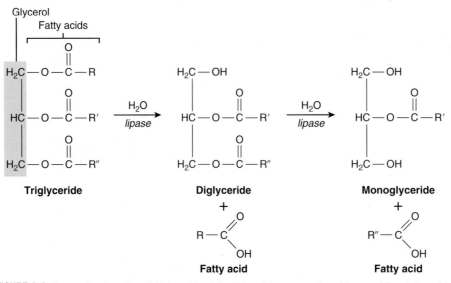

FIGURE 3-9 Enzymatic digestion of triglycerides into diglycerides, monoglycerides, and free fatty acids.

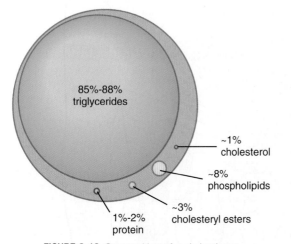

FIGURE 3-10 Composition of a chylomicron.

micelles. The non–water-soluble fat particles (e.g., fatty acids, monoglycerides) are found in the middle of the packaged micelle, whereas the hydrophilic part faces outward. This structure allows the products of lipid digestion to travel to the brush border membrane. Once there, fats are absorbed into the epithelial cells of the intestine. Bile is absorbed and transported by the portal vein to the liver for reuse; this process is called *enterohepatic circulation*. Some medications used to lower blood cholesterol levels work by removing bile acid from this recycling process (see the Drug-Nutrient Interaction box entitled "Questran and Bile").

Monoglycerides and fatty acids that made it into the intestinal cells via micelle transport are now reconstructed to form triglycerides again. Triglycerides are then packaged into a new carrier called a **chylomicron,** along with cholesterol, phospholipids, and proteins (Figure 3-10). This lipoprotein particle formed within the intestinal cell allows the products of fat digestion to enter the circulation. Chylomicrons first enter the

Drug-Nutrient Interaction

Questran and Bile

Bile is produced in the liver and is composed primarily of bile acids, salts, cholesterol, and phospholipids. Each time the liver manufactures bile, cholesterol must be used for this process and is therefore removed from the circulation. However, bile is released by the gallbladder into the small intestine, emulsifies fat, and is then reabsorbed along with the fat and fat-soluble nutrients to be efficiently recycled by the body. Thus, little cholesterol is needed to produce bile.

Questran (cholestyramine) is a bile acid sequestrant. It is also known as an antihyperlipidemic. Questran takes bile out of the recycling loop by binding bile in the gastrointestinal tract and preventing its reabsorption. The bile is then excreted in the feces. Because the body depends on bile for the digestion of dietary fat, the liver will have to make more bile and will use circulating blood cholesterol to produce replacement bile. As such, Questran can be used to lower blood cholesterol levels in individuals at risk for cardiovascular disease by forcing cholesterol out of the circulation to manufacture bile.

Bile acid sequestrants decrease the absorption of bile in addition to other fat-soluble nutrients such as vitamins A, D, E, and K. Individuals taking bile acid sequestrants on a long-term basis may be recommended to take a dietary supplement of fat-soluble vitamins in a water-miscible form to avoid potential nutrient deficiencies.

micelles packages of free fatty acids, monoglycerides, and bile salts; the hydrophobic fat particles are found in the middle of the package, whereas the hydrophilic part faces outward and allows for the absorption of fat into intestinal mucosal cells.
chylomicron a lipoprotein formed in the intestinal cell that is composed of triglycerides, cholesterol, phospholipids, and protein; chylomicrons allow for the absorption of fat into the lymphatic circulatory system before entering the blood circulation.

lacteals, then the lymphatic circulatory system, and then eventually the bloodstream. A summary of fat absorption through the process of micelle production and the formation of chylomicrons is provided in Figure 3-11.

DIGESTIBILITY OF FOOD FATS

The digestibility of fats varies somewhat according to the type of fat, the food source, and the cooking method used. When fried foods are cooked at too high of a temperature, they are more difficult to digest, and substances in the fat break down into carcinogenic materials, thus posing health concerns. Fried foods should be consumed sparingly, and the temperature of the fat should be carefully controlled during frying, grilling, and broiling.

RECOMMENDATIONS FOR DIETARY FAT

DIETARY FAT AND HEALTH

Fats in the diet supply flavor to food, thereby providing a sense of satisfaction and an enhancement of eating pleasure. The American diet has traditionally provided ample fat kilocalories. The current average intake of fat for the total population is 33.7% of kilocalories.[17]

If fat is vital to human health, what then is the concern about fat in the diet?

Health Problems

Research continues to indicate that health problems from excess dietary fat are specific to certain types of fat. And the whole diet must be considered before making any conclusions about the overall health of a diet. In addition, not all individuals metabolize and process fat the same (see the Cultural Considerations box, "Ethnic Differences in Lipid Metabolism").

Amount of fat. Too many kilocalories in the diet, regardless of the source—fat, carbohydrates, or protein—will exceed the requirement of immediate energy needs. The surplus is stored as body fat. Excess body fat is associated with higher rates of all-cause mortality and risk factors for chronic diseases such as diabetes, hypertension, and heart disease.[18,19] How much fat is in your own daily diet? See the Clinical Applications box entitled "How Much Fat Are You Eating?" to assess your fat intake.

Type of fat. As discussed earlier, the type of dietary fat matters. An excess of cholesterol and saturated fat in the diet, which comes from animal food sources, has been historically accepted as a specific risk factor for atherosclerosis, the underlying blood vessel disease that contributes to heart disease (see Chapter 19). However, if saturated fats (from food sources also containing dietary cholesterol) and trans fats are replaced with omega-6 polyunsaturated fatty acids, there appear to be no health benefits.[15] On the other hand, if saturated and trans fats are replaced with omega-3 polyunsaturated fats, there is a favorable result to lipid profiles and risk for heart disease.[15] Monounsaturated fats are also cardio-protective. A diet rich in monounsaturated fats, such as the Mediterranean diet, increases high-density lipoprotein levels, improves the atherogenic index (ratio of total cholesterol to HDL cholesterol), and reduces vascular inflammation, thereby improving the overall cardiovascular health profile.[20-22]

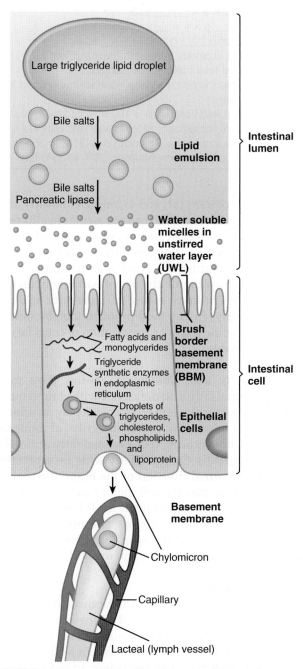

FIGURE 3-11 Summary of fat absorption. (From Mahan LK, Escott-Stump S. *Krause's Food & Nutrition Therapy.* 12th ed. St Louis: Saunders; 2008.)

Cultural Considerations

Ethnic Differences in Lipid Metabolism

Dietary patterns and habits form at an early age as a result of both family influence and environmental factors. The dietary fat intake of some individuals is much lower than that of others simply because of how the individuals were raised. However, since the unveiling of the human genome, we are learning that biologic differences also exist that may affect dietary patterns and determine the ways in which our bodies handle the nutrients we eat. The prevalence of obesity has long been known to differ among ethnic and racial populations, but the exact cause remains uncertain.

Women are often the subjects of study in obesity research. A significant difference in ethnicity exists with regard to the incidence of women 20 years old or older who are overweight in the United States[1]:

- 82.1% of black or African-American women
- 76.9% of Mexican women
- 62.9% of white women

Evidence is accumulating to suggest that biologic differences in lipid metabolism among ethnic groups may contribute to these differences. Researchers have found that obese African-American women uptake fatty acids from circulation into adipose tissue at a higher rate than their white counterparts.[2] In addition, African-American women have an increased capacity to synthesize fat in adipose tissue as compared with white women.[3] Subsequently, African-American women are more efficient at converting excess kilocalories into stored fat.

These types of differences continue to unfold with ongoing genetic studies. Differences such as these will also guide individuals in their dietary choices with regard to how their bodies will respond to specific nutrients. The path from fat in our food to fat on our bodies continues to provide many questions for inspection and evaluation. The science of lipid digestion, metabolism, and use will remain a hot topic for debate and research for years to come.

REFERENCES

1. National Center for Health Statistics. *Health, United States, 2014: with Special Feature of Adults Aged 55-64.* Hyattsville, MD: U.S. Government Printing Office; 2015.
2. Bower JF, et al., Differences in transport of fatty acids and expression of fatty acid transporting proteins in adipose tissue of obese black and white women. *Am J Physiol Endocrinol Metab.* 2006; 290(1):E87-E91.
3. Bower JF, Vadlamudi S, Barakat HA. Ethnic differences in in vitro glyceride synthesis in subcutaneous and omental adipose tissue. *Am J Physiol Endocrinol Metab.* 2002;283(5):E988-E993.

Trans-fatty acids. Observed effects of diets that are high in trans-fatty acids include an increase in low-density lipoprotein (LDL) cholesterol levels, a reduction in the protective high-density lipoprotein (HDL) cholesterol levels, an increase in the atherogenic index and endothelial dysfunction, and an increased production of atherosclerotic inflammatory cytokines.[23] In response to these growing health concerns, beginning in 2003 the FDA required all food manufacturers to identify the amount of trans fats on the nutrition facts label, thereby making the identification of these products much easier (see Figure 3-7). This act motivated the food industry to develop alternative fats and oils to

Clinical Applications

How Much Fat Are You Eating?

Keep an accurate record of everything that you eat and drink for 1 day. Be sure to include all fat or other nutrient seasonings used with your foods (e.g., salad dressing, sugar, mayonnaise). If you want a more representative picture, use the nutrient analysis program that came with this text or another program to which you have access (such as Super Tracker at www.choosemyplate.gov), and evaluate your average intake over a 3- to 7-day period.

Step 1: Calculate the total kilocalories and grams for each of the energy-yielding nutrients (i.e., carbohydrates, fat, and protein) in everything that you eat. Multiply the total grams of each energy nutrient by its respective fuel value:

Fat: _____ g × 9 = _____ kcal

Protein: _____ g × 4 = _____ kcal

Carbohydrate: _____ g × 4 = _____ kcal

Step 2: Add the kcalories from each macronutrient to determine the total kcalories consumed.

Step 3: Calculate the percentage of each energy nutrient in your total diet:

Example: (Fat kcal/Total kcal) × 100 = % fat kcal in diet

Step 4: Compare the amount of fat in your diet with the amount of fat in a typical American diet (31% to 35% fat) and with the DRI recommendations (20% to 35% fat).

avoid the use of trans fats and to improve the fatty acid composition with regard to cardiovascular health risk.

In addition, the FDA has recently removed trans-fatty acids from the list of generally recognized as safe (GRAS) food additives.[24] Food manufacturers have until 2018 to discontinue the use of partially hydrogenated oils (the primary source of trans-fatty acids in the food supply) in any food product, thereby drastically reducing the overall consumption of trans fats in the United States.

Essential fatty acid deficiency. Fat-free diets may lead to essential fatty acid deficiency with clinical manifestations. Because essential fatty acids play an important role in maintaining the integrity of biologic membranes, one indication of essential fatty acid deficiency is dermatitis. Omega-3 fatty acids are especially required for normal function of the brain, the central nervous system, and the cell membranes. Inadequate intake of dietary essential fatty acids is linked to many health problems, such as hair loss, infertility, low blood platelet levels, impaired vision, compromised brain function, and growth retardation in children.

Health Promotion

The ongoing movement in American health care is toward health promotion and disease prevention through the reduction of risk factors related to chronic disease. Heart disease continues to be a leading cause of death, and much attention is given to reducing the various risk factors that lead to this disease. Poor diets contribute to these risk factors, which include obesity, diabetes, elevated levels of triglycerides, and elevated blood pressure. Such risk factors have previously been considered adult-onset, but they are becoming increasingly apparent among obese children and adolescents. The Centers for Disease Control and Prevention reported that 20.3% of all youth between the ages of 12 and 19 years have abnormal lipid levels. Overweight children have a significantly higher prevalence of cardiovascular health risk than normal-weight children.[25] Healthier eating habits are especially important for children in high-risk families (e.g., families with identified lipid disorders and heart disease at young ages).

Additional lifestyle risk factors for chronic disease include smoking, increased stress, and physical inactivity, especially among middle-aged and older individuals. Emphasis is placed on the importance of keeping the body's total daily caloric intake in balance with the total daily energy use to maintain an ideal body weight. Low-fat diets, fad diets, and other issues that affect weight loss are discussed in more detail in Chapter 15.

In addition, changes are apparent in the restaurant industry to reduce the traditional high-fat content of menu items. For example, many restaurants are shifting to using leaner meats; having more variety in food choices (e.g., breakfast items such as fruit, waffles, pancakes, and hot and cold cereals; grilled or broiled chicken and fish; baked potatoes; fresh and packaged salads and fruit); and using vegetable oil for frying.

DIETARY REFERENCE INTAKES

The current DRIs recommend that the fat content of the diet not exceed 35% of the total kilocalories, that less than 10% of the kilocalories come from saturated fats, and that dietary cholesterol be limited to a maximum of 300 mg/day (see Chapter 1). No DRI or Tolerable Upper Intake Level is set for trans-fatty acids. The National Academy of Sciences recommends limiting trans-fat intake to as low as possible while maintaining a nutritionally adequate diet.[4] As mentioned previously, fat is an essential part of the diet; therefore, diets that are completely devoid of fat are equally unhealthy and can result in a deficiency of essential fatty acids.

The DRI for linoleic acid, which is found in polyunsaturated vegetable oils, is set at 17 g/day for men and 12 g/day for women. Alpha-linolenic acid is primarily found in seed oils (flax, canola, and soybean) and dark green leafy vegetables, and it is generally consumed in much lesser quantities than linoleic acid. The recommendation for alpha-linolenic acid intake is 1.6 and 1.1 g/day for men and women, respectively.[4] Some research indicates that consuming more omega-3 fatty acids from vegetables and fish would help to achieve a preferred omega-6 to omega-3 ratio and thus reduce the risk for several chronic diseases.[26]

Dietary Guidelines for Americans

In line with the current national health goal of health promotion through disease prevention by reducing identified risks of chronic disease, the *Dietary Guidelines for Americans* recommend the general control of fat in the diet, especially saturated fat and cholesterol. The following guidelines address dietary fat intake[5]:

- Consume less than 10% of calories from saturated fatty acids by replacing them with unsaturated fatty acids.
- Consume as little dietary cholesterol as possible while consuming a healthy eating pattern.
- Keep trans-fatty acid consumption as low as possible by limiting foods that contain synthetic sources of trans fats (e.g., partially hydrogenated oils) and by limiting other solid fats.
- Choose fat-free or low-fat milk and milk products.
- Choose protein foods that are lean and nutrient-dense.
- Use oils to replace solid fats where possible.

MyPlate

The MyPlate food guidance system provides recommendations for designing a diet that reflects the DRI and *Dietary Guidelines for Americans* recommendations for fat intake within a well-balanced diet. After an individual plan is determined on the basis of age, gender, height, weight, and physical activity level, other helpful tips and resources are available through the free website, www.choosemyplate.gov, such as information about how to choose lean meats, where to find essential fatty acids, tips for eating out, and sample menus.[27]

Putting It All Together

Summary

- Fat is an essential body nutrient that serves important body needs as a backup storage fuel (secondary to carbohydrate) for energy. Fat also supplies important tissue needs as a structural material for cell membranes, a protective padding for vital organs, an insulation source to maintain body temperature, and a covering material for nerve fibers.

- Food fats have different forms and health implications. Saturated fat and cholesterol primarily come from animal food sources. Plant food sources are the richest source of unsaturated fats and may reduce health risks when used in place of trans fats in a well-balanced diet.
- When various foods that contain triglycerides and cholesterol are eaten, specific digestive agents, including bile and pancreatic lipase, prepare and break

down fats. Fatty acids and monoglycerides are incorporated into chylomicrons and absorbed through the lymphatic system into the bloodstream.

- Americans generally consume less omega-3 fatty acids than recommended. Reducing dietary trans-fat intake and maintaining a diet high in monounsaturated fats and omega-3 fats would be more ideal for health promotion and disease prevention.

Chapter Review Questions

See answers in Appendix A.

1. Margaret has been reading information from the Internet regarding the health benefits of coconut oil in the diet. It is important for Margaret to know that coconut oil contains what type of fat?
   a. Saturated
   b. Monounsaturated
   c. Polyunsaturated
   d. Cholesterol

2. Elevated levels of blood fats are referred to as:
   a. Hyperglycemia.
   b. Hyperlipidemia.
   c. Hypertension.
   d. Hypernatremia.

3. A patient has been advised to follow a low saturated fat diet to help reduce the risk of heart disease. Which of the following foods would most likely be recommended as part of this meal plan?
   a. Beef curry made with ghee and whole coconut milk
   b. Skinless chicken and vegetables sautéed with olive oil
   c. Baked potato topped with chili and sour cream
   d. Turkey sausage and egg biscuit

4. Jeremy consumed 1800 calories of which 50 grams were from fat. What percent of calories are provided from fat?
   a. 11
   b. 25
   c. 30
   d. 42

5. Bile from the gallbladder serves as a (an) _____ rather than an enzyme in the chemical digestive process.
   a. Alakali
   b. Acid
   c. Emulsifier
   d. Catalyst

Additional Learning Resources

evolve http://evolve.elsevier.com/Williams/basic/

References and **Further Reading and Resources** in the back of the book provide additional resources for enhancing knowledge.

Proteins

Key Concepts

- Protein in food provides the amino acids that are necessary for building and maintaining body tissue.
- Protein balance within the diet and the body is essential to life and health.

- The quality of the protein within food and its ability to meet the body's needs are determined by the composition of amino acids.

Many different proteins in the body make human life possible. Each of these thousands of specific body proteins has a unique structure that is designed to perform an assigned task. Amino acids are the building blocks of all proteins. People obtain amino acids from a variety of foods. This chapter looks at the specific nature of proteins, both in food and in human bodies; it explains why protein balance is essential to life and health, and it discusses how that balance is maintained.

THE NATURE OF PROTEINS

AMINO ACIDS

Role as Building Blocks

All protein, whether in our bodies or in the food we eat, is composed of building blocks known as amino acids. Amino acids are joined in unique chain sequences to form specific proteins. Each amino acid is joined by a peptide bond (Figure 4-1). Two amino acids joined together are called a *dipeptide*. Three amino acids joined together are called a *tripeptide*. Polypeptides are chains of up to 100 amino acids linked together. Hundreds of amino acids are linked together to form a single protein. When foods rich in protein are eaten, the protein is broken down into amino acids by breaking the peptide bonds during the digestive process. The specific types of protein found in different foods are unique. For example, casein is the protein that is found in milk and cheese; albumin is in egg whites, and gluten is found in wheat products.

Following digestion and absorption into the body, individual amino acids are then reassembled in a specific order to form a variety of new proteins as needed by the body. To maintain its solvency, each protein chain adopts a folded form, which can fold and unfold in accordance with metabolic needs. Because proteins are relatively large, complex molecules, they are occasionally subject to mutations or malformations in structure. For example, protein-folding mistakes are involved in Alzheimer's disease, cystic fibrosis, and other hereditary diseases.

Dietary Importance

Amino acids are named for their chemical nature. The word *amino* refers to compounds that contain nitrogen. Like carbohydrates and fats, proteins have a basic structure of carbon, hydrogen, and oxygen. However, unlike carbohydrates and fats, protein is approximately 16% nitrogen. As such, protein is the primary source of nitrogen in the diet. In addition, some proteins contain small but valuable amounts of the minerals sulfur, phosphorus, iron, and iodine. There are nine essential amino acids that must be supplied to the body through the diet. These amino acids are also known as indispensable and are discussed further below.

CLASSES OF AMINO ACIDS

A total of 20 common amino acids have been identified, all of which are vital to life and health. These amino acids are classified as **indispensable, dispensable,** or **conditionally indispensable** in the diet according to whether the body can make them (Box 4-1).[1]

---

indispensable amino acids the nine amino acids that must be obtained from the diet because the body does not make adequate amounts to support body needs.

dispensable amino acids the five amino acids that the body can synthesize from other amino acids that are supplied through the diet and thus do not have to be consumed on a daily basis.

conditionally indispensable amino acids the six amino acids that are normally considered dispensable amino acids because the body can make them; however, under certain circumstances (e.g., illness), the body cannot make them in high enough quantities, and they become indispensable (cannot do without) in the diet.

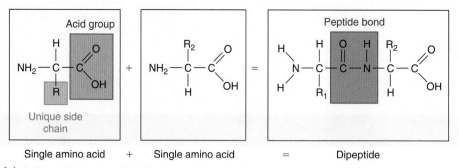

FIGURE 4-1 Amino acid structure. (Modified from Mahan LK, Escott-Stump S. *Krause's Food & Nutrition Therapy.* 12th ed. Philadelphia: Saunders; 2008.)

Box **4-1** | Indispensable, Dispensable, and Conditionally Indispensable Amino Acids

INDISPENSABLE	DISPENSABLE	CONDITIONALLY INDISPENSABLE
Histidine	Alanine	Arginine
Isoleucine	Aspartic acid	Cysteine
Leucine	Asparagine	Glutamine
Lysine	Glutamic acid	Glycine
Methionine	Serine	Proline
Phenylalanine	Tyrosine	
Threonine		
Tryptophan		
Valine		

These classifications were formerly known as *essential, nonessential,* or *conditionally essential,* respectively.

Indispensable Amino Acids

Nine amino acids are classified as indispensable because the body cannot manufacture them in sufficient quantity or at all (see Box 4-1). As the word *indispensable* implies, these amino acids are necessary in the diet and cannot be left out. Under normal circumstances, the remaining 11 amino acids are synthesized by the body to meet continuous metabolic demands throughout the life cycle.

Dispensable Amino Acids

The word *dispensable* can be confusing; all amino acids have essential tissue-building and metabolic functions in the body. However, the term refers to five amino acids (see Box 4-1) that the body can synthesize from other amino acids, provided that the necessary building blocks and enzymes are available. These amino acids are needed by the body for a healthy life, but they are dispensable (i.e., not necessary) in the diet.

Conditionally Indispensable Amino Acids

The remaining six amino acids are classified as *conditionally indispensable* (see Box 4-1). Under certain physiologic conditions, these amino acids, which are normally synthesized in the body (along with the dispensable amino acids), must be consumed in the diet. Arginine, cysteine, glutamine, glycine, proline, and tyrosine are indispensable when endogenous sources cannot meet the metabolic demands. For example, the human body can make cysteine from the essential amino acid methionine. However, when the diet is deficient in methionine, cysteine must be consumed in the diet, thereby making it an indispensable amino acid during that time. Severe physiologic stress, illness, and genetic disorders also may render an amino acid conditionally indispensable.

Phenylketonuria (PKU) is a genetic disorder in which the affected individual lacks the enzyme needed to convert phenylalanine to tyrosine. Therefore, tyrosine becomes an indispensable amino acid for individuals with PKU. In addition, because the conversion of phenylalanine cannot take place, phenylalanine levels in the blood may rise to toxic levels. A specific phenylketonuria diet must be followed and certain foods avoided (see the Drug-Nutrient Interaction box, "Aspartame and Phenylketonuria").

BALANCE

In terms of nutrition, *balance* refers to the relative intake and output of substances in the body to maintain the equilibrium that is necessary for health in various circumstances throughout the life span. This concept of balance can be applied to life-sustaining protein and the nitrogen that it supplies.

Protein Balance

The body's tissue proteins are constantly being broken down into amino acids through **catabolism,** and they are then resynthesized into tissue proteins as needed through **anabolism.** To maintain nitrogen balance, the part of the amino acid that contains nitrogen may be removed by **deamination,** converted into ammonia, and then excreted as urea in the urine. The remaining

catabolism the metabolic process of breaking down large substances to yield smaller building blocks.
anabolism the metabolic process of building large substances from smaller parts; the opposite of catabolism.
deamination the removal of the nitrogen-containing part (amino group) from an amino acid.

non-nitrogen residue will be used to make carbohydrate or fat, or it may be reattached to make another amino acid, if necessary. The rate of this protein and nitrogen turnover varies in different tissues in accordance with the degree of metabolic activity and the available supply of amino acids.

Drug-Nutrient Interaction

Aspartame and Phenylketonuria

SARA HARCOURT

Aspartame is a nonnutritive sweetener (i.e., it does not provide any nutrients or calories) that is composed of two amino acids: aspartic acid and phenylalanine. It is made synthetically, and its structure more closely resembles a protein than a carbohydrate. However, by adding a methanol group, the end product tastes sweet. It is used in foods and beverages as a high-potency sweetener, and it is approximately 200 times sweeter than sucrose (table sugar). Therefore, much less is needed to sweeten a food to the same degree.

Phenylketonuria (PKU) is a disease in which an individual lacks the enzyme phenylalanine hydroxylase. Without this enzyme, phenylalanine cannot be metabolized and thus accumulates in the blood. High levels in the blood are toxic to brain tissue, and this can result in mental degradation and possibly death. Individuals with PKU must follow a strict diet with careful intake of phenylalanine that supports growth but that does not exceed tolerance. Those with PKU should avoid all foods that contain aspartame because of its concentrated phenylalanine content.

Foods that contain phenylalanine, such as aspartame—which is also known by the trade names *NutraSweet* and *Equal*—have warnings on their packages for PKU patients.

Following is a list of common foods that contain aspartame:
- Chewing gum
- Diet sodas
- Frozen desserts
- Gelatins
- Puddings
- Sugar-free candies
- Yogurt

Tissue turnover is a continuous process of reshaping, building, and adjusting to maintain overall protein balance within the body. The body maintains a delicate balance among tissue protein, plasma protein, and dietary protein. With this finely balanced system, healthy individuals have a small dynamic pool of amino acids from tissue protein and dietary protein that is available to meet metabolic needs (Figure 4-2).

Nitrogen Balance

The body's nitrogen balance indicates how well its tissues are being maintained. The intake and use of dietary protein are measured by the amount of nitrogen supplied by food protein and the amount of nitrogen excreted in the urine. For example, 1 g of urinary nitrogen results from the digestion and metabolism of 6.25 g of protein. Thus, if 1 g of nitrogen is excreted in the urine for every 6.25 g of protein consumed, then the body is said to be in nitrogen balance. This balance is the normal pattern in adult health. However, at different times of life or in states of malnutrition or illness, the balance may shift to be either positive or negative.

Positive nitrogen balance. A positive nitrogen balance exists when the body holds on to more nitrogen than it excretes, thus storing more nitrogen in the form of protein (by building tissue) than it is losing (by breaking down tissue). This situation occurs normally during periods of rapid growth, such as infancy, childhood, adolescence, pregnancy, and lactation. A positive nitrogen balance also occurs in individuals who have been ill or malnourished and who are being "built back up" with increased nourishment. In such cases, protein is used to meet increased needs for tissue building and its associated metabolic activity.

Negative nitrogen balance. A negative nitrogen balance occurs when the body excretes more nitrogen

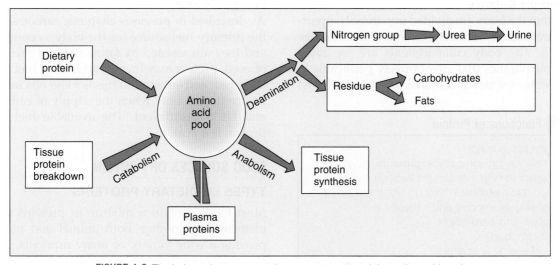

FIGURE 4-2 The balance between protein compartments and the amino acid pool.

than it keeps. This happens when the body has an inadequate dietary supply of protein and/or total energy. In this case, it is necessary for the body to catabolize body tissue containing protein in order to meet other critical functions. Malnutrition, illness, and starvation are examples of periods when negative nitrogen balance may occur.

Negative nitrogen balance is also seen in individuals when protein deficiency—even when kilocalories from carbohydrate and fat are adequate—causes the classic protein deficiency disease kwashiorkor. The failure to maintain the nitrogen balance may not become apparent for some time, but it eventually causes the loss of muscle tissue, the impairment of body organs and functions, and an increased susceptibility to infection. In children, negative nitrogen balance for an extended period causes growth retardation and may be fatal.

FUNCTIONS OF PROTEIN

PRIMARY TISSUE BUILDING

Protein is the fundamental structural material of every cell in the body. In fact, the largest dry-weight portion of the body is protein. Body protein (e.g., the lean mass of muscles) accounts for approximately three fourths of the dry matter in most tissues, excluding bone and adipose tissue. Protein makes up the bulk of the muscles, internal organs, brain, nerves, skin, hair, and nails; and it is also a vital part of regulatory substances such as enzymes, hormones, and blood plasma. All such tissues must be constantly repaired and replaced. The primary functions of protein are to repair worn-out, wasted, or damaged tissue and to build new tissue.

ADDITIONAL BODY FUNCTIONS

In addition to its basic tissue-building function, protein has other critical body functions related to energy, water balance, metabolism, and the body's defense system. Box 4-2 lists the major functions of protein.

Water and pH Balance

Fluids within the body are divided into three compartments: intravascular, intracellular, and interstitial (see Chapter 9). The body compartments are separated with cell membranes that are not freely permeable to protein. Because water is attracted to protein, plasma

---

Box 4-2   Functions of Protein

- Structural tissue building
- Water balance through osmotic pressure
- Buffer agent to help maintain pH balance
- Digestion and metabolism through enzymatic action
- Cell signaling (hormones) and transport (e.g., hemoglobin and transferrin)
- Immunity (antibodies)
- Source of energy (4 kcal/g)

> **osmotic pressure** the pressure that is produced as a result of osmosis across a semipermeable membrane.

proteins such as albumin help to control water balance throughout the body by exerting **osmotic pressure.** This pressure maintains the normal circulation of tissue fluids within the appropriate compartments.

The normal pH of blood is between 7.35 and 7.45. However, constant metabolic functions throughout the body release acidic and alkaline substances, thereby affecting the overall acidity and alkalinity of blood. The unique structure of proteins—a combination of a carboxyl acid group and a base group—allows them to act as buffering agents by releasing or taking up excess acid within the body. If blood reaches a pH in either extreme (i.e., too acidic or too alkaline), plasma proteins denature and can result in death.

Metabolism and Transportation

Protein aids metabolic functions through enzymes, transport agents, and hormones. Digestive and cell enzymes are proteins that control metabolic processes. Enzymes that are necessary for the digestion of carbohydrates (amylase), fats (lipase), and proteins (proteases) are all proteins in structure. Protein also acts as a vehicle in which nutrients are carried throughout the body. Lipoproteins are necessary to transport fats in the water-soluble blood supply. Other examples are hemoglobin, which is the vital oxygen carrier in the red blood cells, and transferrin, which is the iron transport protein in blood. Peptide hormones (e.g., insulin, glucagon) are also proteins that play a major function in the metabolism of glucose (see Chapter 20).

Body Defense System

Protein is used to build special white blood cells (i.e., lymphocytes) and antibodies as part of the body's immune system to help defend against disease and infection.

Energy System

As described in previous chapters, carbohydrates are the primary fuel source for the body's energy system, and they are assisted by fat as a stored fuel. In times of need, protein may furnish additional fuel to sustain body heat and energy, but this is a less-efficient backup source for use only when the supply of carbohydrate and fat is insufficient. The available fuel factor of protein is 4 kcal/g.

FOOD SOURCES OF PROTEIN

TYPES OF DIETARY PROTEINS

Most foods contain a mixture of proteins that complement one another. Both animal and plant foods provide a wide variety of many nutrients, including protein. Dietary proteins are classified as complete or incomplete proteins, depending on their amino acid composition.

Complete Proteins

Protein foods that contain all nine indispensable amino acids in sufficient quantity and ratio to meet the body's needs are called *complete proteins.* These proteins are primarily of animal origin (e.g., egg, milk, cheese, meat, poultry, fish; Figure 4-3). However, there are a couple of exceptions to this rule. Gelatin is an animal protein but is incomplete. And soy is a plant protein but is a complete protein. Gelatin is a relatively insignificant protein because it lacks the three essential amino acids tryptophan, valine, and isoleucine, and it has only small amounts of leucine. And soy products are the only plant sources of complete proteins. This is one reason why it is easy for vegans/vegetarians to maintain a healthy protein balance in their diet without consuming animal products.

Incomplete Proteins

Protein foods that are deficient in one or more of the nine indispensable amino acids are called *incomplete proteins.* These proteins are generally of plant origin (e.g., grains, legumes, nuts, seeds), but they are found in foods that make valuable contributions to the total amount of dietary protein. As mentioned above, the exception is soy protein, which is a complete protein of plant origin.

VEGETARIAN DIETS

Complementary Protein

Current knowledge of protein metabolism and the pooling of amino acid reserves (see Figure 4-2) indicates that a mixture of plant proteins can provide adequate amounts of amino acids when the basic use of various grains is expanded to include soy and other dried legumes (i.e., beans and peas). Because most plant proteins are incomplete and thereby lacking one or more of the indispensable (or essential) amino acids, vegetarians can choose a variety of plant foods so that the amino acids missing in one food are supplied by another. This is the art of combining plant protein foods so that they complement one another and supply all nine indispensable amino acids (see the Cultural Considerations box, "Indispensable Amino Acids and Their Complementary Food Proteins").

A balanced vegetarian eating pattern throughout the day, together with the body's small reserve of amino acids, ensures an overall amino acid balance. The underlying requirement for vegetarians—as for all people—is to eat a sufficient amount of varied foods to meet normal nutrient and energy needs).[2]

Types of Vegetarian Diets

Vegetarian diets differ according to the beliefs or needs of the individuals who are following such food patterns. A survey completed in 2012 estimated that ≅5% of the U.S. adult population (approximately 5 to 12 million people) consistently follow a vegetarian diet.[3] Several reasons lead people to choose a vegetarian diet, including taste preference, environmental and animal cruelty concerns, health incentives, religious adherence (e.g., Buddhists, Hindus, Seventh-Day Adventists), and aversion to the consumption of animal products. Alternatively, a diet that is void of animal products is not always a choice. In some areas in the world, vegetarianism is a result of the lack of resources and availability of animal products.

In general, vegetarians can be described as one of the following four basic types:

1. *Lacto-vegetarians:* These vegetarians accept only dairy products from animal sources to complement their basic diet of plant foods. The use of milk and milk products (e.g., cheese) with a varied mixed diet of whole or enriched grains, legumes, nuts, seeds, fruits, and vegetables in sufficient quantities to meet energy needs provides a balanced diet.
2. *Ovo-vegetarians:* The only animal foods included in the ovo-vegetarian diet are eggs. Because eggs are an excellent source of complete proteins, individuals who are following this diet do not have to be overly concerned with complementary proteins if eggs are consumed consistently.

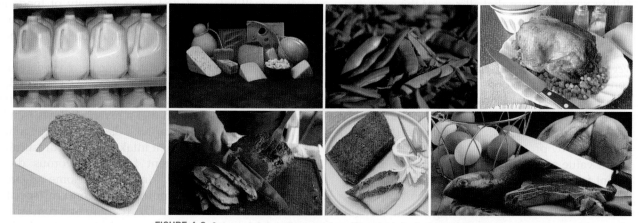

FIGURE 4-3 Sources of complete proteins. (Copyright JupiterImages Corp.)

🌐 Cultural Considerations

Indispensable Amino Acids and Their Complementary Food Proteins

A large percentage of the worldwide population follows various forms of vegetarian diets for religious, traditional, or economic reasons. Many Seventh-Day Adventists follow a lacto-ovo-vegetarian diet, whereas individuals of the Hindu and Buddhist faiths generally are lacto-vegetarian. The Mediterranean diet has such a strong emphasis on grains, pastas, vegetables, and cheese that animal products (i.e., beef, chicken, and fish) are only consumed in small amounts. In other areas of the world, the economic burden of animal products does not allow for the consumption of such foods. Any form of a vegetarian diet can be healthy with a good understanding of how to achieve complete protein balance.

All nine indispensable amino acids must be supplied by the diet. Protein from both animal and plant sources can meet protein requirements. One concern often voiced related to a vegetarian diet is getting a balanced amount of the indispensable amino acids to complement each other and to make complete protein combinations. However, such concerns are usually unnecessary because vegetarian diets that include a variety of plant products provide sufficient high-quality protein to match that of omnivorous diets.

Complementary food combinations are made by mixing families of foods (e.g., grains, legumes, dairy for lacto-vegetarians) to balance the needed amino acids. For example, grains are low in threonine and high in methionine, whereas legumes are just the opposite. Therefore, grains and legumes help to balance one another with regard to the accumulation of all indispensable amino acids. Following are sample food combinations to illustrate complementary protein combinations:

- *Grains and peas, beans, or lentils:* brown rice and beans; whole-grain bread with pea or lentil soup; wheat or corn tortilla with beans; peanut butter on whole-wheat bread; Indian dishes of rice and dal (a legume); Chinese dishes of tofu and rice
- *Legumes and seeds:* falafel; soybeans and pumpkin or sesame seeds; Middle Eastern hummus (garbanzo beans and sesame seeds) or tahini
- *Grains and dairy (for lacto-vegetarians):* whole-wheat pasta and cheese; yogurt and a multigrain muffin; cereal and milk; a cheese sandwich made with whole-grain bread

3. *Lacto-ovo-vegetarians:* These are vegetarians who follow a food pattern that allows for the consumption of dairy products and eggs (Figure 4-4). Their mixed diet consists of plant and animal food sources that exclude meat, poultry, pork, and fish only.
4. *Vegans:* Vegans follow a strict vegetarian diet and consume no animal foods. Their food pattern consists entirely of plant foods (e.g., whole or enriched grains, legumes, nuts, seeds, fruits, vegetables). The use of soybeans, soy milk, soybean curd (tofu), and processed soy protein products enhances the nutritional value of the diet. Careful planning and sufficient food intake ensure adequate nutrition.

The position paper from the Academy of Nutrition and Dietetics states that a vegetarian diet (including the vegan option) can meet the current recommendations for all essential nutrients, including protein.[2] The experts also indicate that the former mindful combination of complementary plant proteins within every given meal is unnecessary; achieving a balance throughout the day with a variety of foods is more important. In addition, vegetarian diets are appropriate throughout all stages of life, including pregnancy, infancy, childhood, adolescence, and older age as well as for those with an athletic lifestyle.

Health Benefits and Risk

Some of the most notable benefits of vegetarianism include the following[2,4-11]:

- Lower levels of dietary saturated fat and cholesterol consumption
- Higher intake of fruits, vegetables, whole grains, nuts, soy products, fiber, and phytochemicals
- Lower prevalence of obesity
- Better lipid profiles and lower rates of death from cardiovascular disease, including ischemic heart disease and hypertension
- Lowered risk of renal disease from high glomerular filtration rates as compared with long-term high animal protein intake
- Effective management of type 2 diabetes and lowering of the risk for developing type 2 diabetes and some forms of cancer (e.g., prostate, gastrointestinal tract, female specific cancer)
- Overall, better quality diet for macronutrient and micronutrient intake as indicated by the Healthy Eating Index
- Other possible benefits include a lowered risk of dementia, diverticulitis, and gallstones

After an extensive review of the effects of vegetarian diets with regard to various medical conditions, some researchers have concluded that "dietary intervention with a vegetarian diet seems to be a cheap, physiologic, and safe approach for the prevention and possible management of modern lifestyle diseases."[12] The preventive mechanism at work in the vegetarian diet is the rich supply of monounsaturated and polyunsaturated fatty acids, fiber, complex carbohydrates, and antioxidants. To reap the benefits of a vegetarian diet, a well-balanced diet from a variety of foods is necessary. It should be noted that not all vegetarians follow an ideal well-balanced diet and therefore do not obtain the health benefits.

Key nutrients to consider for practicing vegetarians are protein, iron, zinc, calcium, vitamin D, vitamin B_{12}, and omega-3 fatty acids.[2,13,14] However, depending on the type of vegetarian diet a person follows (semi-vegetarian, lacto-vegetarian, lacto-ovo-vegetarian, vegan), the overall nutrient intake can vary drastically and may not be different from omnivorous diets for any specific nutrient.[15] In addition, some research shows that these same nutrients of concern (specifically calcium and vitamin D) are more of a concern in individuals who are omnivores but are at risk due

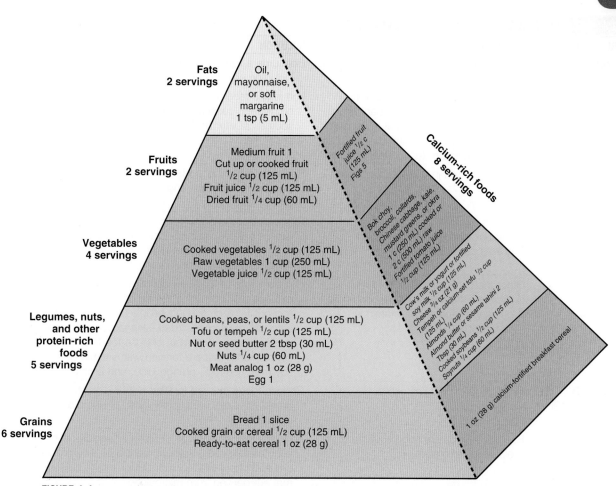

FIGURE 4-4 The lacto-ovo-vegetarian diet pyramid. (Reprinted from Messina V, Melina V, Mangels AR. A new food guide for North American vegetarians. *J Am Diet Assoc.* 2003;103[6]:771-775.)

to income level, overweight status, or ethnicity as opposed to vegetarian status.[16] Reasons for concern and effective ways to overcome these barriers are outlined in Table 4-1.

DIGESTION OF PROTEINS

MOUTH

After a food that contains protein is consumed, the protein must be broken down into the necessary ready-to-use building blocks (i.e., amino acids). This is done through the successive parts of the gastrointestinal tract by mechanical and chemical digestion. The mechanical breaking down of protein begins with chewing in the mouth. The food particles are mixed with saliva and passed on to the stomach as a semi-solid mass.

STOMACH

Because proteins are such large and complex structures, a series of enzymes is necessary for digestion and for the release of individual amino acids, which is the primary form needed for absorption. Unlike the enzymes that are needed for carbohydrate and fat digestion, all enzymes involved in protein digestion

(i.e., proteases) are stored as inactive **proenzymes** called **zymogens**. Zymogens are then activated according to need. The enzymes that are needed for protein digestion cannot be stored in an active form because the cells and organs that produce and store them (which are made of structural proteins) would be digested as well.

The chemical digestion of protein begins in the stomach. In fact, the stomach's chief digestive function is to carry out the first stage of the enzymatic breakdown of protein. The following three agents in the gastric secretions help with this task.

Hydrochloric Acid

Hydrochloric acid begins the unfolding and denaturing of the complex protein chains. This unfolding makes the individual peptide bonds (see Figure 4-1) more available for enzymatic action. Hydrochloric acid

---

proenzyme an inactive precursor (i.e., a forerunner substance from which another substance is made) that is converted to the active enzyme by the action of an acid, another enzyme, or other means.
zymogen an inactive enzyme precursor.

Table 4-1   Nutrient Considerations for Vegetarians

NUTRIENT	PROBLEM	SOLUTION
Protein	Plant protein quality varies; lower bioavailability than animal protein	Consume a variety of plant foods throughout the day, including soy products
Iron	Plant foods contain non-heme iron, which is less bioavailable than the heme iron found in animal foods and which is sensitive to inhibitors such as phytate, calcium, tea, coffee, and fiber	Iron intake recommendations are 1.8 times higher than for omnivores; consume high-iron plant foods with dietary sources of vitamin C, which is an enhancer of iron absorption
Zinc	Plant foods high in phytates bind zinc	Regularly consume foods such as nuts, soy products, zinc-fortified cereals, and soaked and sprouted beans, grains, and seeds
Calcium	Oxalates reduce the absorption of calcium found in spinach, beet greens, and Swiss chard	Regularly consume plant foods that are high in calcium and low in oxalates, such as Chinese cabbage, broccoli, Napa cabbage, collards, kale, okra, and turnip greens in addition to calcium-fortified foods such as orange juice
Vitamin D	Other than endogenously produced vitamin D from sunlight exposure, the primary source of this vitamin is fortified cow's milk	Sun exposure to the face, hands, and forearms for 5 to 15 minutes per day during the summer provides enough sunlight for light-skinned people to produce adequate amounts of vitamin D; dark-skinned people require more sun exposure; otherwise, choose foods or dietary supplements that are fortified with vitamin D, such as soy milk, rice milk, orange juice, and breakfast cereal
Vitamin B_{12}	No plant food contains active vitamin B_{12}	Choose foods that are fortified with B_{12}, such as soy milk, breakfast cereal, nutritional yeast; or use dietary supplements
Omega-3 fatty acid (alpha-linolenic)	Few plant foods are good sources of alpha-linolenic acid	Regularly include sources of alpha-linolenic acid in the diet, such as flaxseeds, walnuts, canola oil, soy products, and breakfast bars fortified with DHA, or take DHA supplements that are derived from microalgae

Adapted from Craig WJ. Health effects of vegan diets. *Am J Clin Nutr.* 2009;89(5):1627S-1633S; Craig WJ, Mangels AR. Position of the American Dietetic Association: vegetarian diets. *J Am Diet Assoc.* 2009;109(7):1266-1282.

also provides the acid medium that is necessary to convert pepsinogen into active **pepsin,** the gastric enzyme specific to proteins.

Pepsin

Pepsin is first produced as an inactive proenzyme called *pepsinogen* by a single layer of chief cells in the stomach wall. The hydrochloric acid within gastric juices then changes pepsinogen to the active enzyme pepsin. Pepsin begins splitting the bonds between the protein's long chain of amino acids, which changes the large protein into short chains of *polypeptides.* If the protein were held in the stomach longer, pepsin could continue this breakdown until only the individual amino acids remained. However, with the normal gastric emptying time, pepsin only completes the first stage of breakdown.

Rennin

The gastric enzyme **rennin** is only present during infancy and childhood, and it is especially important for the infant's digestion of milk. Rennin and calcium act on the casein of milk to produce a curd. By coagulating milk into a more solid curd, rennin prevents the food from passing too rapidly from the infant's stomach to the small intestine.

SMALL INTESTINE

Protein digestion begins in the acidic medium of the stomach, and it is completed in the alkaline medium of the small intestine. Enzymes from the secretions of both the pancreas and the intestine take part in this process.

Pancreatic Secretions

The following three enzymes produced by the pancreas continue breaking down proteins into more and more simple substances:

pepsin the main gastric enzyme specific for proteins; pepsin begins breaking large protein molecules into shorter chain polypeptides, and it is activated by gastric hydrochloric acid.

rennin the milk-curdling enzyme of the gastric juice of human infants and young animals (e.g., calves); rennin should not be confused with renin, which is an important enzyme produced by the kidneys that plays a vital role in the activation of angiotensin.

1. **Trypsin,** which is secreted first as inactive trypsinogen, is activated by the enzyme **enterokinase.** Enterokinase is secreted from the intestinal cells on contact with food entering the duodenum, which is the first section of the small intestine. The active trypsin then works on proteins and large polypeptide fragments that arrive from the stomach. This enzymatic action breaks long protein chains into small polypeptides and dipeptides.
2. **Chymotrypsin,** which is secreted first as the inactive chymotrypsinogen, is activated by trypsin that is already present in the gut. The active enzyme then continues the protein-splitting action of trypsin.
3. **Carboxypeptidase** attacks the acid (i.e., carboxyl) end of the peptide chains, thereby producing small peptides and some free amino acids. Carboxypeptidase is also first released as an inactive proenzyme (procarboxypeptidase), and it is activated by trypsin.

Intestinal Secretions

Glands in the intestinal wall produce the following two protein-splitting enzymes to complete the breakdown of protein and polypeptides and free the remaining amino acids:

1. **Aminopeptidase** attacks the nitrogen-containing (i.e., amino) end of the peptide chain and releases amino acids one at a time, thereby producing peptides and free amino acids.
2. **Dipeptidase,** which is the final enzyme in the protein-splitting system, completes the job by breaking the remaining dipeptides into two individual amino acids.

This finely coordinated system of protein-splitting enzymes breaks down the large, complex proteins into progressively smaller peptide chains and frees each individual amino acid. This is a tremendous overall task. The amino acids are now ready to be absorbed directly into the portal blood circulation for use in the building of body tissues. This remarkable system of protein digestion is summarized in Figure 4-5.

RECOMMENDATIONS FOR DIETARY PROTEIN

INFLUENTIAL FACTORS OF PROTEIN NEEDS

The following three factors influence the body's requirement for protein: (1) tissue growth; (2) the quality of the dietary protein; and (3) the additional needs that result from illness or disease.

Tissue Growth

During rapid growth periods of the human life cycle, more protein per unit of body weight is necessary to build new tissue and to maintain present tissue. Human growth is most rapid during fetal growth throughout gestation, during infant growth the first year of life, and during adolescent growth. Childhood is a sustained time of continued growth, but this occurs at a somewhat slower rate than the three previously mentioned periods. For adults, protein requirements level off to meet tissue-maintenance needs, but individual needs vary.

Dietary Protein Quality

The nature of a protein and its pattern of amino acids significantly influence its dietary quality and value at different stages throughout the life cycle.[17,18] Sufficient energy intake—especially from nonprotein foods—is necessary to conserve protein for tissue structure. In addition, the digestion and absorption of the protein consumed are affected by the complexity of its structure as well as its preparation and cooking. The comparative quality of protein foods may be assessed using several different methods.[19] The following list shows four examples:

1. *Chemical score,* which is derived from the amino acid pattern of the food; a high-quality protein food, such as an egg (with a value of 100), is compared with other foods according to their amino acid ratios
2. *Biologic value,* which is based on nitrogen balance
3. *Net protein utilization,* which is based on the biologic value and the degree of the protein's digestibility

---

trypsin a protein-splitting enzyme secreted as the inactive proenzyme trypsinogen by the pancreas and that is activated and works in the small intestine to reduce proteins to shorter-chain polypeptides and dipeptides.

enterokinase an enzyme produced and secreted in the duodenum in response to food entering the small intestine; it activates trypsinogen to its active form of trypsin.

chymotrypsin a protein-splitting enzyme secreted as the inactive zymogen chymotrypsinogen by the pancreas; after it has been activated by trypsin, it acts in the small intestine to continue breaking down proteins into shorter-chain polypeptides and dipeptides.

carboxypeptidase a specific protein-splitting enzyme secreted as the inactive zymogen procarboxypeptidase by the pancreas; after it has been activated by trypsin, it acts in the small intestine to break off the acid (i.e., carboxyl) end of the peptide chain, thereby producing smaller-chained peptides and free amino acids.

aminopeptidase a specific protein-splitting enzyme secreted by glands in the walls of the small intestine that breaks off the nitrogen-containing amino end (i.e., NH_2) of the peptide chain, thereby producing smaller-chained peptides and free amino acids.

dipeptidase the final enzyme in the protein-splitting system that releases free amino acids from dipeptide bonds.

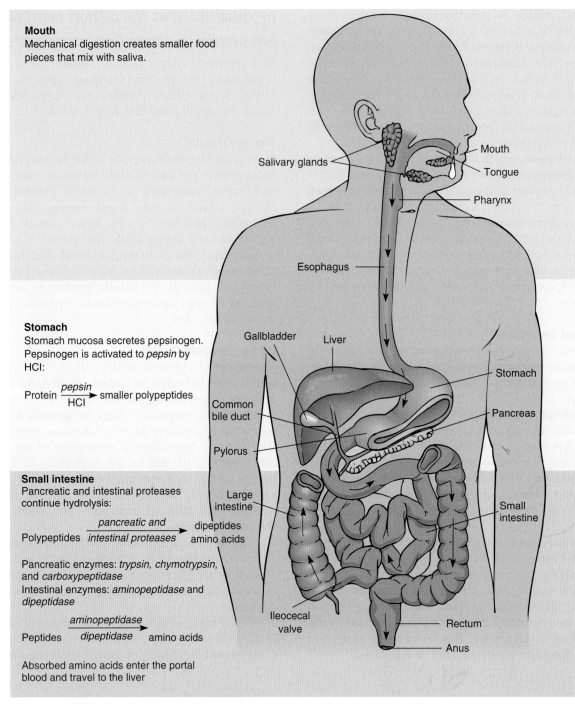

Mouth
Mechanical digestion creates smaller food pieces that mix with saliva.

Stomach
Stomach mucosa secretes pepsinogen. Pepsinogen is activated to *pepsin* by HCl:

$$\text{Protein} \xrightarrow[\text{HCl}]{\textit{pepsin}} \text{smaller polypeptides}$$

Small intestine
Pancreatic and intestinal proteases continue hydrolysis:

$$\text{Polypeptides} \xrightarrow[\textit{intestinal proteases}]{\textit{pancreatic and}} \begin{array}{l}\text{dipeptides}\\\text{amino acids}\end{array}$$

Pancreatic enzymes: *trypsin, chymotrypsin,* and *carboxypeptidase*
Intestinal enzymes: *aminopeptidase* and *dipeptidase*

$$\text{Peptides} \xrightarrow[\textit{dipeptidase}]{\textit{aminopeptidase}} \text{amino acids}$$

Absorbed amino acids enter the portal blood and travel to the liver

FIGURE 4-5 Summary of protein digestion. Note: active enzymes are in *italics*. (Courtesy Rolin Graphics.)

4. *Protein efficiency ratio,* which is based on the weight gain of a growing test animal in relation to its protein intake

Table 4-2 compares various protein food scores on the basis of protein quality. As seen in the table, egg and cow's milk proteins have the highest protein quality score. The quality and digestibility of most plant proteins are significantly lower than those of animal proteins. Therefore, the dietary protein needs of vegans who rely solely on plant foods of lower protein quality (e.g., cereal, legumes) may be slightly higher than those of nonvegetarians.[2] In other words,

because the protein provided by whole-wheat products is only approximately half as bioavailable as the protein that comes from eggs, more protein from whole-wheat products should be eaten to obtain equivalent useable protein. Regardless of dietary preferences for protein foods, a varied and balanced diet is the best way for a healthy person to obtain quality protein.

Illness or Disease

Illness or disease, especially when it is accompanied by fever and catabolic tissue breakdown, raises the

Table 4-2	Comparative Protein Quality of Selected Foods			
FOOD	CHEMICAL SCORE*	BIOLOGIC VALUE	NET PROTEIN UTILIZATION	PROTEIN EFFICIENCY RATIO
Egg	100	100	94	3.92
Cow's milk	95	93	82	3.09
Fish	71	76	—	3.55
Beef	69	74	67	2.30
Unpolished rice	67	86	59	—
Peanuts	65	55	55	1.65
Oats	57	65	—	2.19
Polished rice	57	64	57	2.18
Whole wheat	53	65	49	1.53
Corn	49	72	36	—
Soybeans	47	73	61	2.32
Sesame seeds	42	62	53	1.77
Peas	37	64	55	1.57

Modified from Guthrie H. *Introductory Nutrition.* 6th ed. New York: McGraw-Hill; 1986; and Food and Nutrition Board, Institute of Medicine. *Recommended Dietary Allowances.* 10th ed. Washington, DC: National Academies Press; 1989.
*Amino acid.

body's need for protein and kilocalories for rebuilding tissue and meeting the demands of an increased metabolic rate. Traumatic injury often requires extensive tissue rebuilding. After surgery, extra protein is needed for wound healing and restoring losses. Extensive tissue destruction, such as that which occurs with burns and pressure sores, requires a large increase in protein intake for the healing and grafting processes to be successful.

DIETARY DEFICIENCY OR EXCESS

As with any nutrient, moderation and balance are the keys to health. Too much or too little dietary protein can be problematic for overall body function.

Protein-Energy Malnutrition

Protein-energy malnutrition (PEM) or severe acute malnutrition (SAM) may occur in a variety of situations. The most severe cases are found in areas where all foods—not just protein-rich foods—are in short supply. Children are at the highest risk for experiencing malnutrition because of their high needs during rapid growth and development. However, PEM can affect anyone at any point throughout the life cycle. For example, people with poor nutrient intake (e.g., the elderly, those with eating disorders) may suffer from PEM. PEM is often accompanied with an overall energy deficiency as well. However, individuals with elevated protein needs during infection or disease (e.g., acquired immunodeficiency syndrome, cancer, liver failure) sometimes experience PEM despite seemingly adequate total dietary intake. As previously mentioned, protein has many critical functions in the body. Thus, a dietary deficiency has multiple consequences that are directly related to these functions. Without the amino acid building blocks, the body cannot synthesize needed structural (i.e., muscle) or functional (i.e., enzymes, antibodies, and hormones) proteins.

Two severe forms of PEM are kwashiorkor and marasmus. Characteristics of the two forms of PEM are quite different. Kwashiorkor, which is the more fatal of the two forms, is thought to result from an acute deficiency of protein, whereas marasmus results from a more chronic deficiency of many nutrients, of which protein is one. The end result with either form is stunted growth, a weakened immune system, and poor development.

Kwashiorkor. Kwashiorkor is more common among children who are between the ages of 18 and 24 months, who have been breastfed all their lives, and who are then rapidly weaned, often because of the arrival of a younger sibling. These children are switched from nutritionally balanced breast milk to a dilute diet of mostly carbohydrates and little protein. The children may receive adequate total kilocalories, but they lack enough bioavailable protein sources. The term *kwashiorkor* is a Ghanaian word that refers to the disease that takes over the first child when the second child is born. Characteristics of kwashiorkor include generalized edema and fatty liver as a result of inadequate protein intake to maintain fluid balance and to transport fat from the liver (Figure 4-6).

The exact pathogenesis of kwashiorkor is not well-defined. Research suggests that there may be additional factors involved in the development of the characteristic edema, such as oxidative stress and/or inappropriate antidiuretic hormone response.[20]

Marasmus. Individuals with marasmus have an emaciated appearance with little or no body fat. This

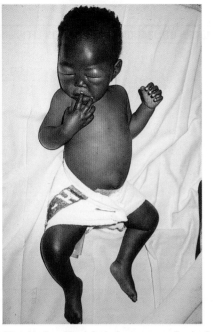

FIGURE 4-6 Kwashiorkor. The infant shows generalized edema, which is seen in the form of puffiness of the face, arms, and legs. (Reprinted from Kumar V, Abbas AK, Fausto N et al. *Robbins Basic Pathology*. 8th ed. Philadelphia: Saunders; 2007.)

is a chronic form of energy and protein deficiency; in other words, it is a result of starvation. Stunted growth and development are more severe with this form of malnutrition. Marasmus can affect individuals of all ages with inadequate food sources.

Excess Dietary Intake

As with most nutrients, one can ingest too much dietary protein. The body has a finite need for protein. When a person has met the dietary protein needs, additional protein is deaminated (i.e., the nitrogen is removed) and the rest is stored as fat or used as energy. Eating excess protein does not build muscle; only exercising with enough protein to support growth can do that. The following problems can occur with diets that are heavily laden with animal protein:

1. Protein foods of animal origin are often also high in saturated fat and cholesterol.
2. If a person fills up on high-protein foods, little room is left for fruits, vegetables, and other whole grains, which are packed with essential vitamins, minerals, and fiber (see the For Further Focus box, "The High-Protein Diet").
3. Excess dietary protein results in inflammation and apoptosis in the glomerular cells of the kidney.[21] This is a risk factor for individuals with kidney disease or diabetes.

Although most protein and amino acid supplements are not harmful in small doses, they are unnecessary in a balanced diet. However, taking excessive single amino acid dietary supplements can be harmful if it is to the exclusion of other essential amino acids, thereby creating an overall imbalance.

DIETARY GUIDES

Dietary Reference Intakes

The Recommended Dietary Allowances (RDAs) continue to be the principal dietary guide for protein consumption, and they are part of the Dietary Reference Intake standards. Similar to carbohydrate and fat recommendations, the DRIs for proteins have been set as a percentage of the total kilocalorie consumption by the National Academy of Sciences. Children and adults should obtain 10% to 35% of their total caloric intake from protein. The RDA standards relate to the age, sex, and weight of the average person, and they are based on the analysis of available nitrogen-balance studies. The RDA for both men and women is set at 0.8 g of high-quality protein per kilogram of desirable body weight per day[1] (i.e., 0.8 g/kg per day; see the Clinical Applications box, "Calculating Dietary Reference Intake for Protein"). Dietary recommendations are higher for infants and for pregnant and breastfeeding women in order to meet metabolic needs.

The RDAs are set to meet the nutritional requirements of most healthy people. Severe physical stress (e.g., illness, disease, surgery) can increase a person's requirement for protein. Of note is that the U.S. Department of Agriculture's "What We Eat in America" report found that the average daily protein intake of men and women 20 years and older is 99 g and 68 g per day, respectively.[22] According to this report, men consume approximately 177% of their Dietary Reference Intakes for protein, and women consume approximately 148% of their protein requirement daily. Thus, additional consumption through protein supplements is unnecessary for the vast majority of the American population because we are already consuming well over our daily requirements. Even if a person needed extra protein, those needs are most likely met if they are consuming the standard American fare.

Dietary Guidelines for Americans

As previously stated, the standard American diet provides more protein than necessary, the majority of which generally comes from animal products. There are potential health risks associated with a diet where excess animal products take the place of other nutrient-dense fruits, vegetables, and whole grains in the meal plan. The key is to create dietary habits that allow for a variety of all food groups, without an excess in any area.

The *Dietary Guidelines for Americans* recommend the following with regard to protein-rich foods[23]:

- Choose a variety of protein foods, including seafood, lean meat and poultry, eggs, beans and peas, soy products, and unsalted nuts and seeds.
- Consume at least 8 oz per week of seafood from a variety of sources.
- Replace protein foods that are high in sodium and solid fat with more nutrient-dense options.

The High-Protein Diet

The per-capita consumption of protein by Americans continues to rise, along with the total caloric intake. In the United States, the per-capita daily consumption of kilocalories and grams of protein rose from 3400 kcal and 101 g of protein in 1909 to 4000 kcal and 120 g of protein in 2010.[1] Not coincidentally, significant weight gains and the health risks associated with obesity (e.g., heart disease, diabetes, hypertension, some forms of cancer) have been noted. The Behavioral Risk Factor Surveillance System results indicate that 33% of men and 46% of women are actively trying to lose weight in the United States at any given time.[2]

Health care professionals are concerned about the rising rate of obesity in this country as well as the methods by which people are trying to battle it. Current surveys report that, of those individuals who are trying to lose weight, only 19% of women and 22% of men reported using the recommended weight-loss strategy of fewer calories and more physical activity.[2] Some of the more popular diets are the high-protein, low-carbohydrate diets.

High-protein diets are often higher in total fat, saturated fat, and cholesterol and lower in fiber and antioxidants. Initial weight loss associated with a high-protein, high-fat diet is caused by the induction of metabolic ketosis and fluid loss from a lack of carbohydrates. Ketosis eventually suppresses the appetite, and this ultimately leads to reduced caloric intake and weight loss.

In terms of recommendations for sustained weight loss, health care professionals turn to research to see what works for most people and has the best results for overall health. There are many studies of various designs in terms of macronutrient composition. Because there are so many papers published on high- versus low-protein weight-loss diets, it is effective to look at large-scale meta-analyses to get a big picture idea of what the results indicate. Interestingly, short-term weight-loss studies (average of 12 weeks) indicate slight beneficial effects of high-protein diets over standard protein diets.[3] However, long-term studies (minimum of 12 months) do not show any health or weight-loss benefits of high-protein diets over diets following the standard macronutrient recommendations.[4]

The Nutrition Committee of the Council on Nutrition, Physical Activity, and Metabolism of the American Heart Association concluded that "high-protein diets are not recommended because they restrict healthful foods that provide essential nutrients and do not provide the variety of foods needed to adequately meet nutritional needs."[5]

The bottom line is that weight loss will require a reduction in total kilocalories consumed. The body still needs all of the essential nutrients to function and those nutrients come from a variety of foods—including fruits, vegetables, grains, and fats, in addition to protein-rich foods. If a weight-loss diet is designed such that most of the energy is supplied by protein-rich foods, there may not be enough kilocalories left to fit in all of the other food groups necessary to meet the body's requirements for essential nutrients.

Weight loss may be accomplished by many methods. However, meeting nutrient needs can only be attained by one method—and that is to eat foods containing those nutrients. A high-protein diet may work well for some people but may not be a good choice for others. Either way, all food groups must be included in order to have an overall healthy diet.

REFERENCES

1. U.S. Department Of Agriculture. *Nutrient Content of the U.S. Food Supply, 1909-2010*. Center For Nutrition Policy And Promotion, 2014. Available From: <Www.Cnpp.Usda.Gov/Usfoodsupply-1909-2010.Htm>.
2. Bish CL, et al. Diet and physical activity behaviors among Americans trying to lose weight: 2000 Behavioral Risk Factor Surveillance System. *Obes Res*. 2005;13(3):596-607.
3. Wycherley TP, et al. Effects of energy-restricted high-protein, low-fat compared with standard-protein, low-fat diets: a meta-analysis of randomized controlled trials. *Am J Clin Nutr*. 2012; 96(6):1281-1298.
4. Schwingshackl L, Hoffmann G. Long-term effects of low-fat diets either low or high in protein on cardiovascular and metabolic risk factors: a systematic review and meta-analysis. *Nutr J*. 2013;12:48.
5. St Jeor ST, et al. Dietary protein and weight reduction: a statement for healthcare professionals from the Nutrition Committee of the Council on Nutrition, Physical Activity, and Metabolism of the American Heart Association. *Circulation*. 2001;104(15):1869-1874.

Calculating Dietary Reference Intake for Protein

There are two ways to calculate a person's dietary recommendation for protein.
1. *Dietary Reference Intakes of Acceptable Macronutrient Distribution Range:* To calculate the protein needs of an individual who is consuming 2200 kcal/day based on the Dietary Reference Intake recommendation of 10% to 35% of total kilocalories, complete the following calculations:
   2200 kcal × 0.10 = 220 kcal/day *and*
   2200 kcal × 0.35 = 770 kcal/day, thus giving a range of 220 to 770 kcal/day from protein
   220 kcal ÷ 4 kcal/g (the fuel factor for protein) = 55 *and*
   770 kcal ÷ 4 kcal/g = 192.5 g of protein per day, thus giving a range of 55 to 192.5 g of protein per day
2. *Recommended Dietary Allowance relative to ideal body weight:* To calculate the protein needs of a woman who is

5 feet, 4 inches tall with an ideal body weight of 120 lb (see Chapter 15) based on the Recommended Dietary Allowance of 0.8 g of protein/kg of body weight per day, perform the following calculations:
Convert weight in pounds to weight in kg (2.2 lb = 1 kg) as follows: 120 lb ÷ 2.2 lb/kg = 54.5 kg
54.5 kg × 0.8 g/kg = 43.6 g of protein per day
Therefore, a woman who measures 5 feet, 4 inches tall and who is consuming 2200 kcal/day with a minimum of 10% of her calories coming from high-quality protein will safely obtain her Recommended Dietary Allowance for protein of 43.6 g per day.

Now, calculate your own dietary needs for protein based on both your total kcal intake and your body weight. Does your usual food intake meet your protein needs?

Table 4-3   Foods That Are High in Protein*

FOOD	APPROXIMATE AMOUNT	PROTEIN (g)
Veal, leg, meat only, braised	3 oz cooked	31.2
Beef, top round, trimmed of fat	3 oz cooked	30.7
Chicken, breast, meat only, roasted	3 oz cooked	26.7
Tuna, fresh, bluefin, cooked with dry heat	3 oz cooked	25.4
Turkey, meat only, roasted	3 oz cooked	24.9
Goose, meat only, roasted	3 oz cooked	24.6
Pork, sirloin, boneless, roasted	3 oz cooked	24.5
Halibut, fresh, cooked with dry heat	3 oz cooked	22.7
Liver, chicken, pan fried	3 oz cooked	21.9
Lamb, shoulder, trimmed to ¼ inch of fat, broiled	3 oz cooked	21.7
Tuna, canned in water, drained	3 oz cooked	21.7
Beef, ground, 70% lean, 30% fat, pan browned	3 oz cooked	21.7
Haddock, cooked with dry heat	3 oz cooked	20.6
Duck, meat only, roasted	3 oz cooked	20
Scallops, steamed	3 oz cooked	19.7
Salmon, Atlantic, cooked with dry heat	3 oz cooked	18.8
Soy burger	3 oz cooked	16.1
Oysters, cooked with moist heat	3 oz cooked	16.1
Tofu, fried	3 oz	14.6
Ham, sliced, 11% fat	3 oz cooked	14.1
Cottage cheese, 2% milk fat	3 oz	11.7
Soy milk	1 cup	11
Milk, 1% fat	1 cup	9.7
Peanut butter, smooth	2 Tbsp	8
Lentils, boiled	3 oz cooked	7.7
Kidney beans, boiled	3 oz cooked	7.4
Cheddar cheese	1 oz	7
Egg, whole, scrambled	1 large	6.8
Yogurt, plain, skim milk	3 oz	4.9

Data from U.S. Department of Agriculture, Agricultural Research Service, Nutrient Data Laboratory. *Nutrient Data Laboratory home page* (website): <http://ndb.nal.usda.gov/>; Accessed September 22, 2011.
*Listed in decreasing order of protein per serving.

Table 4-3 provides a comparison of protein-rich food portions.

MyPlate

As with the other macronutrient recommendations from the MyPlate guidelines, Americans are encouraged to consume a variety of foods to meet all of their nutrient needs (see Figure 1-3).[24] The MyPlate website (www.choosemyplate.gov) includes tips for choosing lean sources of meat, poultry, and fish as well as vegetable protein sources such as beans, nuts, and seeds. A personalized plan can be obtained by entering an individual's age, sex, height, weight, and physical activity level. Sample menus for omnivores and eating tips for vegetarian lifestyles are also available.

Putting It All Together

Summary

- Protein provides the human body with amino acids, which are its primary tissue-building units. Of the 20 common amino acids, 9 are indispensable in the diet, because the body cannot manufacture them as it can the remaining 11.

- Foods that supply all of the indispensable amino acids are called *complete proteins;* these foods are mostly of animal origin. Plant protein foods are considered incomplete proteins, because they lack one or more of the indispensable amino acids. The exception is soy protein, which is of plant origin and provides complete proteins.

- A constant turnover of tissue protein occurs between tissue anabolism and tissue catabolism. Adequate dietary protein and a reserve pool of amino acids help to maintain this overall protein balance. Nitrogen balance is a measure of overall protein balance.
- A mixed diet that includes a variety of foods, together with sufficient nonprotein kilocalories from the primary fuel foods (i.e., carbohydrates), supplies a balance of protein and other nutrients.
- Vegan diets involve only plant proteins. Other vegetarian diets may include dairy products, eggs, and sometimes fish. All vegetarian lifestyles can provide balanced nutrition with planning and variety.
- After protein foods are eaten, a powerful digestive team of six protein-splitting enzymes frees individual amino acids for absorption.
- Protein requirements are principally influenced by growth needs and the nature of the diet in terms of protein quality and energy intake. Clinical influences on protein needs include fever, disease, surgery, and other trauma to body tissues.

Chapter Review Questions

See answers in Appendix A.

1. Amino acids are unique as compared to carbohydrates and fats because of the presence of _____ in their structure.
   a. Carbon
   b. Hydrogen
   c. Phosphorus
   d. Nitrogen

2. Complete proteins can be found in which food source?
   a. Corn
   b. Eggs
   c. Whole-grain bread
   d. Peanuts

3. A substitution to recommend to a patient who is vegan and wants to make a recipe that calls for whole cow's milk would be:
   a. Sour cream.
   b. Egg whites.
   c. Soy milk.
   d. Goat milk.

4. Protein requirements would be the highest for which of the following individuals?
   a. 16-year-old teenager
   b. 25-year-old lawyer
   c. 37-year-old pilot
   d. 62-year-old grandmother

5. A state of negative nitrogen balance is most likely found in which of the following?
   a. A 29-year-old woman who is 6 months' pregnant
   b. A 32 year old on bed rest following severe trauma
   c. A 10-year-old boy who plays soccer every day
   d. A 48-year-old high school math teacher

Additional Learning Resources

evolve http://evolve.elsevier.com/Williams/basic/

References and **Further Reading and Resources** in the back of the book provide additional resources for enhancing knowledge.

Digestion, Absorption, and Metabolism

Key Concepts

- Through a balanced system of mechanical and chemical digestion, food is broken down into smaller substances, and the nutrients are then available for biologic use.
- Special organ structures and functions accomplish these tasks through the successive parts of the gastrointestinal system.

- Absorption, transport, and metabolism allow for the distribution, use, and storage of nutrients throughout the body.

As described in previous chapters, nutrients that the body requires do not come ready to use; rather, they are packaged as foods in a variety of forms. Therefore, whole food must be broken down into smaller substances for absorption and metabolism to meet the body's needs. Digestion of the macronutrients—carbohydrates, fat, and protein—has been discussed in preceding chapters.

This chapter views the overall process of food digestion and nutrient absorption as one continuous whole that involves a series of successive events. In addition, metabolism and the unique body structures and functions that make this process possible are reviewed.

DIGESTION

BASIC PRINCIPLES

Body cells cannot use food as it is eaten. Food must be changed into simpler substances for absorption and then into even more simple constituents that cells can use to sustain life. Preparing food for the body's use involves many steps, including **digestion, absorption, transport,** and **metabolism.**

The different parts of the gastrointestinal (GI) tract and accessory organs are shown in Figure 5-1. The

individual parts of the GI system work systematically together as a whole to complete the process of digestion and metabolism. Food components travel through this system until they ultimately are absorbed and delivered to the cells or excreted as waste.

MECHANICAL AND CHEMICAL DIGESTION

For nutrients to be absorbed, food must go through a series of mechanical and chemical changes. Together, these two actions encompass the overall process of digestion.

The specific mechanical and chemical actions that occur during the digestion of the macronutrients have previously been discussed in Chapters 2 to 4. Of the micronutrients, most vitamins and minerals require little to no digestion. There are some exceptions (e.g., vitamins A and B_{12}, biotin) that require digestion before absorption can take place. Water does not require digestion, and it is easily absorbed into the general circulation. This chapter explores those actions as a whole and then as an interdependent process. Vitamins, minerals, and water will be reviewed again in Chapters 7, 8, and 9, respectively.

Mechanical Digestion: Gastrointestinal Motility

Beginning in the mouth, the muscles and nerves in the walls of the GI tract coordinate their actions to provide the necessary spontaneous motility for digestion to proceed. This automatic response to the presence of food enables the system to break up the food mass swallowed in each bite and move it along the digestive pathway. Muscles and nerves work together to produce constant motility.

Muscles. Layers of smooth muscle in the GI wall interact to provide two general types of movement: (1) muscle tone or tonic contraction, which ensures the continuous passage of the food mass and valve control

---

digestion the process by which food is broken down in the gastrointestinal tract to release nutrients in forms that the body can absorb.

absorption the process by which nutrients are taken into the cells that line the gastrointestinal tract.

transport the movement of nutrients through the circulatory system from one area of the body to another.

metabolism the sum of the vast number of chemical changes in the cell that ultimately produce the materials that are essential for energy, tissue building, and metabolic controls.

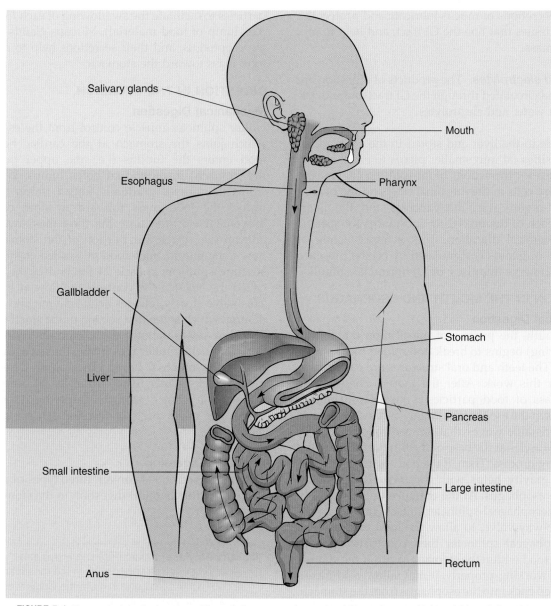

FIGURE 5-1 The gastrointestinal system. Through the successive parts of the system, multiple activities of digestion liberate food nutrients for use. (Courtesy Rolin Graphics.)

along the way; and (2) periodic muscle contraction and relaxation, which are rhythmic waves that mix the food mass and move it forward. These alternating muscular contractions and relaxations that force the contents forward are known as *peristalsis*, a term that comes from the Greek words *peri,* meaning "around," and *stalsis,* meaning "contraction."

Nerves. Specific nerves regulate muscular action along the GI tract. A complex network of nerves in the GI wall called the *intramural nerve plexus* extends from the esophagus to the anus. These nerves do three things: (1) they control muscle tone in the wall; (2) they regulate the rate and intensity of the alternating muscle contractions; and (3) they coordinate all of the various movements. When all is well, these finely tuned movements flow together like those of a great symphony,

without conscience awareness. However, when all is not well, the discord is felt as pain. Such problems and diseases of the GI tract are covered in Chapter 18.

Chemical Digestion: Gastrointestinal Secretions

A number of secretions work together to make chemical digestion possible. Five types of substances are involved.

Hydrochloric acid and buffer ions. Hydrochloric acid and buffer ions are needed to produce the correct pH (i.e., the degree of acidity or alkalinity) that is necessary for enzymatic activity.

Enzymes. Digestive enzymes are proteins produced in the body and are specifically designed to break down other nutrients.

Mucus. Secretions of mucus lubricate and protect the mucosal tissues that line the GI tract, and help to mix the food mass.

Water and electrolytes. The products of digestion are carried and circulated through the GI tract and into the tissues by water and electrolytes.

Bile. Made in the liver and stored in the gallbladder, bile emulsifies fat into smaller pieces to expose more surface area for the actions of fat-splitting enzymes.

Secretory cells in the intestinal tract and the nearby accessory organs (i.e., the pancreas and the liver) produce each of the preceding substances for specific jobs in chemical digestion. The secretory action of these cells or glands is stimulated by (1) the presence of food; (2) nerve impulses; or (3) hormonal stimuli.

DIGESTION IN THE MOUTH AND ESOPHAGUS

Mechanical Digestion

In the mouth, the process of mastication (i.e., biting and chewing) begins to break down food into smaller particles. The teeth and oral structures are particularly suited for this work. After the food is chewed, the mixed mass of food particles is swallowed, and it passes down the esophagus, largely as a result of autonomic peristaltic waves that are controlled by nerve reflexes. Muscles at the base of the tongue facilitate the swallowing process. Then, if the body is in the upright position, gravity helps with the movement of food down the esophagus. At the entrance to the stomach, the gastroesophageal sphincter muscle relaxes, much like a one-way valve, to allow the food to enter. The gastroesophageal sphincter then constricts again to retain the food within the stomach cavity. If the sphincter is not working properly, it may allow acid-mixed food to seep back into the esophagus from the stomach. The result is the discomforting feeling of gastroesophageal reflux, or heartburn.

Heartburn has nothing to do with the heart, but it was so named because the sensations are perceived as originating in the region of the heart. A hiatal hernia is another common cause of heartburn; this occurs when part of the stomach protrudes upward into the chest cavity (i.e., the thorax; see Chapter 18).

Chemical Digestion

The salivary glands secrete saliva that contains **salivary amylase,** which is also called *ptyalin. Amylase* is the general name for any starch-splitting enzyme. Small glands at the back of the tongue (i.e., von Ebner's glands) secrete lingual lipase. *Lipase* is the general name for any fat-splitting enzyme. However, in this case, food does not remain in the mouth long enough for much chemical action to occur. During infancy, lingual lipase is a more relevant enzyme for the digestion of milk fat. The salivary glands also secrete a mucous material that lubricates and binds food particles to facilitate the swallowing of each food bolus (i.e., lump of food material). Mucous glands also line the esophagus, and their secretions help to move the food mass toward the stomach.

DIGESTION IN THE STOMACH

Mechanical Digestion

Under sphincter muscle control from the esophagus, which joins the stomach at the cardiac notch, the food enters the fundus (i.e., the upper portion of the stomach) in individual bolus lumps. Within the stomach, muscles gradually knead, store, mix, and propel the food mass forward in slow, controlled movements. By the time the food mass reaches the antrum (i.e., the lower portion of the stomach), it is now a semiliquid, acid–food mix called **chyme.** A constricting sphincter muscle at the end of the stomach called the *pyloric valve* controls the flow at this point. This valve slowly releases acidic chyme into the duodenum, which is the first section of the small intestine. The slow release allows the alkaline intestinal secretions to quickly buffer the chyme, thus avoiding irritation of the mucosal lining. The caloric density of a meal, which mainly results from its fat composition, influences the rate of stomach emptying at the pyloric valve. The major parts of the stomach are shown in Figure 5-2.

Chemical Digestion

The gastric secretions contain three types of materials that help with chemical digestion in the stomach.

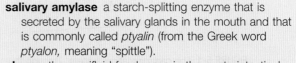

salivary amylase a starch-splitting enzyme that is secreted by the salivary glands in the mouth and that is commonly called *ptyalin* (from the Greek word *ptyalon,* meaning "spittle").
chyme the semifluid food mass in the gastrointestinal tract that is present after gastric digestion.

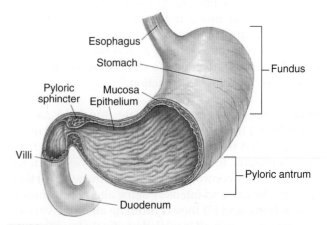

FIGURE 5-2 Stomach. (Reprinted from Raven PH, Johnson GB. *Biology.* 3rd ed. New York: McGraw-Hill; 1992.)

Acid. The hormone **gastrin** stimulates parietal cells within the lining of the stomach to secrete hydrochloric acid. Hydrochloric acid creates the necessary degree of acidity for gastric enzymes to work, and it also activates the first protease, pepsinogen, in the stomach. As you will recall from Chapter 4, protease is the general name for any protein-splitting enzyme. In addition, the acidic environment created by hydrochloric acid secretion in the stomach aids in the absorption of several vitamins and minerals (see the Drug-Nutrient Interaction box, "Acidity for Nutrient Absorption").

Mucus. Mucous secretions protect the stomach lining from the erosive effect of hydrochloric acid. Secretions also bind and mix the food mass and help to move it along the GI tract.

> **gastrin** a hormone that helps with gastric motility, that stimulates the secretion of gastric acid by the parietal cells of the stomach, and that stimulates the chief cells to secrete pepsinogen.

Drug-Nutrient Interaction

Acidity for Nutrient Absorption

The body controls the pH of the gastrointestinal tract contents by secreting acidic or alkaline buffering agents. The release of hydrochloric acid in the stomach decreases the acidity; and bicarbonate, secreted from the pancreas into the small intestines, neutralizes the pH. The release of hydrochloric acid and bicarbonate is controlled by hormones and a feedback system that is constantly fine-tuning the environment of the gastrointestinal tract for optimal performance.

Hydrochloric acid in the stomach has many functions. The acid kills microorganisms, activates pepsinogen, and begins the digestive process of proteins. In addition, the downstream absorption of several vitamins and minerals depends on the exposure to an acidic environment in the stomach. Specifically, the interaction with hydrochloric acid increases the bioavailability of vitamin B_{12}, calcium, iron, zinc, and magnesium further along the GI tract. Therefore, situations that cause a decrease in hydrochloric acid secretion in the stomach can reduce the bioavailability of these vitamins and minerals, slow down the digestive process of protein, and increase the bacterial load.

Proton pump inhibitors are a class of drugs that inhibit the release of acid in the stomach. The use of acid suppressors is one of the most commonly used medications in the United States and they are often used for extended periods of time. While the extent of nutrient deficiency due to the chronic use of proton pump inhibitors is not yet well understood, it is accepted that the clinical implications could be significant and should especially be considered for individuals at risk for nutrient deficiency.[1]

REFERENCE

1. Ito T, Jensen RT. Association of long-term proton pump inhibitor therapy with bone fractures and effects on absorption of calcium, vitamin B_{12}, iron, and magnesium. *Curr Gastroenterol Rep*. 2010; 12(6):448-457.

Enzymes. The inactive enzyme pepsinogen is secreted by stomach cells, and it is activated by hydrochloric acid to become the protein-splitting enzyme pepsin. Other cells produce small amounts of a specific gastric lipase called *tributyrinase*, which works on tributyrin (i.e., butterfat); however, this is a relatively minor activity in the stomach.

Various sensations, emotions, hormones, and foods stimulate the nerve impulses that trigger these secretions. The concept that the stomach is said to "mirror the person within" is not without merit. For example, anger and hostility increase secretions, whereas fear and depression decrease secretions and inhibit blood flow and motility.

DIGESTION IN THE SMALL INTESTINE

Up to this point, the digestion of food has largely been mechanical, and it has resulted in the delivery of a semifluid mixture of fine food particles and watery secretions to the small intestine. Chemical digestion has been minimal. Thus, the major task of digestion and the absorption that follows occur in the small intestine. The structural parts, synchronized movements, and array of specific enzymes of the small intestine are highly developed for the final step of mechanical and chemical digestion.

Mechanical Digestion

Under the control of nerve impulses, the muscular walls of the small intestines stretch from the food mass or hormonal stimuli, and the intestinal muscles produce several types of movement that aid digestion, as follows:

- *Peristaltic waves* slowly push the food mass forward, sometimes with long, sweeping waves over the entire length of the intestine.
- *Pendular movements* from small, local muscles sweep back and forth, thereby stirring the chyme at the mucosal surface.
- *Segmentation rings* from the alternating contraction and relaxation of circular muscles progressively chop the food mass into successive soft lumps and then mix them with GI secretions.
- *Longitudinal rotation* by long muscles that run the length of the intestine rolls the slowly moving food mass in a spiral motion to mix it and expose new surfaces for absorption.
- *Surface villi motions* stir and mix the chyme at the intestinal wall, thereby exposing additional nutrients for absorption.

Chemical Digestion

The small intestines, together with the GI accessory organs (i.e., the pancreas, liver, and gallbladder), supply many secretory materials to accomplish the major chore of chemical digestion. The pancreas and intestines secrete enzymes that are specific for the digestion of each macronutrient.

Pancreatic enzymes.

1. *Carbohydrate:* **Pancreatic amylase** converts starch into the disaccharides maltose and sucrose.
2. *Protein:* Trypsin and chymotrypsin split large protein molecules into smaller and smaller peptide fragments and finally into single amino acids. Carboxypeptidase removes end amino acids from peptide chains.
3. *Fat:* **Pancreatic lipase** converts fat into glycerides and fatty acids.

Intestinal enzymes.

1. *Carbohydrate:* Disaccharidases (i.e., maltase, lactase, and sucrase) convert their respective disaccharides (i.e., maltose, lactose, and sucrose) into monosaccharides (i.e., glucose, galactose, and fructose).
2. *Protein:* The intestinal enzyme enterokinase activates trypsinogen, which is released from the pancreas to become the protein-splitting enzyme trypsin. Amino peptidase removes end amino acids from polypeptides. Dipeptidase splits dipeptides into their two remaining amino acids.
3. *Fat:* Intestinal lipase splits fat into glycerides and fatty acids.

Mucus.   Large quantities of mucus, which are secreted by intestinal glands, protect the mucosal lining from the irritation and erosion that would result from exposure to the highly acidic gastric contents entering the duodenum.

Bile.   Bile is an emulsifying agent and an important part of fat digestion and absorption. It is produced by the liver and stored in the adjacent gallbladder, and it is ready for use when fat enters the intestine.

Hormones.   The hormone **secretin,** which is produced by the mucosal glands in the first part of the intestine, controls the acidity and secretion of enzymes from the pancreas. An alkaline environment in the small intestine, with a pH greater than 8, is necessary for the activity of the pancreatic enzymes. The hormone **cholecystokinin,** which is secreted by intestinal mucosal glands when fat is present, triggers the release of bile from the gallbladder to emulsify fat.

The arrangement of accessory organs to the duodenum, which is the first section of the small intestine, is shown in Figure 5-3. These organs make up the biliary system. The liver is sometimes called the "metabolic capital" of the body, because it performs numerous functions for the metabolism of all converging nutrients (Box 5-1). The liver's many metabolic functions are reviewed in greater detail in Chapter 18.

The various nerve and hormone controls of digestion are illustrated in Figure 5-4. Although small individual summaries of digestion are given in each of the macronutrient chapters, a general summary of the entire digestive process is shown in Figure 5-5 so that

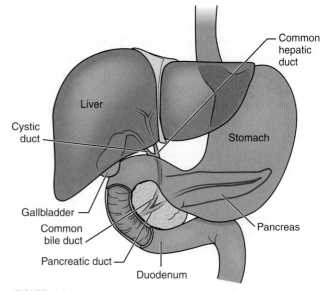

FIGURE 5-3 Organs of the biliary system and the pancreatic ducts.

the overall process can be viewed as it is: one continuous and integrated whole.

ABSORPTION AND TRANSPORT

When digestion is complete, food has been changed into simple end products that are ready for absorption. Carbohydrate foods are reduced to the simple sugars glucose, fructose, and galactose. Fats are reduced into fatty acids and glycerides. Protein is reduced into single amino acids. And vitamins and minerals are liberated. With a water base for solution and transport, in addition to the necessary electrolytes, the whole fluid food-derived mass is now prepared for absorption. For many nutrients, especially certain vitamins and minerals, the point of absorption becomes the vital gatekeeper that determines how much of a given nutrient is available for cellular use. Although the GI tract

pancreatic amylase a major starch-splitting enzyme that is secreted by the pancreas and that acts in the small intestine.

pancreatic lipase a major fat-splitting enzyme produced by the pancreas and secreted into the small intestine to digest fat.

secretin a hormone that stimulates gastric and pancreatic secretions. Secretin secretion is increased in response to a low pH in the duodenum. Secretin stimulates the pancreatic release of bicarbonate to increase the pH to an alkaline environment. Secretin also stimulates the secretion of pepsinogen from the chief cells of the stomach.

cholecystokinin (CCK) a hormone secreted from the mucosal epithelium of the small intestine in response to the presence of fat and certain amino acids in chyme. CCK inhibits gastric motility, increases the release of pancreatic enzymes, and stimulates the gallbladder to secrete bile into the small intestine.

Box 5-1   Functions of the Liver

MAJOR FUNCTIONS
- Bile production
- Synthesis of proteins and blood clotting factors
- Metabolism of hormones and medications
- Regulation of blood glucose levels
- Urea production to remove the waste products of normal metabolism

SPECIFIC METABOLIC FUNCTIONS REGARDING THE MACRONUTRIENTS
- Lipolysis: breaking down lipids into fatty acids and glycerol
- Lipogenesis: building up lipids from fatty acids and glycerol

- Glycolysis: breaking down glucose into pyruvate to enter the Krebs cycle
- Gluconeogenesis: converting noncarbohydrate substances into glucose
- Glycogenolysis: breaking down glycogen into individual glucose units
- Glycogenesis: combining units of glucose to store as glycogen
- Protein degradation: breaking down proteins into single amino acids
- Protein synthesis: building complete proteins from individual amino acids

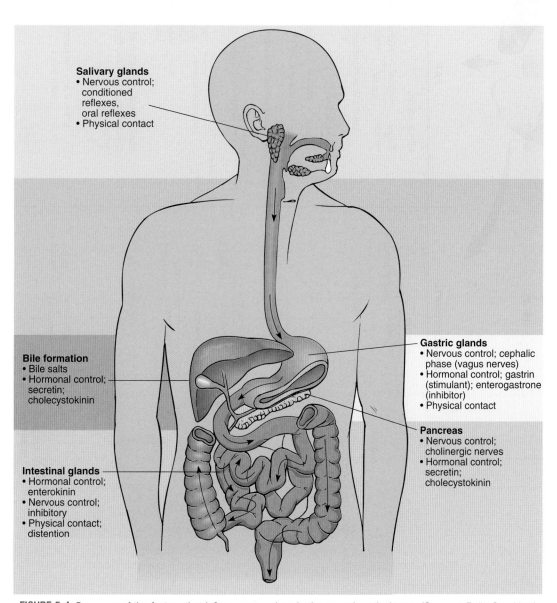

Salivary glands
- Nervous control; conditioned reflexes, oral reflexes
- Physical contact

Bile formation
- Bile salts
- Hormonal control; secretin; cholecystokinin

Intestinal glands
- Hormonal control; enterokinin
- Nervous control; inhibitory
- Physical contact; distention

Gastric glands
- Nervous control; cephalic phase (vagus nerves)
- Hormonal control; gastrin (stimulant); enterogastrone (inhibitor)
- Physical contact

Pancreas
- Nervous control; cholinergic nerves
- Hormonal control; secretin; cholecystokinin

FIGURE 5-4 Summary of the factors that influence secretions in the gastrointestinal tract. (Courtesy Rolin Graphics.)

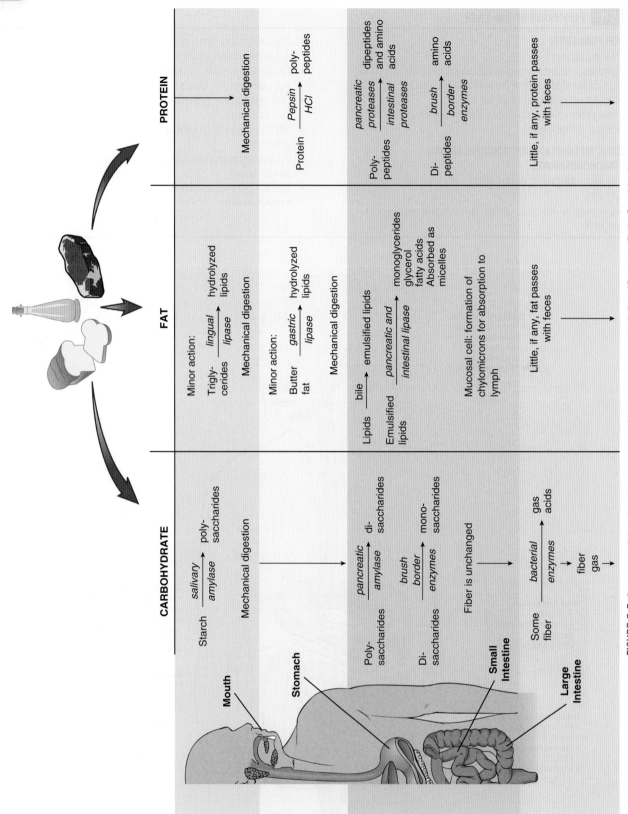

FIGURE 5-5 Summary of the digestive processes. Note: enzymes are in *italics*. (Courtesy Rolin Graphics.)

is quite efficient, 100% of all nutrients consumed are not absorbed as a result of varying degrees of bioavailability. A nutrient's bioavailability depends on the following: (1) the amount of nutrient present in the GI tract; (2) the competition among nutrients for common absorptive sites; and (3) the form in which the nutrient is present (see the Clinical Applications box, "Micronutrient Bioavailability and Competitive Absorption"). This degree of bioavailability is a factor in setting dietary intake standards for all macronutrients and micronutrients.[1-6]

ABSORPTION IN THE SMALL INTESTINE

Absorbing Structures

Three important structures of the intestinal wall surface (Figure 5-6) are particularly adapted to ensure the

Clinical Applications

Micronutrient Bioavailability and Competitive Absorption

Iron and zinc deficiency are two of the most common micronutrient deficiencies worldwide. Subsequently, food fortification/enrichment and dietary supplements containing both iron and zinc are often used as a means for increasing intake. However, just because we consume it, it does not mean we can absorb or use it within the body. Many factors regulate nutrient bioavailability, including the presence of other nutrients.

Iron and zinc enrichment in grain products have several factors working against the absorption of either nutrient. For example, the phytic acid found in grain products decreases the bioavailability of both iron and zinc by binding to the minerals and preventing absorption. In addition, divalent cations compete for absorption throughout the gastrointestinal tract. For example, iron, copper, and zinc compete for binding to transporter molecules during absorption. Thus, a high level of any one divalent metal will reduce the bioavailability of the other

divalent minerals. Grain products are also enriched with folic acid but high intakes of folic acid or calcium may reduce zinc absorption when consumed together.

Does this mean that it is a waste of time to include such products in the diet? No; not at all. Reduced bioavailability is not the same as blocked absorption. Reduced bioavailability only means that a smaller percent of the nutrient consumed is actually absorbed. Fortunately, the body is extremely efficient and does not depend on 100% absorption of all nutrients consumed. If you are working with a patient who is suffering from a nutrient deficiency and he or she has been prescribed a dietary supplement, it would be prudent to check for factors inhibiting or enhancing the bioavailability of that particular nutrient. That way, you can help the patient make ideal choices about when to take their supplement, what foods to take it with or avoid, and what foods to consume to help stabilize the supply of the nutrient of concern.

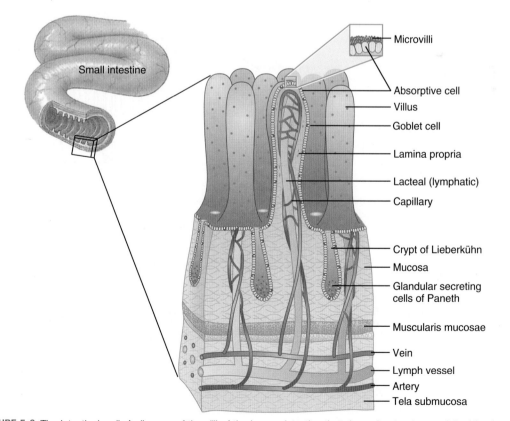

FIGURE 5-6 The intestinal wall. A diagram of the villi of the human intestine that shows its structure and the blood and lymph vessels. (Reprinted from Mahan LK, Escott-Stump S. *Krause's Food & Nutrition Therapy*. 12th ed. Philadelphia: Saunders; 2008.)

maximal absorption of essential nutrients in the digestive process:

- *Mucosal folds:* Like the hills and valleys of a mountain range, the surface of the small intestine piles into many folds. **Mucosal folds** can easily be seen when such tissue is examined.
- *Villi:* Closer examination under a regular light microscope reveals small, finger-like projections that cover the folds of the mucosal lining. These little **villi** further increase the area of exposed surface. Each villus has an ample supply of blood vessels to receive protein, carbohydrate, and water-soluble micronutrient materials. Each villus also has a lymph vessel to receive fat-soluble nutrients. This lymph vessel is called a *lacteal,* because the fatty chyme is creamy at this point and looks like milk.
- *Microvilli:* Even closer examination with an electron microscope reveals a covering of smaller projections on the surface of each tiny villus. The covering of **microvilli** on each villus is called the *brush border,* because it looks like bristles on a brush.

These three unique structures of the inner intestinal wall—folds, villi, and microvilli—combine to make the inner surface nearly 600 times greater than the area of the outer surface of the intestine. The length of the small intestine is approximately 660 cm (22 ft). This remarkable organ is well adapted to deliver nutrients from digested food into the circulation for use within the body's cells. If its entire surface were spread out on a flat plane, the total surface area is estimated to be as large as half of a basketball court. Far from being the lowly gut, the small intestine is one of the most highly developed, exquisitely fashioned, and specialized tissues in the body.

Absorption Processes

A number of absorbing processes complete the task of moving vital nutrients across the inner intestinal wall and into the body circulation. These processes include diffusion, energy-driven active transport, and pinocytosis (Figures 5-7 and 5-8):

---

mucosal folds the large, visible folds of the mucous lining of the small intestine that increase the absorbing surface area.

villi small protrusions from the surface of a membrane; finger-like projections that cover the mucosal surfaces of the small intestine and that further increase the absorbing surface area.

microvilli extremely small, hair-like projections that cover all of the villi on the surface of the small intestine and that greatly increase the total absorbing surface area.

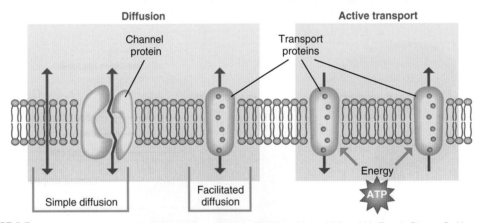

FIGURE 5-7 Transport pathways through the cell membrane. (Reprinted from Mahan LK, Escott-Stump S. *Krause's Food & Nutrition Therapy.* 13th ed. Philadelphia: Saunders; 2012.)

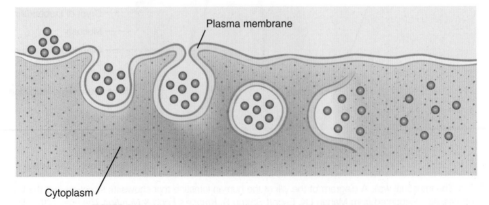

FIGURE 5-8 Pinocytosis; the engulfing of a large molecule by the cell.

- *Simple diffusion* is the force by which particles move outward in all directions from an area of greater concentration to an area of lesser concentration. Small materials that do not need the help of a specific protein channel to move across the mucosal cell wall use this method.
- *Facilitated diffusion* is similar to simple diffusion, but it makes use of a protein channel for the carrier-assisted movement of larger items across the mucosal cell membrane.
- *Active transport* is the force by which particles move against their concentration gradient. Active transport mechanisms usually require some sort of carrier to help transport the particles across the membrane. For example, glucose enters absorbing cells through an active transport mechanism that involves sodium as a partner.
- *Pinocytosis* is the penetration of larger materials by attaching to the thicker cell membrane and being engulfed by the cell (see Figure 5-8).

ABSORPTION IN THE LARGE INTESTINE

Water

The main absorptive task that remains for the large intestine is to absorb water. Most water in the chyme that enters the large intestine is absorbed in the first half of the colon. Only a small amount (approximately 100 mL) remains to form the feces and be eliminated.

Dietary Fiber

Dietary fiber is not digested because humans lack the specific enzymes that are required to break the beta bonds between molecules. However, fiber contributes important bulk to food mass and helps to form feces. The formation and passage of intestinal gas is a normal process of healthy digestion, but it can be problematic for some individuals (see the Clinical Applications box, "The Sometimes Embarrassing Effects of Digestion").

Macronutrients and Micronutrients

Table 5-1 summarizes the major features of intestinal nutrient absorption, including macronutrients and micronutrients. In addition, Figure 5-9 shows the approximate location of absorption of each nutrient as well as the route through which it is absorbed (i.e., lymph or blood).

TRANSPORT

After nutrients have been broken down from food and absorbed, they must be transported to various cells throughout the body. This transportation requires the work of both the vascular and the lymphatic systems.

Vascular System

The vascular system is composed of veins and arteries, and it is responsible for supplying the entire body with

Table 5-1   Intestinal Absorption of Some Major Nutrients

NUTRIENT	FORM	MEANS OF ABSORPTION	CONTROL AGENT OR REQUIRED COFACTOR	ROUTE
Carbohydrate	Monosaccharides (glucose or galactose)	Competitive	—	Blood
		Selective	—	
		Active transport by sodium pump	Sodium	
	Fructose	Facilitated diffusion	Protein carrier	Blood
Protein	Amino acids	Selective	—	Blood
	Some dipeptides	Facilitated diffusion	Pyridoxine (pyridoxal phosphate)	Blood
	Whole protein (rare)	Pinocytosis	Protein carrier	Blood
Fat	Fatty acids	Fatty acid–bile complex (micelles)	Bile	Lymph
	Glycerides (monoglycerides and diglycerides)			
	Few triglycerides (neutral fat)	Pinocytosis	—	Lymph
Vitamins	B_{12}	Facilitated diffusion	Intrinsic factor	Blood
	A, D, E, and K	Bile complex (micelles)	Bile	Blood
	K from bacterial synthesis	From the large intestine to the blood		
Minerals	Sodium	Active transport by sodium pump	—	Blood
	Calcium	Active transport	Vitamin D	Blood
	Iron	Active transport	Ferritin mechanism	Blood (as transferrin)
Water	Water	Osmosis	—	Blood, lymph, and interstitial fluid

The Sometimes Embarrassing Effects of Digestion

After eating certain foods, some people complain of the discomfort or embarrassment of gas. Gas is a normal by-product of digestion, but when it becomes painful or apparent to others, it may become a physical and social dilemma.

The gastrointestinal tract normally holds approximately 3 oz of gas that moves along with the food mass and is silently absorbed into the bloodstream. Sometimes extra gas collects in the stomach or intestine, thereby creating an embarrassing—although usually harmless—situation.

STOMACH GAS

Gas in the stomach results from trapped air bubbles. It occurs when a person eats too fast, drinks through a straw, or otherwise takes in extra air while eating. Burping releases some gas, but the following tips may help to avoid uncomfortable situations:

- Avoid carbonated beverages.
- Do not gulp.
- Chew with the mouth closed.
- Do not drink from a can or through a straw.
- Do not eat while overly nervous.

INTESTINAL GAS

Intestinal gas forms in the colon, where bacteria attack fermentable residues and cause them to decompose and produce gas. Carbohydrates release hydrogen, carbon dioxide, and—in some people with certain types of bacteria in the gut—methane. All three products are odorless (although noisy) gases. Protein produces hydrogen sulfide and volatile compounds such as indole and skatole, which add a distinctive aroma to the expelled air. Changing the diet to include less fermentable residue foods can significantly improve symptoms.[1,2] However, problem foods are specific to individuals and may also depend on the type and quantity of bacteria in the gut.[3]

The following suggestions may help to control flatulence:

- Cut down on simple carbohydrates (e.g., sugars). Especially observe milk's effect, because lactose

intolerance may be the culprit. Substitute cultured forms, such as yogurt or milk treated with a lactase product such as Lactaid (McNeil Nutritionals, Fort Washington, Pa).
- Use a prior leaching process before cooking dry beans to remove indigestible saccharides such as raffinose and stachyose. Although humans cannot digest these substances, they provide a feast for bacteria in the intestines. This simple procedure eliminates a major portion of these gas-forming saccharides. First, put washed, dry beans into a large pot; add 4 cups of water for each pound of beans (approximately 2 cups); and boil the beans uncovered for 2 min. Remove the pot from the heat, cover it, and let it stand for 1 hour. Finally, drain and rinse the beans, add 8 cups of fresh water, bring the water to a boil, reduce the heat, and simmer the beans in a covered pot for 1 to 2 hours or until beans are tender. Season as desired.
- Eliminate known food offenders. These vary from person to person, but some of the most common offenders are beans (if they are not prepared for cooking as described), onions, cabbage, and high-fiber wheat and bran products.

When relief has been achieved, slowly add more complex carbohydrates and high-fiber foods back into the diet. After small amounts are tolerated, try moderate increases. If no relief occurs, medical help may be needed to rule out or treat an overactive gastrointestinal tract.

REFERENCES

1. Azpiroz F, et al. Effect of a low-flatulogenic diet in patients with flatulence and functional digestive symptoms. *Neurogastroenterol Motil.* 2014;26(6):779-785.
2. Serra J. Intestinal gas: has diet anything to do in the absence of a demonstrable malabsorption state? *Curr Opin Clin Nutr Metab Care.* 2012;15(5):489-493.
3. Manichanh C, et al. Anal gas evacuation and colonic microbiota in patients with flatulence: effect of diet. *Gut.* 2014;63(3): 401-408.

---

nutrients, oxygen, and many other vital substances that are necessary for life via the blood. In addition, the vascular system transports waste (e.g., carbon dioxide, nitrogen) to the lungs and kidneys for removal.

Most of the products of digestion are water-soluble nutrients, which therefore can be absorbed into the vascular system (i.e., the blood circulatory system) directly from the intestinal cells. The nutrients travel first to the liver for immediate cell enzyme work before being dispersed to other cells throughout the body. The portion of circulation from the intestines to the liver is called the *portal circulation.*

Lymphatic System

Because fatty materials are not water soluble, another route must be provided. These fat molecules pass into the lymph vessels in the villi (e.g., the lacteals), flow into the larger lymph vessels of the body, and eventually enter the bloodstream through the thoracic duct.

METABOLISM

At this point, the individual macronutrients in food have been broken down through digestion into the basic building blocks (i.e., monosaccharides, amino acids, and fatty acids) and absorbed into the bloodstream or the lymphatic system. Now these nutrients can be converted into needed energy or stored in the body for later use.

In addition, the micronutrients (i.e., vitamins and minerals) have been liberated from any bound proteins, and they are free for absorption. Once inside, the micronutrients are dispersed throughout the body for their many critical functions.

CATABOLISM AND ANABOLISM

Metabolism is the sum of the chemical reactions that occur within a living cell to maintain life. The mitochondrion of the cell is the work center in which all

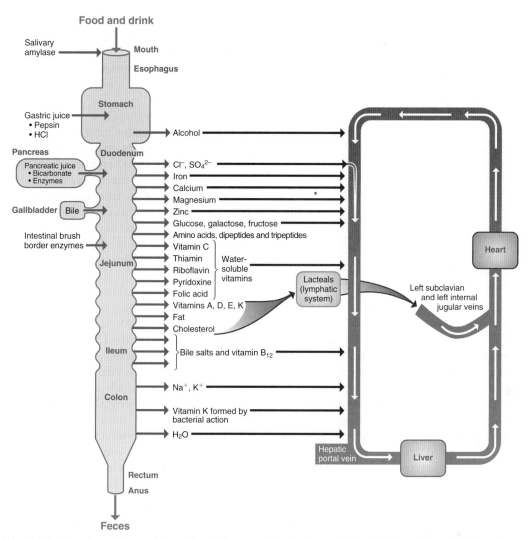

FIGURE 5-9 Sites of secretion and absorption in the gastrointestinal tract. (Mahan LK, Escott-Stump S. *Krause's Food & Nutrition Therapy*. 12th ed. Philadelphia: Saunders; 2008.)

metabolic reactions take place. The two types of metabolism are catabolism and anabolism. Catabolism is the breaking down of large substances into smaller units. For example, breaking down stored glycogen into its smaller building blocks (i.e., glucose) is a catabolic reaction. Anabolism is the opposite; it is the process by which cells build large substances from smaller particles, such as building a complex protein from single amino acids.

The Krebs cycle, which is also known as the *citric acid cycle* or the *TCA* (tricarboxylic acid) *cycle,* is the hub of energy production that occurs in the mitochondria of the cell. It is not so much that energy is *produced* here. Rather, energy is converted into a form that the body can use. The combined processes of metabolism (i.e., catabolic and anabolic reactions) ensure that the body has much needed energy in the form of adenosine triphosphate (ATP). Figure 5-10 illustrates a brief breakdown of the macronutrients and shows how they enter the final step of energy production to ultimately supply cells with ATP.

The rate of ATP production fluctuates, and it speeds up or slows down depending on energy needs at a given time. Energy needs are minimal during sleep, but they increase dramatically during strenuous physical activity. Energy supply and demand are discussed further in Chapter 6.

ENERGY DENSITY

Because carbohydrates have 4 kcal/g and fat has 9 kcal/g, the metabolism of glucose yields less energy (i.e., ATP) than the metabolism of fat, gram for gram. However, the body prefers to use glucose as its primary source of energy. Protein can be used as a source of energy as well, but this is an inefficient use of protein, and it results in extra nitrogen waste. The body only breaks down protein for energy when glucose and fatty acids are in short supply.

STORING EXTRA ENERGY

If the amount of food consumed yields more energy than is needed to maintain voluntary and involuntary

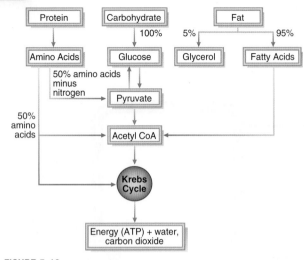

FIGURE 5-10 Metabolic pathways. (Reprinted from Peckenpaugh NJ. *Nutrition Essentials and Diet Therapy*. 10th ed. Philadelphia: Saunders; 2007.)

actions, the remaining energy is stored for later use in the body. The human body is a highly efficient organism. Energy or kilocalories in excess of needs are not wasted. Excess glucose can easily be stored as glycogen in the liver and muscles for quick energy at a later time. The anabolic process of converting extra glucose into glycogen is called glycogenesis.

When the glycogen reserves are full, additional excess energy from carbohydrates, fat, or protein is stored as fat in adipose tissue. Lipogenesis is the building up of triglycerides for storage in the adipose tissue of the body. Both glycogen and stored fat are available for use when energy demands require it. Energy balance and the factors that influence it are discussed further in Chapter 6.

Excess protein intake is not "stored as muscle." The body uses amino acids to build functional and structural proteins as needed, and the liver maintains some free amino acids to meet rapid needs of the body. However, protein intake above and beyond the body's requirements is broken down further so that the nitrogen unit is removed, and the remaining carbon chain can be converted to glucose or fat for storage. The conversion of amino acids to glucose is referred to as gluconeogenesis.

Although alcohol is not a nutrient, it does provide 7 kcal/g. Therefore, alcohol intake adds to the overall supply of energy (see the For Further Focus box, "What About Alcohol?").

ERRORS IN DIGESTION AND METABOLISM

THE GENETIC DEFECT

Certain food intolerances stem from underlying genetic disease. For each genetic disease involving metabolism, the necessary enzyme that controls the cell's use of a specific nutrient is missing, thereby preventing normal nutrient metabolism. Three examples of genetic defects are phenylketonuria (PKU), galactosemia, and glycogen storage diseases.

Phenylketonuria

Phenylalanine hydroxylase is the enzyme that is responsible for metabolizing the essential amino acid phenylalanine. PKU is an autosomal recessive genetic disorder that results when phenylalanine hydroxylase is not produced by the body. Although the disease is not curable, it is treatable through diet. If left untreated, this condition causes permanent mental retardation and central nervous system damage. Other possible symptoms and side effects include irritability, hyperactivity, convulsive seizures, and psychiatric disorders.

PKU affects approximately 1 in every 10,000 to 15,000 live births in the United States. Screening tests began during the 1960s, and they are now mandatory at birth in all areas of the United States. A simple blood test can identify affected infants, and thus treatment can start immediately. With proper treatment, children with PKU grow normally and have healthy lives. The treatment is a low-phenylalanine diet of special formulas and low-protein food products for life (see also the Drug-Nutrient Interaction box titled "Aspartame and Phenylketonuria" in Chapter 4). Unfortunately, the prescribed diet is somewhat unpalatable, and lifelong adherence is low. Intensive family counseling by a metabolic team is needed. Research into cell-directed therapy and more permanent treatment guidelines is ongoing.[7-11]

Galactosemia

Galactosemia is a genetic disease that affects carbohydrate metabolism and that also results from a missing enzyme. Similar to PKU, galactosemia is an autosomal recessive disorder; it affects 1 in every 10,000 to 30,000 live births. The missing enzyme, galactose-1-phosphate uridyltransferase, is one that converts galactose to glucose. Because galactose comes from the breakdown of lactose (milk sugar), all sources of lactose in the diet must be eliminated. When it is not treated, galactosemia causes brain and liver damage. Newborn screening programs, which are required in all states, identify affected infants.[12] If treatment begins immediately, life-threatening damage may be avoided and some complications may be recovered.[13]

Treatment is a strict galactose-free diet, with special formulas for infants and lactose-free food guides. The treatment diet must be followed for life. Despite rigorous treatment, patients with galactosemia generally experience complications at some point in life such as cognitive disability, speech problems, neurologic and/or movement disorders, and ovarian dysfunction for women. Currently there is no globally accepted

For Further Focus

What About Alcohol?

DOES ALCOHOL PROVIDE ENERGY?
Yes. Alcohol contributes to the overall energy intake in the form of calories. Alcohol yields 7 kcal/g. This is more than both carbohydrates and protein, which yield 4 kcal/g each.

IS ALCOHOL A NUTRIENT?
No. Unlike carbohydrates, fats, proteins, vitamins, minerals, and water, alcohol performs no essential function in the body. Alcohol is not stored in the body, but the by-products of metabolism can accumulate to toxic amounts when alcohol is consumed in large quantities.

HOW IS ALCOHOL DIGESTED?
About 85% to 95% of alcohol is absorbed without any chemical digestion. Alcohol is one of the few substances that can be absorbed directly into the circulation from the stomach. Small amounts of alcohol can enter the blood circulation from the mouth and the esophagus. What is not absorbed in the stomach is absorbed in the small intestine and sent directly to the liver for detoxification and metabolism.

HOW IS ALCOHOL METABOLIZED?
Alcohol metabolism takes precedence over the metabolism of any other nutrient in the body because it is a toxin to the liver. The primary by-product of alcohol metabolism is acetaldehyde, which is the culprit for the destruction of healthy tissue that is associated with alcoholism. After detoxifying the alcohol, the liver uses remaining by-products to produce fatty acids.

Fatty acids are combined with glycerol through lipogenesis to form triglycerides, and they are stored in the liver. A single drinking binge can result in an accumulation of fat in the liver. Repeated episodes over time can lead to fatty liver disease, which is the first stage of alcoholic liver disease.

Alcohol metabolism is a priority for the liver. Blood alcohol concentrations peak at approximately 30 to 45 minutes after one drink, which is defined as 12 oz of beer, 5 oz of wine, or 1.5 oz of 80-proof distilled spirits. The liver can only work at a designated speed to metabolize and rid the body of alcohol, regardless of how much has been consumed. When consumption exceeds the rate of metabolism, alcohol and its metabolites begin to accumulate in the blood and circulate throughout the body.

Several factors influence an individual's ability to metabolize alcohol, including gender, food intake, body weight, sex hormones, and medications.

MORE INFORMATION
To find out more about alcohol and its dangers, benefits, and associated diseases, refer to the following websites:
- Mayo Clinic: *site search for alcohol*: www.mayoclinic.org
- Alcoholics Anonymous: www.aa.org
- The National Council on Alcoholism and Drug Dependence: www.ncadd.org
- National Institute on Alcohol Abuse and Alcoholism: www.niaaa.nih.gov

---

treatment protocol that is successful in avoiding all complications.[14]

Glycogen Storage Diseases
Glycogen storage diseases (GSDs) are a group of rare genetic defects that inhibit the normal metabolic pathways of glycogen. This disease occurs in 1 of every 20,000 to 40,000 live births in the United States.[15] Twelve distinct forms of GSD result from the absence of the enzymes that are required for the synthesis or breakdown of glycogen. The specific form of GSD is distinguished by the enzyme that is missing and the tissue affected. The liver is the primary site of glycogen metabolism; therefore, hepatic forms of GSD (e.g., von Gierke's disease or type I glycogenosis) affect the glucose availability of the whole body. Myopathic forms of GSD inhibit normal glycogen metabolism in the striated muscles, and they are less severe than hepatic forms. An example of a myopathic form is McArdle's disease (i.e., type V glycogenosis).

The focus of dietary treatment for patients with GSD is to avoid hypoglycemia through a balanced carbohydrate diet. Because the patients are not able to utilize stored glycogen for blood glucose balance during periods of fasting (e.g., overnight, between meals), a constant and steady intake of available glucose is imperative for cell function throughout the body.

OTHER INTOLERANCES OR ALLERGIES
Other problems with digestion and metabolism are the result of food intolerances or allergies. An example of an error in digestion is lactose intolerance, which results from the inability to digest lactose.

Lactose Intolerance
A deficiency of any one of the disaccharidases (i.e., lactase, sucrase, or maltase) in the small intestine may produce a wide range of GI problems and abdominal pain because the specific sugar involved cannot be digested (see Chapter 2). Lactose intolerance is the most common, and it presents as varying degrees of intolerance. With this condition, there is insufficient lactase to break down the milk sugar lactose; thus, lactose accumulates in the intestine, causing abdominal cramping and diarrhea. Milk and all dairy products containing lactose are carefully avoided. Milk that is treated with a commercial lactase product and milk substitute products (e.g., soy, almond, rice milk) are safe alternatives.

Allergies

Allergies are inappropriate immune responses to substances that are not otherwise harmful. Food allergies are not necessarily problems with digestion or metabolism but can affect the gastrointestinal tract and its normal function. One example would be celiac disease.

Celiac disease is an allergy to the proteins known as gluten. The response is a cellular destruction of the GI tract lining. As a result, digestion of all nutrients is negatively affected. Issues that are specific to GI disorders and allergies are covered in more detail in Chapter 18.

Putting It All Together

Summary

- Nutrients in food must be changed, released, regrouped, and rerouted into forms that body cells can use. The closely related activities of digestion, absorption, and transport ensure that key nutrients are delivered to the cells so that the multiple metabolic tasks that sustain life can be completed.
- Mechanical digestion consists of spontaneous muscular activity that is responsible for the initial mechanical breakdown by mastication and the movement of the food mass along the GI tract by motions such as peristalsis.
- Chemical digestion involves enzymatic action that breaks food down into progressively smaller components and then releases its nutrients for absorption.
- Absorption involves the passage of nutrients from the intestines into the mucosal lining of the intestinal wall. It primarily occurs in the small intestine as a result of the work of highly efficient intestinal wall structures that increase the absorbent surface area.
- Nutrients that are absorbed are then transported throughout the body by the blood circulation.
- The energy-yielding nutrients that we eat are converted into ATP through the cycles of metabolism. Metabolism is the sum of the body processes that change food energy from the macronutrients into various forms of body energy. Metabolism is a balance of both anabolic and catabolic reactions.
- Genetic diseases of metabolism result from missing enzymes that control the metabolism of specific nutrients. Special diets in each case limit or eliminate the particular nutrient involved.

Chapter Review Questions

See answers in Appendix A.

1. If you chew a piece of bread in the mouth for a long time, it begins to taste sweet because of the action of the enzyme:
   a. Pepsin.
   b. Mucus.
   c. Amylase.
   d. Lipase.

2. An example of mechanical digestion is:
   a. Mastication.
   b. Amylase secretion.
   c. Active transport.
   d. Simple diffusion.

3. A 45-year-old female is considering eating $2\frac{1}{2}$ times the recommended protein for her body in order to build more lean muscle. What would you suggest?
   a. Encourage her to proceed since the extra protein will build more muscle.
   b. Explain to her that excess protein intake is broken down and used for energy if needed or stored as fat.
   c. Explain that the extra protein intake will build muscle as long as she increases calorie intake as well.
   d. Encourage her to eat more fruit and vegetables rather than protein, to build muscle mass.

4. A 23 year old who is admitted to the hospital from hypothermia and starvation would most likely be in a state of _____ upon admission.
   a. Catabolism.
   b. Anabolism.
   c. Glycogenesis.
   d. Lipogenesis.

5. A patient who has a large surgical resection of the small intestine would most likely have difficulty with:
   a. Absorbing water.
   b. Secreting pepsin.
   c. Digesting food.
   d. Producing chyme.

Additional Learning Resources

evolve http://evolve.elsevier.com/Williams/basic/

References and **Further Reading and Resources** in the back of the book provide additional resources for enhancing knowledge.

Energy Balance

Key Concepts

- Food energy is changed into energy the body can use to do work.
- The body uses most of its energy supply for basal metabolic needs.
- A balance between the intake of food energy and the output of body work maintains life and health.
- States of being underweight and overweight reflect degrees of energy imbalance.

Our efficient bodies constantly convert energy from food into the energy that is used for work and activity. Fuel is used or stored according to intake and output demands. This chapter looks at the big picture of energy balance among all of the energy-yielding nutrients and demonstrates how energy intake is measured, cycled, and used to meet the body's energy demands.

HUMAN ENERGY SYSTEM

ENERGY NEEDS

The body needs constant energy to do the work that is necessary for maintenance of life and health. Both voluntary and involuntary actions require energy.

Involuntary Body Work

The greatest use of energy in the body is the result of involuntary work, which includes all of the activities that are not consciously performed. These activities consist of such vital processes as circulation, respiration, digestion, and absorption as well as many other internal activities that maintain life. Involuntary body functions require energy in various forms, such as chemical energy (in many metabolic products), electrical energy (in brain and nerve activities), mechanical energy (in muscle contraction), and thermal (i.e., heat) energy to maintain body temperature.

Voluntary Work and Exercise

Voluntary work includes all of the actions related to a person's conscious activities of daily living and physical activity. Although it may seem like we burn more calories performing these intentional actions throughout the day that usually is not the case.

MEASUREMENT OF ENERGY

In common usage, the word **calorie** refers to the amount of energy in food or the amount that is expended in physical actions. However, in human nutrition, the term kilocalorie (i.e., 1000 calories) is used to designate the large calorie unit that is used in nutrition science to avoid dealing with too many zeros. A kilocalorie, which is abbreviated as *kcalorie* or *kcal*, is the amount of heat that is necessary to raise 1 kg of water 1° C. When referring to body or food energy, we will always refer to the kcal in this text. Most people do not realize that there is a difference between a **calorie** and a **kilocalorie**. The terms are used interchangeably in common language but should never be confused in the scientific literature.

The international unit of measure for energy is the joule (J). To convert kilocalories (kcal) into kilojoules (kJ), multiply the number of kilocalories by 4.184 (e.g., 200 kcal × 4.184 = 836.8 kJ). Nutrition facts labels on food products in most of the world express energy in units of kilojoules instead of kilocalories.

FOOD AS FUEL FOR ENERGY

Energy that is needed for voluntary and involuntary body work is in the form of adenosine triphosphate (ATP). ATP is a metabolic end product of the energy-yielding foods consumed (see Figure 5-10). The body must have an adequate supply of fuel to balance energy demands for healthy weight maintenance. As explained earlier in this book, the only three energy-yielding nutrients are the macronutrients carbohydrate, fat, and protein. Carbohydrates are the body's primary fuel, with fat assisting as a storage fuel. Protein is used for energy only when other fuel sources are not available.

calorie a measure of heat; the energy necessary to do work is measured as the amount of heat produced by the body's work; the energy value of a food is expressed as the number of kilocalories that a specified portion of the food will yield when it is oxidized in the body.

Fuel Factors

Fuel factors reflect the quantity of ATP units that will be provided to the body after metabolism of each energy-yielding substance. This may also be referred to as energy density (see Chapter 5). Note that the term *substance* was used instead of energy-yielding *nutrients*. That is because ethanol (i.e., beverage alcohol from fermented grains and fruits) also supplies energy but is not a nutrient. The fuel factors are as follows: carbohydrate, 4 kcal/g; fat, 9 kcal/g; protein, 4 kcal/g; and alcohol, 7 kcal/g.

Energy and Nutrient Density

The term *density* refers to the degree of concentrated material in a given substance. More material in a smaller volume of a given substance increases the density. Thus, the concept of *energy density* refers to a high concentration of energy (i.e., kilocalories) in a small amount of food. Of the three energy-yielding nutrients, foods that are high in fat have the highest energy density. Similarly, foods may be evaluated in terms of their *nutrient density*. A food with a high nutrient density means that it has a relatively high concentration of vitamins and minerals in a smaller volume of a given food. Some foods are both energy and nutrient dense, which means that they provide a lot of both kilocalories and micronutrients. Foods that are referred to as *empty calories* are the direct opposite of a nutrient dense food.

Examples of foods that would fit into each category are:

- Energy dense: butter, oil, French fries, fried meats (e.g., fried chicken), ice cream
- Nutrient dense: vegetables, fruits, legumes, whole grains, lean protein (e.g., non-fatty fish, white chicken), and low-fat dairy/dairy-substitute products
- Energy and nutrient dense: avocados, cheese, seeds (e.g., sunflower seeds), nuts, nut butters (e.g., peanut butter, almond butter)
- Empty calories: soda, pastries, donuts, cakes, sugary drinks

Food guides such as MyPlate and the *Dietary Guidelines for Americans* (see Figures 1-3 and 1-4) recommend foods that are nutrient dense as opposed to only energy dense.

ENERGY BALANCE

Energy—like matter—is neither created nor destroyed. When we refer to energy as "being produced," it really means that it is transformed (i.e., changed in form and cycled through a system). Consider the human energy system as part of the total energy system on Earth. In this sense, two energy systems support life—one within the body and the much larger one surrounding us—as follows:

1. *External energy cycle:* In the environment, the ultimate source of energy is the sun and its vast nuclear reactions. With the use of water and carbon dioxide as raw materials, plants transform the sun's radiation into stored energy (mainly carbohydrate with some fat and protein). The food chain continues as animals eat plants and the products of other animals (e.g., meat, milk, eggs).
2. *Internal energy cycle:* When people eat plant and animal foods, the stored energy of the food changes into body fuels (i.e., glucose and fatty acids) to meet the energy needs within the body. Voluntary and involuntary actions of the body require energy in many forms, such as chemical, electrical, mechanical, and thermal energy. As this internal energy cycle continues, water is excreted, carbon dioxide is exhaled, and heat is radiated, thereby returning these end products to the external environment. The overall energy cycle continually repeats itself to sustain life.

ENERGY INTAKE

The total overall energy balance within the body depends on the energy intake in relation to the energy output. The main source of energy for all body work is food and caloric drinks, and this is supplemented with stored energy in the body tissues.

Estimating Dietary Energy Intake

Personal energy intake can be estimated by recording a day's actual food consumption and calculating its energy value. Nutritrac, which is the nutrition analysis program that is available on the Evolve website for this book (see the front matter for instructions and details), is an excellent tool for evaluating energy intake as well as several other components of an individual's diet (e.g., vitamins, minerals, fat, carbohydrates, sugar, protein). SuperTracker (www.supertracker.usda.gov) is another free software tool that is available through the Internet and that can be used to assess energy intake. SuperTracker may also be used to estimate energy output through physical activity and **basal energy expenditure.** The accuracy of both programs depends on the precision of the food consumption and physical activity recorded and entered into the program by the user.

Stored Energy

When food is not available, such as during sleep, longer periods of fasting, or the extreme stress of starvation, the body draws from its stored energy.

---

basal energy expenditure (BEE) the amount of energy (in kcal) needed by the body for the maintenance of life when a person is at complete digestive, physical, mental, thermal, and emotional rest (i.e., 10 to 12 hours after eating and 12 to 18 hours after physical activity); measured immediately upon waking. Also referred to as basal metabolic rate (BMR).

Glycogen. In a well-nourished person, there is a 12- to 48-hour reserve of glycogen in the liver and muscles. This supply is quickly depleted if it is not replenished by daily food intake. For example, glycogen stores maintain normal blood glucose levels during sleep. The first meal, breakfast (which is so named because it "breaks the fast"), has a significant function for energy intake.

Adipose tissue. Although the amount of fat storage is larger than that of glycogen storage, the supply varies among persons. As an additional energy resource, stored fat provides more kilocalories per gram than any other fuel source.

Muscle mass. Energy derived from protein may be elicited from muscle mass. However, this lean tissue serves important structural functions, and it is ideally not sacrificed for energy use. Only during longer periods of fasting or starvation does the body turn to this tissue for energy.

ENERGY OUTPUT

The necessary activities to sustain life—normal body functions, the regulation of body temperature, and the processes of tissue growth and repair—use energy from food and body reserves. The sum of the total chemical changes that occur during all of these activities is called *metabolism* (see Chapter 5). The following three demands for energy determine the body's total energy requirements: (1) basal energy expenditure; (2) physical activity; and (3) the **thermic effect of food.**

Basal Energy Expenditure

The term *basal energy expenditure* (BEE) or basal metabolic rate (BMR) refers to the sum of all internal working activities of the body while at total rest; it is expressed in kilocalories per day. For example, if an individual's BEE is 1500 kcal, that would represent the amount of energy that this particular person would need to consume, on average, over a 24-hour period to maintain his or her current weight while at complete rest. Sometimes the terms *BEE* and **resting energy expenditure (REE)** are used interchangeably. However, a technical difference exists between BEE and REE. BEE must be measured when an individual is at absolute digestive, physical, mental, thermal, and emotional rest. Maintaining the stringent conditions

required to measure a true BEE is rather difficult; therefore, measurements are most often expressed as REE. The REE is up to 10% higher than a true BEE measurement.[1,2]

For the average person, 60% to 75% of their total energy expenditure (TEE) will be used to meet basal energy demands. And the vast majority of that energy is used by a few small but highly active organs. The combined weight of the brain, heart, liver, and kidneys equals only 5% to 6% of an adult's total body weight. But these highly active organs account for 60% to 70% of the body's REE for the day. Thus, the size of highly metabolically active organs and tissues accounts for the majority of individual variability for REE and total energy needs.[3-5] There are many methods available for predicting a person's REE based on body size and the size of individual organs of high metabolic activity. The evolution of these formulas has been ongoing for more than a century.[6]

Measuring basal energy expenditure or resting energy expenditure. A measure of BEE or REE is sometimes made in clinical practice (e.g., hospital patients with altered metabolism,[2,7,8] athletes, research laboratories) with the use of indirect calorimetry. This method measures the amount of energy that a person uses while at rest. A portable metabolic cart allows the person to breathe into an attached mouthpiece or ventilated hood system while lying down, and the normal exchange of oxygen and carbon dioxide is measured (Figure 6-1). The metabolic rate can be

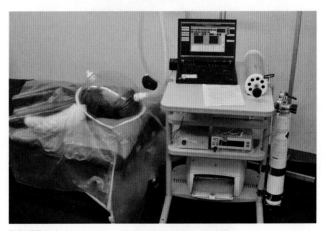

FIGURE 6-1 Measuring resting metabolic rate with a metabolic cart. (Courtesy Susie Parker-Simmons, United States Olympic Committee.)

thermic effect of food an increase in energy expenditure caused by the activities of digestion, absorption, transport, and metabolism of ingested food; a meal that consists of a usual mixture of carbohydrates, protein, and fat increases the energy expenditure equivalent to approximately 10% of the food's energy content (e.g., a 300-kcal piece of pizza would elicit an energy expenditure of 30 kcal to digest the food).

resting energy expenditure (REE) the amount of energy (in kcals) needed by the body for the maintenance of life at rest over a 24-hour period; this is often used interchangeably with the term *basal energy expenditure*, but in actuality it is slightly higher as the protocol for measurement does not put the person at complete rest. Also referred to as resting metabolic rate (RMR).

calculated with a high degree of accuracy from the rate of gas exchange.

The MedGem and BodyGem (Microlife USA, Clearwater, FL) products are alternative, reliable methods for determining REE with fast and portable devices (Figure 6-2).[9-11] Both devices are hand-held and come with disposable mouthpieces and nose clips. The individual being tested holds the device while breathing exclusively into the mouthpiece. Unlike the metabolic cart that measures oxygen and carbon dioxide exchange, the MedGem and BodyGem devices measure only oxygen consumption to determine an individual's REE. The device then predicts REE by using a modified Weir equation with a constant respiratory quotient of 0.85.

Predicting basal energy expenditure or resting energy expenditure. A rudimentary formula for calculating basal energy needs is to multiply 0.9 or 1 kcal/kg body weight by the number of hours in a day. Thus, examples of how the daily basal metabolic needs (in kilocalories) would be calculated for men and women are as follows:

For a 154-lb man:

$$1\,\text{kcal} \times \text{kg body weight} \times 24\,\text{hours}$$
$$(1)\,\text{Convert pounds to kilograms: }154\,\text{lb} \div 2.2 = 70\,\text{kg}$$
$$(2)\,1\,\text{kcal} \times 70\,\text{kg} \times 24\,\text{hr} = 1680\,\text{kcal/24 hr}$$

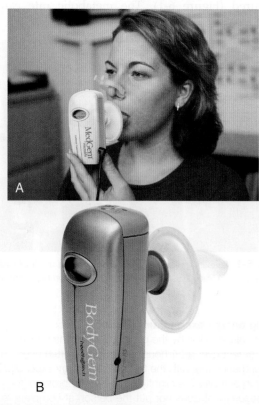

FIGURE 6-2 (A) MedGem and **(B)** BodyGem devices, which are used to determine the resting metabolic rate. (Courtesy Microlife USA, Dunedin, FL.)

For a 121-lb woman:

$$0.9\,\text{kcal} \times \text{kg body weight} \times 24\,\text{hours}$$
$$(1)\,\text{Convert pounds to kilograms: }121\,\text{lb} \div 2.2 = 55\,\text{kg}$$
$$(2)\,0.9\,\text{kcal} \times 55\,\text{kg} \times 24\,\text{hr} = 1188\,\text{kcal/24 hr}$$

Obviously, this simple equation does not take into account age, height, activity level, fitness, or any other factor that would alter energy needs. This formula is useful in determining the energy needs of groups of people to get an overall estimate. For example, if we have a group of individuals going on a backpacking trip and need to determine how much food to take, we could start with this formula. Using the average weight of the group members for the formula, plus additional kilocalories added for activity levels, we could estimate how many kilocalories should be available per person per day. By multiplying that number by the number of people in the group and the number of days for the trip, we could have an approximate estimate of the number of kilocalories the group would need to transport. It is not precise enough to use in a clinical setting or for specific individual needs.

The Mifflin-St. Jeor equations, the Harris-Benedict equations, and the equations that were used for the 2002 Dietary Reference Intake values provide an alternate method of estimating the REE or BEE that is more specific to the individual (Box 6-1). Of these equations, studies found the Mifflin-St. Jeor equation to give the most reliable REE measurement.[12] However, such formulas are not reliable for some patients because of disease state, age (at either end of the spectrum), or obesity status. Therefore, indirect calorimetry measurements are the only accurate methods for reliably calculating energy needs for these patients.[2]

In addition, thyroid function tests may be used as an indicator of BEE because the thyroid hormone plays a significant role in regulating metabolism. Thyroid function tests can measure the activity of the thyroid gland, serum thyroxine levels, thyroid-stimulating hormone levels, serum protein-bound iodine levels, and radioactive iodine uptake levels. Iodine's basic function is in the synthesis of the prohormone **thyroxine.** Such tests are not associated with a kilocalorie amount in terms of total energy needs. However, they can be used as a gauge of normal metabolic function. Abnormal results require the attention of a physician for treatment.

Factors that influence basal energy expenditure. Several factors influence the BEE and should be kept in mind when related test results are interpreted. In addition to the influence from the highly metabolically active organs of the body, other major factors

thyroxine (T₄) thyroid prohormone; the active hormone form is T_3; it is the major controller of basal metabolic rate.

Box 6-1   Equations for Estimating Resting Energy Needs

MIFFLIN-ST. JEOR[1]

Men

TEE (kcal/day) = (10 × weight [kg] + 6.25 × height [cm] − 5 × age [yr] + 5) × PA#

Women

TEE (kcal/day) = (10 × weight [kg] + 6.25 × height [cm] − 5 × age [yr] − 161) × PA#

HARRIS-BENEDICT[2]

Men

TEE (kcal/day) = (66.47 + 5 × Height [cm] + 13.75 × Weight [kg] − 6.755 × Age) × PA#

Women

TEE (kcal/day) = (655.1 + 1.85 × Height [cm] + 9.56 × Weight [kg] − 4.676 × Age) × PA#

#PA Coefficient for Men and Women Applicable to Both Mifflin-St. Jeor and Harris-Benedict Equations

1.200 = Sedentary (little or no exercise; desk job)

1.375 = Lightly active (light exercise/sports 1 to 3 days/wk)

1.550 = Moderately active (moderate exercise/sports 3 to 5 days/wk)

1.725 = Heavy exercise (hard exercise/sports 6 to 7 days/wk)

2002 DIETARY REFERENCE INTAKE ENERGY CALCULATION*,3

EER = TEE + Energy deposition

Children 0 to 36 Months Old

0 to 3 months: (89 × Weight [kg] − 100) + 175 kcal

4 to 6 months: (89 × Weight [kg] − 100) + 56 kcal

7 to 12 months: (89 × Weight [kg] − 100) + 22 kcal

13 to 36 months: (89 × Weight [kg] − 100) + 20 kcal

Boys 3 to 8 Years Old

EER = 88.5 − (61.9 × Age [yr]) + PA × (26.7 × Weight [kg] + 903 × Height [m]) + 20 kcal

Boys 9 to 18 Years Old

EER = 88.5 − (61.9 × Age [yr]) + PA × (26.7 × Weight [kg] + 903 × Height [m]) + 25 kcal

PA Coefficient Used for Boys 3 to 18 Years Old

1.00 if PAL is estimated to be ≥1.0 but <1.4 (sedentary)

1.13 if PAL is estimated to be ≥1.4 but <1.6 (low active)

1.26 if PAL is estimated to be ≥1.6 but <1.9 (active)

1.42 if PAL is estimated to be ≥1.9 but <2.5 (very active)

Girls 3 to 8 Years Old

EER = 135.3 − (30.8 × Age [yr]) + PA × (10.0 × Weight [kg] + 934 × Height [m]) + 20 kcal

Girls 9 to 18 Years Old

EER = 135.3 − (30.8 × Age [yr]) + PA × (10.0 × Weight [kg] + 934 × Height [m]) + 25 kcal

PA Coefficient Used for Girls 3 to 18 Years Old

1.00 if PAL is estimated to be ≥1.0 but <1.4 (sedentary)

1.16 if PAL is estimated to be ≥1.4 but <1.6 (low active)

1.31 if PAL is estimated to be ≥1.6 but <1.9 (active)

1.56 if PAL is estimated to be ≥1.9 but <2.5 (very active)

Men 19 Years Old and Older

EER = 662 − (9.53 × Age [yr]) + PA × (15.91 × Weight [kg] + 539.6 × Height [m])

PA Coefficient for Men 19 Years and Older

1.00 if PAL is estimated to be ≥1.0 but <1.4 (sedentary)

1.11 if PAL is estimated to be ≥1.4 but <1.6 (low active)

1.25 if PAL is estimated to be ≥1.6 but <1.9 (active)

1.48 if PAL is estimated to be ≥1.9 but <2.5 (very active)

Women 19 Years Old and Older

EER = 354 − (6.91 × Age [yr]) + PA × (9.36 × Weight [kg] + 726 × Height [m])

PA Coefficient for Women 19 Years and Older

1.00 if PAL is estimated to be ≥1.0 but <1.4 (sedentary)

1.12 if PAL is estimated to be ≥1.4 but <1.6 (low active)

1.27 if PAL is estimated to be ≥1.6 but <1.9 (active)

1.45 if PAL is estimated to be ≥1.9 but <2.5 (very active)

REFERENCES

1. Mifflin MD, et al. A new predictive equation for resting energy expenditure in healthy individuals. _Am J Clin Nutr_. 1990;51(2): 241-247.
2. Roza AM, Shizgal HM. The Harris Benedict equation reevaluated: resting energy requirements and the body cell mass. _Am J Clin Nutr_. 1984;40(1):168-182.
3. Food and Nutrition Board, Institute of Medicine. _Dietary Reference Intakes for Energy, Carbohydrate, Fiber, Fat, Fatty Acids, Cholesterol, Protein, and Amino Acids_. Washington, DC: National Academies Press; 2002.

EER, Estimated energy requirement; _PA_, physical activity; _PAL_, physical activity level; _TEE_, total energy expenditure.

*Each age-specific and gender-specific equation for the _2002 Dietary Reference Intake Energy Calculations_ has a specific set of PA coefficients. Make sure to use the PA coefficients associated with the specific equation used.

that affect BEE are lean body mass, growth periods, body temperature, hormonal status, and disease state as follows:

- _Lean body mass:_ Lean body mass includes muscles, bones, connective tissue such as ligaments and tendons, and internal organs. One of the largest contributors to overall metabolic rate is the relative percent of lean body mass.[13,14] The more lean body mass a person has, the higher the person's BEE. This is caused by the greater metabolic activity that occurs in lean tissues (i.e., muscles and organs) as compared with adipose tissue. Other factors (e.g., sex, age) are thought to primarily influence the metabolic rate as they relate to the lean body mass.[13]

However, while lean body mass decreases with advanced age, lowered metabolic rate in the elderly population is not entirely explained by changes in body composition.[15,16] In other words, the metabolic rate in the elderly is slower than would be expected according to the amount of their lean tissue. This indicates that the tissue-specific metabolic rate of the lean tissue may also slow with age.[17]

- _Growth periods:_ During rapid growth periods, human growth hormone stimulates cell regeneration and raises BEE to support anabolic metabolism. Thus, growth spurts during childhood and adolescence reflect periods of elevated BEE and energy needs per kilogram of body weight. As growth and the rate of cellular regeneration slow with age, so does BEE. BEE rises significantly during pregnancy, which is a period of rapid growth that requires an additional 340 to 450 kcal/day on average.[1] However, this value is highly variable among women, and it is correlated with total weight gain and prepregnancy percentage of body fat. BEE increases above prepregnancy rates with the progression of pregnancy; average increases with each trimester are 4.5%, 10.8%, and 24%, respectively.[18]

- *Body temperature:* The body's energy expenditure is significantly altered in response to changes in body temperature. Fever increases BEE by approximately 7% for each 1° F rise above normal body temperature. In states of starvation and malnutrition, the process of **adaptive thermogenesis** results in lowered heat production to conserve energy and thus BEE decreases. It has been speculated that a lower core body temperature may be a contributing factor to the efficiency of storing fat in preobese individuals.[19] In cold weather, especially in freezing temperatures, BEE rises in response to the generation of more body heat to maintain normal core temperature.

- *Hormonal status:* Energy expenditure is also influenced by hormonal secretions. As previously mentioned, thyroid hormone plays a significant role in regulating metabolism. Individuals with an underactive thyroid gland may develop hypothyroidism, which results in a decreased metabolic rate. Hypothyroidism is treated with medication (see the Drug-Nutrient Interaction box "Absorption of Levothyroxine" for more information about hypothyroid medication interactions). Conversely, hyperthyroidism occurs when the thyroid gland is overactive (see the Cultural Considerations box "Hypermetabolism and Hypometabolism: What Are They and Who Is at Risk?"). The fight-or-flight reflexes increase metabolic rate in response to the hormone epinephrine. Growth hormone increases metabolism; alternately, a deficiency of normal growth hormone secretions attenuates the metabolic rate and has recently been linked to obesity.[20] Other hormones (e.g., insulin, cortisol) also increase metabolism, and they may fluctuate daily.

- *Disease state:* The presence of disease may alter a patient's total energy expenditure. Depending on the disease, the BEE may be increased or decreased. The best method for obtaining accurate estimates of BEE in such patients is to use direct or indirect calorimetry measurements.[2]

---

adaptive thermogenesis an adjustment to heat production in response to changing environmental influences (e.g., external temperature, diet).

Drug-Nutrient Interaction

Absorption of Levothyroxine

KELLI BOI

Levothyroxine (Synthroid) is a synthetic hormone that is prescribed to treat hypothyroidism and to regulate energy balance. It is absorbed primarily in the jejunum and ileum of the small intestine. Many nutritional factors affect the absorption of the drug[1,2]:

- Levothyroxine absorption is maximized in an empty stomach, which suggests the importance of gastric acid. The presence of food will delay or prevent the drug's absorption.
- Dietary fiber reduces the bioavailability of levothyroxine by binding to the drug and causing it to be eliminated.
- Calcium and iron supplements and soy products interfere with the drug's absorption and reduce its bioavailability.
- Gastrointestinal disorders (celiac disease, lactose intolerance, *Helicobacter pylori* infection, bowel resection, inflammatory bowel disease, and chronic gastritis) all affect the absorptive ability of the digestive system and consequently interfere with the absorption of the drug.

A consistent medication and eating schedule is imperative for normalization of the thyroid hormones through levothyroxine treatment. Levothyroxine should be taken at least 1 hour before or 2 hours after a meal, especially a meal that is high in fiber. Levothyroxine should be taken at least 4 hours before consuming soy products or before taking calcium or iron supplements (however, normal amounts of these minerals in foods do not seem to pose a problem).

The prevalence of celiac disease is higher among patients with autoimmune thyroid disorders.[3] When a patient has celiac disease or lactose intolerance, drug absorption does not improve sufficiently with higher doses of the drug until dietary restrictions for the disorder are followed.[2]

REFERENCES

1. Ruchala M, Szczepanek-Parulska E, Zybek A. The influence of lactose intolerance and other gastro-intestinal tract disorders on L-thyroxine absorption. *Endokrynol Pol.* 2012;63(4):318-323.
2. Liwanpo L, Hershman JM. Conditions and drugs interfering with thyroxine absorption. *Best Pract Res Clin Endocrinol Metab.* 2009;23(6):781-792.
3. Sattar N, et al. Celiac disease in children, adolescents, and young adults with autoimmune thyroid disease. *J Pediatr.* 2011;158(2):272-275 e1.

Physical Activity

The exercise that is involved in work or recreation accounts for wide individual variations in energy output (see Chapter 16). In addition to increasing energy expenditure and reducing the risk of chronic diseases, exercise has positive effects on both physical and mental quality of life.[21,22] Table 6-1 gives some representative kilocalorie expenditures of different types of work and recreation. Although mental work or study does not require additional kilocalories, muscle tension, restlessness, and agitated movements may slightly increase energy needs for some individuals.

The energy expenditure that is used for physical activity goes above and beyond the BEE. Keeping track

Cultural Considerations

Hypermetabolism and Hypometabolism: What Are They and Who Is at Risk?

Hypermetabolism and hypometabolism are conditions in which the metabolic rate is either significantly higher (hyper) or lower (hypo) than normal. Because the thyroid gland is responsible for producing the hormone thyroxine, which controls the metabolic rate, such conditions usually result from malfunctions of the thyroid gland. Clinically, hypermetabolism and hypometabolism involving the thyroid gland are referred to as *hyperthyroidism* and *hypothyroidism,* respectively.

An individual with hyperthyroidism has a significantly higher metabolic rate and higher energy needs than normal. Such increases in energy needs are not explained by lean tissue, age, or gender. This individual has an overactive thyroid gland, which means that he or she produces too much thyroxine. As a result, the normal energy intake recommendations do not meet this patient's needs. For example, a woman who is 25 years old, 5 feet and 5 inches tall, and weighs 125 lb normally needs approximately 2200 kcal/day to maintain her weight if she engages in a moderate level of activity. However, the same woman with hyperthyroidism may need 1.5 to 2.5 times as many kilocalories per day to maintain her current weight.

Hypothyroidism is the opposite of hyperthyroidism. Individuals with hypothyroidism do not produce enough thyroxine for their body size and therefore require less energy than normal to maintain their current body weight. The Dietary Reference Intakes for energy for a patient with hypothyroidism are too high and would result in weight gain. However, effective medications are available for hypothyroidism. Typically, both hyperthyroidism and hypothyroidism are discovered during young adulthood.

Congenital hypothyroidism (CH), which occurs in 4 out of every 10,000 live births in the United States, is a type of hypothyroidism that is present at birth and that can result in mental retardation if it is not treated. Newborn screening for CH began during the 1970s and is now standard. Studies have found that the risk of CH is linked to birth weight, gender, and ethnicity and is common in infants with birth defects such as congenital heart disease.[1] Both male and female infants who weigh less than 4.5 lb or more than 10 lb have a significantly higher risk of developing CH. Females of any weight have 50% more risk than males. The incidence rate of CH in the United States is twice as high in Hispanic newborns and 44% higher in Asian and Native Hawaiian or other Pacific Islander newborns as compared with Caucasian newborns; it is 30% lower in African-American newborns as compared with Caucasian newborns.[2] Improved methods and frequency of testing in the past decade have drastically increased the number of diagnosed and treated cases in the United States.[3,4]

Another risk factor for the development of abnormal thyroid function and, thus, abnormal metabolism is iodine intake. The mineral iodine is an important part of the thyroid hormone thyroxine. The incidence of hyperthyroidism and hypothyroidism has been linked to iodine, with both high and low iodine intakes associated with thyroid disease.[5]

The close monitoring of basal metabolism and total energy expenditure is an important aspect of the treatment of thyroid disease. Medications and energy intake are then modified to control weight and prevent complications.

REFERENCES
1. Monroy-Santoyo S, et al. Higher incidence of thyroid agenesis in Mexican newborns with congenital hypothyroidism associated with birth defects. *Early Hum Dev.* 2012;88(1):61-64.
2. Hinton CF, et al. Trends in incidence rates of congenital hypothyroidism related to select demographic factors: data from the United States, California, Massachusetts, New York, and Texas. *Pediatrics.* 2010;125(suppl 2):S37-S47.
3. Mitchell ML, et al. The increased incidence of congenital hypothyroidism: fact or fancy? *Clin Endocrinol (Oxford).* 2011;75(6):806-810.
4. Wassner AJ, Brown RS. Hypothyroidism in the newborn period. *Curr Opin Endocrinol Diabetes Obes.* 2013;20(5):449-454.
5. Laurberg P, et al. Iodine intake as a determinant of thyroid disorders in populations. *Best Pract Res Clin Endocrinol Metab.* 2010;24(1):13-27.

---

of all energy that is used explicitly for physical activity to calculate the total energy requirement is difficult. Instead, the energy that is used for physical activity can be estimated as a factor of BEE by categorizing the physical activity (PA) level in accordance with standard values (1.0 to 2.5, depending on lifestyle). This factor is then multiplied by the BEE or REE. For example, an individual who works at a desk job and who has little or no leisure activity would have a PA of approximately 1.2 according to the Mifflin-St. Jeor equation. To estimate the total energy expenditure for this individual, you would multiply the person's BEE by a PA factor of 1.2 (see Box 6-1).

Thermic Effect of Food

After eating, extra energy is required for the digestion, absorption, and transportation of nutrients to the cells. This overall stimulating effect is called the *thermic effect of food.* Approximately 5% to 10% of the body's total energy needs for metabolism relate to the digestion and storage of nutrients from food. Another way to think about it is to assume that 5% to 10% of the calories in a food consumed will be used for the digestion of that very food.

Total Energy Expenditure

A person's TEE is comprised of the energy needs for BEE, the physical activities of the person, and the thermic effects of food (Figure 6-3). Total energy requirements vary considerably between individuals. To maintain energy balance, food energy intake must match body energy output as an average over time. An energy imbalance (i.e., when energy intake exceeds energy output) can lead to weight gain (see the Clinical Applications box entitled "Energy Imbalance Over Time"). Treatment should include a decrease in food kilocalories and an increase in physical activity. Extreme and unhealthy weight loss (i.e., anorexia nervosa or starvation) results when food energy intake does not meet body energy requirements for extended

Table 6-1	Energy Expenditure per Pound per Hour during Various Activities	
ACTIVITY		**kcal/lb/hr***
Aerobics, moderate		2.95
Bicycling		
Light: 10 to 11.9 mph		2.72
Moderate: 12 to 13.9 mph		3.63
Fast: 14 to 15.9 mph		4.54
Mountain biking		3.85
Daily Activities		
Cleaning		1.36
Cooking		0.91
Driving a car		0.91
Eating, sitting		0.68
Gardening, general		1.81
Office work		0.82
Reading, writing while sitting		0.70
Sleeping		0.41
Shoveling snow		2.72
Running		
5 mph (12 min/mile)		3.63
7 mph (8.5 min/mile)		5.22
9 mph (6.5 min/mile)		6.80
10 mph (6 min/mile)		7.26
Sports		
Boxing, in ring		5.44
Field hockey		3.63
Golf		2.04
Rollerblading		4.42
Skiing, cross country, moderate		3.63
Skiing, downhill, moderate		2.72
Soccer		3.85
Swimming, moderate		3.14
Tennis, doubles		2.27
Tennis, singles		3.63
Ultimate Frisbee		3.63
Volleyball		1.81
Walking		
Moderate: ≈3 mph (20 min/mile), level		1.50
Moderate: ≈3 mph (20 min/mile), uphill		2.73
Brisk: ≈3.5 mph (17.14 min/mile), level		1.72
Fast: ≈4.5 mph (13.33 min/mile), level		2.86
Weight Training		
Light or moderate		1.36
Heavy or vigorous		2.72

Modified from Nieman DC. *Exercise Testing and Prescription: A Health-Related Approach.* 5th ed. New York: McGraw-Hill; 2003.
*Multiply the activity factor by the weight in pounds by the fraction of hour spent performing the activity: *Example:* A 150-lb person plays soccer for 45 minutes. Therefore, the equation would be as follows: 3.85 (i.e., the factor from the table) × 150 (lb) × 0.75 (hr) = 433.13 calories burned. Energy expenditure depends on the physical fitness of the individual and the continuity of exercise.

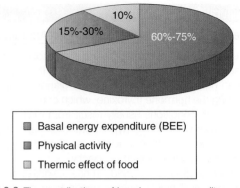

- Basal energy expenditure (BEE)
- Physical activity
- Thermic effect of food

FIGURE 6-3 The contributions of basal energy expenditure, physical activity, and the thermic effect of food to total energy expenditure.

Clinical Applications

Case Study: Energy Imbalance Over Time

You have a 32-year-old female patient with the following anthropometric measurements:

Weight: 120 lb   Height: 5 ft 4 in   BMI: 20.6 kg/m^2

She has been keeping a diet record; and after analyzing it, you find that her average energy intake for each meal/snack is as follows:

Breakfast: 450 kcal
Midmorning snack: 175 kcal
Lunch: 600 kcal
Afternoon snack: 250 kcal
Dinner: 610 kcal
Evening snack: 200 kcal
Thus, her total energy intake averages **2285 kcal/day.**

You calculate her basal energy needs according to the Mifflin-St. Jeor equation and find that her BEE is 1240.5 kcal/day. She reports a very active lifestyle. Therefore, you multiply her BEE by a physical activity factor of 1.725. Her total energy expenditure is: **2140 kcal/day.**

You explain to your patient that she eats more kcals than she is using in a given day; thus she has a positive energy balance of **145 kcal/day.**

QUESTIONS TO CONSIDER:

1. If she continues to consume and burn the same amount of energy, how long will it take for her to gain a pound of fat? (1 lb of fat = 3500 kcal)
2. How would you recommend that she change her lifestyle to maintain her current weight?

periods. Treatment should include a gradual increase in food kilocalories along with moderate activity and rest (see Chapter 15).

The Clinical Applications box entitled "Evaluate Your Daily Energy Requirements" provides a step-by-step example for evaluating your own energy needs. You may also wish to record your food and activities for a day and to calculate your energy intake (i.e., kilocalories) and output (i.e., kilocalorie expenditure in activities). Because it is difficult to keep track of what you are doing 24 hours of the day, the estimate from this method is often quite different from the equations for estimating REE (i.e., Mifflin-St. Jeor,

Harris Benedict). Total your day's activity, and compare it with the general types of similar activities given in Table 6-1. Estimate the total time that you spent on a given activity by adding the total minutes that you spent on that activity at any time and then converting those minutes to hours (or decimal fractions of hours) for the day. Multiply this total time for a given type of activity by the average kilocalories per hour for that activity, and then add them for the day's total kilocalories. Use the following basic steps to calculate your energy expenditure for a day's activities:

1. Total minutes of an activity ÷ 60 = Hours of that activity
2. Total time (hr) × kcal/hr = Total kcal/day for that activity
3. Total kcal/day of all activities = Total energy expenditure for 1 day from activities

Clinical Applications

Evaluate Your Daily Energy Requirements

Your estimated energy requirement (in kcal) per day is the sum of your body's three uses of energy, which are as follows:

1. Basal energy expenditure (also known as basal metabolic rate)
2. Thermic effect of food
3. Physical activity

Let us work through a couple of these calculations together. Then you can plug in your own values to evaluate your daily energy requirements. For our examples, we will use the Estimated Energy Requirement (EER) formula from the 2002 Dietary Reference Intakes. Other formulas are also available in Box 6-1.

EER FORMULA FOR THE 2002 DIETARY REFERENCE INTAKES FOR MEN AND WOMEN OVER 19 YEARS OF AGE:

Men 19 years old and older = 662 − (9.53 × Age [yr]) + Physical activity (PA) × (15.91 × Weight [kg] + 539.6 × Height [m])

Women 19 years old and older = 354 − (6.91 × Age [yr]) + PA × (9.36 × Weight [kg] + 726 × Height [m])

PHYSICAL ACTIVITY

Abbreviated as PA (or PA coefficient) in the formula or sometimes as PAL, meaning physical activity level. The PA level is the ratio of the total energy expenditure to the basal energy expenditure.

LIFESTYLE	PA FACTOR FOR MEN	PA FACTOR FOR WOMEN
Sedentary: Mostly resting with little or no planned strenuous activity and only performing those tasks that are required for independent living	1.0	1.0
Low Active: In addition to the activities of a sedentary lifestyle, the added equivalent of a 1.5- to 3-mile walk at a speed of 3 to 4 mph for the average-weight person*	1.11	1.12
Active: In addition to the activities identified for a sedentary lifestyle, an average of 60 min of daily moderate-intensity physical activity (e.g., walking at 3 to 4 mph for 3 to 6 miles/day) or shorter periods of more vigorous exertion (e.g., jogging for 30 min at 5.5 mph)	1.25	1.27
Very Active: In addition to the activities of a sedentary lifestyle, an activity level equivalent to walking at 3 to 4 mph for 12 to 22 miles/day (approximately 5 to 7 hours per day) or shorter periods of more vigorous exertion (e.g., running 7 mph for approximately 2.5 hours/day)	1.48	1.45

*For example, a man who weighs 70 kg and is 1.77 m tall and a woman who weighs 57 kg and is 1.63 m tall, on the basis of the reference body weights for adults.

Let Us Work Through Our First Example:

We have a 32-year-old woman who weighs 130 lb (59 kg). She is 5 feet and 4 inches tall and is maintaining a regular physical exercise program. She is currently consuming approximately 2600 kcal/day. First we will need to convert all of her measurements into metric terms:

Conversions: 1 pound = 2.2 kg; 39.37 in = 1 m.

Thus our patient is: 130 lb ÷ 2.2 = 59 kg; 5 ft 4 in = 64 inches ÷ 39.37 = 1.626 m.

Now, we will insert her numbers into the formula provided for women using an active PA coefficient:

EER = 354 − (6.91 × 32 yr old) + 1.27 [PA] × (9.36 × 59 kg + 726 × 1.626 meters)

EER = 354 − 221.12 + 1.27 × (552.24 + 1180.5)

EER = 2333.5 kcal/day

Conclusion: According to our calculations and her reported kcal intake of 2600 kcal/day, our patient is likely to gain weight over time. Her energy intake is approximately 266 kcal/day more than her energy output. Because 1 lb of body fat equals approximately 3500 kcal, she could gain about 1 lb every 13 days with her current eating and exercise routine.

Let Us Work One More Example Patient Together:

We have a 41-year-old man who weighs 180 lb (82 kg). He is 6 feet tall and eats an average of 3300 kcal/day while maintaining a very active lifestyle. Work through the calculations on your own to make sure you are getting the order of operations correct. Check your work against the numbers below.

EER = 662 − (9.53 × 41 yr old) + 1.48 [PA] × (15.91 × 82 kg + 539.6 × 1.829 m)

EER = 662 − 390.73 + 1.48 × (1304.62 + 986.93)

EER = 3663 kcal/day

Conclusion: This man will likely lose weight with his current exercise and meal plan, because he is consuming approximately 163 kcal less than he is expending.

Approximately how many pounds will he lose per month?

Now, calculate your own daily energy requirements and estimate your energy balance status. Are you in energy balance?

RECOMMENDATIONS FOR DIETARY ENERGY INTAKE

GENERAL LIFE CYCLE

Growth Periods

During periods of rapid growth, extra energy per unit of body weight is necessary to build new tissue (Table 6-2). The most rapid growth occurs during infancy and adolescence, with continuous but slower growth taking place between these periods. The rapid growth of the fetus and the placenta as well as other maternal tissues makes increased energy intake during pregnancy and lactation highly important.

Adulthood

With full adult growth achieved, energy needs level off to meet requirements for tissue maintenance and usual physical activities. As the aging process continues, a gradual decline in BEE and physical activity decreases the total energy requirement. There is an average decline in BEE of 1% to 2% per decade (assuming that a constant weight is maintained). A more rapid decline occurs around 40 years of age in men and 50 years of age in women. The increase in fat mass and accelerated loss of fat-free mass during menopause among women are associated with a drop in BEE.[23-25] Therefore, food choices should reflect a decline in caloric density and place greater emphasis on increased nutrient density.

Table 6-2	Approximate Caloric Allowances from Birth to the Age of 18 Years	
AGE (yr)		**kcal/lb**
Infants		
Birth to 0.5		33.4
0.6 to 1.0		35.6
Children		
1 to 2		36.2
Boys		
3 to 8		32
9 to 13		26.3
14 to 18		24
Girls		
3 to 8		29.7
9 to 13		23.8
14 to 18		19.3

Data from the Food and Nutrition Board, Institute of Medicine. *Dietary Reference Intakes for Energy, Carbohydrate, Fiber, Fat, Fatty Acids, Cholesterol, Protein, and Amino Acids*. Washington, DC: National Academies Press; 2005.

body mass index the body weight in kilograms divided by the square of the height in meters (kg/m^2); this measurement correlates with body fatness and the health risks associated with obesity.

DIETARY REFERENCE INTAKES

To determine recommendations for energy intake, the Food and Nutrition Board of the Institute of Medicine considered the average energy intake of individuals who were healthy, free living, and maintaining a healthy body weight as determined by **body mass index** measurements (see inside back cover of text for body mass index chart).[1] Table 6-3 gives the mean total energy expenditure throughout the lifecycle. Note the average height, weight, body mass index, and physical activity level within each age and gender group. The DRIs for vitamins and minerals are set at two standard deviations above the mean in order to meet the needs of 97.5% of the population. However, the DRIs for energy are set at the mean for the population so as to not encourage overconsumption of kilocalories.

DIETARY GUIDELINES FOR AMERICANS

The *Dietary Guidelines for Americans* address energy needs by making the following recommendations[26]:

- Choose a healthy eating pattern at an appropriate calorie level to help achieve and maintain a healthy body weight, support nutrient adequacy, and reduce the risk of chronic disease.
- To meet nutrient needs within calorie limits, choose a variety of nutrient-dense foods across and within all food groups in recommended amounts.
- Meet nutritional needs primarily through whole foods.
- Limit calories from added sugars and saturated fats.
- Meet the Physical Activity Guidelines for Americans.

MYPLATE

The MyPlate website (www.choosemyplate.gov) can help you to determine an individualized calorie level and corresponding serving sizes from each of the food groups to meet energy and nutrient density needs on the basis of age, gender, weight, height, and activity level.[27] The site also provides helpful information for maintaining a balance between food intake and energy output through physical activity.

Table 6-3   Median Height, Weight, and Recommended Energy Intake

AGE (yr)	MEAN WEIGHT (kg [lb])	MEAN HEIGHT (m [in])	MEAN BODY MASS INDEX (kg/m²)	BASAL ENERGY EXPENDITURE (kcal/day)	MEAN PHYSICAL ACTIVITY LEVEL	MEAN TOTAL ENERGY EXPENDITURE (kcal/day)
Infants						
Birth to 0.5	6.9 (15)	0.64 (25)	16.9	—	—	501
0.6 to 1.0	9 (20)	0.72 (28)	17.2	—	—	713
Children						
1 to 2	11 (24)	0.82 (32)	16.2	—	—	869
Males						
3 to 8	20.4 (45)	1.15 (45)	15.4	1035	1.39	1441
9 to 13	35.8 (79)	1.44 (57)	17.2	1320	1.56	2079
14 to 18	58.8 (130)	1.70 (67)	20.4	1729	1.80	3116
19 to 30	71 (156)	1.80 (71)	22.0	1769	1.74	3081
31 to 50	71.4 (157)	1.78 (70)	22.6	1675	1.81	3021
51 to 70	70 (154)	1.74 (69)	23.0	1524	1.63	2469
71+	68.9 (152)	1.74 (69)	22.8	1480	1.52	2238
Females						
3 to 8	22.9 (50)	1.20 (47)	15.6	1004	1.48	1487
9 to 13	36.4 (80)	1.44 (57)	17.4	1186	1.60	1907
14 to 18	54.1 (119)	1.63 (64)	20.4	1361	1.69	2302
19 to 30	59.3 (131)	1.66 (65)	21.4	1361	1.80	2436
31 to 50	58.6 (129)	1.64 (65)	21.6	1322	1.83	2404
51 to 70	59.1 (130)	1.63 (63)	22.2	1226	1.70	2066
71+	54.8 (121)	1.58 (62)	21.8	1183	1.33	1564
Pregnant						
First trimester						+0
Second and third trimesters						+300/day
Lactating						
First 12 months						+500/day

Data from Food and Nutrition Board, Institute of Medicine. *Dietary Reference Intakes for Energy, Carbohydrate, Fiber, Fat, Fatty Acids, Cholesterol, Protein, and Amino Acids*. Washington, DC: National Academies Press; 2005.

Putting It All Together

Summary

- In the human energy system, food provides energy. Energy is measured in kilocalories in the United States. Energy from food is cycled through the body's internal energy system in balance with the external environment's energy system, which is ultimately powered by the sun.
- Metabolism is the sum of the body processes that are involved in converting food into various forms of energy available for use within the cells. When food is not available, the body draws on its stored energy, which is in the forms of glycogen, fat, and muscle protein.
- Total energy expenditure is based on the following: (1) basal energy expenditure, which makes up the largest portion of energy needs; (2) energy for physical activities; and (3) the thermic effect of food.
- Energy requirements vary throughout life and are altered in disease states.

Chapter Review Questions

See answers in Appendix A.
1. Which of the following individuals most likely has the highest energy needs per unit of body weight?
   a. 38-year-old male administrative assistant
   b. 72-year-old grandmother
   c. 22-year-old college student
   d. 7-month-old baby boy

2. Which of the following serves to maintain normal blood glucose levels during sleep hours?
   a. Lipid stores
   b. Protein stores
   c. Glycogen stores
   d. Vitamin D stores

3. A measure of a patient's metabolic rate could be determined using:
   a. Glycogen levels.
   b. Indirect calorimetry.
   c. Physical activity records.
   d. Body temperature.

4. Jenny is trying to lose weight and has decreased her energy intake by 250 kcal per day. How long should it take her to lose 1 lb of body fat?
   a. Approximately 8 days
   b. Approximately 14 days
   c. Approximately 27 days
   d. Approximately 32 days

5. Calculate the amount of calories in 1 cup of milk that contains 4 grams of fat, 10 grams of protein, and 15 grams of carbohydrate.
   a. 90 kcal
   b. 120 kcal
   c. 136 kcal
   d. 145 kcal

Additional Learning Resources

evolve Please refer to this text's Evolve website for answers to the Case Study questions.
http://evolve.elsevier.com/Williams/basic/

References and **Further Reading and Resources** in the back of the book provide additional resources for enhancing knowledge.

Vitamins

Key Concepts

- Vitamins are noncaloric, essential nutrients that are necessary for many metabolic tasks.
- Certain health problems are related to inadequate or excessive vitamin intake.
- Vitamins occur in a wide variety of foods and are packaged with the energy-yielding macronutrients.

- The body uses vitamins to make the coenzymes that are required for some enzymes to function.
- The need for particular vitamin supplements depends on a person's vitamin status.

More than any other group of nutrients, vitamins have captured public interest and concern. This chapter answers some of the questions about vitamins: What do they do? How much of each vitamin does the human body need? What foods do they come from? Do we need to take dietary supplements? The scientific study of nutrition, on which the Dietary Reference Intake (DRI) guidelines are based, continues to expand the body of nutrition knowledge. Thus, the answers to these questions have evolved through years of research and discovery.

This chapter looks at the vitamins both as a group and as individual nutrients. It explores general and specific vitamin needs as well as reasonable and realistic dietary supplement use.

THE NATURE OF VITAMINS

DISCOVERY

The study of vitamins and minerals and their many functions in human nutrition remains a subject of interesting scientific investigation.

Early Observations

Vitamins were largely discovered while searching for cures of classic diseases that were suspected to be associated with dietary deficiencies. Such discoveries date back as early as 1753 when British naval surgeon Dr. James Lind observed that many sailors became ill and died on long voyages when they had to live on rations without fresh foods.[1] When Lind provided the sailors with fresh lemons and oranges, no one became ill. Dr. Lind had discovered that **scurvy**, which had been the curse of sailors, was caused by a dietary deficiency of vitamin C and was prevented by adding citrus fruit to the diet. Because British sailors carried limes on these long voyages, they got the nickname *limeys*.

Early Animal Experiments

In 1906 Dr. Frederick Hopkins of Cambridge University began a series of experiments in which he fed a group of rats a synthetic mixture of protein, fat, carbohydrate, mineral salts, and water. All of the rats became ill and died. He then added milk to the purified ration for a separate set of rats, and they maintained normal growth.[2] This important discovery—that additional substances present in natural foods are essential to life—provided the necessary foundation for the individual vitamin discoveries that followed.

Era of Vitamin Discovery

Most of the vitamins that are known today were discovered during the first half of the 1900s. The nature of these vital molecules became more evident over time. A form of the name *vitamin* was first used in 1911, when Casimir Funk, a Polish chemist working at the Lister Institute in London, discovered a nitrogen-containing substance (in organic chemistry, known as an *amine*) that he speculated might be a common characteristic of all vital agents. He coined the word *vitamine*, meaning "vital amine."[3] The final *e* was dropped later, when other vital substances turned out not to be amines, and the name *vitamin* was retained to designate compounds within this class of essential substances. At first scientists assigned letters of the alphabet to each vitamin in the order that they

scurvy a hemorrhagic disease caused by a lack of vitamin C that is characterized by diffuse tissue bleeding, painful limbs and joints, thickened bones, and skin discoloration from bleeding; bones fracture easily, wounds do not heal, gums swell and tend to bleed, and the teeth loosen.

were discovered; however, as more vitamins were discovered, this practice was abandoned in favor of more specific names based on a vitamin's chemical structure or body function. Both letter designation and current name will be used in this text.

DEFINITION

As each vitamin was discovered, the following two characteristics that define a vitamin clearly emerged:
1. It must be a vital organic substance that is not a carbohydrate, fat, or protein; and it must be necessary to perform a specific metabolic function or to prevent a deficiency disease.
2. It cannot be manufactured by the body in sufficient quantities to sustain life, so it must be supplied by the diet.

Because the body only needs vitamins in small amounts, they are considered *micro*nutrients. The total volume of vitamins that a healthy person normally requires each day would barely fill a teaspoon. Thus, the units of measure for vitamins—milligrams or micrograms—are exceedingly small and difficult to visualize (see the For Further Focus box, "Small Measures for Small Needs"). Nonetheless, all vitamins are essential to life.

FUNCTIONS OF VITAMINS

Although each vitamin has its specific metabolic tasks, general functions of vitamins include the following: (1) components of coenzymes; (2) antioxidants; (3) hormones that affect gene expression; (4) components of cell membranes; and (5) components of the light-sensitive rhodopsin molecule in the eyes (i.e., vitamin A).

Metabolism: Enzymes and Coenzymes

Enzymes act as catalysts; catalysts increase the rate at which their specific chemical reactions proceed, but they are not themselves consumed during the reaction. Coenzymes that are derived from vitamins are an integral part of some enzymes, without which these enzymes cannot catalyze their metabolic reactions. For example, several of the B vitamins (i.e., thiamin, niacin, and riboflavin) are part of coenzymes. These coenzymes are, in turn, integral parts of enzymes that metabolize glucose, fatty acids, and amino acids to extract energy.

Tissue Structure and Protection

Some vitamins are involved in tissue or bone building. For example, vitamin C is involved in the synthesis of collagen, which is a structural protein in the skin, ligaments, and bones. In fact, the word *collagen* comes from a Greek word meaning "glue." Collagen is like glue in its capacity to add tensile strength to body structures. Vitamins (e.g., A, C, and E) also act as **antioxidants** to protect cell structures and to prevent damage caused by free radicals.

Small Measures for Small Needs

By definition, vitamins are essential nutrients that are necessary in small amounts for human health. Just how small those amounts truly are is sometimes hard to imagine. Vitamins are measured in the metric system terms of *milligram* and *microgram*. Can you visualize how much that is? Perhaps comparing these amounts with commonly used household measures will be helpful.

Early during the age of scientific development, scientists realized that they needed a common language of measures that could be understood by all nations to exchange rapidly developing scientific knowledge. Thus, the metric system was born. This system was developed in the mid-1800s by French scientists and named *Le Système International d'Unités*, which is abbreviated as *SI units*. The use of these more precise units is now widespread, especially because it is mandatory for all purposes in most countries. The U.S. Congress passed the official Metric Conversion Act in 1975, but America has been slower to apply the metric system to common use as compared with other countries. However, the use of this system in scientific work is explicit worldwide.

Let us compare the two metric measures that are used for vitamins in the United States. Below are the Recommended Dietary Allowances (RDAs) equated with common measures to demonstrate just how small our needs are:
- One *milligram* (mg) is equal to one thousandth of a gram (28 g = 1 oz; 1 g is equal to approximately $\frac{1}{4}$ tsp). RDAs are measured in milligrams for thiamin, riboflavin, niacin, pyridoxine, pantothenic acid, choline, and vitamins C and E.
- A *microgram* (mcg or μg) is equal to one millionth of a gram. RDAs are measured in micrograms for vitamins A (retinol equivalents), B_{12}, D, and K and for folate and biotin.

It is a small wonder that the total amount of vitamins that we need each day would scarcely fill a teaspoon; however, that small amount makes the difference between life and death over time.

Prevention of Deficiency Diseases

When a vitamin deficiency becomes severe, the specific function of that vitamin becomes apparent because the vitamin's function is no longer preformed. For example, the classic vitamin deficiency disease scurvy is caused by insufficient dietary vitamin C. Scurvy is a hemorrhagic disease that is characterized by bleeding in the joints and other tissues and by the breakdown of fragile capillaries under normal blood pressure; these are all symptoms that are directly related to vitamin C's role in producing collagen. Collagen is what makes capillary walls strong. Untreated scurvy leads to internal membrane disintegration and death, as previously mentioned regarding British sailors of earlier centuries. The name *ascorbic*

antioxidant a molecule that prevents the oxidation of cellular structures by free radicals.

acid comes from the Latin word *scorbutus*, meaning "scurvy," and the prefix *a-* means "without"; thus, the term *ascorbic* means "without scurvy." In developed countries today, we do not see frank scurvy often, but we do see vitamin C deficiency in combination with other forms of overt malnutrition.

VITAMIN METABOLISM

The way in which our bodies digest, absorb, and transport vitamins depends on the vitamin's solubility. Vitamins are traditionally classified as either fat soluble or water soluble. The fat-soluble vitamins are A, D, E, and K. The water-soluble vitamins are C and all of the B vitamins. This chapter is divided into the following sections: (1) Fat-Soluble Vitamins; (2) Water-Soluble Vitamins; (3) Plant Nutrients; and (4) Nutrient Supplementation.

Fat-Soluble Vitamins

Intestinal cells absorb fat-soluble vitamins along with dietary fat as a micelle and then incorporate all fat-soluble nutrients into chylomicrons. From the intestinal cells, chylomicrons enter the lymphatic circulation and then the blood (see Chapter 3 for details on fat absorption). The absorption of fat-soluble vitamins is enhanced by the presence of dietary fat. For instance, the vitamin A in a cup of vitamin A–fortified milk is better absorbed from whole or 2% milk than from skim milk, because skim milk contains no fat.

The potential toxicity of each vitamin is determined by the body's capacity to store it and the capacity of the liver and kidneys to clear it. Unlike water-soluble vitamins, fat-soluble vitamins can be stored in the liver and adipose tissue for long periods of time. The body uses this reserve in times of inadequate daily intake. Fat-soluble vitamin accumulation in the body is the reason that excess intake can result in toxicity over time.

Water-Soluble Vitamins

Intestinal cells easily absorb water-soluble vitamins. From these cells, the vitamins move directly into the portal blood circulation. Because blood is mostly water, the transport of water-soluble vitamins does not require the assistance of carrier proteins.

With the exception of cobalamin (vitamin B_{12}) and pyridoxine (vitamin B_6), the body does not store water-soluble vitamins to any significant extent. Therefore, the body relies on the frequent intake of foods that are rich in water-soluble vitamins.

Fat-soluble and water-soluble vitamins are absorbed throughout the small intestines. See Figure 5-9 for the general absorptive sites of nutrients in the gastrointestinal tract.

DIETARY REFERENCE INTAKES

As discussed in Chapter 1, the DRIs are recommendations for nutrient intake by healthy population groups.

Refer back to Chapter 1 for details on the four categories that make up the DRIs. This chapter's discussion of vitamins and the following chapters that discuss minerals, fluids, and electrolytes refer to the various DRI recommendations (especially the RDAs) whenever possible.

SECTION 1 FAT-SOLUBLE VITAMINS

VITAMIN A (RETINOL)

FUNCTIONS

Vitamin A performs the functions of aiding vision, growth, tissue strength, and immunity.

Vision

The chemical name **retinol** was given to vitamin A because of its major function in the retina of the eye. The aldehyde form, retinal, is part of a light-sensitive pigment in retinal cells called *rhodopsin,* which is commonly known as *visual purple.* Rhodopsin enables the eye to adjust to different amounts of available light. A mild vitamin A deficiency may cause night blindness, slow adaptation to darkness, or glare blindness. Vitamin A–related compounds (i.e., the **carotenoids** lutein and zeaxanthin) are specifically associated with the prevention of age-related macular degeneration.[4]

Growth

Retinoic acid and retinol are involved in skeletal and soft-tissue growth through their roles in protein synthesis and the stabilization of cell membranes. The constant need to replace old cells in the bone matrix, the gastrointestinal tract, and other areas requires adequate vitamin A intake.

Tissue Strength and Immunity

The other retinoids (i.e., retinoic acid and retinol) help to maintain healthy epithelial tissue, which is the protective tissue that covers body surfaces (i.e., the skin and the inner mucous membranes in the nose, throat, eyes, gastrointestinal tract, and genitourinary tract). These tissues are the primary barrier to infection. Vitamin A is also important as an antioxidant and in

---

retinol the chemical name of vitamin A; the name is derived from the vitamin's visual functions related to the retina of the eye, which is the back inner lining of the eyeball that catches the light refractions of the lens to form images that are interpreted by the optic nerve and the brain and that makes the necessary light–dark adaptations.

carotenoids organic pigments that are found in plants; known to have functions such as scavenging free radicals, reducing the risk of certain types of cancer, and helping to prevent age-related eye diseases; more than 600 carotenoids have been identified, with β-carotene being the most well-known.

the production of immune cells that are responsible for fighting bacterial, parasitic, and viral attacks.

REQUIREMENTS

Vitamin A requirements are based on its two basic forms in foods and its storage in the body. The established RDAs are listed in the summary table for fat-soluble vitamins (see Table 7-5) and in the DRI tables Appendix B.

Food Forms and Units of Measure

Dietary vitamin A occurs in two forms, as follows:

1. Preformed vitamin A or retinol, which is the active vitamin A found in foods that are derived from animal products.
2. Provitamin A or β-**carotene,** which is a pigment in yellow, orange, and deep green fruits or vegetables that the human body can convert to retinol. Carotenoids are a family of compounds that are similar in structure; β-carotene and lutein are the most common in foods. Box 7-1 lists some of the known carotenoids.

In the typical American diet, a significant amount of vitamin A is in the *pro*vitamin A form (i.e., β-carotene). To account for all food forms, individual carotenoids and preformed vitamin A are measured, and the amounts are converted to retinol equivalents. For the body to make 1 mcg of retinol, 12 mcg of dietary β-carotene, 2 mcg of supplemental β-carotene, or 24 mcg of either α-carotene or β-cryptoxanthin are necessary. An older measure that is sometimes used to quantify vitamin A is the International Unit (IU). One IU of vitamin A equals 0.3 mcg of retinol or 0.6 mcg of β-carotene.

---

carotene a group name for the red and yellow pigments (α-, β-, and γ-carotene) that are found in plant foods; β-carotene is most important to human nutrition because the body can convert it to vitamin A, thus making it a primary source of the vitamin.

Box 7-1   Carotenoids

Carotenes: orange pigments that contain no oxygen
- α-Carotene
- β-Carotene
- γ-Carotene
- δ-Carotene
- Lycopene

Xanthophylls: yellow pigments that contain some oxygen
- α- and β-Cryptoxanthin
- Lutein
- Lycophyll
- Neoxanthin
- Violaxanthin
- Zeaxanthin

Body Storage

The liver can store large amounts of retinol. In healthy individuals, the liver stores approximately 70% of the body's total vitamin A. Thus, the liver is particularly susceptible to toxicity as a result of excessive vitamin A supplementation. The remaining vitamin A stored in the body may be found in tissues such as adipose tissue, the lungs, skin, spleen, eyes, and testes.

DEFICIENCY

Adequate vitamin A intake prevents two eye conditions: (1) xerosis, which involves itching, burning, and red, inflamed eyelids; and (2) xerophthalmia, which is blindness that is caused by severe deficiency. Dietary vitamin A deficiency is the leading cause of preventable blindness in children worldwide (Figure 7-1). The World Health Organization reports that vitamin A deficiency resulting in night blindness currently affects 5.2 million preschool-aged children and 9.8 million pregnant women globally.[5]

As with all nutrients, deficiency symptoms are directly related to vitamin A's functions. Therefore, a lack of dietary vitamin A will also result in epithelial and immune system disorders.

TOXICITY

The condition created by excessive vitamin A intake is called *hypervitaminosis A.* Symptoms include bone pain, dry skin, loss of hair, fatigue, and anorexia. Excessive vitamin A intake may cause liver injury with portal hypertension, which is elevated blood pressure in the portal vein, and ascites, which is fluid accumulation in the abdominal cavity. Because of the potential for toxicity, the upper (intake) level (UL) of retinol for adults has been set at 3000 mcg/day.[6] Toxicity symptoms usually result from the overconsumption of preformed vitamin A rather than of the carotenoids. Excessive vitamin A consumption during pregnancy is

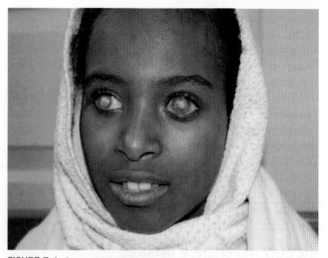

FIGURE 7-1 Corneal blindness from vitamin A deficiency. (Courtesy Lance Bellers In Burton MJ. Prevention, treatment and rehabilitation. *Community Eye Health.* 2009;22(71):33-35.)

a known **teratogen,** which is the reason that acne treatment with medications containing high amounts of vitamin A (e.g., Accutane, Retin-A) is contraindicated during pregnancy.

The absorption of dietary carotenoids is dose dependent at high intake levels. However, the prolonged excessive intake of foods that are high in β-carotene will cause a harmless orange skin tint that disappears when the excessive intakes are discontinued. On the other hand, β-carotene supplements can reach concentrations in the body that promote oxidative damage, cell division, and the destruction of other forms of vitamin A.

FOOD SOURCES AND STABILITY

Fish liver oils, liver, egg yolks, butter, and cream are sources of preformed natural vitamin A. Preformed vitamin A occurs naturally in milk fat. Low-fat and nonfat milks and margarine are significant sources of vitamin A, because they are fortified. Some good sources of β-carotene are dark-green, leafy vegetables such as collard greens, kale, and spinach as well as dark-orange vegetables and fruits such as carrots, sweet potatoes or yams, pumpkins, melon, and apricots. Table 7-1 provides some comparative food sources of vitamin A.

β-Carotene and preformed vitamin A require emulsification by bile salts to be absorbed by the intestine. Preformed vitamin A is efficiently absorbed at a rate of 75% to 100%. The absorption of β-carotene is significantly more variable with an absorption rate of 3% to 90%.[7] The capriciousness of these ranges is attributable to factors such as dietary source, gastric content, nutrient status, and genetic factors. Inside the intestinal cells, both forms are incorporated into chylomicrons with fat, and the chylomicrons pass through the lymphatic system and into the bloodstream. Despite successful absorption, up to 40% of the dietary carotenoids are not metabolized in the enterocytes, further decreasing the bioavailability as compared to preformed vitamin A sources.[8]

Retinol is unstable when it is exposed to heat and oxygen. Quick cooking methods that use little water help to preserve vitamin A in food.

VITAMIN D (CALCIFEROL)

Vitamin D was mistakenly classified as a vitamin in 1922 by its discoverers when they cured rickets with fish oil, which is a natural source of vitamin D.[9] Today, we know that the compounds produced by animals (i.e., **cholecalciferol** or vitamin D_3) and some organisms (i.e., **ergocalciferol** or vitamin D_2) are a **prohormone** rather than a true vitamin. Vitamins D_2 and D_3 are both physiologically relevant to human nutrition, and they are collectively referred to as *calciferol.*

Upon exposure to ultraviolet light, humans are able to convert the precursor 7-dehydrocholesterol, a compound that is found in the epidermal layer of skin, into cholecalciferol. Similarly, organisms such as invertebrates and fungi are capable of converting the precursor ergosterol into ergocalciferol after they receive ultraviolet irradiation.

Cholecalciferol and ergocalciferol must be activated in two successive hydroxylation reactions to yield the active and functional form of vitamin D, **calcitriol.** The first hydroxylation reaction occurs in the liver to produce calcidiol (also known as 25-hydroxycholecalciferol and 25-hydroxyvitamin D_3).

Table 7-1 Food Sources of Vitamin A

ITEM	QUANTITY	AMOUNT (mcg OF RETINOL EQUIVALENTS)
Fruits and Vegetables		
Carrots, raw	½ cup	534
Collard greens, boiled	½ cup	386
Kale, cooked, drained	½ cup	443
Pumpkin, boiled	½ cup	306
Spinach, boiled	½ cup	472
Sweet potato, baked, in skin	1 medium (114 g)	1096
Meat, Poultry, Fish, Dry Beans, Eggs, and Nuts		
Beef liver, pan fried	3 oz	6582
Chicken liver, pan fried	3 oz	3652
Egg yolk, fresh, raw	2 large	130
Milk and Dairy Products		
Cream, heavy, whipping	½ cup	247
Milk, low-fat 2%, fortified	8 oz	134
Milk, skim, fortified	8 oz	149
Fats, Oils, and Sugars		
Fish oil, cod liver	1 Tbsp	4080

Data from the U.S. Department of Agriculture, Agricultural Research Service. Nutrient Data Laboratory. *USDA nutrient database for standard reference* (website): <http://ndb.nal.usda.gov/ndb/>; Accessed September 17, 2014.

teratogen a substance or factor resulting in birth defects or miscarriage of an embryo or fetus.
cholecalciferol the chemical name for vitamin D_3 in its inactive form; it is often shortened to *calciferol.*
ergocalciferol the chemical name for vitamin D_2 in its inactive form; it is produced by some organisms (not humans) upon ultraviolet irradiation from the precursor ergosterol.
prohormone a precursor substance that the body converts to a hormone; for example, a cholesterol compound in the skin is first irradiated by sunlight and then converted through successive enzyme actions in the liver and kidney into the active vitamin D hormone, which then regulates calcium absorption and bone development.
calcitriol the activated hormone form of vitamin D.

1α-hydroxylase the enzyme in the kidneys that catalyzes the hydroxylation reaction of 25-hydroxycholecalciferol (i.e., calcidiol) to calcitriol, which is the active form of vitamin D; 1α-hydroxylase activity is increased by parathyroid hormone when blood calcium levels are low.

resorption the breaking down and releasing of minerals from bones.

The enzyme **1α-hydroxylase** then catalyzes the second hydroxylation reaction in the kidneys to produce calcitriol (also known as 1,25-dihydroxycholecalciferol and 1,25-dihydroxyvitamin D_3). Figure 7-2 illustrates the activation process of vitamin D in the body.

FUNCTIONS

Calcium and Phosphorus Homeostasis

Maintaining calcium homeostasis in the blood is a critical function of vitamin D. Calcitriol acts physiologically with two other hormones—parathyroid hormone and the thyroid hormone calcitonin—to control calcium and phosphorus absorption and metabolism. Calcitriol stimulates the following: (1) the intestinal cell absorption of calcium and phosphorus; (2) the renal reabsorption of calcium and phosphorus; and (3) the osteoclastic **resorption** of calcium and phosphorus from trabecular bone. All of these mechanisms work together to maintain blood calcium and phosphorus homeostasis (see Figure 7-2).

Bone Mineralization

Osteoporosis involves a loss of bone density that leads to brittle bones and spontaneous fractures. Because calcitriol regulates the rate of calcium and phosphorus resorption from bone, it has been clinically used to reduce the risk of osteoporosis.[10-12]

REQUIREMENTS

Establishing requirements for vitamin D is difficult because it is produced in the skin and because the number of food sources are limited. Dietary vitamin D requirements will vary with individual exposure to sunlight, which is affected by the season, the latitude at which people reside, and even a person's skin color.

Research indicates that vitamin D deficiency may be a worldwide nutritional problem, with multifactorial health consequences.[13-15] The primary cause of inadequate circulating serum vitamin D is a lack of sun exposure. In the northern hemisphere, particularly above 35 to 40 degrees latitude, significantly less sunlight is present throughout the winter months. Because the amount of vitamin D produced in the skin is relative to the intensity of the sun, there is an inadequate availability of endogenous vitamin D during the winter at higher latitudes. This also affects the vitamin D requirement of people with darker skin, because melanin absorbs ultraviolet radiation in a way that is similar to that of sunscreen. Thus, less vitamin D is synthesized in darker-skinned people than in

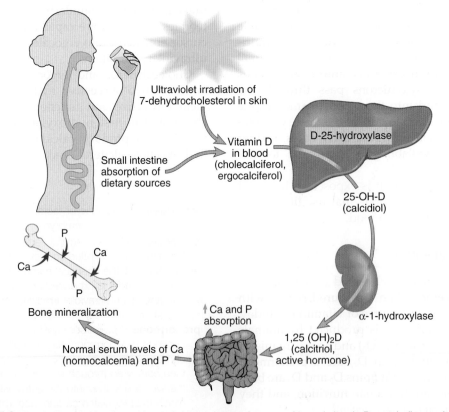

FIGURE 7-2 Vitamin D activation from skin synthesis and dietary sources. Normal vitamin D metabolism maintains blood calcium levels. (Modified from Kumar V, Abbas A, Fausto N, Mitchell R. *Robbins Basic Pathology.* 8th ed. Philadelphia: Saunders; 2007.)

lighter-skinned people who receive the same amount of sun exposure.

A flurry of research over the past decade indicates that the dietary needs of vitamin D are higher than what was previously believed. The DRIs are listed in the summary table for fat-soluble vitamins (see Table 7-5) and in the DRI tables in Appendix B. The American Academy of Pediatrics recommends that infants receive a minimum of 400 IU of vitamin D beginning soon after birth to prevent rickets.[16]

DEFICIENCY

Rickets is caused by chronic calcitriol deficiency during childhood. Children with rickets have soft long bones that bend under the child's weight (Figure 7-3). In addition to causing skeletal malformations, inadequate vitamin D intake prevents children from attaining their peak bone mass, thereby contributing to the development of osteoporosis or osteomalacia as adults. Many other chronic diseases have been linked to vitamin D deficiency, including muscle weakness, several types of cancer, coronary heart disease, hypertension, stroke, tuberculosis, obesity, type 2 diabetes, macular degeneration, neurologic disorders (e.g., Alzheimer and Parkinson disease), and several autoimmune diseases (e.g., type 1 diabetes, multiple sclerosis, rheumatoid arthritis).[14,15]

> **rickets** a disease of childhood that is characterized by the softening of the bones from an inadequate intake of vitamin D and insufficient exposure to sunlight; it is also associated with impaired calcium and phosphorus metabolism.

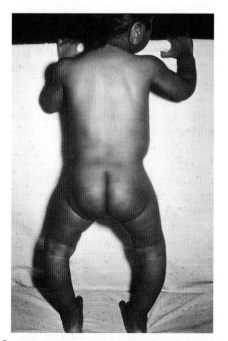

FIGURE 7-3 A child with rickets; note the bowlegs. (Reprinted from Kumar V, Abbas A, Fausto N, Mitchell R. *Robbins Basic Pathology.* 8th ed. Philadelphia: Saunders; 2007.)

There is no universally accepted method for assessing vitamin D status nor a consensus on the vitamin D levels that constitute normal. Bearing that in mind, it is estimated that 50% of Americans have inadequate vitamin D stores when using the deficiency cut-off of ≤20 ng/mL of serum 25-hydroxyvitamin D. There is a disproportionate prevalence occurring among non-Hispanic blacks (81%) and Mexican Americans (58%) as compared to whites (28%).[17] Genetics may account for such large differences between ethnic groups, which calls to question the accuracy of using the same cut-off point of 25-hydroxyvitamin D levels to diagnose deficiency in all racial groups. Researchers believe that despite a lower level of 25-hydroxyvitamin D measured, the bioavailability of vitamin D to the body is the same for black and white individuals.[18] Thus, the cut-off value for defining vitamin D deficiency may be race-specific and is still under investigation.

TOXICITY

Excessive dietary intake of vitamin D can be toxic, especially for infants and children. Symptoms of toxicity or hypervitaminosis D include fragile bones, kidney stones, and the calcification of the soft tissues (e.g., kidneys, heart, lungs). The prolonged intake of excessive cholecalciferol in dietary supplement form may produce elevated blood calcium concentrations (i.e., hypercalcemia) and calcium deposits in the kidney nephrons, which interferes with overall kidney function. The UL for vitamin D among people who are older than 9 years of age is 4000 IU/day (100 mcg).[19] Vitamin D intoxication cannot occur as a result of the cutaneous production of vitamin D. For most people, vitamin D intake from food and dietary supplements is not likely to exceed the UL. However, individuals who consume diets that are high in fatty fish and fortified milk in addition to taking dietary supplements that contain vitamin D may be at risk for toxicity.

FOOD SOURCES AND STABILITY

Fatty fish are one of the only good natural sources of vitamin D. Therefore, a large portion of daily vitamin D intake comes from fortified foods (Table 7-2). Because it is a common food that also contains calcium and phosphorus, milk is a practical food to fortify with vitamin D. The standard commercial practice is to add 400 IU per quart. Butter substitutes such as margarines and dairy substitutes such as soy or rice milk products are often fortified with vitamin D.

Vitamin D is relatively stable under most conditions that involve heat, aging, and storage.

VITAMIN E (TOCOPHEROL)

Early vitamin studies identified a substance that was necessary for animal reproduction.[20] This substance

Table 7-2	Food Sources of Vitamin D	
ITEM	**QUANTITY**	**AMOUNT (INTERNATIONAL UNITS)**
Meat, Poultry, Fish, Dry Beans, Eggs, and Nuts		
Salmon, sockeye, cooked	3 oz	447
Salmon, sockeye, canned, drained solids	3 oz	715
Tuna, light, canned in oil, drained solids	3 oz	229
Tuna, bluefin, fresh	3 oz	193
Milk and Dairy Products		
Milk, low-fat 2%, fortified	1 cup (8 fl oz)	120
Soymilk, vitamin-D fortified	1 cup (8 fl oz)	119
Fats, Oils, and Sugars		
Fish oil, cod liver	1 Tbsp	1360

Data from the U.S. Department of Agriculture, Agricultural Research Service. Nutrient Data Laboratory. *USDA nutrient database for standard reference* (website): <http://ndb.nal.usda.gov/ndb/>; Accessed September 17, 2014.

was named **tocopherol** from two Greek words: *tophos,* meaning "childbirth," and *phero,* meaning "to bring," with the *-ol* ending used to indicate its alcohol functional group. Tocopherol became known as the antisterility vitamin, but it was soon demonstrated to have this effect only in rats and a few other animals and not in people. A number of related compounds have since been discovered. Tocopherol is the generic name for this entire group of homologous fat-soluble nutrients, which are designated as α-, β-, γ-, and δ-tocopherol or tocotrienol. Of these eight nutrients, α-tocopherol is the only one that is significant in human nutrition and thus used to calculate dietary needs.[21]

FUNCTIONS

The most vital function of α-tocopherol is its antioxidant action in tissues. In addition vitamin E has several other important functions, such as cell signalling that drives gene expression and antiproliferative effects in the eye that are seemingly protective against conditions such as glaucoma.[22,23]

Antioxidant Function

α-Tocopherol is the body's most abundant fat-soluble antioxidant. The polyunsaturated fatty acids (see Chapter 3) in the phospholipids of cell and organelle

> **tocopherol** the chemical name for vitamin E, which was named by early investigators because their initial work with rats indicated a reproductive function; in people, vitamin E functions as a strong antioxidant that preserves structural membranes such as cell walls.

membranes are particularly susceptible to free radical oxidation. α-Tocopherol intercepts this oxidation process and protects the polyunsaturated fatty acids from damage.

Relation to Selenium Metabolism

Selenium is a trace mineral that, as part of the selenium-containing enzyme glutathione peroxidase, works with α-tocopherol as an antioxidant. Glutathione peroxidase is the second line of defense for preventing free radical damage to membranes. Glutathione peroxidase spares α-tocopherol from oxidation, thereby reducing the dietary requirement for α-tocopherol. Similarly, α-tocopherol spares glutathione peroxidase from oxidation, thus reducing the dietary requirement for selenium.

REQUIREMENTS

α-Tocopherol requirements are expressed in milligrams per day. The DRIs are listed in the summary table for fat-soluble vitamins (see Table 7-5) and in the DRI tables in Appendix B.

DEFICIENCY

α-Tocopherol stores, along with body fat, are normally accrued in the fetus during the final 1 to 2 months of gestation. Thus, premature infants who missed the period for fat and fat-soluble vitamin accumulation are particularly vulnerable to hemolytic anemia. Without adequate vitamin E for antioxidant protection, the red blood cell membrane phospholipids and proteins are susceptible to oxidation and destruction. Without supplemental vitamin E treatment, the continued loss of functioning red blood cells leads to hemolytic anemia.

A dietary deficiency of vitamin E is rare; the only cases occur in individuals who cannot absorb or metabolize fat. In such cases, the α-tocopherol deficiency disrupts the normal synthesis of myelin, which is the protective phospholipid-rich membrane that covers the nerve cells. The major nerves that are disturbed are the spinal cord fibers that affect physical activity and the retina of the eye, which affects vision.

TOXICITY

α-Tocopherol from food sources has no known toxic effects in people. Supplemental α-tocopherol intakes that exceed the UL of 1000 mg/day may interfere with vitamin K activity and blood clotting. Although the exact mechanism is unknown, this may be particularly problematic for individuals who are deficient in vitamin K or for patients who are receiving anticoagulation therapy.[24]

FOOD SOURCES AND STABILITY

The richest sources of α-tocopherol are vegetable oils (e.g., wheat germ, soybean, safflower). Note that vegetable oils are also the richest sources of polyunsaturated fatty acids, which α-tocopherol protects. Other food sources of α-tocopherol include nuts, seeds, and fortified cereals. Table 7-3 provides a list of food sources of vitamin E.

α-Tocopherol is unstable to heat and alkalis.

VITAMIN K

In 1929 Henrik Dam, a biochemist at the University of Copenhagen, discovered a hemorrhagic disease in chicks that were fed a diet from which all lipids had

Table 7-3	Food Sources of Vitamin E as α-Tocopherol	
ITEM	**QUANTITY**	**AMOUNT (mg OF α-TOCOPHEROL)**
Bread, Cereal, Rice, and Pasta		
Total whole-grain cereal, General Mills	1 cup	18.0
Wheat germ, toasted, plain	1 oz	4.53
Fruits and Vegetables		
Mango, raw	½ medium	1.51
Mustard greens	1 cup	1.13
Nuts and Seeds		
Almonds	1 oz	7.27
Hazelnuts	1 oz	4.26
Sunflower seeds	1 oz	7.40
Fats, Oils, and Sugars		
Cottonseed oil	1 Tbsp	4.80
Safflower oil	1 Tbsp	4.64
Sunflower oil	1 Tbsp	5.59

Data from the U.S. Department of Agriculture, Agricultural Research Service. Nutrient Data Laboratory. *USDA nutrient database for standard reference* (website): <http://ndb.nal.usda.gov/ndb/>; Accessed September 17, 2014.

> **phylloquinone** a fat-soluble vitamin of the K group that is found primarily in green plants.

been removed. Dam hypothesized that an unidentified lipid factor had been removed from the chicks' feed. Dam called it *koagulations vitamin* or *vitamin K,* and the letter that he assigned it is still used today.[25] Dam later succeeded in isolating the agent from alfalfa and identifying it, for which he received the Nobel Prize for physiology and medicine. As with many of the vitamins, several homologous forms of vitamin K make up the group. The major form in plants that was initially isolated from alfalfa by Dam is **phylloquinone,** which is the dietary form of vitamin K. Menaquinone, a second form, is synthesized by intestinal bacteria. Menaquinone contributes approximately half of our daily supply of vitamin K. Menadione is a synthetic precursor of vitamin K, but it has not been used in dietary supplements since the U.S. Food and Drug Administration banned it due to toxicity effects.

FUNCTIONS

Vitamin K has two well-established functions in the body: blood clotting and bone development.

Blood Clotting

The most well-known and the earliest discovered function of vitamin K is in the blood-clotting process. Vitamin K is essential for maintaining the normal blood concentrations of four blood-clotting factors. The first of these vitamin–K-dependent blood factors to be identified and characterized was prothrombin (i.e., clotting factor II). Prothrombin, which is synthesized in the liver, is converted to thrombin upon activation, which then initiates the conversion of fibrinogen to fibrin to form the blood clot (Figure 7-4).

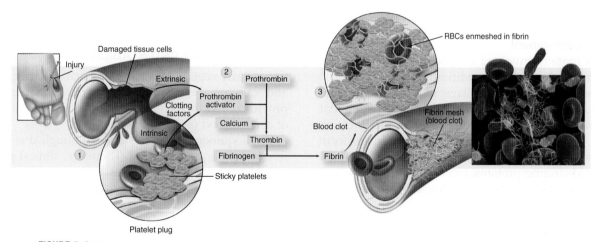

FIGURE 7-4 The blood-clotting mechanism. The complex clotting mechanism can be distilled into three steps: (1) the release of clotting factors from both injured tissue cells and sticky platelets at the injury site, which form a temporary platelet plug; (2) a series of chemical reactions that eventually result in the formation of thrombin; and (3) the formation of fibrin and the trapping of blood cells to form a clot. (Modified from Thibodeau GA, Patton KT. *Anatomy & Physiology.* 8th ed. St Louis: Mosby; 2012.)

Phylloquinone is an antidote for the effects of excessive anticoagulant drug doses, and it is often used to control and prevent certain types of hemorrhages. Fat-soluble vitamins are more completely absorbed when bile is present. Thus, conditions that hinder the release of bile into the small intestine decrease the bioavailability of vitamin K and ultimately increase the length of time that is required for blood to clot. When bile salts are given with vitamin K concentrate, the blood-clotting time returns to normal. See the Drug-Nutrient Interaction box entitled "Vitamin K Considerations with Anticoagulant and Antibiotic Medications" for additional information about special medication-related considerations with vitamin K.

Drug-Nutrient Interaction

Vitamin K Considerations with Anticoagulant and Antibiotic Medications

Anticoagulation medications such as warfarin act to reduce the overall production of blood-clotting factors. Because the primary action of vitamin K is the manufacturing of these same proteins, the amount of vitamin-K–rich foods that a patient eats can affect the medication dose necessary for optimal coagulation control. Many patients have been led to believe that they should completely avoid all foods that are rich in vitamin K while they are taking warfarin. Doing so would lead to an undesirable and unnecessary restriction of many nutrient-rich vegetables and the many vitamins and minerals found within these foods. Alternatively, patients should strive to eat a diet with a relatively consistent amount of vitamin-K–rich foods like dark leafy greens. A dietitian can educate the patient about foods that are rich in vitamin K and help them to achieve a balance between their medication level and their desired vitamin K intake.

One form of vitamin K, menaquinone, is synthesized by healthy bacteria in the gut. This source is significant for meeting overall vitamin K needs. Therefore, the long-term use of medications that destroy gastrointestinal bacteria (e.g., antibiotics) also obliterates a valuable source of vitamin K. Patients should be advised to maintain their daily intakes of food sources of vitamin K (Table 7-4).

Bone Development

Several proteins involved in bone metabolism require vitamin K–dependent modifications to function.[26] The most abundant noncollagenous protein in bone matrix, osteocalcin, is one of the vitamin K–dependent proteins. Vitamin K is involved in the modification of the glutamic acid residues of osteocalcin to form calcium-binding γ-carboxyglutamic acid residues. Like the blood-clotting proteins, osteocalcin binds calcium; unlike the blood-clotting proteins, it forms bone crystals.

REQUIREMENTS

Because intestinal bacteria synthesize menaquinone, a constant supply is normally available to support body needs. Currently not enough scientific evidence is available to establish an RDA; thus, AIs are the

Table 7-4   Food Sources of Vitamin K

VEGETABLES	QUANTITY	AMOUNT (mcg)
Collard greens, cooked, drained	1 cup, chopped	773
Kale, cooked, drained	1 cup, chopped	1062
Mustard greens, cooked, drained	1 cup, chopped	830
Spinach, cooked, drained	1 cup, chopped	889
Swiss chard, cooked, drained	1 cup, chopped	523
Turnip greens, cooked, drained	1 cup, chopped	530

Data from the U.S. Department of Agriculture, Agricultural Research Service. Nutrient Data Laboratory. *USDA nutrient database for standard reference* (website): <http://ndb.nal.usda.gov/ndb/>; Accessed September 17, 2014.

reference values instead. The AIs are listed in the summary table for fat-soluble vitamins (see Table 7-5) and in the DRI tables in Appendix B.

DEFICIENCY

Primary deficiency of vitamin K is not common. However, a deficiency (i.e., hypoprothrombinemia) may present as a secondary result of another clinical condition. Patients who have severe malabsorption disorders (e.g., Crohn's disease) or who are treated chronically with antibiotics that kill intestinal bacteria are susceptible to vitamin K deficiency.

Infants do not have adequate vitamin K stores at birth because vitamin K does not efficiently transfer through the placenta during gestation, and the intestinal tract of a newborn does not yet have vitamin K–producing gut flora. Consequently, vitamin K is routinely given at birth to prevent hemorrhaging.

TOXICITY

Toxicity from vitamin K has not been observed. Therefore, no UL has been established.

FOOD SOURCES AND STABILITY

Green, leafy vegetables such as spinach, collard greens, and kale are the best dietary sources of vitamin K, providing 100 to 1000 mcg of phylloquinone per cup of cooked food (see Table 7-4).

Phylloquinone is fairly stable, although it is sensitive to light and irradiation. Therefore, clinical preparations are kept in dark bottles.

Table 7-5 provides a summary of the fat-soluble vitamins.

primary deficiency deficiency of a nutrient due to inadequate dietary intake. Different from secondary causes where the deficiency is due to malabsorption or other bioavailability hindrances.

Table 7-5   Summary of Fat-Soluble Vitamins

VITAMIN	FUNCTIONS	RECOMMENDED INTAKE (ADULTS)	DEFICIENCY	TOLERABLE UPPER INTAKE LEVEL (UL) AND TOXICITY	SOURCES
Vitamin A (retinol, retinal, and retinoic acid) Provitamin A (carotene)	Vision cycle: adaptation to light and dark; tissue growth, especially skin and mucous membranes; reproduction; immune function	Men, 900 mcg/day; women, 700 mcg/day	Night blindness; xerosis; xerophthalmia; susceptibility to epithelial infection; dry skin; impaired immunity, growth, and reproduction	UL: 3000 mcg/day Hair loss; skin irritation; bone pain, liver damage; birth defects	Retinol (animal foods): cod liver oil, liver, egg yolk, cream, butter, fortified dairy products Provitamin A (plant foods): dark green and deep orange vegetables (e.g., spinach, collard greens, pumpkin, sweet potatoes, carrots)
Vitamin D (cholecalciferol, ergocalciferol)	Maintain calcium and phosphorus homeostasis; calcification of bones and teeth; growth	Between the ages of 1 and 70 years, 600 IU/day; 70 years of age or older, 800 IU/day	Rickets and growth retardation in children; osteomalacia in adults	UL: 1000 to 4000 IU/day Calcification of soft tissue; kidney damage; growth retardation	Synthesized in the skin with exposure to sunlight, fortified milk products, fatty fish, fish oils
Vitamin E (α-tocopherol)	Antioxidant	Adults, 15 mg/day	Breakdown of red blood cells; anemia; nerve damage; retinopathy	UL: 1000 mg/day (from supplements) Inhibition of vitamin K activity in blood clotting	Vegetable oils, vegetable greens, wheat germ, nuts, seeds
Vitamin K (phylloquinone, menaquinone)	Normal blood clotting and bone development	Men, 120 mcg/day; women, 90 mcg/day	Bleeding tendencies; hemorrhagic disease; poor bone growth	UL: Not set Interference with anticoagulation drugs	Synthesis by intestinal bacteria, dark green leafy vegetables

SECTION 2   WATER-SOLUBLE VITAMINS

VITAMIN C (ASCORBIC ACID)

FUNCTIONS

Vitamin C has several critical functions in the body. It acts as an antioxidant and as a cofactor of enzymes, and it plays a role in many metabolic and immunologic activities.

Connective Tissue

Ascorbic acid is necessary to build and maintain strong tissues through its involvement in collagen synthesis. Collagen is especially important in tissues of mesodermal origin, including connective tissues (e.g.,

---

ascorbic acid the chemical name for vitamin C; the vitamin was named after its ability to cure scurvy.

---

ligaments, tendons, bone matrix, other binding lattices that hold together and give tensile strength to tissues) and other tissues that contain connective tissue (e.g., cartilage, tooth dentin, capillary walls).

Every time the amino acids proline or lysine are added during collagen synthesis, they are hydroxylated (i.e., OH is added) to form hydroxyproline and hydroxylysine by the ascorbic acid–dependent enzymes prolyl hydroxylase and lysyl hydroxylase, respectively. Iron is a cofactor for both enzymes, and ascorbic acid is required to maintain the iron atoms in these enzymes in their active ferrous (Fe^{2+}) form. Hydroxyproline and hydroxylysine form covalent bonds with other residues, which strengthen collagen's structure. When ascorbic acid is plentiful, collagen and the connective tissues in which it is integral quickly develop. Blood vessels are particularly dependent on ascorbic acid's role in collagen synthesis to help their walls resist stretching as blood is forced through them.

General Body Metabolism

The more metabolically active body tissues (e.g., adrenal glands, brain, kidney, liver, pancreas, thymus, spleen) contain greater concentrations of ascorbic acid. Ascorbic acid in the adrenal glands is drawn upon when the gland is stimulated. This use of ascorbic acid during adrenal stimulation suggests an increased need for ascorbic acid during stress. Other enzymes that require ascorbic acid perform very diverse functions, including the following: (1) the conversion of the neurotransmitter dopamine to the neurotransmitter norepinephrine; (2) the synthesis of carnitine, a mitochondrial fatty acid transporter that is involved in extracting energy from fatty acids; (3) the oxidation of phenylalanine and tyrosine; (4) the metabolism of tryptophan and folate; and (5) the maturation of some bioactive neural and endocrine peptides. Furthermore, ascorbic acid helps the body to absorb nonheme iron by keeping it in its bioactive reduced ferrous form (Fe^{2+}), thereby making it available for hemoglobin production and helping to prevent iron deficiency anemia.

Antioxidant Function

Similar to vitamin E in function, ascorbic acid is an antioxidant that works to protect the body from damage caused by free radicals. Free radicals lead to oxidative stress, which is associated with increased risks of inflammatory diseases, Alzheimer's disease, cancer, and heart disease.

REQUIREMENTS

The DRIs for vitamin C are listed in the summary table for water-soluble vitamins (see Table 7-14) and in the DRI tables in Appendix B. Because cigarette smoke increases oxidative stress and free radicals in body tissues, the DRI committee recommends an additional 35 mg/day of vitamin C for smokers (see the Clinical Applications box, "Ascorbic Acid Needs in Smokers").

DEFICIENCY

Signs of ascorbic acid deficiency include tissue bleeding (e.g., easy bruising, pinpoint skin hemorrhages; Figure 7-5, *A*), joint bleeding, susceptibility to bone fracture, poor wound healing, bleeding gums, and tooth loss (Figure 7-5, *B*). Extreme deficiency results in the disease scurvy.

TOXICITY

The UL for ascorbic acid is 2000 mg/day. Although most excessive intakes of water-soluble vitamins are efficiently excreted in the urine, levels of more than 2000 mg/day are cleared less efficiently and may result in gastrointestinal disturbances and osmotic diarrhea. The Institute of Medicine states that further research into the toxic effects of ascorbic acid is warranted because of the popularity of high intake of the vitamin in the United States.[21]

FOOD SOURCES AND STABILITY

The best food sources of ascorbic acid include citrus fruits, bell peppers, and kiwis. Additional good sources include berries, broccoli, tomato juice, and other green and yellow vegetables (Table 7-6).

Ascorbic acid is readily oxidized upon exposure to air and heat. Therefore, care must be taken when handling its food sources. Ascorbic acid is not stable in alkaline mediums; thus, baking soda, which often

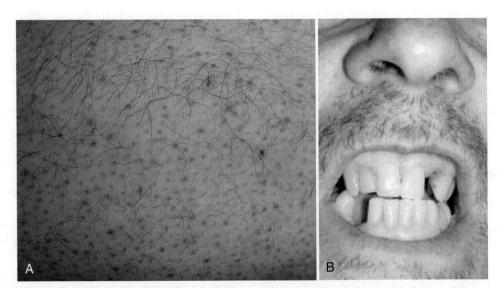

FIGURE 7-5 Scurvy observed on the skin and in the mouth. (*A*, From Al-Dabagh, A., et al., A disease of the present: scurvy in "well-nourished" patients. *J Am Acad Dermatol*, 2013. 69(5): p. e246-7; *B*, Courtesy Nicholas D Magee, Royal Victoria Hospital In Minerva, BMJ: *British Medical Journal* 326(7379):60, 2003.)

Clinical Applications

Ascorbic Acid Needs in Smokers

Free radicals are reactive molecules that can disrupt the normal structure of DNA, proteins, carbohydrates, and fatty acids. Such damage is linked to an increased risk of cancer and cardiovascular disease. Cigarette smoke is one environmental source of free radicals—for both the smoker and anyone inhaling second-hand smoke.[1] The body fights free radicals with antioxidants such as vitamins A, E, and C and minerals such as selenium and zinc. Antioxidants help neutralize free radicals and work to protect the body on a cellular level.

As free radical production increases so does the need for antioxidants. Ascorbic acid is the specific antioxidant essential to the process of breaking down the toxic compounds found in cigarette smoke. Thus, cigarette smokers deplete their supply of ascorbic acid more rapidly than nonsmokers. In addition to the general health recommendation of discontinuing the habit of smoking, it is also recommended that cigarette smokers consume an extra 35 mg of vitamin C per day to help fight the additional free radical damage invoked by smoking.

REFERENCE

1. Moritsugu KP. The 2006 Report of the Surgeon General: the health consequences of involuntary exposure to tobacco smoke. *Am J Prev Med*. 2007;32(6):542-543.

Table 7-6 Food Sources of Vitamin C

ITEM	QUANTITY	AMOUNT (mg)
Vegetables		
Peppers, hot chili, red, raw	½ cup, chopped	108
Red pepper, sweet, raw	½ cup, chopped	95
Tomato, juice, canned	½ cup	85
Fruits, Raw		
Kiwi	½ cup sliced	83
Lemon juice	8 fl oz	94
Orange juice	8 fl oz	124
Orange, navel	1 medium	83
Papaya	1 cup pieces	88

Data from the U.S. Department of Agriculture, Agricultural Research Service. Nutrient Data Laboratory. *USDA nutrient database for standard reference* (website): <http://ndb.nal.usda.gov/ndb/>; Accessed September 17, 2014.

is added to foods to preserve color, destroys the ascorbic acid content. Acidic fruits and vegetables retain their ascorbic acid content better than nonacidic foods, and the vitamin is also highly soluble in water. The more water added for cooking, the more ascorbic acid leaches out of the fruit or vegetable into the cooking water.

THIAMIN (VITAMIN B₁)

The name of the vitamin **thiamin** comes from the presence of the thiazole ring in its structure.

FUNCTIONS

Thiamin is a component of the coenzyme thiamin pyrophosphate, which is involved in several metabolic reactions that ultimately provide the body with energy in the form of adenosine triphosphate (ATP). Thiamin is especially necessary for the healthy function of systems that are in constant action and in need of energy, such as the gastrointestinal tract, the nervous system, and the cardiovascular system.

REQUIREMENTS

The dietary requirement for thiamin is directly related to its function in energy and carbohydrate metabolism. The DRIs are listed in the summary table for water-soluble vitamins (see Table 7-14) and in the DRI tables in Appendix B. Increased thiamin intake is necessary during pregnancy, lactation, and other conditions or lifestyles that increase total kilocalorie needs above the average daily energy requirement. Diseases and conditions that accelerate glucose metabolism, such as fever, also increase the body's use of thiamin and thus the requirement.

DEFICIENCY

Due to thiamin's involvement in the generation of ATP, a deficiency of the nutrient will have downstream effects on energy availability. The gastrointestinal tract relies on a steady supply of energy for muscular activity. Therefore, a lack of dietary thiamin may result in constipation, indigestion, and a poor appetite. The central nervous system also depends on constant energy. Without sufficient thiamin, alertness and reflexes decrease, and apathy, fatigue, and irritability result. If the thiamin deficit continues, nerve irritation, pain, and prickly or numbing sensations may eventually progress to paralysis.

Chronic thiamin deficiency is known as **beriberi**; this paralyzing disease was especially prevalent in Asian countries that relied heavily on polished white rice as a food staple. The name describes the disease well; it is Singhalese for "I can't, I can't," because afflicted people are too ill to do anything. In industrialized societies, thiamin deficiency is largely associated with chronic alcoholism and poor diet. Alcohol inhibits the absorption of thiamin. Alcohol-induced thiamin deficiency causes a debilitating brain disorder known as

thiamin the chemical name of vitamin B₁; this vitamin was discovered in relation to the classic deficiency disease beriberi, and it is important in body metabolism as a coenzyme factor in many cell reactions related to energy metabolism.

beriberi a disease of the peripheral nerves that is caused by a deficiency of thiamin (vitamin B₁) and is characterized by pain (neuritis) and paralysis of legs and arms, cardiovascular changes, and edema.

Wernicke's encephalopathy, which affects mental alertness, short-term memory, and muscle coordination.

TOXICITY

The kidneys clear excess thiamin; therefore, there is no evidence of toxicity from oral intake, and no UL exists.

FOOD SOURCES AND STABILITY

Although thiamin is widespread in most plant and animal tissues, the amount is usually small. Thus, thiamin deficiency is a distinct possibility when food intake is markedly curtailed (e.g., with alcoholism or highly inadequate diets). Good food sources of thiamin include yeast, pork, whole or **enriched** grains (e.g., flour, bread, cereals), and legumes (Table 7-7). Some raw fish contain a thiamin-degrading enzyme (i.e., thiaminase) and consequently are not good sources.

Neutral or alkaline environments will destroy thiamin. As with other water-soluble vitamins, prepared foods retain more thiamin when the cooking water is consumed with the dish rather than discarded.

RIBOFLAVIN (VITAMIN B₂)

The name **riboflavin** comes from the vitamin's chemical nature. It is a yellow-green fluorescent pigment that contains ribose, which is a monosaccharide with five carbons.

FUNCTIONS

Riboflavin is active in its coenzyme forms: flavin adenine dinucleotide (FAD) and flavin mononucleotide (FMN). These two flavin coenzymes are required for macronutrient metabolism to produce ATP via the

> **enriched** a word that is used to describe foods to which vitamins and minerals have been added back to a food after a refining process that caused a loss of some nutrients; for example, iron may be lost during the refining process of a grain, so the final product will be enriched with additional iron.
>
> **riboflavin** the chemical name for vitamin B₂; it has a role as a coenzyme factor in many cell reactions related to energy and protein metabolism.

Krebs cycle and the electron transport chain. Flavoproteins are involved in a number of other metabolic reactions as well. Some examples of riboflavin-dependent reactions include converting the amino acid tryptophan to niacin (vitamin B₃), converting retinal to retinoic acid, and synthesizing the active form of folate.

REQUIREMENTS

Riboflavin needs are related to total energy requirements for age, level of exercise, body size, metabolic rate, and rate of growth. As with thiamin, the RDA is based on average energy use. The DRIs for thiamin are listed in the summary table for water-soluble vitamins (see Table 7-14) and in the DRI tables in Appendix B.

DEFICIENCY

Areas of the body with rapid cell regeneration are most affected by riboflavin deficiency. Symptoms include cracked lips and mouth corners; a swollen, red tongue; burning, itching, or tearing eyes caused by extra blood vessels in the cornea; and a scaly, greasy dermatitis in the skin folds. Riboflavin deficiency usually occurs in conjunction with other B vitamin and nutrient deficiencies (e.g., protein malnutrition) rather than alone. A rare riboflavin-specific deficiency has been given the general name *ariboflavinosis* (i.e., without riboflavin). Its symptoms are tissue inflammation and breakdown and poor wound healing; even minor injuries become easily aggravated and do not heal well.

TOXICITY

No adverse effects of riboflavin intake from food or supplements have been reported. Thus, there is no UL for riboflavin.

FOOD SOURCES AND STABILITY

One of the most frequently consumed natural food source of riboflavin is milk. Each serving of milk contains about 0.5 mg of riboflavin. Other good sources include enriched grains, animal protein sources such as meats (especially beef liver), almonds, and soybeans. Table 7-8 provides a summary of riboflavin food sources.

Riboflavin is destroyed by light; therefore, milk is usually sold and stored in plastic or cardboard cartons instead of glass containers to preserve the vitamin.

Table 7-7	Food Sources of Thiamin	
ITEM	**QUANTITY**	**AMOUNT (mg)**
Bread, Cereal, Rice, and Pasta		
All-Bran Complete cereal, Kellogg's	1 cup	2.0
Product 19 cereal, Kellogg's	1 cup	1.5
Quaker Oat Life cereal, Kellogg's	1 cup	0.54
Total Whole Grain cereal, General Mills	1 cup	2.0
Yeast extract spread	1 tsp	1.4
Meat, Poultry, Fish, Dry Beans, Eggs, and Nuts		
Beans, black, cooked	1 cup	0.42
Ham, sliced, regular (11% fat)	3 oz	0.53
Pork loin, lean, boneless, roasted	3 oz	0.45

Data from the U.S. Department of Agriculture, Agricultural Research Service. Nutrient Data Laboratory. *USDA nutrient database for standard reference* (website): <http://ndb.nal.usda.gov/ndb/>; Accessed September 17, 2014.

Table 7-8	Food Sources of Riboflavin	
ITEM	**QUANTITY**	**AMOUNT (mg)**
Bread, Cereal, Rice, and Pasta		
All-Bran Complete cereal, Kellogg's	1 cup	2.27
Product 19 cereal, Kellogg's	1 cup	1.7
Total Whole Grain cereal, General Mills	1 cup	2.28
Meat, Poultry, Fish, Dry Beans, Eggs, and Nuts		
Beef liver, fried	3 oz	2.9
Chicken liver, simmered	3 oz	1.7
Soybeans, raw	½ cup	0.81
Milk and Dairy Products		
Milk, skim or whole	8 fl oz	0.45
Soy milk	8 fl oz	0.5
Yogurt, low fat	8 fl oz	0.52

Data from the U.S. Department of Agriculture, Agricultural Research Service. Nutrient Data Laboratory. *USDA nutrient database for standard reference* (website): <http://ndb.nal.usda.gov/ndb/>; Accessed September 17, 2014.

NIACIN (VITAMIN B₃)

FUNCTIONS

Niacin is part of two coenzymes. The role of one of the niacin-containing coenzymes (nicotinamide adenine dinucleotide, NAD) is the metabolism of the macronutrients. You should notice the theme among the B vitamin functions with regard to their role in macronutrient metabolism. The function of this niacin-containing coenzyme is similar to that of the coenzymes containing riboflavin and thiamin. The other niacin-containing coenzyme (nicotinamide adenine dinucleotide phosphate, NADP) is involved in DNA repair and steroid hormone synthesis.

REQUIREMENTS

Factors such as age, growth, pregnancy and lactation, illness, tissue trauma, body size, and physical activity —all of which affect energy needs—influence niacin requirements. Because the body can make some of its needed niacin from the essential amino acid tryptophan, the total niacin requirement is stated in terms of niacin equivalents (NEs) to account for both sources. Approximately 60 mg of tryptophan can yield 1 mg of niacin; thus, 60 mg of tryptophan equals 1 NE. The DRIs for niacin are listed in the summary table for water-soluble vitamins (see Table 7-14) and in the DRI tables in Appendix B.

DEFICIENCY

Symptoms of general niacin deficiency are weakness, poor appetite, indigestion, and various disorders of the skin and nervous system. Skin areas that are exposed to sunlight develop a dark, scaly dermatitis. Extended deficiency may result in central nervous system damage with resulting confusion, apathy,

niacin the chemical name for vitamin B₃; this vitamin was discovered in relation to the deficiency disease pellagra; it is important as a coenzyme factor in many cell reactions related to energy and protein metabolism.

pellagra the deficiency disease caused by a lack of dietary niacin and an inadequate amount of protein that contains the amino acid tryptophan, which is a precursor of niacin; pellagra is characterized by skin lesions that are aggravated by sunlight as well as by gastrointestinal, mucosal, neurologic, and mental symptoms.

disorientation, and neuritis. Such signs of nervous system damage are seen in patients with chronic alcoholism. The deficiency disease that is associated with niacin is **pellagra,** which is characterized by the four Ds: *d*ermatitis, *d*iarrhea, *d*ementia, and *d*eath (Figure 7-6). When therapeutic doses of niacin are given, pellagra symptoms improve. Pellagra was common in the United States and parts of Europe during the early twentieth century in regions where corn (which is low in niacin) was the staple food. In the southern United States, more than 3 million cases of pellagra resulted in an estimated 100,000 deaths between 1900 and 1940.[27]

TOXICITY

Excessive niacin intake can produce adverse physical effects, unlike high intakes of thiamin and riboflavin. The UL is 35 mg/day, which is based on the skin flushing caused by high supplemental intakes.[28] Although no evidence exists of adverse effects from consuming

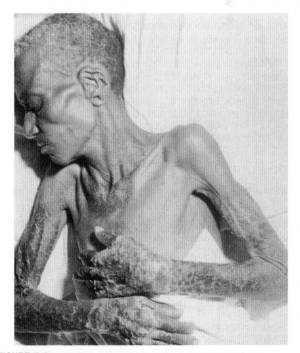

FIGURE 7-6 Pellagra, which results from a niacin deficiency. (Reprinted from McLaren DS. *A Colour Atlas and Text of Diet-Related Disorders.* 2nd ed. London: Mosby–Year Book; 1992.)

niacin that naturally occurs in food, evidence does exist for excessive niacin consumption and adverse effects from nonprescription vitamin supplements and niacin-containing prescription medications. The primary reaction is a reddened flush on the skin of the face, arms, and chest that is accompanied by burning, tingling, and itching. This reaction also occurs in many patients who are therapeutically treated with niacin (see the Clinical Applications box, "Niacin as a Treatment for High Cholesterol").

☁ Clinical Applications

Niacin as a Treatment for High Cholesterol

In addition to the many other important functions of niacin, high-dose niacin supplements can improve blood lipid profiles. At doses of 1500 mg per day, niacin decreases low-density lipoprotein cholesterol and triglyceride levels, both of which are linked with cardiovascular disease. In addition, pharmacologic doses of niacin improve high-density lipoprotein cholesterol levels; this is the "good" cholesterol. When niacin is used in this sense, it is functioning as a drug rather than as a vitamin, and it should be used *only* under medical supervision. Patients with cardiovascular disease who take a statin medication do not benefit further from supplemental niacin; thus, it is not recommended to take both.[1,2]

To understand the potentially beneficial role of niacin at pharmacologic dosing, the potential side effects must also be understood. The RDA for niacin in adult men and women is 16 mg/day and 14 mg/day, respectively. The UL for niacin is 35 mg/day. Therefore, a long-term dose of 1500 mg/day has serious side effects. Adverse effects from pharmacologic dosing are the same as the toxicity effects: flushing of the skin, tingling sensation in the extremities, nausea, and vomiting. Some individuals may even experience liver damage if long-term use is continued unsupervised for months or years at a time. Physicians will periodically check liver enzymes for patients on niacin supplementation or statin medications to monitor any side effects of either medication.

REFERENCES

1. Kolber MR, Ivers N, Allan GM. Niacin added to statins for cardiovascular disease. *Can Fam Physician*. 2012;58(8):842.
2. Keene D, et al. Effect on cardiovascular risk of high density lipoprotein targeted drug treatments niacin, fibrates, and CETP inhibitors: meta-analysis of randomised controlled trials including 117,411 patients. *BMJ*. 2014;349:4379.

FOOD SOURCES AND STABILITY

Meat is a good source of niacin. Most dietary niacin in the United States comes from meat, poultry, or fish (Table 7-9). Enriched and whole-grain breads, bread products, and ready-to-eat cereals have ample levels of niacin. Peanuts are another good source of niacin.

Niacin is stable in acidic mediums and in heat, but it is lost in cooking water unless the water is retained and consumed (e.g., in soup).

VITAMIN B₆

The name **pyridoxine** comes from the pyridine ring in the structure of this vitamin. The term *vitamin*

Table 7-9   Food Sources of Niacin

ITEM	QUANTITY	AMOUNT (mg OF NIACIN EQUIVALENTS)
Bread, Cereal, Rice, and Pasta		
All-Bran Complete cereal, Kellogg's	1 cup	26.7
Product 19 cereal, Kellogg's	1 cup	20.0
Total Whole Grain cereal, General Mills	1 cup	26.7
Wheaties cereal, General Mills	1 cup	13.3
Meat, Poultry, Fish, Dry Beans, Eggs, and Nuts*		
Beef liver, fried	3 oz	14.9
Chicken, light meat, boneless, roasted	3 oz	8.9
Chicken liver, pan-fried	3 oz	11.8
Mackerel, cooked, dry heat	3 oz	9.0
Peanuts, raw	½ cup	8.8

Data from the U.S. Department of Agriculture, Agricultural Research Service. Nutrient Data Laboratory. *USDA nutrient database for standard reference* (website): <http://ndb.nal.usda.gov/ndb/>; Accessed September 25, 2014.
*The amino acid tryptophan can be converted into niacin. Therefore, foods that are high in tryptophan also are significant sources of niacin.

B₆ collectively refers to a group of six related compounds: pyridoxine, pyridoxal, pyridoxamine, and their respective activated phosphate forms. Two of the phosphorylated compounds are the coenzymes pyridoxal 5′-phosphate and pyridoxamine 5′-phosphate.

FUNCTIONS

Pyridoxal 5′-phosphate, which is the metabolically active form of vitamin B₆, has an essential role in protein metabolism and in many cell reactions that involve amino acids. It is involved in neurotransmitter synthesis and, thus, in brain and central nervous system activity. Unlike most water-soluble vitamins, vitamin B₆ is stored in tissues throughout the body, particularly muscle. It participates in amino acid absorption, ATP production, the synthesis of the heme portion of hemoglobin, and niacin formation from tryptophan. Enzymes that make use of vitamin B₆ coenzymes are also involved in carbohydrate and fat metabolism.

REQUIREMENTS

Vitamin B₆ is involved in amino acid metabolism; therefore, needs vary directly in response to protein intake and utilization. The DRIs for vitamin B₆ are

pyridoxine the chemical name of vitamin B₆; in its activated phosphate form (i.e., B_2PO_4), pyridoxine functions as an important coenzyme factor in many reactions in cell metabolism that are related to amino acids, glucose, and fatty acids.

listed in the summary table for water-soluble vitamins (see Table 7-14) and in the DRI tables in Appendix B.

DEFICIENCY

A vitamin B_6 deficiency is unlikely, because more of the vitamin is available in a typical diet than is required. A vitamin B_6 deficiency causes abnormal central nervous system function with hyperirritability, neuritis, and possible convulsions. Vitamin B_6 deficiency is one cause of microcytic hypochromic anemia, because it is required for heme synthesis (part of the red blood cell protein hemoglobin).

TOXICITY

High vitamin B_6 intake from food does not result in adverse effects, but large supplemental doses can cause uncoordinated movement and nerve damage. Symptoms improve when supplemental overdosing is discontinued. The UL for adults is 100 mg/day on the basis of studies that related vitamin B_6 dosage to nerve damage.[28]

FOOD SOURCES AND STABILITY

Vitamin B_6 is widespread in foods. Good sources include grains, enriched cereals, liver and kidney, and other meats (Table 7-10). Limited amounts are found in legumes.

Table 7-10 Food Sources of Vitamin B_6 (Pyridoxine)

ITEM	QUANTITY	AMOUNT (mg)
Bread, Cereal, Rice, and Pasta		
All-Bran cereal, Kellogg's	½ cup	3.72
Complete Wheat Flakes cereal, Kellogg's	1 cup	2.67
Mueslix cereal, Kellogg's	⅔ cup	1.96
Total Whole Grain cereal, General Mills	1 cup	2.67
Fruits and Vegetables		
Banana	1 medium (118 g)	0.43
Potato, baked, with skin	1 medium (173 g)	0.54
Meat, Poultry, Fish, Dry Beans, Eggs, and Nuts		
Beef liver, fried	3 oz	0.87
Chicken, light meat, boneless, roasted	3 oz	0.46
Chicken liver, simmered	3 oz	0.64
Lentils, cooked, boiled	1 cup	0.35
Pistachios, raw	1 oz	0.48
Salmon, cooked, dry heat	3 oz	0.59
Sirloin steak, lean, broiled	3 oz	0.45

Data from the U.S. Department of Agriculture, Agricultural Research Service. Nutrient Data Laboratory. *USDA nutrient database for standard reference* (website): <http://ndb.nal.usda.gov/ndb/>; Accessed September 25, 2014.

Vitamin B_6 is stable to heat but sensitive to light and alkalis.

FOLATE

The given name *folate* comes from the Latin word *folium*, meaning "leaf," because it was originally discovered in dark green, leafy vegetables. In nutrition, the term *folate* refers loosely to a large class of molecules that are derived from folic acid (i.e., pteroylglutamic acid) found in plants and animals. The most stable form of folate is folic acid, which is rarely found naturally in food but which is the form that is usually used in vitamin supplements and fortified food products. In the body, folate is converted to and used as the coenzyme tetrahydrofolic acid (TH_4).

FUNCTIONS

TH_4 participates in DNA synthesis (with the enzyme thymidylate synthetase) as well as cell division. TH_4 is involved in the synthesis of the amino acid glycine, which in turn is required for heme synthesis and thus hemoglobin synthesis.

TH_4 also participates in the reduction of blood homocysteine concentration and indirectly in gene expression (with the enzyme methionine synthase). **Hyperhomocysteinemia** is common in patients with cardiovascular disease. However, whether this contributes to or is merely an effect of cardiovascular disease has not been determined because lowering homocysteine levels through folic acid supplementation does not subsequently lower the risk for cardiovascular events or all-cause mortality.[29]

REQUIREMENTS

Dietary folate equivalencies (DFEs) are used to express the DRI for folate because the bioavailability of naturally occurring food folate differs from that of synthetic folic acid.[30] One mcg of DFE equals 1 mcg of food folate, 0.5 mcg of folic acid taken on an empty stomach, or 0.6 mcg of folic acid taken with food. As a result of the role of folate in cell division during embryogenesis, adequate preconception and pregnancy intakes are linked to reduced neural tube defect occurrences. Thus, the DRIs include a special recommendation that all women who are capable of becoming pregnant take 400 mcg/day of synthetic folic acid from fortified foods or supplements in addition to natural folate found in a varied diet. The DRI recommendations (listed in the summary tables for water-soluble vitamins [see Table 7-14] and in Appendix B) are aimed at providing adequate safety allowances that include specific population groups that are at risk

hyperhomocysteinemia the presence of high levels of homocysteine in the blood; associated with cardiovascular disease.

for deficiency, such as pregnant women, adolescents, and older adults.[28]

DEFICIENCY

Folate deficiency impairs DNA and RNA synthesis. Thus, rapidly dividing cells are affected quickly by folate deficiency. When red blood cells cannot divide, the result is large and immature erythrocytes (i.e., megaloblastic macrocytic anemia). If the deficiency is not corrected, symptoms may progress to poor growth in children, weakness, depression, and neuropathy. Pregnant and lactating women are particularly susceptible to diminished blood folate concentrations and anemia as a result of their higher needs.

Neural tube defects (NTDs) such as spina bifida and anencephaly are some of the most common birth defects in the United States, occurring in approximately 1 in every 1000 pregnancies (Figure 7-7). This defect occurs within the first 28 days after conception, often before a woman realizes that she is pregnant. Although the exact causes of neural tube defects are

> **spina bifida** a congenital defect in the embryonic fetal closing of the neural tube to form a portion of the lower spine, which leaves the spine unclosed and the spinal cord open to various degrees of exposure and damage.
> **anencephaly** the congenital absence of the brain that results from the incomplete closure of the upper end of the neural tube.

not known, adequate stores of folic acid before conception and during early gestation reduce the risk for neural tube defect–affected pregnancies.[31]

TOXICITY

No negative effects have been observed from the consumption of folate from foods. However, some evidence shows that excessive folic acid can mask biochemical indicators of vitamin B_{12} deficiency. Prolonged B_{12} deficiency can result in permanent nerve damage; therefore, the adult UL for supplemental folic acid (not DFE) has been set at 1000 mcg/day.[28]

FOOD SOURCES AND STABILITY

Folate is widely distributed in foods (Table 7-11). Rich sources include green, leafy vegetables; orange juice; legumes; and chicken liver. Since January 1998, as part of an effort to reduce the occurrences of neural tube defects, the U.S. Food and Drug Administration has required all manufacturers of certain grain products

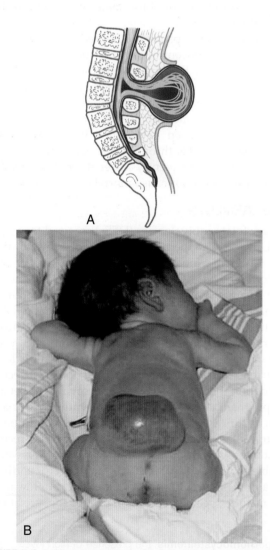

FIGURE 7-7 **A,** Myelomeningocele. **B,** Spina bifida in a child at birth with a cutaneous defect over the lumbar spine. (**B,** Courtesy Dr. Robert C. Dauser, Baylor College of Medicine, Houston, Tex.)

Table 7-11 **Food Sources of Folate**

ITEM	QUANTITY	AMOUNT (mcg OF DFE)
Bread, Cereal, Rice, and Pasta		
All-Bran Complete Wheat Flakes cereal, Kellogg's	1 cup	901
Mueslix cereal, Kellogg's	⅔ cup	674
Product 19 cereal, Kellogg's	1 cup	676
Quaker Oat Life cereal, Kellogg's	1 cup	941
Total Whole Grain cereal, General Mills	1 cup	901
Fruits and Vegetables		
Asparagus, cooked	½ cup	134
Orange juice, fresh	1 cup, 8 oz	74
Spinach, cooked, boiled	½ cup	131
Meat, Poultry, Fish, Dry Beans, Eggs, and Nuts		
Chicken liver, simmered	3 oz	491
Garbanzo beans (chickpeas), cooked, boiled	½ cup	141
Lentils, cooked, boiled	½ cup	179

Data from the U.S. Department of Agriculture, Agricultural Research Service. Nutrient Data Laboratory. *USDA nutrient database for standard reference* (website): <http://ndb.nal.usda.gov/ndb/>; Accessed September 25, 2014.

(e.g., enriched white flour; white rice; corn grits; corn-meal; noodles; fortified breakfast cereals, bread, rolls, and buns) to fortify with folic acid. The fortification of the general food supply has successfully reduced the prevalence of NTDs in the United States by 22.9%.[32] Although there are other non–folate-related causes for NTDs, supplemental folic acid can improve the folate status of women and improve pregnancy outcomes.[33]

The special DRI recommendation that women who are capable of becoming pregnant consume folic acid from supplements or fortified foods is one of only two current RDAs that specifically recommend consuming vitamin sources in addition to those available in a varied diet of natural foods.

Folate is easily destroyed by heat, and it easily leaches into cooking water, especially when the food is submerged in the water. As much as 50% to 90% of food folate may be destroyed during food processing, storage, and preparation.

COBALAMIN (VITAMIN B$_{12}$)

The name **cobalamin** was derived from cobalt, which is the trace mineral that is the single gray atom at the center of cobalamin's corrin ring. The term *vitamin B$_{12}$* originally referred to the synthetic pharmaceutical molecule cyanocobalamin. In nutrition, it has become a term for all cobalamin derivatives, including the two biologically active coenzyme derivatives methylcobalamin and deoxyadenosylcobalamin.

FUNCTIONS

Vitamin B$_{12}$ is essential for DNA synthesis and cell division. There are two cobalamin-dependent coenzymes with critical biologic activity.

Methylcobalamin is a coenzyme that is required for the catalytic activity of two of the same enzymes as tetrahydrofolic acid: methionine synthase and serine hydroxymethyltransferase. Thus, like tetrahydrofolic acid, methylcobalamin participates in the reduction of blood homocysteine concentration and indirectly in gene expression. Methylcobalamin is also involved in the production of the amino acid glycine, which in turn is required for heme synthesis and therefore hemoglobin synthesis.

Deoxyadenosylcobalamin is a coenzyme for the mitochondrial enzyme methylmalonyl-coenzyme A mutase, which is involved in the metabolism of fatty acids that have an odd number of carbon atoms.

cobalamin the chemical name for vitamin B$_{12}$; this vitamin is found mainly in animal protein food sources; it is closely related to amino acid metabolism and the formation of the heme portion of hemoglobin; the absence of hydrochloric acid and intrinsic factor leads to pernicious anemia and degenerative effects on the nervous system.

REQUIREMENTS

The amount of dietary vitamin B$_{12}$ needed for normal human metabolism is quite small, consisting of only a few micrograms per day. A mixed diet that includes animal foods easily provides this much and more. The DRIs for vitamin B$_{12}$ are listed in the summary table for water-soluble vitamins (see Table 7-14) and in the DRI tables in Appendix B. The DRIs include a special recommendation that both men and women who are 50 years old and older meet their RDA with vitamin B$_{12}$–fortified foods or supplements due to decreased absorption with age.[28]

DEFICIENCY

The vast majority of cobalamin deficiency cases are due to poor absorption from food as opposed to inadequate intake. A component of the gastric digestive secretions called *intrinsic factor* is necessary for the absorption of vitamin B$_{12}$ by intestinal cells (Figure 7-8). Gastrointestinal disorders that destroy the cells in the stomach (e.g., atrophic gastritis) disrupt the secretion of intrinsic factor and hydrochloric acid, both of which are needed for vitamin B$_{12}$ absorption. Diseases affecting the small intestine such as Crohn's disease may prevent absorption in the ileum. Long-term use of certain medications also interferes with cobalamin absorption; most notable are the histamine H$_2$ blockers metformin (Glucophage) and protein pump inhibitors.[34]

Primary vitamin B$_{12}$ deficiency from inadequate intake has been reported in vegans (see Chapter 4). Because foods made with animal products are the only natural sources of vitamin B$_{12}$, vegans must rely on dietary supplements or foods fortified with cobalamin to meet their daily requirements. Because many plant-based foods that are vegan friendly have been fortified with vitamin B$_{12}$, a conscientious vegan choosing such foods should not have a problem with inadequate

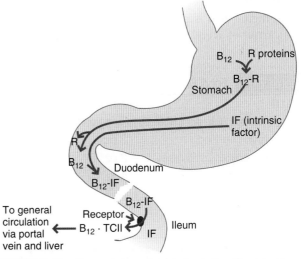

FIGURE 7-8 Digestion and absorption of vitamin B$_{12}$. (Reprinted from Mahan LK, Escott-Stump S. *Krause's Food & Nutrition Therapy.* 13th ed. Philadelphia: Saunders; 2011.)

intake. For example, fortified almond milk has 3 mcg per 8 oz cup.

The general symptoms of vitamin B_{12} deficiency include nonspecific symptoms such as fatigue, anorexia, and nausea. In advanced cases, a multitude of conditions may develop, including hematologic (e.g., **pernicious anemia**), neurologic (e.g., peripheral neuropathy), and digestive (e.g., glossitis) manifestations.[34] In such cases, vitamin B_{12} is most often administered via hypodermic injection to bypass the absorption defect.

TOXICITY

Vitamin B_{12} has not been shown to produce adverse effects in healthy individuals when intake from food or supplements exceeds body needs; therefore, no UL has been established.

FOOD SOURCES AND STABILITY

Vitamin B_{12} is bound to protein in foods. All dietary vitamin B_{12} originates from bacteria that inhabit the gastrointestinal tracts of herbivorous animals. Thus, the only naturally occurring food sources are of animal origin or come from bacteria found on unwashed plants. Human intestinal bacteria also synthesize vitamin B_{12}, but it is not bioavailable. The richest dietary sources are beef liver, lean meat, clams, oysters, herring, and crab (Table 7-12).

Vitamin B_{12} is stable throughout ordinary cooking processes.

PANTOTHENIC ACID

The name **pantothenic acid** refers to this substance's widespread functions in the body and its widespread availability in foods of all types. The name is based on the Greek word *pantothen,* meaning "from every side." Pantothenic acid is present in all living things, and it is essential to all forms of life.

FUNCTIONS

Pantothenic acid is part of coenzyme A (CoA), which is a carrier of acetyl moieties or larger acyl moieties. It is involved in cellular metabolism as well as both protein acetylation and protein acylation.

Acetyl CoA is involved in energy extraction from the fuel molecules glucose, fatty acids, and amino acids. CoA also is involved in the biosynthesis of the following: (1) sphingolipids, which are found in neural tissue; (2) some amino acids; (3) isoprenoid derivatives (e.g., cholesterol, steroid hormones, vitamins A and D); (4) δ-aminolevulinic acid, which is the precursor of the porphyrin rings in hemoglobin, the cytochromes of the electron transport chain, and the corrin ring of vitamin B_{12}; (5) the neurotransmitter acetylcholine; and (6) melatonin, which is a sleep inducer that is derived from the neurotransmitter serotonin.

REQUIREMENTS

The usual intake range of pantothenic acid in the American diet is 4 to 7 mg/day. The AIs for pantothenic acid are listed in the summary table for water-soluble vitamins (see Table 7-14) and in the DRI tables in Appendix B.

DEFICIENCY

Given its widespread natural occurrence, pantothenic acid deficiencies are unlikely. The only cases of deficiency have been in individuals who are fed synthetic diets that contain virtually no pantothenic acid.

TOXICITY

No observed adverse effects have been associated with pantothenic acid intake in people or animals. Therefore, the DRI guidelines have not established a UL for this vitamin.

FOOD SOURCES AND STABILITY

Pantothenic acid occurs as widely in foods as in body tissues. It is found in all animal and plant cells, and it is especially abundant in animal tissues, whole-grain cereals, fortified cereals, and sunflower seeds (Table 7-13). Smaller amounts are found in milk, eggs, and some vegetables.

Pantothenic acid is stable to acid and heat, but it is sensitive to alkalis.

BIOTIN

FUNCTIONS

Biotin is a coenzyme for five carboxylase enzymes. Carboxylase enzymes transfer carbon dioxide moieties

Table 7-12 Food Sources of Vitamin B_{12} (Cobalamin)

ITEM	QUANTITY	AMOUNT (mcg)
Meat, Poultry, Fish, Dry Beans, Eggs, and Nuts*		
Beef liver, pan-fried	3 oz	83
Clams, cooked, moist heat	3 oz	84
Mussels, cooked, moist heat	3 oz	20
Oysters, Pacific, cooked, moist heat	3 oz	25

Data from the U.S. Department of Agriculture, Agricultural Research Service. Nutrient Data Laboratory. *USDA nutrient database for standard reference* (website): <http://ndb.nal.usda.gov/ndb/>; Accessed September 25, 2014.
*Several vegan-friendly meat and dairy substitute products (e.g., soy milk, tofu) are fortified with vitamin B_{12}.

pernicious anemia a form of megaloblastic anemia that is caused by destroyed gastric parietal cells that produce intrinsic factor; without intrinsic factor, vitamin B_{12} cannot be absorbed.
pantothenic acid a B-complex vitamin that is found widely distributed in nature and that occurs throughout the body tissues; it is an essential constituent of the body's main activating agent, coenzyme A.

Table 7-13   Food Sources of Pantothenic Acid

ITEM	QUANTITY	AMOUNT (mg)
Bread, Cereal, Rice, and Pasta		
All-Bran Complete Wheat Flakes cereal, Kellogg's	1 cup	13.34
Total Whole Grain cereal, General Mills	1 cup	13.3
Wheat Flakes, Kellogg's Complete cereal	1 cup	13.5
Fruits and Vegetables		
Avocado, raw	1/4 medium	0.70
Portabella mushroom, grilled	1 cup, sliced	1.53
Potato, baked, with skin	1 medium (173 g)	0.66
Meat, Poultry, Fish, Dry Beans, Eggs, and Nuts		
Beef liver, fried	3 oz	5.90
Chicken liver, simmered	3 oz	5.67
Egg, whole, scrambled	1 large	0.74
Sunflower seeds, dry roasted	1 oz	2
Turkey, breast, roasted	3 oz	0.88
Milk and Dairy Products		
Milk, skim	8 fl oz	0.88
Yogurt, whole milk	8 fl oz	0.88

Data from the U.S. Department of Agriculture, Agricultural Research Service. Nutrient Data Laboratory. *USDA nutrient database for standard reference* (website): <http://ndb.nal.usda.gov/ndb/>; Accessed September 25, 2014.

from one molecule to another in the following biotin enzymes:

1. *α-Acetyl-CoA carboxylase,* which is involved in fatty acid synthesis
2. *β-Acetyl-CoA carboxylase,* which is involved in inhibiting fatty acid breakdown during the hours after starch, sucrose, or fructose is consumed
3. *Pyruvate carboxylase,* which is involved in synthesizing glucose during fasting (gluconeogenesis) or during short bursts of energy (from lactic acid)
4. *Methylcrotonyl-CoA carboxylase,* which is involved in the degradation of the amino acid leucine
5. *Propionyl-CoA carboxylase,* which is involved in the breakdown of the three-carbon fatty acid propionic acid

REQUIREMENTS

The amount of biotin needed for metabolism is extremely small, and it is measured in micrograms. The AIs for biotin are listed in the summary table for water-soluble vitamins (see Table 7-14) and in the DRI tables in Appendix B.

DEFICIENCY

There are no known natural biotin dietary deficiencies. A rare inborn error of metabolism called *biotinidase deficiency* can result in neurologic disturbances if it is left untreated, but it is treatable with lifelong oral biotin supplementation.[35]

Biotin is bound by avidin, a protein that is found in uncooked egg whites. Consequently, consuming raw eggs inhibits biotin absorption.

TOXICITY

No toxicity or other adverse effects from the consumption of biotin by people or animals are known. No data currently support setting a UL for biotin.

FOOD SOURCES AND STABILITY

Biotin is widely distributed in natural foods, but it is not equally absorbed from all of them. For example, the biotin in corn and soy meal is completely bioavailable (i.e., able to be digested and absorbed by the body). However, almost none of the biotin in wheat is bioavailable. The best food sources of biotin are liver, cooked egg yolk, soy flour, cereals (except bound forms in wheat), meats, tomatoes, and yeast. The bacteria that normally inhabit the gut also synthesize biotin, which is available for intestinal cell absorption.

Biotin is a stable vitamin, but it is water soluble. A summary of the water-soluble vitamins is given in Table 7-14.

CHOLINE

Choline is a water-soluble nutrient that is associated with the B-complex vitamins. The Institute of Medicine established an AI of choline for the first time in the 1998 DRIs.[28]

FUNCTIONS

Choline is important for maintaining the structural integrity of cell membranes as a component of the phospholipid lecithin (i.e., phosphatidylcholine). Choline is also involved in lipid transport (i.e., lipoproteins), homocysteine reduction, and the neurotransmitter acetylcholine, which is involved in involuntary functions, voluntary movement, and long-term memory storage, among other things.

REQUIREMENTS

The AIs for choline are listed in the summary table for water-soluble vitamins (see Table 7-14) and in the DRI tables in Appendix B.

DEFICIENCY

Fatty liver disease from choline deficiency has been reported in patients who are administered long-term parental nutrition devoid of choline.[36] There remains speculation about a multitude of other potential effects due to choline deficiency such as cancer, neural tube defects, dementia, and cardiovascular disease.[37]

Table 7-14 Summary of Vitamin C and the B-Complex Vitamins

VITAMIN	FUNCTIONS	RECOMMENDED INTAKE (ADULTS)	DEFICIENCY	TOLERABLE UPPER INTAKE LEVEL (UL) AND TOXICITY	SOURCES
Vitamin C (ascorbic acid)	Antioxidant; collagen synthesis; helps prepare iron for absorption and release to tissues for red blood cell formation; metabolism	Men, 90 mg; women, 75 mg; smokers: an additional 35 mg/day	Scurvy (deficiency disease); sore gums; hemorrhages, especially around bones and joints; anemia; tendency to bruise easily; impaired wound healing and tissue formation; weakened bones	UL: 2000 mg Diarrhea	Citrus fruits, kiwi, tomatoes, strawberries, chili peppers, broccoli, green and red peppers
Thiamin (vitamin B₁)	Normal growth; coenzyme in carbohydrate metabolism; normal function of heart, nerves, and muscle	Men, 1.2 mg; women, 1.1 mg	Beriberi (deficiency disease); gastrointestinal: loss of appetite, gastric distress, indigestion, deficient hydrochloric acid; central nervous system: fatigue, nerve damage, paralysis; cardiovascular: heart failure, edema of the legs	UL not set; toxicity unknown	Pork, whole grains, enriched cereals, legumes, yeast
Riboflavin (vitamin B₂)	Normal growth and energy; coenzyme in protein and energy metabolism	Men, 1.3 mg; women, 1.1 mg	Ariboflavinosis; wound aggravation; cracks at the corners of the mouth; a swollen red tongue; eye irritation; skin eruptions	UL not set; toxicity unknown	Milk; meats, almonds, soybeans, enriched cereals
Niacin (vitamin B₃, nicotinamide, nicotinic acid)	Coenzyme in energy production; normal growth; health of skin	Men, 16 mg of niacin equivalents; women: 14 mg of niacin equivalents	Pellagra (deficiency disease); weakness; loss of appetite; diarrhea; scaly dermatitis; neuritis; confusion	UL: 35 mg Skin flushing	Meat, poultry, fish, whole grains, enriched cereals
Vitamin B₆ (pyridoxine)	Coenzyme in amino acid metabolism: protein synthesis; heme formation; brain activity; carrier for amino acid absorption	Between the ages of 19 and 50 years, 1.3 mg; men 50 years of age or older, 1.7 mg; women 50 years of age or older, 1.5 mg	Anemia; hyperirritability; convulsions; neuritis	UL: 100 mg Nerve damage	Enriched cereals, legumes, meats, poultry, seafood
Folate (folic acid, folacin)	Coenzyme in DNA and RNA synthesis; amino acid metabolism; red blood cell maturation	400 mcg of dietary folate equivalents	Megaloblastic anemia (large immature red blood cells); poor growth; neural tube defects	UL: 1000 mcg Masks vitamin B₁₂ deficiency	Fortified cereals, liver, asparagus, spinach, legumes, orange juice
Cobalamin (vitamin B₁₂)	Coenzyme in synthesis of heme for hemoglobin; myelin sheath formation to protect nerves	2.4 mcg	Pernicious anemia; poor nerve function	UL not set; toxicity unknown	Liver; lean meats, seafood
Pantothenic acid	Formation of coenzyme A; fat, cholesterol, protein, and heme formation	Adequate intake, 5 mg	Unlikely because of widespread distribution in most foods	UL not set; toxicity unknown	Meats, eggs, milk, whole grains, enriched cereals, sunflower seeds, vegetables
Biotin	Coenzyme A partner; synthesis of fatty acids, amino acids, and purines	Adequate intake, 30 mcg	Natural deficiency unknown	UL not set; toxicity unknown	Liver, egg yolk, soy flour, nuts

TOXICITY

Very high doses of supplemental choline have resulted in depressed blood pressure, fishy body odor, sweating, excessive salivation, and reduced growth rate. The UL for adults is 3.5 g/day.[28]

FOOD SOURCES AND STABILITY

Choline is found naturally in a wide variety of foods. Soybean products, eggs, liver, and other meat products are especially rich sources of choline.

Choline is a relatively stable nutrient. It is water soluble, as are all of the B-complex vitamins.

SECTION 3 PLANT NUTRIENTS

PHYTOCHEMICALS

In addition to the vitamins discussed so far in this chapter, there are other bioactive molecules found in plants called *phytochemicals* that have multifaceted health benefits. Phytochemicals are organic molecules. The term *phytochemical* comes from the Greek word *phyton,* meaning "plant." Scientists believe that fruits, vegetables, beans, nuts, and whole grains provide thousands of phytochemicals, many of which have yet to be identified.

What prompted the investigation of phytochemicals were the health differences seen in people who were eating whole foods compared with people who were eating micronutrient-deficient refined foods and relying on dietary supplements for their source of vitamins and minerals. Those individuals obtaining their nutrients from a diet rich in plant foods benefited far more than those who relied on synthetic supplemental forms of nutrients. Such findings have led researchers to conclude that there are other important factors (i.e., phytochemicals) in whole foods beyond the known essential vitamins and minerals.

FUNCTION

Phytochemicals have a wide variety of functions, some of which include antioxidant activity, hormonal actions, interactions with enzymes and DNA replication, and antibacterial effects. Diets that are high in phytochemicals protect against cardiovascular disease, cancer, and other chronic diseases.[38] The beneficial effects of phytochemicals are thought to result from the synergistic actions of multiple constituents as opposed to the actions of isolated compounds,[39] which, in part, explains why taking a dietary supplement with only one of the known phytochemicals (e.g., carotene, lycopene) does not have the same advantageous effects as consuming many phytochemicals in whole food form.

RECOMMENDED INTAKE

There are no established DRIs for phytochemicals. Phytochemicals give fruits and vegetables their specific colors; thus, consuming a colorful variety of fruits, vegetables, whole grains, and nuts will provide a rich supply of phytochemicals. *MyPlate Guidelines* recommend filling half of your plate with fruits and veggies each time you eat. At *www.cdc.gov/nutrition/everyone/fruitsvegetables/index.html,* the Centers for Disease Control and Prevention (CDC) provides recommendations for the servings of fruits and vegetables a person should consume daily on the basis of age, gender, and activity level. One cup of raw or cooked vegetables or vegetable juice or 2 cups of raw leafy greens are equivalent to 1 cup from the vegetable group. One cup of fruit or 100% fruit juice or half a cup of dried fruit is equivalent to 1 cup from the fruit group.[40]

These recommendations are based on research findings indicating that the number of fruits and vegetables a person eats has a direct dose response on their risk for all-cause mortality. In other words, people eating five servings of fruits and vegetables per day have the lowest risk for all-cause mortality.[41] Unfortunately, adolescents and adults in the United States only eat fruits and vegetables on average 2.3 and 2.7 times per day, respectively.[42] This equals approximately half of the recommended amount per day to reap the most health benefits. In fact, with regard to Americans eating according to the dietary recommendations, one group of researchers concluded that "… nearly the entire U.S. population consumes a diet with fewer vegetables and whole grains than recommended and [a] large majority underconsume fruits, milk, and oils relative to recommendations."[43] Thus, it is safe to say that most of us could enhance our phytochemical profile by increasing our fruit and veggie intake each day (see the Cultural Considerations box, "The American Diet").

FOOD SOURCES

Foods derived from animals and those that have been processed and refined are virtually devoid of phytochemicals. Phytochemicals are found in whole and unrefined foods such as vegetables, fruits, legumes, nuts, seeds, whole grains, and certain vegetable oils (e.g., olive oil).

The following is a list of seven typical fruit and vegetable colors along with the specific phytochemical or phytochemical class that these fruits and vegetables usually contain. The specified phytochemical or phytochemical class is generally present in fruits or vegetables of other colors as well. However, color is one prominent indicator that a significant quantity of the specified phytochemical or phytochemical class is present in a food. One specific exception that is worth noting is flavonoids. Although orange-yellow foods are good sources of flavonoids, other significant sources include purple grapes, black tea, olives, onions, celery, green tea, oregano, and whole wheat, none of which have an orange-yellow color.

- *Red* foods provide lycopene.
- *Yellow-green* foods provide zeaxanthin.

Cultural Considerations

The American Diet

By consuming the recommended servings from each food group in accordance with the MyPlate guidelines, an individual's vitamin, mineral, and phytochemical needs should be met. However, the average American does not consume the recommended servings per day of key vitamin-rich foods such as fruits, vegetables, and whole grains. According to the Centers for Disease Control and Prevention, there is not a single state within the United States that reports its citizens average two servings of vegetables per day.[1]

Instead, studies show that the average American overconsumes "nutrient-empty" foods such as added sugars and refined grains. An excess of added sugars and empty calories contribute to weight gain and obesity. Note the high amount of average intake from these empty calorie categories in *italics* below. The average daily foods consumed in the United States for each food group are as follows[2]:

- Fruits   1.05 cups/day
- Vegetables   1.42 cups/day
- Dairy   1.77 cups/day
- Whole grains   0.78 oz/day
- *Refined grains*   *5.68 oz/day*
- Protein-rich foods   5.68 oz/day
- *Added sugars*   *17.73 tsp/day*
- Oils   21.15 g/day
- Solid fats   37.44 g/day

How do you measure up? Can you say that your diet is better than the average American? What about your family and friends? Preventing nutrient deficiency is always preferable to disease treatment. Hence, the old saying, "An apple a day keeps the doctor away."

REFERENCES

1. McGuire S. State indicator report on fruits and vegetables, 2013. Centers for Disease Control and Prevention, Atlanta, Ga. *Adv Nutr.* 2013;4(6):665-666.
2. U.S. Department of Agriculture, Economic Research Service. *Average daily intake of food by food source and demographic characteristics, 2007-10.* Available from: <http://ers.usda.gov/data-products/food-consumption-and-nutrient-intakes.aspx#26667>; Accessed September 16, 2014.

- *Red-purple* foods provide anthocyanin.
- *Orange* foods provide β-carotene.
- *Orange-yellow* foods provide flavonoids.
- *Green* foods provide glucosinolate.
- *White-green* foods provide allyl sulfides.

By consuming one fruit or vegetable from each of these seven color categories regularly, individuals get a variety of phytochemicals. Thousands of other phytochemicals are also widely distributed in fruits, vegetables, grains, soybeans, legumes, and nuts.

SECTION 4 NUTRIENT SUPPLEMENTATION

The Dietary Supplement Health and Education Act (DSHEA) of 1994 officially defined supplements as a product (other than tobacco) that has the following characteristics:

- It is intended to supplement the diet.
- It contains one or more dietary ingredients (including vitamins, minerals, herbs or other botanicals, amino acids, and other substances) or their constituents.
- It is intended to be taken by mouth as a pill, capsule, tablet, or liquid.
- And it is labeled on the front panel as being a dietary supplement.

Dietary supplements are regulated in the United States by the U.S. Food and Drug Administration. The Office of Dietary Supplements (http://ods.od.nih.gov/), which is housed within the National Institutes of Health, has the following mission: "to strengthen knowledge and understanding of dietary supplements by evaluating scientific information, stimulating and supporting research, disseminating research results, and educating the public to foster an enhanced quality of life and health for the U.S. population."[44]

The use of dietary supplements is quite common in the United States. About half of the population regularly takes a dietary supplement. The most commonly used supplement is of the multivitamin or multimineral variety. It is the position of the Academy of Nutrition and Dietetics that "... the best nutrition-based strategy for promoting optimal health and reducing the risk of chronic disease is to wisely choose a wide variety of foods. Additional nutrients from supplements can help some people meet their nutritional needs..."[45] If people eat a healthy and varied diet in accordance with the MyPlate guidelines, adequate nutrients should be provided by whole foods. However, because very few Americans currently eat in the ways that these guidelines recommend, inadequate nutrient consumption is possible.[43] Although dietary vitamin and mineral supplements may be beneficial for bridging this gap, it is also possible to exceed the UL for certain nutrients. Of interest is that the use of dietary supplements is most common among the healthiest people rather than among those who need supplementation the most.

RECOMMENDATIONS FOR NUTRIENT SUPPLEMENTATION

Health care professionals should be aware that people often fail to notify their health care providers about the use of dietary supplements. Drug-nutrient interactions are more common with dietary supplements than with whole foods; thus, it is important to specifically ask patients about their use of vitamin, mineral, macronutrient, or herbal supplements. Although dietary supplements may not be necessary for everyone, there are some instances in which supplemental forms of specific nutrients are recommended on the basis of age, lifestyle, or disease state.

LIFE CYCLE NEEDS

Vitamin needs fluctuate with age and with situations that occur throughout the life cycle.

Pregnancy and Lactation

The DRI guidelines explicitly establish separate recommendations for women during pregnancy and lactation that take into account the increased nutrient demands that occur during this period. To reduce the risk of neural tube defects, the DRI committee recommends that pregnant women and women who are capable of becoming pregnant increase their intake of folic acid from fortified foods and/or dietary supplements in addition to the folate that is already present in their diets. Women may find meeting the increased nutrient needs of pregnancy difficult by diet alone as a result of intolerances, food preferences, or other factors that can marginalize their diet. Supplements may then become a viable way of ensuring adequate intake to meet increased nutrient demands.

Infants, Children, and Adolescents

The American Academy of Pediatrics recommends that all breastfed infants receive 400 IU of supplemental vitamin D daily to help prevent rickets. Infants who are not breastfed, children, and adolescents who do not consume at least 1 quart/day of vitamin D–fortified milk or otherwise have an intake of 400 IU of vitamin D should also receive supplemental vitamin D daily.[16]

Older Adults

The aging process may increase the need for some vitamins because of decreased food intake and less efficient nutrient absorption, storage, and usage (see Chapter 12). The Institute of Medicine recommends that people who are 50 years of age or older take 2.4 mcg/day of supplemental vitamin B_{12}. Advancing age also decreases the ability of the skin to produce vitamin D. Thus, older adults are encouraged to consume extra vitamin D from fortified foods or dietary supplements.[45]

LIFESTYLE AND HEALTH STATUS

Personal lifestyle choices also influence individual needs for nutrient supplementation.

Restricted Diets

People who habitually follow fad diets may find meeting many of the nutrient intake standards difficult, particularly if their meals provide fewer than 1200 kcal/day. Very restrictive diets are not recommended, because they may cause multiple nutrient deficiencies. A wise weight-reduction program should meet all nutrient needs. As mentioned earlier, vegans need supplemental vitamin B_{12} in fortified foods or dietary supplements, because the only natural food sources of this vitamin are of animal origin.

Smoking

Smoking cigarettes adversely affects health in many ways, including reducing the body's vitamin C reserve. Research shows that smokers have significantly less serum vitamin C than nonsmokers.[46] The Institute of Medicine sets the RDA of vitamin C at 35 mg/day higher for smokers to compensate for the oxidative stress that is induced by smoking.[21] The additional vitamin C does not necessarily need to come from a dietary supplement; however, if the person continues to smoke and does not consume additional vitamin C–rich foods, a dietary supplement may be advisable.

Alcohol

The chronic or abusive use of alcohol can interfere with the absorption of B-complex vitamins, especially thiamin, folate, and vitamin B_6. Multivitamin supplements that are rich in B vitamins may partially mitigate the effects. However, decreased alcohol use must accompany this nutrition therapy to rectify the alcohol-induced deficiency.

Disease

Evidence does not support the use of multivitamin and multimineral dietary supplements to prevent chronic disease. However, for patients with certain diseases, dietary supplements may be warranted to help combat specific nutrient deficiencies. In states of disease, malnutrition, malabsorption, debilitation, or hypermetabolic demand, each patient requires careful nutrition assessment. Nutrition support, including therapeutic supplementation as indicated, is part of the total medical treatment. A dietitian plans dietary and supplemental therapy to meet the patient's clinical requirements.

SUPPLEMENTATION PRINCIPLES

BASIC PRINCIPLES

The following basic principles may help to guide nutrient supplementation decisions:

- *Read the labels carefully.* The Nutrition Labeling and Education Act of 1990 standardized and defined label terminology on food products in an effort to ensure that health claims on food packaging are clear and truthful.
- *Vitamins, like drugs, can be harmful in large amounts.* The only time that larger vitamin doses may be helpful is when severe deficiency exists or when nutrient absorption or metabolism is inefficient. A medical provider should be consulted.
- *Professionally determined individual needs govern specific supplement usage.* Each person's need should be the basis for supplementing nutrients. This prevents excessive intake, which may have a cumulative effect over time.

- *All nutrients work together to promote good health.* Consuming large amounts of one vitamin may induce deficiencies of other vitamins or nutrients.
- *Food is the best source of nutrients.* Whole foods are the best "package deals" in nutrition. Foods provide a wide variety of nutrients in every bite as compared with the dozen or so that are found in a dietary supplement. In addition, by itself, a vitamin can do nothing. It is catalytic, so it must have a substrate (i.e., carbohydrate, protein, fat, or their metabolites) on which to work. With the careful selection of a wide variety of foods and with good storage techniques, meal planning, and preparation techniques, most people can obtain ample amounts of essential nutrients from their diets.
- *Evaluate the information.* The Further Reading and Resources section at the end of the chapter provides a list of reliable organizations and resources related to dietary supplements.

MEGADOSES

At high pharmacologic concentrations, vitamins no longer operate strictly as nutritional agents. Nutrients and drugs can do the following: (1) participate in or improve physiologic conditions or illnesses; (2) prevent diseases; or (3) relieve symptoms. However, many people are unaware of the similarities between drugs and vitamins. Most people realize that too much of any drug can be harmful or even fatal and take care to avoid overdosing. However, too many people do not apply this same logic to nutrients and only realize the dangers of vitamin megadoses when they experience toxic side effects.

The liver can store large amounts of fat-soluble vitamins, especially vitamin A. Therefore, the potential toxicity of fat-soluble vitamin megadoses, including liver and brain damage in extreme cases, is well documented.[47-49] Megadoses of one vitamin can also produce toxic effects and lead to a secondary deficiency of another nutrient. In addition, hyperphysiologic levels of one vitamin may increase the need for other nutrients with which it works in the body, thereby effectively inducing a deficiency. The bioavailability of vitamins may be altered by excess supplementation of a vitamin that shares an absorptive site with another vitamin. By overloading these absorptive pathways, the nutrient in highest quantities may render the other vitamin unavailable for absorption. Deficiencies can also occur when a person suddenly stops overdosing, which is known as a *rebound effect.* For example, infants who are born to mothers who took ascorbic acid megadoses during pregnancy may develop rebound scurvy after birth, when their high doses of ascorbic acid are terminated.

FUNCTIONAL FOODS

The term *functional food* has no consistently recognized definition. Generally, "functional foods" include any foods or food ingredients that may provide a health benefit beyond its basic nutritional value. Such foods are also referred to as *nutraceuticals* or *designer foods.* The position of the Academy of Nutrition and Dietetics is that such whole foods—having been fortified, enriched, or enhanced in some way—could be beneficial when regularly consumed as part of a varied diet.[50] The regulation of functional foods is complicated by the fact that the current governing body (the Food and Drug Administration) does not define or recognize functional foods. Box 7-2 gives examples of functional food categories.

Recommendations for functional food intake have not been established because scientific evidence on which to base such recommendations is insufficient. However, over the past decade, much research effort has been focused on determining the clinical efficacy of functional foods. If efficacy is clearly substantiated and reliable assessments for accurately quantifying active constituents in foods are in place, then expert committees will work to establish recommendations for intake. Until such recommendations are established, the daily intake of foods from all food groups—including functional foods—is the best way to meet macronutrient and micronutrient needs.

| Box **7-2** | Functional Food Categories and Selected Food Examples* |

FUNCTIONAL FOOD CATEGORY	SELECTED FUNCTIONAL FOOD EXAMPLES
Conventional foods (whole foods)	Orange juice
Contain natural bioactive food compounds	Soy-based foods Yogurt
Modified foods	Calcium-fortified orange juice
Bioactive ingredients obtained by enrichment or fortification	Folate-enriched breads
Food ingredients that are synthesized	Indigestible carbohydrates

From Crowe KM, et al. Position of the Academy of Nutrition and Dietetics: functional foods. *J Acad Nutr Diet.* 2013;113(8):1096-1103.
*NOTE: Medical foods and dietary supplements are not considered functional foods.

Putting It All Together

Summary

- Vitamins are organic, noncaloric food substances that are necessary in minute amounts for specific metabolic tasks. A balanced diet usually supplies sufficient vitamins. In individually assessed situations, however, vitamin supplements may be indicated.
- The fat-soluble vitamins are A, D, E, and K. They mainly affect body structures (i.e., bones, rhodopsin, cell membrane phospholipids, and blood-clotting proteins).
- The water-soluble vitamins are vitamin C (ascorbic acid), the eight B-complex vitamins (i.e., thiamin, riboflavin, niacin, pyridoxine, folate, cobalamin, pantothenic acid, and biotin), and choline. Their major metabolic tasks relate to their roles in coenzyme factors, except for vitamin C, which is a biologic reducing agent that quenches free radicals and helps with collagen synthesis.
- All water-soluble vitamins—especially vitamin C—are easily oxidized, so care must be taken to minimize the exposure of food surfaces to air or other oxidizers during storage and preparation. With few exceptions, all nutrients in foods are more bioavailable and beneficial to the body than nutrients in supplements.
- Phytochemicals are compounds that are found in whole and unrefined foods derived from plants. A diet that is high in phytochemicals from a variety of sources is associated with a decreased risk for chronic disease.
- Vitamin supplementation is beneficial in some situations. Megadoses of water-soluble or fat-soluble vitamins can have detrimental effects.
- Functional foods are whole foods with added nutrients, such as vitamins, minerals, herbs, fiber, protein, or essential fatty acids that are thought to have beneficial health effects.

Review Questions

See answers in Appendix A.

1. Mary wants to increase her intake of foods rich in β-carotene. Which of the following foods would be the best source?
   a. Whole-wheat bread
   b. Spinach
   c. Scrambled egg
   d. Wheat germ

2. Vitamin D deficiency is more common in people who:
   a. Have darker skin and live at higher latitudes.
   b. Have darker skin and live at lower latitudes.
   c. Have lighter skin and live at higher latitudes.
   d. Have lighter skin and live at lower latitudes.

3. The best menu choice for a patient with a severe wound who needs adequate vitamin C to help promote healing would be:
   a. Stuffed green pepper.
   b. Whole-wheat toast with Swiss cheese.
   c. Chocolate milkshake.
   d. Grilled chicken.

4. Dermatitis, diarrhea, dementia, and death characterize toxic symptoms associated with:
   a. Pellagra.
   b. Scurvy.
   c. Rickets.
   d. Beri-beri.

5. Megaloblastic anemia is associated with:
   a. Vitamin C deficiency.
   b. Selenium deficiency.
   c. Protein deficiency.
   d. Folate deficiency.

Additional Learning Resources

evolve http://evolve.elsevier.com/Williams/basic/

References and **Further Reading and Resources** in the back of the book provide additional resources for enhancing knowledge.

Key Concepts

- The human body requires a variety of minerals to perform its numerous metabolic tasks.
- A mixed diet of varied foods and adequate energy intake is the best source of the minerals that are necessary for life.
- Of the total amount of minerals that a person consumes, only a relatively limited amount is bioavailable to the body.

Over the course of Earth's history, shifting oceans and plate tectonics have deposited minerals throughout its crust. These minerals move from rocks to soil to plants to animals and people. Not surprisingly, the mineral content of the human body is quite similar to that of the Earth's crust.

In nutrition, we focus on mineral elements: single atoms that are simple compared with vitamins, which are large, complex, organic compounds. However, minerals perform a wide variety of metabolic tasks that are essential to human life. This chapter looks at minerals and shows how they differ from vitamins with regard to the variety of their tasks and in the amounts, which range from relatively large to exceedingly small, that are necessary to do those tasks.

NATURE OF MINERALS IN HUMAN NUTRITION

Most living matter is composed of four elements: hydrogen, carbon, nitrogen, and oxygen, which are the building blocks of life. The minerals that are necessary to human nutrition are elements widely distributed in nature. Of the 118 elements on the periodic table, 25 are essential to human life. These 25 elements, in varying amounts, perform a variety of metabolic functions.

CLASSES OF MINERALS

Minerals occur in varying amounts in the body. For example, a relatively large amount (approximately 1.5%) of our total body weight is calcium, most of which is in the bones. An adult who weighs 150 lb has approximately 2.25 lb of calcium in the body. Iron, on the other hand, is found in much smaller quantities. The same adult weighing 150 lb has only approximately 0.11 oz of iron in his or her body. In both cases, the amount of each mineral is specific to its task.

The varying amounts of individual minerals in the body are the basis for classification into two main groups.

Major Minerals

The term *major* describes the amount of a mineral in the body and not its relative importance to human nutrition. Major minerals have a recommended intake of more than 100 mg/day. The seven major minerals are calcium, phosphorus, sodium, potassium, magnesium, chloride, and sulfur. Because the body cannot make minerals, all minerals must be consumed in the foods that we eat.

Trace Minerals

The remaining 18 elements make up the group of trace minerals. These minerals are no less important to human nutrition than the major minerals; however, smaller amounts of them are in the body. Trace minerals have a recommended intake of less than 100 mg/day. Box 8-1 provides a list of all of the minerals that are essential to human nutrition.

FUNCTIONS OF MINERALS

Minerals are involved in most of the body's metabolic processes. They are involved in processes of building tissue as well as activating, regulating, transmitting, and controlling metabolic processes. For example, sodium and potassium are key players in water balance. Calcium and phosphorus are required for osteoblasts to build bone. Iron is critical to the oxygen carrier **hemoglobin.** Cobalt is at the active site of vitamin B_{12}. Thyroid peroxidase in thyroid cells uses iodine to make thyroid hormone, which in turn helps regulate the overall rate of body metabolism.

---

hemoglobin a conjugated protein in red blood cells that is composed of a compact, rounded mass of polypeptide chains that forms globin (the protein portion) and that is attached to an iron-containing red pigment called *heme;* hemoglobin carries oxygen in the blood to cells.

Box 8-1 Major Minerals and Trace Minerals in Human Nutrition

MAJOR MINERALS*	Potassium (K)
Calcium (Ca)	Chloride (Cl)
Phosphorus (P)	Magnesium (Mg)
Sodium (Na)	Sulfur (S)
TRACE MINERALS	Cobalt (Co)
Essential†	Boron (B)
Iron (Fe)	Vanadium (V)
Iodine (I)	Nickel (Ni)
Zinc (Zn)	**Essentiality Unclear**
Selenium (Se)	Silicon (Si)
Fluoride (Fl)	Tin (Sn)
Copper (Cu)	Cadmium (Cd)
Manganese (Mn)	Arsenic (As)
Chromium (Cr)‡	Aluminum (Al)
Molybdenum (Mo)	

*Required intake of more than 100 mg/day.
†Required intake of less than 100 mg/day.
‡Essentiality is currently under review.

MINERAL METABOLISM

Mineral metabolism is usually controlled either at the point of intestinal absorption or at the point of tissue uptake.

Digestion

Minerals are absorbed and used in the body in their ionic forms, which means that they are carrying either a positive or a negative electrical charge. Unlike the macronutrients, minerals do not require a great deal of mechanical or chemical digestion before absorption occurs.

Absorption

The following general factors influence how much of a mineral is absorbed into the body from the gastrointestinal tract: (1) food form—minerals from animal sources are usually more readily absorbed than those from plant sources; (2) body need—more is absorbed if the body is deficient than if the body has sufficient quantities; and (3) tissue health—if the absorbing intestinal surface is affected by disease, its absorptive capacity is greatly diminished.

The absorptive method for each mineral depends on its physical properties. Some minerals require active transport to be absorbed, whereas others enter the intestinal cells by diffusion. Compounds found in foods may also affect the absorptive efficiency. For example, the presence of fiber, phytate, or oxalate—all of which are found in a variety of whole grains, fruits, and vegetables—can bind certain minerals in the gastrointestinal tract, thereby inhibiting or limiting their absorption.

Transport

Minerals enter the portal blood circulation and travel throughout the body bound to plasma proteins or mineral-specific transport proteins (e.g., iron is bound to transferrin in the circulation).

Tissue Uptake

The uptake of some minerals into their target tissue is controlled by hormones, and excess minerals are excreted into the urine. For example, **thyroid-stimulating hormone (TSH)** controls the uptake of iodine from the blood into the thyroid gland depending on the amount that the thyroid gland needs to make the hormone **thyroxine.** When more thyroxine is needed, TSH stimulates the thyroid gland to take up iodine and the kidneys to retain more iodine. When the thyroxine concentration is normal, less TSH is released from the anterior pituitary gland, thereby resulting in less iodine uptake by the thyroid gland and more excretion of iodine into the urine by the kidneys.

Occurrence in the Body

Minerals are found in several forms throughout body tissues. The two basic forms in which minerals occur in the body are as free ions in body fluids (e.g., sodium in tissue fluids, which influence water balance) and as covalently bound minerals that may be combined with other minerals (e.g., calcium and phosphorus in hydroxyapatite) or with organic substances (e.g., iron that is bound to heme and globin to form the organic compound hemoglobin).

MAJOR MINERALS

CALCIUM

The intestinal absorption of dietary calcium depends on the food form and hormonal control. Calcium found in plant forms is sometimes bound to oxalate or phytate and thus not readily available. The interaction of the hormones vitamin D, parathyroid hormone, and calcitonin (from the thyroid gland) directly controls calcium's intestinal absorption and use, along with indirect control by the **estrogen hormones.**

Functions

After it has been absorbed, calcium has four basic functions in the body.

Bone and tooth formation. More than 99% of the body's calcium is found in the bones and teeth. Approximately 1.5% of adult body weight is calcium. When hydroxyapatite is removed from bone, the

thyroid-stimulating hormone (TSH) an anterior pituitary hormone that regulates the activity of the thyroid gland; also known as thyrotropin.
thyroxine an iodine-dependent thyroid gland hormone that regulates the metabolic rate of the body.
estrogen hormones sex hormones produced primarily by the ovaries.

remaining tissue is a collagen matrix. If dietary calcium is insufficient during critical periods (e.g., the initial formation of the fetal skeleton, childhood growth, or the rapid growth of long bones during adolescence), then the construction of healthy bones is hindered. Teeth are calcified before they erupt from the gums; thus, insufficient dietary calcium later in life does not affect tooth structure as it does bone structure.

Blood clotting. Calcium is essential for the formation of fibrin, which is the protein matrix of a blood clot.

Muscle and nerve action. Calcium ions are required for muscle contraction and the release of neurotransmitters from neuron synapses.

Metabolic reactions. Calcium is necessary for many general metabolic functions in the body. Such functions include the intestinal absorption of vitamin B_{12}, the activation of the fat-splitting enzyme pancreatic lipase, and the secretion of insulin by the β cells of the pancreas. Calcium also interacts with the cell membrane proteins that govern the membrane's permeability to nutrients.

Requirements

The Dietary Reference Intake (DRI) for calcium should provide sufficient calcium nourishment for the body while recognizing that a lower intake may be adequate for many individuals. The DRIs for calcium are listed in the summary table for major minerals (see Table 8-3) and in the DRI tables in Appendix B.

Deficiency

Various bone deformities may occur if sufficient dietary calcium is unavailable during growth years. The deficiency disease rickets is related to an inadequate level of vitamin D to support the intestinal absorption of calcium. **Hypocalcemia** relative to blood phosphorus concentration results in tetany, which is a condition that is characterized by muscle spasms. The most common calcium-related clinical issue today is **osteoporosis** (Figure 8-1). Osteoporotic bone fractures have historically been recognized as primarily a problem among postmenopausal women. However, with the increase in life expectancy osteoporotic bone fractures are progressively more common among elderly men as well.[1,2] Each year in the United States, more than 1.5 million bone fractures and $17 to $20 billion in health care costs are linked to osteoporosis (see the Cultural Considerations box, "Bone Health in Gender and

hypocalcemia a serum calcium level that is below normal.
osteoporosis an abnormal thinning of the bone that produces a porous, fragile, lattice-like bone tissue of enlarged spaces that are prone to fracture or deformity.

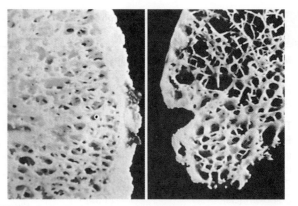

FIGURE 8-1 Osteoporosis. Normal bone *(left)* versus osteoporotic bone *(right)*. (From Maher AB et al: *Orthopaedic nursing*, 3rd ed. Philadelphia, 2002, Saunders.)

Racial Groups").[3] The cost of a single hip fracture has a direct medical cost ranging from $8400 up to $32,000 per person.[4]

Osteoporosis is not a primary calcium deficiency disease as such; rather, it results from a combination of factors that create an overall loss of bone density. These factors include the following: (1) chronic calcium deficiency due to inadequate calcium intake or poor intestinal calcium absorption related to deviations in the amounts of hormones that control calcium absorption and metabolism; (2) a lack of physical activity, which stimulates muscle insertion into bones and significantly influences bone strength, shape, and mass; and (3) side effects of medications such as thiazides (antidiabetic medication) and cyclophosphamide therapy (prostate cancer treatment) that cause bone loss over time. Although not all risk factors are easily modified (e.g., cancer treatment), some risk factors are effectively reduced with lifestyle changes (e.g., diet and exercise). One study found that relatively sedentary men, defined as those participating in less than 33 minutes per day of physical activity, had a 70% increased risk of bone fracture compared to their physically active counterparts.[5] One must realize that there are likely many other factors at play in studies such as this that could contribute to the outcome. However, physical activity is undoubtedly one of the important lifestyle factors involved.

Bone is a dynamic tissue, with both new bone formation and bone resorption occurring constantly. A portion of the skeleton is reabsorbed and replaced with new bone each year; this bone remodeling can affect up to 50% of total bone mass annually in young children and approximately 5% of bone mass in adults. Unfortunately, bone resorption often outpaces bone formation in postmenopausal women and in aging men. The dynamics involved in this process are multifactorial and not fully understood. Increased calcium intake alone—be it via dietary calcium or via supplemental calcium—does not prevent osteoporosis in susceptible adults or successfully treat diagnosed cases of osteoporosis. Therapies that reduce bone loss in

Cultural Considerations

Bone Health in Gender and Racial Groups

The World Health Organization defines low bone mass as a bone mineral density (BMD) of between 1 and 2.5 standard deviations below the mean of a matched reference group. Osteoporosis involves a BMD of 2.5 standard deviations or more below the mean of the reference group.

Osteoporosis affects a significant number of older Americans. Currently, 4.3% of men and 15.4% of women who are 50 years old or older are living with osteoporosis. An additional 43.4 million Americans have low bone mass, which is a significant risk factor for osteoporosis.[1]

Osteoporosis often is thought of as a "white woman's disease." However, this debilitating bone disease is prevalent in men and other racial groups as well. It is well established that there is a disparity between genders, with women carrying more than double the risk for developing osteoporosis. With regard to differences among racial groups, non-Hispanic black men and women have the highest BMD and therefore the lowest risk for osteoporosis throughout life compared with non-Hispanic white and Mexican-Americans.[1-3] The reasons for these observed differences by race are unclear; however, race, gender, and age are all accepted as essential factors when calculating the risk for osteoporosis, which is the most common form of bone disease.

Many factors are involved in BMD and the relative risk for the development of fragile bones, including body weight, physical activity, hormonal influences, and dietary intakes of several vitamins and minerals (not just calcium). Nutrition affects bone health by providing the materials that are needed for tissue deposition, maintenance, and repair. Overall bone strength is determined by BMD and the collagen matrix formation. Collagen, which is a structural protein, accounts for more than 20% of the dry weight of total bone mass and 90% of the organic bone matrix. Collagen degradation is associated with

osteoporosis. As such, the vitamins and minerals that are critical for a strong collagen and bone matrix also are integral to overall bone health. A balance of several nutrients is important for healthy bone building, including protein; calcium; phosphorus; copper; magnesium; manganese; potassium; zinc; and vitamins C, D, and K.

Osteoporosis is largely a preventable disease. It is also a costly disease. Coupled with the general trends of an aging population, this bone disease is a serious national concern. Because BMD reaches a peak mass by the average age of 30 years, the years before this are vital for developing healthy bones and preventing the onset of osteoporosis. Establishing peak bone mass ensures a greater reserve of bone mineral and collagen so that, as age-associated degradation ensues, effects are essentially postponed or abated altogether. A healthy diet following the MyPlate guidelines should provide all of the essential nutrients, and it is imperative during the first three decades of life to establish healthy bones.

For more information about osteoporosis please see the website of the National Institutes of Health Osteoporosis and Related Bone Diseases National Resource Center at www.niams.nih.gov/health_info/bone/osteoporosis/.

REFERENCES

1. Wright NC, et al. The recent prevalence of osteoporosis and low bone mass in the United States based on bone mineral density at the femoral neck or lumbar spine. *J Bone Miner Res.* 2014; 29(11):2520-2526.
2. Looker AC, et al. Lumbar spine and proximal femur bone mineral density, bone mineral content, and bone area: United States, 2005-2008. *Vital Health Stat 11.* 2012;(251):1-132.
3. Looker AC, et al. Age, gender, and race/ethnic differences in total body and subregional bone density. *Osteoporos Int.* 2009;20(7): 1141-1149.

---

osteoporosis include combinations of the various factors that are involved in the building of bones: adequate dietary calcium, the active hormonal form of vitamin D, estrogens, and weight-bearing physical activity. In addition, there are a variety of medications in use for the treatment and prevention of bone loss; however, the long-term compliance of such therapy is poor in the United States.[6]

Food intake studies report that the average calcium intakes of females from adolescence through adulthood are generally well below the DRIs. The period of life during which bone density is reaching its peak is an especially important time to obtain adequate dietary calcium. Teenage girls consume 937 mg/day of calcium on average, whereas the recommended RDA is 1300 mg/day.[7] Deficiencies during this critical period of bone development may have long-term negative outcomes with regard to overall bone strength and risk for osteoporosis.[8]

Toxicity

The toxicity of calcium from food sources is unlikely. However, a tolerable upper intake level (UL) for calcium has been set at 2000 to 3000 mg/day

(depending on age) as a result of the negative effects of excessive calcium supplementation over time. **Hypercalcemia** is associated with the calcification of soft tissue and the decreased intestinal absorption of several other minerals. Excess calcium can interfere with the intestinal absorption of iron, magnesium, phosphorus, and zinc, thereby reducing the bioavailability of these essential nutrients.

Food Sources

Milk and milk products are important dietary sources of readily available calcium.[9] Milk that is used in cooking (e.g., in soups, sauces, or puddings) or in milk products such as yogurt, cheese, and ice cream is an excellent source of calcium. Calcium-fortified soy products, fruit juices, and other food products (e.g., cereals, cereal bars) are also high in bioavailable calcium. In addition, several plants provide a natural source of calcium. Calcium in low-oxalate greens such as bok choy, collard greens, kale, and turnip greens is

hypercalcemia a serum calcium level that is above normal.

absorbed and can be an important source of calcium for vegetarians. Oxalic acid is a compound that is found in plants such as spinach, rhubarb, Swiss chard, beet greens, and certain other vegetables and nuts that forms an insoluble salt with calcium (calcium oxalate), thus interfering with the intestinal absorption of calcium. Phytate, which is another plant compound that is found in grains such as wheat, can also bind with calcium and interfere with its intestinal absorption. Table 8-1 lists food sources of calcium.

In addition to food sources, calcium intake from supplements is widespread. Surveys show that 16% of women and 4% of men in the United States specifically take calcium supplements, whereas 35% of the total population takes a multivitamin and mineral supplement that contains calcium.[10] The bioavailability of calcium from supplements depends on the dose and whether it is taken with a meal. Calcium is best absorbed in doses of 500 mg or less and when taken with food rather than on an empty stomach (see the For Further Focus box, "Calcium from Food or Supplements").

PHOSPHORUS

Functions

The phosphorus atom in nature is most commonly found in combination with four oxygen atoms to form the phosphate molecule. Phosphorus functions in the following metabolic processes.

Bone and tooth formation. The calcification of bones and teeth depends on the deposition of hydroxyapatite $[Ca_{10}(PO_4)_6(OH)_2]$ by osteoblasts in bone's collagen matrix. The ratio of calcium to phosphorus in typical bone is approximately 1.5:1 by weight.

Energy metabolism. Phosphorus in the form of phosphate (PO_4^{3-}) is necessary for the controlled oxidation of carbohydrate, fat, and protein to release the energy in their covalent bonds (as a component of thiamin pyrophosphate), and it captures energy for use in the body as a component of adenosine triphosphate. Phosphate is also involved in protein construction (as a component of RNA), cell function (as a component of cell enzymes activated by phosphorylation), and genetic inheritance (as a component of DNA).

Acid-Base Balance. Phosphate is an important chemical buffer that helps to maintain the pH homeostasis of body fluids.

Requirements

The typical American diet contains enough phosphorus to meet body needs. Surveys indicate that the mean daily phosphorus intake in the United States is approximately 1393 mg/day.[7] Refer to the DRI tables in Appendix B or the summary table for major minerals (see Table 8-3) for the DRIs for phosphorus.

Deficiency

Phosphate (the dietary form of phosphorus) is widely distributed in foods; thus, a deficiency is rare. A person must be completely deprived of food for an extended period to develop a dietary phosphorus deficiency. The only evidence of deficiency has been among people who persistently consumed large amounts of antacids that contained aluminum hydroxide.[11-13] The aluminum ion (Al^{3+}) binds with phosphate, thereby making the phosphate unavailable for intestinal absorption. **Hypophosphatemia** results in bone loss; it is characterized by weakness, loss of appetite, fatigue, and pain.

Table 8-1	Food Sources of Calcium	
ITEM	**QUANTITY**	**AMOUNT (mg)**
Bread, Cereal, Rice, and Pasta		
Cream of Wheat cereal, cooked with water	1 cup	306
Total Whole Grain cereal, General Mills	1 cup	1333
Total Raisin Bran cereal, General Mills	1 cup	1000
Vegetables*		
Collards, cooked	½ cup, chopped	178
Rhubarb, cooked	½ cup, chopped	174
Fruits		
Orange juice, frozen concentrate, fortified with calcium	8 fl oz	364
Meat, Poultry, Fish, Dry Beans, Eggs, and Nuts		
Salmon, pink, canned, drained solids with bone	3 oz	241
Sardines, canned in oil, solids with bone	3 oz	325
Soybeans, green, raw	½ cup	252
Soybeans, green, boiled	½ cup	130
Tofu, raw, firm, prepared with calcium sulfate	½ cup	861
Milk and Dairy Products or Their Substitutes		
Cheese, parmesan, grated, reduced fat	1 oz	314
Milk, skim	8 fl oz	299
Soy milk, calcium fortified	8 fl oz	301
Tofu yogurt	8 fl oz	309
Yogurt, plain, skim milk	8 fl oz	452

Data from the U.S. Department of Agriculture, Agricultural Research Service: Nutrient Data Laboratory. *USDA nutrient database for standard reference* (website): <http://ndb.nal.usda.gov/ndb/>; Accessed October 20, 2014.
*Low bioavailability.

hypophosphatemia a serum phosphorus level that is below normal.

For Further Focus

Calcium from Food or Supplements

Good health is not a simple matter, and our bodies are no simple machines. They require lots of nutrients to function properly, and these must be provided by the diet. One of the major minerals that is needed by our body is calcium. The National Health and Nutrition Examination Study (NHANES) reports that, unfortunately beginning with the adolescent years, the average dietary intake of calcium by females falls below the DRI. The graph below represents the average calcium intake for females by age group.

A variety of factors influence our dietary intake of calcium. Over the past decade, Americans' food choices have changed in ways that directly affect calcium-rich food consumption. For example, many Americans have replaced milk with soft drinks; they are eating out more often at restaurants (which contain less calcium than home-made meals); there is a trend for perpetual dieting (and dairy products are often one of the first foods to go); and there is a lack of risk acknowledgments regarding the importance of calcium-rich foods and health.

Health organizations such as the National Institutes of Health, the Academy of Nutrition and Dietetics, the American Medical Association, and the National Academy of Sciences agree that the best source of calcium is dairy products. The primary reason for this is because, unlike calcium supplements, calcium-rich foods supply the body with other beneficial nutrients as well, including protein; vitamins A, B_{12}, and D (if fortified); magnesium; potassium; riboflavin; niacin; and phosphorus. Some nondairy foods naturally contain calcium, including fish with bones (e.g., canned sardines), soybeans, collards, mustard greens, and rhubarb.* Most people find that meeting the Dietary Reference Intake for calcium exclusively from nondairy foods can be difficult, because the relative amount of calcium in these foods is less than that found in dairy products. For example, half a cup of chopped collards has 178 mg of calcium, whereas 8 oz of skim milk contains 299 mg.[1] Many vegetables contain phytates and oxalates that form insoluble complexes with calcium and thus decrease their bioavailability to the body. This makes the relative amount of calcium meaningfully less from vegetable sources.

Keller and colleagues analyzed the consumer cost and bioavailability of calcium from major sources. They found that Total cereal was the least expensive food source of calcium, with fluid milk and calcium-fortified orange juice being the next least expensive.[2] Calcium from supplements may be found in a variety of forms, including calcium carbonate, citrate, phosphate, lactate, and gluconate. The amount of calcium absorbed into the body from these sources varies considerably. Of the calcium supplements, calcium carbonate in a chewable form (e.g., Tums) or supplement provides the least expensive and most bioavailable source of calcium, with a 34% absorption fraction.[2]

The best way to improve one's overall diet is to consume a variety of foods that are high in calcium, preferably from dairy or fortified dairy substitute sources. However, calcium-fortified foods and supplements may be necessary for some people to meet their recommended intake of calcium.

Regardless of the source of your calcium, take a moment to consider the overall value of your diet, and assess whether improvements are warranted. For more information about the fortification of calcium in the American food supply, please see the paper by Rafferty and colleagues (2007).[3]

REFERENCES

1. U.S. Department of Agriculture, Agricultural Research Service: Nutrient Data Laboratory. *USDA nutrient database for standard reference.* October 11, 2014. Available from <http://ndb.nal.usda .gov/>.
2. Keller JL, Lanou A, Barnard ND. The consumer cost of calcium from food and supplements. *J Am Diet Assoc.* 2002;102(11): 1669-1671.
3. Rafferty J, Walters G, Heaney RP. Calcium fortificants: overview and strategies for improving calcium nutriture of the U.S. population. *J Food Sci.* 2007;72:R152-R158.

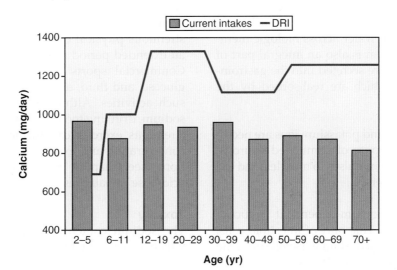

Data from the U.S. Department of Agriculture, Agricultural Research Service. Nutrient intakes from food: mean amounts consumed per female by age. What We Eat in America, NHANES 2009-2010 (website): www.ars.usda.gov/ ba/bhnrc/fsrg. Accessed October 24, 2014; and Food and Nutrition Board, Institute of Health, Dietary Reference Intakes for Calcium and Vitamin D. 2011, National Academy of Sciences: Washington, DC.

*The bioavailability of calcium from some vegetables is very poor.

Toxicity

Hyperphosphatemia from food intake is equally rare. However, if phosphorus intake is significantly higher than calcium intake for a long period, bone resorption may occur. The DRI guidelines list the UL for phosphorus at 4 g/day for people between the ages of 9 and 70 years.[14]

Food Sources

Phosphorus is part of all living tissue, and it is found in all animal and plant cells; therefore, phosphorus is sufficient in the natural food supply of virtually all animals. High-protein foods are particularly rich in phosphorus, so milk and milk products, meat, fish, and eggs are the primary sources of phosphorus in the average diet. The bioavailability of phosphorus from plant seeds (e.g., cereal grains, beans, peas, other legumes, nuts) is much lower, because these foods contain phytic acid, which is a storage form of phosphorus in seeds that humans cannot directly digest. However, a healthy flora of gut bacteria will provide a limited supply of phytase, the enzyme needed to liberate phosphorus from phytic acid.

SODIUM

Sodium is plentiful in the body. Approximately 0.2% of the adult body is sodium.

Functions

The main function of sodium is the maintenance of body water balance, which is discussed further in Chapter 9. Sodium also has important tasks in muscle action and nutrient absorption.

Water balance. Ionized sodium concentration is the major influence on the volume of extracellular water (Figure 8-2). Variations in sodium concentration largely control the movement of water across biologic membranes by osmosis. Sodium is also an integral part of the digestive juices that are secreted into the gastrointestinal tract, most of which are reabsorbed by the intestinal cells.

Muscle action. Sodium and potassium ions are necessary for the normal response of stimulated neurons, the transmission of nerve impulses to muscles, and the contraction of muscle fibers.

Nutrient absorption. Sodium-dependent glucose transporters, which are a vital part of intestinal cells, allow for the passage of glucose and galactose from the intestinal lumen into the intestinal cells.

Requirements

The body is able to function on various amounts of dietary sodium through mechanisms that have been designed to conserve or excrete the mineral as needed. Individual sodium needs vary greatly depending on

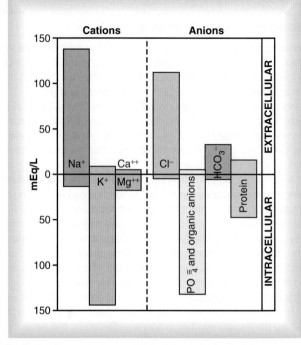

FIGURE 8-2 The ionic composition of the major body fluid compartments. (Reprinted from Guyton AC, Hall JE. *Textbook of medical physiology.* 12th ed. Philadelphia: Saunders; 2006.)

growth stage, sweat loss, and medical conditions (e.g., diarrhea, vomiting). The DRIs for sodium are provided in the summary table for major minerals (see Table 8-3) and in the DRI tables in Appendix B.

Deficiency

Sodium deficiencies are rare, because the body's need is low, and individual intake in the United States is typically high. An exception is during heavy sweating, such as by those who are engaged in heavy labor or strenuous physical exercise in a hot environment for an extended period of time (e.g., more than 2 hours). Commercial sports drinks, which replace sodium, glucose, and fluid, are useful to restore losses during such activities. Although sweat is relatively low in sodium, drinking too much plain water during lengthy strenuous exercise can further dilute blood sodium concentration and exacerbate hyponatremia complications (see Chapter 16). Hyponatremia can result in acid-base imbalances and muscle cramping.

Toxicity

The sodium content of the average American diet, which contains a high amount of processed foods,

hyperphosphatemia a serum phosphorus level that is above normal.
hyponatremia a serum sodium level that is below normal.

usually far exceeds the recommended intake range. The National Health and Nutrition Examination Survey (NHANES) found that women consume an average of 2997 mg/day of sodium and that men have an average intake of 4218 mg/day (approximately 2 to 3 times the recommended amount).[7] Excessive sodium intake has been linked to hypertension in individuals who are salt sensitive (i.e., approximately 30% to 50% of hypertensive patients).[15] However, for most people with healthy kidneys and adequate water intake, the kidneys excrete excess sodium in the urine. The acute excessive intake of sodium chloride (i.e., table salt) causes the accumulation of sodium in the blood (i.e., **hypernatremia**) and extracellular spaces. This sodium can pull water out of cells into the extracellular space by osmosis, thereby causing edema. The current UL for sodium intake is 2.3 g/day but some individuals may have a much lower tolerance.[16]

Food Sources

Common table salt as used in cooking, seasoning, preserving, and processing foods is the main dietary source of sodium. Sodium also occurs naturally in foods, and it is generally most prevalent in foods of animal origin. Enough sodium is found in natural food sources to meet the body's needs. When people regularly consume food from manufacturers that add salt and other sodium compounds to processed foods as a preservative, sodium intake dramatically increases. For example, cured ham has approximately 30 times more sodium than raw pork. Natural unprocessed food sources of sodium include animal products such as milk, meat, and eggs and vegetables such as carrots, beets, leafy greens, and celery (see Appendix C for the sodium and potassium content of foods).

POTASSIUM

The adult body is approximately 0.4% potassium, which is approximately twice the amount of sodium.

Functions

Potassium is involved with sodium in the maintenance of the body water balance, and it also has many other metabolic functions.

Water balance. Potassium is the major intracellular electrolyte. Its osmotic effect holds water inside the cells and counterbalances the osmotic effect of sodium, which draws water out of the cells and into the extracellular fluid compartments (see Figure 8-2).

Metabolic reactions. Potassium plays a role in energy production, the conversion of blood glucose into stored glycogen, and the synthesis of muscle protein.

Muscle action. Potassium ions also play a role in nerve impulse transmission to stimulate muscle action. Along with magnesium and sodium, potassium acts as a muscle relaxant that opposes the stimulating effect of calcium, which allows for muscle contraction. The heart muscle is sensitive to potassium levels; therefore, the blood potassium concentration is regulated within narrow tolerances.

Insulin release. Potassium is necessary for the release of insulin from pancreatic β cells in response to rising blood glucose concentrations.

Blood pressure. Sodium is one of the main dietary factors that are associated with hypertension; however, hypertension may be more related to the sodium and potassium molar ratio than to the amount of dietary sodium alone. A potassium intake that is equal to the sodium intake may help to prevent the development of hypertension, such is the basis for the Dietary Approaches to Stop Hypertension (DASH) diet. (You may visit the National Heart, Lung, and Blood Institute to learn more about the DASH diet, www.nhlbi.nih.gov/health/health-topics/topics/dash/, which will also be covered in Chapter 19.)

Requirements

The average American diet provides significantly less potassium than the established AI (4.7 g/day for adults), with a median daily intake of 2.7 g/day.[7] The *Dietary Guidelines for Americans* encourage the consumption of potassium through an increased daily intake of vegetables and low-fat dairy products.[17] Additional DRIs for potassium are listed in the summary table for major minerals (see Table 8-3) and in the DRI tables in Appendix B.

Deficiency

Symptoms of potassium deficiency are well-defined but seldom related to inadequate dietary intake. **Hypokalemia** is more likely to develop during clinical situations such as prolonged vomiting or diarrhea, severe malnutrition, or surgery. Hypokalemia also is a concern while a person is using antihypertensive medications, particularly diuretics that cause urinary potassium loss. Characteristic symptoms of potassium deficiency include heart muscle weakness with possible cardiac arrest, respiratory muscle weakness with breathing difficulties, poor intestinal muscle tone with resulting bloating, and overall muscle weakness.

Toxicity

As with sodium, the kidneys normally excrete excess potassium so that toxicity does not occur. However, if

---

hypernatremia a serum sodium level that is above normal.

hypokalemia a serum potassium level that is below normal.

oral potassium intake is excessive or if intravenous potassium is given that causes **hyperkalemia**, the heart muscle can weaken to the point at which it stops beating. A UL has not been established for potassium from food sources.

Food Sources

Potassium is an essential part of all living cells; thus, it is abundant in natural foods. The richest dietary sources of potassium are unprocessed foods: fruits such as oranges and bananas, vegetables such as potatoes and leafy green vegetables, fish, whole grains, legumes, seeds, and milk products. Those who eat the recommended number of servings of fruits and vegetables daily usually have an ideal potassium intake. Plant sources of potassium are highly water soluble; therefore, much of the potassium is lost when fruits and vegetables are boiled or blanched (unless the water is retained). Table 8-2 lists food sources of potassium.

CHLORIDE

Chloride is the chemical form of chlorine in the body. Chloride accounts for approximately 0.2% of the body's weight, and it is widely distributed throughout tissues.

Functions

Chloride is predominantly found in the extracellular fluid compartments, where it helps to maintain the water and acid-base balances (see Figure 8-2). Its two significant functions involve digestion and respiration.

Digestion. Chloride (Cl^-) is one element of the hydrochloric acid (HCl) that is secreted in the gastric juices. The action of gastric enzymes requires that stomach fluids have a specific acid concentration (i.e., a pH of approximately 1.0).

Respiration. Carbon dioxide, which is a by-product of cellular metabolism, is transported by red blood cells (RBCs) to the lungs, where it is expelled during respiration. Within the RBCs, the enzyme carbonic anhydrase combines carbon dioxide (CO_2) with water (H_2O) to form carbonic acid (H_2CO_3). Carbonic acid then dissociates into a bicarbonate ion (HCO_3^-) and a proton (H^+). Bicarbonate ions move out of the RBCs and into the plasma, and chloride ions (Cl^-) move into the RBCs and out of the plasma, thereby maintaining the balance of negative charges on either side of the RBC membrane. The exchange of a bicarbonate ion with a chloride ion in the plasma is called the *chloride shift.*

Requirements

The DRIs for chloride are listed in the DRI tables in Appendix B and in the summary table for major minerals (see Table 8-3). Similar to sodium's AI, the need for chloride gradually declines after the age of 50 years.

Deficiency

A dietary deficiency of chloride does not occur under normal circumstances. Because the normal intake and output of chloride from the body parallels that of sodium, conditions that lead to a sodium deficiency also can lead to a chloride deficiency. The primary reason for chloride deficiency is excessive loss of HCl through vomiting, which results in metabolic alkalosis from disturbances in the acid-base balance (see Chapter 9).

Toxicity

The only known dietary cause of chloride toxicity is as a result of severe dehydration, when the concentration of chloride is too great. No ULs are established for chloride.

Table 8-2	Food Sources of Potassium	
ITEM	**QUANTITY**	**AMOUNT (MG)**
Bread, Cereal, Rice, and Pasta		
Wheat germ, toasted cereal	½ cup	535
Vegetables		
Beet greens, boiled	½ cup	654
Potato, russet, baked, with skin	1 medium (173 g)	952
Swiss chard, boiled	½ cup	480
Sweet potato, baked in skin	1 medium (114 g)	542
Fruits		
Apricot, dried	¼ cup	550
Banana	1 medium (118 g)	422
Orange juice, fresh	8 fl oz	496
Prunes, dried, pitted	½ cup	637
Meat, Poultry, Fish, Dry Beans, Eggs, and Nuts		
Beans, white, boiled	½ cup	502
Clams, cooked, moist heat	3 oz	534
Halibut, cooked, dry heat	3 oz	449
Soybean, green, raw	½ cup	794
Soybeans, roasted	½ cup	1264
Milk and Dairy Products		
Milk, skim	8 fl oz	382
Yogurt, plain, low fat	8 fl oz	352

Data from the U.S. Department of Agriculture, Agricultural Research Service: Nutrient Data Laboratory. *USDA nutrient database for standard reference* (website): http://ndb.nal.usda.gov/ndb/. Accessed October 20, 2014.

hyperkalemia a serum potassium level that is above normal.

Food Sources

Dietary chloride is almost entirely provided by sodium chloride, which is the chemical name of ordinary table salt. The kidneys efficiently reabsorb chloride when dietary intake is low.

MAGNESIUM

Approximately 0.1% of the adult body weight is magnesium and 60% of that magnesium is found in the bones.

Functions

Magnesium has widespread metabolic functions, and it is found in all body cells. About 99% of body magnesium is intracellular, with the remaining 1% found in the extracellular space.

General metabolism. Magnesium is a necessary cofactor for more than 300 enzymes that make use of nucleotide triphosphates (e.g., adenosine triphosphate) for activating or catalyzing reactions that produce energy, synthesize body compounds, or help to transport nutrients across cell membranes.

Protein synthesis. Magnesium is a cofactor for enzymes that activate amino acids for protein synthesis and that synthesize and maintain DNA. When cells replicate, they must produce new proteins. The cell replication process requires magnesium to function correctly.

Muscle action. Magnesium ions are involved in the conduction of nerve impulses that stimulate muscle contraction as part of magnesium adenosine triphosphate (MgATP). Calcium is pumped out of the myofibrillar spaces into the sarcoplasmic reticulum by pumps that require MgATP for energy.

Basal energy expenditure. MgATP is involved in the secretion of thyroxine, thus helping the body to maintain a normal metabolic rate and to adapt to cold temperatures.

Requirements

The average American only consumes about 86% of the recommended intake for magnesium, with a median daily intake of 356 mg/day for men and 274 mg/day for women.[7] The DRIs for magnesium are listed in the summary table for major minerals (see Table 8-3) and in the DRI tables in Appendix B.

Deficiency

A primary deficiency of magnesium is quite rare among people who consume balanced diets. Symptoms of hypomagnesemia have been observed in clinical situations such as starvation, persistent vomiting or diarrhea with a loss of magnesium-rich gastrointestinal fluids, and most commonly as a result of renal disorders.

hypomagnesemia a serum magnesium level that is below normal.

Hypomagnesemia is also a symptom of various diseases that involve the cardiovascular and neuromuscular systems as well as in patients with diabetes mellitus, kidney disease, and chronic malnutrition with alcoholism.[18] In severe cases, hypomagnesemia can be life threatening. In cases of magnesium deficiency, it is commonly accompanied with other mineral deficiencies such as hypocalcemia and hypokalemia. Deficiency symptoms include muscle weakness, tetany, and ventricular arrhythmia, which can be fatal.[19]

Toxicity

Magnesium from food has not been observed to have adverse effects at high intake levels. Therefore, the DRI standards give a UL only for magnesium intake from supplements and pharmaceutical preparations. The UL from non-food sources is 350 mg/day for people who are 9 years old and older; it is less for younger children.[14] Individuals who consume excessive amounts of magnesium from supplements or non-food sources (e.g., medications) may experience nausea, vomiting, and diarrhea.

Food Sources

Although magnesium is relatively common in foods, the content is variable. Unprocessed foods have the highest concentrations of magnesium. Major food sources of magnesium include nuts, soybeans, legumes, whole grains, oats, and cocoa. More than 80% of the magnesium in cereal grains is lost with the removal of the germ and outer layers. Significant amounts of magnesium may also be present in drinking water in regions that have hard water with a fairly high mineral content.

SULFUR

Functions

As part of the amino acids cysteine and methionine, sulfur is an essential part of protein structure, and it is present in all body cells. It participates in widespread metabolic and structural functions, and it is also a component of the vitamins thiamin and biotin.

Hair, skin, and nails. Disulfide bonds between cysteine residues in the protein keratin are essential to the structure of the hair, skin, and nails.

General metabolic functions. Sulfhydryl or thiol groups (i.e., sulfur that is covalently bonded to hydrogen) form high-energy bonds that make various metabolic reactions energetically favorable.

Vitamin structure. Sulfur is a component of thiamin and biotin, which act as coenzymes in cell metabolism.

Collagen structure. The disulfide bonding of cysteine residues is necessary for collagen superhelix formation, and it is therefore important in the building of connective tissue.

Requirements

Dietary requirements for sulfur are not stated as such, because sulfur is supplied by protein foods that contain the amino acids methionine and cysteine.

Deficiency

Sulfur deficiency states have not been reported. Such conditions only relate to general protein malnutrition and the deficient intake of the sulfur-containing amino acids.

Toxicity

Sulfur is unlikely to reach toxic concentrations in the body as a result of dietary intake; thus, no UL has been established.

Food Sources

A diet that contains adequate protein contains adequate sulfur. Sulfur is only available to the body as part of the amino acids methionine and cysteine and in the vitamins thiamin and biotin. Thus, animal protein foods are the main dietary sources of sulfur. Sulfur is widely available in meat, eggs, milk, cheese, legumes, and nuts.

Table 8-3 provides a summary of the major minerals.

TRACE MINERALS

IRON

Iron has the longest and best-described history of all of the micronutrients. The human body contains approximately 45 mg of iron per kilogram of body weight. As with several other nutrients, iron is essential for life, but it can be toxic in excess. Thus, the body has developed exquisite systems for balancing iron intake and excretion and for efficiently transporting iron into and out of cells to maintain homeostasis. Iron is transported in the body bound to **transferrin**, and it is stored as **ferritin** in the liver, the spleen, and other tissues (Figure 8-3).

Functions

Iron serves as the functional part of hemoglobin, and it plays a role in the body's general metabolism.

---

transferrin a protein that binds and transports iron through the blood.
ferritin the storage form of iron.
anemia a condition that is characterized by a decreased number of circulating red blood cells, decreased hemoglobin, or both.

Hemoglobin synthesis. Approximately 70% of the body's iron is in hemoglobin within RBCs. Iron is a component of heme, which is the nonprotein part of hemoglobin. Hemoglobin carries oxygen to the cells, where it is used for oxidation and metabolism. Iron also is part of myoglobin, a protein found in muscle cells that is structurally and functionally analogous to hemoglobin in blood.

General metabolism. Iron is necessary for glucose metabolism, antibody production, drug detoxification by the liver, collagen and purine synthesis, and the conversion of β-carotene to active vitamin A.

Requirements

Iron needs vary throughout life, depending on growth and development. The DRIs for iron are listed in the summary table for trace minerals (see Table 8-7) and in the DRI tables in Appendix B. Women require more iron to cover the losses that occur during menstruation. Throughout pregnancy, a woman's RDA for iron increases to 27 mg/day. This increase often requires the addition of an iron supplement, because neither the typical American diet nor the iron stores of many women can meet the increased iron demands of pregnancy. The average iron intake of women in the United States is 13.6 mg/day, which is considerably less than the RDA of 18 mg/day.[7] It should be noted that iron needs are estimated to be 1.8 times higher for vegetarians than for omnivores to accommodate the lower bioavailability of iron from plant sources.[20]

Deficiency

The major condition that indicates a deficiency of iron is **anemia**. Iron-deficiency anemia is commonly evaluated by the percentage of packed RBCs (i.e., hematocrit), the RBC hemoglobin level, or the percentage of transferrin saturation. Iron-deficiency anemia is the most prevalent nutrition problem in the world today (Figure 8-4). The World Health Organization estimates that iron-deficiency anemia affects 24.8% of the population worldwide, with a disproportionate burden among preschool-aged children and pregnant women.[21] The prevalence of iron-deficiency anemia in the United States is significantly lower than that in other regions of the world. For example, the prevalence of anemia in preschool-aged children is estimated as follows per respective region: 64.6% in Africa, 47.7% in Asia, 39.5% in Latin American and the Caribbean, 28% in Oceania, 16.7% in Europe, and 3.4% in North America.[21]

Iron-deficiency anemia may have several causes, including the following: (1) inadequate dietary iron intake (i.e., primary deficiency); (2) excessive blood loss; (3) a lack of gastric hydrochloric acid, which liberates iron for intestinal absorption; (4) the presence of inhibitors of iron absorption (e.g., phytate, phosphate, tannin, oxalate); and (5) the manifestation of intestinal mucosal lesions that affect the absorptive surface area.

Table 8-3   **Summary of Major Minerals**

MINERAL	FUNCTIONS	RECOMMENDED INTAKE (ADULTS)	DEFICIENCY	TOLERABLE UPPER INTAKE LEVEL (UL) AND TOXICITY	SOURCES
Calcium (Ca)	Bone and teeth formation; blood clotting; muscle contraction and relaxation; nerve transmission	Between ages of 19 and 50 years, 1000 mg; between ages of 51 and 70 years, 1200 mg in women and 1000 mg in men; 70 years or older, 1000 mg	Tetany, rickets, osteoporosis	UL: 2500 mg Hypercalcemia; interferes with absorption of other nutrients	Dairy products, canned fish with bones, fortified foods (e.g., orange juice, cereal, tofu products)
Phosphorus (P)	Bone and tooth formation; energy metabolism; DNA and RNA; acid-base balance	700 mg	Unlikely, but can cause bone loss, loss of appetite, and weakness	UL: 4 g Bone resorption (loss of calcium)	High-protein foods (e.g., meat, dairy, fish), soft drinks
Sodium (Na)	Major extracellular fluid control; water and acid-base balance; muscle action; transmission of nerve impulse and resulting contraction; nutrient absorption	Adequate intake: between ages of 19 and 50 years, 1.5 g; between ages of 51 and 70 years, 1.3 g; 71 years or older, 1.2 g	Fluid shifts, acid-base imbalance, cramping	UL: 2.3 g Hypertension in salt-sensitive people; edema	Table salt, processed foods (e.g., luncheon meats, salty snacks)
Potassium (K)	Major intracellular fluid control; acid-base balance; regulation of nerve impulse and muscle contraction; blood pressure regulation; metabolic reactions	Adequate intake: 14 years or older, 4.7 g	Irregular heartbeat, difficulty breathing, muscle weakness	UL not set Cardiac arrest	Fresh fruits and vegetables, meats, dairy, legumes, whole grains
Chloride (Cl)	Acid-base balance (chloride shift); hydrochloric acid (digestion)	Adequate intake: between ages of 19 and 50 years, 2.3 g; between ages of 51 and 70 years, 2.0 g; 71 years or older, 1.8 g	Hypochloremic alkalosis with prolonged vomiting or diarrhea	UL not set Toxicity unlikely	Table salt, processed foods
Magnesium (Mg)	Coenzyme in metabolism, muscle and nerve action; helps with thyroid hormone secretion	Men, 400 to 420 mg; women, 310 to 320 mg	Tremor, spasm, ventricular arrhythmia	UL 350 mg (from supplements) Nausea; vomiting; diarrhea	Whole grains, nuts, seeds, legumes, spinach, cocoa
Sulfur (S)	Essential constituent of cell protein, hair, skin, nails, vitamin, and collagen structure; high-energy sulfur bonds in energy metabolism	Diets that are adequate in protein contain adequate sulfur	Unlikely	UL not set Toxicity unlikely	Meat, eggs, cheese, milk, nuts, legumes

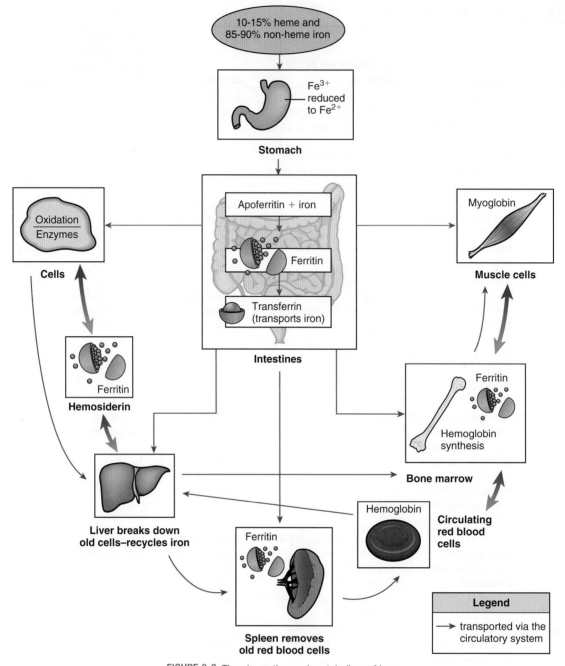

FIGURE 8-3 The absorption and metabolism of iron.

Toxicity

Iron toxicity from a single large dose (20 to 60 mg per kilogram of body weight) results in clinical manifestations that can be lethal.[22] In the United States, iron overdose from supplements is one of the leading causes of poisoning among young children who are less than 6 years old. Symptoms include nausea, vomiting, and diarrhea. If left untreated, the iron toxicity results in free radical damage that overwhelms the body's ability to neutralize the oxidative stress by antioxidants. Symptoms may progress to gastrointestinal bleeding and necrosis, shock, metabolic acidosis, and damage to the myocardium and liver, which may be fatal.[23] The UL for iron is 40 mg/day for children (birth to 18 years) and 45 mg/day for adults.[20]

Hemochromatosis may result from five types of genetic mutations, but it is most commonly the result of a mutation in the hemochromatosis (*HFE*) gene. The congenital disease is an autosomal recessive disorder that results in iron overload even though iron intake is within the normal range. This disorder affects from 1 in 150 to 1 in 250 individuals of northern European

hemochromatosis genetic disease resulting in iron overload

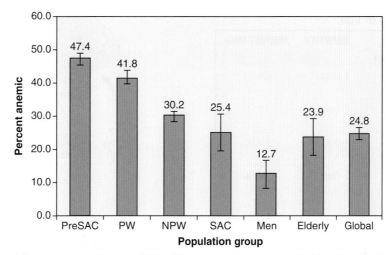

FIGURE 8-4 The global prevalence of anemia (%) in different population groups. *PreSAC,* Preschool-aged children (birth to 4.99 years old); *PW,* pregnant women; *NPW,* nonpregnant women (15 to 49.99 years old); *SAC,* school-aged children (5 to 14.99 years old); *Men,* 15 to 59.99 years old; *Elderly,* includes men who are more than 60 years old and women who are more than 50 years old. (Reprinted from McLean E, Cogswell M, Egil I et al. Worldwide prevalence of anaemia, WHO Vitamin and Mineral Nutrition Information System, 1993-2005. *Public Health Nutr.* 2009;12(4):444-454.)

descent.[24] Afflicted individuals absorb excessive amounts of iron from food; over time, the iron accumulation causes widespread organ damage (usually presenting between the ages of 40 and 60 years). Treatment involves frequent bloodletting (i.e., therapeutic phlebotomy) to reestablish normal serum iron levels; 200 to 250 mg of iron is removed along with each 500-mL unit of whole blood.[24] If treatment begins before pervasive damage occurs, patients may have a normal life expectancy.

Food Sources

The typical Western diet provides an average of 6 mg of iron per 1000 kcal of energy intake. Iron is widely distributed in the U.S. food supply, primarily in meat, eggs, fortified cereals, and some vegetables (Figure 8-5). Liver and fortified cereal products are especially good sources. The body absorbs iron more easily when it is taken along with vitamin C. Iron in food occurs in two forms: heme and nonheme. Heme iron is the most efficiently absorbed form of dietary iron, but it contributes the least to the total iron intake. Heme iron is found in only 40% of the animal food sources and in no plant foods (Table 8-4). Nonheme iron is less efficiently absorbed, because it is more tightly bound in foods, yet most of our food sources (i.e., 60% of the animal food sources and all the plant food sources) contain nonheme iron. To enhance the absorption of nonheme iron, food sources of vitamin C and moderate amounts of lean meats, fish, or poultry should be consumed in the same meal. Enriched and fortified cereal products are a good source of nonheme iron. Table 8-5 lists food sources of iron.

IODINE

The average adult body contains only 15 to 20 mg of iodine.

Functions

Iodine's basic function is as a component of thyroxine (T_4), a hormone that is synthesized by the thyroid gland and that helps to control the basal metabolic rate. T_4 synthesis is ultimately controlled by the hypothalamus and the pituitary gland. A sensitive system

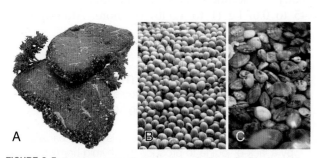

FIGURE 8-5 Food sources of dietary iron. **A,** Beef. **B,** Black-eyed peas. **C,** Oysters and clams. (Copyright JupiterImages Corp.)

Table 8-4	Characteristics of the Heme and Nonheme Portions of Dietary Iron	
	HEME	**NONHEME**
Food sources	None in plant sources; 40% of iron in animal sources	All iron in plant sources; 60% of iron in animal sources
Absorption rate	Rapid; transported and absorbed intact	Slow; tightly bound in organic molecules

Table 8-5	Food Sources of Iron	
ITEM	**QUANTITY**	**AMOUNT (MG)**
Bread, Cereal, Rice, and Pasta		
All Bran Complete Wheat Flakes cereal, Kellogg's	1 cup	24.01
Cream of Wheat, instant, prepared with water	1 cup	11.95
Oatmeal, fortified, instant, prepared with water	1 cup	13.95
Whole Grain Total cereal, General Mills	1 cup	24.00
Fruits and Vegetables		
Seaweed, spirulina, dried	½ cup	15.96
Spinach, boiled, drained*	½ cup	3.21
Meat, Poultry, Fish, Dry Beans, Eggs, and Nuts		
Beef, plate steak, lean only, grilled	3 oz	5.46
Chicken, giblets, simmered	3 oz	5.47
Lamb, liver, pan-fried	3 oz	8.67
Nuts, coconut milk, canned	1 cup	7.46
Oysters, wild, cooked, moist heat	3 oz	7.83
Pork, liver, braised	3 oz	15.23
Soybeans, boiled	½ cup	4.42
Soybeans, mature seeds, raw	½ cup	15.70

Data from the U.S. Department of Agriculture, Agricultural Research Service: Nutrient Data Laboratory. *USDA nutrient database for standard reference* (website): http://ndb.nal.usda.gov/ndb/. Accessed October 21, 2014.
*Low bioavailability.

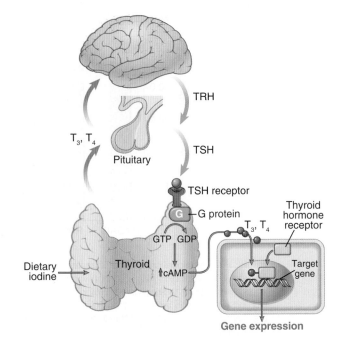

FIGURE 8-6 Uptake of iodine for triiodothyronine and thyroxine production. (Reprinted from Guyton AC, Hall JE. *Textbook of medical physiology.* 12th ed. Philadelphia: Saunders; 2006.)

of feedback mechanisms helps maintain adequate T_4 levels in the body.

The hypothalamus excretes **thyrotropin-releasing hormone (TRH)**. TRH, in turn, stimulates the release of TSH from the anterior pituitary gland. TSH controls the thyroid gland uptake of iodine from the bloodstream and the release of triiodothyronine (T_3) and T_4 into the circulation (Figure 8-6). Blood T_4 concentration acts as a feedback mechanism to determine how much TRH the hypothalamus releases and how much TSH the pituitary gland releases. As blood T_4 concentration decreases, the hypothalamus and the pituitary gland are stimulated to release more TRH and TSH, respectively. The transport form of iodine in the blood is called *serum protein-bound iodine.*

Requirements

To maintain desirable tissue levels of iodine, the adult body's minimal requirement is 50 to 75 mcg/day; therefore, to provide an extra margin of safety, the RDA is 150 mcg/day for all people who are 14 years of age and older.[20] Additional DRIs for iodine are listed in the summary table for trace minerals (see Table 8-7) and in the DRI tables in Appendix B.

Deficiency

The World Health Organization reports that iodine-deficiency disorders are the easiest and least expensive of all nutrient disorders to avert; however, they remain the number one cause of preventable brain damage worldwide.[25] Iodine-deficiency disorders are generally found in geographic locations with mountains or frequent flooding that result in poor soil iodine levels. Access to iodized salt has reduced the global prevalence of iodine deficiency in the last few decades.[26] However, nearly 30% of the world's population still has insufficient iodine intake; these individuals are at high risk for the following deficiency diseases.

Goiter. Goiter is characterized by an enlargement of the thyroid gland (Figure 8-7). When the thyroid gland is starved for iodine, it cannot produce a normal amount of T_4. Because of a low blood T_4 concentration, the pituitary gland continues to release more TSH. Large amounts of TSH overstimulate the nonproductive thyroid gland, thereby causing its size to increase greatly. An iodine-starved thyroid gland may weigh 0.45 to 0.67 kg (1 to 1.5 lb) or more. Although the

thyrotropin-releasing hormone (TRH) a hormone that is produced by the hypothalamus and that stimulates the release of thyroid-stimulating hormone by the pituitary.

goiter an enlarged thyroid gland that is usually caused by a lack of iodine to produce the thyroid hormone thyroxine.

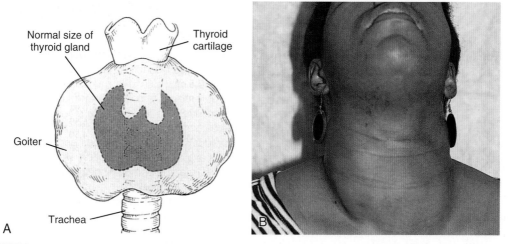

FIGURE 8-7 A, Illustration of a goiter. **B,** The extreme enlargement is a result of an extended duration of iodine deficiency. (**B,** Reprinted from Swartz MH. *Textbook of physical diagnosis.* 7th ed. Philadelphia: Saunders; 2014.)

thyroid is one of the larger endocrine glands, it normally only weighs 10 to 20 g in an adult.

Cretinism and congenital hypothyroidism. Cretinism is a congenital disorder resulting from insufficient thyroid hormone to the fetus during gestation. One reason for unavailable thyroid hormones is maternal iodine deficiency throughout pregnancy. Cretinism is characterized by physical deformity, dwarfism, mental retardation, and auditory disorders. During pregnancy, the mother's need for iodine takes precedence over the iodine needs of the developing fetus. Thus, the fetus suffers from iodine deficiency and continues to do so after birth. The physical and mental development of these children is severely impeded and irreversible.

Congenital hypothyroidism is a disorder resulting from insufficient thyroid hormone during gestation attributable to genetic defects in the metabolic pathways of the thyroid hormones. The severity of defects can vary greatly but early treatment can help prevent further damage (see the Cultural Considerations box, "Hypermetabolism and Hypometabolism: What are they and who is at risk?" in Chapter 6).

Impaired mental and physical development. Studying long-term effects of nutrient deficiencies is difficult. When a person or a population is deficient in one nutrient, they are likely deficient in other nutrients as well. In addition, there are usually other contributing factors that influence the results of the studies (e.g., sociodemographic, ethnic, lifestyle factors). That being said, there are studies indicating that children born to women with even mild iodine deficiency during pregnancy have a significant reduction in their intelligence quotient.[27] Long-term severe iodine deficiency during childhood and adolescence appears to delay growth and the onset of puberty, both of which may be corrected with normalization of dietary iodine levels.[28]

Hypothyroidism. Hypothyroidism occurs when a poorly functioning thyroid gland does not make enough T_4, thereby greatly reducing the basal metabolic rate. There are many causes of hypothyroidism, including both iodine deficiency and iodine toxicity. Iodine deficiency is the most common cause of hypothyroidism worldwide. Symptoms include thin, coarse hair; dry skin; poor cold tolerance; weight gain; and a low, husky voice.[29] In severe and rare cases, hypothyroidism can advance to myxedema coma and death.

Toxicity

When trying to correct for long-term iodine deficiency, practitioners must be careful of over-supplementing. Excess iodine supplementation may lead to thyrotoxicosis or iodine-induced hyperthyroidism.[30] Individuals with underlying thyroid dysfunction are more susceptible to iodine toxicity from chronic or acute doses than are individuals without existing thyroid dysfunction. Iodine toxicity may present as iodine-excess goiter, autoimmune thyroiditis, hypothyroidism, elevated TSH, and ocular damage.

Although the risk of iodine toxicity exists, the continued use of iodized salt is still recommended and widely practiced in several countries, including the United States. The risk for iodine deficiency far outweighs the small potential for iodine toxicity. The UL of iodine in healthy adults is 1100 mcg/day.[20]

Food Sources

The amount of iodine in natural food sources varies considerably depending on the iodine content of the soil in which the food was grown. Seafood consistently provides a good amount of iodine. However, the major reliable source of iodine in U.S. diets is iodized table salt, with each gram containing 77 mcg of iodine. Salt that is used in the preparation of food usually supplies adequate iodine for those people who do not use table salt.

ZINC

Zinc is an essential trace mineral with wide clinical significance. The amount of zinc in the adult body is approximately 1.5 g (0.05 oz) in women and 2.5 g (0.09 oz) in men.

Functions

Zinc is required for the optimal function of more than 300 enzymes. DNA, RNA, and protein synthesis, as well as energy metabolism and food intake regulation, are among the many biochemical and physiologic functions in which zinc is critically involved. Zinc has three major roles in metalloenzymes, including (1) participation in catalytic functions, (2) maintenance of structural stability, and (3) involvement in regulatory functions. These metalloenzymes are active in all major metabolic pathways and are involved in the formation or hydrolysis of proteins, lipids, and carbohydrates. All aspects of the immune system are dependent on adequate zinc availability.[31] Reproduction, optimal activity of growth hormone, and successful synaptic neurotransmission are also among the activities dependent upon zinc. Another critical function of zinc is its role in the structure and function of biomembranes. Zinc functions as a stabilizer of erythrocyte membranes, thus decreasing peroxidation and oxidative damage.

Requirements

Refer to the DRI tables in Appendix B or the summary tables for trace minerals (see Table 8-7) for zinc's RDA. Due to low bioavailability of zinc from plant and grain products, it is estimated that the dietary need for zinc in vegan populations may be as high as 50% greater than their respective DRI.[20]

Deficiency

Adequate zinc intake is imperative for good health during periods of rapid tissue growth, such as childhood and adolescence. Stunted growth, especially in boys, has been observed in some populations in which dietary zinc intake is low.[32] **Hypogeusia** and **hyposmia** are improved with increased zinc intake if dietary zinc intake was previously inadequate. Zinc deficiency commonly causes poor wound healing, hair loss, diarrhea, skin irritation, and overall compromised immune function.[33] Patients with poor appetites, who subsist on marginal diets, or who have chronic wounds or illnesses with excessive tissue breakdown, may be particularly vulnerable to developing zinc deficiency. The For Further Focus box, "Zinc Barriers" discusses other inhibitors to adequate zinc status.

---

hypogeusia impaired taste.
hyposmia impaired ability to smell.

For Further Focus

Zinc Barriers

Inadequate zinc intake, and overt zinc deficiency, is a worldwide nutrition concern, particularly in developing countries.[1] While the prevalence is much lower in developed countries, there remains a risk of inadequate zinc status for some Americans. In a few cases, a primary zinc deficiency may be the cause; however, it is more commonly because susceptible individuals are choosing foods and supplements that reduce zinc's availability for absorption. Here are some examples:

- Dietary fiber may hinder absorption and create a negative zinc balance.
- Vitamin and mineral supplements may contain iron-to-zinc ratios of greater than 3:1 and thus provide enough iron to inhibit zinc absorption.
- Animal foods, which are rich in readily available zinc, are consumed less by cholesterol-conscious individuals.
- Vegetarian diets contain less bioavailable zinc due to high phytic acid consumption.

Low levels of zinc can reduce the amount of carrier-proteins available to transport iron and vitamin A to their target tissues. It can also reduce an individual's immunity and normal appetite and taste for certain foods.

The following suggestions may help to increase dietary zinc bioavailability:

- Include some form of animal food (e.g., meat, milk, and eggs) or vegetarian-acceptable fortified food in the diet each day to ensure an adequate intake of zinc.
- Avoid the excessive use of alcohol.
- Avoid "crash" diets, which are typically low in micronutrients.
- If taking a dietary supplement of zinc, do so separately from iron supplements.

Signs of zinc deficiency are fairly rare in developed countries, but they are becoming more apparent among at-risk people (e.g., older adults who are hospitalized with long-term chronic illnesses, pediatric populations, some vegans).[1-3] However, there is no need for the general public to take megadoses of supplemental zinc. These large doses may compete with other minerals (e.g., iron) and create other micronutrient deficiency problems. Excess zinc can lead to nausea, abdominal pain, anemia, and immune system impairment. As with other nutrients, too much of a good thing can sometimes be as bad as—or even worse than—too little.

REFERENCES

1. Prasad AS. Impact of the discovery of human zinc deficiency on health. *J Trace Elem Med Biol.* 2014;28(4):357-363.
2. Foster M, et al. Effect of vegetarian diets on zinc status: a systematic review and meta-analysis of studies in humans. *J Sci Food Agric.* 2013;93(10):2362-2371.
3. Willoughby JL, Bowen CN. Zinc deficiency and toxicity in pediatric practice. *Curr Opin Pediatr.* 2014;26(5):579-584.

Acrodermatitis enteropathica (AE) is a rare autosomal recessive disorder that results in severe zinc deficiency and death if it is not treated. Patients with this condition are not able to absorb sufficient zinc from the gut. Classic symptoms of acrodermatitis enteropathica begin with skin lesions and progress to severely compromised immune function (Figure 8-8). This inborn error of metabolism is successfully treated with oral

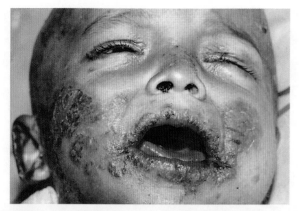

FIGURE 8-8 Skin lesions that are characteristic of severe zinc deficiency in a patient with acrodermatitis enteropathica. (From Kumar V, Abbas AK, Fausto N. *Robbins and Cotran pathologic basis of disease.* 7th ed. Philadelphia: Saunders; 2005.)

zinc supplements at high doses if it is diagnosed during infancy.

Toxicity

As with several other minerals, zinc toxicity from food sources alone is uncommon. However, prolonged supplementation that exceeds the recommended zinc intake can alter lymphocyte function and cause adverse symptoms such as nausea, vomiting, and epigastric pain.[34] The UL for zinc of 40 mg/day was established on the basis of the negative effects of excess zinc supplementation on copper metabolism.[20] Excessive zinc intake inhibits copper absorption, thereby resulting in a zinc-induced copper deficiency.

Food Sources

The greatest source of dietary zinc in the United States is meat, which supplies approximately 70% of the zinc that is consumed. Seafood (particularly oyster) is another excellent source of zinc. Legumes and whole grains are reasonable sources of zinc, but the zinc in these foods is less available for intestinal absorption as a result of phytate binding. A balanced diet usually meets adult needs for zinc. People who consume diets with little or no animal products and who have a high intake of phytate-rich unrefined grains may benefit from zinc-fortified foods or supplements to avoid zinc deficiency.[35] Table 8-6 lists food sources of zinc.

SELENIUM

Functions

Selenium is present in all body tissues except adipose tissue. The highest concentrations of selenium are in the liver, kidneys, heart, and spleen. Selenium is an essential part of the antioxidant enzyme glutathione peroxidase, which protects the lipids in cell membranes from oxidative damage. An abundance of selenium may spare vitamin E to an extent, because both selenium and vitamin E protect against free radical damage. Selenium is also a component of many

Table 8-6 Food Sources of Zinc

ITEM	QUANTITY	AMOUNT (MG)
Bread, Cereal, Rice, and Pasta		
All-Bran Complete Wheat Flakes cereal, Kellogg's	1 cup	20.00
Whole Grain Total cereal, General Mills	1 cup	20.00
Meat, Poultry, Fish, Dry Beans, Eggs, and Nuts		
Beef, chuck, short ribs, lean only, braised	3 oz	10.44
Crab, Alaskan king, cooked, moist heat	3 oz	6.48
Lobster, northern, cooked, moist heat	3 oz	3.44
Oyster, eastern, farmed, cooked, dry heat	3 oz	38.38
Oysters, eastern, wild, cooked, moist heat	3 oz	66.81
Soybean, mature seeds, roasted	½ cup	2.70
Milk and Dairy Products		
Yogurt, plain, skim milk	8 fl oz	2.20

Data from the U.S. Department of Agriculture, Agricultural Research Service: Nutrient Data Laboratory. *USDA nutrient database for standard reference* (website): <http://ndb.nal.usda.gov/ndb/>; Accessed October 21, 2014.

proteins in the body that are referred to as *selenoproteins*. One such selenoprotein is type 1 iodothyronine 5′-deiodinase, which is the enzyme required to convert T_4 to T_3.

Requirements

Refer to the summary table for trace minerals (see Table 8-7) and in the DRI tables in Appendix B for the DRIs of selenium.

Deficiency

Inadequate selenium negatively alters immune function and increases the opportunity for oxidative stress, specifically within the thyroid gland. Selenium intake varies greatly worldwide along with soil selenium availability. Selenium deficiency is generally only found in geographic areas with a poor soil content of selenium. Adequate selenium intake plays a role in preventing *Kashin-Bek disease* and *Keshan disease*. Kashin-Bek disease results in chronic arthritis and joint deformity. Keshan disease, which is named after the area in China where it was discovered, is a disease of the heart muscle that primarily affects young children and women of childbearing age and that can lead to heart failure as a result of cardiomyopathy (i.e., degeneration of the heart muscle).

Toxicity

The most common symptoms of selenium toxicity are hair loss, joint pain, nail discoloration, and gastrointestinal upset (i.e., nausea, vomiting, and diarrhea). Most known cases of dietary selenium toxicity are in isolated regions of the world where the soil has extremely high levels of selenium. However, in 2008 a misformulated dietary supplement resulted in 201 cases of selenium poisoning in the United States, with symptoms that persisted for more than 3 months.[36] The UL for selenium is 400 mcg/day for people who are 14 years old and older.[37]

Food Sources

Most selenium in food is highly available for intestinal absorption. The amount of selenium in food depends on the quantity of selenium in the soil that is used to graze animals and grow plants. Pork, turkey, lamb, chicken, and organ meats (e.g., beef liver) are consistently good sources of selenium. Fish, whole grains, and other seeds are a decent source of selenium, but the quantity will vary. Brazil nuts are an exceptionally good source of selenium with 1275 mg per ½ cup serving.[38] In the United States and Canada, the dietary intake of selenium can vary by the geographic region in which the fruits and vegetables are grown, but these local differences are mostly mitigated by the national food distribution system. The average adult intake of selenium in the United States is 114.5 mcg/day.[7]

The following sections briefly review the remaining essential trace minerals.

FLUORIDE

Fluoride forms a strong bond with calcium; thus, it accumulates in calcified body tissues such as bones and teeth. Fluoride's main function in human nutrition is to prevent the development of dental caries. Fluoride strengthens the ability of teeth to withstand the erosive effect of bacterial acids. The use of fluoridated toothpaste (0.1% fluoride) and improved dental hygiene habits have greatly benefited dental health. Additionally, the fluoridation of the public water supply (for which the optimal level is 1 ppm) is responsible for an added decline in dental caries during recent decades.

The DRIs for fluoride are listed in the summary table for trace minerals (see Table 8-7) and in the DRI tables in Appendix B. The DRI guidelines set the UL for fluoride at 10 mg/day for people who are 9 years old and older to avoid dental **fluorosis** (Figure 8-9).[14]

Crab, shrimp, raisins, grape juice, hot breakfast cereals (Cream of Wheat, grits, and oatmeal), and tea contain the highest concentrations of fluoride. Cooking in fluoridated water raises the fluoride concentration in many foods. People who are using well water should periodically check the fluoride concentration of their water, because well water can contain excessively high natural sources of fluoride.

---

fluorosis an excess intake of fluoride that causes the yellowing of teeth, white spots on the teeth, and the pitting or mottling of tooth enamel.

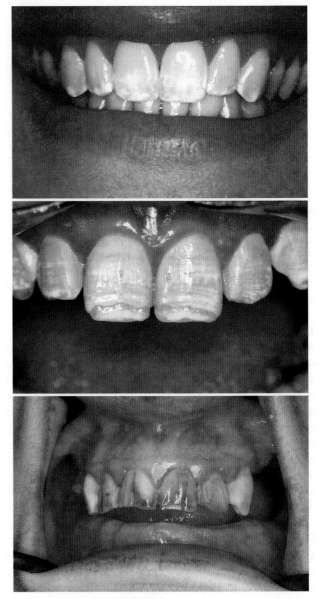

FIGURE 8-9 Fluorosis.

COPPER

Copper has frequently been called the "iron twin," because both iron and copper are metabolized in much the same way, and both are components of cell enzymes. Both of these minerals are also involved in energy production and hemoglobin synthesis. Primary deficiency of copper is rare.

There are two severe inborn errors of metabolism that involve copper. The first is *Menkes' disease*, which is an X-linked genetic disease of copper metabolism that currently has no treatment or cure. Individuals who are affected with Menkes' disease progress through neurodegeneration and connective tissue deterioration, and they usually do not survive past childhood.[39] *Wilson's disease* is a rare autosomal recessive genetic disorder that causes an abnormally high storage of copper in the body. Without treatment,

Wilson's disease can result in liver and nerve damage that leads to death. However, there are treatments for Wilson's disease that may stabilize or even reverse deleterious effects of the disease.[40]

The DRIs for copper are listed in the summary table for trace minerals (see Table 8-7) and in the DRI tables in Appendix B. The UL for copper is 10 mg/day to avoid gastrointestinal upset and liver damage.[20] Copper is widely distributed in natural foods. Organ meats (especially liver), veal, beef, lamb, oysters, soy flour, and legumes are the richest food sources of copper.

MANGANESE

An adult body of approximately 150 lb contains 14 mg of manganese that is found primarily in the brain, bone, liver, pancreas, and pituitary gland. Manganese functions like many other trace minerals: as a component of cell enzymes. Manganese-dependent enzymes catalyze many important metabolic reactions. These metabolic reactions include metabolism of carbohydrates, amino acids, and cholesterol; formation of bone and cartilage; and wound healing through its role in manganese-activated glycosyltransferases. In some magnesium-dependent enzymes, manganese may serve as a substitute for magnesium, depending on the availability of these two minerals. The intestinal absorption and bodily retention of manganese are associated with serum ferritin concentration.

Manganese deficiency has been documented in animal studies, but there are no known manganese deficiencies among humans who are consuming an unrestricted diet. Manganese toxicity occurs as an industrial occupation disease known as *inhalation toxicity* in miners and other workers who are exposed to manganese dust over long periods. The excess manganese accumulates in the liver and the central nervous system, thereby producing severe neuromuscular symptoms that are similar to those of Parkinson's disease. There is also a potential for manganese toxicity among patients who are receiving parenteral nutrition with standard trace element supplementation, because the bioavailability is approximately 95% greater than if it is absorbed enterally. In addition, the normal elimination pathway is often impaired in these patients; thus, manganese accumulates and damages the brain.[41] The UL from dietary sources is 11 mg/day for healthy adults.[20]

The DRIs for manganese are listed in the summary table for trace minerals (see Table 8-7) and in the DRI tables in Appendix B. The most commonly consumed food sources of manganese are of plant origin. Whole grains, cereal products, and soybeans are the richest food sources.

MOLYBDENUM

Molybdenum is better absorbed than many minerals, and inadequate dietary intake is unlikely. The amount of molybdenum in the body is exceedingly small. Molybdenum is the functional catalytic component in several cell enzymes involved in oxidation-reduction reactions. The DRIs for molybdenum are listed in the summary table for trace minerals (see Table 8-7) and in the DRI tables in Appendix B. There is a UL for molybdenum of 2000 mcg/day for adults due to symptoms similar to gout at very high doses (>10 g/day).[20] The amounts of molybdenum in foods vary considerably depending on the soil in which they are grown.

CHROMIUM

Chromium is thought to be an essential component of the organic complex glucose tolerance factor, which stimulates the action of insulin. Chromium supplements were previously thought to reduce insulin resistance (the cause of impaired glucose tolerance) and to improve lipid profiles for at-risk patients. However, a randomized double-blind study that examined the effects of chromium supplements in subjects with impaired glucose tolerance did not find significant improvements in glucose tolerance among those who took chromium compared with the control group.[42] As a result of lack of evidence to the contrary, several researchers believe that chromium should be removed from the list of essential elements for human nutrition because other functions of chromium have not been satisfactorily identified.[43-45]

The AIs for chromium are listed in the summary table for trace minerals (see Table 8-7) and in the DRI tables in Appendix B. No UL has been established.[20] The food content of chromium is difficult to establish and will vary according to soil mineral content where plants are cultivated or animals graze.

Table 8-7 provides a summary of selected trace elements.

OTHER ESSENTIAL TRACE MINERALS

RDAs and AIs were not set for the remaining trace minerals: aluminum, arsenic, boron, nickel, silicon, tin, and vanadium. At the time of the 2002 DRIs, not enough data were available to establish such recommendations.[20] Most of these minerals are deemed essential to the nutrition of specific animals and may be essential to human nutrition as well, although the complete process of their metabolism is not yet fully understood. Because these minerals occur in such small amounts, they are difficult to study, and dietary deficiency is highly unlikely.

The available research data regarding boron, nickel, and vanadium are sufficient to establish a tolerable UL level. The adult ULs for both boron and vanadium were set on the basis of data that were gathered from animal studies: for boron, the UL is 20 mg/day; for vanadium, it is 1.8 mg/day. The adult UL for arsenic was set at 1 mg/day.[20]

Table 8-7   Summary of Selected Trace Elements

MINERAL	FUNCTIONS	RECOMMENDED INTAKE (ADULTS)	DEFICIENCY	TOLERABLE UPPER INTAKE LEVEL (UL) AND TOXICITY	SOURCES
Iron (Fe)	Hemoglobin and myoglobin formation; cellular oxidation of glucose; antibody production	Men, 8 mg; women between ages of 19 and 50 years, 18 mg; women who are 50 years old or older, 8 mg	Anemia, pale skin, impaired immune function	UL: 45 mg Nausea; vomiting; diarrhea; liver, kidney, heart, and central nervous system damage; hemochromatosis	Liver, meats, egg yolk, whole grains, enriched grains, dark green vegetables, legumes, nuts
Iodine (I)	Synthesis of thyroxine, which regulates cell oxidation and basal metabolic rate	150 mcg	Goiter, cretinism, hypothyroidism, hyperthyroidism	UL: 1100 mcg Goiter	Iodized salt, seafood
Zinc (Zn)	Essential enzyme constituent; protein metabolism; storage of insulin; immune system; sexual maturation	Men, 11 mg; women, 8 mg	Impaired wound healing and taste and smell acuity, stunted sexual and physical development	UL: 40 mg Nausea; vomiting; decreased immune function; impaired copper absorption	Meat, seafood (especially oysters), eggs, enriched grains, legumes
Selenium (Se)	Forms glutathione peroxidase; spares vitamin E as an antioxidant; protects lipids in cell membrane	55 mcg	Impaired immune function, Keshan disease, heart muscle failure	UL: 400 mcg Brittleness of hair and nails; gastrointestinal upset	Seafood, kidney, liver, meats, whole grains, Brazil nuts
Fluoride (Fl)	Constituent of bone and teeth; helps prevent dental caries	Adequate Intake: men, 4 mg; women, 3 mg	Increased dental caries	UL: 10 mg Dental fluorosis	Fluoridated water, toothpaste
Copper (Cu)	Associated with iron in energy production, hemoglobin synthesis, iron absorption and transport, and nerve and immune function	900 mcg	Anemia, bone abnormalities	UL: 10 mg Wilson's disease, which results in liver and nerve conduction damage	Liver, seafood, whole grains, legumes, nuts
Manganese (Mn)	Activates reactions in urea synthesis, energy metabolism, lipoprotein clearance, and synthesis of fatty acids	Adequate Intake: men, 2.3 mg; women, 1.8 mg	Clinical deficiency present only with protein-energy malnutrition	UL: 11 mg Inhalation toxicity in miners, which results in neuromuscular disturbances	Cereals, whole grains, soybeans, legumes, nuts, tea, vegetables, fruits
Molybdenum (Mo)	Constituent of many enzymes	45 mcg	Unlikely	UL: 2 mg Toxicity unlikely	Organ meats, milk, whole grains, leafy vegetables, legumes
Chromium (Cr)	Associated with glucose metabolism	Adequate Intake: men, 35 mcg; women, 25 mcg	Impaired glucose metabolism	UL not set Toxicity unlikely	Whole grains, cereal products, brewer's yeast

MINERAL SUPPLEMENTATION

The same principles that were discussed in Chapter 7 for vitamin supplementation apply to mineral supplementation. Special needs during growth periods and in clinical situations may merit specific mineral supplements. Before taking supplements, potential nutrient-nutrient interactions and drug-nutrient interactions should be considered. Several situations can occur in which mineral bioavailability may be hindered (see the Drug-Nutrient Interaction box, "Mineral Depletion").

Drug-Nutrient Interaction

Mineral Depletion

Medications interact with minerals through two major mechanisms: either by blocking absorption or by inducing renal excretion. The following are examples of drug-nutrient interactions that specifically affect mineral status:

- *Diuretics:* People who require the long-term use of diuretic drugs for the treatment of hypertension may need to pay special attention to certain minerals that are also lost. The minerals that are usually excreted with excess water are sodium, potassium, magnesium, and zinc. The intake of foods that are high in these minerals is generally enough to regain homeostasis. Some diuretics (e.g., spironolactone) are potassium sparing and thus extra potassium should not be consumed.
- *Chelating agents:* Chelation therapy is used to remove excess metal ions from the body. Penicillamine is used to treat Wilson's disease and rheumatoid arthritis and to prevent kidney stones. It attaches to zinc and copper, thereby blocking absorption and leading to the excretion and possible depletion of both minerals.
- *Antacids:* The acidic environment of the stomach is required for the absorption of many drugs and nutrients, including minerals. When this environment is altered as a result of the chronic use of antacids, mineral deficiencies can occur. Phosphate deficiency is a concern for individuals who are chronically using over-the-counter antacids. In extreme cases, hypercalcemia may result, causing damage to soft tissues.

LIFE CYCLE NEEDS

Mineral supplements may be warranted in specific situations during rapid growth periods throughout the life cycle.

Pregnancy and Lactation

Women require additional copper, iodine, iron, magnesium, manganese, molybdenum, selenium, zinc, and potentially chromium to meet the demands of rapid fetal growth during pregnancy. DRIs remain elevated for several minerals throughout lactation to meet both mother and infant needs. Not all women will require dietary supplements to meet these increased needs, because they will be met with a healthy, balanced diet. However, iron is regularly supplemented because it is challenging to meet the DRI recommendations through dietary intake alone during pregnancy.

Adolescence

Rapid bone growth during adolescence requires increased calcium, phosphorus, and magnesium.[14,46] If an adolescent's diet is chronically lacking in the minerals critical for bone development at this vital stage, the risk for osteoporosis during the later adult years is intensified.[47] Too little dietary calcium may lead to the resorption of calcium from bone to maintain an appropriate blood calcium concentration. With the major increases in soft-drink consumption coupled with the decreased intake of calcium-containing drinks (i.e., milk or milk substitutes) in the United States, there is reason for concern about poor bone growth during these important years.

Depending on the adequacy of their diet, supplements that combine iron with folate may be indicated for adolescent girls as they begin menstruating.

Adulthood

Healthy adults who consume well-balanced and varied diets do not require mineral supplements. A well-rounded and varied diet in combination with adequate physical activity and exercise maintains optimal bone health in most adults. Studies do indicate that supplemental calcium and vitamin D improve bone health and reduce the risk of fracture among postmenopausal women.[48] However, at any adult age, calcium supplementation alone neither prevents nor successfully treats osteoporosis, the cause of which is multifactorial. In addition to other lifestyle improvements when indicated (e.g., balanced diet, no tobacco products, healthy weight maintenance), calcium supplements may be used as part of a treatment program together with vitamin D, weight-bearing physical activity, and hormone therapy to reduce the risk of osteoporosis.[49]

CLINICAL NEEDS

People with certain clinical problems or those who are at high risk for developing such problems may require mineral supplements.

Iron-Deficiency Anemia

One of the most prevalent health problems encountered in population surveys is iron-deficiency anemia. The need for increased iron intake has long been established for pregnant and breastfeeding women.[20] The following high-risk groups also may need to supplement their diets: adolescent girls and women who are in their childbearing years who consume poor diets; people who are food insecure (i.e., those who are not able to secure enough food on a consistent basis); alcohol-dependent individuals; vegetarians; and elderly people who consume poor diets.

Zinc Deficiency

The increased popularity of vegetarian diets has amplified concern about possible zinc deficiency because of the low zinc content and bioavailability found in plant foods. The position statement of the Academy of Nutrition and Dietetics and the Dietitians of Canada regarding vegetarian diets indicates that zinc requirements for individuals who consume high phytate diets may exceed the current DRIs.[35] Signs of zinc deficiency are slow growth, impaired taste and smell, poor wound healing, and skin irritation; however, 3 to 24 weeks may pass before symptoms appear. Others who are at risk for zinc deficiency include alcohol-dependent individuals; people on long-term, low-calorie diets; and elderly people in long-term institutional care.

Putting It All Together

Summary

- Minerals are elements that are widely distributed in foods. They are absorbed by the intestines and used in building body tissue; activating, regulating, and controlling metabolic processes; and transmitting neurologic messages.
- Minerals are classified in accordance with their relative amounts in the body. Major minerals are necessary in larger quantities than trace minerals, and they make up 60% to 80% of all of the inorganic material in the body. Trace minerals, which are necessary in quantities as small as a microgram, make up less than 1% of the body's inorganic material.
- RDAs have not been set for all minerals because of a lack of scientific data. However, AIs or ULs have been set for almost all essential minerals without RDAs.
- Mineral supplementation—along with vitamin supplementation—continues to be a hot topic of research. There are periods that occur throughout the life cycle and specific disease states that may warrant supplementation. However, in most situations, a balanced diet provides an adequate supply of all of the essential nutrients.

Chapter Review Questions

See answers in Appendix A.

1. It would be beneficial for a 65-year-old woman to consume foods with calcium that are well absorbed such as:
   a. Yogurt.
   b. Baked beans.
   c. Orange slices
   d. Chicken livers.

2. Phosphorus functions in metabolic processes to maintain health by:
   a. Assisting in the formation of fibrin to form clots.
   b. Controlling the uptake of iodine from the blood.
   c. Capturing energy in the form of adenosine triphosphate.
   d. Carrying oxygen to the cells for oxidation and metabolism.

3. A patient has been taking a diuretic medication to manage blood pressure and complains of overall weakness, difficulty breathing, and a feeling of abdominal bloating. These symptoms may be characteristic of:
   a. Sodium toxicity.
   b. Potassium deficiency.
   c. Excess potassium intake.
   d. Iron toxicity.

4. A patient with high blood pressure is recommended to reduce sodium intake in the diet. A food choice that should be limited is:
   a. Whole grain toast with peanut butter.
   b. Pork loin with cranberry sauce.
   c. Beef and bean burrito.
   d. Olive and feta cheese salad.

5. Hypothyroidism is characterized by:
   a. Thin coarse hair, weight gain, poor cold tolerance.
   b. Thin coarse hair, general nervousness, weight loss.
   c. Acne-like skin lesions, weight loss, increased appetite.
   d. Weight gain, heat intolerance, dwarfism.

Additional Learning Resources

evolve http://evolve.elsevier.com/Williams/basic/

References and **Further Reading and Resources** in the back of the book provide additional resources for enhancing knowledge.

Water and Electrolyte Balance

Key Concepts

- Water compartments inside and outside of the cells maintain a balanced distribution of total body water.
- The concentration of various solute particles in water determines the internal shifts and movement of water.

- Water and electrolyte balance has many checks and balances beginning at the cellular level and involves organ and hormonal controls.
- A state of **dynamic equilibrium** among the body's water and acid-base balance system influences the entire body to sustain life.

Water is the most vital nutrient to human existence. Humans can survive far longer without food than without water. Only the continuous need for air is more demanding.

One of the most basic nutrition tasks is ensuring a balanced distribution of water to all body cells. Water is critical for the physiologic functions that are necessary to support life. This chapter briefly looks at the finely developed water and electrolyte balance systems in the body, examines how these systems work, and describes the various parts and processes that maintain them.

BODY WATER FUNCTIONS AND REQUIREMENTS

WATER: THE FUNDAMENTAL NUTRIENT

Basic Principles

Three basic principles are essential to an understanding of the balance and uses of water in the human body.

A unified whole. The human body forms one continuous body of water that is contained by a protective envelope of skin. Water moves to all parts of the body, and it is controlled by solvents within the water and membranes that separate the compartments. Virtually every space inside and outside of cells is filled with water-based body fluids. Within this environment, all processes that are necessary to life are sustained.

Body water compartments. The key word *compartment* is generally used in human physiology to refer to dynamic areas within the body. Body water can be discussed in terms of total body water as well as in separate intracellular or extracellular compartments throughout the body. Membranes separate compartments of water. The body's dynamic mechanisms constantly shift water to places of greatest need and

maintain equilibrium among all parts. The compartments are discussed later in this chapter.

Particles in the water solution. The concentration and distribution of particles in water (e.g., sodium, chloride, calcium, magnesium, phosphate, bicarbonate, protein) determine the internal shifts and balances among the compartments of water throughout the body.

Homeostasis

The body's state of dynamic balance is called **homeostasis**. W.B. Cannon, a physiologist, viewed these principles as "body wisdom."[1] Early in the twentieth century he applied the term *homeostasis* to the capacity that is built into the body to maintain its life systems, despite what enters the system from the outside. The body has a great capacity to use numerous finely balanced homeostatic mechanisms to protect its vital water supply.

BODY WATER FUNCTIONS

Body water performs the following functions:

Solvent

Water provides the basic liquid solvent for all chemical reactions within the body. The **polarity** of water effectively ionizes and dissolves many substances.

---

dynamic equilibrium the process of maintaining balance (i.e., equilibrium) through constant change or motion by energy or action (i.e., dynamic).

homeostasis the state of relative dynamic equilibrium within the body's internal environment; a balance that is achieved through the operation of various interrelated physiologic mechanisms.

polarity the interaction between the positively charged end of one molecule and the negative end of another (or the same) molecule.

Transport

Water circulates throughout the body in the form of blood and various other secretions and tissue fluids. In this circulating fluid, the many nutrients, secretions, metabolites (i.e., products formed from metabolism), and other materials can be carried anywhere in the body to meet the needs of all body cells.

Thermoregulation

Water is necessary to help maintain a stable body temperature. As the body temperature rises, sweat is released and evaporates from the skin, thereby cooling the body.

Lubricant

Water also has a lubricating effect on moving parts of the body. For example, fluid within joints (i.e., synovial fluid) helps to provide smooth movement and prevents damage from constant friction.

BODY WATER REQUIREMENTS

The Dietary Reference Intake (DRI) for water is based on the median total water intake reported by participants in the Third National Health and Nutrition Examination Survey (NHANES), which took place from 1988 to 1994. The amount of total water includes water in both beverages and food. Set as Adequate Intakes (AI), the DRIs for water are the amounts that are required to meet the needs of healthy individuals who are relatively sedentary and living in temperate climates.[2] Recommendations are established to note ideal water intake amounts and to caution against the harmful effects of dehydration, which include metabolic and functional abnormalities. To meet adult fluid needs, the average sedentary woman should consume 2.7 L (91 oz) of total water per day. Because approximately 19% of total water intake comes from food, a woman should aim for 74 oz (≈9.25 cups or 2.2 L) of fluids in the form of beverages per day, with the rest being provided by food. A sedentary man should consume 3.7 L (125 oz) of total water per day. Assuming that approximately 0.7 L of water is consumed within food, a man should aim for 101 oz (≈12.6 cups or 3 L) of fluid in the form of beverages per day.[2] Table 9-1 lists the AI values of fluid for all individuals.

The body's requirement for water varies in accordance with several aspects: environment, activity level, functional losses, metabolic needs, age, and other dietary influences. Therefore any number of these factors will change the individual requirement for fluid intake to offset losses.

Surrounding Environment

Increasing body temperatures may be caused by the climate or by the heat produced by physical work. Whatever the cause, high body temperature results in water loss through sweat and requires fluid intake for replacement. On the opposite end of the spectrum, both cold temperatures and altitude result in elevated respiratory water loss, hypoxia- or cold-induced diuresis, and increased energy expenditure, all of which raise water needs as well.[2]

Activity Level

Heavy work and physical activity increase the water requirement for two reasons: (1) more water is lost in sweat and respiration; and (2) more water is necessary for the increased metabolic demands of physical activity.

Fluid intake needs during activity are highly variable and will depend on body size, sweat rates, and type of activity. Thus, specific hydration plans should be determined on an individual basis. For the average person, fluid balance will be reestablished through normal dietary intake.[3] Athletes may require more specificity to their fluid intake regimen before, during, and after exercise because of prolonged or intense training sessions. The American College of Sports

Table 9-1 Adequate Intake of Water (Liters Per Day)*

AGE	MALE FROM FOOD	MALE FROM BEVERAGES	MALE TOTAL WATER	FEMALE FROM FOOD	FEMALE FROM BEVERAGES	FEMALE TOTAL WATER
Birth to 6 months	0.0	0.7	0.7	0.0	0.7	0.7
7 to 12 months	0.2	0.6	0.8	0.2	0.6	0.8
1 to 3 years	0.4	0.9	1.3	0.4	0.9	1.3
4 to 8 years	0.5	1.2	1.7	0.5	1.2	1.7
9 to 13 years	0.6	1.8	2.4	0.5	1.6	2.1
14 to 18 years	0.7	2.6	3.3	0.5	1.8	2.3
>19 years	0.7	3.0	3.7	0.5	2.2	2.7
Pregnancy, 14 to 50 years				0.7	2.3	3.0
Lactation, 14 to 50 years				0.7	3.1	3.8

Data from the Food and Nutrition Board, Institute of Medicine. *Dietary Reference Intakes for water, potassium, sodium, chloride, and sulfate.* Washington, DC: National Academies Press; 2004.
*1 L = 33.8 oz; 1 L = 1.06 qt; 1 cup = 8 oz.

Medicine, the Academy of Nutrition and Dietetics, and the Dietitians of Canada recommend that athletes drink 5 to 7 mL/kg of body weight of water or sports drink at least 4 hours before exercise to ensure euhydration and at least 16 to 24 oz of fluid for every pound of body weight that is lost during exercise.[4] (See the For Further Focus box entitled "Hydrating with Water, Sports Drink, or Energy Drink" in Chapter 16 for more information about sports drinks.)

Functional Losses
When any disease process interferes with the normal functioning of the body, water requirements are likely affected. For example, with gastrointestinal problems such as prolonged diarrhea, large amounts of water may be lost. Uncontrolled diabetes mellitus causes an excess loss of water through urine as a result of high blood glucose levels. In such cases, the replacement of lost water and electrolytes is vital to prevent dehydration.

Metabolic Needs
Metabolic processes require water. A general rule is that approximately 1000 mL of water is necessary for the metabolism of every 1000 kcal consumed.

Age
Age plays an important role in determining water needs. High fluid intake (via breast milk or formula) is critical during infancy because an infant's body content of water is large (approximately 70% to 75% of their total body weight) and because a relatively large amount of this body water is outside of the cells and thus is more easily lost. As body composition changes throughout the life span, so do relative water needs per kilogram of body weight.

Caffeine and Medications
Certain dietary constituents and medications can affect water requirements because of their natural **diuretic** effects. Caffeine has long been viewed as a diuretic. Although the intake of high concentrations of caffeine (≥300 mg) has an acute diuretic effect, the end result does not appear to be a loss in total body fluid.[5,6] The metabolism of caffeine will vary among individuals; however, the routine intake of caffeine diminishes its influence over time.[5]

Several medications contain diuretics specifically for the purpose of reducing overall body fluid, as in the case of antihypertensive medications (e.g., hydrochlorothiazide [Esidrix], furosemide [Lasix], bumetanide [Bumex], spironolactone [Aldactone]). Individuals who are taking medications that promote water loss should be monitored for dehydration and electrolyte

diuretic any substance that induces urination and subsequent fluid loss.

imbalance, particularly upon beginning the medication (see the Drug-Nutrient Interaction box, "Drug Effects on Water and Electrolyte Balance").

DEHYDRATION
Dehydration is the excessive loss of total body water. Relative severity can be measured in terms of the

Drug-Nutrient Interaction
Drug Effects on Water and Electrolyte Balance
Some medications can affect fluid and electrolyte balance. Drugs with anticholinergic properties, such as the antidepressant amitriptyline (Elavil) and the antipsychotic chlorpromazine (Thorazine), may result in a thickening of the saliva and dry mouth. Individuals who are using these mediations may need to increase their fluid intake to help alleviate such side effects.

Antidepressants are divided into classes on the basis of their activity in the brain. Selective serotonin reuptake inhibitors (SSRIs, such as Paxil, Zoloft, Prozac, Celexa), tricyclics, serotonin–norepinephrine reuptake inhibitors (SNRIs, such as Effexor), and norepinephrine–dopamine reuptake inhibitors (NDRIs, such as Wellbutrin) have oral and gastrointestinal side effects that include taste changes, nausea, vomiting, and dry mouth. Patients can avoid some of the negative side effects by drinking 2 to 3 L of water per day and maintaining a consistent sodium intake.

Corticosteroids are sometimes prescribed to replace the normal hormones that should be released by the adrenal glands. There are a number of conditions that require the administration of corticosteroids. Some examples include inflammation, asthma, arthritis, severe allergies, and intestinal disorders. Corticosteroids such as prednisone, methylprednisolone, and hydrocortisone increase the excretion of several nutrients, including potassium. Patients should be encouraged to increase their daily intake of fluids and of foods that are good sources of potassium to maintain an adequate body balance.

Loop diuretics (e.g., Lasix) and thiazide diuretics (e.g., hydrochlorothiazide) are both used to treat hypertension by increasing the urinary excretion of fluids. Minerals are lost in the urine along with fluid excretion. Patients who are taking these drugs should increase the amount of fresh fruits and vegetables in their diets and eat other foods that are good sources of potassium. Although sodium and chloride also are lost in the urine, it is not necessary to increase the intake of these electrolytes, as long as the individual is consuming a normal varied diet.

Potassium-sparing diuretics (e.g., spironolactone) also work to rid the body of excess fluids, but they do so without wasting potassium in the urine. Therefore, patients should be careful to avoid potassium-based salt substitutes so that they can avoid hyperkalemia (i.e., excessively high potassium levels in the blood).

Antipsychotics (e.g., phenothiazines, chlorpromazine) can cause a condition known as *psychogenic polydipsia*. Patients who are taking these drugs often experience dry mouth, and they will consume large amounts of water. If the patient's fluid consumption exceeds his or her capacity for excretion, this can result in hyponatremia and water intoxication. Symptoms of water intoxication include vomiting, ataxia, agitation, seizures, and coma.

percentage of total body weight loss, with symptoms apparent after 2% of normal weight is lost. Initial symptoms include thirst, headache, decreased urine output, dry mouth, and dizziness. As the condition worsens, symptoms can progress to visual impairment, hypotension, anorexia, muscle weakness, kidney failure, and seizures. Chronic or severe dehydration is associated with risk factors for several adverse health conditions such as kidney infections, kidney stones, gallstones, and constipation.[7] In addition, there is indication that dehydration may adversely influence cognitive function and mood.[8] Without correction, dehydration can advance to coma and death (Figure 9-1). A fluid loss of more than 10% of body weight typically requires medical assistance for a complete recovery.

Dehydration presents special concerns among elderly adults. The hypothalamus is the regulatory center for thirst, hunger, body temperature, water balance, and blood pressure. Physiologic changes in the hypothalamus naturally occur with age and, as a result, elderly individuals exhibit an overall decreased thirst sensation and reduced fluid intake when they are dehydrated compared with younger adults.[9,10] Although this does not always constitute a state of dehydration, it does slow the process of rehydration. Other physiologic changes (e.g., diminishing kidney function) that accompany the aging process may exacerbate body fluid losses.

WATER INTOXICATION

Although it is not nearly as common, water intoxication from overconsumption can occur. The excessive intake of plain water may result in the dangerous condition of hyponatremia (i.e., low serum sodium levels of less than 136 mEq/L). Under normal situations, surplus water consumed is lost by increased urinary output, and this is not likely to pose a problem for a healthy person who is eating an otherwise typical diet. However, individuals with psychiatric disorders such as psychogenic **polydipsia** may consume an excess of water in such a rapid rate that the body cannot correct for the acute dilution of blood and ensuing hyponatremia. If the patient does not receive immediate medical attention, the patient may progress through the subsequent stages of delirium, seizures, coma, and death.[11]

As blood volume is diluted with excess water, the water moves to the intracellular fluid (ICF) spaces to reestablish equilibrium with sodium concentrations there, thereby diluting ICF as well. This movement causes edema (Figure 9-2), lung congestion, and muscle weakness. Individuals who are most at risk for hyponatremia from water intoxication are infants and children (if they are forced to drink water), psychiatric patients with polydipsia, patients who are taking psychotropic drugs, and individuals who are participating in prolonged endurance events without electrolyte replacement.[2]

WATER BALANCE

BODY WATER: THE SOLVENT

Distribution

Normal body water content ranges from 45% to 75% of the total body weight. The relative amount of body water will change throughout the lifecycle with the highest levels occurring during infancy and the lowest levels occurring during the advanced years (Table 9-2). Men usually have about 10% more body water than women for an average of 60% and 50% of total body weight, respectively. Differences are generally

polydipsia excessive thirst and drinking.

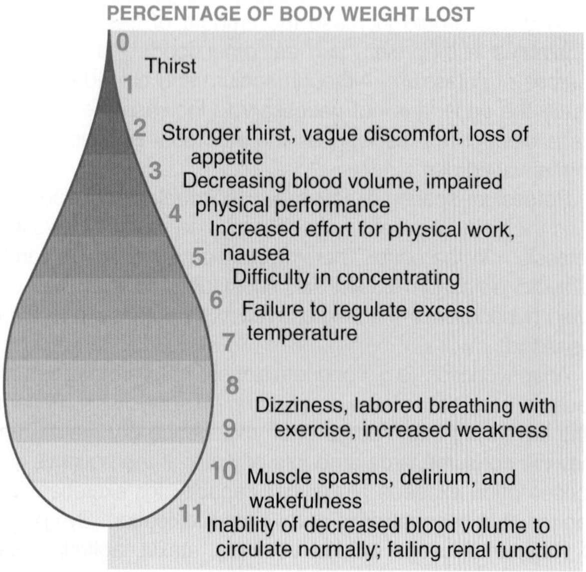

PERCENTAGE OF BODY WEIGHT LOST

0
Thirst
1
2 Stronger thirst, vague discomfort, loss of appetite
3 Decreasing blood volume, impaired physical performance
4 Increased effort for physical work, nausea
5 Difficulty in concentrating
6 Failure to regulate excess temperature
7
8 Dizziness, labored breathing with exercise, increased weakness
9
10 Muscle spasms, delirium, and wakefulness
11 Inability of decreased blood volume to circulate normally; failing renal function

FIGURE 9-1 Adverse effects of progressive dehydration.

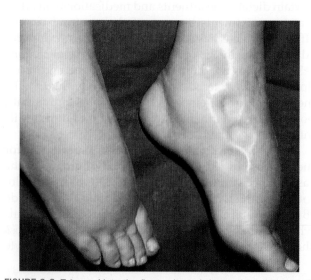

FIGURE 9-2 Edema. Note the finger-shaped depressions that do not rapidly refill after an examiner has exerted pressure. (From Bloom A, Ireland J: *Color Atlas of Diabetes*, 2nd ed. St. Louis, 1992, Mosby.)

attributable to a higher ratio of muscle to fat mass in males. Muscle contains significantly more water compared with adipose tissue. Thus, the more muscle mass and less fat mass a person has, the higher the person's total body water percentage will be. With that in mind, it is very possible that a muscular woman with low body fat would have a higher total body water content than a man of similar weight having less lean tissue and more fat mass.

Total body water is categorized into two major compartments (Figure 9-3).

Extracellular fluid. The total body water outside of the cell is called the *extracellular fluid* (ECF). This water

collectively makes up approximately 20% of the total body weight and 34% of the total body water. One fourth of the ECF is contained in the blood plasma or the intravascular compartment. The remaining ECF is composed of the following: (1) water that surrounds the cells and bathes the tissues (i.e., interstitial fluid); (2) water within the lymphatic circulation; and (3) water that is moving through the body in various tissue secretions (i.e., transcellular fluid).

Interstitial fluid circulation helps with the movement of materials in and out of body cells. Transcellular fluid is the smallest component of ECF (i.e., approximately 2.5% of total body water). Transcellular fluid consists of water within the gastrointestinal tract, cerebrospinal fluid, ocular and joint fluid, and urine within the bladder.

Intracellular fluid. Total body water inside cells is called the *intracellular fluid.* This water collectively amounts to about twice the amount of water that is outside of the cells, thus making up approximately 35% to 45% of total body weight and two thirds of total body water.

Table 9-2 presents the relative amounts of water in the different body water compartments.

Overall Water Balance

Water enters and leaves the body by various routes that are controlled by basic mechanisms such as thirst and hormones. The average adult metabolizes 2.5 to 3 L of water per day in a balance between intake and output.

Water intake. Water enters the body in three main forms: (1) as preformed water in liquids that are consumed; (2) as preformed water in foods that are

Table 9-2	Volumes of Body Fluid Compartments as a Percentage of Body Weight		
BODY FLUID	**INFANT**	**ADULT MALE**	**ADULT FEMALE**
Extracellular fluid			
Plasma	4	4	4
Interstitial fluid	26	16	11
Intracellular fluid	45	40	35
Total	**75**	**60**	**50**

Reprinted from Patton KT, Thibodeau: *Anatomy & Physiology,* 9th ed., St. Louis, Mosby, 2016. Illustration copyright Rolin Graphics.

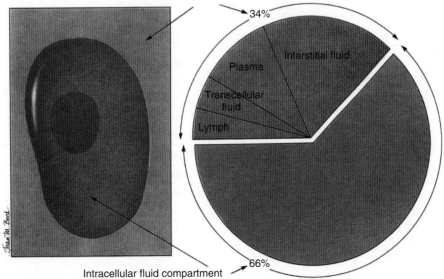

FIGURE 9-3 The distribution of total body water. (From Thibodeau GA, Patton KT. *Anatomy & physiology.* 7th ed. St Louis: Mosby; 2010.)

eaten; and (3) as a product of cell oxidation when nutrients are burned in the body for energy (i.e., metabolic water or "water of oxidation") (Figure 9-4). A variety of foods and their relative water content are listed in Table 9-3.

Older adults are at higher risk for dehydration as a result of inadequate intake and the physiologic changes that are associated with aging. **Xerostomia** is one such physiologic condition that is common in the geriatric population. It is caused by a severe reduction in the flow of saliva; this in turn negatively affects food intake as well as oral health.[12] Xerostomia is also associated with the use of certain medications, with certain diseases or conditions, and with radiation therapy of the head and neck. Conscious attention to adequate fluid intake is an important part of health maintenance and care. Fluid intake should not depend on thirst, because the thirst sensation is an indicator of present dehydration rather than a warning in advance.

Water output. Water leaves the body through the kidneys, skin, lungs, and feces (see Figure 9-4). Of these output routes, the largest amount of water exits through the kidneys. A certain amount of water must be excreted as urine to rid the body of metabolic waste. This is called *obligatory water loss,* because it is compulsory for survival. The kidneys may also process and release an additional amount of water each day, depending on body activities, needs, and intake. This additional water loss varies in accordance with the climate, the physical activity level, and the individual's intake. On average, the daily water output from the body totals approximately 2400 mL, which balances the average intake of water.

Table 9-4 summarizes the comparative intake and output that affect body water balance.

SOLUTE PARTICLES IN SOLUTION

The solutes in body water are a variety of particles in varying concentrations. Two main types of particles control water balance in the body: electrolytes and plasma proteins.

Electrolytes

Electrolytes are small inorganic substances (i.e., either single-mineral elements or small compounds) that can dissociate or break apart in solution and that carry an electrical charge. These charged particles are called *ions.* In any chemical solution, particles are constantly

> **xerostomia** the condition of dry mouth that results from a lack of saliva; saliva production can be hindered by certain diseases (e.g., diabetes, Parkinson's disease) and by some prescription and over-the-counter medications.

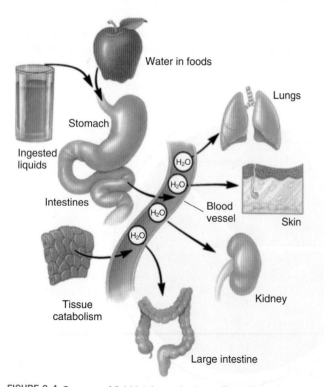

FIGURE 9-4 Sources of fluid intake and output. (From Thibodeau GA, Patton KT. *Anatomy & physiology.* 7th ed. St Louis: Mosby; 2010.)

Table 9-3	Water Content of Selected Food	
FOOD	**WATER CONTENT (%)**	
Apple, raw	86	
Banana, raw	75	
Bread, whole wheat	38	
Broccoli, cooked	89	
Cantaloupe, raw	90	
Carrots, raw	88	
Cheese, cheddar	37	
Chicken, roasted	64	
Corn, cooked	70	
Grapes, raw	81	
Lettuce, iceberg	96	
Mango, raw	82	
Orange, raw	87	
Pasta, cooked	66	
Peach, raw	89	
Pickle	92	
Pineapple, raw	86	
Potato, baked	75	
Squash, cooked	94	
Steak, tenderloin, cooked	50	
Sweet potato, boiled	80	
Turkey, roasted	62	

Modified from the Food and Nutrition Board, Institute of Medicine. *Dietary Reference Intakes for water, potassium, sodium, chloride, and sulfate.* Washington, DC: National Academies Press; 2004.

Table 9-4 Average Daily Adult Intake and Output of Water

INTAKE		OUTPUT	
FORM OF WATER	(mL/day)	BODY PART	(mL/day)
Preformed		Lungs	350
In liquids	1500	Skin	
In foods	700	Diffusion	350
Metabolism (i.e.,	200	Sweat	100
oxidation of food)		Kidneys	1400
		Anus	200
Total	**2400**	**Total**	**2400**

Modified from Thibodeau GA, Patton KT. *Anatomy & physiology.* 7th ed. St Louis: Mosby; 2010.

Table 9-5 Balance of Cation and Anion Concentrations in Extracellular Fluid and Intracellular Fluid*

ELECTROLYTE	EXTRACELLULAR FLUID (mEq/L)	INTRACELLULAR FLUID (mEq/L)
Cation		
Na^+	142	35
K^+	5	123
Ca^{2+}	5	15
Mg^{2+}	3	2
Total	**155**	**175**
Anion		
Cl^-	104	5
PO_4^{3-}	2	80
SO_4^{2-}	1	10
Protein	16	70
CO_3^{2-}	27	10
Organic acids	5	
Total	**155**	**175**

*This balance maintains electroneutrality within each compartment.

in balance between cations and anions to maintain electrical neutrality.

Cations. Cations are ions that carry a positive charge (e.g., concentrations of sodium [Na^+], potassium [K^+], calcium [Ca^{2+}], and magnesium [Mg^{2+}]).

Anions. Anions are ions that carry a negative charge (e.g., concentrations of chloride [Cl^-], bicarbonate [HCO_3^-], phosphate [PO_4^{3-}], and sulfate [SO_4^{2-}]).

The constant balance between electrolytes—specifically sodium and potassium—maintains the electrochemical and cell membrane potentials. Because of their small size, electrolytes can freely diffuse across most membranes of the body, thereby maintaining a balance between the intracellular and extracellular electrical charge. The fluid and electrolyte balances are intimately related, so an imbalance in one creates an imbalance in the other.

Electrolyte concentrations in body fluids are measured in terms of milliequivalents (mEq). Milliequivalents represent the number of ionic charges or electrovalent bonds in a solution. The number of milliequivalents of an ion in a liter of solution is expressed as mEq/L. Table 9-5 outlines the balance between cations and anions in the ICF and ECF compartments, which are exactly balanced.

Plasma Proteins
Plasma proteins—mainly in the form of albumin and globulin—are organic compounds of large molecular size. As such, they are too large to move easily across cell membranes the way that electrolytes do. Therefore, plasma proteins stay inside the blood vessels. Since the body has a constant drive for homeostasis, the proteins (primarily albumin) draw water into the vessels to reestablish equilibrium of the solute concentration between the fluid compartments. In this function, plasma proteins are called *colloids,* which exert **colloidal osmotic pressure (COP)** to maintain the integrity of the blood volume. Without the presence of plasma proteins, fluid leaks from the capillaries and accumulates in the intercellular tissue spaces causing edema

(see Figure 9-2). Cellular proteins help to guard cell water in a similar manner.

Small Organic Compounds
In addition to electrolytes and plasma protein, there are other small organic compounds in body water. Their concentration is ordinarily too small to influence shifts of water. However, in some instances, they are found in abnormally large concentrations that do influence water movement. For example, glucose is a small particle that circulates in body fluids. In the event of uncontrolled diabetes mellitus, the glucose concentration is abnormally high, producing **polyuria** and body water loss.

SEPARATING MEMBRANES
Two types of membranes separate and contain water throughout the body: capillary membranes and cell membranes.

Capillary Membranes
The walls of capillaries are thin and porous. Therefore, water molecules and small particles can move freely

colloidal osmotic pressure (COP) the fluid pressure that is produced by protein molecules in the plasma and the cell; because proteins are large molecules, they do not pass through the separating membranes of the capillary walls; thus, they remain in their respective compartments and exert a constant osmotic pull that protects vital plasma and cell fluid volumes in these areas.
polyuria excessive urination.

across them. Such small particles, having free passage across capillary membranes, include electrolytes and various nutrient constituents. However, larger particles such as plasma protein molecules cannot pass through the small pores of the capillary membrane. These larger molecules remain in the capillary vessel and exert COP to bring water and small molecules back into the capillary.

Cell Membranes

Cell membranes are specially constructed to protect and nourish the cell's contents. Although water is freely permeable, other molecules or ions use channels within the phospholipid bilayer (see Figure 3-6) for passage across the membrane. The membrane channels are highly specific to the molecules that are allowed to pass. For example, sodium channels only allow sodium to pass, and chloride channels only allow chloride to pass.

FORCES MOVING WATER AND SOLUTES ACROSS MEMBRANES

A variety of forces are at work in the cell membrane to allow for the maintenance of dynamic equilibrium.

Osmosis

Osmosis is the movement of water molecules from an area with a low solute concentration to an area with a high solute concentration. When solutions of different concentrations exist on either side of selectively

permeable membranes, the osmotic pressure moves water across the membrane to help equalize the solutions on both sides. Therefore, osmosis can be defined as the force that moves water molecules from an area of greater concentration of water molecules (i.e., with fewer particles in solution) to an area of lesser concentration of water molecules (i.e., with more particles in solution). Figure 9-5 illustrates how water will move from the 10% glucose solution across the semipermeable membrane to the 20% glucose solution to equalize the solute concentrations. Because the membrane is permeable to glucose, the amount of glucose will also change on either side of the membrane to help establish equilibrium.

Diffusion

As osmosis applies to water molecules, diffusion applies to the particles in solution. Simple diffusion is the force by which particles move outward in all directions from an area of greater concentration of particles to an area of lesser concentration of particles (see Chapter 5). The relative movement of water molecules and solute particles by osmosis and diffusion effectively balances solution concentrations—and hence pressures—on both sides of the membrane. Again, refer to Figure 9-5, in which the two balancing forces of osmosis and diffusion are represented.

Facilitated Diffusion

Facilitated diffusion follows the same principles of simple diffusion in that particles passively move down a concentration gradient. The only difference is that, with facilitated diffusion, membrane transporters assist particles with the crossing of the membrane. Some molecules (e.g., glucose) can diffuse across the cell membrane by either simple diffusion or facilitated diffusion, but they move much faster with the help of a transporter.

osmosis the passage of a solvent (e.g., water) through a membrane that separates solutions of different concentrations and that tends to equalize the concentration pressures of the solutions on either side of the membrane.

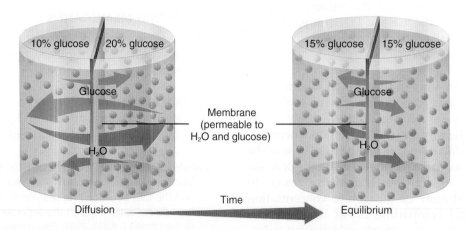

FIGURE 9-5 Osmosis and diffusion through a membrane. Note that the membrane that separates a 10% glucose solution from a 20% glucose solution allows both glucose and water to pass. The container on the left shows the two solutions separated by the membrane at the start of osmosis and diffusion. The container on the right shows the results of osmosis and diffusion after some time. (From Thibodeau GA, Patton KT. *Anatomy & physiology.* 6th ed. St Louis: Mosby; 2007.)

Filtration

Filtration is another form of a passive transport process where water and molecules move down a **hydrostatic pressure** gradient. In this sense, both water and small permeable solute particles are filtered through the pores of capillary membranes from an area of high hydrostatic pressure to an area of low hydrostatic pressure. As fluid pushes against the capillary membrane, the permeable membrane will filter the small particles and allow them to cross through the pores. Meanwhile, the larger particles (e.g., protein) will remain within the capillary. This way, water and small particles can move back and forth between capillaries and cells according to shifting pressures to establish homeostasis.

Active Transport

Particles in solution that are vital to body processes must move across membranes throughout the body at all times, even when the pressure gradients are against their flow. Thus, energy-driven active transport is necessary to carry these particles "upstream" across separating membranes. Such active transport mechanisms usually require a carrier to help ferry the particles across the membrane (see Chapter 5).

Pinocytosis

Sometimes large particles (e.g., proteins, fats) enter cells by the process of pinocytosis (see Chapter 5, Figure 5-8). In this process, large molecules attach themselves to the cell membrane, and they are then engulfed by the cell. In this way, they are encased in a vacuole, which is a small space or cavity that is formed in the protoplasm of the cell. In this cavity, nutrient particles are carried across the cell membrane and into the cell. Once inside the cell, the vacuole opens, and cell enzymes metabolize the particles. Pinocytosis is one of the mechanisms by which fat is absorbed from the small intestine.

CAPILLARY FLUID SHIFT MECHANISM

We have now covered the methods by which water and solutes cross membranes to nourish cells. We must now consider the driving force of order for this movement. The capillary fluid shift mechanism utilizes a combination of the membrane transport methods to perform a balancing act between opposing fluid pressures. It is one of the body's most important controls in maintaining homeostasis throughout the body.

Purpose

Water and other nutrients constantly circulate through the body tissues by way of blood vessels. However, to nourish cells, the water and nutrients must get out of

hydrostatic pressure the force exerted by a fluid pushing against a surface.

the blood vessels (i.e., the capillaries) and into the cells. Water and cell metabolites, which are the products of metabolism that are leaving the cell, must then get back into the capillaries to circulate throughout the body. In other words, water, nutrients, and oxygen must be pushed out of the blood circulation and into the tissue circulation to distribute their goods within the cells; at this point, water and cellular waste products (metabolites and carbon dioxide) must be pulled back into the blood circulation to be disposed through the kidneys and the lungs. The body maintains this constant flow of fluid through the tissues and carries materials to and from the cells by means of hydrostatic pressure and COP.

Process

When blood first enters the capillary system from the larger vessels that come from the heart (i.e., the arterioles), the greater blood pressure from the heart forces water and small particles (e.g., glucose) into the tissues to nourish the cells. This force of blood pressure is an example of hydrostatic pressure. However, plasma protein particles are too large to go through the pores of capillary membranes. When the circulating tissue fluids are ready to reenter the blood capillaries, the initial blood pressure has diminished. The COP of the concentrated protein particles that remain in the capillary vessel is now the greater influence. COP draws water and its metabolites back into the capillary circulation after having served the cells and carries them to larger vessels for blood circulation back to the heart. A small amount of normal turgor pressure from the resisting tissue of the capillary membrane remains the same and operates throughout the system.

Clinical application. This system is dependent upon adequate plasma protein to exert the required osmotic pressure. Without it, there would not be enough osmotic pressure to pull the fluid back into circulation. This is why protein-energy malnutrition results in edema (see Chapter 4).

ORGAN SYSTEM CIRCULATION

In addition to blood circulation, two other major organ systems help to protect the homeostasis of body water: gastrointestinal circulation and renal circulation.

Gastrointestinal Circulation

Fluid secretions involved with digestion and absorption include saliva, gastric juice, bile, pancreatic juice, and intestinal juice. Of these secretions, all but bile are predominantly water. In the latter portion of the intestine, most of the water and electrolytes are then reabsorbed into the blood to circulate over and over again. This constant movement of a large volume of water and its electrolytes among the blood, the cells, and the gastrointestinal tract is called the *gastrointestinal circulation.* The sheer magnitude of this vital gastrointestinal circulation, as shown in Table 9-6, indicates the significance of fluid loss from the upper or lower portion of the gastrointestinal tract. The body works continually to preserve the isotonicity of this circulation with the surrounding extracellular fluid.

Law of isotonicity. The gastrointestinal fluids are part of the ECF compartments, which also includes

Table 9-6	Approximate Total Volume of Digestive Secretions*	
SECRETION		**VOLUME (mL)**
Saliva		1500
Gastric secretions		2500
Bile		500
Pancreatic secretions		700
Intestinal secretions		3000
Total		**8200**

*As produced over the course of 24 hours by an adult of average size.

the blood. These fluids are *isotonic,* which means that they are in a state of equal osmotic pressure that results from equal concentrations of electrolytes and other solute particles. For example, when a person drinks plain water without any solutes or accompanying food, electrolytes and salts enter the intestine from the surrounding blood supply to equalize the pressure and concentration. If a concentrated solution of food is ingested, additional water is then drawn into the intestine from the surrounding blood to dilute the intestinal contents. In each instance, water and electrolytes move among the parts of the ECF compartment to maintain solutions that are isotonic in the gastrointestinal tract with the surrounding fluid (see the Clinical Applications box, "Principles of Oral Rehydration Therapy").

Clinical application. Because of the large amounts of water and electrolytes involved, fluid losses via the upper or lower gastrointestinal tract are the most common cause of clinical hydration and electrolyte

Clinical Applications

Principles of Oral Rehydration Therapy

Diarrhea is usually considered a trivial problem in developed countries; however, it is the second leading cause of death worldwide among children who are younger than 5 years old (pneumonia is the leading cause).[1] Although the vast majority of the deaths from diarrhea are associated with fluid loss, the mere provision of water alone can be dangerous. The principles of electrolyte absorption dictate appropriate rehydration methods for children with diarrhea.

Intravenous therapy, which was developed by Darrow in the 1940s, provided sodium chloride (a base) and potassium in water and proved to be successful.[2,3] Unfortunately, intravenous therapy is often not readily available to those who need it most. A large number of isolated, poor, rural families in both developed and developing countries do not have access to health care facilities. Fortunately, the World Health Organization has developed a means of oral rehydration therapy that is much less expensive and that is being used in the United States as well as in developing countries. If safe drinking water is available, the oral rehydration salt solution packet can be mixed at home and administered by a care provider. The ingredients of the oral rehydration salt packets are[4]:

- 2.6 g of sodium chloride (table salt)
- 2.9 g of trisodium citrate dihydrate
- 1.5 g of potassium chloride (or a salt substitute such as Diamond Crystal or Morton Salt Substitute)
- 13.5 g of glucose

These salts are mixed with 1 L of safe water. (A premade formula such as Pedialyte [Abbott Laboratories, Abbott Park, Ill] is also appropriate.) This combination is based on the principles of sodium absorption that have been observed in the small intestine.

TRANSPORT OF METABOLIC COMPOUNDS

A number of metabolic compounds—principally glucose but also certain amino acids, dipeptides, and disaccharides—depend on sodium to allow them to cross the intestinal wall.

ADDITIVE EFFECTS

The rate at which sodium is absorbed depends on the presence of substances such as glucose or other protein metabolic products. The more substances that are present, the better will be the absorption of sodium.

WATER ABSORPTION

The rate of water absorption is enhanced as sodium absorption improves. Thus, a solution of sodium and potassium salts plus glucose can be given orally.

In addition to oral rehydration therapy, infants and older children with acute diarrhea should continue to eat well-tolerated foods. Fasting practices were based on the former belief that recovery is more effective if the bowel is allowed to rest and heal. To the contrary, children should be fed their regular age-appropriate diets (i.e., breast milk, breast milk substitute, or solid foods), allowed to determine the amount of food that they need, and given extra food as the diarrhea subsides to recover nutritional deficits. Food choices should be guided by individual tolerances. The use of the BRAT diet (**b**ananas, **r**ice, **a**pplesauce, and **t**ea or **t**oast) is not recommended, because it does not include typical foods that are consumed by infants and small children and only worsens the energy and nutrient deficit.

REFERENCES

1. World Health Organization. *End Preventable Deaths: Global Action Plan for Prevention and Control of Pneumonia and Diarrhoea.* Geneva, Switzerland: World Health Organization/The United Nations Children's Fund (UNICEF); 2013.
2. Darrow DC. The retention of electrolyte during recovery from severe dehydration due to diarrhea. *J Pediatr.* 1946;28:515-540.
3. Darrow DC, Pratt EL, et al. Disturbances of water and electrolytes in infantile diarrhea. *Pediatrics.* 1949;3(2):129-156.
4. World Health Organization. *Oral Rehydration Salts: Production of the New ORS.* Geneva: 2006.

problems. Such problems exist, for example, in cases of persistent vomiting or prolonged diarrhea where the patient is unable to replace losses through fluid and food ingestion. Diarrheal disease is the leading cause of preventable child mortality and morbidity in the world.[13] The large concentration of electrolytes involved in the gastrointestinal circulation is shown in Table 9-7. It is not always possible to replace such losses without medical assistance.

Renal Circulation

The kidney's job is to help maintain appropriate levels of all constituents of the blood. This is accomplished by filtering the blood and then selectively reabsorbing water and needed materials to be carried throughout the body. The remaining waste products are concentrated and excreted as urine. Through this continual "laundering" of the blood by the millions of nephrons in the kidneys, water balance and solute balance are maintained. When disease occurs in the kidneys and this filtration process does not operate normally, fluid and solute imbalances occur (see Chapter 21).

HORMONAL CONTROLS

Two hormonal systems help to maintain constant body water balance.

Antidiuretic Hormone Mechanism

The antidiuretic hormone (ADH) mechanism is a first-line defense against **hypovolemia.** ADH, which is also called **vasopressin,** is synthesized by the hypothalamus and stored in the pituitary gland for release. ADH conserves water by working on the kidneys' nephrons to increase the reabsorption of water. In any stressful situation with a threatened or real loss of body water, this hormone is released to rapidly conserve body water and to reestablish the normal blood volume and osmotic pressure (Figure 9-6).

Renin-Angiotensin-Aldosterone System

The renin-angiotensin-aldosterone system is a complex system that corrects for hypovolemia through a negative feedback mechanism. It works to slowly increase blood volume by reabsorbing sodium in the kidneys, which in turn increases water retention. There are many checks and balances within this system to ensure activation is essential.

As blood flow through the kidneys drops below normal, the enzyme **renin** is released from the kidneys into the blood. Renin converts **angiotensinogen** to **angiotensin I.** As the blood flows through the lungs, an

Table 9-7	Approximate Concentration of Certain Electrolytes in Digestive Fluids (mEq/L)			
SECRETION	NA⁺	K⁺	CL⁻	HCO₃⁻

SECRETION	NA^+	K^+	CL^-	HCO_3^-
Saliva	10	25	10	15
Gastric secretions	40	10	145	0
Pancreatic secretions	140	5	40	110
Jejunal secretions	135	5	110	30
Bile	140	10	110	40

hypovolemia low blood volume.
vasopressin a hormone of the pituitary gland that acts on the distal nephron tubule to conserve water by reabsorption; also known as *antidiuretic hormone.*
renin an enzyme released from the kidney due to hypovolemia that converts angiotensinogen to angiotensin I.
angiotensinogen an inactive enzyme produced by the liver that circulates within the blood at all times.
angiotensin I an inactive peptide hormone that is the precursor to angiotensin II.

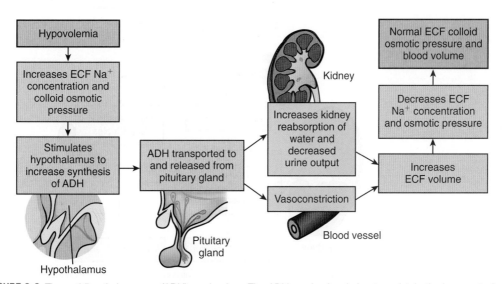

FIGURE 9-6 The antidiuretic hormone *(ADH)* mechanism. The ADH mechanism helps to maintain the homeostasis of extracellular fluid *(ECF)* colloid osmotic pressure by regulating its volume and electrolyte concentration.

enzyme found on the capillaries, called **angiotensin-converting enzyme (ACE),** converts angiotensin I into **angiotensin II.** Angiotensin II does several things: it increases the release of ADH from the pituitary gland, it leads to vasoconstriction, and it circulates to the adrenal glands (located on top of each kidney) where it triggers the release of **aldosterone.** Aldosterone then stimulates the kidneys' nephrons to reabsorb sodium (Figure 9-7). Therefore, the renin-angiotensin-aldosterone system is primarily a sodium-conserving mechanism, but it also exerts a secondary control over water reabsorption, because water follows sodium.

ACID-BASE BALANCE

An acceptable pH must be maintained in body fluids to support life. This balance is achieved with the use of chemical and physiologic buffer systems.

ACIDS AND BASES

The concept of acids and bases relates to hydrogen ion concentration. Acidity is expressed in terms of pH. The abbreviation *pH* is derived from a mathematical term that refers to the power of the hydrogen ion concentration. A pH of 7 is the neutral point between an acid

---

angiotensin-converting enzyme (ACE) the enzyme found on the capillary walls within the lungs that converts angiotensin I to angiotensin II. ACE is also present to a lesser extent in the endothelial cells and the epithelial cells within the kidneys.

angiotensin II an active hormone that constricts blood vessels and stimulates the release of aldosterone. Both actions lead to an increase in blood pressure.

aldosterone a hormone of the adrenal glands that acts on the distal nephron tubule to stimulate the reabsorption of sodium in an ion exchange with potassium; the aldosterone mechanism is essentially a sodium-conserving mechanism, but it also indirectly conserves water, because water absorption follows sodium resorption.

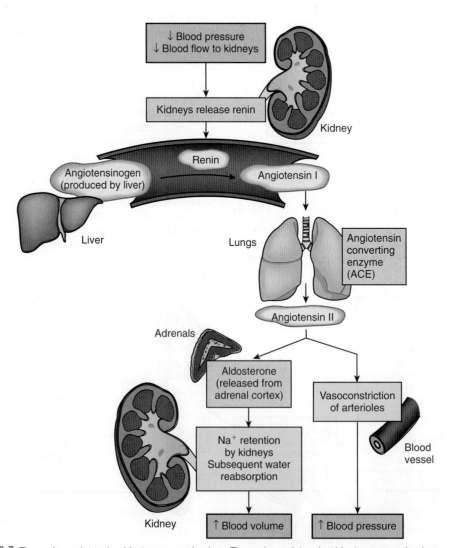

FIGURE 9-7 The renin-angiotensin-aldosterone mechanism. The renin-angiotensin-aldosterone mechanism restores normal extracellular fluid *(ECF)* volume when that volume decreases to less than normal by retaining sodium and water in the kidneys and by promoting vasoconstriction.

and a base. Because pH is a negative mathematic factor, the higher the hydrogen ion concentration (i.e., the more acid), the lower the pH number. Conversely, the lower the hydrogen ion concentration (i.e., the less acid), the higher the pH number. Substances with a pH of less than 7 are acidic, and substances with a pH of more than 7 are alkaline. Box 9-1 lists various sources of acids and bases.

Acids

An acid is a compound that has more hydrogen ions and that also has enough to release extra hydrogen ions when it is in solution.

Bases

A base is a compound that has fewer hydrogen ions. Thus, in solution, it accepts hydrogen ions, thereby effectively reducing the solution's acidity.

Acids and bases are the normal by-products of nutrient absorption and metabolism. As such, mechanisms to reestablish equilibrium within the body are constantly at work.

BUFFER SYSTEMS

The body deals with degrees of acidity by maintaining buffer systems to handle an excess of either acid or base. The human body contains many buffer systems, because only a relatively narrow range of pH (i.e., 7.35 to 7.45) is compatible with life.

Chemical Buffer System

A chemical buffer system is a mixture of acidic and alkaline components. It involves an acid and a base partner that together protect a solution from wide variations in its pH, even when strong bases or acids are added to it. For example, if a strong acid is added to a buffered solution, the base partner reacts with the acid to form a weaker acid. If a strong base is added to the solution, the acid partner combines with it to form a weaker base. The carbonic acid (H_2CO_3)/

bicarbonate ($NaHCO_3$) buffer system is the body's main buffer system for the following reasons.

Available materials. The raw materials for producing carbonic acid (H_2CO_3) are readily available: these are water (H_2O) and carbon dioxide (CO_2).

Base-to-acid ratio. The bicarbonate buffer system is able to maintain this essential degree of acidity in the body fluids because the bicarbonate (base) is approximately 20 times more abundant than the carbonic acid. This 20:1 ratio is maintained even though the absolute amounts of the two partners may fluctuate during adjustment periods. Whether or not additional base or acid enters the system, as long as the 20:1 ratio is maintained, over time, the ECF pH is held constant.

Physiologic Buffer Systems

When chemical buffers cannot reestablish equilibrium, the respiratory and renal systems will respond.

Respiratory control of pH. With every breath, CO_2 (an acid) leaves the body. Therefore, changes in respiration rates can either increase or decrease the loss of acids. Hyperventilation (i.e., increasing the depth and rate of breathing) increases the release of CO_2, thereby combating **acidosis**. Conversely, hypoventilation (i.e., slowing down the depth and pace of breathing) retains CO_2, which ultimately increases the acidity of blood to alleviate **alkalosis**.

Urinary control of pH. In the event that chemical buffer systems and the respiratory buffer system do not reestablish blood pH, the kidneys can adapt by excreting more or less hydrogen ions. If blood pH is too acidic, the kidneys will accept more hydrogen ions from the blood in exchange for a sodium ion. Because sodium ions are basic, blood is losing an acid (i.e., H^+) while gaining a base, thereby increasing blood pH back to normal.

Chemical and physiologic buffer systems are critical for maintaining the blood pH within an acceptable range for life.

Box **9-1**   Sources of Acids and Bases

ACIDS
Carbonic acid and lactic acid: the aerobic and anaerobic metabolism of glucose
Sulfuric acid: the oxidation of sulfur-containing amino acids
Phosphoric acid: the oxidation of phosphoproteins for energy
Ketone bodies: the incomplete oxidation of fat for energy
Minerals: chlorine, sulfur, and phosphorus

BASES
Minerals: potassium, calcium, sodium, and magnesium
Sodium bicarbonate
Calcium carbonate

---

acidosis a blood pH of less than 7.35; *respiratory acidosis* is caused by an accumulation of carbon dioxide (an acid); *metabolic acidosis* may be caused by a variety of conditions that result in the excess accumulation of acids in the body or by a significant loss of bicarbonate (a base).

alkalosis a blood pH of more than 7.45; *respiratory alkalosis* is caused by hyperventilation and an excess loss of carbon dioxide; *metabolic alkalosis* is seen with extensive vomiting in which a significant amount of hydrochloric acid is lost and bicarbonate (a base) is secreted.

Putting It All Together

Summary

- The human body is approximately 45% to 75% water. The primary functions of body water are to provide the water environment that is necessary for cell work, to act as a transporter, to control body temperature, and to lubricate moving parts.
- Body water is distributed in two collective body water compartments: ICF and ECF. The water inside of the cells is the larger portion. The water outside of the cells consists of the fluid that is in spaces between cells (e.g., interstitial and lymph fluid), blood plasma, secretions in transit (e.g., the gastrointestinal circulation), and a smaller amount of fluid in cartilage and bone.
- The overall water balance of the body is maintained by fluid intake and output.
- Two types of solute particles control the distribution of body water: (1) electrolytes, which are mainly charged mineral elements; and (2) plasma proteins, which are chiefly albumin. These solute particles influence the movement of water across cell or capillary membranes, thereby allowing for the tissue circulation that is necessary to nourish cells.
- The acid-base buffer system, which is mainly controlled by the lungs and kidneys, makes use of electrolytes and hydrogen ions to maintain a normal ECF pH of approximately 7.4. This pH level is necessary to sustain life.

Chapter Review Questions

See answers in Appendix A.

1. Elderly adults are at risk for dehydration because of:
   a. Inability to dilute urine.
   b. Decreased serum glucose levels.
   c. Decreased thirst sensation.
   d. Poor intestinal fluid absorption.

2. The easiest way to measure fluid loss during a day of hard work in a hot climate is to:
   a. Measure and compare fluid intake and urine output.
   b. Measure blood pressure throughout the day.
   c. Determine serum sodium levels before and after work.
   d. Measure body weight at the beginning and at the end of the day.

3. A patient with uncontrolled diabetes who is experiencing a high serum blood glucose level may present to the clinic with:
   a. Polyuria.
   b. Anuria.
   c. Oliguria.
   d. Dysuria.

4. Substances that work with electrolytes to help maintain body fluid balance include:
   a. Dietary fiber.
   b. Plasma proteins.
   c. Blood hemoglobin.
   d. Vitamin C.

5. The main electrolyte that surrounds the outside of the cells is:
   a. Sodium.
   b. Calcium.
   c. Potassium.
   d. Calcium.

Additional Learning Resources

evolve http://evolve.elsevier.com/Williams/basic/

References and **Further Reading and Resources** in the back of the book provide additional resources for enhancing knowledge.

Nutrition during Pregnancy and Lactation

Key Concepts

- The mother's food habits and nutritional status before conception—as well as during pregnancy—influence the outcome of her pregnancy.
- Pregnancy is a prime example of physiologic synergism in which the mother, the placenta, and the fetus collaborate to sustain and nurture new life.

- Through the food that a pregnant woman eats, she gives her unborn child the nourishment that is required to begin and support fetal growth and development.
- Through her diet and energy stores, a breastfeeding mother continues to provide nutrition to her nursing baby.

The tremendous growth of a baby from the moment of conception to the time of birth depends entirely on nourishment from the mother. The complex process of rapid human growth and lactation demands a significant increase in nutrients from the mother's diet.

This chapter explores the nutrition needs of pregnancy, as well as nutrition-related risk factors and complications. We will also explore the physiologic process and nutrition demands of lactation. The health and wellness of a pregnant or lactating mother imparts a vital role in the development of a healthy infant.

NUTRITIONAL DEMANDS OF PREGNANCY

Years ago, traditional practices and diet during pregnancy were often restrictive in nature. They were built on assumptions and folklore of the past, and had little or no basis in scientific fact. Early obstetricians even supported the notion that semistarvation of the mother during pregnancy was a blessing in disguise, because it produced a small, lightweight baby who was easy to deliver. To this end, pregnant women were sometimes encouraged to select a diet that was restricted in kilocalories, protein, water, and salt.[1]

Developments in both nutrition and medical science have refuted these ideas and laid a sound base for positive nutrition in current maternal care. It is now known that the mother's and the child's health depend on the pregnant woman eating a well-balanced diet with adequate essential nutrients. In fact, women who have always eaten a well-balanced diet are in a good state of nutrition at conception, even before they know that they are pregnant. Such women have a better chance of having a healthy baby compared with women who have been undernourished before conception and remain so throughout gestation.

The 9 months between conception and the birth of a fully formed baby is a spectacular period of rapid growth and intricate functional development. Such activities require increased energy and nutrient support. General guidelines for these nutrient increases are provided in the comprehensive Dietary Reference Intakes (DRIs) issued by the National Academy of Sciences.[2–7]

The DRIs are based on the general needs of healthy populations. Women who are poorly nourished when becoming pregnant or those with additional risks may require more nutrition support. The *Dietary Guidelines for Americans* also outline specific recommendations for pregnant and lactating women (Box 10-1).[8] This chapter reviews the basic nutrition needs for the positive support of a normal pregnancy, with emphasis placed on critical energy and protein requirements as well as on key vitamin and mineral needs.

ENERGY NEEDS

The metabolic cost of pregnancy is significant over the course of gestation. The exact amount of energy needs will vary greatly among women depending on her prepregnancy weight, health status, and activity level.

Reasons for Increased Need

During the second and third trimesters of pregnancy, the mother needs more kilocalories for two general reasons: (1) to supply the increased fuel demanded by the metabolic workload for both the mother and the fetus; and (2) to spare protein for the added tissue-building requirements. For these reasons, the mother must consider the nutrient and energy density of the food in her diet.

147

Dietary Guidelines for Americans, 2015-2020, for Specific Populations Regarding Pregnancy and Lactation

FOR WOMEN WHO ARE CAPABLE OF BECOMING PREGNANT
- Before becoming pregnant, women are encouraged to achieve and maintain a healthy weight.
- Choose foods that supply heme iron, which is more readily absorbed by the body; additional iron sources; and enhancers of iron absorption, such as vitamin C–rich foods.
- Consume 400 micrograms per day of synthetic folic acid from fortified foods or supplements in addition to food forms of folate from a varied diet.

FOR WOMEN WHO ARE PREGNANT OR BREASTFEEDING
- Women who are pregnant are encouraged to gain weight within the gestational weight gain guidelines.
- Consume 8 to 12 ounces of seafood per week from a variety of seafood types that are lower in methyl mercury. (The U.S. Environmental Protection Agency can advise on low-mercury sources of seafood.)
- Do not drink alcohol while pregnant.

From the U.S. Department of Health and Human Services and U.S. Department of Agriculture. 2015-2020 *Dietary Guidelines for Americans.* 8th Edition. December 2015. Available at http://health.gov/dietaryguidelines/2015/guidelines/.

Amount of Energy Increase

The energy needs of pregnant women remain the same during the first trimester of pregnancy as their kilocalarie needs before conception (i.e., no noticeable difference). The DRIs note an increased need of 340 kcal/day during the second trimester and approximately 452 kcal/day during the third trimester,[6] which is an increase of about 15% to 20% over the energy needs of nonpregnant women. It is important for health care professionals to council women on how this relates to daily life. For example, the increased energy needs of a woman during her second trimester of pregnancy could be met by one additional snack per day consisting of a medium banana (105 kcal), an 8-oz serving of whole milk yogurt (138 kcal), and ⅛ cup of mixed nuts (101 kcal). That snack provides 344 kcal. Providing examples of exactly what "extra energy needs" means is important so that expecting mothers do not misunderstand the message and assume that they need to "eat for two." Increased complex carbohydrates, monounsaturated fats, and polyunsaturated fats are the preferred sources of energy, especially during late pregnancy and throughout lactation.

Active, large, teenage, or nutritionally deficient pregnant women may require more energy than the DRI guidelines. The emphasis always should be on adequate kilocalories to secure the nutrient and energy needs of a rapidly growing fetus. Sufficient weight gain is vital to a successful pregnancy. Gestational weight gain is a predictor of infant birth weight and birth weight is associated with body mass index (BMI) later in life (see back cover of text for BMI table).[9] This translates to each end of the spectrum; both too little and too much weight gain during gestation have implications for the overall health of the infant. Inadequate gestational weight gain increases the risk for preterm deliveries, and for low birth weight babies who have increased risks for poor outcome.[10] Alternatively, excessive weight gain poses both short-term and potentially long-term complications for the mother and fetus.

PROTEIN NEEDS

Reasons for Increased Need

Protein serves as the building block for the tremendous growth of body tissues during pregnancy. Sufficient protein is required to meet the growth needs in the following ways:

Development of the placenta. The placenta is the fetus's lifeline to the mother. A mature placenta requires sufficient protein for its complete development as a vital and unique organ to sustain, support, and nourish the fetus.

Growth of the fetus. The mere increase in size from one cell to millions of cells in a 3.2-kg (7-lb) infant in only 9 months indicates the relatively large amount of protein that is required for such rapid growth.

Growth of maternal tissues. To support pregnancy and lactation, the increased development of uterine and breast tissue is required.

Increased maternal blood volume. The mother's plasma volume increases by 40% to 50% during pregnancy. More circulating blood is necessary to nourish the fetus and to support the increased metabolic workload. However, with extra blood volume comes a need for the increased synthesis of blood components, especially hemoglobin and albumin, which are proteins that are vital to pregnancy. An increase in hemoglobin helps to supply oxygen to the growing number of cells. Meanwhile, albumin production increases to regulate blood volume through osmotic pressure (see Chapter 9). Most women (60% to 75%) will experience some level of edema during the latter part of gestation; however, adequate albumin helps prevent an excessive accumulation of water in tissues.

Amniotic fluid. Amniotic fluid, which contains various proteins, surrounds the fetus during growth and guards it against shock or injury.

Amount of Protein Increase

The protein DRI for nonpregnant women is ≈46 g/day and the DRI for pregnant women is ≈71 g/day.[6] This represents an increase of 25 g/day more than the average woman's protein requirement. However, it should be noted that the average *nonpregnant* woman aged 20 to 39 years old in America already consumes

74 g of protein per day.[11] Thus, individual nutrition counselling for women intending to become pregnant and pregnant women would be beneficial in the early stages to help design personalized dietary advice, because additional protein may or may not be warranted.[12] On the other hand, high-risk or active pregnant women may require more protein than their current diet provides.

Food Sources

Complete protein foods of high biologic value include eggs, milk, beef, poultry, fish, pork, cheese, soy products, and other animal products (e.g., lamb, venison, and so on). Other incomplete proteins from plant sources such as legumes and grains contribute additional valuable amounts of amino acids. Protein-rich foods also contribute other nutrients, such as calcium, iron, zinc, and fat-soluble vitamins. The sample food plan in Table 10-1 demonstrates the amount of food from each food group recommended to supply the daily needed nutrients. See Chapter 4 for more information on dietary sources of protein and protein quality.

KEY MINERAL AND VITAMIN NEEDS

Many nutrients are needed in higher quantities during pregnancy to meet the greater structural and metabolic requirements of gestation. These increases are indicated in the DRI tables in Appendix B. Although all nutrients are important for a successful pregnancy, only the nutrients that pose a specific risk for deficiency are discussed below.

Minerals

The physiologic and metabolic changes that take place during pregnancy are vast and will vary greatly between women.[13] But in all cases, the nutrient needs of the mother must be met before the nutrient needs of the placenta will be met and finally, before the needs of the fetus are fulfilled. As such, all nutrients are of great importance in the mother's diet. **Teratogenic** effects may develop as a result of a maternal diet that is deficient in many of the minerals covered in Chapter 8 (e.g., Kestan disease, goiter, cretinism, fetal growth restriction). We will only cover the more common mineral deficiency concerns in the United States.

Calcium. A good supply of calcium—along with phosphorus, magnesium, and vitamin D—is essential for the fetal development of bones and teeth as well as for the mother's own body needs. Calcium is also necessary for blood clotting. A diet that includes at least 3 cups of milk or milk substitute daily (e.g., calcium-fortified soy milk), generous amounts of green

teratogenic causing a birth defect.

Table 10-1 Daily Food Plan for Pregnant Women*,†

	FIRST TRIMESTER 2200 KCAL	SECOND TRIMESTER 2400 KCAL	THIRD TRIMESTER 2600 KCAL
Grains‡	7 ounces	8 ounces	9 ounces
Vegetables§	3 cups	3 cups	3½ cups
Fruits	2 cups	2 cups	2 cups
Milk	3 cups	3 cups	3 cups
Meat and beans	6 ounces	6½ ounces	6½ ounces
Aim for at least this amount of whole grains per day	3½ ounces	4 ounces	4½ ounces
AIM FOR THIS MUCH WEEKLY			
Dark green vegetables	2 cups	2 cups	2½ cups
Red and orange vegetables	6 cups	6 cups	7 cups
Dry beans and peas	2 cups	2 cups	2½ cups
Starchy vegetables	6 cups	6 cups	7 cups
Other vegetables	5 cups	5 cups	5½ cups
OILS AND DISCRETIONARY CALORIES			
Aim for this amount of oils per day	6 teaspoons	7 teaspoons	8 teaspoons
Limit extras (extra fats and sugars) to this amount per day	266 calories	330 calories	362 calories

From the U.S. Department of Agriculture, Center for Nutrition Policy and Promotion. *USDA's MyPlate home page* (website): www.choosemyplate.gov. Accessed November 4, 2014.
*This particular food plan is based on the average needs of a pregnant woman who is 30 years old, who is 5 feet, 5 inches tall, whose prepregnancy weight was 125 pounds, and who is physically active between 30 and 60 minutes each day. Plans provided by the MyPlate.gov site are specific to each individual woman; however, this is an example for a woman of the described stature and activity level.
†These plans are based on 2200-, 2400-, and 2600-calorie food-intake patterns. The recommended nutrient intake increases throughout the pregnancy to meet changing nutritional needs.
‡Make half of your grains whole.
§Vary your veggies.

vegetables, and enriched or whole grains usually supplies enough calcium. During pregnancy, physiologic changes occur in the mother's absorption capacity to help meet the needs of some nutrients; for example, calcium and zinc are both more bioavailable during pregnancy. This enhanced absorption helps the mother to meet her nutrient needs as well as those of the growing fetus. Calcium supplements may be indicated for cases of poor maternal intake or pregnancies that involve more than one fetus. Because food sources of the two major minerals (i.e., calcium and phosphorus) are almost the same, a diet that is sufficient in calcium also provides enough phosphorus.

Iron. Particular attention is given to iron intake during pregnancy. Iron is essential for the increased hemoglobin synthesis that is required for the greater maternal blood volume as well as for the baby's necessary prenatal storage of iron.

The average intake of iron for women of childbearing age in the United States is 14.5 g/day.[11] Meanwhile, the current DRIs recommend a daily iron intake of 27 mg/day during pregnancy, which is significantly more than both a woman's nonpregnant DRI of 18 mg/day and the current average intake.[5] Iron occurs in small amounts in food sources and much of this intake is not in a readily absorbable form. Even though there is an increased absorptive capacity for iron during pregnancy, the maternal diet alone rarely meets requirements. Consuming foods that are high in vitamin C along with dietary sources of iron enhances the body's ability to absorb and use iron with a low bioavailability. In addition, avoiding foods that inhibit iron absorption (e.g., whole-grain cereals, unleavened whole-grain breads, legumes, tea, coffee) within meals that provide significant iron is recommended.

Because the increased pregnancy requirement is difficult to meet with the iron content of a typical American diet, daily iron supplements are often recommended. Historically, iron supplements given to pregnant women were in excessively high doses (e.g., 100 to 200 mg/day). At this high dose, unpleasant gastrointestinal side effects were common. However, iron supplements that are taken between meals or at bedtime in doses of 20 to 80 mg/day are adequate to prevent iron-deficiency anemia with no clinical gastrointestinal side effects.[14] Although there is limited research available regarding dietary supplement use in pregnant women, one report noted that adherence to iron supplementation is correlated with ethnicity and socioeconomic status.[15] The conclusions of this study indicate that encouragement and education for African-American, Mexican-American, and low-income women to continue taking their iron supplements during pregnancy may benefit both the mother and the fetus.

As with most supplemental forms of nutrients, bioavailability is suboptimal compared with food sources;

hence, the reinforcement of a balanced diet with ample iron is still important. See Table 8-5 for a list of foods that are high in iron.

Vitamins

The DRIs for pregnant women are slightly higher for most vitamins. As total energy intake increases, so do the nutrients contained in the foods consumed. Therefore, the recommended intake for most nutrients is achieved through a selection of nutrient dense foods.

As with the mineral section, we will limit the discussion here to those vitamins that are of specific concern during pregnancy because of inadequate dietary intake. See Chapter 7 for more information on the function of each vitamin.

Folate. Folate is important for both mother and fetus throughout pregnancy. Tetrahydrofolic acid (TH_4) participates in DNA synthesis, cell division, and hemoglobin synthesis. It is particularly relevant during the early periconceptional period (i.e., from approximately 2 months before conception to week 6 of gestation) to ensure adequate nutrient availability in the endometrial lining of the uterus for embryonic tissue development. The neural tube forms during the critical period from 21 to 28 days' gestation, and it grows into the mature infant's spinal column and its network of nerves.

Although the exact mechanism by which folate helps thwart neural tube defects (NTDs) is unknown, it is thought to be a result of a complex relationship between folate availability, genetics, and other environmental factors.[16] While folate intake alone does not guarantee that a pregnancy will be NTD-free, there is enough evidence to support the use of folate supplements and/or food fortification to reduce the overall occurrence. The Centers for Disease Control and Prevention estimates that, before the national fortification of grains with folic acid, there was an annual average of 4130 NTD-affected pregnancies in the United States. Following the 1998 federally mandated food fortification, the national average of NTD-affected pregnancies has declined by 22.9%.[17] An analysis of the worldwide benefit of folate supplementation conservatively estimated that women taking folate supplements during and immediately before pregnancy could reduce the occurrence of NTDs by up to 62%; and that food fortification with folic acid may reduce NTD occurrences by up to 46%.[18]

Spina bifida and *anencephaly* are the two most common forms of NTDs, which are defined as any malformation of the embryonic brain or spinal cord. Spina bifida occurs when the lower end of the neural tube fails to close (see Figure 7-7). As a result, the spinal cord and backbone do not develop properly. The severity of spina bifida varies in accordance with the size and location of the opening in the spine.

Disability ranges from mild to severe, with limited movement and function. Anencephaly occurs when the upper end of the neural tube fails to close. In this case, the brain fails to develop or is entirely absent. Pregnancies that are affected by anencephaly end in miscarriages or death soon after delivery.

The current DRIs recommend a daily folate intake of 600 mcg/day during pregnancy and 400 mcg/day for nonpregnant women during their childbearing years.[3] Women who are unable to achieve such dietary recommendations by eating foods that are fortified with folate may do so with a dietary supplement. All enriched flour and grain products as well as fortified cereals contain a well-absorbable form of dietary folic acid. Other natural sources of folate include liver; legumes (e.g., pinto beans, black beans, kidney beans); orange juice; asparagus; and broccoli.

Vitamin D. As was mentioned in Chapter 7, vitamin D deficiency is thought to be a common worldwide problem, including among pregnant women. There is concern that vitamin D deficiency during pregnancy may be associated with adverse outcomes for both the mother and the fetus, including preeclampsia, gestational diabetes, and preterm birth. However, causality has not yet been determined and research studies investigating the connection between vitamin D deficiency and such pregnancy complications are contradictory.[19,20] The current DRIs recommend pregnant and lactating women consume 15 mcg/d (600 IU) to ensure the absorption and use of calcium and phosphorus for fetal bone growth.[2] Increased vitamin D needs can be met by the mother's intake of at least 3 cups of fortified milk (or milk substitute) in her daily food plan. Fortified milk contains 10 mcg (400 IU) of cholecalciferol (i.e., vitamin D) per quart. The mother's exposure to sunlight increases her endogenous synthesis of vitamin D as well. Lactose-intolerant women or vegetarians can obtain adequate vitamin D from fortified soymilk or rice milk products.

Registered dietitians are an excellent resource for pregnant women who need help planning an individualized balanced diet.

WEIGHT GAIN DURING PREGNANCY

Amount and Quality

Appropriate weight gain is a positive reflection of good nutritional status, and it contributes to a successful course and outcome of pregnancy. The average gestational weight gain is 10 to 16.7 kg (22 to 36.8 lb).[21] Table 10-2 provides an approximation of this weight distribution. The Institute of Medicine recommends setting weight gain goals together with the pregnant woman in accordance with her prepregnancy nutritional status and her BMI.[21] Table 10-3 provides the recommended total gestational weight gain as well as the average rate of weight gain relative to prepregnancy BMI.

Table 10-2	Approximate Weight Gain Distribution during a Normal Pregnancy	
PRODUCT		**WEIGHT (lb)**
Fetus		7.5
Placenta		1.5
Amniotic fluid		2
Uterus		2
Breast tissue		2
Blood volume increase		3
Maternal stores: fat, protein, water, and other nutrients		11
Total		**29**

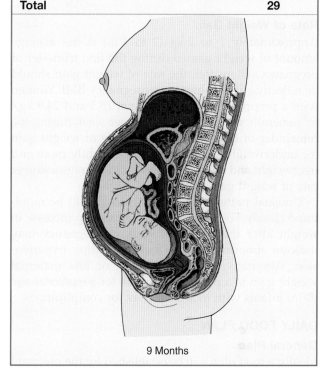

9 Months

Reprinted from Lowdermilk DL, Perry SE. *Maternity & women's health care.* 10th ed. St Louis: Mosby; 2012.

Important considerations in each case are the quantity and quality of weight gain as well as the foods consumed to bring it about, which should involve a nourishing, well-balanced diet. Inappropriate weight gain (i.e., too much or too little) is associated with adverse pregnancy outcomes, such as preterm birth, increased risk of cesarean delivery, low birth weight infant, postpartum weight retention, and failure to initiate breastfeeding.[10,21]

Severe caloric restriction during pregnancy is potentially harmful to the developing fetus and the mother. Such a restricted diet cannot supply all of the energy and nutrients that are essential to the growth process. Thus, weight reduction never should be undertaken during pregnancy. Special care for pregnant women who are suffering from eating disorders (e.g., anorexia nervosa, bulimia nervosa) is essential for the health of both the mother and the fetus.

| Table 10-3 | Recommendations for Total Weight Gain and Rate of Weight Gain during Pregnancy, by Prepregnancy BMI |

PREPREGNANCY BMI	TOTAL WEIGHT GAIN		RATES OF WEIGHT GAIN* 2ND AND 3RD TRIMESTERS	
	RANGE IN kg	RANGE IN lb	MEAN (RANGE) IN kg/week	MEAN (RANGE) IN lb/week
Underweight (<18.5 kg/m²)	12.5-18	28-40	0.51 (0.44-0.58)	1 (1-1.3)
Normal weight (18.5-24.9 kg/m²)	11.5-16	25-35†	0.42 (0.35-0.50)	1 (0.8-1)
Overweight (25.0-29.9 kg/m²)	7-11.5	15-25	0.28 (0.23-0.33)	0.6 (0.5-0.7)
Obese (≥30.0 kg/m²)	5-9	11-20	0.22 (0.17-0.27)	0.5 (0.4-0.6)

From Rasmussen KM, Yaktine AL, editors. *Weight gain during pregnancy: reexamining the guidelines*. Washington, DC: National Academies Press; 2009.
*Calculations assume a 0.5-2 kg (1.1-4.4 lb) weight gain in the first trimester.
†Normal weight women carrying twins: 37 to 54 lb.

Rate of Weight Gain

Approximately 1 to 2 kg (2 to 4 lb) is the average amount of weight gained during the first trimester of pregnancy. Thereafter, the rate of weight gain should be reflective of a woman's prepregnancy BMI. Women with a prepregnancy BMI between 18.5 and 24.9 kg/m² generally gain ≈0.4 kg (14 oz) per week during the remainder of the pregnancy. The rate of weight gain for underweight women should be slightly more and overweight and obese women should average a slower rate of weight gain (see Table 10-3).[21]

Unusual patterns of weight gain should be monitored closely. For example, a sudden sharp increase in weight after the twentieth week of pregnancy may indicate abnormal edema and impending hypertension. Alternatively, an insufficient or low maternal weight gain is a predictor of small for gestational age (SGA) infants with increased risks for complications.

DAILY FOOD PLAN

General Plan

Ideally, a food plan will be established for the pregnant woman on an individual basis to meet her nutrition needs. This core food plan should be a varied and well-rounded diet including all food groups designed to supply the essential nutrients (see Table 10-1).

Alternative Food Patterns

The core food plan provided in Table 10-1 may be only a starting point for women with alternate food patterns. Such food patterns may occur among women with different ethnic backgrounds, belief systems, and lifestyles, thereby making individual diet counseling important. Specific nutrients (not specific foods) are required for successful pregnancies, and these may be found in a variety of foods. Wise health care providers encourage pregnant women to use foods that serve both their personal and their nutritional needs. For example, vegans can meet their dietary protein needs

through the use of soy foods (e.g., tofu, soy milk, soy yogurt, soybeans) and complementary proteins (see Chapter 4 for additional information and resources that address planning a vegetarian diet).

Basic Principles of Diet and Exercise

Whatever the food pattern, two important principles govern the prenatal diet: (1) pregnant women should eat a sufficient quantity of high-quality food; and (2) pregnant women should eat regular meals and snacks and avoid fasting and skipping meals. In addition, pregnant women are encouraged to participate in at least 150 minutes of moderate-intensity aerobic activity spread throughout the week or 30 minutes of moderately intense exercise on most, if not all, days of the week (unless there is a medical reason that prohibits exercise).[12]

GENERAL CONCERNS

GASTROINTESTINAL PROBLEMS

Nausea and Vomiting

Nausea and vomiting affect 69% of women during early pregnancy in the United States.[22] It can be distressing and disruptive to daily life. For the majority of women experiencing nausea and vomiting, it will persist throughout the entire day. As a matter of fact, less than 2% of women experience "morning sickness" (i.e., nausea and vomiting limited to the morning hours).[23] It is likely caused by hormonal adaptations to human chorionic gonadotropin (hCG) during the first trimester, and it generally peaks at about 9 to 11 weeks' gestation.[23] For about half of the women with nausea and vomiting, it will resolve around 14 weeks; and 90% of women will have no additional symptoms after 22 weeks' gestation.[23] In most cases it is self-limiting and does not indicate further complication.

To date, there is inadequate evidence to support the efficacy of any particular pharmacologic or nonpharmacologic intervention for the treatment of nausea and vomiting during pregnancy.[24] Pregnant women often resort to alternative treatments (e.g., acupuncture, accupressure) for the relief of symptoms; however, these methods do not appear to be consistently effective for

---

small for gestational age (SGA) infant is smaller than a gender and gestational age matched infant. Birth weight is below the 10th percentile.

treating nausea and vomiting in this population. Some studies show improvements in symptoms with the use of ginger and vitamin B_6, although findings are inconsistent and high-quality research is limited.[24-26]

Although the data does not indicate any treatment will be effective in all patients, some dietary and lifestyle interventions are worth trying because they have no negative side effects. The following dietary actions *may* help with the relief of symptoms[27,28]:

- Avoid an empty stomach by eating small, frequent meals and snacks that are fairly dry and bland with low-fat and low-fiber.
- Drink liquids between (rather than with) meals.
- Avoid odors, foods, or supplements that trigger nausea.
- Try ginger (125 to 250 mg) or vitamin B_6 supplements (10 to 25 mg).

If nausea and vomiting persist and become severe and prolonged, then the woman should be evaluated for **hyperemesis gravidarum,** a condition in which medical treatment is usually required. Approximately 1% of pregnant women develop hyperemesis gravidarum, and women who have experienced this condition with their first pregnancy are at a greater risk for recurrence during any additional pregnancies (15.2%).[29] Patients with hyperemesis gravidarum should be closely followed for hydration, electrolyte balance, and appropriate weight gain. Pregnancy outcome and fetal growth are both compromised in pregnancies with persistent hyperemeis gravidarum that prevents adequate nutrition and weight gain. Prescription antiemetic medication may benefit some women in this situation (see the Drug-Nutrient Interaction box, "Antiemetic Medications").

Drug-Nutrient Interaction

Antiemetic Medications

KELLI BOI

Hyperemesis gravidarum can compromise the nutritional status of both the mother and the fetus as a result of food aversions or inadequate nutrient intake. In severe cases, a physician may opt to prescribe an antiemetic medication.

One of these medications, Reglan (metoclopramide), may also be prescribed during lactation to stimulate the secretion of prolactin and thus increase the milk supply. Some nutritional implications of taking antiemetics include dry mouth, diarrhea, abdominal pain, and constipation. Phenergan (promethazine), which is another antiemetic option, may increase the patient's need for riboflavin.

---

hyperemesis gravidarum a condition that involves prolonged and severe vomiting in pregnant women, with a loss of more than 5% of body weight and the presence of ketonuria, electrolyte disturbances, and dehydration.

Constipation

Although it is usually a minor complaint, constipation may occur during the latter part of pregnancy as a result of the increasing pressure of the enlarging uterus and the muscle-relaxing effect of progesterone on the gastrointestinal tract, thereby reducing normal peristalsis. Helpful remedies include adequate exercise, increased fluid intake, and consumption of high-fiber foods such as whole grains, vegetables, dried fruits (especially prunes and figs), and other fruits and juices. Pregnant women should avoid artificial and herbal laxatives.

Hemorrhoids

Hemorrhoids are enlarged veins in the anus that often protrude through the anal sphincter, and they are not uncommon during the latter part of pregnancy. This vein enlargement is usually caused by the increased weight of the baby and the downward pressure that this weight produces. Hemorrhoids may cause considerable discomfort, burning, and itching; they may even rupture and bleed under the pressure of a bowel movement, thereby causing the mother anxiety. Hemorrhoids are usually controlled by the dietary suggestions given for constipation. Sufficient rest during the latter part of the day may also help to relieve some of the downward pressure of the uterus on the lower intestine. Hemorrhoids resolve spontaneously after delivery in many women, in which case long-term treatment is not necessary.

Heartburn

Pregnant women sometimes have heartburn or a "full" feeling. These discomforts occur especially after meals, and they are caused by the pressure of the enlarging uterus crowding the stomach. Gastric reflux may occur in the lower esophagus, thereby causing irritation and a burning sensation. The full feeling comes from general gastric pressure, the lack of normal space in the area, a large meal, or the formation of gas. Dividing the day's food intake into a series of small meals and avoiding large meals at any time usually help to relieve these issues. Comfort is sometimes improved by the wearing of loose-fitting clothing.

HIGH-RISK PREGNANCIES

Identifying Risk Factors

Pregnancy-related deaths claim the lives of 600 to 700 women in the United States annually.[30] Identifying risk factors and addressing them early are critical to the promotion of a healthy pregnancy. Nutrition-related risk factors are listed in the Clinical Applications box, "Nutrition-Related Risk Factors In Pregnancy."

To avoid the compounding results of poor nutrition during pregnancy, mothers who are at risk for complications should be identified as soon as possible. Health care professionals should not wait for clinical symptoms of poor nutrition to appear. The best approach is

Clinical Applications

Nutrition-Related Risk Factors in Pregnancy

RISK FACTORS AT THE ONSET OF PREGNANCY

- Age: ≤18 years old or ≥35 years old
- Frequent pregnancies: three or more during a 2-year period
- History of poor obstetric performance or fetal outcome
- Poverty, food insecurity, or both
- Bizarre or trendy food habits or eating disorder
- Abuse of tobacco, alcohol, or drugs
- Therapeutic diet that is required for a chronic disorder
- Poorly controlled preexisting condition (e.g., diabetes, hypertension)
- Weight: ≤85% or ≥120% of ideal body weight

RISK FACTORS DURING PREGNANCY

- Anemia: low hemoglobin level (i.e., less than 12 g) or hematocrit level (i.e., less than 34%)
- Inadequate weight gain: any weight loss or weight gain of less than 1 kg (2 lb) per month after the first trimester
- Excessive weight gain: more than 1 kg (2 lb) per week after the first trimester
- Substance abuse (i.e., alcohol, tobacco, drugs)
- Gestational diabetes, hypertensive disorder of pregnancy, hyperemesis gravidarum, pica, or another pregnancy-related condition
- Poor nutritional status, especially involving folic acid, iron, or calcium
- Multifetal gestation

to identify poor food patterns and to prevent nutrition problems from emerging. Examples of dietary patterns that are not optimal for maternal and fetal nutrition are as follows: (1) insufficient food intake; (2) poor food selection; and (3) poor food distribution throughout the day.

Teenage Pregnancy

Teenage pregnancy rates in the United States are at a record low with an annual rate of 29.4 pregnancies for every 1000 girls between the ages of 15 and 19 years.[31] Pregnancy at this early age is physically and emotionally difficult. From a nutrition standpoint, special care must be given to support the adequate physiologic growth of both the mother and the fetus. The current DRIs distinguish specific vitamin and mineral needs for pregnant females who are younger than 18 years old. See the For Further Focus box, "Pregnant Teenagers," for more information about health and nutrition concerns for adolescent mothers.

Recognizing Special Counseling Needs

Every pregnant woman deserves personalized care and support during pregnancy. Women with risk factors such as those in the following discussion have distinct counseling needs. In each case, the clinician must work with the mother in a sensitive and supportive manner to help her develop a healthy food plan that is both practical and nourishing. Dangerous

practices (e.g., fad dieting, extreme macrobiotic diets, attempted weight loss) should be identified early and amended. In addition to avoiding dangerous practices, several topics require sensitive counseling, including those related to age and parity, detrimental lifestyle habits, and socioeconomic problems.

Age and parity. Pregnancies at either age extreme of the reproductive cycle carry special risks. Adolescent pregnancy adds many social and nutritional risks as its social upheaval and physical demands are imposed on an immature teenage girl. Sensitive counseling necessitates both helpful information and emotional support with good prenatal care throughout. Alternatively, pregnant women who are older than 35 years old and having their first child also require special attention. Pregnancy rates among women who are more than 35 years old continue to rise in the United States.[32] These women are at a higher risk for obstetric and perinatal complications such as preeclampsia, gestational diabetes, and cesarean delivery.[33-35] In addition, women with an extremely high parity rate (i.e., those who have had several pregnancies within a limited number of years) are at an increased risk for poor pregnancy outcomes[36,37] and are often facing the increasing physical and economic pressures of child care.

Obesity. Obesity poses health concerns at any stage of life, including pregnancy. Excessive gestational weight gain, particularly in normal and overweight women, increases the risk for adiposity in the offspring and perhaps the complications of obesity later in life.[38] Thus, individual and specific person-centered counselling for pregnant women is ideal to help improve overall pregnancy outcome.[12]

Alcohol. Alcohol use during pregnancy can lead to **fetal alcohol spectrum disorders (FASDs),** of which **fetal alcohol syndrome (FAS)** is the most severe form (Figure 10-1). Fetal alcohol spectrum disorders comprise the leading causes of *preventable* mental retardation and birth defects in the United States. It is difficult to determine the exact prevalence of FAS; however, one study estimated that between 2 and 7 per 1000 live births in the United States are affected by FAS.[39] Alcohol is a

---

fetal alcohol spectrum disorders a group of physical and mental birth defects that are found in infants who are born to mothers who used alcohol during pregnancy; the physical and mental disabilities vary in severity; there is no cure.

fetal alcohol syndrome (FAS) a combination of physical and mental birth defects that are found in infants who are born to mothers who used alcohol during pregnancy; this is the most severe of the fetal alcohol spectrum disorders; there is no cure.

Pregnant Teenagers

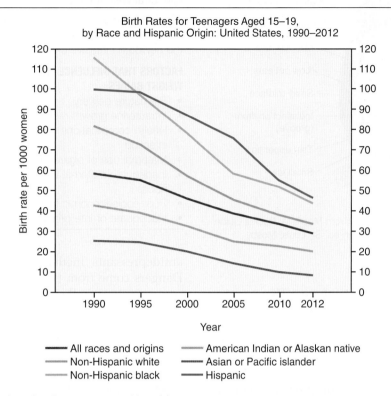

Birth Rates for Teenagers Aged 15–19,
by Race and Hispanic Origin: United States, 1990–2012

- All races and origins
- Non-Hispanic white
- Non-Hispanic black
- American Indian or Alaskan native
- Asian or Pacific islander
- Hispanic

Few situations are as life-changing for a teenage girl and her family as an unintended pregnancy. Depending on how she and her family—as well as her partner—deal with the situation, lifelong consequences may occur for them as well as for the broader community. Adolescent pregnancy rates have historically been higher among African-American and Hispanic teens than among whites in the United States, but rates are gradually declining in all ethnic groups.[1]

Teen pregnancy is associated with a high risk for complications and poor outcome, with increased rates of low birth weight, preterm delivery, and infant mortality.[1] The following problems *may* contribute to pregnancy complications with teens: the physiologic demands of the pregnancy, which compromise the teenager's needs for her own unfinished growth and development; the psychosocial influences of a low income; inadequate diet; and experimentation with alcohol, smoking, and other drugs. Little or no access to appropriate prenatal care may also significantly contribute to a lack of support, including nutrition support, for the pregnancy. Early nutrition intervention is essential, and it can change the course of events and the pregnancy outcome. Changes from the inconsistent and often poor food pattern of teenagers may be difficult to achieve. Experienced and sensitive health care workers in teen clinics emphasize the need for supportive individual and group nutrition counseling. The following suggestions may help to secure a positive and healthy environment for the teen.

KNOW EACH CLIENT PERSONALLY

All nutrition services must be tailored to the unique needs and characteristics of each pregnant teenager. Many of these girls have lower educational levels to which informative material must be adapted. Low-income teens lack the financial resources to maintain an adequate diet, and those who are living at home may have little control over the food that is available to them. Personal stress regarding the pregnancy is paramount, and nutrition concerns are often not a priority.

SEEK WAYS TO MOTIVATE CLIENTS

If clients are participating in the Women, Infants, and Children (WIC) Food and Nutrition Services program, schedule meetings on days that clients are coming in for their supplemental food vouchers or other health care appointments. Invite the teen's mother and her friends to accompany her to group counseling sessions so that they can support the recommendations that are made. Make each recommendation concrete and reasonable. Avoid scare tactics.

MAKE APPROPRIATE ASSESSMENTS

Use simple and concrete forms to evaluate dietary intake (e.g., the basic food groups of the MyPlate.gov guidelines). A traditional model can be used, with increased amounts indicated for pregnancy, as both an educational and an assessment tool.

PLAN PRACTICAL INTERVENTIONS

Plan short, enjoyable, and active learning sessions. Use positive reinforcement liberally. Provide specific suggestions for carrying out changes at home. Review progress during follow-up sessions, and always maintain a supportive atmosphere.

SUPPORT THE TEENAGER'S RESPONSIBILITY

Help the teenager learn to be responsible. Pregnant teenagers must take on responsibility, often for the first time, for their own nourishment and the nourishment of others. Helping them in a supportive manner to understand and carry out this responsibility—which ultimately only they can do—is a primary objective of nutrition counseling. Nutrition consultants must be skillful so that they can establish the kind of rapport and relationship in which these responsibilities can develop and grow.

REFERENCE

1. Ventura SJ, Hamilton BE, Matthews TJ. National and state patterns of teen births in the United States, 1940-2013. *Natl Vital Stat Rep.* 2014;63(4):1-34.

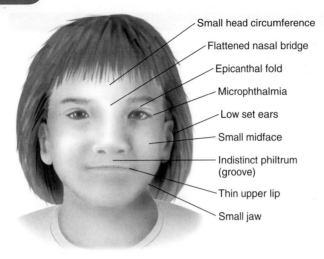

Small head circumference

Flattened nasal bridge

Epicanthal fold

Microphthalmia

Low set ears

Small midface

Indistinct philtrum (groove)

Thin upper lip

Small jaw

FIGURE 10-1 Fetal alcohol syndrome. (From Moore M: Pocket Guide to Nutritional Assessment and Care, 6th ed. St. Louis, Mosby, 2009.)

potent and well-documented **teratogen.** There are no safe amounts, types, or times during pregnancy that are acceptable for the consumption of alcohol. FAS is 100% preventable by abstaining from alcohol during pregnancy.

Nicotine. An estimated 12.3% of pregnant women continue to smoke cigarettes during pregnancy.[40] Maternal cigarette smoking or exposure to second-hand smoke (also known as environmental tobacco smoke) during pregnancy is associated with placental complications, preterm delivery, fetal growth restriction, congenital abnormalities, and sudden infant death syndrome (SIDS).[41-45] Women who stop smoking at the onset of pregnancy have similar pregnancy outcomes as nonsmokers, meaning that they are able to avoid such smoking-related complications for their infant.[45]

See the Clinical Applications box, "Low Birth Weight Baby" for more information regarding risk factors for fetal growth restriction.

Drugs. Drug use, whether medicinal or recreational, poses problems for both the mother and the fetus, especially when it involves the use of illicit substances. Drugs cross the placenta and enter the fetal circulation, thereby creating a potential addiction in the unborn child. *Neonatal abstinence syndrome* (NAS) is a condition from which the infant suffers after birth because of the abrupt discontinuation of a drug chronically used throughout gestation. Substances that may result in NAS include opioids (heroin, methadone, buprenorphine, and prescription opioid medications), selective serotonin reuptake inhibitors (SSRIs), tricyclic

teratogen a substance that causes a birth defect.

Clinical Applications

Low Birth Weight Baby

Infants who weigh less than 2500 g (5 lb, 8 oz) at birth often present with medical complications and require special care in the newborn intensive care unit.

FACTORS THAT INFLUENCE THE TREND TOWARD LOW BIRTH WEIGHT BABIES
- Premature delivery
- Intrauterine growth restriction
- Health complications of the mother, including disease or infection
- Maternal use of cigarettes, alcohol, and drugs
- Inadequate maternal weight gain and/or poor dietary habits
- Poor socioeconomic factors
- Inadequate or late prenatal care

---

antidepressants, methamphetamines, and inhalants.[46] Dangers come from the drugs themselves, the use of contaminated needles, and the impurities that are contained in illicit substances. Self-medication with over-the-counter drugs also may present adverse effects. Pregnant women should always check the label for safety notices of use during pregnancy or speak with their doctor or pharmacist regarding medications.

Medications made from vitamin A compounds (e.g., retinoids such as tretinoin [Accutane], which are prescribed for severe acne) have caused birth defects and the spontaneous abortion of malformed fetuses by women who conceived during acne treatment. Thus, the use of this medication without contraception is contraindicated.[47]

Caffeine. Caffeine use is common during pregnancy. Caffeine crosses the placenta and enters fetal circulation. Studies on caffeine use and pregnancy risks have been controversial with conflicting results over the past several decades. Three large-scale reviews of the available literature did not find consistent evidence that either normal or high intakes (defined as ≥300 mg/d) of caffeine during pregnancy posed a risk for congenital malformations, growth restriction, or spontaneous abortion (miscarriage).[48-50] Of note, two of the reviews were funded by the Caffeine Committee of the International Life Sciences Institute and the National Coffee Association. The use of caffeine and safety during pregnancy is difficult to study; however, it will continue to be a hot topic of research for years to come.

Pica. Pica is the craving for and the purposeful consumption of nonfood items (e.g., chalk, laundry starch, clay). It is a practice that is sometimes seen in pregnant or malnourished individuals. Although the etiology is unknown, pica is significantly associated with iron-deficiency anemia as well as other contributing factors, such as poor zinc status, hunger, and psychologic stress.[51-53] Although pica may occur in any population group, worldwide it is most common among pregnant women. The practice of eating nonfood substances can introduce pathogens (e.g., bacteria, worms) and inhibit micronutrient absorption, thereby resulting in various deficiencies. Most patients do not readily report the practice of pica; therefore, practitioners should always ask patients directly about their consumption of any nonfood substance.

Socioeconomic difficulties. Special counseling is often needed for women and young girls who live in low-income situations. Poverty particularly puts pregnant women in grave danger, because they need resources for food, medical care, and shelter. Dietitians and social workers on the health care team can provide special counseling and referrals. Community resources include programs such as the Special Supplemental Nutrition Program for Women, Infants and Children, known as *WIC*, which has helped to improve the health and well-being of many children in the United States. WIC also provides nutrition education counseling regarding the nutrition needs of both the mothers and their babies.

COMPLICATIONS OF PREGNANCY

For the majority of pregnant women, their gestation will progress without complication. However, for others, preexisting conditions or health problems that develop along with the pregnancy will present difficulties. One such example is *hyperemesis gravidarum,* which was discussed earlier in this chapter. Other issues may affect only the fetus, such as *neural tube defects.* Although there are a large number of obstacles that may complicate pregnancy, we will focus only on the more common conditions here.

Anemia

Iron-deficiency anemia is the most common nutritional deficiency worldwide and is a risk factor for delivering low birth weight infants.[54,55] Approximately 42% of pregnant women worldwide experience iron-deficiency anemia (Hb <110 g/L). Although a disproportionate amount of these cases occur in underdeveloped countries, the prevalence ranges greatly, from about 6% in North America to 55.8% in Africa.[56] Anemia is more prevalent among poor women, many of whom live on marginal diets that lack iron-rich foods, but it is by no means restricted to lower socioeconomic groups.

Dietary intake must be improved and supplements used as necessary to avoid the long-term detrimental effects on the fetus of iron deficiency during gestation. As a result of the severe complications of both iron- and folate-deficiency anemia, the World Health Organization currently recommends an intermittent (once, twice, or three times weekly on nonconsecutive days) iron and folic acid dietary supplement as a safe, effective, and inexpensive way to prevent anemia during pregnancy for women living in areas with a high risk for anemia.[57]

Intrauterine Growth Restriction

Women with high-risk pregnancies have an elevated risk of **intrauterine growth restriction (IUGR).** A fetus with IUGR is at risk for preterm birth and being small for gestational age,[58] both of which are associated with increased infant morbidity and mortality. Many factors contribute to IUGR, but low prepregnancy weight, inadequate weight gain during pregnancy, inadequate folate and iron status, and the use of cigarettes, alcohol, and other drugs are modifiable risk factors. Furthermore, infants who suffer from IUGR are at higher risk for the development of chronic diseases as adults, including cardiovascular disease and hypertension.[59]

Hypertensive Disorders of Pregnancy

The etiology of hypertension development during pregnancy is unknown, but it is a leading cause of pregnancy-related deaths worldwide. Hypertension is defined as a blood pressure of ≥140 mm Hg systolic or ≥90 mm Hg diastolic. Hypertensive disorders of pregnancy include several classifications[60]:

- *Chronic hypertension:* preexisting hypertension or hypertension that appears before 20 weeks' gestation.
- *Gestational hypertension:* high blood pressure diagnosed after 20 weeks' gestation. Blood pressure returns to normal within 6 weeks' postpartum. Affects 5% to 10% of all pregnancies.
- *Preeclampsia:* gestational hypertension plus proteinuria (≥300 mg/d of protein in the urine). Affects 2% to 5% of all pregnancies.
- *Eclampsia:* preeclampsia plus seizures.
- *Preeclampsia superimposed on chronic hypertension:* preexisting hypertension with the development of proteinuria during gestation. Affects 20% to 25% of women with chronic hypertension.

Hypertension is called the *silent disease* because it has no symptoms. However, there are other indicators that alert patients to report to their doctor if they experience signs such as severe headaches, blurred vision, chest pain, nausea, or a sudden weight gain (i.e., edema). Specific treatment varies according to individual severity and presentation;[61] however, in any case, optimal nutrition is important, and prompt medical attention is required. Salt restriction is not advised because it does not prevent preeclampsia or

intrauterine growth restriction (IUGR) a condition that occurs when a newborn weighs less than 10% of predicted fetal weight for gestational age.

help to treat the symptoms. An overall healthy diet before and during pregnancy with a high intake of plant foods, antioxidants, and high fiber is thought to be helpful.

Women with mild preexisting hypertension or gestational hypertension, without additional co-morbidities, are usually not at risk for poor pregnancy outcome.[60] Complications of severe hypertensive and preeclampsia/eclampsia often require hospitalization and, in advanced cases, induced labor. Preeclampsia is thought to be a disorder of the placenta and there are currently no known cures. Preeclampsia/eclampsia is associated with poor fetal outcomes such as maternal and fetal morbidity and mortality, IUGR, low birth weight, and preterm delivery.[60] Thus, early and consistent prenatal care is imperative in order to identify symptoms early.

Gestational Diabetes

Gestational diabetes is defined as glucose intolerance with onset during pregnancy, and the definition applies regardless of whether medication (e.g., oral hypoglycemic agents, insulin) or only diet modification is used for treatment. Women found to have diabetes at their initial prenatal visit (usually by fasting or random blood glucose test) are assumed to have had undiagnosed diabetes before becoming pregnant and are therefore diagnosed with overt diabetes and not gestational diabetes.[62] The prevalence of gestational diabetes in the United States is approximately 7% of all pregnancies annually.[62] The treatment for gestational diabetes follows a similar protocol as that for type 2 diabetes, with diet and exercise of paramount importance as a first-line treatment plan.

Prenatal clinics routinely screen pregnant women between 24 and 28 weeks' gestation with either a **"One-Step"** or a **"Two-Step"** oral glucose tolerance test for diagnosis. Particular attention is given to women who are at higher risk for the development of gestational diabetes, including those who are 30 years old and older who are overweight (i.e., those with a BMI of $\geq 26 \text{ kg/m}^2$) and who have a history of any of the following predisposing factors:

- Previous history of gestational diabetes
- Family history of diabetes
- Ethnicity associated with a high incidence of diabetes (Asian, Hispanic, African Americans, and Native Americans)
- Glucosuria
- Obesity
- Previous delivery of a large baby weighing 4.5 kg (10 lb) or more

Women with gestational diabetes are at higher risk for caesarean delivery and fetal damage such as birth defects, **stillbirth**, **macrosomia**, and neonatal hypoglycemia. Additionally, these women have a 7-fold increased risk of developing type 2 diabetes later in life.[63] Therefore, identifying and providing close

follow-up testing and treatment with a well-balanced diet, exercise, and medication (as needed) are important interventions.

Preexisting Disease

Preexisting diseases (e.g., cardiovascular diseases, hypertension, type 1 or 2 diabetes, HIV, eating disorders) can cause complications during pregnancy. Inborn errors of metabolism (e.g., phenylketonuria) and food allergies or intolerances (e.g., celiac disease, lactose intolerance) must also be taken into consideration and maintained under good control to mitigate any flare-ups or compromised nutrient intake. All potential preexisting diseases will not be discussed here, because pregnant women may have any combination of preexisting conditions.

In each case, a woman's pregnancy is managed—usually by a team of specialists—in accordance to the principles of care related to pregnancy and the particular disease involved. See Chapters 18 through 23 for major nutrition-related diseases that require medical nutrition therapy.

LACTATION

Breastfeeding is "an unequalled way of providing ideal food for the healthy growth and development of infants."[64] Breastfeeding is recommended for at least 1 year with iron-fortified solid foods added to the exclusive diet of breast milk at about 6 months of age.

TRENDS

Approximately 37% of infants worldwide are **exclusively breastfed** for the first 6 months of life, compared with only 18.8% in the United States.[65,66] Although the rates are still low in the United States compared with other countries, breastfeeding has been on the rise

---

"One-Step" a method for diagnosing diabetes using a 75-g oral glucose tolerance test. The patient's fasting plasma glucose level is measured; then the patient drinks a solution with 75 mg of glucose and plasma glucose is measured again at 1-hour and 2-hour postconsumption. Diagnostic criteria are based on the levels of plasma glucose at each measurement.

"Two-Step" a method for diagnosing diabetes using a two-step method of oral glucose tolerance test in a nonfasting patient. Step 1: The patient drinks a 50-g glucose solution and plasma glucose is measured at 1-hour postconsumption. If the patient's plasma glucose level is ≥ 140 g/dL then the patient must return for Step 2, which is a fasting 100-g glucose tolerance test.

stillbirth the death of a fetus after the twentieth week of pregnancy.

macrosomia an abnormally large baby.

exclusively breastfed feeding the infant only breast milk with no supplemental liquids or solid foods, other than necessary medications or vitamin/mineral supplements.

in the last few decades (Figure 10-2). Breastfeeding initiation and continuation are highest among well-educated, older women (see the Cultural Considerations box, "Breastfeeding Trends in the United States").[67]

The *Healthy People 2020* report lists specific goals to increase the prevalence and duration of breastfeeding in the United States[68]:

- Increase the proportion of infants who are breast-fed at least 1 year to 34%.
- Increase the proportion of employers that have worksite lactation support programs to 38%.
- Increase the proportion of live births that occur in facilities that provide recommended care for lactating mothers and their babies to 8%.
- Reduce the proportion of breastfed newborns who receive breast milk substitutes within the first 2 days of life to 14% or less.

THE BABY-FRIENDLY HOSPITAL INITIATIVE

The Baby-Friendly Hospital Initiative, which was launched by the World Health Organization and the United Nations Children's Fund, has worked to promote breastfeeding rates worldwide since 1991. Box 10-2 outlines the 10 steps for successful breast-feeding that are recommended by the Baby-Friendly Hospital Initiative. Almost all women who choose to breastfeed their infants can do so, provided they have the necessary information and support from their family, community, and health care system.[64] Well-nourished mothers who exclusively breastfeed provide adequate nutrition to their infants, as well as a host of other beneficial components.

PHYSIOLOGIC PROCESS OF LACTATION

Mammary Glands and Hormones

The female breasts are highly specialized secretory organs (Figure 10-3). Throughout pregnancy, the mammary glands are preparing for lactation. The mammary glands are capable of extracting certain nutrients from the maternal blood in addition to synthesizing other compounds. The combined effort results in the nutrient-complete breast milk.

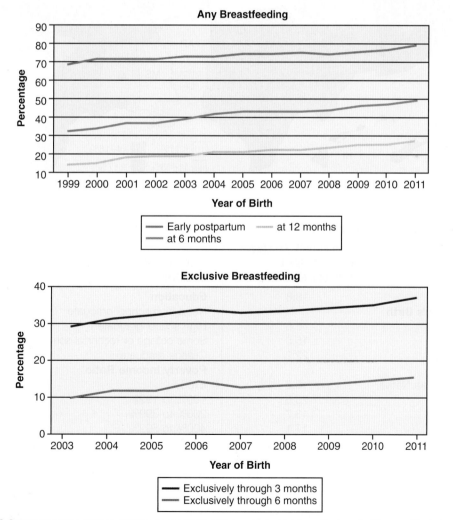

FIGURE 10-2 Breastfeeding among children in the United States. (Adapted from Centers for Disease Control and Prevention. *Breastfeeding among U.S. children born 2001–2011, CDC National Immunization Survey, 2011*. Cited November 14, 2014. Available from www.cdc.gov/breastfeeding/data/NIS_data.)

Breastfeeding Trends in the United States

Increasing the prevalence of breastfeeding continues to be a health goal both nationally and internationally. In the United States, breastfeeding is most common among women who have a higher socioeconomic and education level; and are 30 years old or older. A higher prevalence of breastfeeding is also noted among married women, and it is more common in the Western states (see map).[1,2]

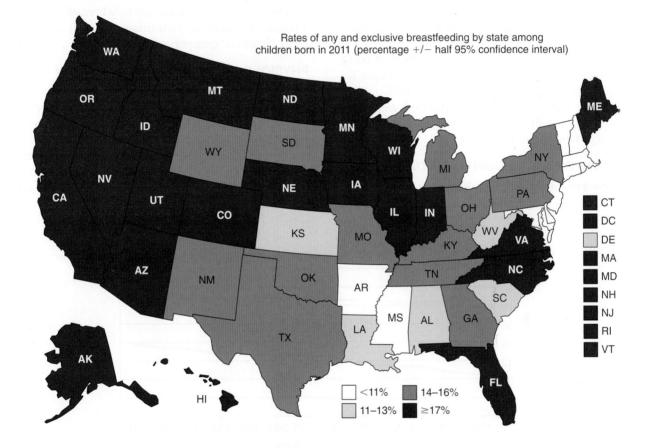

Rates of any and exclusive breastfeeding by state among children born in 2011 (percentage +/− half 95% confidence interval)

Legend:
- <11%
- 11–13%
- 14–16%
- ≥17%

CT, DC, DE, MA, MD, NH, NJ, RI, VT

PREVALENCE OF BREASTFEEDING IN THE UNITED STATES	
SELECTED CHARACTERISTICS OF MOTHER	PERCENTAGE *EXCLUSIVE* BREASTFEEDING THROUGH 6 MONTHS
Total	18.8
Mother's Age at Baby's Birth	
≤20 years	5.6
20 to 29 years	15.5
≥30 years	22.2
Race or Ethnicity	
American Indian or Alaska Native	15.6
Asian	26.6
Black	13.7
Hispanic	17.1
Hawaiian or Pacific Islander	21.0
White	20.3

PREVALENCE OF BREASTFEEDING IN THE UNITED STATES	
SELECTED CHARACTERISTICS OF MOTHER	PERCENTAGE *EXCLUSIVE* BREASTFEEDING THROUGH 6 MONTHS
Education	
Not a high school graduate	13.5
High school graduate	15.8
Some college or technical school	16.5
Collage graduate	25.5
Poverty Income Ratio*	
<100%	14.2
100% to 199%	18.0
200% to 399%	22.0
400% to 599%	25.2
≥600%	23.1

Cultural Considerations—cont'd

As a health care provider, be sure to note the perceived obstacles to the initiation and continuation of breastfeeding so that education and alternatives may be presented at the appropriate time (i.e., before delivery). The American Academy of Pediatrics notes the following potential obstacles[3]:

- Insufficient prenatal education about breastfeeding
- Disruptive hospital policies and practices
- Inappropriate interruption of breastfeeding
- Early hospital discharge in some populations
- Lack of timely routine follow-up care and postpartum home health visits
- Maternal employment (especially in the absence of workplace facilities that support breastfeeding)
- Lack of family and broad societal support
- Media portrayal of bottle-feeding as normal
- Commercial promotion of infant formula through the distribution of hospital discharge packs containing breast milk substitutes

- Coupons for free or discounted formula
- Misinformation about what medical conditions may be contraindications for breastfeeding
- Lack of guidance and encouragement from health care professionals

REFERENCES

1. National Center for Chronic Disease Prevention and Health Promotion. *Rates of any and exclusive breastfeeding by socio-demographics among children born in 2011.* Atlanta, Ga: Centers for Disease Control and Prevention; 2014. Available at: <www.cdc.gov/breastfeeding/data/nis_data/rates-any-exclusive-bf-socio-dem-2011.htm>.
2. Centers for Disease Control and Prevention. *Rates of any and exclusive breastfeeding by state among children born in 2011.* Atlanta, Ga: Department of Health and Human Services; 2014. Available at: <www.cdc.gov/breastfeeding/data/nis_data/rates-any-exclusive-bf-state-2011.htm>.
3. Gartner LM, et al. Breastfeeding and the use of human milk. *Pediatrics.* 2005;115(2):496-506.

*The poverty income ratio is the self-reported family income compared with the federal poverty threshold value. It depends on the number of people in the household.

Box 10-2   Ten Steps to Successful Breastfeeding

1. Have a written breastfeeding policy that is routinely communicated to all health care staff.
2. Train all health care staff in the skills that are necessary to implement this policy.
3. Inform all pregnant women about the benefits and management of breastfeeding.
4. Help mothers to initiate breastfeeding within 30 minutes after birth.
5. Show mothers how to breastfeed and maintain lactation, even if they may be separated from their infants.
6. Give newborn infants no food or drink other than breast milk unless it is medically indicated to do so.
7. Practice rooming in: allow mothers and infants to remain together 24 hours a day.
8. Encourage breastfeeding on demand.
9. Give no artificial teats or pacifiers to breastfeeding infants.
10. Foster the establishment of breastfeeding support groups, and refer mothers to these groups when they are discharged from the hospital or clinic.

From the World Health Organization, United Nations Children's Fund. *The Baby-Friendly Hospital Initiative* (website): www.unicef.org/programme/breastfeeding/baby.htm#10. Accessed November 16, 2014.

After the delivery of the baby, milk production and secretion are stimulated by the two hormones **prolactin** and **oxytocin,** respectively. The stimulation of the nipple from infant suckling sends nerve signals to the brain of the mother (Figure 10-4); this nerve signal then causes the release of prolactin and oxytocin.

prolactin hormone released from the anterior pituitary gland that stimulates milk production.
oxytocin hormone released from the posterior pituitary gland that stimulates milk let-down.

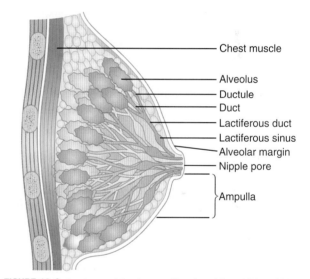

FIGURE 10-3 Anatomy of the breast. (Reprinted from Mahan LK, Escott-Stump S. *Krause's food & nutrition therapy.* 12th ed. Philadelphia: Saunders; 2008.)

Let-down is the process of the milk moving from the upper milk-producing cells down to the nipple for infant suckling.

Supply and Demand

Milk production is a supply-and-demand procedure. The mammary glands are stimulated to produce milk each time that the infant feeds. Therefore, the more milk that is taken from the breast (i.e., during breastfeeding or pumping), the more milk the mother produces, thereby always meeting the infant's needs. As a result of this supply-and-demand production, mothers of multiple infants (e.g., twins, triplets) are able to produce more milk with the additional stimulation. Some mothers of multiples choose to pump and

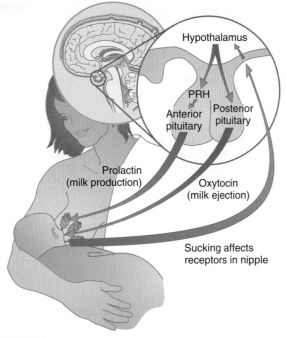

FIGURE 10-4 Physiology of milk production and the let-down reflex. *PRH*, Prolactin-releasing hormone. (Reprinted from Mahan LK, Escott-Stump S. *Krause's food & nutrition therapy.* 13th ed. Philadelphia: Saunders; 2012.)

Table 10-4	Nutrition Composition of Human Milk versus Cow's Milk*		
	HUMAN MILK		**COW'S MILK, WHOLE**
NUTRIENT	**COLOSTRUM**	**MATURE**	
Kilocalories	55	73	63
Protein (g)	2.0	1.07	3.25
Carbohydrate (g)†	7.4	7.2	4.95
Fat (g)	2.9	4.56	3.35
Fat-Soluble Vitamins			
A (IU)	296	221	167
D (IU)	—	3	53‡
E (mg)	0.8	0.08	0.07
K (mcg)	—	0.3	0.3
Water-Soluble Vitamins			
Thiamin (mg)	0.02	0.015	0.05
Riboflavin (mg)	0.029	0.037	0.17
Niacin (mg)	0.075	0.18	0.09
Vitamin C (mg)	6	5.2	0
Folate (mcg)	0.05	5	5
Minerals			
Calcium (mg)	31	33	116
Phosphorus (mg)	14	15	87
Iron (mg)	0.09	0.03	0.03
Zinc (mg)	0.5	0.18	0.38
Magnesium (mg)	4.2	3	10
Sodium (mg)	48	18	44
Potassium (mg)	74	53	136

*Per 100 mL.
†Lactose.
‡Fortified.

then bottle-feed the infants the breast milk so that other members of the family can help with feedings.

Composition

Breast milk changes in composition to meet the specific needs of infants as they grow. **Colostrum** is the first milk that is produced after birth. It is a yellowish fluid that is rich in antibodies, and it gives the infant his or her first immune boost. Mature breast milk comes in within a few days after delivery. The terms foremilk, midmilk, and hindmilk are used to recognize the changing milk composition throughout each feeding. As the breast is emptied, the milk becomes more concentrated in fat. Hence hindmilk is a good source of essential fatty acids for the infant. As you can see from Table 10-4, the composition of mature human milk is quite different from that of cow's milk. Cow's milk is an inappropriate food source for infants younger than 1 year old because of its high protein and electrolyte levels.

Complications

Although breastfeeding is a natural physiologic process, it is not without complications. Many women find breastfeeding difficult and these problems rapidly

> **colostrum** fluid first secreted by the mammary glands for the first few days after birth, preceding the mature breast milk. Colostrum contains up to 20% protein, including a large amount of lactalbumin, more minerals, and immunoglobulins that represent the antibodies found in material blood. It has less lactose and fat than mature milk.

lead to the cessation of breastfeeding. Not all issues are physiologic in nature though; some problems women face are psychologic and perception-based.[69] For example, the two most common reasons women stop breastfeeding are (1) their perception that the baby is not satisfied with breast milk alone and (2) they do not think they are making enough milk. Mothers have reported discontinuation of breastfeeding within the first month of the infant's life because of the following common reasons[70]:

- Physiologic and nutritional: Sore, cracked, or bleeding nipples; engorged breast; the baby had trouble latching on; breastfeeding was too painful; breast milk alone did not satisfy my baby; I did not have enough milk; and I had trouble getting the milk flow to start.
- Psychosocial: Breastfeeding was too tiring or inconvenient; I did not want to breastfeed in public.
- Medical and infant self-weaning: My baby lost interest; I was sick and had to take medicine; my baby weaned himself.

Almost all of the complications encountered during breastfeeding could either be prevented or be treated by motivated and educated health care practitioners and mothers. A thorough understanding of the physiology of lactation and the psychosocial factors influencing the success of breastfeeding are imperative to effectively support a nursing mother. The article by Bergmann and colleagues (full reference provided in the reference section for this chapter at the back of the book.) is an excellent resource for understanding the common medical problems of breastfeeding.[69]

NUTRITION AND LIFESTYLE NEEDS

The basic diet recommended for the mother during pregnancy, as well as any prenatal supplements used, should be continued through the lactation period. The MyPlate food guide system provides specific nutrient information for pregnant and lactating women at www.choosemyplate.gov/pregnancy-breastfeeding.html. The Daily Food Plan for Moms takes into account the mother's age, height, weight, and physical activity level; the infant's age; and the amount of breast milk the mom is producing to offer individualized recommendations. The website also provides help with menu planning for mothers with an easy-to-use interactive site.

Diet

Energy and nutrients. Lactation requires energy for both the process and the product. Some of this energy will be met by the extra fat that is stored in the mother during pregnancy. The increased calorie recommendations are 330 kcal/day (plus 170 kcal/day from maternal stores) during the first 6 months of lactation and 400 kcal/day during the second 6 months of lactation over the woman's nonpregnant, nonlactating energy requirements. The requirement for protein during lactation is 25 g/day more than a woman's average need of 46 g/day, for a total of 71 g/day (i.e., 1.1 g/kg body weight per day).[6]

An example of a core food plan for meeting the nutrient needs of pregnant and lactating women is presented in Table 10-1. When considering the energy requirement for the development of a zygote to a 7.5-lb infant, it is no surprise that energy intake is a critical part of a healthy pregnancy. Likewise, providing that infant with enough nutrition through exclusive breastfeeding to double their birthweight in about 5 months will require a substantial amount of energy and nutrients provided by the mother through her diet and stored body fat.

Fluids. Because milk is a fluid, breastfeeding mothers need ample fluids for adequate milk production; their fluid intake should be approximately 3 L/day. Water and other sources of fluid such as juices, milk, and soup contribute to the fluid that is necessary to produce milk. Beverages that contain alcohol and caffeine should be avoided, because these substances pass into the breast milk.

Lifestyle

In addition to the increase in overall diet and fluid intake, breastfeeding mothers require rest, moderate exercise, and relaxation. Because the production and let-down reflexes of lactation are hormonally controlled, negative environmental and psychologic factors may contribute to the early cessation of breastfeeding.[71] Such factors are called *prolactin inhibitors,* and they include stress, fatigue, medical complications, lack of support, poor self-efficacy, and irregular breastfeeding. A lactation specialist can help by counseling mothers about their new family situations and by helping them to develop a plan to meet their personal needs.

LONG-TERM IMPACTS OF FEEDING METHODS

Risks of Using Breast Milk Substitutes

Medical professionals agree that breastfeeding is the normal means by which an infant should be fed and that other feeding methods carry risks for the infant. For decades, the literature has presented many "benefits of breastfeeding." However, many researchers believe that it is more useful to present the *risks of formula feeding* as opposed to the benefits of feeding in a normal manner.[72] Another way to look at it is to assume that the many "benefits of breastfeeding" are only the normal expectations of infant feeding; therefore, infants who are receiving other forms of breast milk substitutes are suffering a loss.

Advantages of Breastfeeding

Many physiologic and practical advantages of breastfeeding are gained by both the mother and the infant. Several such benefits are listed in Box 10-3.

The antibodies in human milk that are passed to the nursing infant make a significant contribution to the infant's immune system. This accounts for the reduced risk of many diseases and infections. In addition, research indicates that breastfed infants are cognitively advanced compared with formula-fed infants, despite differences in environments, with a positive relationship seen between the duration of breastfeeding and the intelligence quotient of the child.[73] In a recent publication on the long-term advantages of breastfeeding, the World Health Organization concluded that "there is strong evidence of a causal effect of breastfeeding on IQ".[74]

The mother receives many health benefits as well. Some noted advantages of breastfeeding for the

---

lactation specialist health care professionals with specialized knowledge and clinical expertise in breastfeeding and human lactation. Also known as a lactation consultant.

Box 10-3	Benefits of Breastfeeding Compared with Using Breast Milk Substitutes (i.e., Formula)

BENEFITS FOR INFANTS	BENEFITS FOR MOTHERS
• Optimal nutrition for infant • Strong bonding with mother • Safe, fresh milk • Enhanced immune system • Reduced risk for acute otitis media, nonspecific gastroenteritis, severe lower respiratory tract infections, and asthma • Protection against allergies and intolerances • Promotion of the correct development of the jaw and teeth • Association with higher intelligence quotient and school performance through adolescence as a function of parental skill • Reduced risk for sudden infant death syndrome • Reduced risk for chronic diseases such as obesity, type 1 and 2 diabetes, heart disease, and childhood leukemia • Reduced risk for infant morbidity and mortality	• Strong bonding with infant • Increased energy expenditure, which may lead to faster return to prepregnancy weight • Faster shrinking of the uterus • Reduced postpartum bleeding • Delayed return of the menstrual cycle • Decreased risk for chronic diseases such as type 2 diabetes and breast and ovarian cancer • Improved bone density and decreased risk for hip fracture • Decreased risk for postpartum depression; enhanced self-esteem in the maternal role • Time saved by not having to purchase, prepare, and mix formula • Money saved by not buying formula and from not having to pay the increased medical expenses associated with formula feeding

From James DC, Lessen R. Position of the American Dietetic Association: promoting and supporting breastfeeding. *J Am Diet Assoc*. 2009;109(11):1926-1942.

mother are decreased bleeding; an earlier return to prepregnancy weight; and decreased risks of breast cancer, ovarian cancer, and osteoporosis.[75]

ADDITIONAL RESOURCES

The Academy of Nutrition and Dietetics and the American Academy of Pediatrics encourage and strongly support breastfeeding for all able mothers for the first 12 months of life and continued thereafter for as long as mutually desired.[75,76] The American Academy of Pediatrics keeps updated breastfeeding information available for the public at www.healthychildren.org.

The World Health Organization has written and posted an entire chapter entitled "Infant and Young Child Feeding" for medical students and allied health professionals that is freely available online at whqlibdoc.who.int/publications/2009/9789241597494_eng.pdf. A multitude of additional resources about this topic are available from the World Health Organization at www.who.int/topics/breastfeeding/en/.

Putting It All Together

Summary

- Pregnancy involves the fundamental interaction of the following three distinct yet unified biologic entities: the mother, the placenta, and the fetus. Maternal needs also reflect the increasing nutritional needs of the placenta and the fetus.
- Optimal weight gain during pregnancy varies with the normal nutritional status and weight of the woman, with a goal of 25 to 35 lb for a woman of normal prepregnancy weight. Sufficient weight gain is important during pregnancy to support the rapid growth that is taking place. However, the nutritional quality of the diet is as significant as the quantity of weight gain.
- Common problems during pregnancy include nausea and vomiting associated with hormonal adaptations and, later, constipation, hemorrhoids, or heartburn that result from the pressure of the enlarging uterus. These problems are usually relieved without medication by simple and often temporary changes in the diet.

- Unusual or irregular eating habits, age, parity, inadequate weight gain, and low socioeconomic status are among the many related conditions that put pregnant women at risk for complications.
- The ultimate goal of prenatal care is a healthy infant and a healthy mother who can breastfeed her child if she chooses to do so. Breast milk provides essential nutrients in quantities that are uniquely suited for optimal infant growth and development.

Chapter Review Questions

See answers in Appendix A.

1. Complete protein sources that can help meet increased nutrient needs during pregnancy are:
   a. Cow's milk and soy milk.
   b. Baked beans and green beans.
   c. Orange juice and grapefruit juice.
   d. Whole-grain cereal and whole-grain bread.

2. An increase of 340 kcal/day is recommended during pregnancy during the:
   a. Second trimester.
   b. Third trimester.
   c. First and second trimesters.
   d. Second and third trimesters.

3. It is important to counsel women of childbearing age to consume adequate amounts of folic acid to reduce the risk of:
   a. Developing type 2 diabetes mellitus.
   b. Developing hyperemesis gravidarum.
   c. Malformation of the neural tube during the gestation period.
   d. Poor absorption of calcium and phosphorus during fetal bone growth.

4. Benefits of breastfeeding include:
   a. More flexibility in the mother's schedule.
   b. Enhanced immune system in the infant.
   c. Reduced risk of iron deficiency in the infant.
   d. Decreased energy needs for the mother.

5. Gestational diabetes is more common in women who have:
   a. Anemia.
   b. Hyperemesis.
   c. Obesity.
   d. Hypertension.

Additional Learning Resources

evolve http://evolve.elsevier.com/Williams/basic/

References and **Further Reading and Resources** in the back of the book provide additional resources for enhancing knowledge.

11 Nutrition during Infancy, Childhood, and Adolescence

Key Concepts

- The normal growth of individual children varies within a relatively wide range of measures.
- Human growth and development require both nutritional and psychosocial support.

- A variety of food patterns and habits supply the energy and nutrient requirements of normal growth and development, although basic nutritional needs change with each growth period.

In any culture, food nurtures both the physical and the emotional process of "growing up" for each infant, child, and adolescent. Food and eating during these significant years of childhood do not exist apart from the overall process of psychosocial development and physical growth. The entire process plays a role in creating and shaping the whole person.

This chapter outlines the nutritional needs and food patterns of each age group and briefly discusses some of the more common health problems that have nutrition implications.

GROWTH AND DEVELOPMENT

LIFE CYCLE GROWTH PATTERN

The normal human life cycle follows four general stages of overall growth, with individual variation along the way. The nutrition needs of an individual will depend more on the person's **biologic age** than his or her **chronologic age.** For example, if two infants were born yesterday and one infant was 6 weeks premature and the other infant was born at full term, they will both be 1 day old but will have different nutritional needs relative to their physiologic development (i.e., their biologic age). The differences in nutrition needs, based on biologic age, are most important during key growth periods of life. Most notably, this is during infancy and the growth spurts surrounding puberty.

Infancy

Growth is rapid during the first year of life, with the rate tapering off somewhat during the latter half of the year. Most infants more than double their birth weight

by the time they are 6 months old, and they triple it by the time they reach about 12 to 15 months of age. Growth in length is not quite as rapid, but infants generally increase their birth length by 50% during the first year and double it by 4 years of age.

Childhood

Between infancy and adolescence, the childhood growth rate slows and becomes irregular. Growth occurs in small spurts during which children have increased appetites and eat accordingly. Appetites usually taper off during periodic plateaus. Parents who recognize the ebb and flow of normal growth patterns during the latent period of childhood can relax and enjoy this time. Alternatively, unawareness of or inexperience with this normal flux in growth and appetite can result in stress and battles over food between parents and children.

Adolescence

The onset of puberty begins the second stage of rapid growth, which continues until adult maturity. Levels of growth hormone and sex hormones rise, which brings multiple and often bewildering body changes to young adolescents. During this period, long bones grow quickly, sex characteristics develop, and fat and muscle mass increase significantly.

Adulthood

With physical maturity comes the final phase of a normal life cycle. Physical growth levels off during adulthood and then gradually declines during old age. However, mental and psychosocial development lasts a lifetime.

MEASURING CHILDHOOD GROWTH

Individual Growth Rates

Children grow at widely varying rates. Therefore, the best counsel for parents is that children are individuals. A child's growth is not inadequate because the rate

biologic age age of the body relative to physiologic and maturity developmental standards.
chronologic age amount of time a person has lived.

does not equal that of another child. Growth can be measured in children as it relates to physical development as well as mental, emotional, social, and cultural growth.

Physical Growth Measurement

Growth charts. Growth charts, such as those developed by the World Health Organization (WHO) and the Centers for Disease Control and Prevention (CDC), provide an assessment tool for measuring height, weight, and head circumference growth patterns in infants, children, and adolescents. These charts are based on large numbers of well-nourished children who represent the national population. They are used as guides to follow an individual child's pattern of physical growth in relation to the standard growth curves of healthy children.

The current recommendation is for clinicians to use the WHO growth charts for infants from birth to 2 years old and the CDC growth charts for children who are more than 2 years old.[1] The combined use of the WHO and CDC growth charts allows practitioners to plot the growth patterns for height (or length), weight, and head circumference from birth to the age of 20 years. The body mass index (BMI)-for-age charts for children can be used continuously from 2 years of age into adulthood. Because the BMI during childhood is an indicator of the adult BMI, the risk of obesity can be identified and addressed early.

Growth charts are not used to identify "short" or "tall" children. They are used as a means for the continuous assessment of a child's growth rate. Measurements are plotted as a percentile of the population in terms of a specific **anthropometric measurement.** For example, if a child has a height-for-age at the 70th percentile, then 29% of age-matched and gender-matched children are taller, and 70% are shorter. With adequate nutrition and in the absence of disease, this child should continue to grow on about the 70th percentile curve.

There are specific growth charts for boys and girls. Figure 11-1 demonstrates two examples of the growth charts. The Evolve site for this book includes a full set of the WHO and CDC growth charts, which are also available at www.cdc.gov/growthcharts/who _charts.htm. To assess a child's growth accurately, the following three things are essential: (1) an appropriate growth chart (girl vs. boy, appropriate age group, and WHO vs. CDC); (2) an accurate measurement; and (3) an accurate calculation of the child's age. Small errors in measurement can easily lead to a false alarm

regarding a child's growth pattern. See the Clinical Applications box "Use and Interpretation of Growth Charts" for a step-by-step demonstration of how to accurately use and interpret the standard charts.

Growth charts for children with special health care needs. Specialized growth charts are available for several conditions that affect standard childhood growth. Examples include low or very low birth weight infants, achondroplasia, Down syndrome, fragile X syndrome, Prader-Willi syndrome, sickle cell disease, and spastic quadriplegia. Specialty growth charts are developed by collecting anthropometric data of children with a particular condition and using that information to design a chart reflecting expected growth patterns. Although the amount of data used to create such charts is much less than that used to establish the standard CDC charts, these charts are usually still more appropriate to use for children with special health care needs. For example, children with Down syndrome are generally shorter in stature than age-matched controls. Thus, plotting them on a CDC growth chart will indicate that they are below average in height. On the other hand, by plotting them on a specialized chart for children with Down syndrome, their height will be compared to other age-matched children with the same condition and expected growth pattern. Specialized growth charts are not available for all special health care needs.

Psychosocial Development

Various assessments can be used to measure mental, emotional, social, and cultural growth and development. Food is intimately related to these aspects of psychosocial development as well as to physical growth. The growing child does not learn food attitudes and habits in a vacuum but rather as a part of close personal and social relationships. Such relationships begin very early in life.

NUTRITIONAL REQUIREMENTS FOR GROWTH

Growth requires an ample supply of macronutrients and micronutrients. Food intake must meet the daily demands of life and physical activity, while also providing for additional nutrients to build bones, supply tissues and organs, and increase the blood supply to feed and nourish that growth.

ENERGY NEEDS

The demand for energy as measured in kilocalories per kilogram (kg) of body weight per day (kcal/kg/d) is relatively large throughout infancy and childhood. During the first 3 years of life, children need somewhere between 80 and 120 kcal/kg/d to support rapid growth.[2] Although the exact energy needs of premature infants are highly variable and not well-defined, they are thought to range from 110 to 135 kcal/kg/d.[3,4]

---

anthropometric measurements physical measurements of a person's body. Examples include height, weight, body composition; and head, hip, and waist circumferences.

Birth to 24 months: Girls
Head circumference-for-age
and Weight-for-length percentiles

NAME _____

RECORD # _____

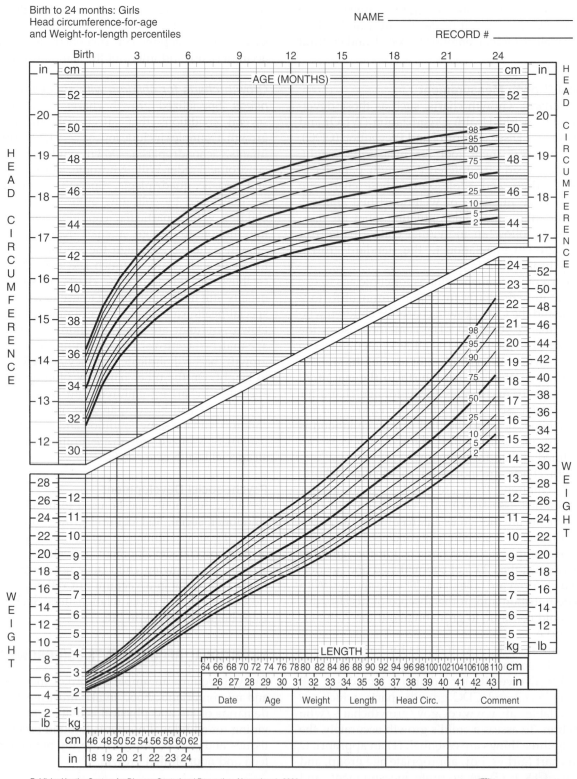

Published by the Centers for Disease Control and Prevention, November 1, 2009
SOURCE: WHO Child Growth Standards (http://www.who.int/childgrowth/en)

A

FIGURE 11-1 Example of a CDC and WHO growth chart. (Courtesy National Center for Health Statistics, National Center for Chronic Disease Prevention and Health Promotion, Hyattsville, Md.)

2 to 20 years: Boys
Body mass index-for-age percentiles

NAME _____

RECORD # _____

Date	Age	Weight	Stature	BMI*	Comments

*To Calculate BMI: Weight (kg) ÷ Stature (cm) ÷ Stature (cm) × 10,000
or Weight (lb) ÷ Stature (in) ÷ Stature (in) × 703

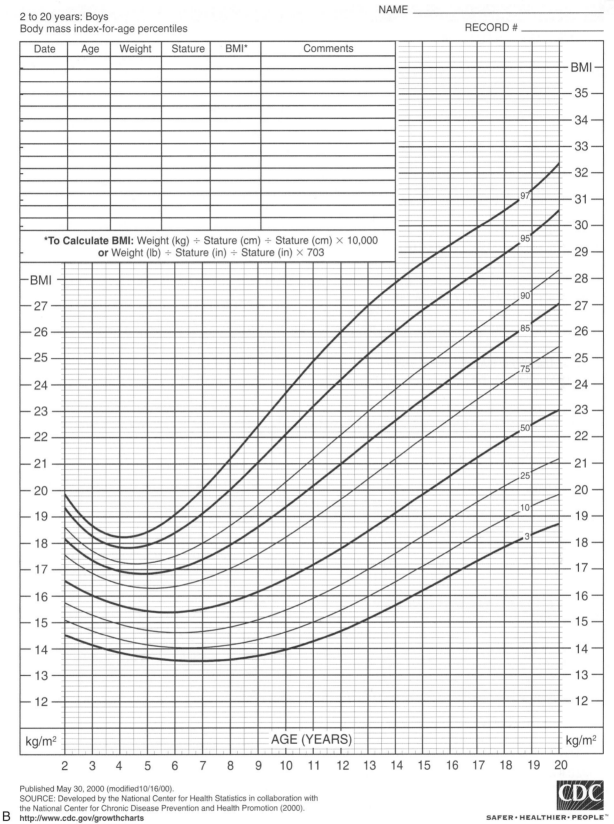

Published May 30, 2000 (modified10/16/00).
SOURCE: Developed by the National Center for Health Statistics in collaboration with
the National Center for Chronic Disease Prevention and Health Promotion (2000).
http://www.cdc.gov/growthcharts

B

CDC
SAFER · HEALTHIER · PEOPLE™

FIGURE 11-1, cont'd

⬧ **Clinical Applications**

Use and Interpretation of Growth Charts

PURPOSE

This guide instructs health care providers how to use and interpret the Centers for Disease Control and Prevention (CDC) and World Health Organization (WHO) growth charts. With the use of these charts, health care providers can assess growth in infants, children, and adolescents and compare it with a nationally representative reference that is based on children of all ages and ethnic groups.

During a routine screening, health care providers assess physical growth by using the child's weight, stature or length, and head circumference. When plotted correctly, a series of measurements offers important information about a child's growth pattern and possible nutrition risks. Contributing factors such as parental stature and the presence of acute or chronic illness should also be considered when making health and nutrition assessments.

STEP 1: OBTAIN ACCURATE WEIGHTS AND MEASURES

When weighing and measuring children, follow procedures that yield accurate measurements, and use equipment that is well maintained.

STEP 2: SELECT THE APPROPRIATE GROWTH CHART

Select the growth chart to use on the basis of the age and gender of the child:
- Use the WHO growth standards to monitor growth for infants and children who are between the ages of birth and 2 years.
- Use the CDC growth charts for children who are 2 years old and older.

STEP 3: RECORD DATA

First, record information about factors obtained at the initial visit that may influence growth.
- Enter the child's name and the record number, if appropriate.
- Enter the mother's and father's statures, as reported.
- Enter the child's gestational age in weeks and date of birth.
- Enter the child's birth weight, length, and head circumference.
- Add any notable comments (e.g., breastfeeding, illnesses, biologic parent anthropometrics unknown).
  Record information obtained during the current visit.
- Enter today's date.
- Enter the child's age.
- Enter the child's weight, stature, and head circumference (if appropriate) immediately after taking the measurement.
- Add any notable comments (e.g., child was not cooperative in getting measurements).

STEP 4: CALCULATE THE BODY MASS INDEX

The body mass index (BMI) is calculated by using weight and stature measurements. The BMI-for-age chart compares a child's weight relative to stature with that of other age- and gender-matched children.
- Determine the BMI with the following calculation:
  BMI = Weight (kg)/Stature (m^2)
  Weight and stature measurements must be converted to the appropriate decimal value.

Example: 37 lb 4 oz = 37.25 lb; 41½ in. = 41.5 in.
Enter the BMI to one place after the decimal point (e.g., 15.204 = 15.2).

STEP 5: PLOT THE MEASUREMENTS

On the appropriate growth chart, plot the measurements recorded in the data entry table for the current visit.
- Find the child's age on the horizontal axis. When plotting weight for length, find the length on the horizontal axis. Use a straight edge or a right-angle ruler to draw a vertical line up from that point.
- Find the appropriate measurement (i.e., weight, length, stature, head circumference, or BMI) on the vertical axis. Use a straight edge or a right-angle ruler to draw a horizontal line across from that point until it intersects the vertical line.
- Make a small dot where the two lines intersect.

STEP 6: INTERPRET THE PLOTTED MEASUREMENTS

- The curved lines on the growth chart show selected percentiles that indicate the rank of the child's measurement. For example, when the dot is plotted on the 95th percentile for BMI-for-age, it means that 5% of age- and gender-matched children in the reference population have a higher BMI and 94% have a lower BMI.
  1. Determine the percentile rank.
  2. Determine if the percentile rank suggests that the anthropometric index is indicative of nutritional risk on the basis of the percentile cutoff value.
     The 2nd and 98th percentile values are the cut-off for indicating nutritional or overall health concern.
     Measurements involving weight (BMI-for-age, weight-for-length/height, and weight-for-age) that are ≥85th and ≤97th percentiles indicate an *at risk status* that should be monitored.
  3. Compare today's percentile rank with the rank from previous visits to identify any major shifts in the child's growth pattern and the need for further assessment.

The WHO recommends using the 2nd and 98th percentiles as cut-off points at which children who fall outside of this range are screened for potential health- or nutrition-related problems. Children and adolescents with a BMI-for-age above the 85th percentile are at risk for being overweight as adults. The 95th percentile on the BMI-for-age charts correlates with a BMI of 30 in adults, which is considered obese. Because the BMI-for-age charts correlate with the adult BMI index, they can be used from childhood into adulthood, thereby providing a lifelong assessment tool that indicates risk factors for chronic disease associated with obesity.

For additional information on the use and interpretation of growth charts, please see: World Health Organization Growth Chart Training; available at: www.cdc.gov/nccdphp/dnpao/growthcharts/who/index.htm.

Source: World Health Organization. Training Course on Child Growth Assessment. Geneva: WHO.2008

To put the enormity of these energy needs into context, adults usually need between 30 and 40 kcal/kg/d.

The Dietary Reference Intake values (see Appendix B) present general recommendations for energy and protein needs at different ages. However, specific individual needs vary with biologic age and condition. The total daily caloric intake of an average 5-year-old child is spent in the following way:

- Basal metabolism: 50%
- Physical activity: 25%
- Tissue growth: 12%
- Fecal loss: 8%
- Thermic effect of food: 5%

However, some children are more physically active than others and have a higher daily caloric expenditure. Likewise, a child who is growing rapidly has higher tissue growth needs and a higher basal metabolism compared with a similar child who is not going through a growth spurt.

Carbohydrates are the preferred energy source of total kilocalories by the body. Carbohydrates also spare protein so that it may be used for the vital task of growth instead of burned as energy. Fat is a backup energy source, and it supplies the essential fatty acids that are necessary for growth.

PROTEIN NEEDS

Protein is the fundamental tissue-building substance of the body. It supplies the essential amino acids for tissue growth and maintenance. As a child gets older and the growth rate slows, the protein requirements per kilogram of body weight gradually decline. For example, for the first 6 months of life, the protein requirements of an infant are 1.52 g/kg; however, the protein needs of a fully grown adult are only 0.8 g/kg.[2] A healthy, active, growing child usually eats enough of a variety of foods to supply the necessary protein and kilocalories for overall growth.

WATER REQUIREMENTS

Water is an essential nutrient that is second only to oxygen for life. Metabolic needs, especially during periods of rapid growth, demand adequate fluid intake. Infants require more water per unit of body weight than adults for the following three important reasons: (1) a greater percentage of the infant's total body weight is composed of water; (2) a larger proportion of the infant's total body water is in the extracellular spaces; and (3) infants have a larger proportional body surface area and metabolic rate compared with adults. In 1 day, an infant generally consumes an amount of water that is equivalent to 10% to 15% of his or her body weight, whereas an adult consumes a daily amount that is equivalent to 2% to 4% of his or her body weight. Table 11-1 provides a summary of the estimated daily fluid needs during the years of growth.

MINERAL AND VITAMIN NEEDS

All minerals and vitamins have important roles in tissue growth and maintenance as well as in overall energy metabolism. Positive childhood growth depends on adequate amounts of all essential substances. Some nutrients of special concern are discussed in the following sections.

Calcium

Calcium needs are critical during the most rapid growth periods of infancy through adolescence. During infancy, the mineralization of the skeleton is taking place while the bones are growing larger and the teeth are forming. Many factors influence bone development in infants and toddlers, including genetics, the maternal nutritional status during pregnancy, preterm birth, the type of infant feeding, the calcium and phosphorus content of breast milk or of a breast milk substitute (i.e., commercial formula), and the diet and physical activity during the toddler and preschool years.[5]

Approximately 40% of adult peak bone mineral density is deposited during the short period of adolescence. The development of good bone density requires an ample dietary supply of calcium, phosphorus, vitamin D, protein, and several other nutrients. In fact, both research and clinical experience indicate that as a preventive measure to reduce the risk for fractures and osteoporosis, appropriate calcium intake and weight-bearing activity must be emphasized during adolescence more so than at any other time throughout the life span.[6,7]

Calcium absorption, calcium deposition in bone, and calcium retention peak just before puberty and coincide with linear bone growth periods. Researchers have found significant differences in calcium retention

Table 11-1   Approximate Daily Fluid Needs during Growth Years

AGE	MALES AND FEMALES (L/day)	AGE	MALES (L/day)	FEMALES (L/day)
Birth to 6 months	0.7	9 to 13 years	2.4	2.1
7 to 12 months	0.8	14 to 18 years	3.3	2.3
1 to 3 years	1.3	>19 years	3.7	2.7
4 to 8 years	1.7			

Data from the Food and Nutrition Board, Institute of Medicine. *Dietary Reference Intakes for water, potassium, sodium, chloride, and sulfate.* Washington, DC: National Academies Press; 2004.

among ethnic groups.[8] The Cultural Considerations box entitled "Racial Differences in Calcium Retention and Peak Bone Mass" discusses this issue further.

Iron

Iron is essential for hemoglobin formation and cognitive development during the early years of life. Infants of mothers with iron-deficiency anemia during gestation are at risk for iron-deficiency anemia at birth. Iron deficiency during this critical time of life is negatively associated with long-term cognitive and behavioral performance in children.[9,10]

The iron content of breast milk is highly absorbable and fully meets the needs of an infant for the first 6 months of life.[11] At that point, the infant's nutrition needs for iron typically exceed that provided exclusively by breast milk, and the addition of solid foods (e.g., enriched cereal, egg yolk, meat) at approximately 6 months of age supplies additional iron. Infants who are not breastfed need an iron-fortified breast milk substitute.

Vitamin Supplements

Much debate has occurred over the years about dietary supplementation of vitamins and minerals for infants and children. The American Academy of Pediatrics recognizes only two vitamins that are potentially needed in supplemental form: vitamins K and D.[12]

Nearly all infants who are born in the United States and Canada receive a one-time prophylactic injection of 1 mg of vitamin K at birth. Vitamin K is critical for blood clotting. A major contributor to the daily supply of vitamin K is provided by bacterial production in the gut. Because infants are born without bacterial flora, their vitamin K synthesis and stores are minimal.

The concern for a high prevalence of vitamin D deficiency, and subsequent low vitamin D levels in breast milk, led to the recommendation that breastfed infants receive oral vitamin D drops (400 IU) beginning at hospital discharge and continuing until the infant is drinking 16 oz of vitamin D–fortified milk, or dairy substitute, daily.[13] Recent studies indicate that mothers supplemented with vitamin D produce breast milk that is adequate to meet the infant's needs; however, more research is necessary to determine if supplementation recommendations should change.[14] Formula-fed infants receive supplemental vitamin D in the breast milk substitute.

Excessive supplementation in infants and children is not unusual, and, as with adults, toxicity is a danger. Excess amounts of vitamins A and D are of special concern in children (see Chapter 7). Excess intake may occur over prolonged periods as a result of carelessness or misunderstanding. Parents should take care to provide only the amount that they are directed to give and no more. Vitamin supplements in the form of gummy bears or other candy-type treat should be kept out of children's reach.

🌐 Cultural Considerations

Racial Differences in Calcium Retention and Peak Bone Mass

As discussed in the Cultural Considerations box in Chapter 8, "Bone Health in Gender and Racial Groups," noted disparities exist among the genders and ethnic groups regarding bone density. African Americans have significantly higher bone mineral density and strength than their Caucasian counterparts throughout life. Two studies involving adolescent girls provided insight into the mechanism behind racial differences in peak bone mass. Bryant and colleagues found that, during the period of peak calcium retention and development of bone mass, African-American girls were able to retain 57% more dietary calcium than Caucasian girls, and they had a higher rate of bone formation.[1] The authors concluded that adult differences in bone mass originate during adolescence, thereby making the dietary intake of calcium-rich foods throughout the teen years a critical component of lifelong bone health.

A follow-up study that compared calcium retention with a range of calcium intake in a similar cohort of subjects obtained similar results. African-American girls retain more calcium at all intake levels than do their Caucasian counterparts; and retention peaks for both ethnic groups just before the onset of puberty.[2] This difference in calcium retention is apparent in conjunction with lower 25(OH)-vitamin D levels, higher 1,25(OH)-vitamin D levels, and higher parathyroid hormone (PTH) levels among African-American girls, all of which influence calcium absorption efficiency.[3,4]

Because adolescence is such a pivotal point for bone health via calcium retention, factors that affect the body's ability to maintain dietary calcium are equally as important. Dietary sodium promotes the loss of calcium through urinary excretion. Wigertz and colleagues were interested in comparing the differences in this effect between adolescent African-American and Caucasian girls. Those authors found that urinary calcium excretion increased along with increased sodium intake among Caucasian girls much more so than among African-American girls.[5] This indicates that high intakes of sodium in Caucasian girls will intensify the loss of calcium and further weaken potential bone mass.

Health care providers should impress upon adolescent girls—especially Caucasian girls—that high calcium intake, limited sodium consumption, and regular weight-bearing physical activity will have long-lasting benefits for their bone health.

REFERENCES

1. Bryant RJ, et al. Racial differences in bone turnover and calcium metabolism in adolescent females. *Clin Endocrinol Metab.* 2003; 88(3):1043-1047.
2. Braun M, et al. Racial differences in skeletal calcium retention in adolescent girls with varied controlled calcium intakes. *Am J Clin Nutr.* 2007;85(6):1657-1663.
3. Weaver CM, et al. Vitamin D status and calcium metabolism in adolescent black and white girls on a range of controlled calcium intakes. *J Clin Endocrinol Metab.* 2008;93(10):3907-3914.
4. Warden SJ, et al. Racial differences in cortical bone and their relationship to biochemical variables in Black and White children in the early stages of puberty. *Osteoporos Int.* 2013;24(6): 1869-1879.
5. Wigertz K, et al. Racial differences in calcium retention in response to dietary salt in adolescent girls. *Am J Clin Nutr.* 2005; 81(4):845-850.

NUTRITION REQUIREMENTS DURING INFANCY

Food is intimately related to each stage of development. Physical growth and personal psychosocial development go hand in hand.

INFANT CLASSIFICATIONS

Infants may be classified according to several different terms depending on their maturity, gestational age, and weight. Nutritional needs of the infant and feeding methods will vary accordingly.

Maturity

Term infants. Full-term infants are born between 37 and 42 weeks' gestation. Mature newborns have finely developed body systems and grow rapidly. Provided with adequate nutrition, they will gain approximately 168 g (6 oz) per week during the first 6 months.

Premature infants. Premature infants are defined as having been born before 37 weeks' gestation. Special care is crucial for tiny premature babies, who are generally categorized further into two groups that are defined by weight or size for gestational age.

Weight Classification

Although both term and preterm infants may be classified as low birth weight, it is more common among premature infants. *Low birth weight* (LBW) infants weigh less than 2500 g (5 lb 8 oz); *very low birth weight* (VLBW) infants weigh less than 1500 g (3 lb 5 oz); *extremely low birth weight* (ELBW) babies weigh less than 100 g (2 lb 3 oz). The lower the birth weight, the higher the risks for complications and poor infant outcome.

Size for Gestational Age Classification

This classification is relative to gestational age; therefore, infants who are born full term or preterm may also be categorized according to their expected size. The categories are as follows:

Appropriate for gestational age (AGA). The infant's weight, length, and head circumference are all within the normal range on a growth chart (i.e., between the 10th and 90th percentiles) relative to the infant's gestational age.

Large for gestational age (LGA). Birth weight is ≥90th percentile for their age and gender, also known as *macrosomia*.

Small for gestational age (SGA). Birth weight is ≤10th percentile for their age and gender. This category is further divided into:
- *Proportionately small for gestational age (pSGA):* birth weight, length, and head circumference are all ≤10th percentile for age and gender.

- *Disproportionately small for gestational age (dSGA):* length and head circumference are of normal size but weight is ≤10th percentile.

CONSIDERATIONS REGARDING FEEDING PREMATURE INFANTS

The feeding process is an important component of the bonding relationship between the parent and the child. In the event that an infant is premature or otherwise has complications surrounding the process of feeding, there are trained health care professionals who can assist parents to bridge the gap for optimal nourishment for the child.

Physiologic Delays Relevant to Feeding

Premature infants are subject to problems with growth and nutrition. Because their bodies are not fully formed, they differ from term infants of normal weight in the following ways: (1) they have more body water, less protein, and fewer mineral stores; (2) there is little subcutaneous fat to maintain body temperature; (3) they have poorly calcified bones; (4) their nerve and muscle development is incomplete, thus making their sucking reflexes weak or absent; (5) they have a limited ability for digestion, absorption, and renal function; and (6) they have immature livers that lack developed metabolic enzyme systems or adequate iron stores. To survive, these tiny babies require special attention to their nutrition and method of feeding.

Milk Content for Premature Infants

The American Academy of Pediatrics recommends the normal feeding of breast milk to premature and other high-risk infants. Infants of mothers who are not able to breastfeed are encouraged to consider using human milk from milk banks.[12] Mothers of preterm infants produce milk that is significantly higher in energy, carbohydrates, protein, and fat to meet the elevated needs of preterm infants.[15] If the energy provided in the breast milk alone is not meeting the energy demands of a preterm infant, **human milk fortifiers** may be used in addition to breast milk to increase the nutrient content.

Methods of Milk Delivery

For most premature infants, nursing or bottle-feeding can be successful with care and support. Infants who have not yet developed the sucking reflex, which is acquired between 32 and 34 weeks' gestation, can still benefit from breast milk, provided that the mother is

---

human milk fortifiers powder or liquid mixed with breast milk to increase the concentration of calories and protein in the milk for premature and low birth weight infants who need more kilocalories than provided in breast milk.

willing and able to pump her breast milk for delivery to the baby by tube or cup feeding.

If the infant cannot tolerate enteral feedings through the gastrointestinal tract then peripheral or central vein feedings are required. Parenteral nutrition is used in special cases to nourish the infant directly through the vascular system, but carries significant risks and thus is avoided if possible.

WHAT, HOW, AND WHEN TO FEED THE MATURE INFANT

Breast Milk

Human milk is the ideal first food for infants, and it is the primary recommendation of pediatricians and dietitians.[12,16] As the infant grows, breast milk adapts in composition to match the needs of the developing child, and the fat content of breast milk changes from the beginning to the end of a single feeding (see Chapter 10).

The newborn's **rooting reflex**, his or her oral needs for sucking, and basic hunger help to facilitate breastfeeding for healthy, relaxed mothers (Figure 11-2). Mothers who are away from their infant for several hours at a time and want to breastfeed their babies can do so by using manual expression or a breast pump while away. The milk can be stored and frozen in

> **rooting reflex** reflex that occurs when an infant's cheek is stroked or touched. The infant will turn toward the stimuli and make sucking (or rooting) motions in an effort to nurse.

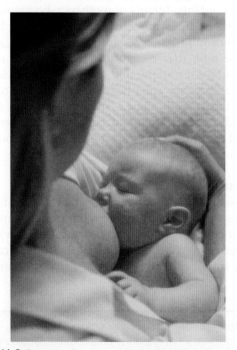

FIGURE 11-2 Breastfeeding the newborn infant. Note that the mother avoids touching the infant's outer cheek so as not to counteract the infant's natural rooting reflex at the touch of the breast. (Copyright JupiterImages Corp.)

sealed plastic baby bottle liners for later use. Breastfeeding mothers can find support and guidance through local groups of the national La Leche League or professional certified lactation counselors. For additional information about successful breastfeeding, see Chapter 10.

Breast Milk Substitute

If a mother chooses not to breastfeed or if some condition in either the mother or the baby prevents it, bottle-feeding of an appropriate breast milk substitute is an acceptable alternative. Research shows that many mothers do not adhere to recommended safety precautions when preparing infant formula, which can increase the risk for infant food-borne illness and scalding.[17,18] The type of commercial infant formula chosen, sterile procedures in formula preparation, and the amount of formula consumed are some aspects that must be addressed to ensure the safety of the child.

Choosing a commercial infant formula. Most mothers who use breast milk substitutes use a standard commercial formula. In some cases of milk allergy or intolerance, a soy-based formula (not soy milk) is used. For infants who are allergic to cow's milk and soy-based formulas, amino acid–based formulas may be medically advised. Examples include Nutramigen (Mead Johnson Nutrition, Evansville, Ind), EleCare (Abbott Nutrition, Columbus, Ohio), and Neocate (Nutricia North America, Gaithersburg, Md). Table 11-2 compares the nutrient composition of breast milk with those of standard and specialty formulas.

Preparing the formula. With any commercial formula, the manufacturer's instructions for mixing concentrated or powdered formula with water should be precisely and consistently followed, and the formula should be refrigerated until use. Throughout the process, scrupulous cleanliness and accurate dilution are essential to prevent infection and illness. A ready-to-feed formula only requires a sterile nipple and bypasses many problems, but it is substantially more expensive. Bottles should be heated in a bowl of warm water (not in a microwave) to prevent uneven heating and scalding the infant's mouth.

Feeding the formula. Babies usually drink formula either cold or warm; they primarily want it to be consistent. Tilting the bottle to keep the nipple full of milk can prevent air swallowing, and the baby's head should be slightly elevated during feeding to facilitate the passage of milk into the stomach. Caregivers should be encouraged to never prop the bottle or leave the baby alone to feed, especially as a pacifier at sleep time. This practice deprives the infant of the cuddling that is a vital part of nurturing, and it also allows milk to pool in the mouth, which can cause choking, earache,

Table 11-2 Nutritional Values of Human Milk and Breast Milk Substitutes

NUTRITIONAL COMPONENT PER LITER	HUMAN MILK, MATURE	STANDARD FORMULAS* ENFAMIL, WITH IRON, READY TO FEED	SPECIAL FORMULAS FOR INFANTS WHO ARE NOT BREASTFED OR WHO CANNOT TOLERATE STANDARD FORMULAS	
			NUTRAMIGEN (CASEIN HYDROLYSATE AND FREE AMINO ACIDS)	PURAMINO (FREE AMINO ACIDS)
Kilocalories	729	649	687	676
Protein (g)	10.7	14.2	19.05	18.9
Fat (g)	45.6	36	36.4	35.8
Carbohydrate (g)	71.7	74	70.9	71.7
Calcium (mg)	333	526	645	635
Phosphorus (mg)	146	361	437	351
Sodium (mg)	177	186	323	318
Potassium (mg)	533	732	750	743
Iron (mg)	0.31	12[†]	12.28[†]	12.17[†]

*Most standard formulas are very similar. This represents an average of Enfamil (Mead Johnson Nutrition, Evansville, Ind).
[†]With added iron.

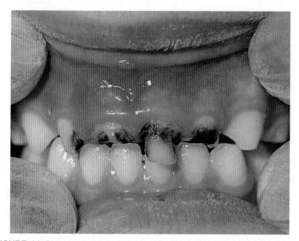

FIGURE 11-3 Baby bottle tooth decay. (From Swartz MH. *Textbook of physical diagnosis, history, and examination*. 5th ed. Philadelphia: Saunders; 2006.)

or **baby bottle tooth decay**. Children should never be put to sleep with a bottle of milk or fruit juice or any other caloric liquid that is capable of pooling in the mouth. Natural bacteria found in the mouth feed on carbohydrates, thereby producing enamel-damaging acid. Baby bottle tooth decay (Figure 11-3) is a serious and completely avoidable problem that results from this practice.

Cleaning bottles and nipples. Whether preparing a single bottle for each feeding or an entire day's batch, scrub, rinse, and sterilize all equipment with the use of the *terminal sterilization method*. Rinse bottles and nipples after each feeding with special bottle and nipple brushes that force water through nipple holes to prevent formula from crusting in them.

Weaning

Throughout the feeding process, observant parents quickly learn to recognize their baby's signs of hunger and satiety and to follow the baby's lead. Babies are individuals who set their own particular needs according to age, activity level, growth rate, and metabolic efficiency. A newborn has a very small stomach that holds only 1 to 2 fluid ounces (fl oz), but he or she will gradually take in more as his or her stomach capacity enlarges relative to overall body growth. The amounts of increased intake during the first 6 months vary and reflect growth patterns. By 6 to 9 months of age, as increasing amounts of other foods are introduced, **weaning** from bottle-feeding takes place. For some children, growing physical capacities and the desire for independence lead to self-weaning, but many children need a little added encouragement from their parents.

Cow's Milk

An infant should never be fed cow's milk during the first year of life. Unmodified cow's milk is not suitable for infants; it provides too heavy a load of solutes for the infant's gastrointestinal tract and renal system. Infants can drink cow's milk after 1 year of age. However, children between the ages of 1 and 2 years

baby bottle tooth decay the decay of the baby teeth as a result of inappropriate feeding practices such as putting an infant to bed with a bottle; also called *nursing bottle caries, bottle mouth,* and *bottle caries.*
weaning the process of gradually acclimating a young child to food other than the mother's milk or a breast milk substitute as the child's natural need to suckle wanes.

old should not be fed reduced-fat cow's milk (e.g., skim or low-fat milk), because insufficient energy is provided and because linoleic acid, which is the essential fatty acid for growth that is found in the fat portion of the milk, is lacking.

Solid Food Additions

When to introduce. Iron-fortified solid foods should be added to the infant's basic diet of breast milk (or breast milk substitute) at approximately 6 months of age. Age is one of the basic indicators of readiness for solid foods. However, each infant will develop motor skills at his or her own rate. The American Academy of Pediatrics note that other signs of readiness to begin solid foods include the following:

- Can the infant hold his or her head up? Infants should have good head control before solids are introduced.
- Does the infant open his or her mouth in anticipation of food coming his or her way? Infants ready for solid foods will show signs such as reaching for the food and eagerness to be fed.
- Can the infant move the food from the spoon to his or her throat to swallow? The infant should have controlled movement of the tongue. The ability to swallow solids is a reflex that will develop when the infant is capable of this task. If the infant pushes food out of his or her mouth when served, then he or she may not be ready for solids.
- Is the infant large enough? Generally, infants should have doubled their birth weight before being offered any solid foods.

The most effective prevention regimen against allergic disease is to provide breast milk and to avoid all solid foods and cow's milk for a minimum of 17 weeks after birth.[19] Thereafter, one new food every 3 to 5 days, as the infant tolerates, may be introduced.[20] It is equally important that parents and other caregivers are able to understand feeding cues from the infant (e.g., hunger, satiety) for a mutually pleasant experience.

What to introduce. When solid foods are started, no specific sequence of food additions must be followed. Some organizations promote the introduction of vegetables or even meat before fruits or grains. The root of this recommendation lies in the following two theories: (1) fruits are sweeter than vegetables, and infants may develop a preference for a sweet taste first and then not like the more bitter taste of vegetables (although this theory lacks strong support); and (2) infants who were given meat before cereal had better zinc intake.

Table 11-3 provides a general schedule for the introduction of solid foods, but individual needs and responses vary, and the suggestions of individual practitioners should be the guide for a specific child. Introduce foods one at a time (starting with iron-fortified cereal) and in small amounts so that if an

Table 11-3	Guideline for Adding Solid Foods to an Infant's Diet during the First Year
WHEN TO ADD	**FOODS ADDED***
6 months	Iron-fortified infant cereal made from rice, barley, or oats (these are offered one at a time) Pureed baby food (vegetables or strained fruit)
8 months	Whole-milk yogurt Pureed baby food (meats)
8 to 10 months	Introduce more grain products one at a time, including wheat, various crackers and breads, pasta, and cereal Add more vegetables and fruits in various textures (e.g., chopped, mashed, cooked, raw) Egg yolks, beans, and additional types of pureed meats Cottage cheese and hard cheeses (e.g., cheddar, Colby-Jack)
10 to 12 months	Infants should be able to tolerate a large variety of grain products and textures Chopped fruits and vegetables Finger foods
12 months	Whole eggs Whole milk

*Semisolid foods should be given immediately before milk feeding. First, 1 or 2 tsp should be given. If the food is accepted and tolerated well, then the amount should be increased 1 to 2 Tbsp per feeding.

adverse reaction occurs the offending food can be easily identified. The highly allergenic foods (e.g., peanuts, tree nuts, cow's milk) can be given as complementary foods once a few traditional first foods (e.g., rice and oat cereal) have been tolerated. Highly allergenic foods should first be given at home rather than at a day care center or a restaurant.[20]

Commercial or homemade complementary foods. Some parents prefer to prepare their own baby food. Baby food can be prepared at home by cooking and straining vegetables and fruits, freezing a batch at a time in ice cube trays, and then storing the cubes in plastic bags in the freezer. A single cube can later be reheated for feeding. Good food-safety practices should always be used. A variety of commercial baby foods are also available and are now prepared without added sugar or unnecessary seasonings.

Throughout the early feeding period, whatever plan is followed, there are a few basic principles that should guide the feeding process: (1) necessary nutrients—not any specific food or sequence—are needed; (2) food is a basis for learning; and (3) normal physical development guides an infant's feeding behavior (see the For Further Focus box, "How Infants Learn to Eat"). Good food habits begin early during life and continue as the child grows. By 8 or 9 months of age, infants should

How Infants Learn to Eat

Guided by reflexes and the gradual development of muscle control during their first year of life, infants learn many things about living in their particular environments. A basic need is food, which infants obtain through a normal developmental sequence of feeding behaviors during the process of learning to eat.

1 TO 3 MONTHS

Rooting, sucking, and swallowing reflexes are present at birth in term infants, along with the tonic neck reflex. Infants secure their first food, milk, with a suckling pattern in which the tongue is projected during a swallow. In the beginning, head control is poor, but it develops by the third month of life.

4 TO 6 MONTHS

The early rooting and biting reflex fades. Infants now change from a suckling pattern with a protruded tongue to a mature and stronger suck with liquids, and a munching pattern begins. Infants are now able to grasp objects with a palmar grip, bring them to the mouth, and bite them.

7 TO 9 MONTHS

The gag reflex weakens as infants begin chewing solid foods. They develop a normal controlled gag along with control of the choking reflex. A mature munching increases their intake of solid foods while chewing with a rotary motion. These infants can sit alone, secure items, release and resecure them, and hold a bottle alone. They begin to develop a pincer grasp to pick up small items between the thumb and forefinger and put the items into the mouth.

10 TO 12 MONTHS

Older infants can now reach for a spoon. They bite nipples, spoons, and crunchy foods; they can grasp a bottle or food and bring it to the mouth; and, with assistance, they can drink from a cup. These infants have tongue control to lick food morsels off of the lower lip, and they can finger-feed themselves with a refined pincer grasp. These normal developmental behaviors are the basis for the progressive pattern of introducing semisolid and table foods to older infants.

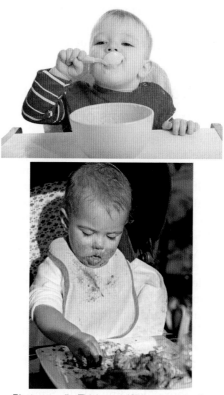

Photos credit: Thinkstock/Collection: Istock.

be able to eat soft table foods (i.e., cooked, chopped, and simply seasoned foods) without requiring special infant foods.

Summary Guidelines

The guidelines for infant feeding are as follows:

- *Breastfeeding* should be continued for at least the first full year of life, and it should be supplemented with a vitamin K shot at birth and daily vitamin D drops.
- *Iron-fortified formula* should be used for any infant who is not breastfeeding.
- *Water and juice* are unnecessary for breastfed infants during the first 6 months of life.
- *Solid foods* may be introduced at approximately 6 months of age, after the **extrusion reflex** of early infancy disappears and the ability to swallow solid food is established.
- *Whole cow's milk,* or milk substitute, may be introduced at the end of the first year (if the infant is consuming one third of his or her kilocalories as a balanced mixture of solid foods, including cereals, vegetables, fruits, and other foods). Reduced-fat or fat-free cow's milk is not recommended until after the age of 2 years.
- **Allergens** such as wheat, egg white, citrus juice, and nuts should not be given as the first solid foods but should be introduced soon after traditional solid foods are tolerated. See Chapter 18 for more information about food allergies and intolerances.
- *Honey* should not be given to an infant who is younger than 1 year old, because botulism spores have been reported in honey, and the immune system capacity of the young infant cannot resist this infection.
- *Foods with a high risk for choking and aspiration* such as hot dogs, nuts, grapes, carrots, popcorn, cherries, peanut butter, and round candy are best delayed for

extrusion reflex the normal infant reflex to protrude the tongue outward when it is touched.

allergens food proteins that elicit an immune system response or an allergic reaction; symptoms may include itching, swelling, hives, diarrhea, and difficulty breathing as well as anaphylaxis in the worst cases.

careful use only with the older child and not given to an infant.

- Beginning at age 6 months, fluoride supplementation should be provided to infants residing in communities where the fluoride concentration in the water is ≤0.3 ppm.[21]

Throughout the first year of life, the requirements for physical growth and psychosocial development are met by breast milk or a breast milk substitute, a variety of solid food additions, and a loving and trusting relationship between the parents or caregivers and the child.

NUTRITION REQUIREMENTS DURING CHILDHOOD

TODDLERS (1 TO 3 YEARS OLD)

When children learn to walk at approximately 1 year of age, these toddlers are off and running, exploring everything and learning new skills. This dawning sense of self, which is a fundamental foundation for ultimate maturity, carries over into many areas, including that of food and eating. After parents become accustomed to the rapid growth and resulting appetite of the first year of life, they may be concerned when they see their toddler eating less food and at times having little appetite while being easily distracted from food to another activity. Increasing the variety of foods available helps children to develop good food habits. The food preferences of young children grow directly from the frequency of a food's use in pleasant surroundings and the increased opportunity to become familiar with a number of foods (see the Clinical Applications box, "Feeding Made Simple"). Sweets should be reserved for special occasions and not used habitually or as bribes.

Energy and protein needs are still high (per kilogram of body weight) compared with adult needs. Toddlers have a wide range of energy needs during this time, and these are related to their velocity of growth and level of physical activity. Muscle mass, bone structure, and other body tissues continue to grow rapidly and require an adequate dietary supply of protein, minerals, and vitamins. The Food and Nutrition Board recommends a daily intake of 19 g of fiber to prevent constipation and to promote a healthy gastrointestinal tract.[2]

PRESCHOOL-AGED CHILDREN (3 TO 5 YEARS OLD)

Physical growth and appetite continue in spurts during this period. Mental capacities develop, and the expanding environment is gradually explored. Children continue to form patterns, attitudes, and basic eating habits as a result of social and emotional experiences involving food. **Food jags** are not uncommon in this age group. A jag may last a few days or weeks but they are usually self-limiting and of no major long-term concern. Again, the key to happy and healthy eating is food variety, appropriately sized portions, and a big dose of parental patience.

Group eating becomes a significant means of socialization. For example, during preschool, food preferences trend toward what the group is eating. In such situations, a child learns a variety of food habits and establishes new relationships with food and with their meal-time companions. A solid foundation of healthy eating habits developed during this time with the supervision and encouragement from caregivers will set the stage for eating behaviors throughout childhood. Likewise, unhealthy habits established during this time will be long-lived.

The U.S. Department of Agriculture published a child-friendly version of MyPlate, with dietary and physical activity recommendations and messages designed to appeal to young children (Figure 11-4). The USDA Food and Nutrition Information Center's "Lifecycle Nutrition" page has resources for educators, families, parents, and kids as well as much more information about improving the overall nutritional health of children (fnic.nal.usda.gov, go to "Lifecycle Nutrition").

SCHOOL-AGED CHILDREN (5 TO 12 YEARS OLD)

The generally slow and irregular growth rate continues during the early school years, and it is accompanied by overall body changes. During the year or two before adolescence reserves are being laid for the rapid growth period ahead. This is the last lull before the storm of growth. By this time, body types are established, and growth rates vary widely. Girls' development usually bypasses that of boys during the latter part of this stage. With the stimulus of school and a variety of learning activities, children experience increasing mental and social maturity; they develop the ability to problem-solve and participate in competitive activities; and they discover a growing sense of autonomy.

Parental food habits continue to have the most influence on a child's eating behavior[22]; however, the process of moving toward independence during this influential stage of life introduces other stimuli that impact food choices. One such persuasive factor is the amount and type of **screen time** to which children are exposed. High-risk television behaviors, in particular, are correlated to long-term negative effects on food habits and risk for obesity.[23-25] Product marketing for foods with low nutritional value is commonplace in television advertisements. One study concluded that

---

food jag brief sprees or binges of eating one particular food.

screen time time spent in front of any electronic screen—television, computer, smart phone, DVD players, portable gaming devices, etc.

Clinical Applications

Feeding Made Simple

BIRTH TO 2 YEARS OLD

A study of parental adherence to infant and toddler feeding recommendations—the Feeding Infant and Toddlers Study (FITS)—found that the early introduction of solid foods, cow's milk, and juices persists despite recommendations from the American Academy of Pediatrics to delay the introduction of such foods until infants are developmentally ready (approximately 6 months of age for solid foods and juices and 1 year of age for cow's milk). The FITS study also found the following inappropriate infant feeding patterns: high-calorie foods with low nutrient densities (e.g., candy, soda, dessert) are being consumed by children younger than 1 year old, infants are being fed grains other than iron-rich infant cereals, and up to 30% of children are not eating vegetables.[1,2] Although the results of the most recent FITS study showed marked improvements over previous data, parents should be reminded that nutrient needs of children this young do not allow for empty calories in the diet.

2 TO 5 YEARS OLD

Some parents spend a lot of time coaxing, begging, and even threatening their 2- to 5-year-old children to eat more than two peas at dinnertime. You can help save parents' time, tears, and energy by helping them to develop child-feeding strategies that are based on the normal developmental needs of their children. Some gentle reminders for parents include the following:

- Children are not growing as fast as they did during the first year of life. Consequently, they need less food.
- Children's energy needs are irregular. Note their activity level, and provide food as needed to help their bodies keep up with the many activities planned for each day.

The following suggestions may make feeding children easier:

- *Offer a variety of foods.* After a taste, put a new food aside if it is not taken, and then try it again later to help the child develop broad tastes. Children often need 10 to 20 exposures to a food before accepting it.
- *Serve small portions.* Let children ask for seconds if they are still hungry.
- *Guide children to serve themselves appropriate portions.* Like adults, children's eyes tend to be bigger than their stomachs. Gentle reminders help them pay attention to satiety cues.
- *Avoid overseasoning.* Let a child's tastes develop gradually. If a food is too spicy, no amount of cajoling will make him or her eat it.

- *Do not force foods that the child dislikes.* Individual food dislikes usually do not last long. If the child shuns one food, offer a similar one if it is available at that meal (e.g., offer a fruit if the child rejects a vegetable) so that little chance of nutrient deficiency occurs.
- *Keep quick-fix nutritious foods around for off-hour snacks.* To keep parents from turning into permanent short-order cooks, keep foods such as fresh and dried fruit, 100% fruit or vegetable juice, cheese, peanut butter, whole-grain bread, and crackers available to serve between meals to provide essential nutrients.
- *Respect eating schedules in a nursery school or preschool program.* Because food is not always available in the classroom, young students learn to eat at regular times. They also tend to try foods that they rejected at home, probably because of peer influence or a desire to impress a new authority figure such as a teacher.
- *Be patient.* Remember that, although adults may discuss world events over broccoli, toddlers are just now learning how to pick up food with a fork.

Toddlers may take longer to eat, or they may not even eat at all. Nevertheless, with flexibility, time, patience, and a sense of humor, most parents find that they can get enough nutrients into their children to keep them healthy and happy throughout the preschool years. When presented with nutritious food choices, preschoolers tend to self-regulate their intake to meet energy needs without adult intervention. Children's food preferences are strongly influenced by familial and environmental factors, which can create either a healthy or an unhealthy eating dynamic.[3]

For more information about healthy feeding patterns for children, see the following resources:

- Ellen Satter Institute: www.ellynsatterinstitute.org—see *How to Feed*
- Ogata BN, Hayes D. Position of the Academy of Nutrition and Dietetics: nutrition guidance for healthy children ages 2 to 11 years. *J Acad Nutr Diet.* 2014;114(8):1257-1276.

REFERENCES
1. Siega-Riz AM, et al. Food consumption patterns of infants and toddlers: where are we now? *J Am Diet Assoc.* 2010;110 (12 suppl):S38-S51.
2. Saavedra JM, et al. Lessons from the feeding infants and toddlers study in North America: what children eat, and implications for obesity prevention. *Ann Nutr Metab.* 2013;62(suppl 3):27-36.
3. Scaglioni S, et al. Determinants of children's eating behavior. *Am J Clin Nutr.* 2011;94(6 suppl):2006S-2011S.

every hour spent in front of a television was associated with a decrease in the overall quality of the child's diet (i.e., more junk food and less fruits and vegetables).[25] Although this is a powerful correlation, it is not causative. There are several factors and decisions involved (by both the child and the parent or caregiver) when it comes to what foods are actually consumed. In other words, turning on the TV did not put junk food into the hands of a child; someone had to purchase the food and make it available.

Peer food habits and the school environment are two other examples of important facets that impact childhood eating behaviors. Some children bring their lunch to school whereas others make food purchasing decisions within the provisions available. Each school will provide a variety of healthy food options, but it is ultimately up to the child to decide what and how much to eat, hence the reason that good food habits cultivated during the younger years are so important.

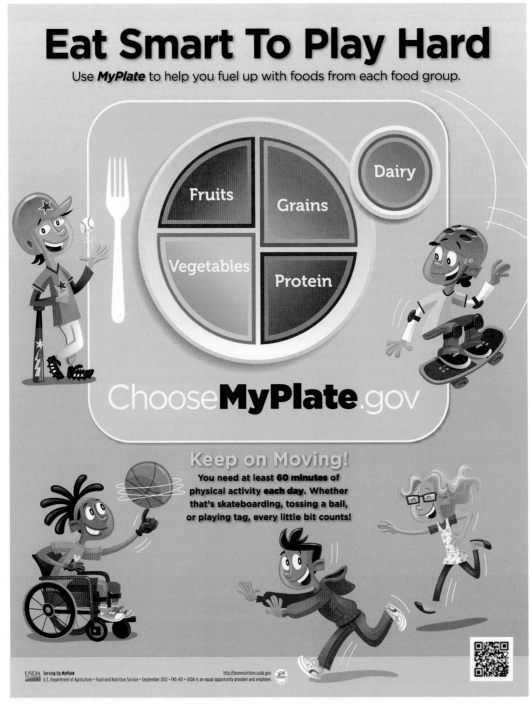

FIGURE 11-4 Eat Smart to Play Hard MyPlate Poster for Kids, which is targeted to meet the needs of children between the ages of 6 and 11 years. (Reprinted from the U.S. Department of Agriculture, Food and Nutrition Service. *Serving up MyPlate.* Washington, DC: U.S. Government Printing Office; 2012. Available at: <www.fns.usda.gov/tn/myplate>.)

For some children the *School Breakfast and Lunch Programs* provide the only nourishing meals of their day. These are federally assisted meal programs that operate in public and nonprofit private schools as well as residential child-care institutions. The meals are provided free or at a low-cost to the students and meet the *U.S. Dietary Guidelines* recommendations for children. The school breakfast and lunch programs and

other community nutrition programs are discussed further in Chapter 13.

NUTRITION PROBLEMS DURING CHILDHOOD

There are several health problems that kids will endure throughout childhood, many of which have nutrition implications (e.g., diarrhea, vomiting, fever). Although these issues are distressing for both children and

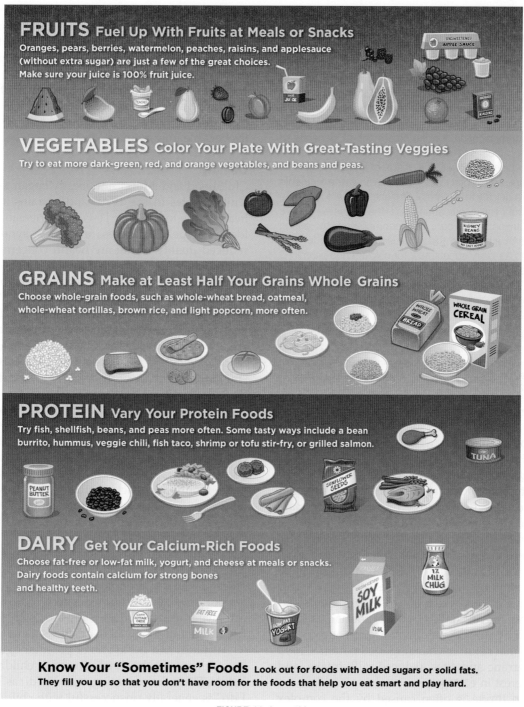

FRUITS Fuel Up With Fruits at Meals or Snacks
Oranges, pears, berries, watermelon, peaches, raisins, and applesauce
(without extra sugar) are just a few of the great choices.
Make sure your juice is 100% fruit juice.

VEGETABLES Color Your Plate With Great-Tasting Veggies
Try to eat more dark-green, red, and orange vegetables, and beans and peas.

GRAINS Make at Least Half Your Grains Whole Grains
Choose whole-grain foods, such as whole-wheat bread, oatmeal,
whole-wheat tortillas, brown rice, and light popcorn, more often.

PROTEIN Vary Your Protein Foods
Try fish, shellfish, beans, and peas more often. Some tasty ways include a bean
burrito, hummus, veggie chili, fish taco, shrimp or tofu stir-fry, or grilled salmon.

DAIRY Get Your Calcium-Rich Foods
Choose fat-free or low-fat milk, yogurt, and cheese at meals or snacks.
Dairy foods contain calcium for strong bones
and healthy teeth.

Know Your "Sometimes" Foods Look out for foods with added sugars or solid fats.
They fill you up so that you don't have room for the foods that help you eat smart and play hard.

FIGURE 11-4, cont'd

caregivers, they usually do not have long-term repercussions. Here we will focus only on the problems that have the potential to have chronic complications.

Failure to Thrive

The term *failure to thrive* has been used in pediatrics to describe infants, children, or adolescents who do not grow and develop normally. Failure to thrive most commonly affects young children between the ages of 1 and 5 years. Careful nutrition assessment is essential for identifying underlying feeding problems. The following factors may be involved:

- *Clinical disease:* central nervous system disorders, endocrine disease, congenital defects, or intestinal obstruction (see the Drug-Nutrient Interaction box, "Anticonvulsants and Nutrient Metabolism")
- *Neuromotor problems:* poor sucking or abnormal muscle tone from the retention of primitive reflexes that should have already faded; eating, chewing, and swallowing problems
- *Dietary practices:* parental misconceptions or inexperience regarding what constitutes a normal diet for infants; inappropriate formula-feeding or

Anticonvulsants and Nutrient Metabolism

KELLI BOI

Epilepsy is a chronic neurologic condition that affects 2 million people in the United States. Children who are younger than 2 years old and adults older than the age of 65 years are most likely to be affected by epilepsy.[1] Carbamazepine (Tegretol) is a widely-used medication for the treatment of generalized tonic-clonic and focal seizures.

Carbamazepine increases the metabolism of vitamin D, calcium, folate, and biotin, which means that the nutrients are used more quickly than normal. Patients who are receiving this drug should make adjustments to their diets to ensure adequate nutrition. This can be accomplished by eating more foods that are rich in these nutrients, including fortified dairy products, or dairy substitutes, for calcium and vitamin D and green leafy vegetables for folate and biotin. For those who require the long-term use of carbamazepine, dietary supplements—especially of calcium and vitamin D—may be necessary.

REFERENCE

1. National Center for Chronic Disease Prevention and Health Promotion. *Targeting Epilepsy: Improving the Lives of People with One of the Nation's Most Common Neurological Conditions: At a Glance 2011.* Atlanta, Ga: Centers for Disease Control and Prevention; 2011.

improper dilutions when mixing breast milk substitutes

- *Unusual nutrient needs or losses:* adequate diet for growth but inadequate nutrient absorption and thus excessive fecal loss; hypermetabolic state that requires increased dietary intake
- *Psychosocial problems:* family environment and relationships that result in emotional deprivation of the child and require medical and nutritional intervention; similar problems also may occur between 2 and 4 years of age when parents and children have conflicts about normal changes caused by slowed childhood growth and energy needs that result in changing food patterns, food jags, erratic appetites, reduced milk intake, and disinterest in eating

Failure to thrive is often caused by the complex interaction of factors, and no easy solutions exist. Vigilant history taking, supportive nutritional guidance, and warm personal care are necessary to influence growth patterns in these infants. The careful and sensitive correction of the social and environmental issues that surround the problem is crucial.

Anemia

The fortification of cereals and breads with iron has considerably reduced the cases of iron-deficiency anemia in the United States. However, anemia remains a concern for children with **food insecurity** and poor diets. Children should begin eating iron-rich foods around 6 months of age. *Milk anemia* is a term that is sometimes used for toddlers (≥1 year old) who excessively consume cow's milk to the exclusion of other iron-rich foods. Although milk is an important source of several nutrients, it is a poor source of iron. Even if these children eat some iron-rich foods, their high calcium intake can inhibit the absorption of iron. Iron-deficiency anemia has been linked to delayed cognitive development in children, and it can have irreversible long-term effects.[26]

Obesity

Childhood and adolescent obesity began to rise in the United States in the 1970s and remains a significant health issue today (Box 11-1). Hypertension, hyperlipidemia, type 2 diabetes, metabolic syndrome, and reduced quality of life are health concerns that have traditionally been associated with older, overweight adults; however, they are increasingly becoming a problem among school-aged children.[27,28] Although there are many issues involved, some factors during gestation and early infancy that increase the risk for childhood obesity include inadequate or excessive gestational weight gain, gestational diabetes, maternal smoking, and the use of breast milk substitutes (i.e., formula-feeding).[29-31]

Both genetics and environment play major roles in the risk for obesity and are likely covariables. Although overweight parents are more likely to have overweight children, there are modifiable risk factors that, if addressed, may reduce the risk for obesity for the entire family. Such factors include poor food selection, restrictive feeding practices that contribute to binging behaviors, and low physical activity. Infants and children are innately capable of recognizing satiety and self-regulating energy balance. However, this inherent awareness seems to decline between the ages of 3 and 5 years, when environmental factors (e.g., inappropriate portion sizes, encouragement to "clean the plate," caregivers using food as a reward) start to influence the amount of food eaten, despite satiety.

Attitudes and behaviors of parental figures are key determinants in the development of childhood eating habits. Thus, the parenting style of "do as I say, not as I do" is generally unsuccessful with children. Parents must lead by example. In addition to the guidelines for feeding children given earlier in the Clinical Applications box entitled "Feeding Made Simple," the following recommendations are helpful for guiding parents toward appropriate eating environments and for helping them to lower the risk of obesity in their children[32]:

food insecurity limited or uncertain availability of nutritionally adequate and safe foods or limited or uncertain ability to acquire acceptable foods in socially acceptable ways.

Box 11-1 Childhood Overweight and Obesity Facts

PREVALENCE OF OBESITY

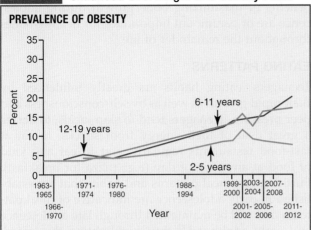

NOTE: Overweight is defined as BMI greater than or equal to sex- and age-specific 95th percentile from the 2000 CDC Growth Charts.
SOURCES: CDC/NCHS, National Health Examination Surveys II (ages 6-11), III (ages 12-17), and National Health and Nutrition Examination Surveys (NHANES) I-III, and NHANES 1999-2000, 2001-2002, 2003-2004, 2005-2006, 2007-2008, and 2011-2012.

Contributing Factors
- Genetics
- Behavioral factors: excessive energy intake, physical inactivity
- Environmental factors: parental role models, child-care atmosphere, and lack of exposure to health, wellness, and nutrition at home and/or school

Consequences
- Health risks: asthma, sleep apnea, cardiovascular disease, liver disease, and type 2 diabetes
- Psychosocial risks: low self-esteem and social discrimination

The Centers for Disease Control and Prevention's website about childhood obesity (www.cdc.gov/obesity/childhood/index.html) has up-to-date information regarding the prevalence, current treatment recommendations, and information about state-based programs to help alleviate the health burden of childhood overweight and obesity.

- Choose specific meal times.
- Provide a wide variety of nutrient-dense foods (e.g., fruits, vegetables) rather than "junk" foods with high energy density and poor nutrient content.
- Offer an age-appropriate portion size.
- Limit nonnutritive snacking and the use of juice or sweetened beverages.
- Encourage children to regulate their own food intake based on intuitive eating principles.
- Have regular family meals to promote social interaction and to role model healthy food-related behavior.
- Limit screen time.
- Make physical activity a daily family affair.

Physical activity is an important part of a healthy lifestyle from birth to death. By developing an appreciation for and an enjoyment of regular physical activity during childhood, the risk for obesity may be reduced along with the health problems associated with it.

Lead Poisoning

Lead poisoning in children can be extremely damaging to the central nervous system, and it can negatively alter both cognitive and motor skills. The CDC estimates that more than 535,000 American children between the ages of 1 and 5 years have high blood lead levels (≥5 mcg/dL)[33] (see the Cultural Considerations box in Chapter 13 titled "The Continued Burden of Lead Poisoning"). The majority of lead exposure among children is the result of lead-based paint. Lead-containing paint chips from deteriorating buildings or renovations result in high levels of lead-contaminated dust. Children explore with their hands and mouths at this age, thereby making the oral intake and inhalation of lead highly likely. Lead-based paint was banned in the United States in 1978; however, many millions of homes still contain lead paint. Children who live below the poverty line and in homes built before 1950 are at the greatest risk.[33] One of the *Healthy People 2020* targets is the complete elimination of lead exposure in children.[34]

NUTRITION REQUIREMENTS DURING ADOLESCENCE (12 TO 18 YEARS OLD)

PHYSICAL GROWTH

Body Composition

The final growth spurt of childhood occurs with the onset of puberty. This rapid growth is evident in increasing body size and the development of sex characteristics in response to hormonal maturation. Because the velocity of growth and onset of puberty can vary greatly among individual boys and girls, biologic age is a better indicator of nutritional needs than chronologic age throughout adolescence.

There are distinct patterns of body composition changes. Girls store more subcutaneous fat in the abdominal area. The pelvis widens in preparation for future childbearing, and the size of the hips also increases, which causes much anxiety for many figure-conscious young girls. In boys, physical growth is seen more in increased muscle mass and long-bone growth. At first a boy's growth spurt is slower than that of a girl, but he soon surpasses her in both weight and height.

Obese children are likely to progress through puberty at an earlier age than normal weight children.[35] Moreover, early sexual maturation increases the risk of adult-onset chronic disease (e.g., metabolic syndrome, cardiovascular disease, some types of cancer).[36,37] Girls who reach sexual maturation early (<12 years old) are more likely to become overweight or obese as adults than girls who do not mature until later.[38] In addition, recent research indicates an association between sexual abuse, interpersonal violence, and bullying with excess body fatness in adolescents.[39] Differences in biologic age, as defined by stage of puberty and body composition, are important when assessing growth on a growth chart (see the Cultural Considerations box, "Growth Charts: Can You Use Them for All Children?").

Bone Mineral Density

Bone mineral density reaches its peak velocity of accumulation during the preadolescent years (≈8 years old) through about age 20.[40] Linear growth reaches its peak at about 16 years of age for females and 21 years of age for males. Adolescents consuming a balanced diet with calcium containing dairy or dairy substitutes achieve higher peak bone mass and linear growth than do their counterparts who do not eat a balanced diet. Even when females on a low dairy and calcium diet are supplemented with calcium, their bone mineral density does not reach the same level as those girls who

naturally have a high calcium diet.[41] The long-term benefits of maximizing bone growth during adolescence are of paramount importance for healthy bones throughout the remainder of life.

EATING PATTERNS

Teenagers' eating habits are greatly influenced by their rapid growth as well as by self-consciousness and peer pressure. Teenagers tend to skip meals, to derive a great deal of their energy from snacks, to eat at fast-food restaurants regularly, and to eat any kind of food at any time of day (e.g., pizza for breakfast). Furthermore, meal patterns and habits that are established in early adolescence are indicative of meal patterns that will be maintained through late adolescence and early adulthood,[42] thus highlighting the importance of establishing well-balanced healthy meals and eating schedules during the childhood and early adolescence years. Unfortunately, some teenagers begin to experiment with alcohol. Even a mild form of alcohol abuse in combination with the elevated nutrition demands of adolescence can easily undermine a teen's nutritional status. Boys usually fare better than girls in general overall nutrition. Their larger appetite and the sheer volume of food consumed usually ensure an adequate intake of nutrients. Alternatively, because they are under a greater social pressure for thinness, girls may tend to restrict their food and have an inadequate nutrient intake.

EATING DISORDERS

Social, family, and personal pressures concerning figure control strongly influence many young girls and an increasing number of young boys. As a result, they sometimes follow unwise self-imposed crash diets for weight loss. In some cases complex eating disorders such as anorexia nervosa and bulimia nervosa may develop. Psychologists have traditionally identified mothers as the main source of family pressure to remain thin. However, fathers may also contribute to the problem if they are emotionally distant and do not provide important feedback to build self-worth and self-esteem in their young children. Parents must help their children to see themselves as loved no matter what they weigh so that these children are not as vulnerable to social influences that equate extreme thinness with beauty.

Eating disorders involve a distorted body image and a morbid and irrational pursuit of thinness. Such disordered eating often begins during the early adolescent years, when many girls see themselves as fat even though their average weight is often below the normal weight for their height. The longer the duration of the illness, the less likely it is that a full recovery will be achieved. Thus, early detection and intervention are critical for restoration of overall health. Warning signs, treatment options, and diagnostic criteria are covered in Chapter 15.

🌐 Cultural Considerations

Growth Charts: Can You Use Them for All Children?

HUMAN MILK OR BREAST MILK SUBSTITUTES

Breastfed infants have a slightly different growth curve than formula-fed infants. Breastfed infants grow slightly more rapidly than formula-fed infants during the first 2 months of life, and then the rate of growth declines to a level that is slower than that of infants receiving breast milk substitutes. The original CDC growth charts were predominantly based on formula-fed infants, which is why it is no longer recommended to use those charts for children under the age of 2 years.

The WHO charts used infants that were exclusively breastfed in accordance with feeding recommendations (i.e., breastfeed for at least 12 months, with solid foods introduced between 4 and 6 months) to obtain the standard growth curves. All infants should be plotted on the WHO growth charts, regardless of feeding method.

GROWTH CHARTS IN RELATION TO VARIATIONS IN SEXUAL MATURATION

With regard to charting the growth patterns of an adolescent, practitioners should be aware of the differences in the timing of sexual maturation and how that relates to overall weight and body fat. Black girls and boys begin the process of sexual maturity before Mexican-American or white children do.[1] Such differences between racial groups are potentially important when assessing growth on a growth chart. More sexually mature children are expected to be taller and heavier than their less mature peers.

USING GROWTH CHARTS FOR VARIOUS RACES

Currently, there are not enough available data to create growth charts that are racial/ethnic-specific. Therefore, the CDC and the WHO promote the use of the standard growth charts for all racial and ethnic groups. Future studies will determine if significant differences exist and warrant the development of charts that are specific to different racial and ethnic backgrounds.

REFERENCE

1. Ramnitz MS, Lodish MB. Racial disparities in pubertal development. *Semin Reprod Med*. 2013;31(5):333-339.

Putting It All Together

Summary

- The growth and development of healthy children depends on optimal nutrition support. In turn, good nutrition depends on many social, psychologic, cultural, and environmental influences that affect individual growth potential throughout the life cycle.
- The nutrition needs of children change with each unique growth period.
- Social and cultural factors influence the developing food habits of all children and these habits often last a lifetime.
- Infants experience rapid growth. Human milk is the natural first food, with solid foods introduced around 6 months of age, when digestive and physiologic processes have matured.
- Toddlers, preschoolers, and school-aged children experience slowed and irregular growth as compared with infancy. During this period, their energy demands are less per kilogram of body weight, but they require a well-balanced diet for continued growth and health.
- Adolescents undergo a large growth spurt during puberty. This rapid growth involves both physical and sexual maturation. A well-balanced diet should supply adequate nutrients to support bone mineralization and tissue growth.
- There are several nutrition-related health concerns that affect children and adolescents, of which obesity is the most common.

Chapter Review Questions

See answers in Appendix A.

1. Which of the following foods would most likely be appropriate for an 8-month-old infant?
   a. Whole milk
   b. Scrambled egg
   c. Chopped apples
   d. Regular yogurt

2. It is not recommended to introduce which of the following foods as the first solid food for an infant?
   a. Infant oat cereal
   b. Egg white
   c. Pureed carrots
   d. Applesauce

3. Appropriate feeding tips to convey to parents of toddlers include:
   a. Season food more than usual so the child will eat.
   b. Offer a variety of foods but do not force the child to eat.
   c. Serve small portions and ensure that the child finishes them.
   d. Do not allow the child to serve themselves small portions.

4. Parents can help school-age children develop healthy eating habits by:
   a. Teaching how to restrict food intake to avoid weight gain.
   b. Leading by example and eating a diet that provides nutrient-dense foods.
   c. Ensuring that children never eat high-fat or energy-dense snack foods.
   d. Encouraging children not to adopt parents' unhealthy eating habits.

5. Teenage girls more often respond to social and peer pressure to restrict food intake and control weight, which can lead to:
   a. Obesity.
   b. Epilepsy.
   c. Disordered eating.
   d. Type 1 diabetes mellitus.

Additional Learning Resources

evolve http://evolve.elsevier.com/Williams/basic/

References and **Further Reading and Resources** in the back of the book provide additional resources for enhancing knowledge.

12

Nutrition for Adults: The Early, Middle, and Later Years

Key Concepts

- Gradual aging throughout the adult years is a unique process that is based on an individual's genetic heritage and life experience.
- Aging is a total life process that involves biologic, nutritional, social, economic, psychologic, and spiritual aspects.

- Nutrition requirements change along with progressive physiologic changes of the body.

The rapid growth and development of adolescence leads to physical maturity as adults. Physical growth in size levels off, but the constant cell growth and regeneration that are necessary to maintain a healthy body continue. Other aspects of growth and development—mental, social, psychologic, and spiritual—continue for a lifetime.

Food and nutrition continue to provide essential support during the adult aging process. Life expectancy is increasing; thus, health promotion and disease prevention are even more important to ensure quality of life throughout these extended years.

This chapter explores the ways in which positive nutrition can help adults to lead healthier, disease-free lives.

ADULTHOOD: CONTINUING HUMAN GROWTH AND DEVELOPMENT

COMING OF AGE IN AMERICA

Americans are experiencing tremendous change in the composition of the population. The report from the U.S. Department of Health and Human Services entitled *Healthy People 2020* presents national goals for helping all people to make informed decisions about their health. One of the primary goals set for 2020 is to attain high-quality, longer lives that are free of preventable disease, disability, injury, and premature death.[1] Achieving this goal requires proper nutrition, among other healthy lifestyle habits.

Population and Age Distribution

The U.S. Census Bureau predicts that the U.S. population will increase by 30% from 2015 to 2060 to a total of 416 million people.[2] Older segments of the population will grow significantly during this period. The number of people who are older than 65 years old will double, for a record high of 23% of the total

population.[3] The median age will increase from 36 years old to 42 years old by 2060. Figure 12-1 shows population growth and projections from 1900 to 2060 for older adults. Growth rates for various ethnic subgroups continue to rise as well (see the Cultural Considerations box, "The Aging Composition of the U.S. Population"). A changing age distribution in the population results in changes in the health care system as well as job demands in geriatric health care. Healthy nutrition and lifestyle factors adopted early in life help ensure these years are spent in a disease-free state.

Life Expectancy and Quality of Life

Life expectancy has dramatically increased during the past century, from only 47 years in 1900 to a projected average of 85.6 years in 2060 (84 years for men and 87.1 for women).[4] However, there are notable differences in life expectancy among various population groups and among those with different household incomes.[5] Americans consistently value health-related quality of life, which is one's personal sense of physical and mental health and ability to act within the environment. Quality of life is a major focus of the *Healthy People 2020* initiative.[1]

Impact on Health Care

Career opportunities in the fields of disease prevention and health promotion are at an all-time high. Community and private classes about healthy lifestyles and nutrition target the prime concerns for a growing adult population. Weight management and diabetes management are two of the most popular

> **life expectancy** the number of years that a person of a given age may expect to live; this is affected by environment, lifestyle, gender, and race.

topics. Dietitians, nurses, life coaches, personal trainers, psychologists, and other members of the health care team may be involved at various levels of such programs. A dire need exists for individuals to adopt healthy lifestyles in an effort to safeguard their health. The health care system in America cannot continue to finance the ever increasing expense of disease treatment, particularly when most chronic diseases are preventable.

SHAPING INFLUENCES ON ADULT GROWTH AND DEVELOPMENT

The overall process of human aging has the unique potential for growth and fulfillment at every stage. The periods of adulthood (i.e., the young, middle, and older years) are no exception. Many individual and group events mark the course; however, at each stage, the four basic areas of adult life—physical,

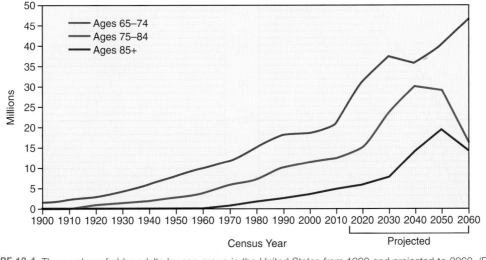

FIGURE 12-1 The number of older adults by age group in the United States from 1900 and projected to 2060. (From U.S. Census Bureau, Population Division: *Projections of the population by sex and age for the United States: 2015 to 2060 (NP2014-T9); release date December 2014.*)

🌐 Cultural Considerations

The Aging Composition of the U.S. Population

Shifting racial and ethnic patterns continue to reshape the American population as a whole, particularly in the older segment of the population. With respect to U.S. adults older than age 65, the non-Hispanic population is expected to increase by about 60% by 2050. Meanwhile, the Hispanic population is expected to increase by a factor of five, from 3.1 million to 15.4 million. It is projected that the aggregate minority population will become the majority population by 2043.[1]

The current life expectancy varies among ethnic groups. For example, Caucasians have a life expectancy of 80 years, whereas African Americans have a life expectancy of 76.1 years.[2] Living arrangements, household income, educational attainment, type of medical insurance, and many other variables fluctuate among ethnic groups, all of which influence life expectancy.

Health care providers should understand and address the cultural and ethnic needs of an elderly individual when providing nutrition education. All areas of social, socioeconomic, and available health care play significant factors when designing the best care plan. Cookie-cutter meal plans for one ethnic group are not particularly useful for another culturally diverse population. Given the rapidly changing ethnic diversity of the

elderly population in the United States, it will be increasingly important to understand and practice cultural sensitivity.

In addition, the growth structure of the population presents specific concerns with regard to health, medical, and financial dependency. Note the horizontal black lines on the figure on the next page: the population between those lines represents the working class. The populations below and above those lines represent individuals who are largely dependent upon the working class for financial support either directly or indirectly via income taxes. In 2012 only 13.7% of the population was older than age 65. By 2030, that percentage will increase to 20.3%.[1] Over this same time frame, the working class population will decrease from 62.8% to 57.3%. Essentially, there will be a smaller percent population of providers to support the increasing percentage of elderly dependents. Healthy aging will be imperative to sustain the health care system.

REFERENCES

1. Ortman JM, Velkoff VA, Hogan H. *An aging nation: the older population in the United States, current population reports, P25-1140.* Washington, DC: U.S. Census Bureau; 2014.
2. U.S. Census Bureau, Population Division. *Projected life expectancy at birth by sex, race, and hispanic origin for the United States: 2015 to 2060.* Washington, DC: U.S. Government Printing Office; 2014.

Continued

Age and Sex Structure of the Population for the United States: 2012, 2030, and 2050

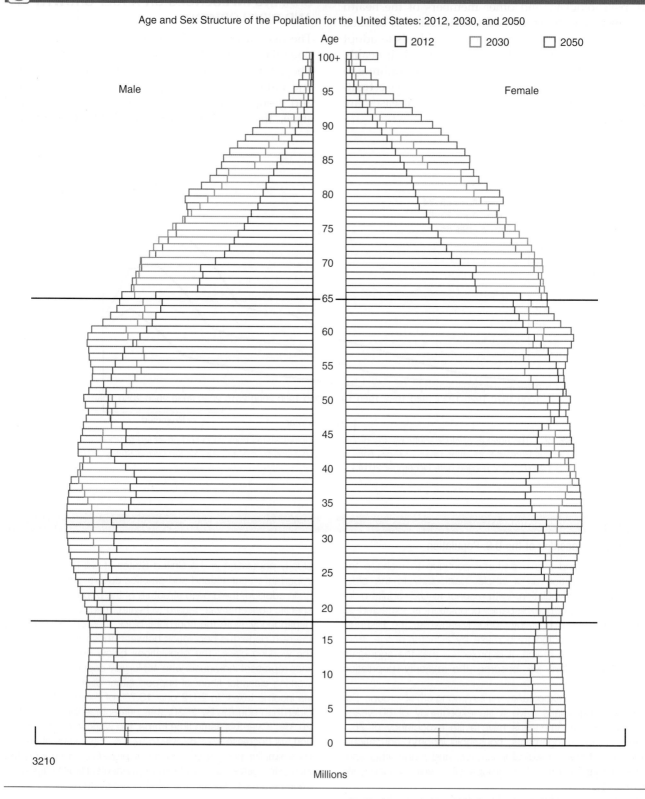

psychosocial, socioeconomic, and nutritional—shape general growth and development.

Physical Growth

The overall physical growth and maturity of the human body, which are governed by the genetic potential, level off during the early adult years. Physical growth is no longer a process of increasing numbers of cells; rather, it involves the vital growth of new cells to replace old ones. After physical maturity is established, energy requirements decrease. Adjustment to a gradually declining metabolic rate and thus the need for fewer kilocalories is important for weight management. At older ages, individual vigor reflects the health status of the preceding years.

Psychosocial Development

Human personality development continues throughout the adult years. Three unique stages of personal psychosocial growth progress through the young, middle, and older years. It should be noted that the exact chronologic age at which an adult enters each stage will vary. For example, the designation of "middle adults" as aged 45 to 64 years old is an estimation. Individuals will progress through each stage at their own rate.

Young adults (20 to 44 years old). With physical maturity, young adults become increasingly independent. They form many new relationships; adopt new roles; and make many choices about continued education, career, jobs, marriage, and family. Young adults often experience considerable stress but also significant personal growth. These are years of developing professionally, establishing a home community, and deciding whether to have children, all of which are part of early personal struggles to make one's way in the world. Sometimes health problems relate to these early stressful periods. The firm establishment of healthy lifestyle behaviors during this period (e.g., engaging in regular exercise, choosing balanced meals that promote and preserve health) is important for maintaining quality of life for the long term.

Middle adults (45 to 64 years old). The middle years often present an opportunity to expand personal growth. In most cases of middle-aged adults who had children, their children have grown and are beginning to make their own lives, and parents may have a sense of "it's my turn now." This also is a time of coming to terms with what life has offered with a refocusing of ideas, life directions, and activities. Early evidence of chronic disease appears in some middle-aged adults. Wellness, health promotion, and the reduction of disease risks continue to be major focuses of health care.

Older adults (65 years old and older). Adults vary widely with regard to their personal and physical resources for dealing with older age. They may have a sense of wholeness and completeness, or they may increasingly withdraw from life. If the outcome of their life experiences is positive, they arrive at an older age rich in the wisdom of their years; they enjoy life and health, and they enrich the lives of those around them. However, some elderly people arrive at these years poorly equipped to deal with the adjustments associated with aging and the health problems that may arise. As this population continues to grow, the subdivisions of young-old (65 to 74 years old), elderly (75 to

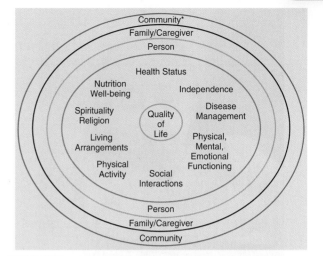

FIGURE 12-2 Factors that influence the quality of life of adults who are 60 years old and older. *The term *community* includes health and supportive services at local, state, and federal levels as well as health professionals and researchers. (Reprinted from Kuczmarski MF, Weddle DO, American Dietetic Association. Position paper of the American Dietetic Association: nutrition across the spectrum of aging. *J Am Diet Assoc.* 2005;105:616-630.)

84 years old), and old-old (85 years old and older) have become a widespread way to characterize individuals as general health and quality of life continue to improve. Many factors that influence perceived and actual quality of life are integrally associated with nutritional status (Figure 12-2).

Socioeconomic Status

All human beings grow up and live their lives in a social and cultural context. The rapidly changing world continues to experience major social and economic shifts. Most adults and their families feel the strain in some way, and these pressures directly influence food security and health. Economic insecurity creates added stress and often leads to the need for food assistance (Figure 12-3). Sometimes social and financial pressures along with a decreasing sense of acceptance and productivity cause elderly people to feel unwanted and unworthy.

Depression is a clinical syndrome that is not part of normal aging, and it is closely related to poor overall health, increased cost of health care, poor financial resources, feelings of loneliness, and mortality.[6-8] The use of antidepressive medications by adults in the United States has increased by fourfold in the past two decades.[9] Elderly patients with declining health are particularly susceptible to depression, which is a common psychiatric condition seen in the elderly population and is a leading cause of **unintentional weight loss**.[10] *Failure to thrive* in the geriatric population, which

unintentional weight loss weight loss of 5% of body weight over a 6- to 12-month period that is not intentional.

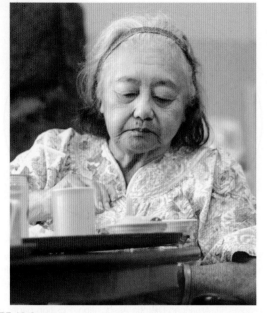

FIGURE 12-3 Elderly woman assisted by the Supplemental Nutrition Assistance Program (SNAP) to obtain needed food. (Copyright JupiterImages Corp.)

is generally multifactorial and caused by a combination of chronic diseases, is associated with impaired physical function, malnutrition, depression, and cognitive impairment.[11] All people need a sense of belonging, achievement, and self-esteem. Unfortunately, many elderly people suffer from loneliness, uncertainty, and depression, all of which increase mortality.

Some basic needs that are common to all people are economic security, adequate nutrition, personal effectiveness, suitable housing, constructive and enjoyable activities, satisfying social relationships, and spiritual freedom. An increasing number of healthy, motivated, young-old adults are continuing to contribute to the workforce; they are redefining what it means to be a senior citizen.

Nutrition Needs

The energy and nutrient needs of individual adults in each age group vary in accordance with living and working situations. The Dietary Reference Intake (DRI) recommendations for healthy adults meet most needs, but the aging process influences individual nutritional requirements. Only in the most recent DRIs have scientists distinguished the nutrient needs of the 50- to 70-year-old adults from those who are ≥71 years old. In previous publications of the DRIs there was not a large enough population of healthy elderly adults to study their nutrient requirements. With the aging of the population in recent decades, there are enough data on nutrient requirements of the elderly to warrant a separate category for those older than 71 years.

THE AGING PROCESS AND NUTRITION NEEDS

GENERAL PHYSIOLOGIC CHANGES

Biologic Changes

Throughout life, every experience makes an imprint on one's individual heritage. Everyone ages in different ways, depending on his or her personal makeup and available resources.

Metabolism. Beginning at about the age of 30 years, a gradual loss of functioning cells occurs, which results in reduced cell metabolism and changes in body composition. This change in metabolic rate reflects both lean muscle mass loss as well as a loss of high metabolically active organ tissues such as the brain, liver, heart, and kidneys.[12,13] The rate of this decline accelerates during the later years. Not all skeletal muscle mass loss is mandatory though. A contributing factor to **sarcopenia** is inadequate dietary protein metabolism and physical activity.[14]

Regular physical activity helps to maintain muscle mass and thus the metabolic rate. However, 25% of Americans do not participate in any leisure-time physical activity.[15] The current *Physical Activity Guidelines for Americans* recommend 150 minutes of moderate-intensity physical activity (or 75 minutes of vigorous-intensity physical activity) per week to reduce the risk of chronic disease (see Chapter 16). For more extensive health benefits, adults should participate in twice as much activity per week (i.e., 300 minutes of moderate-intensity activity or 150 minutes of vigorous-intensity activity).[16]

Hormones. Hormonal changes during the aging process have many repercussions in general health. The common decline in insulin production or insulin sensitivity results in elevated blood glucose levels and diabetes. Decreases in the level of **melatonin** may interfere with normal sleep cycles. Part of the normal changes in body composition is attributed to decreases in the levels of growth hormone and the sex hormones estrogen and testosterone. **Menopause** involves the cessation of estrogen and progesterone production by the ovaries. This dramatic change in a woman's life, which usually occurs between the ages of 45 and 55 years, represents the most significant hormonal change associated with age. Menopause is accompanied by an increase in body fat, a decrease in lean tissue, and an increase in the risk of chronic disease (specifically heart disease and osteoporosis). Despite these changes,

sarcopenia loss of lean tissue mass associated with aging.
melatonin the hormone responsible for regulating body rhythms.
menopause the end of a woman's menstrual activity and capacity to bear children.

women today are better equipped than ever before with both social and medical support to embrace this period of life and to maintain health for many decades to come.

Effect on Food Patterns

Some of the physical changes of aging affect food patterns. For example, the secretion of digestive juices lessens and the motility of gastrointestinal muscles gradually weaken, which causes decreased absorption and bioavailability of nutrients. Decreased taste, smell, thirst, and vision also affect appetite and reduce food and fluid intake. Several other conditions that commonly afflict elderly adults are not so obviously related to food intake but should be considered. For example, decreased hand function, which is especially common in the elderly, can reduce hand-eye coordination and the ability to prepare and cook food. Older people may experience increased concern about body functions, more social stress, personal losses, and fewer social opportunities to maintain self-esteem; all of these concerns can affect food intake. A lack of sufficient nourishment is the primary nutrition problem of older adults.

Individuality of the Aging Process

Although the biologic changes of senescence are generally similar, each person is unique, and people show a wide variety of individual responses. Individuals age at different rates and in different ways, depending on their genetic heritage and the health and nutrition resources of their prior years. For example, some individuals are in the best shape of their lives after retirement when given the extra time to eat and exercise freely and without stressful time constraints. Thus, specific needs vary with functional ability.

NUTRITION NEEDS

Macronutrients and Fluids

The basal metabolic rate declines an average of 1% to 2% per decade, with a more rapid decline occurring at approximately 40 years of age for men and 50 years of age for women.[17] This correlates with a gradual loss of functioning body cells and reduced physical activity, as discussed earlier. The current national standard is based on estimates of 5% decreased metabolic activity during the middle and older years. The mean energy expenditure for women who are between the ages of 51 and 70 years and have an ideal body mass index (BMI) of 18.5 to 25 kg/m² is 2066 kcal/day; for women who are older than 71 years, it is 1564 kcal/day. For men of the same age and BMI, energy expenditure averages 2469 kcal/day and 2238 kcal/day, respectively.[17] These recommendations are based on the averages of the population, and they may vary greatly

among individuals. Physical and health statuses as well as living situations influence overall energy and nutrient requirements. Obesity throughout the adult years, and especially in the elderly, has a significant association with an increased prevalence of disability.[18] Thus, health promotion that includes weight control and disease prevention is an important aspect of healthy living throughout the entire life span.

The basic fuels that are necessary to supply these energy needs are the same as they are for all stages of life: primarily carbohydrate, along with moderate fat.

Carbohydrate. Approximately 45% to 65% of total kilocalories should come from carbohydrate, with an emphasis on complex carbohydrates (e.g., whole grains, vegetables). Easily absorbed sugars (i.e., the simple sugars in soft drinks, candy, and sweets) may also be used for energy, but they should be used in limited amounts and comprise no more than 10% of total kilocalorie intake. As a person's metabolic rate declines, so does the room for empty calories. An absolute minimum of 130 g of carbohydrates per day is necessary to maintain normal brain function in both children and adults.[17]

Fat. High quality dietary fat provides a backup energy source, important fat-soluble vitamins, and essential fatty acids. A reasonable goal is to aim for a diet consisting of about 30% fat, with an emphasis on monounsaturated and polyunsaturated fat sources. Fat digestion and absorption may be delayed in elderly people, but these functions are not greatly disturbed. Sufficient fat for taste enhancement better aids appetite and in some cases provides needed kilocalories to prevent unintentional weight loss.

Protein. The DRIs recommend a protein intake of 0.8 g per kilogram of body weight for adults. Thus, the average weight man (154 lb) would need 56 g/day and the average weight woman (127 lb) would need to consume 46 g/day. Protein should provide approximately 10% to 35% of the total kilocalories (see Chapter 4).[17] The average adult in the United States consumes approximately 1.5 times this amount of protein on any given day.[19] However, the protein needs of older adults (≥65 years) are higher per kilogram of body weight because of decreased metabolic performance and sarcopenia. In addition, the requirement for protein may rise during illness or convalescence or in the presence of a wasting disease. In any case, protein needs are related to two basic factors: (1) the protein quality (i.e., the quantity and ratio of its amino acids); and (2) an adequate number of total kilocalories in the diet. The most recent protein recommendations from the European Society for Clinical Nutrition and Metabolism are that adults ≥65 years old consume between 1.0 and 1.5 g of protein/kg/day depending on their health status (Table 12-1).[20]

---

senescence the process or condition of growing old.

Fluid. Water needs (relative to total energy needs) do not decline with age. See Table 9-1 for fluid intake recommendations for adults.

Micronutrients and Health Concerns

A diet that includes a variety of foods should supply adequate amounts of most vitamins and minerals for healthy adults. However, some essential nutrients may require special attention because of their relationship with possible health problems in the aging adult and morbidity or medication interactions.

Bone health. Vitamin D and calcium are essential nutrients for growth and for the maintenance of healthy bone tissue. Osteoporosis (porous bone) is a disorder in which bone mineral density is low and bones become brittle, with a high risk of breaking (Figure 12-4). The prevalence of osteopenia and osteoporosis, along with resultant disability, increases significantly with age (Figure 12-5). Race and sex are also influential factors in overall bone health (see the

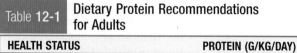

osteopenia a condition that involves low bone mass and an increased risk for fracture.

Table 12-1	Dietary Protein Recommendations for Adults	
HEALTH STATUS	**PROTEIN (G/KG/DAY)**	
Healthy Adults ≤65 years old	0.8	
Healthy Adults ≥65 years old	1.0 to 1.2	
Older adults with acute or chronic illness	1.2 to 1.5	

Cultural Considerations box "Bone Health in Gender and Racial Groups" in Chapter 8). Contributing factors to poor bone health for all populations include the following: (1) inadequate calcium and vitamin D intake; (2) physical inactivity; (3) smoking and alcohol use; (4) decreased estrogen level after menopause in women; (5) thin body frame; and (6) certain disease states and the use of medications that alter mineral bioavailability and bone turnover. Chapters 7 and 8 present good food sources of calcium and vitamin D.

Food safety. Safe food handling practices are important throughout the life cycle. In the event that an elderly individual begins to lose eyesight, hand-eye coordination, or taste and smell acuity, the risk for food-borne illness increases. The loss of such skills alters the ability to taste and smell spoiled food, see properly to prepare food, or have the coordination

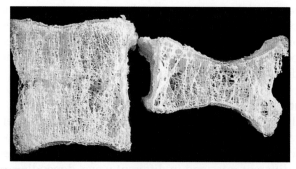

FIGURE 12-4 Osteoporotic vertebral body *(right)* shortened by compression fractures compared with a normal vertebral body. Note that the osteoporotic vertebra has a characteristic loss of horizontal trabeculae and thickened vertical trabeculae. (Reprinted from Kumar V, Abbas AK, Fausto N, Mitchell R. *Robbins basic pathology.* 8th ed. Philadelphia: Saunders; 2007.)

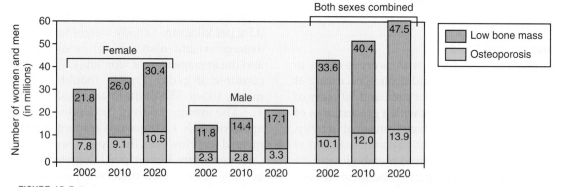

FIGURE 12-5 Projected prevalence of osteoporosis and low bone mass of the hip among women, men, and both sexes who are 50 years old or older. Note that the National Health and Nutrition Examination Survey is conducted by the National Center for Health Statistics, which is a part of the Centers for Disease Control and Prevention. This survey is conducted on a nationally representative sample of Americans. As a part of the study, bone mineral density of the hip was measured in 14,646 men and women who were 20 years old or older throughout the United States from 1988 until 1994. These values were compared with the World Health Organization definitions to derive the percentage of individuals who were older than 50 years and have osteoporosis and low bone mass. These percentages were then applied to the total population of men and women who were older than 50 years old to estimate the absolute number of men and women in the United States with osteoporosis and low bone mass. Projections for 2010 and 2020 are based on population forecasts for these years; they are significantly higher than current figures because of the expected growth in the overall population and the expected aging of the population. (Reprinted from U.S. Department of Health and Human Services. *Bone health and osteoporosis: a report of the surgeon general.* Rockville, Md: 2004.)

necessary to cut and chop food—all of which pose a potentially dangerous health risk. Specific food-borne illnesses and food safety practices are discussed at length in Chapter 13.

Nutrient Supplementation

The use of dietary supplements by elderly adults—usually on a self-prescribed basis—is common. Although such routine use may not be necessary, supplements are often recommended for people in debilitated states or to overcome malabsorption conditions. Physiologic changes associated with aging are known to alter the bioavailability of vitamin B_{12} and the endogenous synthesis of vitamin D. Therefore, dietary intake alone may not provide an adequate intake of certain nutrients.

Vitamin B_{12}. The DRIs specify that individuals who are ≥50 years old should consume vitamin B_{12} in supplemental form or through fortified foods because of the high risk of deficiency that results from decreased gastric acid production.[21] Hydrochloric acid is secreted from the gastric mucosal cells, and it is necessary for vitamin B_{12} digestion, along with intrinsic factor (see Figure 7-8). However, as people age, the production and secretion of hydrochloric acid often decrease and may result in inadequate vitamin B_{12} absorption. In this case, oral supplements would not overcome the lack of hydrochloric acid and/or intrinsic factor. Thus, subcutaneous vitamin B_{12} injections, which bypass the digestive tract and are not dependent on such factors for absorption, are necessary.

Vitamin D. Some researchers believe that about half of the elderly population worldwide is deficient in vitamin D and warrants supplementation.[22] Yet, as discussed in Chapter 7, the measurement tools for assessing vitamin D status and the parameters for normal versus deficient status are not universally accepted. It is routine to screen individuals at risk for vitamin D deficiency; however, it is not recommended to screen for vitamin D deficiency in asymptomatic adults because the cost of doing so is not justified.[23]

The DRIs for vitamin D are 600 IU/day for individuals who are between 1 and 70 years old and 800 IU/day for individuals who are older than 70 years of age.[24] To meet the dietary recommendation for vitamin D, elderly individuals should consume foods that are fortified with vitamin D or take a dietary supplement to overcome the reduced ability to endogenously synthesize vitamin D. Individuals living in nursing homes or other situations with little to no sunlight exposure, who avoid dairy products (which are good sources of vitamin D), or who are obese may benefit from vitamin D evaluation to determine the need for supplementation. Supplementing with vitamin D in older or institutionalized adults *may* reduce the risk of falls, although not necessarily the

risk of fracture, but other health benefits are inconclusive.[25] As with all fat-soluble vitamins, there is a risk of toxicity from excessive supplementation of vitamin D.[24]

Excess supplementation. As with most things, too much is counterproductive. The subset of the population that is most likely to take dietary supplements are older, white, educated, active women, who do not smoke and have annual incomes above the poverty line.[26] Not coincidentally, the adults most likely to take dietary supplements are also the ones who are likely to have the best overall diet and healthy lifestyle. Most people do not talk to their primary care physicians about what and how much of a dietary supplement they take, unless specifically asked. While it is rare that a multivitamin/mineral supplement, or the previously mentioned individual supplements of vitamins B_{12} or D, would result in toxicity it is always recommended to report and discuss the use of dietary and herbal supplements to health care providers.

CLINICAL NEEDS OF THE ELDERLY

HEALTH PROMOTION AND DISEASE PREVENTION

Reducing Risk for Chronic Disease

The emphasis of adult health care is on reducing individual risks for chronic disease as people grow older. This approach has always been used for the development of the *Dietary Guidelines for Americans* and the national health objectives. These guidelines outline lifestyle changes that people can make to live healthier lives (see Figure 1-4, *Dietary Guidelines for Americans*). The guidelines emphasize individual needs and good eating habits that are based on moderation and variety. Health care providers are encouraged to promote healthy lifestyles among all patients and to relay the importance of disease prevention.

Nutritional Status

Many of the health problems experienced by elderly adults result from the physiologic changes of aging and progressive states of malnutrition. Malnutrition is multifactorial. Some of the following reasons may be involved:
- Poor food habits
  - Lack of appetite or loneliness and not wanting to eat alone
  - Lack of food availability as a result of economic or social issues
- Poor oral health (e.g., missing teeth, poorly fitting dentures)
- General gastrointestinal problems
  - Declining salivary secretions and dry mouth, with diminished thirst and taste sensations
  - Inadequate hydrochloric acid secretion in the stomach

- Decreased enzyme and mucus secretion in the intestines
- General decline in gastrointestinal motility

Individual medical symptoms range from vague indigestion or irritable colon to specific diseases such as peptic ulcer or diverticulitis (see Chapter 18). The Mini Nutritional Assessment (MNA) is one of the standard assessment tools routinely used to evaluate nutritional risk in elderly individuals residing in nursing homes (Figure 12-6).[27] The MNA is a reliable tool that is highly sensitive and can detect the risk of malnutrition early. Other assessment tools that are used in the geriatric population include the Malnutrition Screening Tool, the Nutritional Risk Screening 2002, the Malnutrition Universal Screening Tool, and the Subjective Global Assessment.[28]

Dental. Poor oral health–related quality of life is associated with malnutrition in the elderly.[29] The number of healthy teeth remaining; the ability to chew food; the presence of xerostomia (dry mouth), periodontal disease, or dental caries; the degree of taste perception; the ability to swallow; and the perception of oral health are all important aspects in one's ability to eat, speak, and socialize comfortably. Elderly individuals who are institutionalized and have no remaining teeth (i.e., edentulous) have a specific need for individualized nutrition care (see the Clinical Applications box, "Feeding Older Adults with Sensitivity").

Dehydration. Dehydration, which can be a problem in any age group, is common in the elderly population. Physiologic changes in the hypothalamus naturally occur with age, and, as a result, elderly individuals exhibit an overall decreased thirst sensation and reduced fluid intake compared with younger adults.[30,31]

In addition, other physiologic changes associated with aging, such as diminishing kidney function, may exacerbate losses of body fluid. Although this combination does not necessarily guarantee dehydration in elderly adults, it does lead to slower rates of rehydration. If a sickness causing vomiting or diarrhea is added to this scenario, these conditions could push an elderly patient into a state of dehydration. Another example would be a patient choosing to avoid fluids because he or she needs assistance with getting water or getting to the bathroom; so the patient rationalizes that if he or she does not drink as much, he or she will not have to get up as often.

Weight Management and Physical Activity

Unintentional weight loss and weight gain can be signs of malnutrition. Many of the same depressed living situations and emotional factors that result in unhealthy weight loss also may lead to excessive weight gain. Overeating or undereating may be a coping mechanism for the stressful conditions that are encountered by some individuals. Obesity among adults has been on the rise in all subgroups of the population for decades (Figure 12-7).[32] Not surprisingly, so have obesity-related chronic diseases.

Regular physical activity and adequate dietary protein intake should be a part of life through the adult and elderly years in order to maintain lean tissue and anabolic processes.[33] Physical activity is a major factor in weight management, and it can help prevent many of the debilitating conditions of old age by maintaining strength, functionality, independence, and overall quality of life.[34] The *Physical Activity Guidelines* and the *Dietary Guidelines for Americans* specifically note the long-term benefits of regular cardiovascular and strength-training exercises

---

⬔ Clinical Applications

Feeding Older Adults with Sensitivity

Many older adults have eating and/or feeding problems that could lead to malnutrition. Each person is a unique individual with particular needs requiring sensitive support to meet his or her nutritional and personal necessities.

BASIC GUIDELINES
- *Analyze food habits carefully.* Learn about the attitudes, situations, and desires of the older person. Nutrition needs can be met with a variety of foods, so make suggestions in a practical, realistic, and supportive manner.
- *Never moralize.* Never say, "Eat this because it is good for you." This approach has little value for anyone, especially for those who are struggling to maintain their personal integrity and self-esteem in a youth-oriented, age-fearing culture.
- *Encourage food variety.* Mix new foods with familiar comfort foods. New tastes and seasonings often encourage appetite and increase interest in eating. Many

people think that a bland diet is best for all elderly persons, but this is not necessarily true. The decreased taste sensitivity of aging necessitates added attention to variety and seasoning. Smaller amounts of food and more frequent meals may also encourage better nutrition.

ASSISTED FEEDING SUGGESTIONS
- Make no negative remarks about the food that is served.
- Identify the food that is being served.
- Allow the person to have at least three bites of the same food before going on to another food to allow time for the taste buds to become accustomed to the food.
- Give sufficient time for the person to chew and swallow.
- Give liquids throughout the meal and not just at the beginning and end.
- Keep attention focused on the patient. Do not carry on a conversation with another person, read, use a cell phone, or otherwise disrespect the patient who is relying on you for support.

Mini Nutritional Assessment

MNA®

Nestlé
Nutrition Institute

Last name:		First name:		
Sex:	Age:	Weight, kg:	Height, cm:	Date:

Complete the screen by filling in the boxes with the appropriate numbers. Total the numbers for the final screening score.

Screening

A   Has food intake declined over the past 3 months due to loss of appetite, digestive problems, chewing or swallowing difficulties?
0 = severe decrease in food intake
1 = moderate decrease in food intake
2 = no decrease in food intake   ☐

B   Weight loss during the last 3 months
0 = weight loss greater than 3 kg (6.6 lbs)
1 = does not know
2 = weight loss between 1 and 3 kg (2.2 and 6.6 lbs)
3 = no weight loss   ☐

C   Mobility
0 = bed or chair bound
1 = able to get out of bed / chair but does not go out
2 = goes out   ☐

D   Has suffered psychological stress or acute disease in the past 3 months?
0 = yes   2 = no   ☐

E   Neuropsychological problems
0 = severe dementia or depression
1 = mild dementia
2 = no psychological problems   ☐

F1 Body Mass Index (BMI) (weight in kg) / (height in m)^2
0 = BMI less than 19
1 = BMI 19 to less than 21
2 = BMI 21 to less than 23
3 = BMI 23 or greater   ☐

IF BMI IS NOT AVAILABLE, REPLACE QUESTION F1 WITH QUESTION F2.
DO NOT ANSWER QUESTION F2 IF QUESTION F1 IS ALREADY COMPLETED.

F2 Calf circumference (CC) in cm
0 = CC less than 31
3 = CC 31 or greater   ☐

Screening score   ☐☐
(max. 14 points)

12-14 points:	Normal nutritional status
8-11 points:	At risk of malnutrition
0-7 points:	Malnourished

Ref.   Vellas B, Villars H, Abellan G, et al. *Overview of the MNA® - Its History and Challenges.* J Nutr Health Aging 2006;10:456-465.

Rubenstein LZ, Harker JO, Salva A, Guigoz Y, Vellas B. *Screening for Undernutrition in Geriatric Practice: Developing the Short-Form Mini Nutritional Assessment (MNA-SF).* J. Geront 2001;56A: M366-377.

Guigoz Y. *The Mini-Nutritional Assessment (MNA®) Review of the Literature - What does it tell us?* J Nutr Health Aging 2006; 10:466-487.

Kaiser MJ, Bauer JM, Ramsch C, et al. *Validation of the Mini Nutritional Assessment Short-Form (MNA®-SF): A practical tool for identification of nutritional status.* J Nutr Health Aging 2009; 13:782-788.

® Société des Produits Nestlé, S.A., Vevey, Switzerland, Trademark Owners

© Nestlé, 1994, Revision 2009. N67200 12/99 10M

For more information: www.mna-elderly.com

FIGURE 12-6 Mini Nutritional Assessment. (Copyright Nestle USA, Inc., Glendale, Calif, 2009.)

Continued

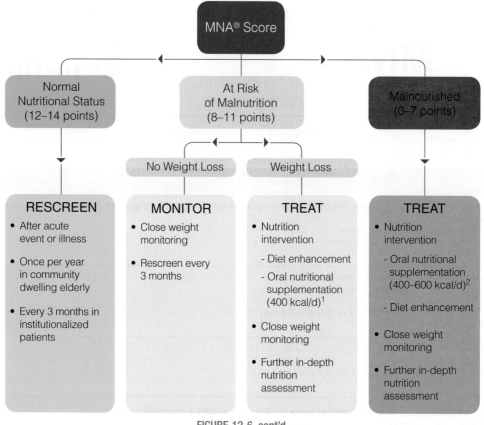

FIGURE 12-6, cont'd

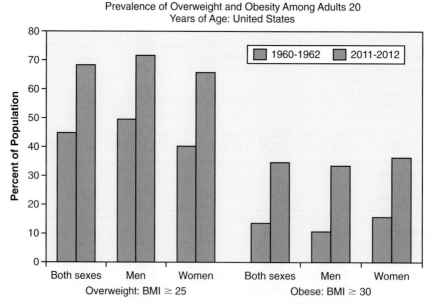

FIGURE 12-7 Prevalence of overweight and obesity among adults between the ages of 20 and 74 years in the United States. (Data from Ogden CL et al. Prevalence of childhood and adult obesity in the United States, 2011-2012. *JAMA*. 2014;311[8]:806-814.)

in adults.[16,35] As the population continues to age, health care facilities are adapting to the increased need for aerobic and balance classes that are aimed specifically at older adults who enjoy and benefit from daily exercise. Box 12-1 lists the benefits of physical activity as indicated by the Centers for Disease Control and Prevention (CDC).

One specific example of how exercise can help prevent disease is with type 2 diabetes. Decreased glucose tolerance is the *prediabetes syndrome* in which the insulin response to glucose in the bloodstream is inadequate to maintain blood glucose levels within a normal range but not high enough for a diagnosis of diabetes (see Chapter 20). Weight management through

Box 12-1 **Benefits of Physical Activity**

- Help maintain weight control
- Reduce the risk of cardiovascular disease, type 2 diabetes, metabolic syndrome, and some cancers
- Strengthen bones and muscles
- Improve mental health and mood
- Improve one's ability to perform daily activities and prevent falls, especially among older adults
- Increase the chance of living longer

For more information see the Centers for Disease Control and Prevention. *The benefits of physical activity* (website): www.cdc.gov/physicalactivity/everyone/health/index.html. Accessed July 14, 2015.

regular physical activity along with balanced meals and snacks can help individuals to avoid excessively high blood glucose concentrations and potentially delay or avoid the onset of diabetes.[36] The reason physical activity is important in this equation is that exercise increases the skeletal tissue glucose uptake independent of insulin.[37] Thus, even though insulin sensitivity is declining with age, regular exercise will improve blood glucose levels by shuttling glucose into the tissues and out of the blood.

Individual Approach

Effective health promotion and disease prevention requires individualized and realistic planning. All personalities and problems are unique, and specific needs vary widely. An adult suffering from malnutrition or any of the chronic diseases discussed below will need a sensitive person-centered approach addressing all aspects of health and well-being (see the Clinical Applications box, "Case Study: Situational Problem of an Elderly Woman").

CHRONIC DISEASES OF AGING

Chronic diseases of aging (e.g., hypertension, heart disease, stroke, emphysema, diabetes, cancer, arthritis, asthma) occur more frequently with advancing age, but they may present at a younger age in individuals with a strong family history of disease. Health experts believe that chronic disease is not an inevitable consequence of aging and estimate that 80% of all cases of heart disease, stroke, and type 2 diabetes and 40% of cancer cases could have been prevented by lifestyle modifications.[38] The CDC recommends the following lifestyle changes to promote health and prevent chronic disease in adulthood: (1) participate in regular physical activity; (2) maintain a healthy weight by choosing a balanced diet rich in fruits and vegetables; (3) stop smoking; and (4) limit alcohol intake.

Diet Modifications

In the presence of chronic disease, diet modifications and nutrition support are an important part of therapy. Details of these modified diets per disease are given in Chapters 17 through 23. In any situation, individual-

Clinical Applications

Case Study: Situational Problem of an Elderly Woman

Mrs. Johnson, a recently widowed 78-year-old woman, lives alone in a three-bedroom house in Atlanta, Georgia. A fall 1 year ago resulted in a broken hip, and she now depends on a walker for limited mobility. Her only child, a daughter, lives in Portland, Oregon, and does not want to bear the burden of responsibility for her mother. Mrs. Johnson's only income is a monthly Social Security check for $1100. Her monthly mortgage payment, property taxes, insurance payments, and utility and phone bills amount to $907.

A recent medical examination revealed that Mrs. Johnson has iron-deficiency anemia and that she has lost 12 pounds during the past 3 months. Her current weight is 80 pounds, and she is 5 feet, 2 inches tall. Mrs. Johnson states that she has not been hungry, and her daily diet is repetitious: broth, a little cottage cheese and canned fruit, saltine crackers, and hot tea. She lacks energy, she rarely leaves the house, and she appears to be emaciated and generally distraught.

QUESTIONS FOR ANALYSIS

1. Identify Mrs. Johnson's personal problems, and describe how they might be influencing her eating habits. How could her physical problems have influenced her food intake?
2. What nutritional improvements could she make in her diet (include food suggestions), and how are these related to her physical needs at this stage of her life?
3. What practical suggestions do you have for helping Mrs. Johnson to cope with her physical and social environment? What resources, income sources, food, and companionship can you suggest? How do you think these suggestions would benefit her nutritional status and overall health?

ized food plans relative to needs are essential for successful therapy.

Medications

Because people are living longer (many with one or more chronic disease), older adults may be taking several prescription drugs in addition to over-the-counter medications. **Polypharmacy** can affect overall nutritional status when drug-nutrient interactions occur (see Chapter 17). Many of the medications that are often used by the elderly (e.g., blood pressure medication, antacids, anticoagulation medications, laxatives, diuretics, decongestants) can directly affect fluid balance, appetite, and the absorption and use of nutrients, thereby possibly contributing to malnutrition or dehydration. When questioning patients about medication use, health care providers should specifically ask about the use of dietary supplements and herbs. Toxicities from supplements can be dangerous, even though many of these products are considered

polypharmacy the use of multiple medications by the same patient.

to be "natural." Each person requires the careful evaluation of all of his or her drug use and instructions about how to take medications in relation to meals (see the Drug-Nutrient Interaction box, "Medication Use in the Adult").

COMMUNITY RESOURCES

GOVERNMENT PROGRAMS FOR OLDER AMERICANS

Adults who are living below the national poverty level have a higher incidence of multiple chronic diseases than any other socioeconomic group.[9] Health care providers must be aware of community resources and refer patients when appropriate. Many older adults who are at risk for malnutrition and who are eligible for nutrition assistance programs are not partaking in the available services. In many cases, participation

could be improved through the help of an advocate who is willing to make application and help set up their involvement.

Older Americans Act

The Administration on Aging of the U.S. Department of Health and Human Services (www.aoa.gov) manages programs for older adults. Nutrition Services Incentive Programs provide cash and/or commodities to supplement meals offered at congregate and home-delivered nutrition programs. These services are focused on reaching the elderly with the greatest social and economic need.

Congregate nutrition services. This program provides adults who are older than 60 years of age and their spouses (particularly those with low incomes) with nutritionally sound meals in senior centers and

Drug-Nutrient Interaction

Medication Use in the Adult

Half of adults older than age 45 take at least one prescription medication, and this percentage increases with age. Polypharmacy is common in the United States; 39% of adults ≥65 years old take five or more prescription drugs regularly.[1] Polypharmacy is significantly more prevalent in the non-Hispanic white population than in any other segment of the population.

The most commonly prescribed medications in the United States for adults ≥65 years old are cardiovascular agents (to treat high blood pressure, high cholesterol level, heart disease, and kidney disease), anti–acid reflux drugs, antidiabetic agents, anticoagulants, and analgesics.[1]

In addition to prescription drugs, nonprescription (i.e., over-the-counter) medications, dietary supplements (i.e., vitamins and minerals), and herbal supplements are also commonly used by these individuals. Several potential drug-nutrient interactions may occur with commonly used medications,

particularly with antidepressants, antihyperlipidemics, hypertensive medications, nonsteroidal antiinflammatory drugs, and antihistamines. Because such a high percentage of patients are taking at least one medication, diet interactions with common medications must be considered.

Many medications have side effects that can affect appetite, weight, or the ability to absorb nutrients from food. Residents in skilled nursing facilities are at higher risk for polypharmacy and nutrition-related effects. It is crucial for the multidisciplinary team to communicate openly about changes in the patient's appetite, eating habits, and medication regimen so that potential risks can be identified. Foods and nutrients that should be avoided when taking common medications are listed below.

REFERENCE
1. National Center for Health Statistics. *Health, United States, 2014: with special feature of adults aged 55-64.* Hyattsville, MD: U.S. Government Printing Office; 2015.

DRUG CLASS	FOOD/NUTRIENT INTERACTION	HOW TO AVOID AN ADVERSE REACTION
Certain antidepressants (i.e., monoamine oxidase inhibitors)	Alcohol and foods that contain tyramine	Avoid beer, red wine, and tyramine-containing foods such as cheese, yogurt, sour cream, liver, cured meats, caviar, dried fish, avocados, bananas, raisins, soy sauce, miso soup, ginseng, and caffeine-containing products
	Fluids	Drink 2 to 3 L of water per day and take the drugs with food; keep sodium intake consistent
Antihyperlipidemics	Food and alcohol	Take with the evening meal, and avoid more than one alcoholic drink per day
	Fat-soluble vitamins, folate, B_{12}, and iron	Include rich sources of these vitamins and minerals in the diet
	Grapefruit juice	Avoid grapefruit juice
Antihypertensives	Licorice and tyramine-rich foods	Avoid licorice and tyramine-containing foods
	Grapefruit juice	Avoid taking with grapefruit juice
Nonsteroidal antiinflammatory drugs	Alcohol	Limit alcohol intake
	Vitamin C, folate, and vitamin K	Increase intake of foods that are high in these vitamins and minerals
	Fluid balance	Take with water
Antihistamines	Alcohol	Avoid alcohol
	Grapefruit juice	Avoid taking with grapefruit juice

other public or private community facilities. In these settings, older adults can gather for a hot noon meal and have access to both wholesome food and social support. In addition to meals, other services include nutrition screening, education, assessment, and counseling, as needed.

Home-delivered meals. For those older adults who are ill or disabled and who cannot travel to the community centers, meals are delivered by couriers to their homes (i.e., Meals on Wheels). This service meets nutrition needs and provides human contact and support. The couriers are usually volunteers who are concerned about other people and their needs. A courier is often the only person a homebound individual will interact with during the day.

United States Department of Agriculture
The U.S. Department of Agriculture provides both research and services for older adults.

Research centers. Research centers for studies on aging have been established in various areas of the United States and are supported by the U.S. Department of Agriculture. For example, the Human Nutrition Research Center on Aging at Tufts University in Boston is the largest research facility in the world dedicated to the study of nutrition in aging. Studies there involve research on topics such as nutrition and its interactions with cardiovascular disease, cancer, inflammation, immunity, and obesity. Much more knowledge about the nutritional requirements of older adults is needed to provide better care.

Extension services. The U.S. Department of Agriculture operates agricultural extension services in state land grant universities, including food and nutrition education services. County home advisers help communities with practical materials and counseling for elderly people and community workers.

Supplemental nutrition assistance program (SNAP). SNAP, which was formerly known as the Food Stamp Program, issues electronic benefits transfer cards to the primary care provider in households with a monthly income ≤130% of the federal poverty line, regardless of age. The cards are similar to debit cards, and they can be used at authorized food retail outlets to purchase eligible food items. About 42 million low-income individuals benefit from SNAP services every month. Elderly adults (≥60 years old) have the lowest participation rates at 42% of those eligible for services

participating in SNAP. This is significantly less than other age groups, whose participation rates are up to 90%.[39] SNAP promotes the consumption of fruits, vegetables, whole grains, fat-free or low-fat milk products, lean meats, poultry, and fish.

Commodity supplemental food program. Individuals who are older than 60 years of age with a household income ≤130% of the federal poverty line are also eligible for assistance in the form of food packages. These food packages are not intended to provide a complete diet but rather to supplement the diet with foods that are high in the nutrients that are typically lacking in the diet of an elderly person.

Senior farmers' market nutrition program. This is a grant-based program that provides low-income older adults (i.e., ≥60 years of age with an income that is ≤185% of the federal poverty income guidelines) with coupons that they can exchange for fresh fruits, vegetables, and herbs obtained from farmers' markets, community-supported agriculture programs (CSAs), and roadside stands. This program has increased the average servings of fruits and vegetables among participants, and it helps support local farmers.

Public Health Departments
Public health departments throughout the United States are an outreach division of the U.S. Department of Health and Human Services. Skilled health professionals work in the community through local and state public health departments. Public health nutritionists are important members of this health care team; they provide nutrition counseling and education, and they help with various food assistance programs.

PROFESSIONAL ORGANIZATIONS AND RESOURCES
National Groups
The American Geriatrics Society and the Gerontological Society of America are national professional organizations of physicians, nurses, dietitians, and other interested health care workers. These societies publish journals and promote community and government efforts to meet the needs of aging individuals.

Community Groups
Senior centers in local communities are valuable resources for both well and disabled adults. Local medical societies, nursing organizations, and dietetic associations sponsor various programs to help meet the needs of elderly people. Often times these programs are held within the local senior centers. The Commission on Dietetics offers a Board Certification as a Specialist in Gerontological Nutrition. Similar certifications are offered within other health care professional licensing bodies. There are registered dietitians in private practice in most communities, and they can

state land grant universities an institution of higher education that has been designated by the state to receive unique federal support as a result of the Morrill Acts of 1862 and 1890.

supply a variety of individual and group services as well.

Volunteer Organizations

Many volunteer activities of health organizations (e.g., the American Heart Association, the American Diabetes Association) relate to the needs of older people and may serve as both rewarding opportunities for young-old adults and important sources of health-sustaining activities and information for old-old adults.

Chapter 13 discusses additional resources for nutritional assistance.

ALTERNATIVE LIVING ARRANGEMENTS

There are a multitude of alternative living arrangements for seniors of all levels of independence. For example, independent living facilities are for independently functioning individuals who do not need medical attention and who enjoy recreational and social events with other seniors. Other housing options provide more services, may be staffed with health care workers, and provide different levels of care in accordance with needs. Examples include congregate care, continuing care retirement communities, and assisted living facilities. Nursing homes are fully staffed with medical professionals and are able to provide for most medical needs in the absence of an acute episode that requires hospitalization. The next sections of this chapter discuss only the types of alternative living arrangements that provide food and health care (i.e., not independent living facilities). Several organizations that provide helpful information about alternative living arrangements for seniors are listed in the Further Reading and Resources section at the back of the book.

CONGREGATE CARE ARRANGEMENTS

Congregate care arrangements are focused on keeping the elderly living in their own homes for as long as possible with outside assistance available to meet specific needs. Some congregate care services were mentioned previously: congregate community meals, nutrition education through extension services, and home-delivered meals. Other services include personal care aides, adult day services, transportation, respite care, and more. Personal care aides may shop for groceries, cook, and even help with feeding, if necessary.

The emphasis on modified diets in such settings varies. Congregate meals and home-delivered meals are not likely to be specific to diets for individuals with highly particular needs. For example, individuals with diabetes who count carbohydrates, those with food intolerances or allergies, or those who have difficulty swallowing certain food consistencies (e.g., dysphagia) may require additional assistance. Most congregate care programs are regulated at the state level.

Public programs (e.g., congregate meals and home-delivered meals) are required to offer meals that meet the *Dietary Guidelines for Americans* and each meal should provide one third of the DRIs for select nutrients.

CONTINUING CARE RETIREMENT COMMUNITIES

Continuing care retirement communities provide a continuum of residential long-term care, from independent living with community-organized events to nursing care facilities. Dietary assistance varies by the needs of the resident. Seniors can move into the community as independent living residences and participate in community activities and meals as they so choose. When their functional statuses indicate, seniors receive more care. Continuing care retirement communities usually have assisted living facilities and nursing homes in a campus-style setting. Nutritional involvement within these facilities is discussed in the next sections of this chapter, and it applies within this continuum-of-care approach as well.

ASSISTED LIVING FACILITIES

Assisted living facilities can go by several names, including *board and care, domiciliary care, sheltered housing, residential care,* and *personal care.* Assisted living arrangements may also exist within continuing care communities. Individual state governments regulate licensure for assisted living facilities. Most assisted living facilities provide all meals and snacks; housekeeping; laundry; and help with dressing, bathing, and personal hygiene. Some facilities provide social activities, limited transportation, and basic medication administration, but they may not provide medical or nursing care. Living areas vary from full apartments with kitchens, to studio-type apartments with small kitchenettes, to rooms with baths. The functional status of the individual helps to determine the most appropriate setting.

Meals are generally served in a cafeteria or restaurant setting. Some facilities provide menus with several options at each meal, and others serve a set menu for all residents, with attention given to special needs. Most assisted care facilities cater to basic dietary requests and the therapeutic diet needs of their residents. States vary widely with regard to regulations and standards for nutrition policies and services. Most states require that a registered dietitian review and approve the meal plans.

NURSING HOMES

Nursing homes or long-term care facilities provide the most medical, nursing, and nutrition support of the alternative living arrangements. Approximately 1.37 million people reside in nursing homes in the United States.[9] Many nursing homes also provide a residential rehabilitation site outside of the hospital for patients to recover from injuries, acute illnesses, and operations. Most patients in nursing homes need help with activities of daily living (e.g., bathing, toileting, transferring), and many need assistance with eating.

Nursing homes have dietitians on staff who are able to design meal plans to meet specific dietary requirements of individual patients. However, much less emphasis on therapeutic diets is given for this population, because a less-restrictive diet model is thought to be more beneficial at this life stage.[40]

Additionally, family-style eating arrangements (e.g., a cafeteria with a server) benefit individuals who are at high risk for malnutrition, especially those with cognitive impairment and below-optimal BMI.[41] Researchers believe that the autonomy, ambiance, and social interaction of family-style eating (compared with plated tray delivery) contribute to the significant increase in energy and nutrient intake. Many of these factors are depicted in Figure 12-2, which demonstrates how such issues relate to overall quality of life.

Putting It All Together

Summary

- Meeting the nutrition needs of adults—especially older adults—may present a challenge for several reasons. Current and past social, economic, and psychologic factors influence needs, and the biologic process of aging differs widely among individuals.
- As the average life expectancy continues to increase, research and recommendations regarding the needs of an aging population are updated.
- Many illnesses in older adults are the result of malnutrition rather than the effects of aging. Health promotion and disease prevention during early adulthood are key elements to sustain functionality throughout the later years.
- When working with older people, health care professionals must analyze food habits carefully and approach clients with encouragement for positive changes to be made. Individual supportive guidance and patience are necessary when administering nutrition resources and support.
- A variety of assisted living arrangements and nutrition services are available for seniors of all functional levels.

Chapter Review Questions

See answers in Appendix A.

1. The best way for older adults to maintain their muscle mass and metabolic rate is:
   a. Ensuring ample protein intake.
   b. Engaging in regular physical activity.
   c. Using multivitamin/multimineral supplements.
   d. Maintaining adequate fluid intake.

2. The risk of osteoporosis can be reduced by eating foods containing adequate amounts of:
   a. Protein and vitamin C.
   b. Vitamins B_{12} and B_6.
   c. Iron and zinc.
   d. Calcium and vitamin D.

3. A patient has been taking an antihistamine medication with a glass of grapefruit juice each morning. The health care professional should encourage the patient to:
   a. Continue this practice.
   b. Replace the grapefruit juice with water.
   c. Take the medication at bedtime with grapefruit juice.
   d. Take the medication with only a half glass of grapefruit juice.

4. A typical physiologic change in older adults that can affect nutrient intake is:
   a. An increase in metabolism requiring more calories to meet energy needs.
   b. A decline in intestinal motility that can lead to constipation.
   c. More hydrochloric acid secretion in the stomach.
   d. A general increase in appetite, especially toward the end of the day.

5. The Older American Act provides programs for older adults for meal assistance that includes:
   a. Support groups with counselors who eat meals together.
   b. Delivery of groceries to participants at home.
   c. Home-delivered meals and congregate meals.
   d. Vouchers for purchasing energy-dense foods.

Additional Learning Resources

evolve Please refer to this text's Evolve website for answers to the Case Study questions. http://evolve.elsevier.com/Williams/basic/

References and **Further Reading and Resources** in the back of the book provide additional resources for enhancing knowledge.

chapter

13

Community Food Supply and Health

Key Concepts

- Modern food production, processing, and marketing have both positive and negative influences on food safety.
- A variety of organisms in contaminated food can transmit disease.
- Poverty often prevents individuals and families from having adequate access to their community food supply.
- There are several aid programs available to help individuals secure food for themselves and their family.

The health of a community largely depends on the safety of its available food and water supply. The American system of government control agencies and regulations, along with local and state public health officials, works diligently to maintain a safe food supply. The food supply in the United States has undergone dramatic changes during the past several decades.

This chapter explores the factors that influence the safety of food. Potential health problems related to the food supply can arise from several sources, such as the lack of sanitation, food-borne disease, and poverty.

FOOD SAFETY AND HEALTH PROMOTION

Keeping the enormous food supply in the United States safe is no small task. Several federal agencies help to control food safety and quality. In addition to the agencies listed in Table 13-1, there are multiple other federal, state, and local agencies that participate in education and research to promote the safety of the food supply.

THE U.S. FOOD AND DRUG ADMINISTRATION

Although several agencies are involved in the overall food safety of products sold in the United States, only the diverse roles of the U.S. Food and Drug Administration (FDA) are discussed here because they are responsible for the majority of the food supply.

Enforcement of Federal Food Safety Regulations

The FDA is a law-enforcement agency that has been charged by the U.S. Congress with ensuring that America's food supply is safe. The agency enforces federal food safety regulations through various activities that ensure the safety of most food products, including the following: (1) enforcing food sanitation and quality control; (2) controlling food additives;

(3) regulating the movement of foods across state lines; (4) maintaining the nutrition labeling of foods; and (5) ensuring the safety of public food service. The agency's methods of enforcement are recall, seizure, injunction, and prosecution. The use of recall is the most common method, and this is followed by seizures of contaminated food. Injunction involves a court order to stop the sale and production of a food item. This procedure is not common, and it generally occurs in response to a claim that a food item is potentially harmful or that it has not undergone appropriate testing or acquired adequate approval for sale.

Consumer Education and Research

The FDA's Center for Food Safety and Applied Nutrition maintains an online library with educational materials intended for educators, health professionals, and the general public. Pamphlets, books, posters, and other materials are available to download, distribute, or print from their website. Food Safety.gov (www.foodsafety.gov) is an organization that serves as the liaison between the public and all government agencies that are involved in food safety.

Along with the U.S. Department of Agriculture's (USDA) Agricultural Research Service, the FDA scientists continually evaluate foods and food components through their own research. The following is a list of some of the current research projects involving nutrition: consumer behavior research (e.g., food safety surveys, health and diet surveys), risk and safety assessment of high-risk foods and food contaminants, safe practices for food processors, the Whole Genome Sequencing Program, and the **Total Diet Study**. The

---

Total Diet Study FDA program beginning in 1961 that evaluates the levels of nutrients and contaminants in foods.

Table 13-1   Agencies Involved in Food Safety Regulation

AGENCY	RESPONSIBILITIES
U.S. Food and Drug Administration (FDA)	Primary governing body of the American food supply, with the exception of commercial meat, poultry, and egg products. Also governs dietary supplements, bottled water, food additives, and breast milk substitute infant formulas
Food Safety and Inspection Service of the U.S. Department of Agriculture (USDA)	Responsible for the food safety of both domestic and imported meat, poultry, and processed egg products
National Oceanic and Atmospheric Administration (NOAA) Seafood Inspection Program	Governs the safety of seafood and fisheries
Environmental Protection Agency	Regulates the use of pesticides and other chemicals and ensures the safety of public drinking water
Federal Trade Commission	Regulates the advertising and truthful marketing of food products
Centers for Disease Control and Prevention	Monitors and investigates cases of food-borne illness, and is proactive with regard to education and prevention

Healthy People Initiative is an FDA project that set the goals and objectives for the *Healthy People 2020*.

FOOD LABELS

Early Development of Label Regulations

During the mid-1960s, the FDA established "truth in packaging" regulations that dealt mainly with food standards of identity. As food processing advanced and the number of available food items grew, the labels included nutrition information as well. Both types of label information—standards and nutrition facts—are important to consumers.

Food standards. The basic standards of identity require that labels on foods that do not have an established reference standard must list all of the ingredients in order of relative amount found in the product. Other food standard information on labels relates to food quality, fill of container, and enrichment or fortification. Major food allergens must also be noted on the food label, although some exceptions apply. For example, a container of milk does not have to include a notice of "this product contains milk." Major food allergens are defined by the FDA as milk, egg, fish (e.g., bass, flounder, or cod), crustacean shellfish (e.g., crab, lobster, or shrimp), tree nuts (e.g., almonds, pecans, or walnuts), wheat, peanuts, and soybeans.

Nutrition information. Under regulations that were adopted in 1973, the FDA began developing a labeling system that describes a food's nutritional value. Some producers began to add limited information on their own to meet this increasing market demand. Many people became concerned that nutrition labeling was inadequate, but the real difficulty was what and how much was being labeled and in what format. Information about nutrients and food constituents that consumer groups believed should be listed on labels included the amount of macronutrients and their total energy value, the key micronutrients (e.g.,

calcium, iron, vitamin A), and the levels of sodium, cholesterol, trans fat (as of 2006), and saturated fat. Concerned public and professional groups also want nutrients to be identified in terms of percentages of the current Dietary Reference Intake standards per defined portion.

Approximately half of shoppers consult the food label, review the ingredients' list, or read the health claims printed on the food package before purchasing a food product.[1] Women with a higher education and higher income are the most likely demographic to use the food label to make purchasing decisions. Individuals who use and understand the food labels also have an overall healthier diet pattern than those individuals who do not.[1] Obviously, there are many factors that contribute to healthy dietary choices, not just food labels. However, if the labels are to invoke a positive influence on the dietary choices of the population as a whole, the presentation and information must be clear, concise, and easily understandable.[2]

Background of Present U.S. Food and Drug Administration Label Regulations

Two factors have fueled rapid progress toward better food labels: (1) an increase in the variety of food products entering the U.S. marketplace; and (2) changing patterns of American eating habits. Both factors led many health-conscious consumers and professionals alike to rely increasingly on nutrition labeling to help attain health goals.

Despite the initial regulations, a number of labeling problems persisted such as misleading health claims, vague terms such as "natural," and varying serving sizes. These problems indicated a need to reorganize the entire food-labeling system. This need was reinforced by three landmark reports that related nutrition and diet to national health goals: *The Surgeon General's Report on Nutrition and Health,* the National Research Council's *Diet and Health Report,* and the Public Health Service's national health goals and objectives, *Healthy*

People 2000. On the basis of these reports, the Institute of Medicine of the National Academy of Sciences established a Committee on the Nutrition Components of Food Labeling to study and report on the scientific issues and practical needs involved in food-labeling reform. The committee's report provided basic guidelines for the rule-making process conducted by the FDA, the USDA, and the U.S. Department of Health and Human Services for submission to Congress to achieve the needed reforms. Three areas formed the basis of the recommendations from the Institute of Medicine: (1) foods for mandatory regulations; (2) the format of label information; and (3) the education of consumers. This report became the basic guideline for the Nutrition Labeling and Education Act of 1990.

Current Food Label Format

Nutrition facts label. Figure 13-1, represents the changes that the FDA recently approved for the updated Nutrition Facts Label.[3] As noted in the new label, there are significant changes. Some specific changes include the following:

- The font size will be significantly increased to draw attention to the *number of servings per container* and the total calories per serving.
- Calories from fat will no longer be printed below the total calories.
- An alternate format suggests separating nutrients into categories of *Quick Facts, Avoid Too Much,* and *Get Enough* to bring attention to the pros and cons to each food's nutrient quality.
- *Vitamin D and Potassium* will replace *Vitamin A and Vitamin C* as required nutrients on the label. Current research indicates that vitamins A and C are no longer of public health concern as nutrient deficiencies. However, surveys indicate that the average person does not consume enough vitamin D and potassium.
- *Added Sugars* will be a required nutrition fact to distinguish between naturally occurring sugar in a food from added sugar. Additionally, the FDA now requires a declaration of the percent daily value (%DV) for added sugars.
- The *Daily Reference Values* will be updated according to current DRI values.
- *Serving sizes* will be updated to reflect typical consumption. For example, a 20-oz soda will now be 1 serving instead of 2.5 servings (previously 8 oz = 1 serving).

Food manufacturers have 2 years to comply with the new format. This label is typically displayed on the side or on the back of the food package. The serving size (i.e., the amount of the food that is customarily consumed at one time) must be given and expressed in household measures; this is followed by the metric weight in parentheses and the total number of servings per container. The nutrients listed on the label in Figure 13-1 are the bare essentials

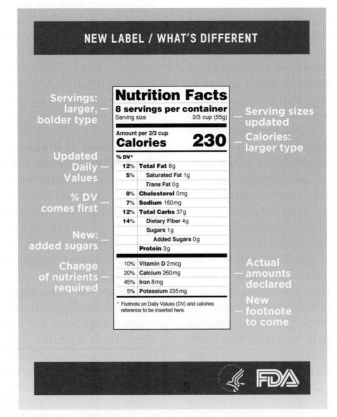

FIGURE 13-1 The new Nutrition Facts Label approved by the U.S. Food and Drug Administration. (Courtesy U.S. Food and Drug Administration, Washington, DC.)

for the information that must be provided. Manufacturers may choose to include additional information, such as amounts of polyunsaturated fat, monounsaturated fat, soluble and insoluble fiber, sugar alcohol (e.g., sorbitol), other carbohydrates, other vitamins and minerals, and caffeine.[4]

The FDA established 2000 calories as the reference amount for calculating the *percent daily value* (% DV), although individuals may vary greatly with regard to their specific needs. As a reference tool, the % DVs can be used to determine the overall value of a specific nutrient in the food (see the For Further Focus box,

"Glossary of Terms for Nutrition Facts Labels"). For example, if the % DV for fiber in one serving of whole-grain bread is 10%, a person who is eating the bread acquires one tenth of the recommended total fiber intake for his or her day.

Front-of-package labeling. Many food manufacturers use front-of-package labeling to propagate nutrition information. Figure 13-2 presents several examples of such labels. Currently, there are few U.S. federal regulations in place to standardize front-of-package labels. However, most developed countries

---

For Further Focus

Glossary of Terms for Nutrition Facts Labels

To improve communication between producers and consumers, all producers must use the standard wording supplied by the U.S. Food and Drug Administration (FDA). Whether these terms are used in the Nutrition Facts box or elsewhere as part of the manufacturer's product description, all producers must use the commonly accepted terms. The following is a sampling of these terms.

NUTRITION FACTS BOX
Daily Values
Daily values (DVs) are reference values that relate the nutrition information to a total daily diet of 2000 kcal, which is appropriate for most women and teenage girls as well as for some sedentary men. The footnote indicates the daily values for a 2500-kcal diet, which meets the needs of most men, teenage boys, and active women. To help consumers determine how a food fits into a healthy diet, Figure 13-1 shows the nutrients that must be listed on the label. Other vitamins and minerals may be listed if the manufacturers choose to do so, but this is not required.

Daily Reference Value
As part of the DVs listed, the daily reference values are a set of dietary standards for the following nutrients: total fat; saturated fat; cholesterol; total carbohydrate; dietary fiber; iron; calcium; and sodium. The current label also provides the daily reference value for vitamins A and C but the proposed label will include the daily reference value for vitamin D and potassium instead. No % DV is provided for trans fat, sugar, or protein. There is no recommendation or need to include any added sugar or trans fat in the diet and protein is not a public health concern because most individuals older than 4 years of age consume more than enough protein daily. The % DVs are based on a 2000-kcal diet. The daily reference values do not appear on the label, because they are part of a food's DV.

Descriptive Terms on Products
The FDA has specifically defined many terms. Manufacturers must follow these definitions if they use these terms on their product. The following are examples:
- *Fat free:* Less than 0.5 g of fat per serving.
- *Low cholesterol:* ≤20 mg of cholesterol per serving and per 100 g; 2 g of saturated fat or less per serving. Any label claim about low cholesterol is prohibited for all foods that contain more than 2 g of saturated fat per serving.

- *Light* or *Lite:* At least a one-third reduction in kilocalories. If fat contributes 50% or more of total kilocalories, fat content must be reduced by 50% compared with the reference food.
- *Less sodium:* At least a 25% reduction; 140 mg or less per reference amount per serving.
- *High:* 20% or more of the DV per serving.
- *Reduced saturated fat:* At least 25% less saturated fat than an appropriate reference food.
- *Lean:* Applied to meat, poultry, and seafood; less than 10 g of fat, 4 g of saturated fat, and 95 mg of cholesterol per serving.
- *Extra lean:* Applied to meat, poultry, and seafood; less than 5 g of fat, 2 g of saturated fat, and 95 mg of cholesterol per serving.
- For more information, see "How to Understand and Use the Nutrition Facts Label" on the FDA website at www.fda.gov/food/ingredientspackaginglabeling/labelingnutrition/ucm274593.htm.

HEALTH CLAIMS
- The FDA guidelines indicate that any health claim on a label must be supported by substantial scientific evidence. The following claims are examples:
  - Low sodium and the prevention of hypertension
  - Calcium and vitamin D and the prevention of osteoporosis
  - Low dietary fat and a reduced risk of cancer
  - Low dietary cholesterol and saturated fat and a reduced risk of coronary heart disease
  - Fiber-containing grain products, fruits, and vegetables and a reduced risk of cancer
  - Grain products and fruits and vegetables that contain fiber, especially soluble fiber, and the prevention of coronary heart disease
  - Fruits and vegetables that are rich in vitamins A or C and a lowered risk of cancer
  - Folate and the prevention of neural tube defects
  - Soy protein and a reduced risk of coronary heart disease
  - Stanols/sterols and a reduced risk of coronary heart disease
- For more information, refer to "Health Claims Meeting Significant Scientific Agreement" on the FDA website at www.fda.gov/food/ingredientspackaginglabeling/labelingnutrition/ucm2006876.htm.

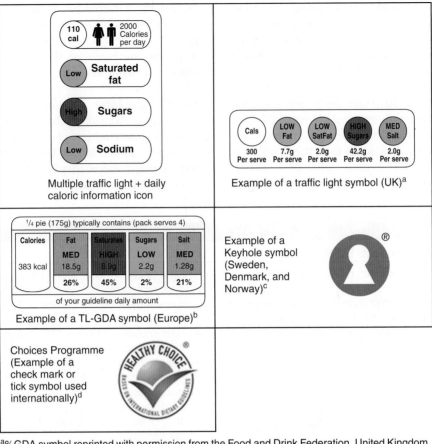

Multiple traffic light + daily caloric information icon

Example of a traffic light symbol (UK)[a]

Example of a TL-GDA symbol (Europe)[b]

Example of a Keyhole symbol (Sweden, Denmark, and Norway)[c]

Choices Programme (Example of a check mark or tick symbol used internationally)[d]

[a]%GDA symbol reprinted with permission from the Food and Drink Federation, United Kingdom.
[b]TL-GDA symbol reprinted with permission from the Food Standards Agency, United Kingdom.
[c]Keyhole symbol reprinted with permission from the National Food Administration, Sweden.
[d]Choices logo reprinted with permission from the Choices International Foundation, Belgium.

FIGURE 13-2 Examples of front-of-packaging labels. (Hersey JC et al. Effects of front-of-package and shelf nutrition labeling systems on consumers. *Nutr Rev.* 2013;71[1]:1-14; Roberto, C.A., et al., Evaluation of consumer understanding of different front-of-package nutrition labels, 2010-2011. Prev Chronic Dis, 2012. 9: p. E149.)

are currently in deliberation to establish standardized regulations for such labels. Ideally, front-of-package labels would be symbolic (instead of text-heavy) and easy to visually interpret. Such icons should be understandable despite education level or native language. Studies indicate that using the multiple traffic light plus caloric intake label (see Figure 13-2) is the most well accepted and comprehensive way to help individuals identify healthier food options.[5,6]

Since front-of-package and shelf-tag labeling is voluntary and at the discretion of the food manufacturer, there are many limitations with this method of consumer nutrition education. Consumers may be confused and frustrated with the inconsistencies of nutrition information printed on processed food packages. Much to the chagrin of nutrition professionals and the public in general, the labels food manufacturers choose to use on their products may or may not be helpful in deciphering the foods that are the most wholesome. The inherit problem is that there is not a uniformly accepted method for defining a food's overall *diet quality*.[7] The oscillation of these messages tends to discredit the intent instead of instill trust in

the public. Some experts believe that front-of-package labeling should be banned altogether because the focus should remain on the Nutrition Facts Label alone.[8]

Health claims. Health claims that link nutrients or food groups with a risk for disease are strictly regulated. To make an association between a food product and a specific disease, the FDA must approve the claim, the food must meet the criteria set forth for that specific claim, and the wording used on the package must be approved. Health claims can often be found on the front, side, or back of a food package.

A list of nutrients that are currently approved for use in the United States and the specific diseases with which they are associated is given in the For Further Focus box entitled "Glossary of Terms for Nutrition Facts Labels." An example of such a health claim would be the link between a diet that is low in saturated fat and cholesterol and a reduced risk of coronary heart disease. For a food to carry this label, it must be low in saturated fat, low in cholesterol, and low in total fat. If the food is fish or game meat, it must be deemed "extra lean." The specific wording of this example claim must include the following: *saturated fat and cholesterol, coronary heart disease,* or *heart disease;* there must also be a physician's statement about the claim that defines high or normal total cholesterol level. The FDA also provides model claim statements from which food producers may choose. For this specific claim, the model statement is as follows: *"Although many factors affect heart disease, diets low in saturated fat and cholesterol may reduce the risk of this disease."*[4]

FOOD TECHNOLOGY

America's food supply has radically changed over the years. These changes, which have swept the food marketing system, are rooted in widespread social changes and scientific advances. The agricultural and food processing industries have developed various methods and chemicals to increase and preserve the food supply. However, critics voice concerns about how these changes have affected food safety and the overall environment. Such concerns are frequently focused on pesticide use and food additives.

AGRICULTURAL PESTICIDES

Reasons for Use

Large American agricultural corporations as well as individual farmers use a number of chemicals to improve their crop yields. These materials have made possible the advances in food production that are deemed necessary to feed a growing population. For example, farmers use certain chemicals to control a wide variety of destructive insects that reduce crop yield.

Problems

Concerns and confusion continue regarding the use and effects of such chemicals. The four general areas of concern are as follows: (1) pesticide residues on foods; (2) the gradual leaching of the chemicals into groundwater and surrounding wells; (3) the increased exposure of farm workers to these strong chemicals; and (4) the increased amount of chemicals necessary as insects develop tolerance. Over time, the use of these chemicals has created a pesticide dilemma, and there is currently no clear answer regarding what to do in the face of conflicting interests. Thousands of pesticides are in use, and assessing the risks of specific pesticides is an important but complicated task.

Alternative Agriculture

An increasing number of concerned farmers, with help from soil scientists, are turning away from heavy pesticide use toward alternative agricultural methods.

Organic farming. Organic plant foods are grown without synthetic pesticides, fertilizers, sewage sludge, genetically modified organisms, or ionizing radiation.

Organic meat, poultry, eggs, and dairy products are from animals that have been raised without antibiotics or growth hormones. In 2002 the USDA enacted a set of nationally recognized standards to identify certified organic food. For a food to carry the USDA Organic Seal (Figure 13-3), the farm and processing plant where the food was grown and packaged must have undergone government inspections and met the USDA organic standards (see the For Further Focus box, "Organic Food Standards").[9] All foods that are produced organically are not required to use the organic label; it is a voluntary program. Companies that use the label on their food without certification face a large fine. Sales of organic foods are rapidly growing and an increasing number of farmers—especially in California, which is the major supplier of U.S. fruits and vegetables—are using organic farming.

There are many studies available in the literature comparing specific nutritional parameters of individual foods grown either in an organic or in a conventional manner. When looking at the available evidence as a whole, organic foods are not recognized as being safer or more nutritious than conventionally produced foods.[10] However, organic foods are 30% less likely to contain pesticide residues and may be less likely to contain antibiotic-resistance bacteria. There

> **organic farming** the use of farming methods that employ natural means of pest control and that meet the standards set by the National Organic Program of the U.S. Department of Agriculture; organic foods are grown or produced without the use of synthetic pesticides or fertilizers, sewage sludge, genetically modified organisms, or ionizing radiation.

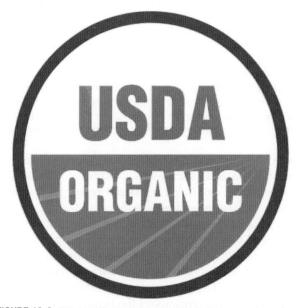

FIGURE 13-3 Official U.S. Department of Agriculture organic seal, which is available at www.ams.usda.gov/AMSv1.0/nop. (Courtesy National Organic Program, Agricultural Marketing Service, U.S. Department of Agriculture, Washington, DC.)

Organic Food Standards

The National Organic Program, which is a constituent of the U.S. Department of Agriculture (USDA), was established to ensure standards for organic foods. In response to the growing market, the National Organic Program has set strict standards for the growth, production, and labeling of organic foods. Although many methods prohibited by the organic standards (e.g., irradiation, genetic modification) are deemed safe by the USDA, these methods of farming have been banned in certified organic foods because of public concern.

Organic foods have four labeling categories with specific guidelines for each, as follows:

1. *100% organic:* Products that carry this label must be made or produced exclusively with certified organic ingredients, and they must have passed a government inspection. These products may use the USDA Organic Seal on their labels and advertisements.

2. *Organic:* Products labeled as *organic* must contain 95% to 100% organic ingredients and also must have passed a government inspection. The National Organic Program must approve all other ingredients for use as nonagricultural substances or as products not commercially available in organic form. These products may also use the USDA Organic Seal with the percentage of organic ingredients listed.

3. *70% organic ingredients:* Products made with at least 70% certified organic ingredients may state on the product label *"made with organic ingredients"* and list up to three ingredients or food groups. These foods also must meet the National Organic Program guidelines for growth or production without synthetic pesticides, fertilizers, sewage sludge, bioengineering, or ionizing radiation. The USDA Organic Seal may not be displayed on these products or used in any advertising.

4. *Less than 70% organic ingredients:* Foods made with less than 70% certified organic ingredients may not use the USDA Organic Seal or make any organic claims on the front panel of the package. They can list the specific organic ingredients on the side panel of the package.

All food products made with at least 70% organic ingredients must also supply the name and address of the government-approved certifying agent on the product.

For more information about the USDA organic standards, visit the National Organic Program website at www.ams.usda.gov/AMSv1.0/nop.

---

are no significant differences in the risk of contamination with bacteria such as *Escherichia coli*, *Salmonella*, *Campylobacter*, or *Listeria* between organic vs. conventionally grown meat products.[10]

Organic farmers can still use natural pesticides and fertilizers; therefore, they are not producing pesticide-free foods. Other common points of confusion are with the use of the following terms: *natural*, *hormone free*, and *free range*. These terms are not synonymous with *organic*. Truthful terms about the production of a food can appear on the food label, but they do not mean that the product is organic. The term *natural* may be used on products that contain no artificial ingredients (e.g., coloring, chemical preservatives) and if the product and its ingredients are only minimally processed. The Food Safety and Inspection Service of the USDA does not approve use of the terms *hormone free* or *antibiotic free*. Instead, the phrases *raised without added hormones* and *raised without added antibiotics* are allowed, provided that the producer is able to supply an affidavit that attests to the production practices that are used to support the claim. One important note about the use of hormones is that they are approved for use only in beef cattle and lamb production. Therefore, any such claim on a poultry product would be allowed only if it were immediately followed by this statement: "Federal regulations prohibit the use of hormones in poultry."

Organic farming may be more beneficial for the environment and safer for the agricultural workers; however, methods for assessing the differences are currently lacking.[11] Regardless of environmental and nutritional impact, organic farming has lower crop yields, requires more land, and is more expensive than conventional crops. Nevertheless, the consumer demand for organic food in the United States continues to thrive and provides encouragement for the development of sustainable systems to support organic agriculture.

Biotechnology. Biotechnology is a broad term that has application in human nutrition, medications, agriculture, and environmental sciences. Biotechnology is the use of biologic processes or organisms to make or modify products. In its most basic form, selective breeding of plants or animals with desired traits is an example of biotechnology that has been in use for many millenniums. Two commonly used medications produced through means of biotechnology are insulin and penicillin. Two examples of biotechnology in agriculture and nutrition are the development of corn that expresses a specific protein that serves as an insecticide and the synthesis of rice with increased levels of β-carotene.

While genetic manipulation in various forms has been used to improve crop yields for thousands of years, most U.S. consumers are unaware of the extent to which these foods have entered the marketplace. In the United States, 94% of soybean crop acreage and 93% of corn crops are genetically modified (GM) varieties (Figure 13-4).[12] Thus, most people in the United States have consumed some form of GM foods because corn and soy are pervasive in grocery store products.

Plant physiologists have developed strains of plants that reduce the need for toxic pesticide and herbicide application. Other GM products are developed for qualities such as drought resistance; enhanced protein, oil, or vitamin content; and viral/fungal resistance. Approved genetic modifications are currently used to protect against virus infections and insects on tomatoes, potatoes, squash, papayas, rice, sugarbeets, and

Rapid Growth in Adoption of Genetically Engineered Crops Continues in the U.S.

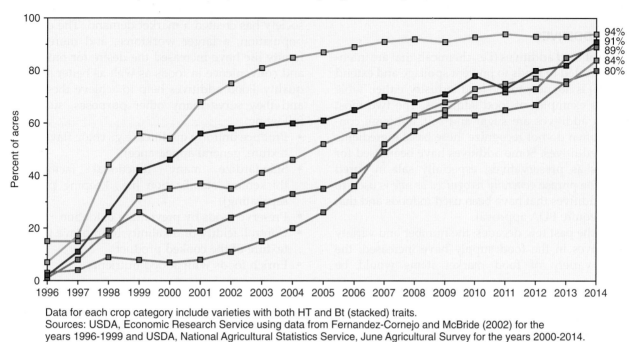

Data for each crop category include varieties with both HT and Bt (stacked) traits.
Sources: USDA, Economic Research Service using data from Fernandez-Cornejo and McBride (2002) for the years 1996-1999 and USDA, National Agricultural Statistics Service, June Agricultural Survey for the years 2000-2014.

—— HT soybeans   —— HT cotton   —— Bt cotton   —— Bt corn   —— HT corn

FIGURE 13-4 Adoption of genetically engineered crops continues to grow rapidly in the United States. *Bt, Bacillus thuringiensis* bacterium; *HT, herbicide tolerant.* (Reprinted from U.S. Department of Agriculture, Economic Research Service. *Adoption of genetically engineered crops in the U.S., 2014.* Washington, DC: 2014.)

other crops. GM crops are tested for their composition, safety, and environmental effects. The National Institutes of Health, the Animal Plant Health Inspection Service of the USDA, the FDA, and the Environmental Protection Agency are all involved in the regulation of GM foods in commercial use, which are the most heavily regulated foods.

Such forms of agriculture remain controversial around the world because of many unknown factors regarding the long-term effects on the environment and overall human health. Research that was completed with soybeans revealed that wild-type and GM soybean varieties had exactly the same allergenicity, thus concluding that genetic modification did not increase the likelihood of allergies in this crop.[13] This type of research will be important for all types of GM crops to ensure safety and improve consumer acceptability.

Irradiation. Food irradiation is the use of ionizing radiation to kill bacteria and parasites that are on food after harvest. Irradiation helps to prevent food-borne illness caused by *Escherichia coli, Salmonella, Campylobacter, Listeria, Shigella,* and *Salmonella*. Three different methods of irradiation are used, all of which are approved by the World Health Organization, the Centers for Disease Control and Prevention (CDC), the USDA, and the FDA.

The use of irradiation is not a new science; wheat flour and white potatoes were approved for irradiation

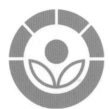

FIGURE 13-5 Radura symbol of irradiation. (Courtesy Food Safety and Inspection Service, U.S. Department of Agriculture, Washington, DC.)

during the early 1960s. In addition to reducing or eliminating disease-causing germs, irradiation can be used to increase the shelf-life of produce. Foods that are irradiated have unaltered nutritional value; they are not radioactive, they have no harmful substances introduced as a result of irradiation, but they may taste slightly different.[14] A variety of foods have been approved for irradiation in the United States, including meat, poultry, grains, some seafood, fruits, vegetables, herbs, and spices. The FDA requires that all irradiated foods be appropriately labeled either with the radura symbol for irradiation (Figure 13-5) or with a written description that states that the food has been exposed to irradiation.

Consumer rejection in the United States and around the world is mainly the result of altered taste and a fear of the unknown long-term effects of irradiation on human health. The U.S. government continues to support the use and safety of such foods; however, without consumer acceptance, companies that are using such procedures have limited success.

FOOD ADDITIVES

The use of food additives (i.e., chemicals that are intentionally added to foods to prevent spoilage and extend shelf-life) is not new to the food industry, either. Table 13-2 lists examples of food additives. The two most common additives are sugar and salt, although consumers often do not recognize these basic ingredients as food additives. Some additives have been used for centuries as preservatives, especially salt in cured meats. The phrase *generally recognized as safe* is used to define additives that have been used in foods and that do not require FDA approval.

Over the past few decades, the number and variety of additives in the food supply have increased; the current variety of food market items would be

impossible without them. Scientific advances have created processed food products, and the changing society has created a market demand. The expanding population, a larger workforce, and more complex family life have increased the desire for more variety and convenience in foods as well as better safety and quality. Food additives help to achieve these desires, and they serve many other purposes, such as the following:

- Produce uniform qualities (e.g., color, flavor, aroma, texture, general appearance)
- Standardize many functional factors (e.g., thickening, stabilization [i.e., keeping parts from separating])
- Preserve foods by preventing oxidation
- Control acidity or alkalinity to improve flavor and texture of the cooked product
- Enrich foods with added nutrients

Table 13-2	Examples of Food Additives

The following summary lists the types of common food ingredients, the reasons they are used, and some examples of the names that can be found on product labels that refer to them. Some additives are used for more than one purpose.

TYPES OF INGREDIENTS	WHAT THEY DO	EXAMPLES OF USES	NAMES FOUND ON PRODUCT LABELS
Preservatives	Prevent food spoilage from bacteria, mold, fungi, or yeast (antimicrobials); slow or prevent changes in color, flavor, or texture and delay rancidity (antioxidants); maintain freshness	Fruit sauces and jellies, beverages, baked goods, cured meats, oils and margarines, cereals, dressings, snack foods, packaged fruits, and vegetables	Ascorbic acid, citric acid, sodium benzoate, calcium propionate, sodium erythorbate, sodium nitrite, calcium sorbate, potassium sorbate, BHA, BHT, EDTA, tocopherols (vitamin E)
Sweeteners	Add sweetness with or without extra calories (nutritive or non-nutritive)	Beverages, baked goods, confections, table-top sugar, sugar substitutes, many processed foods	Sucrose (sugar), glucose, fructose, sorbitol, mannitol, corn syrup, high fructose corn syrup, saccharin, aspartame, sucralose, acesulfame potassium (acesulfame-K), neotame
Color additives	Offset color loss due to exposure to light, air, temperature extremes, moisture and storage conditions; correct natural variations in color; enhance colors that occur naturally; provide color to colorless foods	Many processed foods, (candies, snack foods, margarine, cheese, soft drinks, jams and jellies, gelatins, pudding and pie fillings)	FD&C Blue Nos. 1 and 2, FD&C Green No. 3, FD&C Red Nos. 3 and 40, FD&C Yellow Nos. 5 and 6, Orange B, Citrus Red No. 2, annatto extract, beta-carotene, grape skin extract, cochineal extract or carmine, paprika oleoresin, caramel color, fruit and vegetable juices, saffron (NOTE: Exempt color additives are not required to be declared by name on labels but may be declared simply as colorings or color added)
Flavors and spices	Add specific flavors (natural and synthetic)	Pudding and pie fillings, gelatin dessert mixes, cake mixes, salad dressings, candies, soft drinks, ice cream, BBQ sauce	Natural flavoring, artificial flavor, and spices

Table 13-2   Examples of Food Additives—cont'd

TYPES OF INGREDIENTS	WHAT THEY DO	EXAMPLES OF USES	NAMES FOUND ON PRODUCT LABELS
Flavor enhancers	Enhance flavors already present in foods (without providing their own separate flavor)	Many processed foods	Monosodium glutamate (MSG), hydrolyzed soy protein, autolyzed yeast extract, disodium guanylate or inosinate
Fat replacers (and components of formulations that are used to replace fats)	Provide expected texture and a creamy "mouth-feel" in reduced-fat foods	Baked goods, dressings, frozen desserts, confections, cake and dessert mixes, dairy products	Olestra, cellulose gel, carrageenan, polydextrose, modified food starch, microparticulated egg white protein, guar gum, xanthan gum, whey protein concentrate
Nutrients	Replace vitamins and minerals lost in processing (enrichment), add nutrients that may be lacking in the diet (fortification)	Flour, breads, cereals, rice, macaroni, margarine, salt, milk, fruit beverages, energy bars, instant breakfast drinks	Thiamine hydrochloride, riboflavin (vitamin B_2), niacin, niacinamide, folate or folic acid, β-carotene, potassium iodide, iron or ferrous sulfate, α-tocopherols, ascorbic acid, vitamin D, amino acids (L-tryptophan, L-lysine, L-leucine, L-methionine)
Emulsifiers	Allow smooth mixing of ingredients, prevent separation, keep emulsified products stable, reduce stickiness, control crystallization, keep ingredients dispersed, and help products dissolve more easily	Salad dressings, peanut butter, chocolate, margarine, frozen desserts	Soy lecithin, mono- and diglycerides, egg yolks, polysorbates, sorbitan monostearate
Stabilizers, thickeners, binders, and texturizers	Produce uniform texture, improve "mouth-feel"	Frozen desserts, dairy products, cakes, pudding and gelatin mixes, dressings, jams and jellies, sauces	Gelatin, pectin, guar gum, carrageenan, xanthan gum, whey
pH control agents and acidulants	Control acidity and alkalinity, prevent spoilage	Beverages, frozen desserts, chocolate, low-acid canned foods, baking powder	Lactic acid, citric acid, ammonium hydroxide, sodium carbonate
Leavening agents	Promote rising of baked goods	Breads and other baked goods	Baking soda, monocalcium phosphate, calcium carbonate
Anti-caking agents	Keep powdered foods free-flowing, prevent moisture absorption	Salt, baking powder, confectioner's sugar	Calcium silicate, iron ammonium citrate, silicon dioxide
Humectants	Retain moisture	Shredded coconut, marshmallows, soft candies, confections	Glycerin, sorbitol
Yeast nutrients	Promote growth of yeast	Breads and other baked goods	Calcium sulfate, ammonium phosphate
Dough strengtheners and conditioners	Produce more stable dough	Breads and other baked goods	Ammonium sulfate, azodicarbonamide, L-cysteine
Firming agents	Maintain crispness and firmness	Processed fruits and vegetables	Calcium chloride, calcium lactate
Enzyme preparations	Modify proteins, polysaccharides and fats	Cheese, dairy products, meat	Enzymes, lactase, papain, rennet, chymosin
Gases	Serve as propellant, aerate, or create carbonation	Oil cooking spray, whipped cream, carbonated beverages	Carbon dioxide, nitrous oxide

Reprinted from International Food Information Council and U.S. Food and Drug Administration. *Food ingredients and colors, 2010.* Available at: <www.fda.gov/downloads/Food/IngredientsPackagingLabeling/ucm094249.pdf>; Accessed January 2015.

A number of micronutrients and antioxidants are used as additives in processed foods not for their ability to increase nutrient content but rather for their technical effects either during processing or in the final product.

FOOD-BORNE DISEASE

Tracking the prevalence, food origin, and pathogen responsible for food-borne illness is an extremely difficult task. The symptoms of food-borne illness are often difficult to distinguish from other forms of illness and are often thought of as a "stomach bug" or "flu." Furthermore, most forms of food-borne illness are short-lived and self-limiting, and the victim does not visit a physician. Or, even if the person does see a physician, the pathogen responsible may not be identified. The CDC tracks, investigates, and reports the incidence of food-borne illness in the United States but their ability to do so is dependent upon the illness first being reported to them. Local, state, and tribal health departments voluntarily report food-borne illness to the CDC. **Outbreaks of food-borne illness** are more likely to be reported to the CDC than individual instances of illness. Thus, the estimated cases of food-borne illness are extrapolations of actual reported cases using the assumption that most cases are not reported.

> **outbreak of food-borne illness** defined by the CDC as the occurrence of two or more similar illnesses resulting from ingestion of a common food.

PREVALENCE

The CDC estimates that 1 in 6 people gets sick each year from food-borne illness. Many disease-bearing organisms inhabit the environment and can contaminate food and water. Much has been learned about the pathogens that commonly contaminate food and water and about ways to prevent food-borne illness outbreaks. However, lapses in control still occur, and these can result in high incidences of illness and hospitalization as well as economic burden. The estimated annual incidence of food-borne illness continues to be a public health concern since rates are well above *Healthy People 2020* targets.[15] Figure 13-6 presents the relative rates of confirmed cases of certain pathogens in 2014 compared to those from 2006. Of the identified causes of food-borne illness in the United States, 54% are due to bacteria, 36% are due to viruses, 8% are the result of chemical or toxic agents, and 2% are due to parasites.[16]

FOOD SAFETY

Buying and Storing Food

The control of food-borne disease focuses on strict sanitation measures and rigid personal hygiene. First, the food itself should be of good quality and not defective or diseased. Second, dry or cold storage should protect it from deterioration or decay, which is especially important for products such as refrigerated convenience foods; this is the fastest growing segment of the convenience food market, and it is potentially the most dangerous because these foods are not sterile. These vacuum-packaged or modified-atmosphere chilled food products are only minimally processed

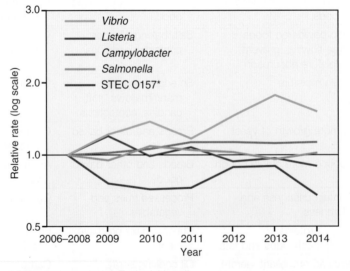

* Shiga toxin-producing Escherichia coli

FIGURE 13-6 Relative rates of culture-confirmed infections with known pathogens compared with 2006-2008 rates, by year. The actual incidences of these infections cannot be determined from this figure. (From Crim SM et al. Preliminary incidence and trends of infection with pathogens transmitted commonly through food - Foodborne Diseases Active Surveillance Network, 10 U.S. sites, 2006-2014. *MMWR Morb Mortal Wkly Rep.* 2015;64[18]: 495-499.)

and not sterilized, and they are at risk of temperature abuse. Home refrigerator temperatures should be held at ≤40° F. At temperatures ≥45° F, any precooked or leftover foods are potential reservoirs for bacteria that survive cooking and that can then recontaminate cooked food. Food safety depends on the following critical actions (Figure 13-7):

- *Clean:* Wash hands and surfaces often.
- *Separate:* Do not cross-contaminate.
- *Cook:* Cook to proper temperatures.
- *Chill:* Refrigerate promptly.

All food preparation areas must be scrupulously clean, and foods must be washed or cleaned well. Cooking procedures and temperatures must be followed as directed. All utensils, dishes, and anything else that comes in contact with food must be clean. Leftover food should be stored and reheated appropriately or discarded (Table 13-3). Food does not need to be cooled to room temperature before refrigerating; this practice allows food to sit in a temperature range that is perfect for bacterial growth. Leftovers should be refrigerated within 2 hours. Garbage must be contained and disposed in a sanitary manner. Safe methods of food handling, cooking, and storage are simple and mostly common sense; however, they often are neglected, and this may lead to food-borne illness.

Food safety publications for all types of foods and populations can be found at the Food Safety and Inspection Service website at www.fsis.usda.gov.

Preparing and Serving Food

All people who handle food—especially those who work in public food services—should follow strict measures to prevent contamination. For example, washing hands properly and wearing clean clothing,

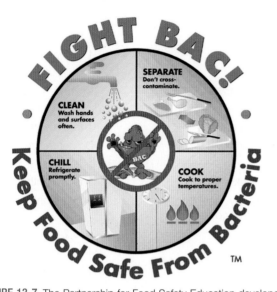

FIGURE 13-7 The Partnership for Food Safety Education developed the "Fight BAC!" (i.e., bacteria) campaign to prevent food-borne illness. Campaign graphics are available at www.fightbac.org. (Courtesy Partnership for Food Safety Education, Washington, DC.)

Table 13-3 Cold Storage		
PRODUCT	**REFRIGERATOR (40° F)**	**FREEZER (0° F)**
Eggs		
Fresh, in shell	3 to 5 weeks	Do not freeze
Raw yolks and whites	2 to 4 days	1 year
Hard cooked	1 week	Does not freeze well
Liquid Pasteurized Eggs, Egg Substitutes		
Opened	3 days	Does not freeze well
Unopened	10 days	1 year
Mayonnaise, Commercial		
Refrigerate after opening	2 months	Do not freeze
Frozen Dinners and Entrees		
Keep frozen until ready to heat	—	3 to 4 months
Deli and Vacuum-Packed Products		
Store-prepared (or homemade) egg, chicken, ham, tuna, and macaroni salads	3 to 5 days	Does not freeze well
Hot Dogs and Luncheon Meats		
Hot Dogs		
Opened package	1 week	1 to 2 months
Unopened package	2 weeks	1 to 2 months
Luncheon Meat		
Opened package	3 to 5 days	1 to 2 months
Unopened package	2 weeks	1 to 2 months

Continued

Table 13-3   Cold Storage—cont'd

PRODUCT	REFRIGERATOR (40° F)	FREEZER (0° F)
Bacon and Sausage		
Bacon	7 days	1 month
Sausage, raw—from chicken, turkey, pork, beef	1 to 2 days	1 to 2 months
Smoked breakfast links, patties	7 days	1 to 2 months
Hard sausage—pepperoni, jerky sticks	2 to 3 weeks	1 to 2 months
Summer Sausage Labeled "Keep Refrigerated"		
Opened	3 weeks	1 to 2 months
Unopened	3 months	1 to 2 months
Corned Beef		
Corned beef, in pouch with pickling juices	5 to 7 days	Drained, 1 month
Ham, Canned, Labeled "Keep Refrigerated"		
Opened	3 to 5 days	1 to 2 months
Unopened	6 to 9 months	Do not freeze
Ham, Fully Cooked		
Vacuum sealed at plant, undated, unopened	2 weeks	1 to 2 months
Vacuum sealed at plant, dated, unopened	"Use-By" date on package	1 to 2 months
Whole	7 days	1 to 2 months
Half	3 to 5 days	1 to 2 months
Slices	3 to 4 days	1 to 2 months
Hamburger, Ground, and Stew Meat		
Hamburger and stew meat	1 to 2 days	3 to 4 months
Ground turkey, veal, pork, lamb, and mixtures of them	1 to 2 days	3 to 4 months
Fresh Beef, Veal, Lamb, and Pork		
Steaks	3 to 5 days	6 to 12 months
Chops	3 to 5 days	4 to 6 months
Roasts	3 to 5 days	4 to 12 months
Variety meats—tongue, liver, heart, kidneys, chitterlings	1 to 2 days	3 to 4 months
Prestuffed, uncooked pork chops, lamb chops, or chicken breasts stuffed with dressing	1 day	Does not freeze well
Soups and stews, vegetable or meat added	3 to 4 days	2 to 3 months
Fresh Poultry		
Chicken or turkey, whole	1 to 2 days	1 year
Chicken or turkey, pieces	1 to 2 days	9 months
Giblets	1 to 2 days	3 to 4 months
Cooked Meat and Poultry Leftovers		
Cooked meat and meat casseroles	3 to 4 days	2 to 3 months
Gravy and meat broth	1 to 2 days	2 to 3 months
Fried chicken	3 to 4 days	4 months
Cooked poultry casseroles	3 to 4 days	4 to 6 months
Poultry pieces, plain	3 to 4 days	4 months
Poultry pieces in broth, gravy	3 to 4 days	6 months
Chicken nuggets, patties	3 to 4 days	1 to 3 months
Other Cooked Leftovers		
Pizza, cooked	3 to 4 days	1 to 2 months
Stuffing, cooked	3 to 4 days	1 month

Reprinted from Food Safety and Inspection Service. *Basics for handling food safely.* Available at <www.fsis.usda.gov/wps/portal/fsis/topics/food-safety-education/get-answers/food-safety-fact-sheets/safe-food-handling>; Accessed January 2015.

gloves, and aprons are imperative. Basic rules of hygiene should apply to all people who are handling food, whether they work in food processing and packaging plants, process and package foods in markets, or prepare and serve food in restaurants. In addition, people with infectious diseases should have limited access to direct food handling.

The following are the minimal internal temperatures to be reached when cooking various foods:

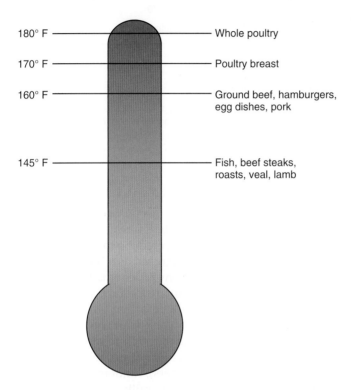

180° F — Whole poultry

170° F — Poultry breast

160° F — Ground beef, hamburgers, egg dishes, pork

145° F — Fish, beef steaks, roasts, veal, lamb

The Hazard Analysis & Critical Control Point (HACCP) food safety system focuses on preventing food-borne illness by identifying critical points and eliminating hazards. Many organizations, including the USDA and the FDA, use the HACCP standards. For more information about HACCP, visit www.fda.gov/Food/GuidanceRegulation/HACCP/default.htm.

FOOD CONTAMINATION

Food-borne illness usually presents with flu-like symptoms, but it can advance to a lethal illness. Not all bacteria found in foods are harmful, and some are even beneficial (e.g., the bacteria in yogurt). Bacteria that are harmful to people are referred to as *pathogens*. Certain subgroups of the population are at higher risk for the development of food-borne illness as a result of age and physical condition. Groups with the highest risks are young children, pregnant women, elderly individuals, and people with compromised immune systems.

Food-borne illness generally results from the ingestion of bacteria, viruses, or parasites. Illness that results from bacteria is caused either by an infection or by toxins that are produced by the bacteria. All types of foods can be carriers of food-borne illness. Figure 13-8

shows the relative existence of food-borne illness due to various food sources.

Bacterial Food Infections

Bacterial food infections result from eating food that is contaminated by large colonies of bacteria. Specific diseases result from specific bacteria (e.g., salmonellosis, shigellosis, listeriosis).

Salmonellosis. Salmonellosis is caused by *Salmonella*, a bacterium that was named for the American veterinarian pathologist Daniel Salmon (1850-1914), who first isolated and identified the species that commonly cause food-borne infections: *Salmonella typhi* and *Salmonella paratyphi*. *Salmonella* can be found in the gastrointestinal tracts of most animals, including humans and birds. These organisms readily grow in raw or unpasteurized milk or foods containing raw or undercooked eggs, poultry, or meat. Seafood from polluted waters—especially shellfish such as oysters and clams—may also be a source of infection. The unsanitary handling of foods and utensils can spread the bacteria. Resulting cases of gastroenteritis may vary from mild to severe diarrhea. Immunization, pasteurization, and sanitary regulations that involve community water and food supplies as well as food handlers help to control outbreaks.

Approximately 40,000 cases of salmonellosis are reported in the United States each year, although thousands of other cases likely are unreported.[17] Because the incubation and reproduction of the bacteria take time after the food is eaten, symptoms of food infection develop relatively slowly (i.e., up to 48 hours later). Symptoms include diarrhea, fever, vomiting, and abdominal cramps. The illness usually lasts 4 to 7 days, with most affected individuals recovering completely. Severe dehydration from diarrhea and vomiting may require intravenous fluids.

Shigellosis. Shigellosis is caused by the bacteria *Shigella,* which was named for the Japanese physician Kiyoshi Shiga (1870-1957), who first discovered a main species of the organism, *Shigella dysenteriae,* during a dysentery epidemic in Japan in 1898. *Shigella* is in the feces of infected individuals and is transmitted to other people or food through means of poor hygiene. The boiling of water or the pasteurization of milk kills the organisms, but the food or milk may easily be reinfected through unsanitary handling. The disease is spread similarly to how salmonella is transmitted: by feces, fingers, and flies and by foods that are handled by unsanitary carriers. Shigellosis, similar to salmonellosis, is more common during the summer, and it most often occurs in young children.

Approximately 14,000 cases are reported annually, but because many cases are not diagnosed, the CDC estimates that the actual number of cases may be as much as 20 times higher.[18] Shigellosis is usually

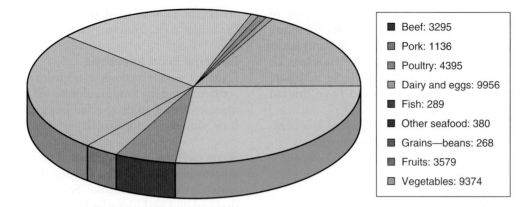

Source: Interagency Food Safety Analytics Collaboration (IFSAC) Project.
Foodborne Illness Source Attribution Estimates for Salmonella, Escherichia coli O157 (E. coli O157),
Listeria monocytogenes (Lm), and Campylobacter using Outbreak Surveillance Data, 2015.)

FIGURE 13-8 The number of illnesses attributed to each food category during 2008-2012. Includes total illnesses caused by a single confirmed case of either *Salmonella, E. coli O157, Campylobacter,* or *Listeria* and attributed to a food that can be assigned to a single food category. (Source: Interagency Food Safety Analytics Collaboration [IFSAC] Project. *Foodborne illness source attribution estimates for Salmonella, Escherichia coli O157 [E. coli O157], Listeria monocytogenes (Lm), and Campylobacter using outbreak surveillance data,* 2015.)

confined to the large intestine; it may vary from a mild, transient intestinal disturbance in adults to fatal dysentery in young children. Symptoms appear within 4 to 7 days and include cramps, diarrhea, fever, vomiting, and blood or mucus in the stool. Because of the long incubation period, it is exceptionally difficult to identify the food source.

Listeriosis. Listeriosis is caused by the bacteria *Listeria,* which was named for the English surgeon Baron Joseph Lister (1827-1912), who first applied knowledge of bacterial infection to the principles of antiseptic surgery in a benchmark 1867 publication that led to "clean" operations and the development of modern surgery. However, only within the past 30 years has knowledge of bacteria's role as a direct cause of foodborne illness increased and the major species to cause human illness, *Listeria monocytogenes,* been identified. Before 1981, *Listeria* was thought to be an organism of animal disease that was transmitted to people only by direct contact with infected animals. However, this organism occurs widely in the environment and in high-risk individuals, such as the elderly, pregnant women, infants, and patients with suppressed immune systems.

Listeriosis can produce a rare but fatal illness with severe symptoms such as diarrhea, flu-like fever and headache, pneumonia, sepsis, meningitis, and endocarditis. Pregnant women are 10 times more likely to get listeriosis than the general public.[19] Listeriosis has been traced to a variety of foods, including soft cheese, poultry, seafood, raw milk, refrigerated raw liquid whole eggs, and meat products (e.g., pâté). *Listeria* is capable of growing in some foods despite being refrigerated.

Escherichia coli. *Escherichia coli* was discovered by Theodor Escherich (1857-1911), a German pediatrician and bacteriologist who discovered the rod-shaped bacteria in 1885. It was not recognized as a human pathogen until 1982. There are many types of *E. coli,* and not all types are harmful to humans. In fact, some strains are part of the healthy gut flora that survive in the intestines and produce a valuable supply of vitamin K. *E. coli* is most often spread through fecal contamination (e.g., contaminated foods, not properly washing hands after changing diapers), undercooked meat, and unpasteurized foods (e.g., milk, apple cider, soft cheeses).

An estimated 265,000 infections from Shiga toxin–producing strains of *E. coli* occur annually in the United States and 36% of those are from the O157:H7 strain.[20] This strain is most dangerous to young children and elderly adults (see the Drug-Nutrient Interaction box, "Drug-Resistant *Escherichia coli* and the Food Supply"). Most cases involve diarrhea, stomach cramps, and low-grade fevers that start within 2 to 8 days after ingestion and that usually resolve within 7 days. About 5% to 10% of individuals infected with *E. coli* will develop **hemolytic uremic syndrome**, which is a potentially deadly condition.

Vibrio. Filippo Pacini (1812-1883) first isolated microorganisms that he called "vibrions" from cholera patients in 1854. Prevalence of infection from these

hemolytic uremic syndrome a condition that results most often from infection with *Escherichia coli* and that presents with a breaking up of red blood cells (i.e., hemolysis) and kidney failure.

Drug-Nutrient Interaction

Drug-Resistant *Escherichia coli* and the Food Supply

KELLI BOI

The agricultural use of antimicrobial drugs is suspected in the development of drug-resistant bacterial strains that are transmitted to humans via the food supply.[1] Drug-resistant strains of *Escherichia coli* bacteria are prevalent in the retail meat and poultry supply businesses. Resistance to first-line antibiotics by these bacteria represents a major cause of illness, death, and increased health care costs. Researchers have found that drug-resistant *E. coli* infections in humans were more closely related to the strains of bacteria found in chickens than to those found in the gut flora of humans, which suggests that drug-resistant *E. coli* strains are likely transmitted to humans via poultry that is carrying the infection.[2]

A classic example is the 2006 outbreak of *E. coli* infection in the United States that was traced to commercially grown spinach. This prompted a nationwide recall of bagged spinach and of products that had been made with the contaminated spinach. Upon investigation, the U.S. Food and Drug Administration found several environmental risk factors, including proximity to waterways that were exposed to cattle and wildlife feces.[3] Although the washing of the spinach would not have prevented the *E. coli* outbreak, the U.S. Food and Drug Administration recommends the employment of safe food-handling practices among all consumers to prevent contamination from many causes.

Populations that are at risk for infection with drug-resistant strains of bacteria include children, elderly adults, and those who are immunocompromised. In health care settings, proper food safety practices are especially important. Drug-resistant strains of bacteria necessitate the long-term use of powerful antibiotics. Nausea, vomiting, and diarrhea are common with antibiotic use as a result of the destruction of the natural gut flora. Some antibiotics such as ciprofloxacin (Cipro) can bind to calcium, magnesium, iron, and zinc, thereby interfering with their absorption. Thus, the long-term use of this antibiotic can result in poor bioavailability of these minerals.

REFERENCES

1. Mellata M. Human and avian extraintestinal pathogenic *Escherichia coli*: infections, zoonotic risks, and antibiotic resistance trends. *Foodborne Pathog Dis*. 2013;10(11):916-932.
2. Johnson JR, et al. Antimicrobial drug-resistant *Escherichia coli* from humans and poultry products, Minnesota and Wisconsin, 2002-2004. *Emerg Infect Dis*. 2007;13(6):838-846.
3. U.S. Department of Health and Human Services. FDA finalizes report on 2006 spinach outbreak. Available from: <www.fda.gov/NewsEvents/Newsroom/PressAnnouncements/2007/ucm108873.htm>; 2007. Cited January 2015.

particular bacteria continues to rise in the United States.[15] It is a salt-requiring organism that inhabits the salt-water coastal regions of North America, and it is usually ingested by humans via contaminated seafood. Immunocompromised individuals are most susceptible to *Vibrio* infection. Thoroughly cooking seafood—especially shellfish such as oysters—reduces the risk of infection.[21]

Bacterial Food Poisoning

Food poisoning is caused by the ingestion of bacterial toxins that have been produced in food as a result of the growth of specific kinds of bacteria before the food is eaten. The powerful toxin is directly ingested, so symptoms of food poisoning develop rapidly. Two types of bacterial food poisoning, staphylococcal and clostridial, are most commonly responsible.

Staphylococcal food poisoning. Staphylococcal food poisoning was named for the causative organism, which is mainly *Staphylococcus aureus*, a round bacterium that forms masses of cells. *S. aureus* results in powerful toxins in the contaminated food that rapidly produce illness (i.e., 1 to 6 hours after ingestion). The symptoms appear suddenly, and they include severe cramping and abdominal pain with nausea, vomiting, and diarrhea, usually accompanied by sweating, headache, fever, and sometimes prostration and shock. However, recovery is fairly rapid, and symptoms ordinarily subside within 1 to 3 days (see the Clinical Applications box, "Case Study: A Community Food Poisoning Incident").[22] The amount of toxin ingested and the susceptibility of the individual eating it determine the degree of severity.

The source of the food contamination could be something as minor as a small, or even unnoticed, staphylococcal infection on the hand of a worker preparing the food. Foods that are particularly effective carriers of staphylococci and their toxins include custard or cream-filled bakery goods, processed meats, ham, tongue, cheese, ice cream, potato salad, sauces, chicken and ham salads, and combination dishes such as spaghetti and casseroles. The toxin causes no change in the normal appearance, odor, or taste of the food, so the victim has no warning. A careful food history helps to determine the source of the poisoning, and portions of the food are obtained for examination, if possible. Bacteria may not be found, because heating kills the organisms but does not destroy the toxins that have been produced.

Clostridial food poisoning. Clostridial food poisoning was named for spore-forming, rod-shaped bacteria, mainly *Clostridium perfringens* and *Clostridium botulinum*, which can also form powerful toxins in infected foods.

C. perfringens spores are widespread in the environment, including soil, water, dust, and refuse. This organism is frequently located on raw meat and poultry, and it multiplies rapidly when food is held at temperatures between 109° F and 117° F for extended periods of time. In many cases, cooked meat is improperly prepared, refrigerated, or reheated. Control depends on careful preparation and adequate cooking of meats, prompt service, and immediate refrigeration at sufficiently low temperatures. Once ingested, the

Clinical Applications

Case Study: A Community Food Poisoning Incident

John and Eva Wesson agreed that their lodge dinner had been the best they had ever had, especially the dessert: custard-filled cream puffs, John's favorite. He had eaten two of them, despite Eva's protests; and thought maybe that was why he began to feel ill shortly after they arrived home. Eva's stomach felt a little upset, too, so they both took some antacid pills, thinking that their "stomachaches" were from eating more rich food than they were accustomed to eating. They went to bed early.

However, by 11:00 PM, Eva woke up alarmed. John was vomiting, and he had diarrhea and increasingly severe stomach cramps. He complained of a headache, and his pajamas were wet with sweat. He had a fever and appeared to be in shock. Eva began to have similar pains and symptoms, although they were not as severe as John's pains.

One of their friends who had also been at the lodge dinner telephoned; she and her husband had the same symptoms.

By now, John was prostrate and unable to move. Eva immediately called 911, and they were both taken to the hospital. After treatment in the emergency department for shock, followed by observational care and rest the following day, John's symptoms had subsided, and he was allowed to go home. The physician advised John and Eva to eat lightly for a few days and to get more rest. He said that he would investigate the cause in the meantime. During the next few days, John and Eva learned that almost all their friends who had been at the lodge dinner had an experience that was similar to their own.

The physician contacted the public health department to report the incident. His was one of several similar calls, a public health officer said, and the department was already investigating.

The following week, the public health officer returned the physician's call to report his findings. The cream puffs that the lodge restaurant had served that evening had been purchased from a local bakery. At the bakery, health officials had located a worker with an infected cut on his little finger—"a small

thing," the worker said. He could not understand what all the fuss was about.

The health officials also located the delivery truck driver, who had started out at midmorning to make his rounds and to take the cream puffs to the lodge. When they questioned the driver, they learned that the delivery truck had broken down during his afternoon deliveries, before he had reached the lodge. The driver said that he had been irritated by a 3-hour wait at the garage while the truck was being fixed, but he still got the order to the lodge restaurant in time for the dinner.

At the lodge, the chef said that everyone was so busy with the dinner that, when the cream puffs finally arrived, no one had time to give them much notice. They had decided not to put the cream puffs in the refrigerator because they were about to be served.

When John and Eva's physician called them afterward to report the story, John and Eva decided that they would not eat at the lodge restaurant again. Besides, by then, John had lost his taste for cream puffs.

QUESTIONS FOR ANALYSIS

1. Why is the control of the community's food supply an important responsibility of the health department?
2. Which disease agents may be carried by food or water?
3. What agent caused John and Eva's illness? Was this a food infection or a food poisoning? Why?
4. While the investigation was occurring and before John and Eva learned the real cause of their illness, John thought it must have been caused by "those things farmers and food processors put into food these days." What substances did John mean? Give some examples.
5. Why are these materials used for growing and processing food?
6. What are some ways in which food is protected from its point of production to the table? How can food be preserved for later use?
7. Which agency controls food safety and quality? How does it do so?

---

bacteria produce toxins within the gastrointestinal tract, resulting in poisoning and illness.

The bacterium *C. botulinum* causes a more serious type of food poisoning than *C. perfringens* but occurs much less frequently. Food-borne botulism results from the ingestion of food that contains the powerful paralyzing toxin produced from this strain of *Clostridium*. Depending on the dose of toxin consumed and the individual response, symptoms will appear within 18 to 36 hours. Nausea, vomiting, weakness, blurred vision, and slurred speech are typical initial symptoms. The toxin progressively irritates motor nerve cells and blocks the transmission of neural impulses at the nerve terminals, thereby causing a gradual paralysis. In severe cases, a sudden respiratory paralysis with airway obstruction may result in death.

C. botulinum spores are widespread in soil throughout the world and may be carried on harvested food to the food processing plant. Canned foods are a high-risk food for botulism contamination. Like all *Clostridia*, this species is **anaerobic** or nearly so. The relatively air-free can and canning temperatures ($\geq 27°$ C [$80°$ F]) provide good conditions for toxin production. The development of high standards in the commercial canning industry has eliminated this source of botulism, but cases still result each year, mainly from the ingestion of home-canned foods. Boiling food for 10 minutes destroys the toxin, although not the spore.

anaerobic a microorganism that can live and grow in an oxygen-free environment.

Therefore, all home-canned food—no matter how well preserved it is considered to be—should be boiled for at least 10 minutes before it is eaten.

Viruses

Food-borne disease outbreaks resulting from norovirus contamination are estimated to be the most common cause of food-borne illness in the United States. However, norovirus is much less likely to cause hospitalization than other forms of food-borne illness such as *Salmonella* or *E. coli* contamination.[16] Other viral forms of food-borne illness include **hepatitis** A and rotavirus. Hepatitis A is much less common in the United States and other areas that routinely utilize hepatitis A vaccines than in less developed countries. Again, the stringent control of community water and food supplies as well as the personal hygiene and sanitary practices of food handlers are essential for the prevention of food-borne disease.

Parasites

Giardiasis (from the parasite *Giardia lamblia*) is the most common form of parasitic food-borne illness in the United States. It is usually transmitted through water although it can also be transmitted through food, person-to-person contact, or animal-to-person contact. *Giardia* lives in the intestines of infected individuals and is passed on through their feces. *Giardia* can live outside of the body for a long time (weeks or even months) and thus reinfection is a risk. Symptoms begin 1 to 3 weeks after becoming infected and include gastrointestinal disturbances such as diarrhea, stomach cramps, gas, and greasy stools.

Two types of parasitic worms are of concern in relation to food: (1) roundworms, such as the *trichina (Trichinella spiralis)* worm found in pork; and (2) flatworms, such as the common tapeworms found in beef and pork. The following control measures are essential: (1) laws controlling hog and cattle food sources and pastures to prevent the transmission of the parasites to the meat produced for market; and (2) the avoidance of rare beef and undercooked pork as an added personal precaution. Table 13-4 summarizes examples of common food contamination.

Environmental Food Contaminants

Lead. Heavy metals such as lead may contaminate food and water as well as the air and environmental objects. Although lead poisoning in the United

States has dramatically declined since the removal of lead from gasoline and paint, it continues to plague certain subgroups of the population (see the Cultural Considerations box, "The Continued Burden of Lead Poisoning"). Children are especially vulnerable to lead poisoning, particularly those of poor families who live in older homes or impoverished areas with peeling lead paint.[23] No levels of lead in the blood are safe. While the prevalence of lead poisoning has declined significantly since the 1980s, 2.6% of all children (more than $\frac{1}{2}$ million) between the ages of 1 and 5 years old in the United States still have blood lead levels ≥5 mcg/dL.[24] Eliminating high blood lead levels in children is one of the *Healthy People 2020* goals.[25]

Of all sources of lead, lead paint (which was banned in the United States in 1978) is the most problematic source of contamination for children. Millions of homes in the United States have lead in their paint surfaces. Children who live in these homes face lead exposure as a result of breathing airborne particles of paint dust created by disturbed or deteriorating walls or by abrasive paint removal before remodeling. The amount of lead-containing dust on the floor of a home is significantly associated with the blood lead level in children.[26] Drinking water may be an important source of lead in high-risk households with water that comes through lead service pipes or plumbing joints that have been sealed with lead solder. Current Environmental Protection Agency rules for public drinking water, however, have lowered the controlled lead exposure levels even further.

Children with elevated blood lead levels have lower intellectual performance compared with similar children who do not suffer from lead toxicity.[27,28] This same high-risk population group is also at risk for iron deficiency. Iron-deficiency anemia can increase the risk for lead poisoning fourfold to fivefold, it has a similar deleterious effect on neurology, and it can thus further complicate lead toxicity and long-term neurologic damage.[29]

Natural toxins. Toxins that are produced by plants or microorganisms also contaminate the food and water supply. Mercury, which is found naturally in the environment in addition to being a by-product of human production, is converted to methyl mercury by bacteria. Methyl mercury is a toxin that contaminates large bodies of water and the fish within that water. This contamination can pass through the food chain to people who regularly consume large fatty fish. Aflatoxin, which is another natural toxin, is produced by fungi. It may contaminate foods such as peanuts, tree nuts, corn, and animal feed.

Other food contaminants and pollutants that may pose a risk to human health come from a variety of sources (e.g., factories, sewage, pesticides, fertilizers) but end up leaching into the ground, thereby contaminating food production areas and the water supply.

hepatitis the inflammation of the liver cells; symptoms of acute hepatitis include flu-like symptoms, muscle and joint aches, fever, nausea, vomiting, diarrhea, headache, dark urine, and yellowing of the eyes and skin; symptoms of chronic hepatitis include jaundice, abdominal swelling and sensitivity, low-grade fever, and ascites.

Table 13-4   Examples of Food-Borne Disease

ORGANISM	COMMON NAME OF ILLNESS	ONSET TIME AFTER INGESTING	SIGNS AND SYMPTOMS	DURATION	FOOD SOURCES
Bacillus cereus	B. cereus food poisoning	10 to 16 hours	Abdominal cramps, watery diarrhea, nausea	24 to 48 hours	Meats, stews, gravies, vanilla sauce
Campylobacter jejuni	Campylobacteriosis	2 to 5 days	Diarrhea, cramps, fever, and vomiting; diarrhea may be bloody	2 to 10 days	Raw and undercooked poultry, unpasteurized milk, contaminated water
Clostridium botulinum	Botulism	12 to 72 hours	Vomiting, diarrhea, blurred vision, double vision, difficulty swallowing, muscle weakness; can result in respiratory failure and death	Variable	Improperly canned foods, especially home-canned vegetables; fermented fish, baked potatoes in aluminum foil
Clostridium perfringens	Perfringens food poisoning	8 to 16 hours	Intense abdominal cramps, watery diarrhea	Usually 24 hours	Meats, poultry, gravy, dried or precooked foods, time- and/or temperature-abused foods
Cryptosporidium	Intestinal cryptosporidiosis	2 to 10 days	Diarrhea (usually watery), stomach cramps, upset stomach, slight fever	May be remitting and relapsing over weeks to months	Uncooked food or food contaminated by an ill food handler after cooking, contaminated drinking water
Cyclospora cayetanensis	Cyclosporiasis	1 to 14 days, usually at least 1 week	Diarrhea (usually watery), loss of appetite, substantial loss of weight, stomach cramps, nausea, vomiting, fatigue	May be remitting and relapsing over weeks to months	Various types of fresh produce (imported berries, lettuce, basil)
Escherichia coli producing toxin	E. coli infection (common cause of "travellers' diarrhea")	1 to 3 days	Watery diarrhea, abdominal cramps, some vomiting	3 to 7 or more days	Water or food contaminated with human feces
Escherichia coli O157:H7	Hemorrhagic colitis or E. coli O157:H7 infection	1 to 8 days	Severe (often bloody) diarrhea, abdominal pain and vomiting; usually little or no fever is present; more common among children 4 years old or younger; can lead to kidney failure	5 to 10 days	Undercooked beef (especially hamburger), unpasteurized milk and juice, raw fruits and vegetables (e.g., sprouts), contaminated water
Hepatitis A	Hepatitis	28 days average (15 to 50 days)	Diarrhea, dark urine, jaundice, flu-like symptoms (i.e., fever, headache, nausea, abdominal pain)	Variable, usually 2 weeks to 3 months	Raw produce, contaminated drinking water, uncooked foods and cooked foods that are not reheated after contact with an infected food handler, shellfish from contaminated waters

Organism	Some common names of the illness	Onset time after ingesting	Signs & symptoms	Duration	Food sources
Listeria monocytogenes	Listeriosis	9 to 48 hours for gastrointestinal symptoms, 2 to 6 weeks for invasive disease	Fever, muscle aches, and nausea or diarrhea; pregnant women may have a mild flu-like illness, and infection can lead to premature delivery or stillbirth; elderly or immunocompromised patients may develop bacteremia or meningitis	Variable	Unpasteurized milk, soft cheeses made with unpasteurized milk, ready-to-eat deli meats
Noroviruses	Variously called viral gastroenteritis, winter diarrhea, acute nonbacterial gastroenteritis, food poisoning, and food infection	12 to 48 hours	Nausea, vomiting, abdominal cramping, diarrhea, fever, headache; diarrhea is more prevalent among adults, vomiting is more common among children	12 to 60 hours	Raw produce, contaminated drinking water, uncooked foods and cooked foods that are not reheated after contact with an infected food handler, shellfish from contaminated waters
Salmonella	Salmonellosis	6 to 48 hours	Diarrhea, fever, abdominal cramps, vomiting	4 to 7 days	Eggs, poultry, meat, unpasteurized milk or juice, cheese, contaminated raw fruits and vegetables
Shigella	Shigellosis or bacillary dysentery	4 to 7 days	Abdominal cramps, fever, diarrhea; stools may contain blood and mucus	24 to 48 hours	Raw produce, contaminated drinking water, uncooked foods and cooked foods that are not reheated after contact with an infected food handler
Staphylococcus aureus	Staphylococcal food poisoning	1 to 6 hours	Sudden onset of severe nausea and vomiting, abdominal cramps; diarrhea and fever may be present	24 to 48 hours	Unrefrigerated or improperly refrigerated meats, potato, and egg salads; cream pastries
Vibrio parahaemolyticus	*V. parahaemolyticus* infection	4 to 96 hours	Watery (occasionally bloody) diarrhea, abdominal cramps, nausea, vomiting, fever	2 to 5 days	Undercooked or raw seafood, such as shellfish
Vibrio vulnificus	*V. vulnificus* infection	1 to 7 days	Vomiting, diarrhea, abdominal pain, bloodborne infection, fever, bleeding within skin, ulcers that require surgical removal; can be fatal to persons with liver disease or weakened immune systems	2 to 8 days	Undercooked or raw seafood, such as shellfish (especially oysters)

Reprinted from U.S. Department of Health and Human Services and U.S. Food and Drug Administration. *Foodborne illness-causing organisms in the U.S. What you need to know.* Available at <www.fda.gov/Food/ResourcesForYou/Consumers/ucm103263.htm>; Accessed January 2015.

Cultural Considerations

The Continued Burden of Lead Poisoning

Exposure to lead continues to be a problem in the United States. Among all age groups, children between the ages of 1 and 5 years have the highest risk for elevated blood lead levels (BLLs). Among racial groups, non-Hispanic black children have the highest incidence rates. Following are the percentages of children between the ages of 1 and 5 years with elevated BLLs of 5 mcg/dL or more[1]:

- All children between the ages of 1 and 5 years: 2.6%
- Non-Hispanic black children: 5.6%
- Mexican-American children: 1.9%
- Non-Hispanic white children: 2.4%

The accumulation of lead in the blood results in oxidative stress and interferes with the normal physiologic functions of calcium, zinc, and iron. In addition to neurologic damage, prolonged elevated lead in the body can cause anemia, kidney damage, seizures, encephalopathy, and eventually paralysis.

The figures depict the BLLs of children by race beginning in 1988. Note the successful decrease in severely affected children over time and the disparity of minority groups with elevated blood lead levels. In January 2012, the CDC's Advisory Committee on Childhood Lead Poisoning recommended that BLLs in children be kept below 5 mcg/dL. Thus, Figure A represents the percent of children with blood lead levels ≥10 mcg/dL for the years measured and Figure B represents the percent of children with blood lead levels ≥5 mcg/dL from 1999 to date.

REFERENCE

1. Centers for Disease Control and Prevention. Blood lead levels in children aged 1-5 years - United States, 1999-2010. *MMWR Morb Mortal Wkly Rep*. 2013;62(13):245-248.

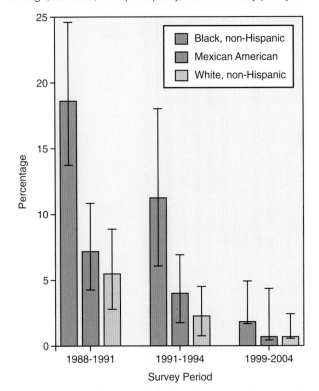

A. Percentage of children between the ages of 1 and 5 years with blood lead levels of ≥10 mcg/dL by race or ethnicity and survey period according to the National Health and Nutrition Examination Surveys. 95% confidence interval. (Data from Jones RL, Homa DM, Meyer PA et al. Trends in blood lead levels and blood lead testing among US children aged 1 to 5 years, 1988-2004. *Pediatrics*. 2009;123[3]:e376-e385.)

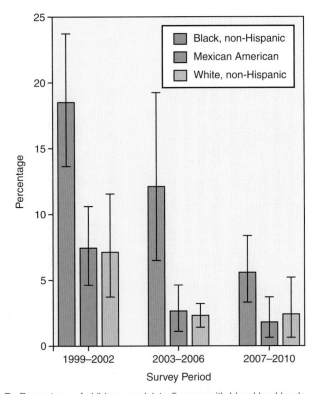

B. Percentage of children aged 1 to 5 years with blood lead levels ≥5 mcg/dL, by selected characteristics—United States, National Health and Nutrition Examination Survey, 1999-2002, 2003-2006, and 2007-2010. (Data from Centers for Disease Control and Prevention. Blood lead levels in children aged 1-5 years—United States, 1999-2010. MMWR Morb Mortal Wkly Rep. 2013;62(13): 245-248.)

FOOD NEEDS AND COSTS

HUNGER AND MALNUTRITION

Worldwide Malnutrition

Hunger, famine, and death exist in many countries of the world today. Lack of sanitation, cultural inequality, overpopulation, and economic and political structures that do not appropriately use resources are all factors that may contribute to malnutrition. Figure 13-9 demonstrates the complicated interaction of the many factors that lead to malnutrition.

Chronic food or nutrient shortages within a population perpetuate the cycle of malnutrition, in which undernourished pregnant women give birth to low birth weight infants. These infants are then more susceptible to infant death or growth retardation during childhood. When high nutrient needs throughout childhood and adolescence are not met, the incidence of malnourished or growth-stunted adults with shorter life expectancies and reduced work capacities continues to rise. Figure 13-10 illustrates the two drastically different outcomes that occur depending on whether a child has access to education, financial needs, and health care. Malnutrition may result from total kilocalorie deficiency or single-nutrient deficiencies. The most common deficiencies in the world today are iron-deficiency anemia, protein-energy malnutrition, vitamin A deficiency, and iodine deficiency.

The United Nations Committee on World Food Security was formed to address the 840 million people worldwide who do not have enough food to meet their basic nutritional requirements. The long-term goals of this committee are to eliminate world hunger by raising the level of overall nutrition, improving agricultural productivity, and enhancing the lives of the rural populations.[30,31] The plan is composed of several commitments that are focused on stabilizing the social, economic, and environmental production and distribution of nutritionally adequate food. Information and updates about the progress of this committee can be found at www.fao.org/monitoringprogress/index_en.html.

Malnutrition in America

In the United States, which is one of the wealthiest countries on earth, hunger and malnutrition among the poor persist. More than 49 million individuals experience **food insecurity** regularly.[32] Individuals who are at the highest risk for food insecurity are those who live below the income-to-poverty ratio, households

> **food insecurity** limited or uncertain availability of nutritionally adequate and safe foods or limited or uncertain ability to acquire acceptable foods in socially acceptable ways.

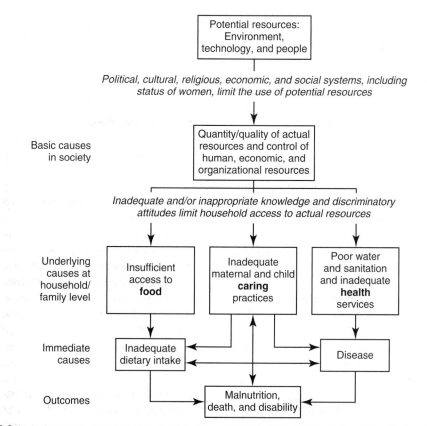

FIGURE 13-9 Multiple causes of malnutrition. (Adapted from United Nations Children's Fund, The State of the World's Children, 1998, New York, NY UNICEF/Oxford University Press, 1998.)

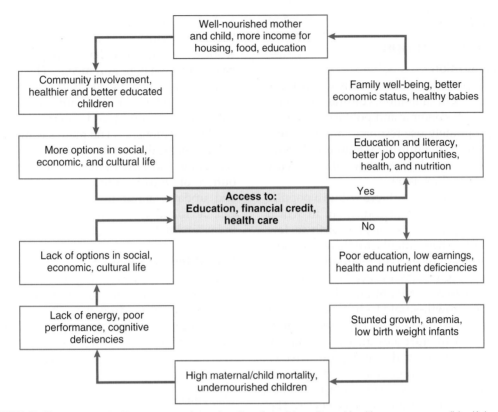

FIGURE 13-10 Differences in life outcomes when education, financial credit, and health care are accessible. (Adapted from Cohen MJ et al.: Hunger 1995: Causes of Hunger: The State of World Hunger, Silver Springs, MD, Bread for the World Institute, 1994.)

with children headed by a single woman, African Americans and Hispanics, and households in central city areas.[32] At both the government and the personal levels of any society, food availability and use involve money and politics. Various factors are implicated, such as land management practices, water distribution, food production and distribution policies, and food assistance programs for individuals and families in need.

FOOD ASSISTANCE PROGRAMS

In situations of economic stress and natural disasters, individuals and families may need help with acquiring resources, including food. Many people experience hunger every day. Dietitians, nurses, and other health care providers should be aware of the available food assistance programs to make appropriate referrals.

Commodity Supplemental Food Program

Under the Commodity Supplemental Food Program (CSFP), the USDA purchases food items that are good sources of nutrients but that are often lacking in the diets of the target population (i.e., low-income elderly ≥60 years old). The USDA then distributes the food to state agencies and tribal organizations. From there, the food is dispersed to local agencies for public allocation. Local agencies (e.g., departments of health, social services, education, or agriculture) are responsible for

evaluating eligibility, providing nutrition education, and dispersing food. This program is not currently available in every state. The most recent report noted that an average of 579,000 people participate in the CSFP services each month.[33] Information about CSFP can be found at www.fns.usda.gov/csfp.

Supplemental Nutrition Assistance Program (SNAP)

SNAP, which was formerly known as the food stamp program, began during the late depression years of the 1930s and was expanded during the 1960s and 1970s. This program has helped many people to purchase food, the majority of which are children and elderly adults. The USDA estimated that 45.7 million people participated in SNAP services in the United States each month during 2015 at an annual cost of $73.9 billion.[34] With this program, electronic benefits transfer cards are issued to the primary care provider of the household. These cards are used in a way that is similar to a debit card in approved retail stores to supplement the household's food needs for 1 month. Households must have a monthly income that is below the program's eligible poverty limit to qualify. SNAP is a federal program and operates in all states and U.S. territories. It is administered at the local level. More information about this program can be found at the USDA's Food and Nutrition Service website at www.fns.usda.gov/snap.

Special Supplemental Food Program for Women, Infants, and Children

The Special Supplemental Food Program for Women, Infants, and Children (WIC) provides nutrition supplementation, education, and counseling in addition to referrals for health care and social services to women who are pregnant, postpartum, or breastfeeding and to their infants and children who are younger than 5 years old. WIC has established criteria for participation, and each applicant must be income-eligible and determined to be at nutritional risk. The food packages provided through WIC meet the *Dietary Guidelines for Americans* and promote the consumption of fruits, vegetables, and whole grains. The average monthly food cost per participant as reported for fiscal year 2015 was $43.58.[35] Participants are provided with vouchers that are exchanged for foods such as milk, eggs, cheese, juice, fortified cereals, fruits, and vegetables at participating retailers. These foods supplement the diet with rich sources of protein, iron, and certain vitamins to help reduce risk factors such as poor growth patterns, low birth weight, prematurity, preeclampsia, miscarriage, and anemia.

WIC was established in 1972, and it currently has more than 8 million participants. WIC offices are established in every state and U.S. territory. Approximately half of all participants are children between the ages of 1 and 5 years.[36] More information can be found at www.fns.usda.gov/wic.

School Meals Program

The **school breakfast and lunch programs** provide meals that meet the *Dietary Guideline* recommendations for many children who otherwise would lack balanced meals. The Academy of Nutrition and Dietetics has voiced concerns about the lack of nutritional standards with à la carte and **competitive foods** offered at many schools.[37] Competitive foods historically contributed to the overconsumption of calories, plate waste of nutritionally balanced school lunches, and the decreased intake of nutrients by students. Fortunately, regulations enacted in 2012 are intended to eliminate the sale of foods of minimal nutritional value by setting nutritional requirements for any food sold on school grounds during breakfast or lunch periods.[38]

There are several programs available to assist low-income children with receiving healthy food while at school. Current programs in the United States include the National School Lunch, Fresh Fruit and Vegetable, School Breakfast, Special Milk, and Summer Food Service programs. The National School Lunch program includes subprograms for children from low-income families that provide nutritionally balanced meals and snacks after school and during the summer months, when school is not in session. The USDA supports the program by reimbursing schools for each meal served and by donating food from surplus agricultural stocks.

Children eat for free or at reduced rates, and these meals often comprise their main food intake for the day. The meals provided must fulfill approximately one third of a child's Recommended Dietary Allowance for protein, vitamin A, vitamin C, iron, calcium, and calories, and it must meet the *Dietary Guidelines for Americans,* which call for diets that are lower in total fat and that contain more fruits, vegetables, and whole grains. The Special Milk Program provides milk to children who do not have access to the other meal programs. More information about School Meal programs can be found at www.fns.usda.gov/school-meals/child-nutrition-programs.

Nutrition Services Incentive Program

The Nutrition Services Incentive Program, which was formerly known as the Nutrition Program for the Elderly, is operated through the U.S. Department of Health and Human Services Administration on Aging. The purpose of the program is to promote socialization, health and well-being for older individuals by reducing hunger and food insecurity.

This program provides cash or commodities from the USDA for the delivery of nutritious meals to the elderly. Regardless of income, all people who are older than 60 years old can eat hot lunches at a community center under the Congregate Meals Program; if they are ill or disabled, they can receive meals at home by using the services of the Home-Delivered Meals Program. The act specifies that economically and socially needy people be given priority. Both programs accept voluntary contributions for meals. More information can be found at www.fns.usda.gov/nsip.

FOOD BUYING AND HANDLING PRACTICES

For many American families, the problem is spending their limited food dollars wisely. Even on a low-cost plan for food purchasing, an average family of four can expect to spend $720 to $855 per month on food alone.[39] Shopping for food can be complicated, especially when each item in a supermarket's overabundant supply shouts, "Buy me!" Food marketing is big business, and producers compete for prize placement and shelf space. A large supermarket stocks many thousands of different food items. A single food item may be marketed a dozen different ways at as many different prices. In diet counseling, clients and families typically

---

school breakfast and lunch programs federally assisted meal programs that operate in public and nonprofit private schools and residential child-care institutions; these programs provide nutritionally balanced, low-cost, or free meals to children each school day.

competitive foods any food or beverage that is served outside of a federal meal program in a food-program setting, regardless of nutritional value.

express their greatest need as help with buying food. The following wise shopping and handling practices help with the provision of healthy foods as well as with controlling food costs.

Planning Ahead

Use sales' circulars in newspapers, plan general menus, and keep a checklist of basic pantry supplies. Make a list ahead of time according to the location of items in a regularly used grocery store. Such planning controls impulse buying and reduces extra trips. Plan a time to food shop without children in tow.

Buying Wisely

Understanding packaging, carefully reading labels, and watching for sale items help to improve purchasing power. Only buy in quantity if it results in real savings and if the food can be adequately stored or used. Be cautious when selecting so-called "convenience foods"; the time saved may not be worth the added cost. For fresh foods, try alternative food sources such as farmers' markets, community supported agriculture (CSAs), and gardens.

Storing Food Safely

Control food waste and prevent illness caused by food spoilage or contamination. Conserve food by storing items in accordance with their nature and use. Use dry storage, covered containers, and correct-temperature refrigeration as needed. Keep opened and partly used food items at the front of the shelf for timely use. Avoid waste by preparing only the amount needed. Use leftovers in creative ways or freeze for quick meals later.

Cooking Food Well

Use cooking processes that retain maximal food value and that maintain food safety. Cooking vegetables for shorter periods (e.g., stir frying, steaming) and with as little water as possible helps to retain their vitamin and mineral nutritive quality. Prepare food with imagination and good sense. Give zest and appeal to dishes with a variety of seasonings, combinations, and serving arrangements. No matter how much they know about nutrition and health, people usually eat because they are hungry and because the food looks and tastes good, not necessarily because it is healthy.

Putting It All Together

Summary

- Common public concerns about the safety of the community food supply center on the use of chemicals such as pesticides and food additives. These substances have produced an abundant food supply, but they have also raised concerns, and they require close monitoring.
- The FDA is the main government agency that was established to maintain the control of the food supply. It conducts activities related to areas such as food safety, food labeling, food standards, consumer education, and research.
- Numerous organisms such as bacteria, viruses, and parasites that can contaminate food may cause food-borne disease. Rigorous public health measures control the sanitation of food handling areas and the personal hygiene of food handlers. The same standards should apply to home food handling preparation and storage.
- Families who are under economic stress may benefit from counseling about financial assistance. Various U.S. food assistance programs help families in need, and referrals can be made to appropriate agencies. Families may also benefit from assistance with the buying and use of food.

Chapter Review Questions

See answers in Appendix A.

1. When purchasing packaged foods, consumers with food allergies should pay particular attention to:
   a. The Nutrition Facts Label.
   b. Any health claims.
   c. Symbols on the package.
   d. The list of ingredients.

2. Addition of nutrients to refined grains that were previously lost during processing is called:
   a. Enrichment.
   b. Fortification.
   c. Replacement.
   d. Enhancement.

3. One of the most important ways to prevent contamination while handling food is to:
   a. Wash hands and wear disposable gloves.
   b. Wash all poultry items with warm water.
   c. Cook all meat and egg dishes to 120° F.
   d. Always remove peelings from fruit.

4. Jenny finds some leftover pizza that has been in the refrigerator for 7 days. She is wondering if she could still eat it. Your response would be:
 a. Yes, as long as it is thoroughly reheated.
 b. Yes, as long as it does not have an odor or mold.
 c. No, it should be discarded after 3 to 4 days if it was refrigerated.
 d. No, it should be discarded after 24 hours if it was refrigerated.

5. Improperly home-canned green beans can result in:
 a. Tapeworms.
 b. Botulism.
 c. Listeriosis.
 d. Rotavirus.

Additional Learning Resources

evolve Please refer to this text's Evolve website for answers to the Case Study questions.
http://evolve.elsevier.com/Williams/basic/

References and **Further Reading and Resources** in the back of the book provide additional resources for enhancing knowledge.

Food Habits and Cultural Patterns

Key Concepts

- Personal food habits develop as part of a person's social and cultural heritage as well as his or her individual lifestyle and environment.

- Social and economic changes often result in alterations in food patterns.
- American eating patterns are influenced by many different cultures.

Why do people eat what they eat? Food is necessary to sustain life and health, but people eat certain foods for many reasons other than good health and nutrition, although these are important factors. As noted in Chapter 13, the broader food environment from which we have to choose is often influenced by factors such as politics and poverty, which limit personal control and choice.

A variety of connotations are attached to food. All food habits are intimately related to people's way of life: their values, beliefs, and situations. However, sometimes these food patterns change over time with more exposure to other cultural patterns.

SOCIAL, PSYCHOLOGIC, AND ECONOMIC INFLUENCES ON FOOD HABITS

SOCIAL IMPACT

Human behavior reveals activities, processes, and structures that comprise social life. In any society, social groups are largely formed by factors such as economic status, education, residence, occupation, and family. Accordingly, values and practices differ among groups. Subgroups also develop on the basis of region, religion, age, sex, social class, health issues, special interests, ethnic backgrounds, politics, and other common traits such as group affiliations.

Food habits, like any other form of human behavior, are gradually established with influences from every direction.

Food is a symbol of acceptance, warmth, and friendliness in social relationships. People tend to accept food or food advice readily from friends, acquaintances, and people who they view as trusted authorities. This guidance is especially strong in family relationships. Food habits that are closely associated with family sentiments often stay with people throughout their lives. During adulthood, certain foods may even trigger a flood of childhood memories and are valued for reasons apart from any nutritional importance.

FACTORS THAT INFLUENCE PERSONAL FOOD CHOICES

Ethnic patterns and regional cultural habits are strong influences that establish food traditions early in life. However, shifts within a society result in changes in food consumption patterns for better or worse (e.g., globalization of the food supply). See Box 14-1 for a list of several factors involved in personal food choices.

Psychologic Influences

Understanding dietary patterns begins with the recognition of the psychologic influences that are involved (see Box 14-1). Many of these psychologic factors are rooted in childhood experiences. For example, when a child is hurt or disappointed, parents may offer a cookie or a piece of candy to distract the child. Then, when adults feel hurt, they may turn to similar comfort foods to help them cope. Certain foods, especially sweets and other pleasurable flavors, stimulate "feel good" body chemicals in the brain called *endorphins* that give a mild "high" that may actually help ease pain.

Food and Psychosocial Development

From infancy to old age, emotional maturity grows along with physical development. At each stage of human growth, food habits are part of both physical and psychosocial development. For example, a 2-year-old toddler who is taking his first steps toward eventual independence from his parents may learn to control his parents through food by refusing to eat at meal times or otherwise being a picky eater. Psychologists believe that **food neophobia** may also be involved. This normal developmental trait may be an instinct from the evolutionary past that protected children from eating harmful foods when they were just becoming independent from their mothers.

food neophobia the fear of new food.

Box 14-1 Factors That Determine Food Choices

PHYSICAL FACTORS	PHYSIOLOGIC FACTORS
Available food supply	Allergies
Food technology	Disability
Geography, agriculture, and distribution	Health and disease status
Sanitation and housing	Heredity
Season and climate	Nutrient and energy needs
Storage and cooking facilities	Therapeutic diets

SOCIAL AND ECONOMIC FACTORS	PSYCHOLOGIC FACTORS
Advertising and marketing	Habits
Culture	Preferences
General and nutrition education	Emotions
Income	Cravings
Political and economic policies	Personal food acceptance
Religion and social class	Positive or negative experiences and associations
Social problems, poverty, alcoholism, and drug abuse	

Marketing and Environmental Influences

Food habits are also manipulated by television, radio, magazines, and other media messages. Influences from peers, availability of convenience items, marketing at the local grocery store, and many other factors of persuasion may sway the decision-making process for food choices throughout life. Advertising strategies that make use of brand mascots and cartoon media characters on food packages greatly impact children's eating patterns by increasing the preference for products baring the known character logo.[1,2] Because fresh fruits and vegetables are not processed or packaged, such logos are consequently not used on these healthier snack items. Foods that are routinely endorsed on American television are heavy in the very food components that are discouraged by the dietary guidelines (i.e., trans fat, saturated fat, sugar, and sodium).[3,4]

Marketing trends and media also influence what a culture views as beautiful. In the United States, a very thin figure is valued, and such provocations may dictate food choices, meal composition, lifestyle, and body-image expectations.

Economic Influences

Many American families live under socioeconomic pressures, especially during periods of recession and inflation. The problems of middle-income families differ in relative terms, but low-income families—especially those in poverty situations—often suffer extreme needs. These families may lack adequate housing and have little or no access to educational opportunities. As a result, they may be poorly prepared for jobs, only make a day-to-day living at low-paying work, or may be unemployed. Approximately 14.8% of Americans live with an income that is below

the federal poverty level, with the highest burden on African-American and Hispanic families.[5]

The cost of a healthy diet composed of whole grains, lean meats, fruits, vegetables, and low-fat dairy is difficult to achieve for some families that are living at or below the federal poverty line. Thus, it is not surprising that people with low incomes bear the greater burden of unnecessary illness and malnutrition. In an effort to make healthy food more affordable, some organizations have suggested an additional taxation on selected foods with little or no nutritional quality as a means of subsidizing the cost of healthy choices, such as fruits and vegetables.[6-8] Such taxation would thereby make "junk food" a more expensive option than buying fruits and vegetables.

CULTURAL DEVELOPMENT OF FOOD HABITS

Each particular society that identifies itself with a common denominator (e.g., ethnicity, religion, geographic location, lifestyle) has its own unique cultural food pattern.

STRENGTH OF PERSONAL CULTURE

Culture involves much more than the major and historic aspects of a person's communal life (e.g., language, religion, politics, location). It also develops from all of the habits of everyday living and family relationships, such as preparing and serving food. In a gradual process of conscious and unconscious learning, cultural values, attitudes, customs, and practices become a deep part of individual lives. Although part of this heritage may be revised or rejected as adults, people are ultimately responsible for shaping their own lives and passing traditions on to the subsequent generations as they see fit. Americans have a broad range of food habits that have been shaped by a world of cultural diversity.

Food habits are among the oldest and most deeply rooted aspects of a culture. An individual's cultural background largely determines what is eaten as well as when and how it is eaten. All types of customs, whether rational or irrational or beneficial or injurious, are found in every part of the world. Many foods take on symbolic meanings related to major life events (e.g., birth, death, weddings). From ancient times, ceremonies and religious rites involving food have surrounded certain events and seasons. Food gathering, preparing, and serving have followed specific customs, many of which remain intact today.

TRADITIONAL CULTURE-SPECIFIC FOOD PATTERNS

The United States has long been considered a "melting pot" of ethnic and racial groups. In more recent years, however, this image no longer seems appropriate. America's diversity has come to be recognized and even celebrated as a basis for its national strength. This recognition is particularly demonstrated by the diversity of America's cultural food availability. Pockets of ethnic groups in which native lifestyles are somewhat retained are apparent in many American cities (e.g., "Chinatown," "Little Italy").

Many different cultural food patterns are part of American family and community life. These patterns have contributed special dishes or modes of cooking to American eating habits. In turn, many of these cultural food habits have been Americanized. Older members of the family use traditional foods more regularly, with younger members of the family using them mainly on special occasions or holidays. Nevertheless, traditional foods have strong meanings and bind families and cultural communities in close fellowship. Individual tastes and geographic patterns will vary, but general food patterns are connected with culture and have a strong influence on how people eat.

In the sections that follow, some of the specific cultural food patterns that have shaped the American food supply are briefly discussed. It should be noted that individuals of any heritage may consume typical American foods as well as the examples provided here; or may not follow customary dietary patterns at all. Assumptions about dietary patterns cannot be made, but knowledge of the variety of unique traditional foods provides a rudimentary understanding of the range of possible food choices. Such an understanding of various cultural food patterns is valuable when providing dietary guidance as a health care professional.

Spanish and Native American Influences

Mexican. The food habits of the early Spanish settlers and Native American nations form the basis of the current food patterns among people of Mexican heritage who live in the United States, chiefly in the South and Southwest. The following foods are basic to this pattern: dried beans, tomatoes, corn, and squash. Variations and additions may be found in different places or among those of different income levels. Relatively small amounts of meat are used, and eggs are occasionally eaten. A high prevalence of lactose intolerance limits large intakes of milk products. Fruit (e.g., mango, papaya, avocado) is consumed in varying amounts, depending on availability and price. For centuries, corn has been the basic grain used for bread in the form of tortillas, which are flat cakes that are baked on a hot surface or griddle. Wheat is also used when making tortillas, and rice and oats are added cereals. Major seasonings are chili peppers, onions, and garlic; the basic fat has historically been lard. See Table 14-1 for representative foods from each food group within a traditional Mexican cuisine.

Acculturation to the typical Western diet of Americans is a significant concern for Hispanic and Latino immigrants. Adopting such dietary habits is associated with reduced quality of life due to chronic disease (see the

Cultural Considerations box, "Acculturation to an American Diet").

Puerto Rican. The largest population of Puerto Ricans residing in the United States lives in New York City. The Puerto Rican people share a common heritage with many Hispanic Caribbean countries, so many of

Cultural Considerations

Acculturation to an American Diet*

Immigration from one part of the world to another is usually accompanied by changes with regard to dietary intake, lifestyle, and disease risk to match the new culture; this is referred to as *acculturation*. Several studies have evaluated the changes that occur over time, specifically with Hispanic or Latino immigrants, because this population encompasses the fastest-growing ethnic group in the United States. One such systematic review evaluated the relationship between ethnicity, acculturation, and overall diet quality among Latinos who were living in the United States. Researchers noted that Latinos who exhibited more acculturation consistently scored worse in overall diet quality by eating less fruit, rice, and beans and by consuming more sugar and sugar-sweetened beverages than their less accultured counterparts (i.e., those Latinos who maintained their cultural diet rather than adopting poor dietary habits in America).[1]

Acculturation has been linked to an increased risk for chronic diseases such as diabetes, obesity, and cardiovascular disease in the Hispanic/Latino populations.[2,3] The risk for diabetes increases even when demographic factors, socioeconomic status, and BMI are controlled. In other words, the increased prevalence of diabetes in highly acculturated Latino individuals was not exclusively due to these adjusted factors; the more acculturated, the higher the prevalence of diabetes.[3] Another study that evaluated the diets of Latinos with diabetes showed that, as more acculturation takes place for the immigrants in their new environment, their diets include less dietary fiber and more saturated fat, both of which are contraindicated for good health.[4]

REFERENCES

1. Ayala GX, Baquero B, Klinger S. A systematic review of the relationship between acculturation and diet among Latinos in the United States: implications for future research. *J Am Diet Assoc.* 2008; 108(8):1330-1344.
2. Daviglus ML, et al. Prevalence of major cardiovascular risk factors and cardiovascular diseases among Hispanic/Latino individuals of diverse backgrounds in the United States. *JAMA.* 2012;308(17): 1775-1784.
3. O'Brien MJ, et al. Acculturation and the prevalence of diabetes in US Latino Adults, National Health and Nutrition Examination Survey 2007-2010. *Prev Chronic Dis.* 2014;11:E176.
4. Mainous AG 3rd, Diaz VA, Geesey ME. Acculturation and healthy lifestyle among Latinos with diabetes. *Ann Fam Med.* 2008;6(2): 131-137.

*For more information about acculturation, see the following paper: Satia JA. Dietary acculturation and the nutrition transition: an overview. *Appl Physiol Nutr Metab.* 2010;35(2):219-223.

acculturation the process of an individual or group of people adopting the behaviors and lifestyle habits of a new culture.

Table 14-1   Historical Dietary Patterns of Spanish and Native American Cultures

ETHNIC GROUP	BREAD, CEREAL, RICE, AND PASTA GROUP	VEGETABLE GROUP	FRUIT GROUP	MILK, YOGURT, AND CHEESE GROUP	MEAT, POULTRY, FISH, DRY BEANS, EGGS, AND NUTS GROUP	FATS, OILS, AND SWEETS GROUP
Mexican	Corn and related products, taco shells, corn or flour tortillas, rice, white bread	Chili peppers, tomatoes and salsa, squash, yam bean root (jicama), prickly pear cactus, yucca root (cassava or manioc)	Avocado, guacamole, citrus fruits, papaya	Cheese, flan, sour cream and aged cheese	Black or pinto beans, refried beans, Mexican sausage (chorizo), beef, chicken, pork, goat, eggs	Lard
Caribbean persons (includes Puerto Rican and Cuban individuals)	Rice, sweet potatoes, chayote squash, plantains (usually fried)	Beets, eggplant, corn, tubers (yucca), white yams (boniato)	Tropical fruits, avocado, breadfruit, grapefruit, lemons, limes, mango	Flan, hard cheese (queso de mano)	Chicken, fish, pork, legumes, sausage (chorizo)	Lard, olive and peanut oil
Native American (each tribe may have specific foods; commonly consumed foods are listed here)	Blue corn flour used to make cornbread, mush dumplings; fruit dumplings (walakshi); fry bread (biscuit dough deep fried); ground sweet acorns; tortillas; wheat or rye used to make cornmeal and flour	Cabbage, carrots, cassava, dandelion greens, eggplant, milkweed, onions, pumpkin, squash, sweet and white potatoes, turnips, wild tullies (a tuber), yellow corn	Dried wild cherries and grapes; wild bananas, berries, and yucca	Not heavily used in traditional dishes	Duck, eggs, fish eggs, geese, venison, beef, pork, chicken, mutton, smoked or processed meat, wild rabbit, dried beans, lentils, nuts (all)	Lard and shortening

Modified from Grodner M, Roth S, Walkingshaw B. *Nutritional Foundations and Clinical Applications: A Nursing Approach.* 5e, St. Louis: Mosby; 2012.

their food patterns are similar (Figure 14-1).[9] However, Puerto Ricans add tropical fruits and vegetables, many of which are available in their neighborhood markets in the United States. Starchy vegetables and fruits such as plantains and green bananas, are popular foods. Two other basic foods are rice and beans. Milk, meat, yellow and green vegetables, and other fruits are used in limited quantities, but dried codfish is a staple (see Table 14-1). The traditional cooking fat is lard.

Native American. The Native American population of American Indians and Alaska Natives is composed of 566 federally recognized diverse groups that live in small rural communities, in metropolitan cities, and on reservations.[10] Despite their individual diversity, the various groups share a spiritual attachment to the land and a determination to retain their culture. Food has great religious and social significance in these groups. Serving food is an integral part of celebrations, ceremonies, and everyday hospitality. Foods may be

prepared and used in different ways from region to region. Variation reflects what can be grown locally, harvested, or hunted on the land or fished from its rivers; it also reflects what is available in food markets (see Table 14-1).

Among the American Indian groups of the Southwest United States, the food pattern of the Navajo people—whose reservation extends over a 25,000 square mile area at the junction of New Mexico, Arizona, and Utah—is one example. The Navajos learned farming and established corn and other crops as staples. They later learned herding from the Spaniards, which made sheep and goats available for food and wool. Some families also raise chickens, pigs, and cattle. Today, Native American food habits combine traditional dietary staples (e.g., corn/maize, beans, rice) with modern food products from available supermarkets and fast-food restaurants (Figure 14-2). However, health concerns are growing as a result of the increased use of modern convenience or snack foods that are

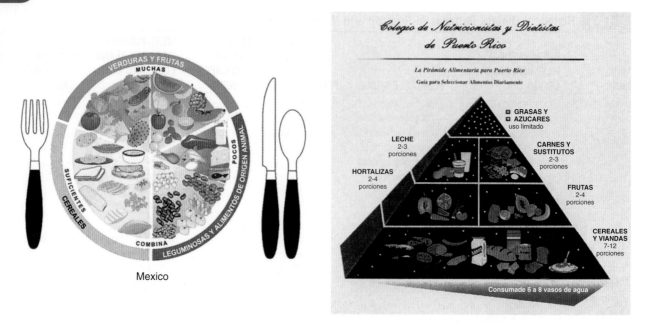

Mexico

Puerto Rico

FIGURE 14-1 National food guides for Mexico and Puerto Rico. (Reprinted from Painter J, Rah JH, Lee YK. Comparison of international food guide pictorial representations. *J Am Diet Assoc*. 2002;102:483-489, with permission from the Academy of Nutrition and Dietetics.)

Dairy Group
1 cup low-fat, skim, or acidophilus milk
1 cup low- or non-fat yogurt
1-1/2 ounces natural cheese (or 2 ounces processed), low- or non-fat preferred
*Breast milk for babies, goat's milk, bone soup, fish head soup, or canned salmon with bones

Vegetable Group
1 cup raw leafy greens
1/2 cup other vegetables, cooked or raw
3/4 cup vegetable juice, green beans, squash, kale, broccoli, or zucchini
*Sprouts or new shoots, wild mushrooms, nopalitos, wild onion, amaranth leaves (wild spinach), fresh or dried squash, lambsquarter (kappa), wild mustard, peeled stems, purslane or jicama

Bread Group
1 6-inch corn tortilla
1 7-1/2-inch flour tortilla**
4-6 crackers**
1 slice bread**
1/2 hamburger bun**
1/2 cup cooked cereal**
1 ounce ready-to-eat cereal**
1/2 cup rice or pasta (cooked)**
*Indian biscuits (bannock bread), popcorn, Indian wheat or psyllium (plantago), barley, wild oats, wild rice, amaranth and mesquite flour, popped amaranth seeds, wild peas, or corn (fresh, frozen or cooked)

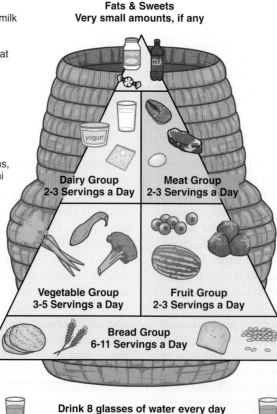

Fats & Sweets
Very small amounts, if any

Dairy Group
2-3 Servings a Day

Meat Group
2-3 Servings a Day

Vegetable Group
3-5 Servings a Day

Fruit Group
2-3 Servings a Day

Bread Group
6-11 Servings a Day

Drink 8 glasses of water every day unless your doctor has advised limited fluids.

Fats & Sweets
Butter or margarine, lard, gravy, fried foods, mayonnaise, ranch dressing, chips, sugar, candy, jelly, desserts, soda pop, sports drinks, or fruit flavored juice.
*Fry bread, animal fat, fish oil, honey, chucata (mesquite gum), atole (sweetened liquid corn or mesquite), or Mexican cheese

Meat Group
2-3 ounces cooked meat, poultry, or fish
Count as one ounce of meat:
1 medium egg or 1 low-fat hotdog
1/2 cup cooked dried beans, peas or tuna
2 Tbsp peanut butter, nuts or seeds
*Deer, rabbit, squirrel, pigeon, lamb, mariscos, fish (fresh or frozen), fowl, quail, eggs of birds or salmon, chia seeds, garbanzo or tepary beans, wild acorns, hazelnuts, or pine nuts

Fruit Group
1/2 - 3/4 cup 100% fruit juice
1 small piece fresh fruit
1/2 cup canned or fresh chopped fruit or melon
1/4 cup dried fruit
*Blueberries, huckleberries, or blackberries, choke cherries, wild crabapples, wild black cherries, prickly pear or saguaro fruit, strawberries, plums, melons

FIGURE 14-2 Southern Arizona Native American Food Guide: Choices for a Healthy Life. *Traditional foods. **Whole-grain products recommended. (Osterkamp LK, Longstaff L. Development of a dietary teaching tool for American Indians and Alaskan Natives in Southern Arizona. *Nutr Educ Behav*. 2004;36:272-274.)

high in fat, sugar, calories, and sodium, especially among children and teenagers.

Other Native American tribes in the United States have their own heritages and distinct dietary habits relative to customs and the regions in which they live.

Influences of the Southern United States

Black or African American. Black or African-American individuals make up the largest minority group in the United States. According to the U.S. Census, 14% of Americans are black or African American.[11] The majority of black people in the United States arrived from West Africa through enslavement during the 1600s and 1700s. Approximately 11 million Africans were sold into slavery, with nearly 6% of those individuals ending up in the United States (the remaining individuals were sold in the West Indies and South America).[12] Although the majority of black people in the United States have African heritage, some individuals originated later from the Caribbean and Central America. Thus, some Americans with black or brown skin are not African Americans.

African-American cultures, especially in the Southern states, have contributed a rich heritage to American food patterns, particularly to Southern cooking as a whole. Similar to their moving music styles (e.g., spirituals, blues, gospel, jazz), the food patterns of Southern African Americans developed through a creative ability to turn staples at hand into

memorable food. Although regional differences occur, as with any basic food pattern, the representative uses of foods from the basic food groups are outlined in Table 14-2. Unique foods such as spoonbread (a soufflé-like dish of cornmeal with beaten eggs) and "hoppin John" (black-eyed peas served over rice, traditionally served on New Year's Day to bring good luck for the new year) are two examples of foods specific to this region. African American's have a high prevalence of lactose intolerance. Consequently, some cheese is used in meals but not much milk. Pork, corn, green leafy vegetables, and fried foods are common staples in the traditional fare. Sunday dinner feasts provide time for social and family gathering where traditional comfort foods are in high demand (particularly in the South).

French American. The **Cajun** people, who are concentrated in the southwestern coastal waterways of

> **Cajun** a group of people with an enduring tradition whose French-Catholic ancestors established permanent communities in southern Louisiana after being expelled from Acadia (now Nova Scotia, Canada) by the reigning English during the late eighteenth century; they developed a unique food pattern from a blend of native French influence and the Creole cooking that was found in the new land.

Table 14-2   Historical Dietary Patterns of the African-American and Cajun American Cultures

ETHNIC GROUP	BREAD, CEREAL, RICE, AND PASTA GROUP	VEGETABLE GROUP	FRUIT GROUP	MILK, YOGURT, AND CHEESE GROUP	MEAT, POULTRY, FISH, DRY BEANS, EGGS, AND NUTS GROUP	FATS, OILS, AND SWEETS GROUP
African American (particularly in the Southern states)	Biscuits, cornbread as spoonbread, cornpone, or hush puppies; grits	Leafy greens (dandelion greens, kale, mustard greens, collard greens), butter beans, cabbage, corn, green beans, okra, sweet and white potatoes, tomatoes, turnips	Peaches, bananas, watermelon, melon, fruit juice	Buttermilk	Eggs, ground beef, pork and pork products (chitterlings, bacon, pig's feet, pig ears), poultry, organ meats, venison, rabbit, catfish, buffalo fish, flounder, legumes, peanuts	Lard, shortening, and vegetable oils; pies and cakes
French/Cajun	French bread, hushpuppies, cornbread muffins, cush-cush (cornmeal mush cooked with milk), grits, rice	Onions, bell peppers, celery, okra, parsley, shallots, tomatoes, yams	Ambrosia (freshly peeled orange segments and orange juice with sliced bananas and freshly grated coconut), blackberries, lemons, limes, strawberries	Not heavily used in traditional dishes	Catfish, red snapper, shrimp, blue crab, oysters, crawfish, chicken, pork sausage, legumes	Poultry fat; pies, bread pudding, pecan pralines

southern Louisiana, have contributed a unique cuisine and food pattern to America's rich and varied fare. This pattern continues to provide a unique model for the rapidly expanding forms of American ethnic food. The Cajuns are descendants of the early French colonists of Acadia, which is a peninsula on the eastern coast of Canada. During the pre-Revolutionary wars between France and Britain, both countries contended for the area of Acadia. However, after Britain won control of Canada, the fear of an Acadian revolt led to a forcible deportation of the French colonists in 1755. After traveling down the Atlantic coast and then westward along the Gulf of Mexico, a group of the impoverished Acadians settled along the bayou country of what is now Louisiana. To support themselves, they developed their distinctive food pattern from the seafood at hand and from what they could grow and harvest. Over time, Cajuns blended their own French culinary background with the Creole cooking that they found in their new homeland around New Orleans.

Cajun foods are strong flavored and spicy, with the abundant seafood as a base and usually cooked as a stew and served over rice. The well-known hot chili sauce Tabasco, which is made from crushed and fermented red chili peppers blended with spices and vinegar, is still made by generations of a Cajun family on Avery Island on the coastal waterway of southern Louisiana. Other popular seasonings include cayenne pepper, crushed black pepper, white pepper, bay leaves, thyme, and **filé powder.** The most popular shellfish native to the region is the crawfish, which is now grown commercially in the fertile rice paddies of the bayou areas. The low-country boil or **crawfish boil** originated from this region. See Table 14-2 for other representative foods.

Wine is a typical drink for people with French heritage, but this is true more so in France than in the United States; however, wine is considered a staple for drinking and cooking for the Cajuns and French Canadians. While the Canadian Food Guide does not necessarily demonstrate specific French inclinations, it is presented in Figure 14-3. Note the similarities between Canada's Food Guide and the MyPlate recommendations from the United States (see Figure 1-3).

---

filé powder a substance that is made from ground sassafras leaves; it seasons and thickens the dish into which it is added.
crawfish boil traditional Louisiana Cajun festive meal. Typically includes crawfish, crab, shrimp, small ears of corn, new potatoes, onions, garlic and seasonings such as cayenne pepper, hot sauce, salt, lemons, and bay leaf. Smoked sausage links are occasionally added. All ingredients are added to a large pot and boiled. The contents are then spread out on newspaper-covered tables for everyone to eat from directly.

Asian Food Patterns

There are many distinct cultures and food patterns throughout Asia. The most commonly encountered cultural food patterns from Asia found within the United States are influenced from China, Japan, and some of the Southeast Asian countries (Vietnam, Laos, Cambodia, and the Philippines).

Chinese. The Chinese include a large array of fruits and vegetables. Chinese cooks believe that refrigeration diminishes natural flavors, so they select the freshest foods possible, hold them for the shortest time possible, and cook them quickly at a high temperature in a *wok* (a round-bottom pan) with small amounts of fat and liquid. The wok allows heat to be controlled with a quick stir-frying method that preserves natural flavor, color, and texture. Vegetables that are cooked just before serving are still crisp and flavorful when served. Meat is used in small amounts in combined dishes, more so than as a single main entree. A small amount of milk is used as well as eggs and soybean products (e.g., tofu), which add other sources of protein. Foods that have been dried, salted, pickled, spiced, candied, or canned may be added as garnishes or relishes to mask some flavors or textures or to enhance others. Rice is the staple grain that is used at most meals. The traditional beverage is unsweetened green tea. Seasonings include soy sauce, ginger, almonds, and sesame seeds. Peanut oil is the main cooking fat. Figure 14-4 illustrates the pictorial food guides for China, Japan, and Korea. Table 14-3 provides representative foods from each culture.

Japanese. In many ways, Japanese food patterns are similar to those of the Chinese. Rice is the basic grain served at meals, soy sauce is used for seasoning, and tea is the main beverage. The Japanese diet contains more seafood, especially in the form of sushi, than the Chinese diet does (see Table 14-3). The term *sushi* does not necessarily mean raw fish; some sushi is prepared with only vegetables or with cooked fish. Short-grain sticky rice mixed with vinegar and a little sugar is used for sushi. Many varieties of fish, shellfish, and fish eggs are used. Vegetables are often steamed or pickled. Fresh fruit is eaten in season, and a tray of fruit is a typical dessert after a main meal. Soybean products are common in the Japanese diet, as is the use of seaweed. Aesthetic appeal is an important part of food preparation and presentation in Japanese culture. Soup is frequently served as part of both lunch and dinner meals. The overall Japanese diet is high in sodium content and low in milk products because of the high prevalence of lactose intolerance.

Southeast Asian. The largest groups of refugees from Southeast Asia are Vietnamese, but others have come from the adjacent war-torn countries of Laos and Cambodia. Since 1975, in the wake of the Vietnam War,

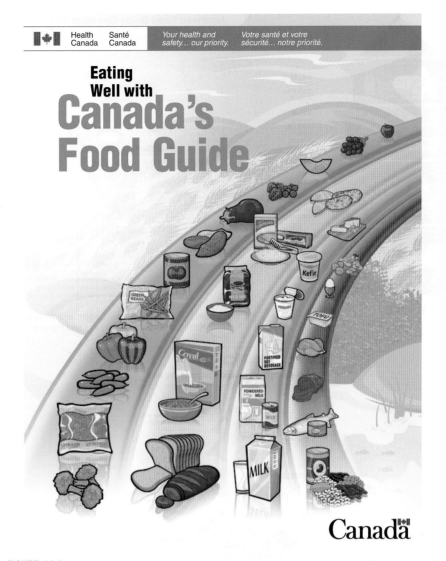

FIGURE 14-3 Canada's Food Guide. (www.hc-sc.gc.ca/fn-an/food-guide-aliment/index-eng.php.)

more than 700,000 Vietnamese have immigrated to the United States. A significant number of Filippinos immigrated to America during the early 1900s when the Philippines were an American territory. Refugees from Southeast Asia mainly settled in California, with other groups located in New York, Florida, Texas, Illinois, and Pennsylvania.

As a whole, the food patterns from the various Southeast Asian countries have similar characteristics to one another and have an effect on American diet and agriculture. Asian grocery stores throughout the country stock many traditional Asian food items. Rice (both long grain and glutinous) forms the basis of the Southeast Asian food pattern and is eaten at most meals. The Vietnamese usually eat their rice plain in a separate rice bowl and not mixed with other foods, whereas other Southeast Asians may eat rice in mixed dishes. Soups are also commonly served with meals. Many fresh fruits and vegetables are eaten along with fresh herbs and other seasonings such as chives, spring onions, chili peppers, ginger root, coriander, turmeric,

and fish sauce. Many kinds of seafood (i.e., fish and shellfish) are included in the diet, as well as chicken, duck, and pork (see Table 14-3). Red meat is usually eaten only in small quantities. In a traditional Asian diet, nuts and legumes are the primary sources of protein. Stir-frying in a wok with a small amount of lard or peanut oil is a common method of cooking.

Third and fourth generation immigrants and refugees have acculturated to American food choices. These changes include the use of more eggs, beef, pork, dairy products, candy and other sweet snacks, bread, fast foods, soft drinks, butter, margarine, and coffee.

Mediterranean Influences

Many countries border the Mediterranean Sea. The specifics of the food culture in these countries vary; however, the general dietary patterns of this region are believed to have protective qualities against the development of certain chronic diseases (see the Clinical Applications box, "Mediterranean Diet and Heart

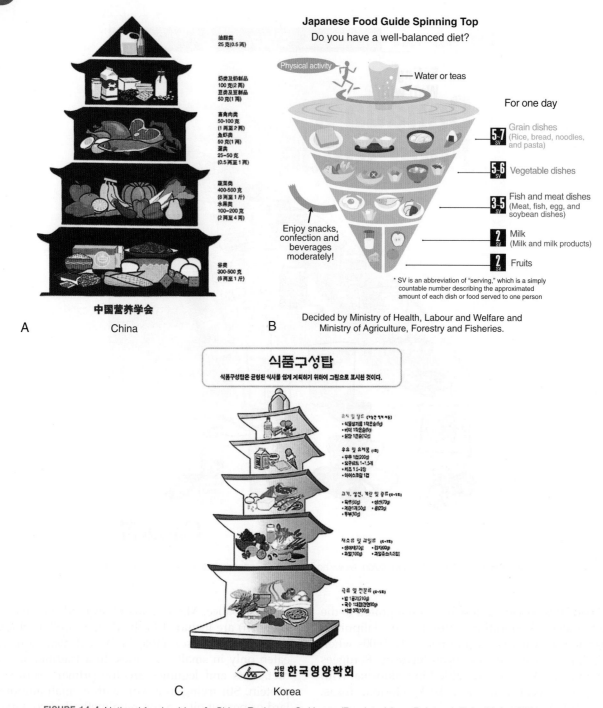

FIGURE 14-4 National food guides. **A,** China; **B,** Japan; **C,** Korea. (Reprinted from Painter J, Rah JH, Lee YK. Comparison of international food guide pictorial representations. *J Am Diet Assoc.* 2002;102:483-489, with permission from the Academy of Nutrition and Dietetics; and Yoshiike N, Hayashi F, Takemi Y, et al. A new food guide in Japan: the Japanese food guide Spinning Top. *Nutr Rev.* 2007;65[4]:149-154.)

Disease"). We will only focus on the influences that have the largest impact within the United States and those that are most closely associated with the Mediterranean Diet Pyramid (Figure 14-5).

Italian. The sharing of food is an important part of Italian life. Meals are associated with warmth and fellowship, and special occasions are shared with families and friends. Bread and pasta are the basic ingredients of most meals. Milk, which is seldom used alone, is

typically mixed with coffee in equal portions. Cheese is a favorite food, with many popular varieties available. Meats, poultry, and fish are used in many ways, and the varied Italian sausages and cold cuts are famous worldwide. Vegetables are used alone, in mixed main dishes, or in soups, sauces, and salads. Seasonings include herbs and spices, garlic, wine, olive oil, tomato puree, and salted pork. Main dishes are prepared by initially browning vegetables and seasonings in olive oil; adding meat or fish; covering with

Table 14-3   Cultural Dietary Patterns of Asian Influence

ETHNIC GROUP	BREAD, CEREAL, RICE, AND PASTA GROUP	VEGETABLE GROUP	FRUIT GROUP	MILK, YOGURT, AND CHEESE GROUP	MEAT, POULTRY, FISH, DRY BEANS, EGGS, AND NUTS GROUP	FATS, OILS, AND SWEETS GROUP
Chinese	Rice, noodles, wheat products, stuffed noodles (wonton) filled buns (boa); stuffed dumplings	Asparagus, bamboo shoots; bean sprouts, cabbage, Chinese celery, Chinese parsley (coriander), Chinese turnips (lo bok), cucumbers, dry fungus (black Judas ear), leafy green vegetables, Chinese broccoli (gai lan), lotus tubers, okra, snow peas, taro root, white radish	Kumquats	Not heavily used in traditional dishes	Fish, seafood, legumes, nuts, organ meats, pigeon eggs, pork and pork products, tofu	Peanut, soy, sesame, and rice oil; lard
Japanese	Short-grain rice and rice products, rice flour (mochiko), noodles (somen, soba)	Artichokes, bamboo shoots, broccoli, beets, burdock (gobo) cabbage, dried mushrooms (shiitake), eggplant, horseradish (wasabi), ginger, green onion, Japanese parsley (seri), lotus root (renkon), mustard greens, pickled vegetables, seaweed, white radish	Pear-like apples (nasi), dates, figs, persimmons, plums, pineapple	Not heavily used in traditional dishes	Fish and shellfish including dried fish with bones, raw fish (sashimi), fish cake (kamaboko); soybeans and soybean products (tofu), red beans (adzuki)	Soy and rice oil
Filipino	Noodles, rice, rice flour (mochiko), stuffed noodles (wonton), white bread	Bamboo shoots, dark green leafy vegetables (malunggay and salyot), eggplant, sweet potatoes, okra, palm, peppers, turnips, root crop (gabi), pickled vegetables	Avocado, banana, bitter melon (ampalaya), breadfruit, guavas, jackfruit, limes, mango, papaya, pod fruit (tamarind), pomelos, rhubarb, tangelo (naranghita), strawberries, pickled fruits	Custards, evaporated milk	Fish in all forms; dried fish (dilis); egg roll (lumpia); fish sauce (alamang, bagoong); legumes, organ meats, pork with chicken in soy sauce (adobo), pork sausage, tofu	None
Southeastern Asians (i.e., Laos, Cambodia, Thailand, Vietnam, the Hmong, and the Mien)	Rice (long and short grain) and related products such as noodles; Hmong cornbread or cake	Artichoke, bamboo shoots, beans, broccoli, Chinese parsley (coriander), cabbage, Chinese chard and radish, mustard greens, mushrooms, peppers, pickled vegetables, water chestnuts, Thai chili peppers	Apple pear (Asian pear), bitter melon, dates, durian, figs, grapefruit, guava, jackfruit, mango, papaya	Sweetened condensed milk	Beef, chicken, duck, eggs; fish and shellfish, legumes, peanuts, soybeans, organ meats, pork, tofu	Lard, peanut oil

Modified from Grodner M, Roth S, Walkingshaw B. *Nutritional Foundations and Clinical Applications: A Nursing Approach.* 5e. St. Louis: Mosby; 2012.

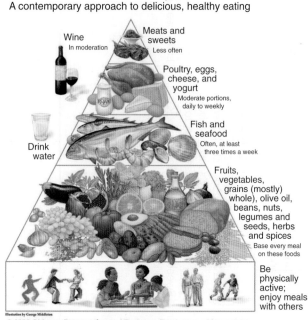

Mediterranean Diet Pyramid
A contemporary approach to delicious, healthy eating

Wine
In moderation

Meats and sweets
Less often

Poultry, eggs, cheese, and yogurt
Moderate portions, daily to weekly

Fish and seafood
Often, at least three times a week

Drink water

Fruits, vegetables, grains (mostly) whole), olive oil, beans, nuts, legumes and seeds, herbs and spices
Base every meal on these foods

Be physically active; enjoy meals with others

Illustration by George Middleton

© 2009 Oldways Preservation and Exchange Trust • www.oldwayspt.org

FIGURE 14-5 Mediterranean Diet Pyramid. (Copyright 2009, Oldways Preservation & Exchange Trust, Boston, Mass; www.oldwayspt.org/mediterranean-diet-pyramid.)

such liquids as wine, broth, or tomato sauce; and simmering on low heat for several hours. Fresh fruit is often eaten as dessert or as a snack (Table 14-4).

Greek. The largest population of immigrants from the Balkans was from Greece. Everyday meals are simple, but Greek holiday meals are occasions for serving many delicacies. Bread is always the center of every meal, with other foods considered accompaniments. Milk is seldom used as a beverage but instead served in the cultured form of yogurt. Cheese is a favorite food, especially *feta,* which is a white cheese that is made from sheep's milk and preserved in brine. Lamb is the preferred meat, but other sources of protein, especially fish, also are eaten. Eggs are sometimes a main dish, but they are rarely a breakfast food. Many vegetables are used, often as a main entree, and they are cooked with broth, tomato sauce, onions, olive oil, and herbs such as parsley. A typical salad of thinly sliced raw vegetables and feta cheese, dressed with olive oil and vinegar, is often served with meals; the traditional Greek salad also is a favorite at many American restaurants. Rice is a main grain in many dishes. Fruit is an everyday dessert, but rich pastries such as *baklava* are served on special occasions (see Table 14-4).

RELIGIOUS DIETARY LAWS

The dietary practices within Christianity (e.g., Catholic, Protestant, and Eastern Orthodox churches), Judaism, Hinduism, Buddhism, and Islam fluctuate in accordance with each follower's independent understanding and interpretation of what constitutes a healthy and proper diet. Such dietary laws may apply to what, how, and when specific foods are allowed or avoided. Some dietary laws are applicable at all times (e.g., no pork at any time for Islamic followers), whereas other laws apply only during religious ceremonies (e.g., during Lent for Roman Catholics). Following are examples of two such religions and their dietary laws.

Jewish

Basic food pattern. All Jewish festivals are religious in nature and have historic significance, but the observance of Jewish food laws differs among the three basic groups within Judaism: (1) orthodox, with strict observance; (2) conservative, with less strict observance; and (3) reform, with less ceremonial emphasis and minimal general use. The basic body of dietary laws is called the *Rules of Kashrut* as established in the Torah. Foods that are selected and prepared in accordance with these rules are called *kosher,* from the Hebrew word meaning "fit, proper." These laws originally had special ritual significance. Current Jewish dietary laws govern the slaughter, preparation, and serving of meat; the combining of meat and milk; and the use of fish and eggs. The following are some of the Jewish food restrictions:

- *Meat:* Appropriate meats should come from animals that chew their cud and that have cloven hooves. Pork, rabbits, and birds of prey are avoided at all times. All forms of meat are thoroughly cleansed of blood.
- *Meat and milk:* Meat and milk products are both part of the kosher Jewish diet; however, they are not to be eaten at the same meal or prepared with the use of the same dishes. Orthodox homes maintain two sets of regular dishes: one for serving meat and the other for meals that contain dairy products. An additional two sets of dishes are maintained especially for use during Passover.
- *Fish:* Only fish with fins and scales are allowed. These may be eaten with either meat or dairy meals. Shellfish and crustaceans are avoided.
- *Eggs:* No egg with a blood spot may be eaten. Eggs may be used with either meat or dairy meals.

Representative foods and influence of festivals. Many traditional Jewish foods relate to festivals of the Jewish calendar that commemorate significant events in Jewish history; examples include the Sabbath, Rosh Hashanah, Yom Kippur, Sukkot, Hanukkah, Purim, and Passover. A few representative foods, mostly of Eastern European influence, include the following:

- *Bagels:* doughnut-shaped hard yeast rolls
- *Blintzes:* thin, filled, rolled pancakes
- *Borscht (borsch):* a soup of meat stock, beaten egg or sour cream, beets, cabbage, or spinach that is served hot or cold

Clinical Application

Mediterranean Diet and Heart Disease

The Mediterranean Diet reflects the traditional dietary patterns of the cultures surrounding the Mediterranean Sea. This specific dietary pattern was more pronounced in Greece and Italy before the globalization of the food market in the 1960s.[1] There are many variations on what specifically constitutes the Mediterranean Diet, because the region encompasses many countries (see map below) and diverse cultural food traditions. However, it may loosely be defined as a diet high in fruits, vegetables, legumes, nuts, whole-grain cereals, fatty fish, and olive oil. The diet is low in added sugar and saturated fat from meat and dairy products. Compared to the typical Western diet, the Mediterranean Diet is relatively low in total protein (≈10% of total kilocalories) and much higher in monounsaturated fat. Another key component of the Mediterranean Diet is daily moderate intake of wine with meals, predominantly red wine. According to the Mediterranean Diet Score,* *moderate alcohol intake* is defined as 10 to 50 g per day for men and 5 to 25 g per day for women.[1]

As with any study involving diet and disease, it remains difficult to elucidate the specific factors of the Mediterranean Diet that provide cardio-protective attributes. Nevertheless, it is well accepted that individuals and populations following a Mediterranean-type diet and lifestyle have a reduction in the risk for cardiovascular disease.[2,3] Consuming a diet rich in plant foods provides ample antioxidants, phytochemicals, fiber, vitamins, and minerals. Avoiding processed foods also reduces the intake of trans fats, added sugar, and high-glycemic foods. Moderate intake of red wine provides antioxidant polyphenols that are protective against atherogenesis. A high intake of olive oil and a low consumption of animal products provide a favorable unsaturated to saturated lipid ratio. Taken as a whole, the diet is antiinflammatory, palatable, and easy to follow long-term, and is indicated as an effective method for cardiovascular disease prevention.

REFERENCES

1. Trichopoulou A, et al. Definitions and potential health benefits of the Mediterranean diet: views from experts around the world. *BMC Med.* 2014;12:112.
2. Ros E, et al. Mediterranean diet and cardiovascular health: Teachings of the PREDIMED study. *Adv Nutr.* 2014;5(3):330S-336S.
3. Martinez-Gonzalez MA, Bes-Rastrollo M. Dietary patterns, Mediterranean diet, and cardiovascular disease. *Curr Opin Lipidol.* 2014;25(1):20-26.

Countries that border the Mediterranean Sea

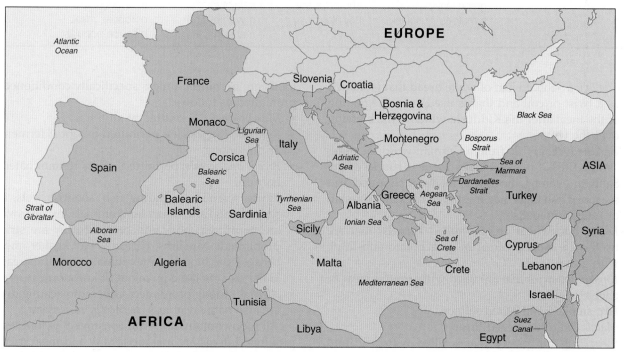

*Mediterranean Diet Score: a method for assessing a person's adherence to the Mediterranean Diet.

Table 14-4   Historical Dietary Patterns of the Mediterranean

ETHNIC GROUP	BREAD, CEREAL, RICE, AND PASTA GROUP	VEGETABLE GROUP	FRUIT GROUP	MILK, YOGURT, AND CHEESE GROUP	MEAT, POULTRY, FISH, DRY BEANS, EGGS, AND NUTS GROUP	FATS, OILS, AND SWEETS GROUP
Italian	Bread, pasta, polenta, risotto	Artichokes, asparagus, cabbage, capers, chicory, corn, eggplant, endive, fennel, garlic, golden onion, green leafy vegetables, mushrooms, peppers, potatoes, radicchio, tomatoes, truffles	Apricots, cherries, dates, figs, grapes, pomegranates, oranges	Many rich cheeses made from cow, sheep, and goat milk such as asiago, mozzarella, taleggio, gorgonzola, ricotta, provolone, ragusano	Beef, goat, lamb, pork (prosciutto, salami, sausage), poultry, fish (including anchovies, sardines, and a variety of other seafood and shellfish), legumes (chickpeas, fava beans, lentils)	Olive oil, lard
Greek	Bread, pita bread, rice	Artichokes, beets, Brussels sprouts, cabbage, cucumber, eggplant, garlic, green beans, leeks, bell peppers, spinach, stuffed grape leaves, tomatoes, zucchini	Apricots, avocado, cherries, currants, dates, figs, grapes, pomegranates, oranges, olives, jams and chutneys are popular	Buttermilk, cream, a variety of cheeses made from goat, sheep, and cow's milk such as feta, graviera, kefalotyri myzithra, and manouri	Lamb, beef, veal, rabbit, poultry, eggs, snails, legumes (chickpeas, fava beans, lentils, red beans), seafood (fish eggs, mussels, squid, octopus); meat pies are popular	Olive oil

- *Challah:* a Sabbath loaf of white bread that is shaped as a twist or coil and that is used at the beginning of the meal after the Kiddush, which is the blessing over the wine
- *Gefüllte (gefilte) fish:* from a German word meaning "stuffed fish," this is usually the first course of the Sabbath evening meal; it is made of chopped and seasoned fish filets that are stuffed back into the skin or rolled into balls
- *Kasha:* buckwheat groats (hulled kernels) that are used as a cooked cereal or as a potato substitute with gravy
- *Knishes:* pastries that are filled with ground meat or cheese
- *Lox:* smoked and salted salmon
- *Matzo:* flat, unleavened bread
- *Strudel:* a thin pastry that is filled with fruit and nuts, rolled, and baked

Muslim

Basic food pattern. Muslim dietary laws are based on the restriction or prohibition of some foods and the promotion of others, and they are derived from the Islamic teachings found in the Quran. The laws are binding and must be followed at all times, even during pregnancy, hospitalization, and travel. In the most strict and observant areas, these laws are also binding for visitors in the host Muslim country. Almost all

foods are permitted unless specifically conditioned or prohibited as follows:

- *Milk products:* permitted at all times
- *Fruits and vegetables:* permitted except if fermented or poisonous
- *Breads and cereals:* permitted unless contaminated or harmful
- *Meats:* seafood (including fish, shellfish, eels, and sea animals) and many land animals (except swine) are permitted; pork and birds of prey are strictly prohibited. Muslims typically eat kosher meats, because the blood of the animal is not to be eaten. Halal meat is the equivalent of kosher meat.
- *Alcohol:* strictly prohibited. Other intoxicating drugs are also banned unless medically necessary.

All food combinations are consumed as long as no prohibited items are included. Milk and meat may be eaten together, which is in contrast with Jewish kosher laws. The Quran mentions certain foods as being of special value to physical and social health, including figs, olives, dates, honey, milk, and buttermilk. Foods that are prohibited by the Muslim dietary laws may be eaten when no other sources of food are available.

Representative foods in the Middle East. Specific food choices will reflect not only the Muslin dietary law but also the geographic region in which people live. Following are a number of typical foods and dishes that may be used as appetizers, main dishes, snacks, or salads for individuals in the Middle East:

- *Bulgur (or burghel):* partially cooked and dried cracked wheat that is available in a coarse grind as a base for pilaf or in a fine grind for use in tabouli and kibbeh
- *Falafel:* a "fast food" that is made from a seasoned paste of ground, soaked beans that is formed into shapes and fried
- *Fatayeh:* a snack or appetizer that is similar to a small pizza, with toppings of cheese, meat, or spinach
- *Kibbeh:* a meat dish that is made of cracked wheat shell filled with small pieces of lamb and fried in oil
- *Pilaf:* sautéed and seasoned bulgur or rice that is steamed in a bouillon, sometimes with poultry, meat, or shellfish
- *Pita:* a flat circular bread that is torn or cut into pieces and stuffed with sandwich fillings or used as a scoop for a dip such as *hummus,* which is made from chickpeas
- *Tabouli:* a salad made from soaked bulgur that has been combined with chopped tomatoes, parsley, mint, and green onion and then mixed with olive oil and lemon juice

Influence of festivals. The fourth pillar of Islam as commanded by the Quran is fasting. Among the Muslim people, a 30-day period of daylight fasting is required during **Ramadan.** Ramadan was chosen for the sacred fast because that was when Muhammad received the first of the revelations that were subsequently compiled to form the Quran, and it is also the month when Muhammad's followers first drove their enemies from Mecca in 624 AD. During the month of Ramadan, Muslims all over the world observe daily fasting by taking no food or drink from dawn until sunset. However, nights are often spent at special feasts. First, an appetizer such as dates or a fruit drink is served, and then followed by the family's "evening breakfast," which is called the *iftar.* At the end of Ramadan, a traditional feast that lasts up to 3 days concludes the observance. Special dishes that include delicacies such as thin pancakes dipped in powdered sugar, savory buns, and dried fruits mark this occasion (see the Cultural Considerations box, "Id al-Fitr: The Post-Ramadan Festival").

All Muslims past the age of puberty, regardless of medical condition, observe the fast of Ramadan. Individuals with diabetes, who are taking certain medications, or who are pregnant or breastfeeding may experience complications during this time. Individuals may be exempt from fasting in certain situations but should make up the days of fasting before the next

> **Ramadan** the ninth month of the Muslim year, which is a period of daily fasting from sunrise to sunset.

Id al-Fitr: The Post-Ramadan Festival

At the conclusion of Ramadan, Islam's holy month of prayer and fasting, wealthy merchants and princes in Muslim countries traditionally hold public feasts for the needy. This is known as the Festival of Id al-Fitr.

Over the years, many delicacies have been served to symbolize the joy of returning from fasting and the heightened sense of unity, brotherhood, and charity that the fasting experience has brought to the people. Among the foods served are chicken or veal sautéed with eggplant and onions and then simmered slowly in pomegranate juice and spiced with turmeric and cardamom seeds. The highlight of the meal is usually *kharuf mahshi,* which is a whole lamb (i.e., a symbol of sacrifice) that is stuffed with a rich dressing made of dried fruits, cracked wheat, pine nuts, almonds, and onions and seasoned with ginger and coriander. The stuffed lamb is baked in hot ashes for many hours so that it is tender enough to be pulled apart and eaten with the fingers.

At the conclusion of the meal, rich pastries and candies are served; these may be flavored with spices or flower petals. Some of the sweets are taken home and savored for as long as possible as a reminder of the festival.

Ramadan fast. Health care professionals must be sensitive to such religious practices when counseling patients.

Table 14-5 outlines other common religions with specific dietary practices and their food or beverage restrictions.

CHANGING AMERICAN FOOD PATTERNS

The stereotype of the all-American family of two parents and two children eating three meals a day with no snacks in between is no longer the norm. Far-reaching changes have occurred with regard to Americans' ways of living and, subsequently, their food habits. Modifying one's own personal eating patterns is difficult enough; helping clients and patients to make needed changes for positive health reasons can be even more challenging. Such guidance requires a culturally sensitive and flexible understanding of the complex factors that are involved.

HOUSEHOLD DYNAMICS

What constitutes a typical American household has changed dramatically over the past several decades. A growing proportion of households involve groups of unrelated people living together. Beginning in the 1960s, the number of women in the workforce rose rapidly and this trend was not restricted to any social, economic, or ethnic group. The number of women in the workforce reached its peak in 1999 with 60% of all women employed. Currently, approximately 58% of women participate in the workforce in the United States. Women of all racial and ethnic groups hold half of all management and professional positions in the

Table 14-5   Religious Dietary Practices

	SEVENTH-DAY ADVENTIST	BUDDHIST	EASTERN ORTHODOX	HINDU	JEWISH	MORMON	MUSLIM	ROMAN CATHOLIC
Beef		Avoided by most devout		Prohibited or strongly discouraged				
Pork	Prohibited or strongly discouraged	Avoided by most devout		Avoided by most devout	Prohibited or strongly discouraged		Prohibited or strongly discouraged	
All meat	Avoided by most devout	Avoided by most devout	Permitted but some restrictions apply	Avoided by most devout				Permitted but some restrictions apply
Eggs, dairy	Permitted but avoided at some observances	Permitted but avoided at some observances	Permitted but some restrictions apply	Permitted but avoided at some observances	Permitted but some restrictions apply			
Fish	Avoided by most devout	Avoided by most devout	Permitted but some restrictions apply	Permitted but some restrictions apply	Permitted but some restrictions apply		Permitted but some restrictions apply	
Shellfish	Prohibited or strongly discouraged	Avoided by most devout	Permitted but avoided at some observances	Permitted but some restrictions apply	Prohibited or strongly discouraged			
Meat and dairy at same meal					Prohibited or strongly discouraged			
Leavened foods					Permitted but some restrictions apply			
Ritual slaughter of animals					Practiced		Practiced	
Alcohol	Prohibited or strongly discouraged			Avoided by most devout		Prohibited or strongly discouraged	Prohibited or strongly discouraged	
Caffeine	Prohibited or strongly discouraged					Prohibited or strongly discouraged	Avoided by most devout	

Modified from Kittler PG, Sucher KP. Food and Culture. 4th ed. Belmont, Calif: Brooks/Cole; 2004.

American labor market.[13] Working parents increasingly rely on food items and cooking methods that save time, space, and labor. Compared to the mid-1960s, more meals are consumed away from the home now and significantly less time is spent preparing and cooking meals.[14]

WITH WHOM AND WHERE WE EAT

Family meals, as they have been known, have changed. Breakfasts and lunches are seldom eaten in a family setting. Although research shows that frequent family meals are positively associated with improved nutritional value and beneficial developmental assets and that they are inversely related to high-risk behaviors among adolescents (e.g., substance abuse, violence), family meal time is on the decline.[15,16] Furthermore, when meals are consumed away from the home, the overall diet quality is inferior to typical meals consumed at home.[17]

HOW OFTEN AND HOW MUCH WE EAT

Frequency

Americans' habits have also changed with regard to when they eat. Mid-morning and mid-afternoon breaks at work usually involve food or beverages; evening television snacks and midnight refrigerator raids are not uncommon. Americans are increasing the number of times a day that they eat to as many as 11 "eating occasions"; this pattern has been termed *grazing*. This shift is not necessarily bad, depending on the nature of the periodic snacking or grazing. In fact, frequent small meals may be better for the body than three larger meals per day, especially when healthy snacking and grazing contribute to needed nutrient and energy intake (see the For Further Focus box, "Snacking: An All-American Food Habit").

Portion Sizes

Growing portion sizes are a concerning trend in typical American meals and snacks. Portion sizes and energy consumption from low-nutrient quality foods such as salty/savory snacks and sugar-sweetened beverages have increased substantially from that of the 1970s.[18,19] Despite many reports about the "portion distortion" issues in American eating patterns, serving sizes remain unnecessarily large, and most consumers continue to eat and drink relative to the amount of food and beverage served instead of in response to their actual hunger and energy needs.[20,21]

In 2003 researchers compared portion sizes of selected foods from fast-food restaurants to the sizes available the year those same foods were introduced.[22] In 1954, a regular order of french fries from Burger King was 2.6 oz. Fifty years later, a medium order of Burger King fries averaged 4.1 oz. In 1955, the only size of fries that McDonald's offered was a 2.4-oz portion. At the time of this study, the McDonald's portions range from small (2.4 oz) to Supersize (7.1 oz).

For Further Focus

Snacking: An All-American Food Habit

The snack market in the United States continues to grow. Consumer spending for all foods has increased, with a large portion of the increase being spent on snacks. Snacking is said to "ruin your appetite," and perhaps the consumption of excess soft drinks and other sources of "junk food" does, but is snacking altogether bad? Not necessarily. Many people snack on foods that are essential contributions to total nutritional adequacy (e.g., fruit, cheese, eggs, bread, crackers). The following represents the average percent of daily nutrients that Americans age 2 years and older obtain through snacking[1]:

- 24% of total energy
- 14% of protein
- 16% of vitamin A
- Between 16% and 23% of the B vitamins
- 28% of vitamin C
- 18% of vitamin D
- 24% of vitamin E
- 25% of calcium
- 28% of magnesium
- 17% of iron and zinc
- 22% of potassium

These are relatively significant contributions to the overall daily nutrient intake of key vitamins and minerals. Thus, not all snack foods are junk food. Snacking—or grazing, as some people do, which involves more frequent nibbling—is clearly a significant component of food behavior. Rather than rule against the practice, dietitians should promote snack foods that enhance nutritional well-being.

REFERENCE

1. U.S. Department of Agriculture, Agricultural Research Service. *Snacks: Percentages of Selected Nutrients Contributed by Food and Beverages Consumed at Snack Occasions, by Gender and Age, What We Eat in America, NHANES 2011-2012*. Washington, DC: 2014.

Hamburger sizes have likewise increased by 3-4-fold in the same amount of time for both fast-food chains. Despite this knowledge, very little has changed in the last decade to reduce portion sizes to pre-supersized proportions[23] (other than the discontinuation of the Supersize serving at McDonald's in 2004 after the release of the documentary *Super Size Me*).

Such sizes dwarf the standard serving sizes on the U.S. Department of Agriculture's MyPlate food guide. According to MyPlate, a standard serving of soda is 12 fl oz. However, the average size of a soda served at a fast-food eatery is 23 fl oz.[22] The Academy of Nutrition and Dietetics' position paper titled *"Total Diet Approach to Healthy Eating"* emphasizes the importance of portion control as a part of an overall healthy eating style.[24] The U.S. Department of Health and Human Services created an interesting Portion Distortion Quiz that depicts serving size changes over the past 20 years and it is worth checking out as an educational tool and eye opener (www.nhlbi.nih.gov/health/educational/wecan/eat-right/portion-distortion.htm).

ECONOMICAL BUYING

Many Americans are making diet changes to save money, and no-frills grocery stores are becoming more and more popular across the country. With a warehouse-type store, the cost of overhead is significantly reduced, and store owners can pass that savings on to consumers. Many Americans also are members of bulk-food chains such as Costco and Sam's Club. Buying in bulk (i.e., economy size or family size) can save money, but only if the quantity can be efficiently used; no savings are incurred if the food is not properly stored or not eaten before it spoils. Grocery stores also provide cost-per-unit pricing on the shelves to make comparing the prices of similar foods in different-sized containers or packages easier for the consumer.

Tempting advertisements often lure consumers into ordering or purchasing more food than they need at both restaurants and grocery stores. Deals such as "two for one" and "value meals" could be a great bargain, but they supply more food than is necessary for one person. Educating patients and clients on understanding proper portion sizes, buying in bulk, and knowing how to properly store food for later use (see Chapter 13) may be helpful in promoting a healthy lifestyle for them and their family.

Putting It All Together

Summary

- All people grow up and live in a social setting. Each person inherits a culture and a particular social structure, complete with its food habits and attitudes about eating.
- The effects on health that are associated with major social and economic shifts should be understood—as well as the current social forces, including cultural, religious, and psychologic—to help people make dietary changes that will benefit their health.
- Food patterns of Americans are changing. People who live fast-paced, complex lives increasingly rely on new forms of convenience food.
- Eating away from the home and at fast-food restaurants continues to increase energy intake and oversized portions.

Chapter Review Questions

See answers in Appendix A.

1. A dish that would most likely not be included on a meal plan for a patient who practices Muslim dietary law would be:
   a. Stuffed pork loin.
   b. Chicken parmesan.
   c. Bulgur pilaf with lamb.
   d. Pita bread and hummus.

2. Which of the following would most likely be found within a traditional diet for individuals of Mexican heritage?
   a. Meats, fish, eggs.
   b. Dried beans, tomatoes, corn.
   c. Corn, wheat, fish.
   d. Challah, lox, strudel.

3. A meal consisting of turnip greens, fried chicken, black-eyed peas, and cornbread is most typical of which region of the United States?
   a. Southern
   b. Northeastern
   c. Southwestern
   d. Midwestern

4. A blend of French culinary and Creole cooking is found among which cultural group?
   a. Jewish
   b. Italian
   c. Cajun
   d. Chinese

5. Changes in American food patterns have been influenced by:
   a. More women choosing to be homemakers.
   b. More families eating together at home.
   c. People eating fewer meals at restaurants.
   d. An increase in standard portion sizes.

Additional Learning Resources

evolve   http://evolve.elsevier.com/Williams/basic/

References and **Further Reading and Resources** in the back of the book provide additional resources for enhancing knowledge.

Weight Management

Theresa Dvorak, MS, RDN, CSSD, ATC

Key Concepts

- Underlying causes of obesity include a host of various genetic, environmental, and psychologic factors.
- Short-term food patterns or fads often stem from food misinformation that appeals to some human psychologic need; however, these fads do not necessarily meet physiologic needs.

- Realistic weight management focuses on individual needs and health promotion, including meal pattern planning and regular physical activity.
- Severe underweight carries physiologic and psychologic risk to the body.

Currently 68.5% of adults in the United States are overweight, of which 35% are obese and 6.4% are extremely obese. This epidemic—which results in large part from poor diet, physical inactivity, and genetics—is not limited to adults.[1] The National Center for Health Statistics reported that 17% of children and adolescents between the ages of 2 and 19 years are also obese.[1] Weight-loss diets are abundant and do not lack in variety with regard to the philosophy of the methods used to shed unwanted pounds. This variety also leads to greater confusion about weight-loss methods and expectations. Despite an apparent obsession with weight and the multibillion dollar industry of weight-loss diets and products, Americans continue to grow in undesirable directions (Figure 15-1). This chapter examines the problem of weight management and seeks a more positive and realistic health model that recognizes personal needs and sound weight goals.

OBESITY AND WEIGHT CONTROL

BODY WEIGHT VERSUS BODY FAT

Obesity develops from many interwoven factors—including personal, physical, psychologic, and genetic—and is difficult to pinpoint. As used in the traditional medical sense, *obesity* is a clinical term for excess body fat, and it is generally used to describe people who are at least 20% above a desired weight for height. The terms *overweight* and *obesity* are often used interchangeably, but they technically have different meanings. *Overweight* denotes a body weight that is above a population weight-for-height standard. Meanwhile, the word *obesity* is a more specific term that refers to the degree of fatness (i.e., the relative excess amount of fat in the total **body composition**). Over the past 5 decades, the percentage of obese adults (i.e., those with a **body mass index [BMI]** of 30 or greater) 20 years of age and older has increased from 13.4% of the

population to 35.3%.[2] Although the relative prevalence of overweight and obesity among adults in America has not increased in the past decade, it still remains at epidemic proportions.

Box 15-1 provides the classifications of BMI and the BMI chart is located on the inside back cover of the text. BMI can be tracked from childhood to adulthood with the Centers for Disease Control and Prevention growth charts (see Chapter 11). BMI is a reliable method of predicting the relative risk of becoming an overweight adult on the basis of the presence or absence of excess weight at various times throughout childhood. Children and adolescents who are overweight or obese are significantly more likely to continue to suffer from obesity as they age.[3]

Every person is different, and normal weight ranges vary in healthy people. Until recently, the important factor of age for setting a reasonable body weight for adults had been overlooked. With advancing age, body weight usually increases until approximately the age of 50 years for men and the age of 70 years for women, after which it declines.

The exclusive use of BMI to define obesity has undergone criticism because it does not measure body fat per se but rather total body weight relative to height. This method classifies some individuals as obese when they do not have excess body fat. For example, a football player in peak condition can be extremely "overweight" according to standard height/weight charts. In other words, he can weigh

---

body composition the relative sizes of the four body compartments that make up the total body: lean body mass (muscle mass), fat, water, and bone.
body mass index (BMI) the body weight in kilograms divided by the square of the height in meters (i.e., kg/m^2).

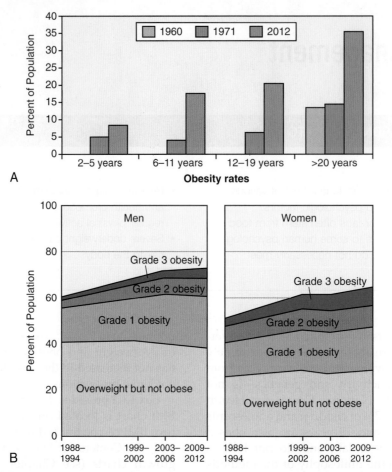

FIGURE 15-1 (A) Trends in obesity, by age: United States, 1960-2012. Estimates for adults are age adjusted. For adults: obesity is defined as a BMI of 30 or more. For children: obesity is defined as a BMI ≥95th percentile of the CDC sex-specific BMI-for-age growth charts from 2000. (B) Trends in overweight and obesity among adults, by sex: United States 1988-1994 through 2009-2012. Estimates are age adjusted for adults 20 years and older. Grade 1 obesity: BMI ≥30 and <35; Grade 2 obesity: BMI ≥35 and <40; Grade 3 obesity: BMI ≥40. (A, Modified from Fryar CD, Carroll MD. *Prevalence of Overweight, Obesity, and Extreme Obesity Among Adults: United States, Trends 1960–1962 through 2011–2012.* Atlanta, Ga: National Center for Health Statistics; 2014. Ogden CL, et al. Prevalence of childhood and adult obesity in the United States, 2011-2012. *JAMA.* 2014;311[8]:806-814. **B,** Reprinted from National Center for Health Statistics. *Health, United States, 2014: With Special Feature of Adults Aged 55-64.* Hyattsville, MD: U.S. Government Printing Office; 2015.)

Box 15-1 Body Mass Index Classifications	
BODY MASS INDEX RANGE (KG/M²)	**CLASSIFICATION**
18.5 to 24.9	Normal
25 to 29.9	Overweight
30 to 35	Obese
>35	Clinically or extremely obese

considerably more than the average man of the same height, but much more of his weight is likely lean muscle mass rather than excess fat. Thus, for individuals with more muscle mass than the average person, BMI may not be the most ideal means of assessing risks associated with weight. In order to increase accuracy of assessing chronic disease risk, the use of waist circumference is included because it is well-known that the greater the amount of adipose tissue stored within the abdominal region the higher the risk for disease.[4]

WAIST CIRCUMFERENCE AND INCREASED RISK

Men: ≥40 inches

Women: ≥35 inches

Thus for the vast majority of the population, BMI coupled with waist circumference is closely associated with health risks stemming from excess body fat.

BODY COMPOSITION

Given that BMI and waist circumference are much easier to assess than body composition, they are recommended as the standard for assessing health relative to weight. BMI is related to body fat percentages for most individuals (Figure 15-2). However, body composition assessment provides an additional measure of overall health and fitness. Health professionals can measure body fatness with the use of a variety of methods:

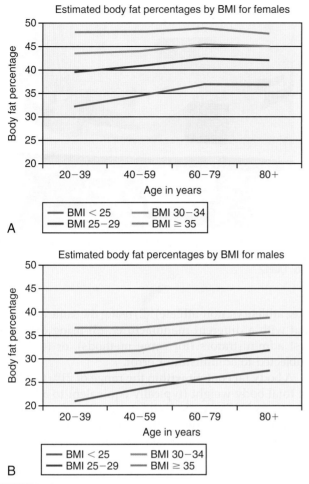

FIGURE 15-2 Body fat percentage as it correlates with body mass index (BMI): **A,** females; **B,** males. (Adapted from Li C, Ford ES, Zhao G, et al. Estimates of body composition with dual-energy x-ray absorptiometry in adults. *Am J Clin Nutr.* 2009;90[6]:1457-1465.)

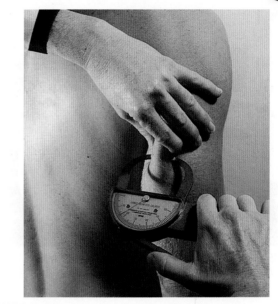

FIGURE 15-3 Assessment tools include skin fold calipers, which measure the relative amount of subcutaneous fat tissue at various body sites. (Reprinted from Mahan LK, Escott-Stump S. *Krause's Food & Nutrition Therapy.* 13th ed. Philadelphia: Saunders; 2011.)

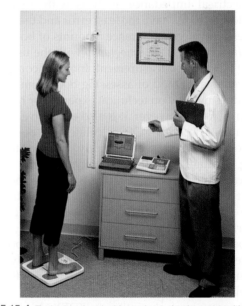

FIGURE 15-4 Tanita bioelectrical impedance body composition measurement tool. (Courtesy Tanita Corp., Arlington Heights, Ill.)

- *Body fat calipers* measure the width of skin folds at precise body sites, because most of the body fat is deposited in layers just under the skin. These measures are then used in specific formulas to calculate an estimated body fat composition (Figure 15-3). Calipers are an easy, portable, inexpensive, and noninvasive way to measure body fat. However, the reliability of the test depends on the skill of the technician, which can vary greatly.
- *Hydrostatic weighing* is a more precise method and is often used in athletic programs and research studies; although with advancing technologies it is not used as frequently now. Hydrostatic weighing requires the complete submersion of an individual in water. The person must exhale as much air as possible and then stay underwater for a few seconds for an accurate reading to be obtained. Although this method is relatively accurate, it is not easy, portable, or inexpensive, and many patients are not willing or able to perform the test.
- *Bioelectrical impedance analysis* (BIA) is an easy, portable, inexpensive, and noninvasive body composition measurement tool. One type, a foot-to-foot

analyzer, requires that the person stand on a modified scale with bare feet while an undetectable electrical current travels through his or her body (Figure 15-4). The analyzer determines the individual's body fat percentage on the basis of gender, age, height, weight, total body water, and the rate at which the electrical current travels. Fat impedes the current; therefore, a lower total body fat composition results in a faster travel time of the current. Such analyzers have both a standard adult setting and an athletic setting. Although this method does not require any special skill on either the client's part or the technician's part, discrepancies in some people have been noted between total body fat percentages

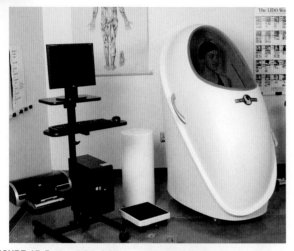

FIGURE 15-5 The BOD POD uses air displacement technology to measure body composition. (Courtesy Life Measurements, Inc., Concord, Calif.)

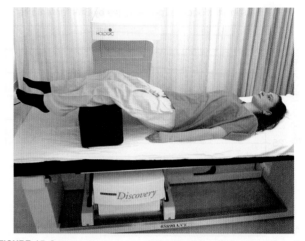

FIGURE 15-6 Dual-energy x-ray absorptiometry. (Courtesy University of Utah, Division of Nutrition and Integrative Physiology, Salt Lake City, Utah.)

as measured by bioelectrical impedance versus dual-energy x-ray absorptiometry.[5,6] Bioelectrical impedance machines that use a multiple-frequency bioelectrical impedance analysis with eight-point tactile electrodes have the least error and the highest correspondence to reference amounts of body fat.[5,7]

- *Air displacement plethysmography* with the use of the BOD POD (Life Measurement, Inc., Concord, Calif) is a reliable method of assessing body composition that does not rely on technical expertise or radiation (Figure 15-5). However, it is also expensive and not portable. The BOD POD calculates the percentage of body fat using weight, body volume, thoracic lung volume, and body density. Current studies indicate that the BOD POD is a reliable measurement tool for most subgroups of the population, but discrepancies may arise when measuring children, elderly, and morbidly obese individuals.[8-11] However, it does offer a reliable means of assessing body fat percentage in overweight and non–morbidly obese populations, whereas other methods are often not as reliable.[6]

- *Dual energy x-ray absorptiometry* (DEXA) is a highly accurate way to assess body composition using radiation to distinguish bone, muscle, water, and fat density (Figure 15-6).[12] Although this method is less intimidating than hydrostatic weighing for some people, it is substantially more expensive than other methods. DEXA is currently used as the gold standard to validate all other body composition analysis methods.

Even though the aforementioned methods of measuring body composition are valuable assessments for determining a person's body fatness, caution should be taken because there is inherent error within all of them and to date there are insufficient data to determine population norms. It is also important to note that even within the same method of analysis different results may be obtained by (1) using different settings (i.e., athlete vs. non-athlete), (2) using the same machine but with a different manufacturer, (3) using different test administrators (for some methods), or (4) being subjected to administrator error.

A body fat content within the range of 21% to 25.8% of total body weight (typically equivalent to a BMI of ≤25 kg/m^2) is associated with the lowest risk of chronic disease for men between the ages of 20 and 79 years. For women of the same age, the ideal range is somewhat higher: 32.2% to 36.9%.[13] Body fat percentage ranges that are associated with fitness are slightly lower than those associated with a healthy BMI and chronic disease prevention. The American College of Sports Medicine (ACSM) classifies men as having "Very lean" and "Excellent" body fatness levels when their body fat percentages are between 4.2% and 10.5%, for 20- to 29-year-old men and when they are between 11.4% and 18.8% for women of the same age group (Figure 15-7).[4] Note that these levels are ACSM categories associated with fitness and are not recommendations for the general public.

MEASURES OF WEIGHT MAINTENANCE GOALS

Standard Height/Weight Tables

Height/weight tables are general population guides and should be regarded only as such. Individual needs must be considered. One of the standard tables used in the United States is the Metropolitan Life Insurance Company's ideal weight-for-height chart. These charts are based on life expectancy information gathered since the 1930s from the company's population of life insurance policyholders. Many people have questioned how well these tables represent the total current population, because the data are based on such a select group of individuals (most of whom were Caucasian, middle- to upper-class men for the first few decades of data gathering) and may not consider the wide variety of individuals who are found within a diverse community.

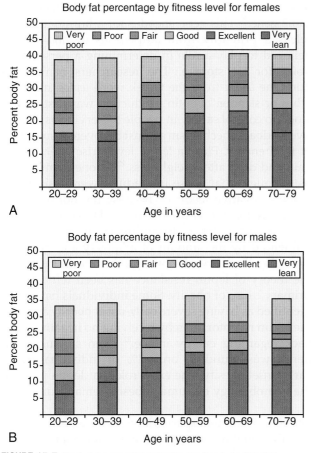

FIGURE 15-7 Body fat percentage by fitness level: **A,** females; **B,** males. (Adapted from American College of Sports Medicine. *ACSM's Health-Related Physical Fitness Assessment Manual.* 4th ed. Philadelphia, Pa: 2014.)

More recent height/weight tables rely on BMI calculations and are based on the National Research Council data for weight and health, the current *Dietary Guidelines for Americans,* and recent medical studies. These guidelines directly relate height and weight ranges to relative risks for chronic diseases (see the BMI table on the inside back cover). Within each age group, obesity is significantly associated with higher all-cause mortality rates.[14]

Healthy Weight Range

Following are general calculations that make use of the Hamwi method for determining healthy or ideal weight goals:

- *Men:* 106 lb for the first 5 feet, then add or subtract 6 lb for each inch above or below 5 feet, respectively. A range is then taken by adding and subtracting 10% to account for small and large body frames.
- *Women:* 100 lb for the first 5 feet, then add or subtract 5 lb for each inch above or below 5 feet,

---

Hamwi method a formula for estimating the ideal body weight on the basis of gender and height.

---

respectively. A range is then taken by adding and subtracting 10% to account for small and large body frames.

For example, a 5-foot, 6-inch woman would have an ideal body weight range of 100 lb + (6 in × 5 lb) = 130 ± 10%. Therefore, her ideal body weight is 130 lb with an acceptable range of 117 to 143 lb.

As with BMI, this calculation does not account for usual changes that are associated with age (i.e., a loss of stature and slight increases in weight) or for individuals with very high muscle mass. A person's ideal weight may give him or her an approximate number for a healthy weight goal. Three important considerations must be taken into account when relying on ideal body weight calculations: frame size, variation, and essentiality of body fat.

Body frame. Height (in centimeters) divided by wrist circumference (in centimeters) provides an estimate of body frame size. For an accurate measurement, the patient's arm should be flexed at the elbow with the palm facing up and the hand relaxed. With a flexible measuring tape, measure the wrist circumference at the joint distal (i.e., toward the hand) to the styloid process (i.e., the bony wrist protrusion). Individuals with a small frame size would have an ideal body weight at the lower end of their ideal body weight range and vice versa for individuals with a large frame size. The following example indicates the standards for body frame size, which are useful for interpreting ideal body weight:

$$\text{Height: 5 ft, 4 in} = 64 \text{ in} \times 2.54 \text{ cm/in} = 162.56 \text{ cm}$$

$$\text{Wrist circumference} = 15.8 \text{ cm}$$

$$162.56/15.8 = 10.29 = \text{Medium frame}$$

FRAME SIZE	MALE RATIO	FEMALE RATIO
Small	>10.4	>10.9
Medium	10.4 to 9.6	10.9 to 9.9
Large	<9.6	<9.9

Individual variation. Ideal weight varies with time and circumstance throughout life. A person's ideal weight depends on many factors, including gender, age, body shape, metabolic rate, genetics, and physical activity. Just as everyone varies in shoe size, so too do we vary in body weight. Specific individual situations govern needs.

Necessity of body fat. Some body fat is essential for survival. Every cell membrane in the body has fat molecules within it. Fat is used for insulation, temperature regulation, the cushioning of vital organs, and many other functions. The estimated essential body fat level (i.e., the minimal amount required for health) is approximately 3% for men and 12% for women. It should be noted that these are *minimal* amounts of body fat and not optimal levels. Health and hormonal regulation is negatively affected by inadequate body fat and severe caloric restriction.[15,16]

OBESITY AND HEALTH
Weight Extremes
Clinically severe or significant obesity is a health hazard in itself and creates other medical problems by placing strain on all body systems. Both extremes of weight—fatness and extreme thinness—pose health problems.

Overweight and Health Problems
Obesity increases the risk of related conditions such as hypertension, type 2 diabetes, heart disease, arthritis, and certain types of cancer.[17] Weight loss can reduce elevated blood glucose levels and blood pressure in obese people.[18,19] In turn, these improvements reduce risks related to heart disease and diabetes.

CAUSES OF OBESITY
Basic Energy Balance
How does a person become overweight? Although some people have congenital obesity, a major contributor to obesity in Americans is physical inactivity. A recent review article found that a simple and well-defined walking program of more than 5000 steps per day (<5000 steps/day is considered sedentary) can help to reduce total body weight, BMI, waist circumference, and resting heart rate and to improve glucose tolerance among people independent of changes to dietary intake.[20] Regular exercise has a significant effect on increasing lean body mass and reducing the risk of the chronic diseases associated with obesity.

The overall energy imbalance (e.g., more energy intake from food and drink than energy output through physical activity and basal metabolic needs) is the primary cause of excess weight accumulation. Excess intake of macronutrients is stored in the body as fat. Approximately 3500 kcal is stored in each 1 lb (0.45 kg) of body fat. A minor daily imbalance in which energy intake exceeds output by a mere 100 kcal (approximately 14 almonds) can result in a significant weight gain in 1 year, as follows:

$$100 \text{ kcal/day} \times 365 \text{ days/year} = 36,500 \text{ extra kcal/year}$$
$$36,500 \text{ kcal} \div 3500 \text{ kcal/lb} = 10.4 \text{ lb/year (4.7 kg)}$$

However, some overweight people only eat moderate amounts of food, and some people of average weight eat much more but never seem to gain unwanted pounds. Because many individual differences exist, factors other than energy balance are involved in maintaining a healthful weight.

Hormonal Control
Leptin. A research group at Rockefeller University first reported to have found the "obesity gene" in an overweight strain of laboratory mice. Soon thereafter, these researchers located the human equivalent of the same gene.[21] This gene encodes for a hormone that is released primarily from adipose tissue and that is believed to play a role in determining a person's set point for fat storage. The researchers named the hormone *leptin* from the Greek word *leptos,* meaning "thin or slender." Leptin production was first understood to control satiety in people by serving as a negative feedback mechanism against the overconsumption of total energy. Plasma leptin levels rise after weight gain and drop after weight loss.[22] At one point, scientists thought that obese individuals were resistant to leptin's negative feedback because the hormone did not cross the blood-brain barrier. However, studies indicate that leptin is also produced in the brain and influenced by the amount of adiposity and gender.[23] With the discovery of leptin production in the brain, the theory of leptin resistance has been refuted as a primary cause of obesity. Some individuals have been identified as having severe **early-onset obesity** and lack the leptin receptor, thereby receiving no negative feedback regarding energy intake.[22] Even so, such incidence was found in only 3% of individuals with early-onset obesity. The exact role that leptin plays in the neurobiology of human obesity remains unclear.

Ghrelin. The counterpart to leptin is the enteric peptide ghrelin. Ghrelin is an appetite stimulant that is secreted from the stomach to activate the **appetite-regulating network.** When administered exogenously, ghrelin increases appetite and promotes adiposity.[24] Such a discovery has led to investigations of the use of a ghrelin antagonist to fight obesity.[25] Despite years of research, many questions remain unanswered about the roles of leptin and ghrelin and with regard to how some individuals do not respond to fluctuations of these substances in their plasma levels.

Genetic and Environmental Factors
Genetic inheritance probably influences a person's chances of obesity more than any other factor. Family food and lifestyle patterns provide an environment that allows this genetic trait to present itself.

Genetic control. The predisposition for obesity is highly associated with genetics, thereby making certain people highly susceptible to becoming obese in an environment that allows for such a genetic expression

---

clinically severe or significant obesity a BMI of 40 or more or a BMI of 35 to 39 with at least one obesity-related disorder; also referred to as extreme obesity and morbid obesity.

early-onset obesity a genetically associated obesity that occurs during early childhood.

appetite-regulating network a hormonally controlled system of appetite stimulation and suppression.

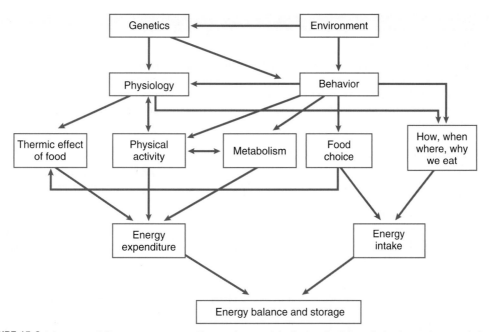

FIGURE 15-8 Interwoven influence among genetics, environmental effects, physiology, behavior, and energy balance.

(see the Cultural Considerations box, "Genetics and the Predisposition for Obesity").[26] Genetic regulation may control the amount of body fat that an individual has the potential to carry. A person then eats to gain or lose whatever amount of fat the body is naturally set or programmed for in accordance with the weight below or above this internally regulated set point. Thus, people who have lost body fat below their pro-grammed level will eat to regain to their genetic set point when food is again available. Similarly, people with lower programmed fat levels who have gained excess body fat will lose weight when they resume their regular food intake. This is not to say that a person has no control over his or her own body weight: the genetic influence is the predisposing factor but not the determining factor. The daily life, environment, and habits that a person chooses influence the expression of this genetic trait (Figure 15-8). In one thorough review of genetic and epigenetic influences on obesity, the author states that, "nutritional and exercise inter-ventions have been shown to be able to counteract acquired (or imprinted) epigenetic patterns to normal-ize expression of these [obesity] genes."[26]

Family reinforcement. An individual's genetic pre-disposition for increased body fat is reinforced by inappropriate family food patterns. Studies show that if a child is obese it greatly increases the risk of over-weight or obesity as an adult.[3,27] In addition to genetic influence, families also exert social pressure and teach children habits and attitudes toward food. Thus, the development of healthy eating and physical activity habits during childhood and teenage years with emphasis on decreasing the energy density of foods, increasing healthful food choices (such as fruits and

vegetables), and increasing physical activity are highly encouraged to establish balanced food and lifestyle patterns.[27]

Physiologic factors. The amount of body fat that a person carries is related to the number and size of fat cells in the body. Critical periods for becoming obese occur during early growth periods, when cells are mul-tiplying rapidly during childhood and adolescence. After the body has added extra fat cells for more fuel storage, these cells remain for a person's lifetime and can store varying amounts of fat. Basal metabolic rate, physical activity, and lean muscle mass are major physiologic factors for determining individual fat storage. Women store more fat during pregnancy and after menopause in response to hormonal changes.

Psychologic factors. Work, family, and social envi-ronments may cultivate emotional stress, which many people respond to by eating for comfort. Media mes-sages and societal pressures to maintain the cultural "ideal" thin body type contribute to the strain of con-stant dieting. These messages are often dichotomous (e.g., good versus bad food; eat this, not that) and convey negative and oversimplified ideas, which in turn can perpetuate the chronic dieters' dilemma of yo-yo dieting (e.g., weight loss followed by weight gain) and cause reductions in metabolic rate and lean body mass.

Other environmental factors. Many environmental factors add to the ever-increasing problem of obesity in the United States. The following are only a few: an increase in energy-dense food availability; low-cost fast and convenient foods; increase in portion sizes;

Cultural Considerations

Genetics and the Predisposition for Obesity*

When comparing the prevalence of obesity among various racial and ethnic groups in the United States, researchers have found significant differences with regard to the risk for obesity in women (see graph below).[1] Few differences are seen among different racial and ethnic groups of men. According to the National Center for Health Statistics, the female prevalence of adolescent and adult obesity per racial and ethnic group is as follows:

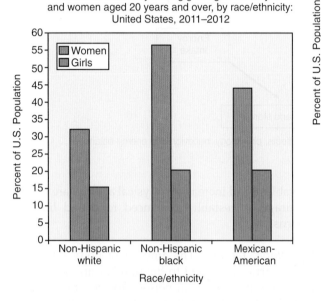

Prevalence of obesity among girls aged 12–19 years and women aged 20 years and over, by race/ethnicity: United States, 2011–2012

An even more dramatic trend noted throughout the National Center for Health Statistics data for the past few decades is the significant increase in obesity in both genders. Summarized below are the findings from these surveys, which include all racial and ethnic groups together. The numbers show the prevalence of obesity in both genders among adults who are 20 years old and older as percentages of the population[1,2]:

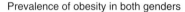
Prevalence of obesity in both genders

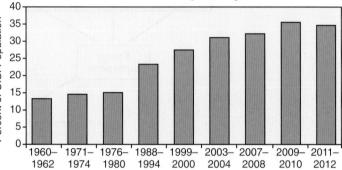

Although genetics does play a role in the prevalence of and predisposition for obesity, such influences cannot explain such an increase in obesity among the entire population.

REFERENCES

1. Ogden CL, Carroll MD, Kit BK, Flegal KM. *National Health and Nutrition Examination Survey, 2011-2012. Prevalence of Obesity Among Adults: United States, 2011-2012*. NCHS data brief, no 131. Hyattsville, MD: National Center for Health Statistics; 2013.
2. Fryar CD, Carroll MD, Ogden CL. *NCHS Health E-Stat: prevalence of overweight, obesity, and extreme obesity among adults: United States, 1960-1962 through 2011-2012*. Retrieved December 8, 2014, from <cdc.gov>, 2014.

*With contributions from Caiti Christensen.

---

decrease in food preparation time and skills; decrease in physical activity; increase in screen time (e.g., television, computer, video games); less active leisure time; and decreased physical requirements of activities of daily living (e.g., domestic appliances such as washing machines, vacuum cleaners, and dishwashers; central heating, cars, delivery services, elevators).

INDIVIDUAL DIFFERENCES AND EXTREME PRACTICES

Individual Energy Balance Levels

Several factors influence a person's energy balance. Estimating energy requirements is a useful starting point for practitioners to assess an individual's calorie needs.

Energy out. Factors such as the basal metabolic rate (BMR), body size, lean body mass, age, gender, and physical activity influence the total daily calorie expenditure (see Chapter 6). Some people have more

genetic-based metabolic efficiency (i.e., the ability to "burn" energy more readily than others do).

Energy in. When calculating a person's energy intake, Nutrition Facts labels and dietary analysis software indicate only an estimated value. Reported food and drink values represent the averages of many similar samples of that type of food. Thus, determining the exact amount of kilocalories consumed by a person throughout the day is difficult.

Extreme Practices

Desperate attempts to lose weight may drive people to extreme measures, which sometimes worsen health risks.

Fad diets. A constant array of diet books and weight-loss supplements that promise to "melt the fat away" continue to flood the American market (Table 15-1). These books and supplements usually sell briefly and

Table 15-1 Comparison of Select Common Weight-Loss Diets

DIET	PHILOSOPHY	FOODS TO EAT	FOODS TO AVOID	DIET COMPOSITION (AVERAGE FOR 3 DAYS)	RECOMMENDED SUPPLEMENTS	HEALTH CLAIMS SCIENTIFICALLY PROVEN?	PRACTICALITY	LOSE AND MAINTAIN WEIGHT?
Atkins*	Eating too many carbohydrates causes obesity and other health problems; ketosis leads to decreased hunger; carbohydrates prevent your body from burning fat	Meat, fish, poultry, eggs, cheese, high-fiber vegetables, butter, oil, nuts, seeds	Carbohydrates, specifically bread, pasta, most fruits and high-carbohydrate vegetables, milk, alcohol	Protein: 27% Carbohydrates: 5% Fat: 68% (saturated, 26%)	Atkins supplement that includes chromium picolinate, carnitine, coenzyme Q10	No long-term validated studies published	Limited food choices; difficult to eat in restaurants, because only plain protein sources and limited vegetables and salads allowed	Yes, but initial weight loss is mostly water; does not promote a positive attitude toward food groups; difficult to maintain for the long term because the diet restricts food choices
Eat Right 4 Your Type†	Blood type determines the way your body absorbs nutrients and dictates the diet and exercise plan that will suit you best	Type O: meat, seafood, fruits, vegetables Type A: fruits, vegetables, beans, most seafood, grains Type B: meat, beans, fruits, vegetables, seafood, low-fat dairy Type AB: seafood, dairy, fruits, vegetables	Type O: wheat, beans Type A: meat, dairy, wheat Type B: chicken, wheat, lentils Type AB: meat	Not applicable (diet varies according to blood type, ancestry, and so on)	Depends on your blood type and overall health, which includes immune, skin, digestive, bone, joint, circulation, mental, and hormonal health as well as concurrent medications	No; theories and long-term results not validated	Not applicable (diet varies according to blood type, ancestry, and so on)	Possibly, if caloric intake is less than energy output

Continued

Table 15-1 Comparison of Select Common Weight-Loss Diets—cont'd

DIET	PHILOSOPHY	FOODS TO EAT	FOODS TO AVOID	DIET COMPOSITION (AVERAGE FOR 3 DAYS)	RECOMMENDED SUPPLEMENTS	HEALTH CLAIMS SCIENTIFICALLY PROVEN?	PRACTICALITY	LOSE AND MAINTAIN WEIGHT?
hCG[‡]	Daily injections of human chorionic gonadotropin hormone keep the body in an anabolic state and reduce appetite; combined with a very low calorie diet that promotes weight loss	500 calories per day. Breakfast: Tea or coffee without sugar. Lunch and Dinner: 100 g of lean meat, vegetable, breadstick, and either an apple, an orange, or ½ a grapefruit	Oils, butter, dressing. Also avoid cosmetics, lotions, medications, massages	Protein: 53% Carbohydrates: 36% Fat: 11%	125 IU of hCG administered daily	No long-term validated studies published to support the claim. Studies have found dangers such as thromboembolism, hypothyroidism, bone mineral loss, and anxiety	Very limited food choices and caloric intake	Yes, by caloric restriction; limited food choices are not practical for the long term; diet is only meant to be followed for 26-40 days
Paleo[§]	Eating the diet we are genetically adapted to based on our hunter-gatherer ancestry; high protein, low carbohydrate intake will reduce risk of chronic disease and promote weight loss	Meat, seafood, fruits, vegetables, eggs, nuts, seeds, plant oils	Grains, legumes, dairy, refined sugars, potatoes, processed foods, salt	Protein: 46% Carbohydrates: 28% Fat: 28%	None	No; theories and long-term results not validated	Deficient in calcium and vitamin D	Possibly if caloric intake is less than output
The South Beach Diet[‖]	Switching to the "right" carbohydrates stops insulin resistance, reduces cravings, and causes weight loss	Seafood, chicken breast, lean meat, low-fat cheese, nut oils, most vegetables, low-fat dairy; later, most whole grains and beans	Fatty meats, full-fat cheese, refined grains, sweets, juice, potatoes	Phase 1: Protein: 34% Carbohydrates: 14.8% Fat: 50%	Multivitamins and omega-3 fatty acids; Metamucil recommended during phase 1	Evidence does exist to link the avoidance of saturated fats with the reduced risk of heart disease	First phase is more difficult; later phases are mostly healthy foods and more practical	Yes, although initial weight loss is mostly water; sustained weight loss through reduced calorie intake

Diet	Description	Foods to eat	Foods to avoid	Supplements	Long-term studies	Practicality	Macronutrient composition	Effective for weight loss
Whole30¶	Eliminating processed foods for a 30-day period allows your metabolism to reset and rebalances hormone levels	Meat, seafood, eggs, vegetables, some fruit	Added sugars, alcohol, grains, legumes, dairy	None	No long-term validated studies published	Not practical for long term; difficult to eat in restaurants due to restrictions	Protein: 53% Carbohydrates: 30% Fat: 19%	Possibly, if caloric intake is less than output
Zone 1-2-3 Program**	Eating the right combination of foods leads to a metabolic state at which the body functions at peak performance and stabilizes hormonal communication, thereby leading to decreased hunger, increased energy, and increased control of cellular inflammation	Protein, fat, and carbohydrates in exact proportions only (40/30/30); alcohol in moderation	Fruit (some types), saturated fats	200 IU of vitamin E	No; theories and long-term results not validated	Food must be eaten in required proportions of protein, fat, and carbohydrates; menus are plain and unappealing; vegetable portions are very large; difficult to calculate portions	Protein: 34% Carbohydrates: 36% Fat: 29% (saturated, 9%) Alcohol: 1%	Yes, by caloric restriction; could result in weight maintenance if carefully followed; diet is rigid and difficult to maintain

With contribution from Caiti Christensen.

*Atkins RC. Dr. Atkins' New Diet Revolution. New York: Avon Books; 1999.

†D'Adamo PJ, Whitney C. Eat Right 4 Your Type. New York: Riverhead Books; 2002.

‡Simeons DA. Pounds & Inches: A New Approach to Obesity. Rome, Italy: Popular Publishing; 2010. Goodbar N, Foushee J, Eagerton D, Haynes K, Johnson A. Effects of the human chorionic gonadotropin diet on patient outcomes. Ann Pharmacother. 2013;47:E23-E23.

§Cordain L PhD. The Paleo Diet™—live well, live longer. Retrieved December 3, 2014, from http://thepaleodiet.com/.

‖Agatston A. The South Beach Diet. Emmaus, Pa: Rodale Inc; 2003.

¶Hartwig M, Hartwig D. It Starts with Food. Riverside, NJ: Victory Belt Publishing; 2014.

**Sears B. The Zone. New York: HarperCollins; 1995.

then fade away, largely because their quick fixes either do not work or are not sustainable. They lead individuals to believe that weight loss is easy and effortless when the reality is very different. Such a complex problem has no simple answers. Most of the fad diets fail on the following two counts:

1. *Scientific inaccuracies and misinformation:* Fad diets and supplements are often nutritionally inadequate and based on false claims.
2. *Failure to address the necessity of changing long-term habits and behaviors:* People are often set up for failure regarding the maintenance of a healthy weight once it is achieved. The basic behavioral problem involved in changing food and exercise habits for life—thereby developing a new lifestyle—is unrecognized.

With some diets, the degree of energy restriction is impossible to maintain long term. Many fad dieters find themselves caught in a vicious cycle of **chronic dieting syndrome** and its harmful physical and psychologic effects.

Fasting. The drastic approach of fasting takes many forms, from literal fasting to the use of very-low-calorie diets (e.g., 800 kcal or less per day). Possible effects of a semistarvation diet include acidosis, low blood pressure, electrolyte imbalance, a loss of lean muscle mass, and decreased BMR. Such programs cannot be maintained for the long term without deleterious effects on health. The regaining of body fat mass is often overshot after a semistarvation diet; in other words, when the individual resumes normal eating, he or she gains back more fat mass than he or she initially possessed.[28]

Specific macronutrient restrictions. Avoiding any food group or macronutrient (e.g., carbohydrates, fats, or proteins) as a means for weight loss is unfounded. Such diets that are extremely low fat or extremely low in carbohydrates are too restrictive to maintain for extended periods, and they also carry health risks.

Clothing and body wraps. Special "sauna suits" and body wrapping have been claimed to help weight loss in certain body areas or to reduce cellulite tissue. Some people endure mummy-like body wrapping in an attempt to reduce body size. However, the resulting small weight loss is a result of temporary water loss. Fat mass cannot be melted away without using the stored energy (i.e., burning the calories) in the **adipocytes.**

Weight-loss drugs. Diuretics and exogenous hormones should never be used to alter body weight or lean tissue mass without strict medical indication and supervision. Various amphetamine compounds were once popular for the medical treatment of obesity, but they are no longer used because of their dangerous health consequences. Common over-the-counter drugs have included phenylpropylamine (Accu-trim, Dexatrim), which is a stimulant that is similar to amphetamine; and ephedra, which is currently banned in the United States. In addition, there are many herbs that claim weight-loss benefits. The U.S. Food and Drug Administration (FDA) maintains an updated list of contaminated and potentially dangerous over-the-counter drugs and supplements on its website at www.fda.gov/Drugs/ResourcesForYou/Consumers/default.htm.

A pair of related weight-loss drugs—fenfluramine and phentermine—were prescribed to be used together in the popular "fen-phen" combination for weight loss. Shortly thereafter, physicians found that one in eight patients who were using fen-phen developed valvular regurgitation, which is a sometimes fatal condition.[29] The FDA, with the support of the medical community, quickly removed these drugs from the market in 1997. Likewise, in 2010 the FDA withdrew sibutramine (Meridia) from the U.S. market as a result of an increased risk of heart attack and stroke with its use. Sibutramine was another weight-loss medication that worked by increasing the heart rate and thus increasing energy expenditure. Although the pursuit of pharmacotherapy for the treatment of obesity is intense, few safe options are currently available.

Drugs that are used to treat obesity generally work in one of the following four ways:

1. Reducing energy intake by suppressing the appetite
2. Increasing energy expenditure by stimulating the BMR
3. Reducing the absorption of food in the gut
4. Altering lipogenesis and lipolysis

The FDA approved orlistat (Alli, Xenical) for the treatment of clinically significant obesity in 1999. Orlistat inhibits dietary fat absorption. Orlistat has been successful with weight loss, but reports indicate that maximal benefits occur only when it is combined with lifestyle changes that induce a **negative energy balance.**[30] As with many medications, unpleasant side effects are associated with this medication, including diarrhea, gas, and abdominal pain (see the Drug-Nutrient Interaction box, "Orlistat: An Over-the-Counter Weight-Loss Aid"). These medications may be effective in promoting weight loss; however, without

chronic dieting syndrome a cyclic pattern of weight loss by dieting followed by rapid weight gain; this abnormal psychophysiologic food pattern becomes chronic, changing a person's natural body metabolism and relative body composition to the abnormal state of a metabolically obese person of normal weight.
adipocytes fat cells.
negative energy balance more total energy is expended than consumed.

Drug-Nutrient Interaction

Orlistat: An Over-the-Counter Weight-Loss Aid*

In February 2007, the U.S. Food and Drug Administration approved the drug orlistat (Alli) as an over-the-counter weight-loss aid for overweight adults. When combined with a low-fat diet, the drug can be an effective adjunct to a weight-loss program. Orlistat works by inhibiting the absorption of fat in the intestine by up to 30%, thereby reducing the caloric impact of food.[1]

However, as a result of its mechanism of action, orlistat also inhibits the absorption of fat-soluble vitamins. A multivitamin taken at least 2 hours before or after a dose of orlistat is recommended to prevent the suboptimal absorption of vitamins A, D, E, and K. Even with vitamin supplementation, vitamin D and E absorption may be significantly decreased.[2]

In addition, orlistat can cause uncomfortable gastrointestinal side effects such as flatulence and loose stools. Eating large amounts of fat can increase these side effects, whereas fiber supplements that contain psyllium may help to reduce them.[3]

Orlistat is not approved for use by children who are younger than 18 years old, and it is contraindicated for people with absorptive disorders (e.g., pancreatitis, gallbladder disorders) and for those who are not overweight. Because this drug is now available over-the-counter, patients may take orlistat irresponsibly. It is important for clinicians to inquire about all medications and nutritional supplements that their patients are taking so that they may accurately advise these individuals about potential interactions and negative health consequences.

REFERENCES

1. Bragg R, Crannage E. Review of pharmacotherapy options for the management of obesity. *J Am Assoc Nurse Pract.* 2015;1-9.
2. Filippatos TD, Derdemezis CS, Gazi IF, et al. Orlistat-associated adverse effects and drug interactions: a critical review. *Drug Saf.* 2008;31(1):53-65.
3. Sumithran P, Proietto J. Benefit-risk assessment of orlistat in the treatment of obesity. *Drug Saf.* 2014;37(8):597-608.

*With contributions from Kelli Boi.

adequate nutritional and lifestyle changes, weight regain is likely when the medication is discontinued.

Surgery. Surgical techniques are usually reserved for the medical treatment of clinically severe obesity among patients who have not had success with other methods of long-term weight loss. Studies show that *bariatric surgery* provides significant and sustained weight loss and a reduced relative risk of death as a result of a decrease in several conditions and co-morbid diseases associated with obesity.[31,32] Although surgery historically has been the most successful method of permanent weight loss among patients with severe obesity, it is not without risks and complications.

Two primary types of surgical procedures are performed for weight loss: restrictive (e.g., making the stomach smaller) and combination restrictive and malabsorptive procedures (e.g., making the stomach smaller and inducing malabsorption). Gastric restriction involves the creation of a small stomach pouch

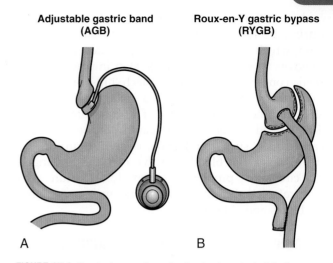

Adjustable gastric band (AGB) **Roux-en-Y gastric bypass (RYGB)**

A B

FIGURE 15-9 Surgical procedures for the treatment of clinically severe obesity: **A,** gastric banding; **B,** Roux-en-Y.

that is designed to reduce the space available for food in the stomach, thereby limiting appetite and eating. Adjustable gastric bands can be placed by laparoscopic surgery, and the band is subcutaneously adjusted as needed with the use of a small port (Figure 15-9, *A*). Malabsorptive procedures rearrange the small intestine to decrease the length and efficiency of the gut for nutrient absorption.[33] The most commonly performed and considered the 'gold standard' is the Roux-en-Y bariatric procedure (Figure 15-9, *B*). This procedure restricts the stomach to about 20 to 30 mL, reconfigures the small intestine, and may lead to neuron and hormone changes within the gut. Because of the reconfiguration of the small intestine, vitamin and mineral supplements are prescribed for the rest of the patient's life. The most common nutrient deficiencies include iron, calcium, vitamin D, and vitamin B_{12}. The inherent risks of surgery and postsurgical malnutrition are critical issues that should be thoroughly addressed with the patient.[33]

Following either procedure counseling by a dietitian is imperative to avoiding **dumping syndrome.** This is done by decreasing simple carbohydrate intake, avoiding fluid with food, and determining portion size and an eating plan, while providing instruction on how to avoid malnutrition. Weight-loss surgeries require a skilled team of specialists, nutrition care, careful patient selection, and continuous follow-up in partnership with the patient and his or her family. Long-term success is dependent on the patient being able to maintain nutritional, physical activity, and behavioral changes.

dumping syndrome condition in which there is a quick emptying of the stomach of a hyperosmolar content into the small intestine, causing fluid to shift into the intestinal lumen from the intravascular compartment.

A more limited type of cosmetic surgery developed during the 1980s is a form of local fat removal, **lipectomy,** which is commonly called *liposuction.* Lipectomy removes fat deposits under the skin in places of cosmetic concern, such as the stomach, hips, or thighs. A thin tube is inserted through a small incision in the skin, and the desired amount of fat is suctioned away. This procedure can be quite painful, however, and it carries risks such as infection, large disfiguring skin depressions, and blood clots that can lead to dangerous circulatory problems or even kidney failure. Any surgical procedure carries risk and may cause other problems and side effects.

A SOUND WEIGHT-MANAGEMENT PROGRAM

ESSENTIAL CHARACTERISTICS

There are no shortcuts to successful long-term weight control or weight loss. Weight loss requires hard work and strong individual motivation. Weight management requires a personalized program that focuses on changing lifestyle factors such as food and exercise behaviors. Choices that build a healthy mental and physical state with ample positive social support are desirable. The most recent position paper by the Academy of Nutrition and Dietetics regarding weight management makes note of the following: "A healthful lifestyle requires significant planning, proficiency in making appropriate choices and estimating portion sizes, and diligence in monitoring energy intake and activity, all of which take time to develop and maintain."[34]

BEHAVIOR MODIFICATION

Basic Principles

Food behavior is rooted in many human experiences. Behavior-oriented therapies are designed to help change patterns that contribute to excessive weight and that can help empower individuals to plan constructive actions to meet personal health goals. This behavioral approach must begin with a detailed examination of the following three basic aspects of each undesirable eating behavior:

1. *Cues or antecedents:* What stimulates the behavior?
2. *Response:* What happens during the eating or sedentary behavior after the cue?
3. *Consequences:* What happens after the response to the eating or sedentary behavior that reinforces it?

Basic Strategies and Actions

A program of personal behavior modification for weight management is directed toward the following:

---

lipectomy the surgical removal of subcutaneous fat by suction through a tube that is inserted into a surface incision or by the removal of larger amounts of subcutaneous fat through a major surgical incision.

---

(1) the control of eating behavior (e.g., a food diary that includes when, where, why, how, and how much); (2) the promotion of physical activity to increase energy output; and (3) the pursuit of emotional (stress), social, and psychologic health. Three progressive actions follow for the planning of individual strategies as outlined below.

Defining problem behavior. Specifically define the problem behavior, potential barriers to the new behavior, and the desired behavior outcome. This process clearly establishes goals and contributing objectives.

Recording and analyzing baseline behavior. Record eating and exercise behavior, and carefully analyze it in terms of physical setting and people involved. What types of patterns emerge? How often do these patterns occur? What conditions seem to trigger desirable and undesirable behaviors? What consequent events seem to maintain the habits (e.g., time, place, people, social responses, hunger before and after, emotional state, other factors)?

Planning a behavior management strategy. Set up controls of the external environment that involves the situational forces related to each of the three behavior areas involved: (1) the stimulus that occurs before the behavior; (2) the response to the behavior; and (3) the results of the behavior. The goal is to break the identified links to old and undesirable behaviors and to recondition them to the desired new eating and exercise behaviors. The Clinical Applications box entitled "Breaking Old Links: Strategies for Changing Food Behavior" provides a few examples of reconditioning personal food and exercise habits to more positive behaviors.

DIETARY MODIFICATION

Basic Principles

The central dietary approach in a weight-management program that may achieve a degree of lasting success must be based on the following five characteristics:

1. *Realistic goals:* Goals must be realistic in terms of overall weight loss and rate of loss, averaging ½ to 1 lb per week (or no more than 2 lb per week for clinically severe obese patients). Even minor amounts of weight loss (e.g., 10% of body weight) can reduce the health risks that are associated with obesity.[34] Therefore, patients do not need to focus on achieving their ideal body weight but rather a relative weight loss on the basis of current weight.

2. *Negative energy balance:* The most important factor that affects weight loss is the establishment of a negative energy balance with a reduction of 500 to 1000 kcal/day.[34] The negative energy balance should be achieved through a combination of reduced energy in and increased energy out.

Clinical Applications

Breaking Old Links: Strategies for Changing Food Behavior*

Old habits die hard. They are never easy to change, but the effort is worthwhile in the case of undesirable eating behaviors that contribute to excess body fat and that are thus harmful to health. Following are some behavioral suggestions.

1. Deal with Behavioral Cues

Minimize as many cues for the problem behavior as possible. Anticipate situations that are associated with problem foods, and then put temptation out of reach, and make the problem behavior as difficult as possible to perform. Freeze leftovers, remove problem food items from the kitchen or store them in hard-to-reach places, or take a route home other than by the familiar bakery or fast-food restaurant.

Suppress the cues that cannot be entirely eliminated. Control social situations that maintain the behavior, reward the alternate desired behavior, have a trusted person monitor your eating patterns, manage stress without the use of food, minimize contact with excessive food, use smaller plates to make smaller food portions appear larger, and make use of positive nonfood "treat" activities (e.g., hiking, bowling, or a massage).

Strengthen cues for desirable behaviors. Follow the MyPlate guidelines and the *Dietary Guidelines for Americans* for appropriate food choices and amounts. Use food behavior aids (e.g., records, a diary or journal). Distribute appropriate foods among meal and snack patterns. Make desirable food behavior as attractive and as enjoyable as possible.

2. Deal with Actual Food Behavior in Response to Cues

Slow the pace of eating. Take one bite at a time, and place the utensil on the plate between bites. Chew each bite slowly. Sip water. Consciously plan conversation with meal companions for between bites. Visualize eating in slow motion. Enhance the social aspect of eating.

Savor the food. Eat slowly, and sense the taste, smell, and texture of the food. Develop and practice these sensory feelings to the extent that they can be described and brought to mind afterward. Look for food seasonings and combinations that will enhance this process and bring to mind positive feelings about the food experience.

3. Deal with the Follow-up Behavior

Decelerate the problem behavior. Slow down its frequency, and respond neutrally when it occurs rather than with negative talk or thoughts. Give social reinforcement to the decreasing number of times that the problem behavior occurs. Acknowledge the ultimate consequences of the undesirable behavior in the development of health problems.

Accelerate the desired behavior. Update the progress records or personal journal daily. Respond positively to all desired behavior, and provide material reinforcement for positive behavior. Provide social reinforcement by enlisting the help of close friends or family for constructive efforts to modify behavior.

Such a program requires patience, motivation, and work. Continuously evaluate progress toward desired behavior while maintaining a realistic goal, and then plan individual or group maintenance and support activities during an extended follow-up period.

*With contribution from Caiti Christensen.

3. *Nutritional adequacy:* The diet must be nutritionally adequate. Consuming less food requires conscious choices of nutrient-dense foods. In addition, the ratio of macronutrients should have an appropriate balance that is based on a wide variety of food sources.
4. *Cultural appeal:* The food plan must be similar enough to an individual's cultural eating patterns to form the basis for a permanent alteration of eating habits.
5. *Energy readjustment to maintain weight:* When the desired weight level is reached, the kilocalorie level is adjusted in accordance with maintenance needs.

Energy Balance Components

The two sides of energy balance are energy intake in the form of food and drink and energy output in the form of metabolic work and physical activity. For successful weight reduction, both components must be addressed.

Energy input: food behaviors. Clinicians should not assign arbitrary serving sizes and numbers of servings without knowledge of the patient's actual eating patterns. Food diaries are helpful for establishing the patient's normal food choices, the amounts typically eaten, and the distribution of meals throughout the day. From this baseline information, clinicians can help to identify minor changes to initiate, such as eating smaller portions, replacing soda with water, decreasing the overall energy density of foods consumed, and encouraging patients to eat slowly to savor the food's taste and to improve satiety.[34,35] Whole foods should be emphasized and processed foods minimized. Ideally, calories should be evenly distributed throughout the day. The use of fat, sugar, salt, and fiber should be quantified and modified, if necessary, to meet the *2015-2020 Dietary Guidelines for Americans*. Table 15-2 provides suggested servings of the food groups and subgroups to meet recommended nutrient intakes. These guides can serve as a focal point for sound nutrition education. Some additional suggestions are provided in the Clinical Applications box "Practical Suggestions for Changing Food Behaviors."

Energy output: exercise behaviors. Energy output as physical activity must be increased relative to normal activity. For someone who has no planned physical activity, a regular daily exercise schedule that starts with simple walking for approximately a half hour each day and building up to a brisk pace is a great way to begin. Some form of aerobic exercise (e.g., swimming, running, biking) or resistance exercise should be added (see the For Further Focus box, "Benefits of Aerobic Exercise in Weight Management"). An exercise class may be helpful to maintain motivation. Encourage patients to experiment with various

Table 15-2   U.S. Department of Agriculture Food Patterns

For each food group or subgroup,[a] recommended average daily intake amounts[b] at all calorie levels. Recommended intakes from vegetable and protein food subgroups are per week. For more information and tools for application, go to MyPlate.gov.

CALORIE LEVEL OF PATTERN[c]	1000	1200	1400	1600	1800	2000	2200	2400	2600	2800	3000	3200
Fruits	1 c	1 c	1½ c	1½ c	1½ c	2 c	2 c	2 c	2 c	2½ c	2½ c	2½ c
Vegetables[d]	1 c	1½ c	1½ c	2 c	2½ c	2½ c	3 c	3 c	3½ c	3½ c	4 c	4 c
Dark-green vegetables	½ c/wk	1 c/wk	1 c/wk	1½ c/wk	1½ c/wk	1½ c/wk	2 c/wk	2 c/wk	2½ c/wk	2½ c/wk	2½ c/wk	2½ c/wk
Red and orange vegetables	2½ c/wk	3 c/wk	3 c/wk	4 c/wk	5½ c/wk	5½ c/wk	6 c/wk	6 c/wk	7 c/wk	7 c/wk	7½ c/wk	7½ c/wk
Beans and peas (legumes)	½ c/wk	½ c/wk	½ c/wk	1 c/wk	1½ c/wk	1½ c/wk	2 c/wk	2 c/wk	2½ c/wk	2½ c/wk	3 c/wk	3 c/wk
Starchy vegetables	2 c/wk	3½ c/wk	3½ c/wk	4 c/wk	5 c/wk	5 c/wk	6 c/wk	6 c/wk	7 c/wk	7 c/wk	8 c/wk	8 c/wk
Other vegetables	1½ c/wk	2½ c/wk	2½ c/wk	3½ c/wk	4 c/wk	4 c/wk	5 c/wk	5 c/wk	5½ c/wk	5½ c/wk	7 c/wk	7 c/wk
Grains[e]	3 oz-eq	4 oz-eq	5 oz-eq	5 oz-eq	6 oz-eq	6 oz-eq	7 oz-eq	8 oz-eq	9 oz-eq	10 oz-eq	10 oz-eq	10 oz-eq
Whole grains	1½ oz-eq	2 oz-eq	2½ oz-eq	3 oz-eq	3 oz-eq	3 oz-eq	3½ oz-eq	4 oz-eq	4½ oz-eq	5 oz-eq	5 oz-eq	5 oz-eq
Enriched grains	1½ oz-eq	2 oz-eq	2½ oz-eq	2 oz-eq	3 oz-eq	3 oz-eq	3½ Oz-eq	4 oz-eq	4½ oz-eq	5 oz-eq	5 oz-eq	5 oz-eq
Protein Foods[d]	2 oz-eq	3 oz-eq	4 oz-eq	5 oz-eq	5 oz-eq	5½ oz-eq	6 oz-eq	6½ oz-eq	6½ oz-eq	7 oz-eq	7 oz-eq	7 oz-eq
Seafood	3 oz/wk	5 oz/wk	6 oz/wk	8 oz/wk	8 oz/wk	8 oz/wk	9 oz/wk	10 oz/wk	10 oz/wk	11 oz/wk	11 oz/wk	11 oz/wk
Meat, poultry, eggs	10 oz/wk	14 oz/wk	19 oz/wk	24 oz/wk	24 oz/wk	26 oz/wk	29 oz/wk	31 oz/wk	31 oz/wk	34 oz/wk	34 oz/wk	34 oz/wk
Nuts, seeds, soy products	1 oz/wk	2 oz/wk	3 oz/wk	4 oz/wk	4 oz/wk	4 oz/wk	4 oz/wk	5 oz/wk	5 oz/wk	5 oz/wk	5 oz/wk	5 oz/wk
Dairy[f]	2 c	2½ c	2½ c	3 c	3 c	3 c	3 c	3 c	3 c	3 c	3 c	3 c
Oils[g]	15 g	17 g	17 g	22 g	24 g	27 g	29 g	31 g	34 g	36 g	44 g	51 g
Maximum SoFAS[h] **Limit, Calories (% of Calories)**	137 (14%)	121 (10%)	121 (9%)	121 (8%)	161 (9%)	258 (13%)	266 (12%)	330 (14%)	362 (14%)	395 (14%)	459 (15%)	596 (19%)

Fruits	All fresh, frozen, canned, and dried fruits and fruit juices: for example, oranges and orange juice, apples and apple juice, bananas, grapes, melons, berries, raisins
Vegetables	
• Dark-green vegetables	All fresh, frozen, and canned dark-green leafy vegetables and broccoli, cooked or raw: for example, broccoli; spinach; romaine lettuce; collard, turnip, and mustard greens
• Red and orange vegetables	All fresh, frozen, and canned red and orange vegetables, cooked or raw: for example, tomatoes, red peppers, carrots, sweet potatoes, winter squash, and pumpkin
• Beans and peas (legumes)	All cooked beans and peas: for example, kidney beans, lentils, chickpeas, and pinto beans; does not include green beans or green peas (see additional comment under protein foods group)
• Starchy vegetables	All fresh, frozen, and canned starchy vegetables: for example, white potatoes, corn, green peas
• Other vegetables	All fresh, frozen, and canned other vegetables, cooked or raw: for example, iceberg lettuce, green beans, and onions
Grains	
• Whole grains	All whole-grain products and whole grains used as ingredients: for example, whole-wheat bread, whole-grain cereals and crackers, oatmeal, and brown rice
• Enriched grains	All enriched refined-grain products and enriched refined grains used as ingredients: for example, white breads, enriched grain cereals and crackers, enriched pasta, white rice
Protein Foods	All meat, poultry, seafood, eggs, nuts, seeds, and processed soy products; meat and poultry should be lean or low-fat and nuts should be unsalted; beans and peas are considered part of this group as well as the vegetable group, but should be counted in one group only
Dairy	All milks, including lactose-free and lactose-reduced products and fortified soy beverages, yogurts, frozen yogurts, dairy desserts, and cheeses; most choices should be fat-free or low-fat; cream, sour cream, and cream cheese are not included because of their low calcium content

From U.S. Department of Agriculture and U.S. Department of Health and Human Services. *Dietary Guidelines for Americans, 2010.* Washington, DC: U.S. Government Printing Office; 2010.

aAll foods are assumed to be in nutrient-dense forms, lean or low-fat, and prepared without added fats, sugars, or salt. Solid fats and added sugars may be included up to the daily maximum limit identified in the table. Food items in each group and subgroup are:

bFood group amounts are shown in cup(s) (c) or ounce-equivalents (oz-eq). Oils are shown in grams (g). Quantity equivalents for each food group are:
- Grains, 1 ounce-equivalent is 1 ounce of sliced bread; 1 ounce of uncooked pasta or rice; ½ cup of cooked rice, pasta, or cereal; 1 tortilla (6-inch diameter); 1 pancake (5-inch diameter); 1 ounce of ready-to-eat cereal (about 1 cup of cereal flakes).
- Vegetables and fruits, 1 cup equivalent is 1 cup of raw or cooked vegetable or fruit; ½ cup of dried vegetable or fruit; 1 cup of vegetable or fruit juice; 2 cups of leafy salad greens.
- Protein foods, 1 ounce-equivalent is 1 ounce of lean meat, poultry, seafood; 1 egg; 1 Tbsp of peanut butter; ½ ounce of nuts or seeds. Also, ¼ cup of cooked beans or peas may be counted as 1 ounce-equivalent.
- Dairy, 1 cup equivalent is 1 cup of milk, fortified soy beverage, or yogurt; 1½ ounces of natural cheese (e.g., cheddar); 2 ounces of processed cheese (e.g., American).

cSee the *Dietary Guidelines for Americans, 2010,* for estimated calorie needs per day by age, gender, and physical activity level. Food intake patterns at 1000, 1200, and 1400 calories meet the nutritional needs of children ages 2 to 8 years. Patterns from 1600 to 3200 calories meet the nutritional needs of children ages 9 years and older and adults. If a child aged 4 to 8 years needs more calories and, therefore, is following a pattern at 1600 calories or more, the recommended amount from the dairy group can be 2½ cups per day. Children aged 9 years and older and adults should not use the 1000-, 1200-, or 1400-calorie patterns.

dVegetable and protein food subgroup amounts are shown in this table as weekly amounts, because it would be difficult for consumers to select foods from all subgroups daily.

eWhole-grain subgroup amounts shown in this table are minimums. More whole grains up to all of the grains recommended may be selected, with offsetting decreases in the amounts of enriched refined grains.

fThe amounts of dairy foods in the 1200- and 1400-calorie patterns have increased to reflect new Recommended Dietary Allowances for calcium that are higher than previous recommendations for children aged 4 to 8 years.

gOils and soft margarines include vegetable, nut, and fish oils and soft vegetable oil table spreads that have no trans fats.

hSoFAS are calories from solid fats and added sugars. The limit for SoFAS is the remaining amount of calories in each food pattern after selecting the specified amounts in each food group in nutrient-dense forms (forms that are fat free or low fat and with no added sugars). The number of SoFAS is lower in the 1200-, 1400-, and 1600-calorie patterns than in the 1000-calorie pattern. The nutrient goals for the 1200- to 1600-calorie patterns are higher and require that more calories be used for nutrient-dense foods from the food groups.

Clinical Applications

Practical Suggestions for Changing Food Behaviors

GOALS
Set SMART goals: Specific, Measurable, Attainable, Realistic, and Timely. Do not set your goals too high. Keep them focused.

KILOCALORIES
Do not be an obsessive calorie counter. Instead, learn the general values of some of your home-prepared meals, modify recipes or make occasional substitutes, and read labels often.

PLATEAUS
Anticipate plateaus; they happen to everyone. As the body adjusts to a new energy balance, lean-to-fat body mass ratio, and metabolic rate, weight-loss rates can slow down. Increase amount or intensity of exercise during these periods to help get started again.

BINGES
Do not be discouraged if you binge. Individuals who have previously struggled with binge eating behavior may have an occasional setback. Try to keep these binges infrequent and, when possible, plan ahead for special occasions. Adjust the following day's diet or the remainder of the same day accordingly. Changing binge eating behavior is not easy. The assistance of a psychologist and a dietitian may be helpful.

STRESS EATING
Avoid eating in response to stress; eating because of stress only causes guilt and added calories but does nothing for the stressor. Instead try doing a combination of things to better cope: work on a journal, talk to someone, go for a walk, hug a friend, do a hobby, take 10 deep breaths, or drink a glass of water.

HOME MEALS
Try to avoid making a separate menu for yourself (or another person on a weight-loss program). Adapt your needs to the family meal, and then adjust the seasonings or method of preparation to involve fewer kilocalories, especially by reducing or omitting fat. Everyone deserves to be healthy.

EATING AWAY FROM HOME
Watch your portions. When you are a guest, limit extras such as sauces and dressings, and trim your meat well. In restaurants, select singly prepared items rather than combination dishes. Avoid items with heavy sauces or fat seasonings as well as fried foods. Select fruit or sherbet for dessert rather than pastries. Focus more on the social aspect rather than the food.

MEAL PATTERN
Eat three or more small meals a day. If snacks between meals help you, then plan part of your day's allowance to account for them. The point is to spread your daily energy allowance throughout the day. Avoid the common pattern of no breakfast, little or no lunch, and a huge dinner.

GET TO THE WHY?
If you can stay focused on 'Why is this change important to me?' or 'Why do I want to make this change?' you will be able to find intrinsic motivation for when it gets really hard. Some find it helpful to repeat it as a mantra daily.

For Further Focus

Benefits of Aerobic Exercise in Weight Management

The goal of weight management is to reduce excess body fat and, in most cases, build lean body mass (muscle). However, both tissues may be lost when a person tries to reach a weight goal merely by reducing food intake.

Optimal body composition can be achieved by combining food restriction with aerobic exercise. Aerobic exercise consists of activities sustained long enough to draw on the body's fat reserve for fuel while oxygen intake is increased (thus the term *aerobic*). Lean body tissue burns fats in the presence of oxygen. Therefore aerobic activity is best suited for achieving the ideal balance of high lean body mass and low fatty tissue in the body.

The benefits of aerobic exercise to an overweight person in a weight management program include the following:
- Suppressed appetite
- Reduced total body fat
- Higher BMR
- Increased circulatory and respiratory function
- Increased energy expenditure
- Retention of tissue protein and building of lean body mass levels

Some individuals complain about the slow rate of weight loss, difficulty in controlling appetite, and consistent "flabbiness" despite continuing diet management. These individuals may welcome the suggestion of aerobic activity to help manage weight loss. Suggestions include a brisk daily walk, jumping rope, swimming, bicycling, jogging, running, aerobic or spinning classes, or another activity that increases the heart rate enough to have an aerobic effect and can be maintained for 20 to 30 minutes. Carefully note the physical stress this activity may place on individuals who have not exercised for some time or who have medical problems related to exertion. These individuals should have a medical check-up before beginning such a program on their own or at a fitness center. And then the program should start slowly and incrementally increase in time and intensity.

---

activities until they find one that they enjoy and that they feel they can maintain for the long term. Following are current recommendations by the *2015-2020 Dietary Guidelines for Americans*, regarding exercise and weight maintenance or weight loss[36]:

- Choose a healthy eating pattern at an appropriate calorie level to help achieve and maintain a healthy body weight, support nutrient adequacy, and reduce the risk of chronic disease.
- Increase the amount of physical activity engagement each week.
- Limit screen time and decrease the amount of time spent being sedentary.

Specific physical activity recommendations are discussed in greater detail in Chapter 16.

Principles of a Sound Food Plan

A careful diet history (see Chapter 17) can be the basis for a sound personalized food plan and should involve the principles of energy and nutrient balance, distribution balance and portion control, a food guide, and a preventive approach.

Energy balance. Under normal circumstances, when energy expenditure is greater than energy intake, weight loss occurs. Because 1 lb of fat is equal to approximately 3500 kcal, an energy deficit of 500 kcal/day results in a weight loss of about 1 lb per week; a deficit of 250 kcal equals a ½-lb weight loss per week (Box 15-2). All people who are pursuing weight loss should determine their current total energy needs as a basis for diet planning (Box 15-3). Modifications to energy intake and energy output can then be adjusted to produce a negative energy balance. As discussed throughout this text, individual energy needs vary greatly. Therefore, assuming that all people on a weight-loss program should limit caloric intake to 1400 kcal/day (or any other prefabricated amount) is not appropriate. For a person who normally consumes 2000 kcal/day, the ideal scenario is a deficit of approximately 500 kcal/day. The total of those 500 kcal should not all come from diet. Reducing calorie intake by 25%

(2000 × 25% = 500 kcal) would likely leave a person hungry and constantly thinking about food. Instead, the weight-loss program could include a 250-kcal reduction in energy intake and a 250-kcal increase in energy expenditure for a total deficit of 500 kcal (see the Clinical Applications box, "Case Study: Sara's Energy Balance and Weight-Management Plan").

Nutrient balance. Basic diet components are needed to achieve the following nutrient balance:
- *Carbohydrate:* Approximately 45% to 65% of the total kilocalories, with emphasis on complex forms such as whole grains and fruits and vegetables that are good sources of fiber. Limit simple sugars.
- *Protein:* Approximately 10% to 35% of the total kilocalories, with emphasis on lean foods and small portions.
- *Fat:* Approximately 15% to 25% of the total kilocalories, with emphasis on essential fatty acids from plant foods and minimal animal and trans fats.
- The food plan should meet the recommendations of the *2015-2020 Dietary Guidelines for Americans* (see Figure 1-4).

The use of special diet foods is not necessary because they are often more expensive. All foods can fit into a sound weight-loss plan with moderation and put into the context of the overall plan.

Distribution balance and portion control. Spreading food fairly evenly throughout the day with four to five meals or snacks, including breakfast, along with avoiding the practice of skipping meals are advised.[34] Hunger usually peaks every 4 to 5 hours. If

---

Box 15-2 Kilocalorie Adjustment Necessary for Weight Loss

To lose 454 g (1 lb) per week there needs to be a 500-kcal energy deficit per day.

BASIS OF ESTIMATION:
1 lb of body fat = 454 g
1 g of pure fat = 9 kcal
1 g of body fat = 7.7 kcal (differences due to water in fat cells)
454 g × 7.7 kcal/g = 3496 kcal/454 g of body fat (or ≈3500 kcal)
500 kcal energy deficit × 7 days = 3500 kcal = 454 g of body fat = 1 lb

---

Box 15-3 Estimation of Adult Energy Needs

MIFFLIN-ST. JEOR EQUATION
Men
Total Energy Expenditure (kcal/day) = (Weight [kg] × 10 + Height [cm] × 6.25 − Age × 5 − 5) × Physical activity coefficient
Women
Total Energy Expenditure (kcal/day) = (Weight [kg] × 10 + Height [cm] × 6.25 − Age × 5 − 161) × Physical activity coefficient

PHYSICAL ACTIVITY COEFFICIENT
1.200 = Sedentary (little or no exercise)
1.375 = Lightly active (light exercise or sports 1 to 3 days per week)
1.550 = Moderately active (moderate exercise or sports 3 to 5 days per week)
1.725 = Very active (hard exercise or sports 6 to 7 days per week)
1.900 = Extra active (very hard exercise or sports and physical job)

Clinical Applications

Case Study: Sara's Energy Balance and Weight-Management Plan

Sara is a 34-year-old accountant who leads a more or less sedentary life due to her long work hours and 3-year-old son at home. She wants to work on losing her pregnancy weight and get back in shape. She was a college athlete and never struggled with her weight until now.

Sara begins to look carefully at her energy balance. She weighs 175 lb, and is 5 feet, 7 inches tall. Sara's average food intake is approximately 2500 kcal/day. She wants to lose weight in a healthy, long-term way by adjusting her energy balance.

QUESTIONS FOR ANALYSIS
1. What are Sara's present daily total energy needs in kilocalories according to the Mifflin-St. Jeor equation?
2. How does this total energy need compare with her food energy intake?
3. To lose approximately 1 lb per week, how much should Sara reduce the caloric value of her daily diet?
4. In addition to reducing her dietary kilocalories, what else could Sara do to help create a negative energy balance and improve her body condition?

an individual has certain "problem times" of the day, planning simple snacks for those periods helps to maintain balance. Long periods without refueling can result in low blood glucose level and intense hunger followed by subsequent periods of overeating, usually of whatever can be found at the time, which is often "junk foods" with empty calories from vending machines. Balanced meals and healthful snacks require the foresight of planning and preparation.

Inappropriately large portion sizes continue to contribute to the energy intake imbalance for many Americans. Meals eaten both at home and away from home may be problematic so try to use smaller plates/cups, order a half serving, or pack half of the entrée to go at the start of the meal. Portion sizes and portion control are important factors in a sound food plan. See Chapter 14 for a discussion of portion control.

Food guide. The Academy of Nutrition and Dietetics publishes the "Choose Your Foods: Weight Management" food exchange list (available from www.eatright.org) that follows the general *Dietary Guidelines for Americans*. This basic food exchange system is a good general reference guide for comparative food values and portions, variety in food choices, and basic meal planning. Table 15-2 provides examples of food plans that meet nutrient needs at 12 different calorie levels. A simple plan also can be outlined by using the food groups of the MyPlate guidelines (see Figure 1-3). The overall food guide should consist of plenty of fruits and vegetables, whole grains, and lean proteins, while reducing the energy density of foods eaten, with water as the ideal beverage. Given the complexity of the variables associated with weight loss and maintenance the most effective food guide should be individualized for the patient by a dietitian.

Preventive approach. The most positive work with weight management is aimed at prevention. Current trends indicate that the U.S. population of children and adolescents continues to gain excess weight, and these overweight children are becoming obese adults. Major culprits in this health epidemic are inappropriate eating patterns and inadequate physical activity. Support for young parents and children before obesity develops can help to prevent many problems later in adulthood. This support and guidance should include early nutrition counseling and education, which can help to build positive health habits, especially in the forms of healthful eating behaviors and increased exercise through active play and physical activities for the entire family. Many programs for young children—such as Head Start, school breakfast and lunch programs, and the Special Supplemental Nutrition Program for Women, Infants and Children (WIC) (see Chapter 13)—address obesity issues through education and prevention for both parents and children.

FOOD MISINFORMATION AND FADS

A fad is any popular fashion or pursuit that is embraced with fervor. Food fads are scientifically unsubstantiated beliefs about certain foods that may persist for a short time in a given community or society. The word *fallacy* means "a deceptive, misleading, or false notion or belief." Food fallacies are false or misleading beliefs that underlie food fads. The jargon term *quack* is a shortened form of *quicksalver,* a term that was invented centuries ago by the Dutch to describe the pseudophysician or pseudoprofessor who sold worthless salves, magic elixirs, and cure-all tonics. He proclaimed his wares in a patter that skeptical people compared with the quacking of a duck. In medicine, nutrition, and allied health fields, a quack is a fraudulent pretender who claims to have skill, knowledge, or qualifications that he or she does not truly possess. The motive for such quackery is usually money, and the quack uses a hoax to feed on the physical and emotional needs of his or her victims.

Unscientific statements about food often mislead consumers and contribute to poor food habits. False information may come from folklore or fraud. Food choices should be based on sound scientific knowledge from responsible authorities; misinformation should be recognized as such.

FOOD FADS

Types of Claims

Food faddists make exaggerated claims about certain types of food. These claims generally fall into the following four basic groups:

1. *Food cures:* Certain foods cure specific conditions.
2. *Harmful foods:* Certain foods are harmful and should be omitted from the diet.
3. *Food combinations:* Special food combinations restore health and are effective for reducing weight.
4. *Natural foods:* Only "natural" foods can meet body needs and prevent disease. The term *natural* may be used on unprocessed or minimally processed products that contain no artificial ingredients, coloring ingredients, or chemical preservatives. Some people consider all processed foods unhealthy, including those that are enriched or fortified.

Erroneous Claims

Claims that are simply erroneous require careful examination. On the surface, they seem to be simple statements about food and health. However, further observation reveals that they focus on a food itself and not on the specific nutrients that are in the food, which are the actual physiologic agents of life and health. Some individuals may be allergic to specific foods and should avoid them. In addition, certain foods may supply relatively large amounts of individual nutrients and therefore are good sources of those nutrients. Each nutrient is found in a wide variety of different foods. Remember that people require specific nutrients and not necessarily specific foods.

Dangers

Why should health care workers be concerned about food fads and their effect on food habits? What harm do food fads cause? Food fads generally involve four possible negative effects.

Danger to health. Responsibility for one's health is fundamental. However, self-diagnosis and self-treatment can be dangerous, especially when such action follows questionable sources. By following such a course, people with real illness may fail to seek appropriate medical care. Many ill and anxious people have been misled by fraudulent claims of cures and have postponed proven effective therapy.

Cost. Some foods and supplements used by faddists are harmless, but many are expensive. Money spent for useless items is wasted. When dollars are scarce, a family may neglect to buy foods that fill basic needs in an attempt to purchase a "miracle cure."

Lack of sound knowledge. Misinformation hinders the development of individuals and society and ignores scientific progress. The perpetuation of certain superstitions can counteract sound teaching about health.

Distrust of the food market. America's food environment is changing. People should be watchful, but a blanket rejection of all modern food production is unwarranted. People must develop intelligent concerns and rational approaches to meet their nutrition needs.

WHAT IS THE ANSWER?

What can be done to counter food habits that are associated with food fads, misinformation, or even outright deception? Helpful instruction is based on personal conviction, practice, and enthusiasm. The following approaches to positive teaching can be used.

Using Reliable Sources

Sound background knowledge is essential and should include the following:

1. Knowing the product being pushed and the people or company behind it
2. Knowing how human physiology and biochemistry work
3. Knowing the scientific method of problem solving (e.g., collect the facts, identify the problem, determine a reasonable solution or action, carry it out, and evaluate the results)

Sound community resources include the following:

- Extension educators work in the community through state and county Extension Service offices and direct highly successful community nutrition activities, such as their Expanded Food and Nutrition Education Program. These specialists develop many food and nutrition guides, especially for those with limited education or who speak English as a second language. Information about the program can be found at www.csrees.usda.gov/nea/food/efnep/efnep.html.
- The FDA and U.S. Department of Agriculture (USDA) produce many educational materials related to food and nutrition (see Chapter 13). Requests for these mostly free materials can be directed to FDA and USDA agency offices.
- "Cultural and Ethnic Food and Nutrition Education Materials: A Resource List for Educators" is provided by the USDA at www.nal.usda.gov/fnic/pubs/ethnic.pdf.
- Public health nutritionists and dietitians located in county and state public health offices and as part of special programs (e.g., WIC) can provide information. WIC state agencies are listed at www.fns.usda.gov/wic/Contacts/statealpha.htm.
- Dietitians in local medical care centers who serve hospitalized patients, outpatient clinics, and private practice also are valuable resources. The Academy of Nutrition and Dietetics nationwide nutrition network can be accessed at www.eatright.org/find-an-expert.

Recognizing Human Needs

Consider the emotional needs that food and food rituals help to fulfill. These needs are a part of life, and they should be used in a positive way in nutrition teaching. Even if a person is using food as an emotional crutch, the emotional need is still real. Never take away crutches without offering a better and wiser form of support. Food and all the associations that go along with it compose a basic enjoyment of life. Maintaining a balance between food as entertainment and food as fuel is the challenge of identifying the human needs that are being met by certain foods. The establishment of a healthy diet must consider all such human needs; it may involve specialized help, such as that provided by behavioral therapists.

Remaining Alert to Teaching Opportunities

Use any opportunity that arises to present sound nutrition and health information, whether formally or informally. Learn about the available resources described previously. Develop communication skills, avoid monotony, and use a well-disciplined imagination.

Thinking Scientifically

Even very young children can be taught to use the problem-solving approach to everyday situations. Children are naturally curious. With their eternal questioning—"Why?"—they often seek evidence to support the statements that they hear. Three basic questions help with the evaluation of claims in any

| Box 15-4 | The Food and Nutrition Science Alliance's 10 Red Flags of Junk Science |

1. Recommendations that promise a quick fix
2. Dire warnings of danger from a single product or regimen
3. Claims that sound too good to be true
4. Simplistic conclusions drawn from a complex study
5. Recommendations based on a single study
6. Dramatic statements that are refuted by reputable scientific organizations
7. Lists of "good" and "bad" foods
8. Recommendations made to help sell a product
9. Recommendations based on studies published without peer review
10. Recommendations from studies that ignore differences among individuals or groups

Reprinted from the Food and Nutrition Science Alliance (FANSA). *10 Red Flags of Junk Science.* Chicago: 1995.

situation: (1) "What do you mean?"; (2) "How do you know?"; and (3) "What is your evidence?"

The Food and Nutrition Science Alliance is a partnership of seven professional scientific societies that have joined together to disseminate sound nutrition information. This organization issued a list of 10 red flags to help guide consumers toward making educated decisions about nutrition and health issues (Box 15-4). This list is an excellent guide when evaluating reports and claims about various diets, supplements, and other nutrition-related fads.

Knowing Responsible Authorities

The FDA is legally responsible for controlling the quality and safety of food and drug products marketed in the United States. However, this is a tremendous task that requires public help. Other government, professional, and private organizations can provide additional resources (see the Further Reading and Resources list at the end of the chapter).

UNDERWEIGHT

GENERAL CAUSES AND TREATMENT

Extremes in underweight—just as in overweight—can pose health problems. Although general malnutrition and excessive thinness is a less-common problem in the U.S. population than overweight and obesity, it does occur, and it is usually associated with poor living conditions or long-term disease. A person who is more than 10% below the average weight for height and age is considered underweight; someone who is 20% or more below the average weight has cause for significant health concerns. Physiologic and psychologic effects may occur, especially among young children. Their resistance to infection is lowered, their general health is poor, and their strength is reduced.

Causes

Underweight is associated with conditions that cause general malnutrition, including the following:
- *Wasting disease:* long-term disease with chronic infection and fever that raise the BMR
- *Poor food intake:* diminished food intake that results from psychologic factors that cause a person to refuse to eat, loss of appetite, or personal poverty and limited available food supply
- *Malabsorption:* poor nutrient absorption that results from chronic diarrhea, a diseased gastrointestinal tract, the excessive use of laxatives, or drug-nutrient interactions
- *Hormonal imbalance:* hyperthyroidism or a variety of other hormonal imbalances that increase the caloric needs of the body
- *Low energy availability:* condition that results from greatly increased physical activity without a corresponding increase in food or a lack of available food supply
- *Poor living situation:* an unhealthy home environment that results in irregular and inadequate meals, where eating is considered unimportant, and where an indifferent attitude toward food exists

Dietary Treatment

Special nutrition care to rebuild body tissues and to regain health is necessary for underweight and undernourished patients. Food plans should be adapted to each person's unique situation, whether it involves his or her personal needs, living situation, economic needs, or any underlying disease. The dietary goal, in accordance with each person's tolerance, is to increase energy and nutrient intake, with adherence to the following needs:
- *High-caloric diet:* above the standard requirement for that individual
- *High protein:* to rebuild tissues
- *High carbohydrate:* to provide the primary energy source in an easily digested form
- *Moderate fat:* to provide essential fatty acids and add energy without exceeding tolerance limits
- *Good sources of vitamins and minerals:* provided by a variety of nutrient-dense foods and dietary supplements when individual deficiencies require them

A variety of foods attractively served may help to revive the appetite and increase the desire to eat more. Nourishing meals and snacks should be spread throughout the day and should include favorite foods often. A basic aim is to help build good food habits so that improved nutritional status and weight can be maintained. Residents in long-term care facilities are especially vulnerable to weight-loss problems, and they have special needs (see the Clinical Applications box, "Problems of Weight Loss among Older Adults in Long-Term Care Facilities"). In addition, several medications that are often prescribed to elderly individuals

Clinical Applications

Problems of Weight Loss among Older Adults in Long-Term Care Facilities

The American population of adults who are 65 years old and older is rapidly increasing. The most rapid population increase over the next decade will be among those who are older than 85, and many of these elderly people will require long-term care in nursing homes.

One of the problems that is encountered among elderly residents is low body weight and rapid unintentional weight loss. These conditions can become serious health problems, and they are a sensitive indicator of malnutrition that can contribute to illness and death. Because weight loss is such a strong predictor of morbidity and mortality in clinical settings, early and continuing observation to assess needs is important, especially in relation to factors that contribute to weight loss.

In general, weight loss in this population can be caused by the following: (1) the physical effects of the metabolic changes of aging; (2) the physical effects of disease; or (3) certain factors that alter the amount and type of food eaten. Physical disease (e.g., cancer) can cause extreme weight loss as a result of metabolic abnormalities, taste changes, loss of appetite, nausea, and vomiting. Other diseases that affect weight include gastrointestinal problems; uncontrolled diabetes; cardiovascular disorders (e.g., congestive heart failure); pulmonary disease; infection; and alcoholism. Psychologic factors or psychiatric disorders may also contribute to malnutrition and weight loss from depression, memory loss, disorientation, apathy, and appetite disturbance. Some altered mental states may be caused by nutritional deficiencies (e.g., low levels of folate and B-complex vitamins) as well as by protein-energy malnutrition. These conditions can be corrected with specific nutritional support.

The following additional physiologic, psychologic, and social factors may influence food intake and body weight and thus contribute to malnutrition among elderly people:

- *Body composition changes:* Height and body weight gradually decline as people age. Body weight usually peaks between the ages of 34 and 54 years in men and between 55 and 75 years in women, and it decreases thereafter. Body fat losses are generally not significant. One cause of weight loss is a decline in body water, which is caused in part by the weakening of the normal thirst mechanism. Therefore, a feeling of thirst cannot be relied upon to secure adequate water intake, so water must frequently be offered and encouraged. More constant attention to fluid intake also helps with the common problem of xerostomia (i.e., dry mouth) in older adults. Xerostomia results from inadequate salivary secretions, which makes eating difficult, thereby contributing to malnutrition. Lean body mass also declines with age, and this results in a lower basal metabolic rate and decreased physical activity and energy requirements. Thus, any possible increase in physical activity and the use of nutrient-dense foods are encouraged.
- *Taste changes:* The regeneration of taste bud cells slows with age, but the extent and effect on food intake vary widely. The sense of smell also declines with age and may negatively affect taste. The increased use of appropriate seasoning and flavoring in food preparation is needed.
- *Dentition:* About half of Americans have lost some or all of their teeth by the age of 65 years. Many have dentures, but chewing problems are often present. Nursing home residents frequently report chewing, biting, and swallowing problems that interfere with eating and adequate food intake. The assessment of specific needs and dental care solutions helps to correct eating problems.
- *Gastrointestinal problems:* Delayed gastric emptying may contribute to distention and lack of appetite. A decrease in gastric secretions, including hydrochloric acid, may hinder the absorption of vitamin B_{12}, folate, and iron, thereby contributing to anemia and a loss of appetite. Constipation is a common complaint that often leads to laxative abuse and that results in interference with nutrient absorption. An increase in dietary fiber, liquids, and physical activity can help to provide a more natural approach to establishing normal bowel movements.
- *Drug-nutrient interactions:* Elderly people often take a number of prescribed and over-the-counter medications, some of which are the direct cause of anorexia, nausea, and vomiting. Other drugs are indirect causes in that they induce nutrient malabsorption; this leads to deficiencies that in turn cause anorexia and weight loss. Drug therapy for elderly patients should involve constant medical, nutrition, and nursing attention to ensure appropriate use.
- *Functional disabilities:* Difficulty with eating may prevent or alter the capacity of elderly people to take in sufficient food. These problems may vary from more difficult functional disabilities that interfere with putting food into the mouth and swallowing (e.g., problems that often require a trained therapist) to dependence on feeding assistance that can be provided by sensitive nursing care.
- *Social problems:* Socioeconomic problems are often involved in the care of the elderly. A specially trained geriatric social worker can help to secure possible sources of financial assistance. A sense of social isolation can also lead to decreased food intake. Family support, sensitive contact with nursing home staff and residents, and as much involvement as possible in group activities are necessary.

Health care workers in geriatric settings need continuing education and sensitization to the potential dangers of low body weight and weight loss among their patients. Older individuals with acute and chronic illnesses and functional disabilities are at the greatest risk for nutrition-related problems. These people require continual nutrition assessment and the monitoring of their body weight. Some of the restrictions of "special diets" should be relaxed or discontinued when the risk of malnutrition is evident, with the goal of increasing nutrient intake and making eating as enjoyable as possible.

may result in anorexia or weight loss. This rehabilitation process requires creative counseling for the patient and the family along with practical guides and support. In some cases, tube feeding or intravenous feeding (e.g., parenteral nutrition) may be necessary (see Chapter 22).

Ideal weight gain includes both lean and fat tissue. To gain muscle, physical exercise must be part of the treatment. Resistance training increases lean tissue and, in turn, boosts appetite. A variety of weight-lifting and strength-training programs can be designed, depending on the desires of the individual, and they should be encouraged as an important part of healthy weight gain.

DISORDERED EATING

To discuss disordered or abnormal eating, we must first define "normal eating." Normal eating is when an individual is capable of the following:

- Eating when he or she is hungry and stopping when full
- Demonstrating moderate restraint with regard to food selection
- Recognizing that overeating and undereating are sometimes acceptable and trusting his or her body to establish a balance
- Having the ability to be flexible with his or her eating schedule

Disordered eating is defined as any eating pattern that is not normal, and it can include a variety of subclinical problems. This type of eating or thought patterns can be in a range from infrequent episodes, to more often such as with **eating disorder not otherwise specified,** or consistent enough to meet diagnostic criteria for an eating disorder. Disordered eating can range from an insurmountable fear of eating fat to an inability to eat in public. Family and personal tensions as well as social pressures for thinness may result in serious body image disturbances and eating problems that push the disordered eating behavior to the point of becoming a clinical eating disorder. The three most common eating disorders are **anorexia nervosa (AN), bulimia nervosa (BN),** and **binge eating disorder (BED)** (Box 15-5).

The most recent position paper from the Academy of Nutrition and Dietetics regarding eating disorders states that eating disorders are "psychiatric disorders with diagnostic criteria based on psychologic, behavior, and physiologic characteristics."[37] Death rates from eating disorders are significant compared with other psychologic diseases: 4.37% for anorexia nervosa and 2.33% for bulimia nervosa.[38] Eating disorders are secretive in nature; therefore, establishing a true estimate of population prevalence is difficult. However, research indicates that eating disorders occur less frequently among males than females and that homosexual and bisexual males are at higher risk than their heterosexual counterparts.[39]

Clinical eating disorders all have similar risk factors, all of which may be influenced by genetic and/or environmental factors.

These risk factors include the following[40]:

- *Sociocultural influences:* media exposure for idealization of thinness, perceived pressure for thinness, and thin-ideal internalization
- *Personality traits:* negative emotionality (anxiety, anger), perfectionism; negative urgency/impulsivity especially when distressed in patients specifically with BN and BED
- *Neurocognitive processes:* decreased cognitive flexibility (inability to move between multiple tasks), motor or cognitive inhibitory control, and serotonin disturbances

Anorexia Nervosa

The estimated lifetime prevalence of anorexia nervosa is 0.9% in women and 0.3% in men.[41] This complex psychologic disorder results in self-imposed starvation. In addition to the diagnostic criteria provided in Box 15-5, Table 15-3 outlines the clinical signs that are associated with both anorexia nervosa and bulimia nervosa. Features of anorexia nervosa include the following[42]:

- Genetic predisposition
- Dieting behavior
- High level of exercise
- **Body dysmorphic disorder**
- Obsessive-compulsive disorder
- Acculturation
- Perfectionism
- Negative self-evaluation

All forms of eating disorders require an interdisciplinary team for treatment success. Nutrition therapy

---

eating disorder not otherwise specified subthreshold disordered eating that is not consistent with the diagnostic criteria for bulimia nervosa or anorexia nervosa.

anorexia nervosa an extreme psychophysiologic aversion to food that results in life-threatening weight loss; a psychiatric eating disorder that results from a morbid fear of fatness in which a person's distorted body image is reflected as fat when the body is malnourished and extremely thin as a result of self-starvation.

bulimia nervosa a psychiatric eating disorder related to a person's fear of fatness in which cycles of gorging on large quantities of food are followed by compensatory mechanisms (e.g., self-induced vomiting, the use of diuretics and laxatives) to maintain a "normal" body weight.

Binge eating disorder a psychiatric eating disorder that is characterized by the occurrence of binge eating episodes at least twice a week for a 6-month period.

body dysmorphic disorder an obsession with a perceived defect of the body.

Box 15-5 American Psychiatric Association Diagnostic Criteria

ANOREXIA NERVOSA

A. Restriction of energy intake relative to requirements, leading to a significantly low body weight in the context of age, sex, developmental trajectory, and physical health. *Significantly low weight* is defined as a weight that is less than minimally normal or, for children and adolescents, less than that minimally expected.

B. Intense fear of gaining weight or becoming fat or persistent behavior that interferes with weight gain, even though at a significantly low weight.

C. Disturbance in the way in which one's body weight or shape is experienced; undue influence of body weight or shape on self-evaluation, or persistent lack of recognition of the seriousness of the current low body weight.

1. *Restricting type:* During the last 3 months, the individual has not engaged in recurrent episodes of binge eating or purging behavior (i.e., self-induced vomiting or the misuse of laxatives, diuretics, or enemas). The subtype describes presentations in which weight loss is accomplished primarily through dieting, fasting, and/or excessive exercise.

2. *Binge eating/purging type:* During the last 3 months, the individual has engaged in recurrent episodes of binge eating or purging behavior (i.e., self-induced vomiting or the misuse of laxatives, diuretics, or enemas).

BULIMIA NERVOSA

A. Recurrent episodes of binge eating. An episode of binge eating is characterized by both of the following:

1. Eating, during a discrete period of time (e.g., within any 2-hour period), an amount of food that is definitely larger than most individuals would eat during a similar period of time and under similar circumstances.

2. A sense of a lack of control over eating during the episode (e.g., a feeling that one cannot stop eating or control what or how much one is eating).

B. Recurrent inappropriate compensatory behavior in order to prevent weight gain, such as self-induced vomiting; the misuse of laxatives, diuretics, or other medications; fasting; or excessive exercise.

C. The binge eating and inappropriate compensatory behaviors both occur, on average, at least once a week for 3 months.

D. Self-evaluation is unduly influenced by body shape and weight.

E. The disturbance does not occur exclusively during episodes of anorexia nervosa.

EATING DISORDER NOT OTHERWISE SPECIFIED

This category applies to presentations in which symptoms characteristic of feeding and eating disorder that cause clinically significant distress or impairment in social, occupational, or other important areas of functioning predominate but do not meet the full criteria for any of the disorders in the feeding and eating disorders diagnostic class. The other specified feeding or eating disorder category is used in situations in which the clinician chooses to communicate the specific reason that the presentation does not meet the criteria for any specific feeding and eating disorder. This is done by recording "other specified feeding or eating disorder"

followed by the specific reason (e.g., "bulimia nervosa of low frequency").

Examples of presentations that can be specified using the "other Specified" designation include the following:

A. **Atypical anorexia nervosa:** All of the criteria for anorexia nervosa are met, except that despite significant weight loss, the individual's weight is within or above the normal range.

B. **Bulimia nervosa (of low frequency and/or limited duration):** All of the criteria for bulimia nervosa are met, except that the binge eating and inappropriate compensatory behaviors occur, on average, less than once a week and/or for less than 3 months.

C. **Binge-eating disorder (of low frequency and/or limited duration):** All of the criteria for binge-eating disorder are met, except that the binge eating occurs, on average, less than once a week and/ or for less than 3 months.

D. **Purging disorder:** Recurrent purging behavior to influence weight or shape (e.g., self-induced vomiting; misuse of laxatives, diuretics, or other medications) in the absence of binge eating.

E. **Night eating syndrome:** Recurrent episodes of night eating, as manifested by eating after awakening from sleep or by excessive food consumption after the evening meal. There is awareness and recall of the eating. The night eating is not better explained by external influences such as changes in the individual's sleep-wake cycle or by local social norms. The night eating causes significant distress and/or impairment in functioning. The disordered pattern of eating is not better explained by binge-eating disorder or another mental disorder, including substance use, and is not attributable to another medical disorder or to an effect of medication.

BINGE EATING DISORDER

A. Recurrent episodes of binge eating. An episode of binge eating is characterized by both of the following:

1. Eating, in a discrete period of time (e.g., within any 2-hour period), and amount of food that is definitely larger than what most people would eat in a similar period of time under similar circumstances.

2. A sense of lack of control over eating during the episode (e.g., a feeling that one cannot stop eating or control what or how much one is eating).

B. Binge eating episodes are associated with three (or more) of the following:

1. Eating much more rapidly than normal.
2. Eating until feeling uncomfortably full.
3. Eating large amounts of food when not physically hungry.
4. Eating alone because of feeling embarrassed by how much one is eating.
5. Feeling disgusted with oneself, depressed, or very guilty afterward.

C. Marked distress regarding binge eating is present.

D. Binge eating occurs, on average, at least once a week for 3 months.

E. The binge eating is not associated with the recurrent use of inappropriate compensatory behavior as in bulimia nervosa and does not occur exclusively during the course of bulimia nervosa or anorexia nervosa.

From the American Psychiatric Association. *Diagnostic and statistical manual of mental disorders.* 5th ed. text revision, Washington, DC: American Psychological Association Press; 2013.

Table 15-3 | Nutrition-Related Clinical Signs Commonly Associated with Anorexia Nervosa and Bulimia Nervosa

CLINICAL SIGNS	ANOREXIA NERVOSA	BULIMIA NERVOSA
Electrolyte abnormalities	Hypokalemia with refeeding syndrome; hypomagnesemia; hypophosphatemia	Hypokalemia accompanied by hypochloremic alkalosis; hypomagnesemia
Cardiovascular effects	Hypotension; irregular, slow pulse; orthostasis; sinus bradycardia	Cardiac arrhythmias; palpitations; weakness
Gastrointestinal effects	Abdominal pain; bloating; constipation; delayed gastric emptying; feeling of fullness; vomiting	Constipation; delayed gastric emptying; dysmotility; early satiety; esophagitis; flatulence; gastroesophageal reflux disease; gastrointestinal bleeding
Endocrine imbalances— reproductive, metabolic	Cold sensitivity; diuresis; fatigue; hypercholesterolemia; hypoglycemia; menstrual irregularities	Menstrual irregularities; rebound fluid retention with edema
Nutrient deficiencies	Protein-energy malnutrition; various micronutrient deficiencies	Variable
Skeletal and dental effects	Bone pain with exercise; osteopenia; osteoporosis	Dental caries; erosion of the surface of the teeth
Muscular effects	Wasting; weakness	Weakness
Weight status	Underweight state	Variable
Cognitive status	Poor concentration	Poor concentration
Growth status	Arrested growth and maturation	Typically not affected

From American Dietetic Association. Position of the American Dietetic Association: nutrition in the treatment of anorexia nervosa, bulimia nervosa, and other eating disorders. *J Am Diet Assoc.* 2006;106(12):2073-2082.

goals that are specific to anorexia nervosa are focused on restoring a healthy weight and normalizing eating patterns.

Bulimia Nervosa

The estimated lifetime prevalence of bulimia nervosa is 1.5% in women and 0.5% in men.[41] Bulimia is an eating disorder that involves repeated episodes of binge eating followed by one or more compensatory mechanisms to rid the body of excess calories. Compensatory mechanisms include self-induced vomiting, laxative abuse, strict dieting or fasting, and excessive exercise. The constituents of a binge will vary among patients, but it generally involves the consumption of excessive quantities of food during a short period of time. Oral and dental problems from the purging behavior may involve oral mucosal irritation, decreased salivary secretions (xerostomia), and irreversible tooth enamel erosion. Table 15-3 provides other clinical signs of bulimia nervosa.

Individuals with bulimia nervosa often go unnoticed and undiagnosed compared with individuals with anorexia nervosa. Their body weights are generally within a normal range, but they may fluctuate. Features of bulimia nervosa include the following[42]:
- Negative self-evaluation
- Parental influences such as comments about weight
- Parental obesity
- Childhood obesity
- High use of escape-avoidance coping
- Low perceived social support

- "All or none" perceptions about eating
- Impulsive personality

Nutrition therapy goals for patients with bulimia nervosa are focused on eliminating episodes of binging and purging.

Binge Eating Disorder

The estimated lifetime prevalence of binge eating disorder is 2.9% for women and 3.0% for men.[41] This eating disorder has the highest prevalence rate of all eating disorders; it is described as binging episodes without compensatory behaviors. This reactive type of eating often follows stress or anxiety as an emotional eating pattern to soothe or relieve painful or tense feelings. The binges may be triggered by psychologic factors that involve the self and body image. Patients with binge eating disorder are most often overweight or obese. Features of binge eating disorder include the following[42]:
- Repeated exposure to negative comments about shape, weight, and eating
- Negative self-evaluation
- Perfectionism
- Childhood obesity
- Low self-esteem
- High levels of body concern
- High use of escape-avoidance coping
- Low levels of perceived social support

Nutrition therapy goals for patients with binge eating disorder are focused on eliminating binge episodes and often involve psychotherapy, behavioral weight-loss treatment, and psychopharmacology.

Treatment

These psychologic disorders require therapy from a team of skilled professionals, including physicians, psychologists, and dietitians. Even with the best of care, recovery is slow, and the word *cure* is seldom used. Many patients with eating disorders have persistent food and weight preoccupations throughout their lives.

Patients with eating disorders often have neurologic disturbances. These chemical disturbances were first considered the cause of disordered eating behavior. However, researchers have found that when a normal weight and eating pattern are reestablished in the patient, the neurologic chemistry returns to normal. Therefore, one of the first issues to address for the treatment of an eating disorder is establishing a healthy weight in the patient. Psychologic therapy is more successful when neurologic disturbances are reduced. Next, the team of professionals must work together to restore eating habits and attitudes toward food, to optimize physical and mental health, and to heal intrapersonal and interpersonal problems. Continuing support groups that include friends, family, and health care professionals are critical for long-term treatment.

Putting It All Together

Summary

- In the traditional medical model, obesity has been viewed as an illness and a health hazard, which may be true in some cases. Current approaches view moderate overweight differently, however; in terms of the important aspects of fatness, leanness, and body composition they propose a more person-centered positive health model.
- Planning a weight-management program for either an overweight or an underweight person must involve the metabolic and energy needs of the individual. Personal food choices and habits as well as fatty tissue needs during different stages of the life cycle must be considered.
- Important aspects of a weight-reduction program include changing food behaviors and increasing physical activity. A sound program is based on reduced energy intake for gradual weight loss and nutrient balance, with meals distributed throughout the day for energy needs. The ideal plan begins with prevention and stresses the formation of positive food and exercise habits during early childhood to prevent major problems later in life.
- Food fads and misinformation are increasingly popular within all facets of American society. Identifying harmful practices and providing accurate information are basic functions of the health care provider.
- Excessive thinness is a cause for health concern. Malnutrition may result in underweight individuals for a variety of medical and psychologic reasons.
- Eating disorders require professional team therapy that includes medical, psychologic, and nutritional care.

Chapter Review Questions

See answers in Appendix A.

1. An ideal weight range for a female who is 5 feet, 3 inches tall is:
   a. 90 to 100 lb.
   b. 100.5 to 115.2 lb.
   c. 103.5 to 126.5 lb.
   d. 126.5 to 136.8 lb.

2. Susie is about 20 lb overweight and wants to lose 10 lb of body weight for her high school reunion. When should she begin to change her diet and exercise habits to promote healthy weight loss and reach her goal?
   a. At least 10 months before the reunion
   b. At least 10 weeks before the reunion
   c. At least 4 weeks before the reunion
   d. At least 10 days before the reunion

3. A sound weight-management program includes:
   a. Gradual weight loss and adequate nutrient intake.
   b. Periods of fasting to cleanse the body of toxins.
   c. Minimal carbohydrate intake.
   d. Use of portion-controlled commercial products.

4. Reducing excess body fat and the ability to build lean body mass are benefits of:
   a. A low carbohydrate diet.
   b. Aerobic exercise.
   c. Protein supplements.
   d. Bariatric surgery.

5. A meal plan for a patient who is underweight as a result of malabsorption incorporates:
   a. High protein, high fat foods.
   b. High protein, low carbohydrate foods.
   c. High protein, moderate fat foods.
   d. Low protein, high fat foods.

Additional Learning Resources

evolve Please refer to this text's Evolve website for answers to the Case Study questions. http://evolve.elsevier.com/Williams/basic/

References and **Further Reading and Resources** in the back of the book provide additional resources for enhancing knowledge.

16 Nutrition and Physical Fitness

Kary Woodruff, MS, RD, CSSD

Key Concepts

- Regular physical activity is an important part of a healthy lifestyle, and it relies on healthy muscle structure.
- Different levels of physical activity draw on a variety of body fuel sources.
- Sedentary lifestyles are a contributing factor to poor health.
- A healthy personal exercise program combines both strengthening and aerobic activities.

This chapter demonstrates that balanced nutrition and physical fitness are essential interrelated parts of an overall healthy lifestyle. Both reduce risks associated with chronic diseases, and both are important therapies for the treatment of chronic conditions. Health care workers should provide their patients with sound guidelines for nutrition and physical fitness while setting good examples.

PHYSICAL ACTIVITY RECOMMENDATIONS AND BENEFITS

GUIDELINES AND RECOMMENDATIONS

Technology is rapidly reducing the necessity for physical activity as part of everyday life. Many modern conveniences (e.g., moving sidewalks, escalators) contribute to sedentary lifestyles and the overall health issues that accompany them. Only 21% of Americans are meeting the recommended guidelines for aerobic and muscle-strengthening activity, and half (50%) of adults participate in 30 minutes of moderate physical activity five or more times per week, which is the minimum recommendation.[1]

Increased participation in regular physical activity is a national health goal. The U.S. Department of Health and Human Services has set nutrition and physical fitness goals for Americans—among many other health-related goals—in its *Healthy People 2020* report.[2] The 2020 targets for participation in physical activity are listed in Box 16-1. In addition to these goals, the *Physical Activity Guidelines for Americans*, the *Dietary Guidelines for Americans*, the MyPlate guidelines, and the Dietary Reference Intakes all address the need to participate in physical activity on a regular basis.

Physical activity differs from exercise according to the following definition[3]:

- *Physical activity:* bodily movement produced by the contraction of skeletal muscles that substantially increases energy expenditure above the basal level

- *Exercise:* a subcategory of physical activity that is planned, structured, repetitive, and with the purpose of improving or maintaining one or more component of physical fitness

The *Physical Activity Guidelines for Americans* are based on the following three components[3]:

- *Intensity:* how hard a person works to do the activity
  - Moderate intensity is equivalent in effort to brisk walking.
  - Vigorous intensity is equivalent in effort to running or jogging.
- *Frequency:* how often a person performs aerobic activity
- *Duration:* how long a person performs an activity during any one session

The *Physical Activity Guidelines for Americans* are as follows[3]:

- *Children and adolescents:* Children and adolescents should engage in 60 minutes or more of physical activity each day.
  - *Aerobic:* Most of the 60 or more minutes per day should be either moderate- or vigorous-intensity aerobic physical activity and should include vigorous-intensity physical activity at least 3 days a week.
  - *Muscle strengthening:* As part of their 60 or more minutes of daily physical activity, children and adolescents should include muscle-strengthening physical activity on at least 3 days of the week.
  - *Bone strengthening:* As part of their 60 or more minutes of daily physical activity, children and adolescents should include bone-strengthening physical activity on at least 3 days of the week.
- *Adults:* Adults should avoid inactivity on all days of the week. Some physical activity is better than none, and adults who participate in any amount of physical activity gain some health benefits. (Note that the following recommendations for adults are given as minutes per week.)

Healthy People 2020 Physical Activity Objectives

- Reduce the proportion of adults who engage in no leisure-time physical activity. Target: 32.6%.
- Increase the proportion of adults who meet current federal physical activity guidelines for aerobic physical activity and for muscle-strengthening activity.
  - Increase the proportion of adults who engage in aerobic physical activity of at least moderate intensity for at least 150 minutes per week, 75 minutes per week of vigorous-intensity exercise, or an equivalent combination. Target: 47.9%.
  - Increase the proportion of adults who engage in aerobic physical activity of at least moderate intensity for more than 300 minutes per week, more than 150 minutes per week of vigorous-intensity exercise, or an equivalent combination. Target: 31.3%.
  - Increase the proportion of adults who perform muscle-strengthening activities on 2 or more days of the week. Target: 24.1%.
  - Increase the proportion of adults who meet the objectives for aerobic physical activity and muscle-strengthening activity. Target: 20.1%.
- Increase the proportion of adolescents who meet current federal physical activity guidelines for aerobic physical activity and for muscle-strengthening activity.
  - Aerobic physical activity. Target: 20.2%.
  - Muscle-strengthening activity. Target not yet set.
  - Aerobic physical activity and muscle-strengthening activity. Target not yet set.

From U.S. Department of Health and Human Services. *Healthy People 2020.* Washington, DC: U.S. Government Printing Office; 2010.

- For substantial health benefits, adults should perform at least 150 minutes a week of moderate-intensity aerobic physical activity, 75 minutes a week of vigorous-intensity aerobic physical activity, or an equivalent combination of moderate- and vigorous-intensity aerobic activity. Aerobic activity should be performed in episodes of at least 10 minutes and should ideally be distributed throughout the week.
- For additional and more extensive health benefits, adults should increase their aerobic physical activity to 300 minutes a week of moderate-intensity aerobic activity, 150 minutes a week of vigorous-intensity aerobic physical activity, or an equivalent combination of moderate- and vigorous-intensity activity. Additional health benefits are gained by engaging in physical activity beyond this amount.
- Adults should also perform moderate- or high-intensity muscle-strengthening activities that involve all major muscle groups on 2 or more days a week, because these activities provide additional health benefits.

- *Older adults:* The guidelines given for adults also apply to older adults. In addition, the following guidelines are specific to older adults:
  - When older adults cannot perform 150 minutes of moderate-intensity aerobic activity a week because of chronic conditions, they should be as physically active as their abilities and conditions allow.
  - Older adults should do exercises that maintain or improve balance if they are at risk of falling.
  - Older adults should determine their level of effort for physical activity relative to their level of fitness.
  - Older adults with chronic conditions should understand whether and how their conditions affect their ability to perform regular physical activity safely.

Figure 16-1 provides suggestions on how to incorporate recommended activities into daily life.

HEALTH BENEFITS

With a personalized program that has been designed to meet individual needs, all people can develop healthy lifestyles. The longer that people follow some form of regular exercise routine, the more committed they become. Water aerobics, walking, and other low-impact workouts are becoming more and more popular in health clubs and have enabled more people to participate (e.g., those who cannot lift heavy weights or participate in high-intensity aerobic activities). Several of these new gym members are older adults who have health problems that may improve with moderate exercise. Regular exercise helps with the management of health, reduces the risk of chronic disease, promotes independence, and increases quality of life (Box 16-2).

For most people, physical activity should not pose any problem or hazard. The Physical Activity Readiness Questionnaire has been designed to identify the small number of adults for whom physical activity may be inappropriate or those who should have medical advice regarding the type of activity that is most suitable for them (Figure 16-2). All practitioners in the health care field should be well informed with regard to their scope of practice for exercise recommendations and prescriptions. This chapter discusses general recommendations. Much like in the field of dietetics where the registered dietitian is recognized as the nutrition expert, exercise scientists, physiologists, and certified personal trainers are the experts in exercise.

The sense of fitness achieved by exercise helps people to feel good physically, emotionally, and psychologically. In addition to this general sense of well-being, exercise (especially aerobic exercise) has special benefits for people with certain health problems, such as those that follow.[4,5]

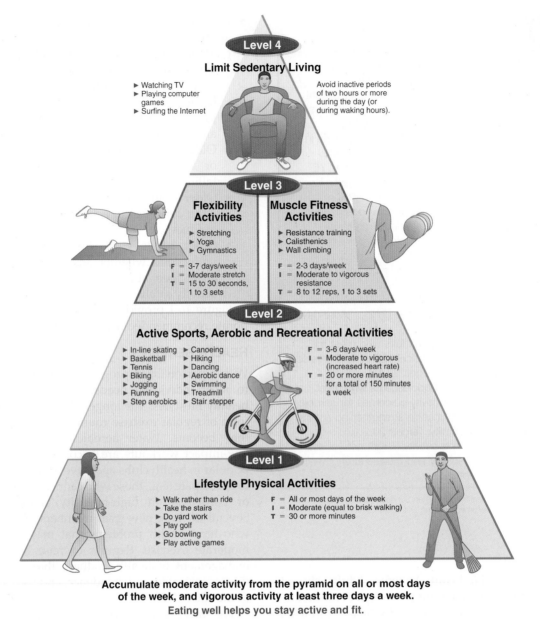

FIGURE 16-1 Physical activity pyramid.

Coronary Heart Disease

Exercise reduces the risk for heart disease in several ways, including improved heart function, decreased blood cholesterol levels, and improved oxygen transport.

Heart muscle function. The heart is a four-chambered organ that is approximately the size of an adult fist. Exercise—especially aerobic conditioning—strengthens the heart muscle, thereby enabling it to pump more blood per beat (i.e., stroke volume). A heart that has been strengthened by exercise has an increased aerobic capacity; in other words, the heart can pump more blood per minute without an undue increase in the heart rate. Therefore, exercises that rely primarily on the aerobic oxygen system for energy (e.g., walking, jogging, workouts using cardiopulmonary exercise machines) improve heart function.

Blood lipid levels. Resistance training programs have improved blood lipid profiles by significantly raising high-density lipoprotein level and by lowering the total cholesterol level, the low-density lipoprotein level, the total cholesterol to high-density lipoprotein ratio, and the triglyceride level.[6] Additionally, moderate intensity aerobic exercise has been shown to increase high-density lipoprotein levels, and when intensity level is increased, low-density lipoprotein and triglyceride levels were lowered.[6] Both exercise effects (i.e., improved heart function and cholesterol profile) lower the risks for diseased arteries.

Box 16-2 Health Benefits Associated with Regular Physical Activity*

CHILDREN AND ADOLESCENTS
Strong Evidence
- Improved cardiorespiratory and muscular fitness
- Improved bone health
- Improved cardiovascular and metabolic health biomarkers
- Favorable body composition

Moderate Evidence
- Reduced symptoms of depression

ADULTS AND OLDER ADULTS
Strong Evidence
- Lower risk of early death
- Lower risk of coronary heart disease
- Lower risk of stroke
- Lower risk of high blood pressure
- Lower risk of adverse blood lipid profile
- Lower risk of type 2 diabetes
- Lower risk of metabolic syndrome
- Lower risk of colon cancer
- Lower risk of breast cancer
- Prevention of weight gain
- Weight loss, particularly when combined with reduced calorie intake
- Improved cardiorespiratory and muscular fitness
- Prevention of falls
- Reduced depression
- Better cognitive function (for older adults)

Moderate to Strong Evidence
- Better functional health (for older adults)
- Reduced abdominal obesity

Moderate Evidence
- Lower risk of hip fracture
- Lower risk of lung cancer
- Lower risk of endometrial cancer
- Improved weight maintenance after weight loss
- Increased bone density
- Improved sleep quality

From U.S. Department of Health and Human Services. *2008 Physical activity guidelines for Americans.* Washington, DC: 2008.
*NOTE: The Advisory Committee rated the evidence of health benefits of physical activity as strong, moderate, or weak. To do so, the Committee considered the type, number, and quality of studies available, as well as the consistency of findings across studies that addressed each outcome. The Committee also considered evidence for causality and dose response in assigning the strength-of-evidence rating.

Oxygen-carrying capacity. Exercise also enhances the circulatory system by increasing the oxygen-carrying capacity of the blood. As training continues, a person's efficiency of oxygen use and uptake (**VO₂max**) will improve.

Hypertension

Cardiovascular complications increase along with rising levels of blood pressure. According to the American Heart Association, approximately one in three adults in the United States has **hypertension**.[7] People with stage 1 hypertension (i.e., a systolic

pressure of 140 to 159 mm Hg or a diastolic pressure of 90 to 104 mm Hg) represent the overwhelming majority of hypertensive individuals in the general population, and exercise has become one of the most effective nondrug treatments for this condition.[8] Even for people with higher levels of blood pressure, exercise has proven to be an important adjunct to drug therapy by offsetting adverse drug effects and lowering medication requirements.

Normal rises in blood pressure occur during both aerobic and resistance-type exercises and both forms of exercise are beneficial for individuals with hypertension. However, exercisers with diagnosed hypertension should avoid excess exertion to prevent severe stress on the cardiovascular system. An example would be holding your breath during the exertion phase of the exercise, such as with the lifting of heavy weights.

Diabetes
Physically active lifestyles are especially beneficial for individuals with type 2 diabetes to improve overall health and to reduce the risk of the chronic complications associated with diabetes.[9] Exercise improves the action of a person's naturally produced insulin by increasing the sensitivity of insulin receptor sites. Exercise also enhances glucose uptake without requiring insulin by skeletal muscle cells clearing glucose from the blood. When managing type 1 diabetes mellitus, the type of exercise and timing must be balanced with food and insulin injections to prevent reactions caused by drops in blood glucose levels (see Chapter 20 for a more detailed discussion of diabetes).[10]

Weight Management
Exercise is extremely beneficial for weight management in the following ways: (1) it helps to regulate appetite; (2) it increases the basal metabolic rate; (3) it reduces the genetic fat deposit set point level; and (4) it is critical for weight-loss maintenance. Together with a well-planned diet, physical exercise improves the energy balance in favor of increased energy output (see Chapter 15). Fat is used efficiently as the primary fuel source during lower-intensity aerobic exercise such as walking, jogging, swimming, and light cycling, though moderate to higher intensity excise will result in higher caloric expenditure within the same time frame (Table 16-1).

VO₂max the maximal uptake volume of oxygen during exercise; this is used to measure the intensity and duration of exercise that a person can perform.
hypertension chronically elevated blood pressure; systolic blood pressure is consistently 140 mm Hg or more or diastolic blood pressure is consistently 90 mm Hg or more.

Physical Activity Readiness
Questionnaire - PAR-Q
(revised 2002)

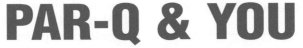

PAR-Q & YOU

(A Questionnaire for People Aged 15 to 69)

Regular physical activity is fun and healthy, and increasingly more people are starting to become more active every day. Being more active is very safe for most people. However, some people should check with their doctor before they start becoming much more physically active.

If you are planning to become much more physically active than you are now, start by answering the seven questions in the box below. If you are between the ages of 15 and 69, the PAR-Q will tell you if you should check with your doctor before you start. If you are over 69 years of age, and you are not used to being very active, check with your doctor.

Common sense is your best guide when you answer these questions. Please read the questions carefully and answer each one honestly: check YES or NO.

YES	NO	
☐	☐	**1. Has your doctor ever said that you have a heart condition <u>and</u> that you should only do physical activity recommended by a doctor?**
☐	☐	**2. Do you feel pain in your chest when you do physical activity?**
☐	☐	**3. In the past month, have you had chest pain when you were not doing physical activity?**
☐	☐	**4. Do you lose your balance because of dizziness or do you ever lose consciousness?**
☐	☐	**5. Do you have a bone or joint problem (for example, back, knee or hip) that could be made worse by a change in your physical activity?**
☐	☐	**6. Is your doctor currently prescribing drugs (for example, water pills) for your blood pressure or heart condition?**
☐	☐	**7. Do you know of <u>any other reason</u> why you should not do physical activity?**

If you answered

YES to one or more questions

Talk with your doctor by phone or in person BEFORE you start becoming much more physically active or BEFORE you have a fitness appraisal. Tell your doctor about the PAR-Q and which questions you answered YES.

- You may be able to do any activity you want — as long as you start slowly and build up gradually. Or, you may need to restrict your activities to those which are safe for you. Talk with your doctor about the kinds of activities you wish to participate in and follow his/her advice.
- Find out which community programs are safe and helpful for you.

NO to all questions

If you answered NO honestly to <u>all</u> PAR-Q questions, you can be reasonably sure that you can:

- start becoming much more physically active – begin slowly and build up gradually. This is the safest and easiest way to go.
- take part in a fitness appraisal – this is an excellent way to determine your basic fitness so that you can plan the best way for you to live actively. It is also highly recommended that you have your blood pressure evaluated. If your reading is over 144/94, talk with your doctor before you start becoming much more physically active.

DELAY BECOMING MUCH MORE ACTIVE:

- if you are not feeling well because of a temporary illness such as a cold or a fever – wait until you feel better; or
- if you are or may be pregnant – talk to your doctor before you start becoming more active.

PLEASE NOTE: If your health changes so that you then answer YES to any of the above questions, tell your fitness or health professional. Ask whether you should change your physical activity plan.

<u>Informed Use of the PAR-Q</u>: The Canadian Society for Exercise Physiology, Health Canada, and their agents assume no liability for persons who undertake physical activity, and if in doubt after completing this questionnaire, consult your doctor prior to physical activity.

FIGURE 16-2 Physical Activity Readiness Questionnaire. (Courtesy Canadian Society for Exercise Physiology. Copyright 2002.)

Table 16-1	Source of Energy for Varying Exercise Intensity
EXERCISE INTENSITY	FUEL USED BY MUSCLE
<30% VO$_2$max (easy walking)	Mainly muscle fat stores
40% to 65% VO$_2$max (jogging, brisk walking)	Fat and carbohydrate in similar proportions
75% VO$_2$max (running)	Mainly carbohydrate
>80% VO$_2$max (sprinting)	Nearly 100% carbohydrate

VO$_2$max, Peak oxygen uptake.

Table 16-2	Aerobic Exercises for Physical Fitness	
TYPE OF EXERCISE	AEROBIC FORMS*	
Ball playing	Handball Racquetball Squash	
Bicycling	Stationary biking Touring or mountain biking	
Dancing	Aerobic routines Ballet Disco	
Jumping rope	Brisk pace	
Running or jogging	Brisk pace	
Skating	Ice skating Roller skating	
Skiing	Cross country	
Swimming	Steady pace	
Walking	Brisk pace	

*Maintained at an aerobic level for at least 30 minutes.

Bone Disease

Weight-bearing exercises (e.g., walking, running) help to strengthen bones by increasing **osteoblast** activity. The weight-bearing load increases calcium deposits in bone, thereby increasing bone density and reducing the risk for osteoporosis. While the benefits of exercise on bone density are most notable during the peak bone growth periods of adolescents and young adults, older adults are encouraged to engage in weight-bearing exercise regularly to prevent further decreases in bone mineral density. However, excessive forms of training can have a destructive effect in which bone density is lost as a result of overtraining or undernutrition, or both.

Mental Health

Exercise stimulates the production of *endorphins*. These natural chemicals decrease pain and improve mood, which may include an exhilarating type of "high." Mental health benefits from physical activity are persistent throughout life. Recent studies have shown not only that exercise can lower one's risk for depression and anxiety disorders but also, as individuals age, that physical activity is associated with a lower risk of Alzheimer's disease, dementia, and Parkinson's disease, and can increase one's overall quality of life.[11,12]

TYPES OF PHYSICAL ACTIVITY

A well-balanced exercise program incorporates resistance training, aerobic activities, flexibility and stretching exercises, and an assortment of activities of daily living. A good fitness plan is a combination of different enjoyable activities that most effectively reduce the risk of several chronic diseases.

Resistance Training

Resistance training creates and maintains muscle and bone strength, improves blood pressure in prehypertensive/hypertensive individuals, and increases insulin sensitivity. An ideal resistance program should

> **osteoblast** cells that are responsible for the mineralization and formation of bone.

include 8 to 10 separate exercises (with 8 to 12 repetitions of each) focusing on all major muscle groups and that are performed 2 to 3 days per week. A more progressive model incorporates gradual load increases to stimulate muscle overload, greater muscle specificity and variation, and a training regimen of 4 to 5 days per week.[13] For an individual whose primary goal is to gain strength and power, the repetitions should be of high intensity, with fewer than 6 repetitions before muscle fatigue occurs. For improved endurance, a lower weight should be used that will allow at least 15 repetitions before muscle fatigue occurs.

Aerobic Exercise

Forms of exercise that can be sustained at a necessary level of intensity to provide aerobic benefits include activities such as swimming, running, jogging, bicycling, and aerobic dancing routines and similar workouts (Table 16-2). Perhaps the simplest and most popular form of stimulating exercise is walking. Figure 16-3 illustrates how aerobic walking can fit into almost anyone's lifestyle. If the pace is fast enough to elevate the pulse rate and if it is maintained for at least 20 minutes, then walking can be an excellent form of aerobic exercise. It is convenient, and it requires no equipment other than good walking shoes. Table 16-3 provides information about energy expenditure per hour for various activities at a given body weight.

Weight-Bearing Exercise

Both aerobic and resistance-type exercises may fit into this category. Weight-bearing exercises such as walking, jogging, aerobic dancing, and jumping rope are important for bone structure and strength. In these exercises, muscles are working against gravity. The load put on bones during weight-bearing exercises stimulates them to become more dense. This decreases

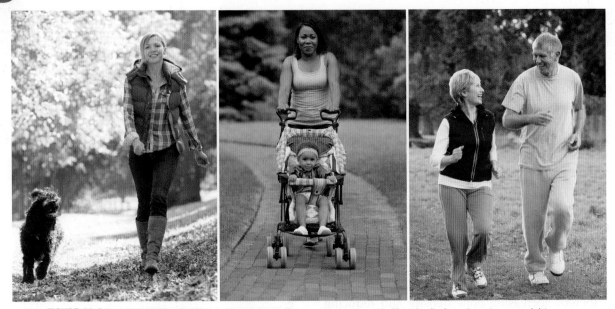

FIGURE 16-3 Aerobic walking is an exercise that can fit into almost anyone's lifestyle. (Left and center, copyright JupiterImages Corp.; right, copyright PhotoDisc.)

Table 16-3	Approximate Energy Expenditure Per Hour during Various Activities	
ACTIVITY	**KILOCALORIES PER HOUR***	
Sleeping	63	
Lying or sitting, awake	70	
Standing, relaxed	84	
Rapid typing, sitting	105	
Dressing and undressing	140	
Walking slowly (24 min/mile)	210	
Water aerobics	280	
High-impact aerobics	490	
Football, flag or touch	560	
Walking quickly (12 min/mile)	560	
Stair, treadmill	630	
Swimming, vigorous effort	700	
Running (8 min/mile)	875	

*For an adult who weighs 70 kg (154 lb).

the risk of falls, which can be very debilitating for aging individuals.

Activities of Daily Living

Many activities of daily living do not reach aerobic levels (e.g., walking to work or to the store, walking the dog, playing catch with children) but are enjoyable and should be incorporated into daily life. The more the activity is appreciated and enjoyed, the more likely it is to be continued and thus provide greater benefit. Activities of daily living create opportunities to be active throughout the day regardless of structured exercise, therefore contributing to greater daily energy

expenditure. Activities of daily living may also help break up sedentary behavior, which itself increases risk for metabolic disease. Even if one is exercising according to the recommendations, sedentary behavior (such as long periods of sitting) can have detrimental health effects.[13]

MEETING PERSONAL NEEDS

Health Status and Personal Gains

When planning a personal exercise program, first assess an individual's health status, present level of fitness, personal needs, and resources necessary for equipment or cost. Discussing an exercise program with a medical practitioner is always recommended, and getting medical clearance before beginning an exercise program is especially important for older persons and those with chronic diseases (see Figure 16-2). Seeking advice and guidance from a certified personal trainer or an exercise physiologist will be of great benefit. There are many organizations that certify personal trainers, but some are more reputable than others. The American College of Sports Medicine is one of the leading authorities for certifying professionals as Health Fitness Specialists, Certified Personal Trainers, Clinical Exercise Specialists, and Registered Clinical Exercise Physiologists (visit www.acsm.org).

The exercise that is chosen should be something that is both enjoyable and of aerobic value. In addition, the individual should start slowly and build gradually to avoid burnout and injury. Moderation and regularity are the chief guides.

Achieving Aerobic Benefits

To build aerobic capacity, the level of exercise must raise the pulse rate to within 60% to 90% of an individual's maximal heart rate. An acceptable way

Table 16-4	Target Zone Heart Rate According to Age to Achieve Aerobic Physical Effect of Exercise		
AGE (YEARS)	MAXIMAL ATTAINABLE HEART RATE (PULSE = 220 – AGE)	TARGET ZONE 70% MAXIMAL RATE	85% MAXIMAL RATE
20	200	140	170
25	195	136	166
30	190	133	161
35	185	129	157
40	180	126	153
45	175	122	149
50	170	119	144
55	165	115	140
60	160	112	136
65	155	108	132
70	150	105	127
75	145	101	124

produce a smooth symphony of action through simultaneous and alternating contraction and relaxation. Muscular activity requires oxygen and energy.

Oxygen

The most profound limit to exercise is the person's ability to deliver oxygen to his or her tissues and to then use that oxygen for energy production. This vital ability depends on the fitness of the pulmonary and cardiovascular systems. Fitness level—and thus oxygen and fuel use—is influenced by two major factors: (1) the fitness of the lungs, heart, and blood vessels; and (2) body composition.

Cardiovascular fitness. Cardiovascular fitness is defined in terms of aerobic capacity, which depends on the body's ability to deliver and use oxygen in sufficient quantities to meet the demands of increasing levels of exercise. Oxygen uptake increases with exercise intensity until either the demand is met or the ability to supply it is exceeded. The maximum rate at which the body can take in oxygen (i.e., aerobic capacity) is the VO_2max. This capacity determines the intensity and duration of exercise that a person can perform.

Body composition. Body composition is a reflection of the four body compartments that make up the total body weight: lean body mass, fat, water, and bone (see Chapter 15). Lean body mass is more metabolically active (i.e., requires more fuel) than other body tissues such as adipose tissue. Thus, a person's fitness level and oxygen use is influenced by the amount of energy-demanding lean body mass relative to total fat mass.

Fuel Sources

The fuel sources required for energy are the basic energy nutrients: primarily carbohydrate (glucose and glycogen) and some fat. Protein is only used as an energy source when the other fuels are exhausted and it is not a very efficient energy source.

The relative use of stored fat for energy during exercise depends on the level of fitness of the person and the intensity of the exercise. Trained endurance athletes are more efficient at using fat for energy than are their untrained counterparts. Regardless of training status, as exercise intensity increases, so will reliance upon carbohydrate as a fuel source. It can be thought of as a dimmer switch. Sustained, low-intensity exercises (i.e., 25% to 65% VO_2max) rely primarily on muscle

to estimate the maximal heart rate is to subtract the person's age from 220. For aerobic benefits, 70% of maximal heart rate should then be maintained for ≥10 minutes, accumulating 150 minutes per week (Table 16-4). Resting pulse rate should be checked before starting the exercise period and then again during and immediately afterward to monitor progress toward the target exercising heart rate and aerobic capacity. Heart rate monitors are a convenient way to monitor and keep track of the heart rate.

Exercise Preparation and Care

Whatever the choice of exercise, preparation and continuing care are important. It is not in the scope of this nutrition text to explore the details of various exercise programs. However, some very basic guidelines include warming up the muscles to prevent stress or injury and taking time to cool down after exercising. Do not go beyond tolerance limits; instead, listen to the body. Rest when tired, and stop when hurting. Contact a physician if symptoms do not subside. When more challenge is desired, gradually increase the exercise level by number of repetitions, weight intensity, or endurance—not all three at the same time.

DIETARY NEEDS DURING EXERCISE

MUSCLE ACTION AND FUEL

Structure and Function

The synchronized action of millions of specialized cells that make up our skeletal muscle mass makes possible all forms of physical activity. A finely coordinated series of small bundles within the muscle fibers

aerobic capacity a state in which oxygen is required to proceed; milliliters of oxygen consumed per kilogram of body weight per minute as influenced by body composition.

fat stores for energy through the aerobic pathway and uses relatively smaller amounts of carbohydrate.[14] As intensity increases, so does the relative contribution of carbohydrate for energy. When exercise intensity exceeds 65% VO2max, carbohydrate becomes the predominant fuel source and fat contributes less. This is due in part to the relative rate in which each macronutrient is broken down to render ATP. Because fat is a more dense nutrient, fat metabolism is slower and requires more oxygen than does the metabolism of carbohydrates.

FLUID AND ENERGY NEEDS

Fluid

Blood is primarily water and thus fluid status directly impacts the body's ability to distribute oxygen and nutrients to working muscle cells. Dehydration limits performance and exercise capacity, especially in untrained individuals.[15,16] It is believed that dehydration of 2% or more of one's body weight will impair athletic performance, though emerging evidence indicates this may not always be the case, especially in well-trained athletes. The extent of dehydration depends upon the intensity and duration of the exercise, the environmental conditions, the level of fitness, and the pre-exercise hydration status. With continued exercise, the body temperature rises in response to heat that is released during energy production. To control this temperature rise, the body sends as much heat as possible to the skin, where it is released in sweat to evaporate on the skin. Over time—and especially in hot weather—this excessive sweating can lead to dehydration. If dehydration continues, athletes may experience problems such as cramps, delirium, vomiting, hypothermia, or hyperthermia. By providing fluid replacement throughout periods of exercise, many of these problems can be prevented.

Regular fluid intake should be planned for all types of athletes where there will be considerable fluid loss. Athletes who are engaged in longer and more demanding endurance events (i.e., more than 1 hour), especially in a warm environment, may benefit from an electrolyte and glucose sports drinks that has optimal gastric emptying and intestinal absorption times (see the For Further Focus box, "Hydrating with Water, Sports Drink, or Energy Drink").[17]

Energy and Nutrient Stores

Exercise raises energy needs and helps regulate appetite to meet this need. See Table 16-3 for some examples of the amount of kilocalories expended by general activities. For athletes and other active individuals, proper dietary choices are essential for daily energy needs, nutrient reserves, and optimal performances. Without adequate energy during prolonged exercise, nutrient levels fall too low to sustain the body's continued demands. Fatigue follows, and exhaustion may result.

For Further Focus

Hydrating with Water, Sports Drink, or Energy Drink

Sports drinks began with a solution called *Gatorade*, a beverage that its developers named for their university's football team. They reasoned that, if they analyzed the sweat of their players, they could then replace the lost minerals and water in a drink that contained some flavoring, coloring, and sugars to make it acceptable; it would taste better and have more benefits than plain water. Although Gatorade proved beneficial for some athletes, most do not need it during general nonendurance exercise.

The ideal fluid to prevent dehydration depends on how demanding the exercise is and how long it lasts. For exercise less than 60 to 90 minutes, physically fit athletes can maintain hydration with plain water. However, endurance athletes need both water and fuel (i.e., carbohydrate), especially during hot weather for exercise lasting more than 60 to 90 minutes. For athletes who lose substantial amounts of water and sodium through sweat, electrolyte replacement is also an important consideration. Although rare, hyponatremia (i.e., a plasma sodium concentration of less than 135 mEq/L) can be fatal. The most common cause of hyponatremia among endurance athletes is excess sodium loss through sweat in combination with fluid replacement by plain water. Water dilutes the plasma sodium even more, thereby exacerbating the condition. Thus, sports drinks that contain sodium (0.5 to 0.7 g/L) and potassium (0.8 to 2.0 g/L) as well as carbohydrate are recommended for athletes during endurance events that last 2 hours or more.[1]

Other products entering the sports-drink market claim to have no added sugar but supply ample amounts of fructose and glucose from their fruit-juice bases. Fructose does not leave the stomach rapidly, and it is absorbed more slowly from the intestine compared with glucose, potentially causing bloating or diarrhea. Another category of sports drinks on the market adds large amounts of vitamins and minerals to their solutions. These extra vitamins do not help an athlete's performance; on a hot day, a perspiring athlete could easily consume a megadose of vitamins after drinking four or five bottles of such a product.

Energy drinks and energy shots have become quite popular, especially among adolescent and young adult athletes. The potential performance benefit from these products primarily comes from the caffeine and/or carbohydrate content.[2] Because the safety and efficacy of many of the added ingredients, such as taurine, guarana, gingko biloba, etc. are not well established, and the actual amount of these ingredients contained in the product is typically unknown, athletes should be encouraged to use a sports nutrition product with better established research, such as traditional sports drinks.

Although sports drinks may meet the needs of athletes who are competing in physically demanding endurance events, they are not required by those who are participating in less-demanding sports activities. Water is the best solution for regular needs, and it costs far less.

REFERENCES

1. Rodriguez NR, et al. Position of the American Dietetic Association, Dietitians of Canada, and the American College of Sports Medicine. Nutrition and athletic performance. *J Am Diet Assoc.* 2009;109(3): 509-527.
2. Campbell B, et al. International Society of Sports Nutrition position stand: energy drinks. *J Int Soc Sports Nutr.* 2013;10(1):1.

Energy and nutrient needs for most individuals who participate in physical activity are discussed in this chapter under the following heading. Specific dietary recommendations for meeting energy needs and maximizing nutrient stores for athletic performance during training and competition are discussed separately, because the needs of athletes are greater than what most people need for daily physical activity.

MACRONUTRIENT AND MICRONUTRIENT RECOMMENDATIONS

Carbohydrate

Carbohydrate is the preferred fuel and critical energy source for an active person both before exercise and during the recovery period. Complex carbohydrates sustain energy needs and supply necessary fiber, vitamins, and minerals. Carbohydrate fuels come from two sources: circulating blood glucose and glycogen stored in muscle and liver tissue. Complex carbohydrates (i.e., starches) are preferable to simple carbohydrates (i.e., monosaccharides and disaccharides) when consumed as part of the diet. Starches break down gradually, help to maintain blood glucose levels more evenly (thus avoiding hypoglycemia), and maintain glycogen stores as a constant primary fuel.

Diets that are low in carbohydrate are unable to meet energy demands and result in poor performance and increased fatigue, especially during prolonged bouts of intense exercise.[18] A low-carbohydrate diet decreases the body's capacity for work, which intensifies over time. Physically active individuals on low-carbohydrate diets are susceptible to fatigue, ketoacidosis, and dehydration. Conversely, a moderate- to high-carbohydrate diet enhances muscle glycogen concentrations and exercise performance.[18] In addition, consuming small amounts of carbohydrates during exercise improves whole-body carbohydrate oxidation and metabolic efficiency, especially when a high-carbohydrate meal has not been consumed immediately before exercise.[19,20] Therefore, eating foods with adequate carbohydrates before and during exercise helps to maintain the glucose concentrations that are necessary to exercise strenuously and delay fatigue.

Fat

Dietary recommendations for fat intake to support physical activity do not vary from standard guidelines. In the presence of oxygen, fatty acids serve as a fuel source from stored fat tissue. No evidence supports improved physical performance with a dietary fat intake of more than 30% of the total daily energy intake. However, an extremely low fat intake can be dangerous if the diet is deficient in the essential fatty acids (i.e., linoleic and α-linolenic acids). A moderate level of fat is necessary in the diet for the absorption of fat-soluble vitamins and to ensure the adequate intake of the essential fatty acids.

Protein

Under normal circumstances, protein provides a relatively insignificant contribution to energy resources during exercise. Therefore, no more than the usual adult requirement (i.e., 0.8 g/kg body weight) is needed to meet the general protein needs of a healthy, moderately active adult, though some current research is examining whether moderately active individuals have higher protein needs. For endurance and strength-trained athletes, the protein requirement may increase (see "Athletic Performance" later in this chapter). Protein requirements are influenced by sex, age, and intensity, duration, and type of exercise as well as by energy intake and carbohydrate availability.[21]

Vitamins and Minerals

Vitamins and minerals are not oxidized during the process of energy production. However, vitamins and minerals are essential as catalytic cofactors in enzyme reactions (see Chapters 7 and 8). Increased physical exertion during exercise does not require a greater intake of vitamins and minerals beyond currently recommended intakes. A well-balanced diet supplies adequate amounts of vitamins and minerals, and exercise may improve the body's efficient use of them. Because athletes have an increased dietary need for energy, a larger kilocalorie intake from nutrient-dense foods would automatically boost their general intake of vitamins and minerals.

Multivitamin and mineral supplementation does not improve physical performance in healthy people who are eating well-balanced diets, and the potential side effects from megavitamin supplements are well-known. However, therapeutic iron supplements may be necessary for some individuals who are experiencing iron-deficiency anemia (see the Drug-Nutrient Interaction box, "Iron Supplementation"). For indoor athletes and/or athletes with limited sun exposure, assessment of vitamin D status may also be warranted. In addition, the special assessment of nutrient-energy status is needed for amenorrheic female athletes. Chronic negative energy balance is not uncommon among athletes such as gymnasts, ballet dancers, and runners, who may also suffer from disordered eating. Disordered eating patterns may include low calcium and energy intake, which can have serious consequences for bone development (see the Clinical Applications box, "The Female Athlete Triad: How Performance and Social Pressure Can Lead to Low Bone Mass").

---

hypoglycemia an abnormally low blood glucose level that may lead to muscle tremors, cold sweat, headache, and confusion.

amenorrheic the absence or abnormal cessation of the menses.

Iron Supplementation*

Iron plays an essential role in oxygen transport and energy metabolism, which are crucial during exercise. Injury, excessive losses in sweat, inadequate nutrient intake, periods of rapid growth, hemolysis, and menstrual losses all increase the risk for iron depletion in athletes. Iron deficiency—with or without anemia—can affect performance especially when the individual is symptomatic, so athletes should aim to meet the Dietary Reference Intakes for iron from the diet: 18 mg for women and 8 mg for men.[1] This can be accomplished by eating iron-rich foods such as red meat, legumes, dark green leafy vegetables, dried fruits, and fortified grains.

Research supports the importance of the periodic screening of athletes to monitor iron status before clinical symptoms of deficiency occur.[2] Groups that are at higher risk for low iron stores are females, adolescents, vegetarians, and long-distance runners.[3] The most common blood indices for iron status are as follows:

- *Hemoglobin:* a protein structure that contains iron that is needed for oxygen transport
- *Hematocrit:* the proportion of packed red blood cells with regard to total blood volume
- *Ferritin:* a protein that stores iron for later use

During periods of intense training, athletes may benefit from supplemental iron, particularly in the presence of iron-deficiency anemia or iron deficiency with physical symptoms including fatigue.[2,3] When iron supplements are prescribed, the following precautions should be taken:

- Most oral iron supplements provide nonheme iron including iron salts. The absorption of nonheme iron is increased in the presence of vitamin C. Taking supplements with vitamin C–rich foods will enhance absorption.

- Supplemental iron may cause nausea, constipation, abdominal pain, and blackened stools.[1,3] Taking supplements with meals and drinking plenty of fluids can help to alleviate these symptoms.
- Iron and calcium compete for absorption. Avoid taking iron supplements with milk or other calcium-containing products.
- Other dietary components that inhibit iron absorption include polyphenols (found in tea and coffee), oxalic acid (found in spinach, chard, and berries), and phytates (found in whole grains and legumes).

At the initiation of a training program, individuals commonly experience a transient decrease in hemoglobin and serum ferritin levels as a result of increased plasma volume. This is sometimes referred to as "sports anemia," and it is not true iron deficiency.[4] Iron supplementation is not appropriate in these cases.

REFERENCES

1. Goodman C, et al. A to Z of nutritional supplements: dietary supplements, sports nutrition foods and ergogenic aids for health and performance—Part 21. *Br J Sports Med*. 2011;45(8):677-679.
2. Reinke S, et al. Absolute and functional iron deficiency in professional athletes during training and recovery. *Int J Cardiol*. 2012; 156(2):186-191.
3. DellaValle DM. Iron supplementation for female athletes: effects on iron status and performance outcomes. *Curr Sports Med Rep*. 2013;12(4):234-239.
4. Ottomano C, Franchini M. Sports anaemia: facts or fiction? *Blood Transfus*. 2012;10(3):252-254.

*With contributions from Kelli Boi.

ATHLETIC PERFORMANCE

GENERAL TRAINING DIET

All individuals who regularly participate in physical activity must apply the general principles of exercise and energy balance that have been previously described. At what point does a person who regularly exercises become an athlete? It is often difficult to determine exactly when someone's nutrient needs require additional attention. From a nutrition standpoint, one of the main differences in an athlete's diet compared with that of the general public is that athletes require more fluid and energy to cover their needs during exercise. However, it is well accepted that physical activity, athletic performance, and exercise recovery are enhanced by optimal nutritional strategies for everyone.[22]

Athletes who are involved in heavy training are more susceptible to immunosuppression because of the extreme demands that are placed on the body. A well-balanced diet with plenty of carbohydrates and protein from a variety of foods helps to prevent exercise-induced malnutrition and the risk for injury and infection.[23,24]

It should be noted that the nutrient and energy needs of child and adolescent athletes should be adjusted according to their specific developmental needs; thus recommendations for adults may not apply to this population. A Certified Specialist in Sports Dietetics (CSSD) or sports dietitian can customize nutrient recommendations for these athletes.

Total Energy

When exercise levels rise from mild or moderate amounts up to strenuous levels, caloric needs also rise to supply adequate fuel. Exact energy needs vary depending on sex, age, body size, genetics, body composition, and the type of training involved. Adequate total energy intake allows athletes to maintain appropriate weight and body composition while maximizing performance.[25] Methods for calculating basic energy needs are discussed in Chapter 6. Total energy needs should first be estimated with the use of the Cunningham equation (Box 16-3), the Harris-Benedict equation, or the DRIs; energy requirements specific to the duration, frequency, and intensity of the exercise performed can then be added to the basic needs. A CSSD is a qualified nutrition professional who can

Clinical Applications

The Female Athlete Triad: How Performance and Social Pressure Can Lead to Low Bone Mass

The female athlete triad is a medical condition comprised of three interrelated components faced by women who are very physically active: (1) low energy availability with or without disordered eating; (2) menstrual dysfunction; and (3) low bone mineral density. Each component of the Triad can be highly variable, so we consider each along a spectrum. At the 'healthy' end of the continuum there is adequate energy availability, ovulatory menstrual cycles, and normal bone mineral density. At the other end of the continuum we identify clinical endpoints of low energy availability with or without disordered eating, amenorrhea, and osteoporosis. The goal of the practitioner is early attention and intervention to prevent any of the Triad's components from advancing to pathologies exhibited at the clinical end of the spectrum.

Energy availability is defined as the amount of dietary energy remaining after subtracting the energy required for exercise training.[1] Adequate energy is required for all metabolic processes; if after accounting for exercise, the remaining energy balance is too low, normal metabolism suffers. Low energy availability results from an inadequate dietary intake to meet both the training and the physiologic needs of the female athlete. This may be the result of restrained eating, dieting, disordered eating/eating disorder behaviors (see Chapter 15), or simply the athlete's lack of knowledge regarding how much energy she should be consuming. Regardless of the cause, prolonged low energy availability may ultimately lead to menstrual dysfunction. The combination of a hypoestrogenic environment and energy deficiency can play a causal role in low bone mineral density.[1]

Women who participate in competitive endurance sports (e.g., rowing, long-distance running) or who are judged partially on physical appearance (e.g., ice skating, diving, or dancing) are more likely to be preoccupied with their weight and to have self-image issues. Social and competitive pressure to be thin can contribute to her sense of imperfection. These demands can lead some women to develop disordered eating patterns that, in combination with strenuous exercise, result in low energy availability. Performance may deteriorate as the athlete loses focus and concentration and as she becomes fatigued. Some women develop psychologic eating disorders, such as binge eating disorder, bulimia nervosa, or anorexia nervosa (see Chapter 15), which in turn may progress to additional health problems, including depression, low self-esteem, seizures, cardiac arrhythmia, myocardial infarction, and other health complications. The severity of the eating disorder is linked to the amount of stress and concern the woman feels about her body image coupled with the emphasis placed on her weight by herself, her trainers, and her coaches. Athletes often believe that leanness enhances performance, and some are willing to take health risks to satisfy their perfectionist needs and habits.

Inadequate caloric intake and disordered eating can cause menstrual irregularity. Amenorrhea is the cessation of previously regular menses for 3 months; primary amenorrhea is the repression of all menstrual cycles until the age of 15 years. This condition may be seen in young female gymnasts who, in the most competitive circles, may strive to delay the onset of puberty to maintain their small, child-like physiques. Some women may have oligomenorrhea, which are sporadic cycles occurring 3 to 9 times a year. The levels of estrogen and progesterone that regulate menses are affected by metabolism, intensive exercise, dieting, or stress.

Bone density reaches its peak before the age of 30 years; therefore, young women must strive for dense bones during early adulthood to have healthy bone density later in life. If the density of the bones is diminished early, osteopenia occurs; if it is severe enough, this can be a sign of future osteoporosis. In active young women with inadequate diets and menstrual irregularities, cases of bone density 25% lower than normal have been reported, which can increase the likelihood of stress fractures and injuries.

Some studies indicate that weight-bearing activities (e.g., gymnastics) seem to improve BMD and may help to prevent decreases in bone density later in life. Yet the problem facing female athletes who eat improperly is that the rate of decline in BMD intensifies as menstrual cycles continue to be erratic. Weight-bearing sports will not overcome the tendency toward low BMD if diet and exercise levels are not carefully monitored. In today's weight-conscious society, the emphasis must not be on a perfect image, size, or body but rather on the balance of health and training. The female athlete's skeletal integrity suffers as she resorts to drastic measures in her aspiration for an overly lean physical image.

The primary treatment for the Triad is to address the underlying cause, that is, low energy availability. Energy status must be normalized through adjusting dietary intake and modifying exercise training.[1] Restoration of body weight is the most effective way to support resumption of menses and improve bone health. The cause of inadequate intake must be assessed—if it is due to lack of knowledge, athlete education is required; if there is concurrent disordered eating/eating disorders, then psychologic treatment must be included as well.

The need to educate trainers, athletes, and health professionals about the consequences of neglected nutrition is imperative. Young female athletes must understand that depriving themselves of life's essential nutrients does significant bodily harm.

REFERENCE
1. De Souza MJ, et al. 2014 Female Athlete Triad Coalition Consensus Statement on Treatment and Return to Play of the Female Athlete Triad: 1st International Conference held in San Francisco, California, May 2012, and 2nd International Conference held in Indianapolis, Indiana, May 2013. Br J Sports Med. 2014;48(4):289.

assess an athlete's energy needs based upon the details of an athlete's training and competition needs and provide appropriate energy recommendations.

Athletes' nutrient needs are best met by consuming a variety of foods to meet energy needs; these are represented by the MyPlate guidelines (see Figure 1-3).

Carbohydrate

Athletes who are competing in prolonged endurance events should increase their energy intake from carbohydrates. General training needs are usually met with 5 to 7 g/kg body weight per day of carbohydrate. Endurance athletes have higher needs of 7 to 10 g/kg

Box 16-3	Cunningham Equation[26]
	kcal/day = 500 + 22 × FFM (kg)

body weight per day, with ultra-endurance athletes requiring up to 12 g/kg body weight per day.[27]

Fat

Dietary fat is needed to meet energy needs, to supply essential fatty acids, and to maintain weight. No performance benefit occurs from consuming a diet that is less than 20% or greater than 35% of calories in the diet coming from fat.

Protein

For highly trained endurance and strength-trained athletes, the protein requirement may increase to 1.2 to 1.7 g/kg/day.[21] Protein needs, even for highly trained athletes, can usually be met through diet alone. For example, a 170-lb (77-kg) strength-training male athlete may have protein needs of 1.5 g/kg body weight: 77 kg × 1.5 g of protein/kg = 115.5 g of protein per day. The average daily protein intake by U.S. men and women who are 20 years old and older is nearly 100 g and 68 g per day, respectively.[28] Thus, even for an athlete who is heavily building muscle mass, a slight increase of 15 g of protein per day over the average American intake would meet his needs. Some athletes choose to consume protein supplements to help meet increased protein needs. Consumption of small to moderate amounts of these products may be safe, but excess consumption of whole protein or amino acid supplements may cause dehydration and could ultimately put a taxing load on the kidneys as a result of excess nitrogen excretion and therefore is not recommended.

COMPETITION

Carbohydrate Loading

To prepare for an endurance event, athletes sometimes follow a dietary process called *carbohydrate* or *glycogen loading* (see the For Further Focus box, "Carbohydrate Loading for Endurance Performance"). The current practice—which has been modified from earlier, more stressful protocols—takes place the week before the event. The protocol includes a moderate and gradual tapering of exercise while increasing total carbohydrate intake in the diet (Table 16-5).

Pregame Meal

The ideal pregame meal depends on the tolerance of the athlete. It usually is a light to moderate meal eaten 3 to 4 hours before the event. This meal should be high in carbohydrates (approximately 1-4 grams of carbohydrate per kilogram of body weight), low in fat and fiber, and moderate in protein; it should also provide sufficient fluid and be familiar to the athlete.[29,30] Fat

For Further Focus

Carbohydrate Loading for Endurance Performance

Glycogen is the body storage form of carbohydrate in the liver and skeletal muscle that provides an immediate source of fuel and protects blood glucose levels. Glycogen is restored with each day's food intake, but, during heavy exercise, normal glycogen stores are quickly depleted. Without glucose available from oral intake or glycogen breakdown, not even stored fat can be used effectively as an energy source. Glycogen depletion can become the limiting factor for performance, especially in endurance performance.

During the 1960s, trainers and coaches began to explore ways of avoiding this state of exhaustion in their athletes during endurance events. They reasoned that, if the athletes exercised heavily and ate a low-carbohydrate diet for 3 days to use up the stored glycogen, and then only exercised lightly and ate a high-carbohydrate diet for the next 3 days, glycogen stores would become supersaturated and therefore enable them to perform at a higher level. When this practice was tested, the increase in glycogen stores in muscle and the athletes' performance was significantly improved compared with their previous work capacity.

This practice has become known as *carbohydrate loading*, and it is specifically designed for endurance athletes. Carbohydrate loading is only effective when total energy intake is adequate; athletes consuming low-calorie diets do not benefit from carbohydrate loading.[1]

Today, less-stressful and modified versions of tapered depletion are used to prevent possible injury to muscle tissue. These methods can be individualized in accordance with the training program, and are more productive for the athlete. See Table 16-5 for an example of an exercise and carbohydrate regimen.

REFERENCE

1. Sedlock DA. The latest on carbohydrate loading: a practical approach. *Curr Sports Med Rep.* 2008;7(4):209-213.

Table 16-5	Example of a Precompetition Program for Carbohydrate Loading	
DAY	**EXERCISE**	**DIET**
1	90-minute period at 70% VO₂max	Mixed diet; 5 g of carbohydrate/kg body weight
2 and 3	Gradual tapering of time and intensity: <40-minute period	Same as day 1
4 and 5	Continuation of tapering: <20-minute period	Mixed diet; 10 g of carbohydrate/kg body weight
6	Complete rest	Same as days 4 and 5
7	Day of competition	High-carbohydrate preevent meal

and protein slow the rate of emptying in the stomach and thus should not be consumed in high quantities immediately before a workout or competition.

This schedule gives the body time to digest, absorb, and transform the meal into stored glycogen.

Box 16-4 Sample Pregame Meal

This sample pregame meal includes approximately 229 g of carbohydrates; it is high in complex carbohydrates and low to moderate in protein, fat, and fiber:

- 1½ cups of cooked rice (325 kcal, 67 g of carbohydrate)
- Vegetable + tofu stir-fry (375 kcal, 36 g of carbohydrate)
- 1 yam, medium (177 kcal, 42 g of carbohydrate)
- 1 banana, medium (105 kcal, 27 g of carbohydrate)
- 1½ cups of grape juice (210 kcal, 57 g of carbohydrate)

Appropriate food choices include pasta, bread, bagels, lowfat muffins, and cereal with nonfat milk. Box 16-4 outlines a sample pregame meal. Of most importance, however, is planning the pregame meal in accordance with what works well for the specific athlete.

Hydration Before, During, and After Exercise

Adequate hydration is an important consideration for athletes. Fluid needs depend on the following: (1) the intensity and duration of the exercise; (2) the surrounding temperature, altitude, and humidity; (3) the individual's fitness level and metabolic rate; and (4) the pregame or preexercise state of hydration. The thirst mechanism may not be an accurate gauge for fluid replacement; therefore, athletes are advised to make specific plans for fluid intake relative to individualized needs. In addition to water loss, which can be as much as 2.4 L/hr in extreme conditions, sweat also contains sodium and small amounts of other minerals (e.g., potassium, magnesium, chloride), which may need to be replaced depending upon the amount of sweat lost.

To maximize performance and to avoid the complications of dehydration, athletes are advised to do the following:

Before exercise: Establish euhydration at least 4 hours before exercise by drinking 5 to 7 mL/kg body weight of water or a sports beverage. Void excess fluid before competition, and do not attempt hyperhydration.

During exercise: Drink during exercise to avoid excessive water loss, which is defined as a loss of more than 2% of body weight from water. The amount of fluid that is necessary to accomplish this will be highly individualized.

After exercise: Replace fluid loss after the completion of exercise by drinking 16 to 24 oz of fluid for every pound of body weight that is lost.[29]

A number of sports drinks with added sugar, electrolytes, and flavorings are available, but questions have been raised about their use or misuse (see the For Further Focus box, "Hydrating with Water, Sports Drink, or Energy Drink"). Except for endurance events that last more than 1 hour, plain water usually is the rehydration fluid of choice. Electrolytes are replaced during the athlete's next meal. For events that last longer than 60 to 90 minutes, beverages with 6% to 8% carbohydrate concentrations may be beneficial.

Energy During Exercise

For activities lasting 1 hour or less, most athletes do not require dietary sources of energy during the exercise period. However, performance is enhanced during longer endurance or higher intensity events with the interval consumption of carbohydrate. For high-intensity or endurance exercise lasting more than 1 hour, 30 to 60 grams of carbohydrate per hour are recommended; for ultra-endurance events longer than 2.5 hours, up to 90 grams of carbohydrate per hour may be needed.[29] Consuming equal amounts of the preferred food or drink every 15 to 20 minutes throughout the event is ideal compared with consuming the entire amount at once. Athletes should experiment with various forms of carbohydrate before a competition to determine what is best tolerated. Athletes can choose from a large variety of sports drinks, gels, and other forms of carbohydrates. The food of choice should provide carbohydrates primarily from glucose, with little or no fat, protein, or fiber.

Energy After Exercise: Recovery

Proper nutrition is important to the athlete before and during exercise, and it also plays a significant role in recovery after the event. Fluid and carbohydrate replacement beverages consumed immediately after a glycogen-depleting endurance event result in higher glycogen synthesis and muscle recovery than if replacement beverages are delayed for 2 hours or more.[30] Beverages with added sodium help minimize insensible fluid losses. For athletes taking only a short break between events (e.g., triathletes), foods and beverages that are ingested should primarily contain simple carbohydrates. Athletes with at least 24 hours to recover should consume at least 1.2 g of carbohydrate per kilogram of body weight (taken over several hours) from foods or fluids to optimize the rate of muscle glycogen recovery.[31] Muscle protein synthesis will be maximized with the addition of 20 to 25 g of intact protein, or the equivalent of 9 g of essential amino acids (such as from supplements) within the first few hours.

ERGOGENIC AIDS AND MISINFORMATION

Since ancient times, athletes have been seeking and experimenting with "magic" substances or treatments to gain a competitive edge. Nutritional supplements and **ergogenic** aids are highly prevalent in the athletic world, though very few of these substances have been proven to demonstrate even a slight increase in

ergogenic the tendency to increase work output; various substances that increase work or exercise capacity and output.

performance, and several are questionable with regard to safety. Most of the marketed ergogenic aids do not work as claimed but they are relatively harmless (see the Drug-Nutrient Interaction box, "Nutritional Ergogenic Supplements").

The use of androgens is of great concern; it is dangerous, and, in competitive sports, it is illegal. The use of steroids is widespread among athletes and bodybuilders, sometimes starting as early as high school or even junior high school. Steroids are synthetic sex hormones that have two actions: (1) anabolic (i.e., tissue growth) and (2) androgenic (i.e., **masculinization**). Athletes have

> **masculinization** a condition marked by the attainment of male characteristics (e.g., facial hair) either physiologically as part of male maturation or pathologically by either sex.

Drug-Nutrient Interaction

Nutritional Ergogenic Supplements

Athletes and other individuals who are interested in improving their athletic performance often seek the help of ergogenic aids. Supplement manufacturers can make health claims about the effect of a substance on the structure or function of the body, but they are not required to demonstrate safety or efficacy. Therefore, a myriad of nutritional supplements are targeted to those who seek to enhance performance. Ergogenic aids can be classified into four categories on the basis of their efficacy and safety: (1) those that perform as claimed; (2) those that *may* perform as claimed; (3) those that do *not* perform as claimed; and (4) those that are dangerous, banned, or illegal.

THOSE THAT PERFORM AS CLAIMED

- *Creatine* is the most commonly used ergogenic aid. At moderate doses, it is considered safe, but high doses and creatine "loading" can cause a rapid increase in body mass that likely relates to increased water content in the muscle. Instances of gastrointestinal distress (e.g., cramping, diarrhea, nausea) may be associated with ingesting other substances along with creatine.[1]
- *Caffeine* was removed from the World Anti-Doping Agency's restricted list in 2004, but it is still a restricted substance for the National Collegiate Athletic Association. Caffeine's ergogenic benefit comes from acting directly on the skeletal muscle during endurance exercise, and by acting on the central nervous system, resulting in decreased ratings of exertion.[1] High-dose caffeine intake may cause gastrointestinal distress and could interfere with the ergogenic effects of creatine. Using caffeine-containing energy drinks can be ergolytic (i.e., performance impairing), especially in combination with other stimulants, alcohol, or other supplements.[2]
- *Alkalizing agents* such as sodium bicarbonate and sodium citrate may cause abdominal pain, nausea, cramps, and diarrhea. Excessive doses can cause severe metabolic acidosis. Performance benefits are less likely to occur in trained than in untrained individuals.[3]
- *Protein and amino acid supplements* are as effective as food for promoting lean body mass, but supplements may contain banned ingredients that are not listed on the label. These supplements should be used with caution.[4]

THOSE THAT MAY PERFORM AS CLAIMED

- *β-Hydroxymethylbutyrate* (HMB) has been shown to enhance recovery especially in resistance exercise through slowing protein degradation and increasing protein synthesis. HMB is thought to be relatively safe but should only be taken as recommended.[5]

- *Nitrate (beet juice)* has some support in its performance-enhancing effects on endurance performance through increasing the availability of nitric oxide. This can improve blood flow and efficiency of oxygen use at submaximal exercise.
- *Beta-alanine* has similar pH buffering effects as sodium bicarbonate however through different mechanisms. Research is promising and few side effects are noted.
- *Bovine colostrum, human growth hormone, and sodium phosphate* have been studied for potential ergogenic benefits, and the research is inconclusive. Serious adverse effects have been demonstrated in some studies if taken in high amounts, especially with human growth hormone. More research is needed before safe recommendations can be made.[6]

THOSE THAT DO NOT PERFORM AS CLAIMED

- *Branched-chain amino acids* are essential amino acids that are oxidized in skeletal muscle. Exercise increases the oxidation of these substances in the muscle, but there is little evidence that ingestion of supplemental branched-chain amino acids improves exercise performance, though some research supports its promise for immune support. High doses may cause gastrointestinal distress and interfere with the absorption of other essential amino acids.[7]
- Other substances in this category include *ribose, carnitine, chromium picolinate, conjugated linoleic acid, medium-chain triglycerides,* and *pyruvate*. Research has not conclusively determined that these substances have any ergogenic benefit, and some may have adverse effects.

THOSE THAT ARE DANGEROUS, BANNED, OR ILLEGAL

- A limited list of banned substances is found on Evolve.

REFERENCES

1. Tarnopolsky MA. Caffeine and creatine use in sport. *Ann Nutr Metab*. 2010;57(suppl 2):1-8.
2. Eudy AE, et al. Efficacy and safety of ingredients found in preworkout supplements. *Am J Health Syst Pharm*. 2013;70(7):577-588.
3. Peart DJ, Siegler JC, Vince RV. Practical recommendations for coaches and athletes: a meta-analysis of sodium bicarbonate use for athletic performance. *J Strength Cond Res*. 2012;26(7):1975-1983.
4. Maughan RJ. Quality assurance issues in the use of dietary supplements, with special reference to protein supplements. *J Nutr*. 2013;143(11):1843S-1847S.
5. Wilson JM, et al. International Society of Sports Nutrition Position Stand: beta-hydroxy-beta-methylbutyrate (HMB). *J Int Soc Sports Nutr*. 2013;10(1):6.
6. Liddle DG, Connor DJ. Nutritional supplements and ergogenic AIDS. *Prim Care*. 2013;40(2):487-505.
7. Bishop D. Dietary supplements and team-sport performance. *Sports Med*. 2010;40(12):995-1017.

been known to take steroids in megadoses of 10 to 30 times their normal body hormonal output to increase muscle size, strength, and performance. However, the physiologic side effects can be devastating, including masculinization and **gynecomastia**; liver abnormalities such as dysfunction, tumor, and hepatitis; an increased risk of atherosclerosis; and the atrophy of the testicles and decreased sperm production. Psychologic effects vary from mood swings to depression and mania or hypomania.

> **gynecomastia** the excessive development of the male mammary glands, frequently as a result of increased estrogen levels.

Athletes and their coaches are particularly susceptible to claims and myths about foods and dietary supplements. All athletes, particularly those who are involved in highly competitive sports, constantly search for the competitive edge. Knowing this, manufacturers sometimes make distorted or false claims about their products. Athletes should know that there are no quick fixes. When it comes to supplements and ergogenic aids, there are five questions to ask: Is it safe? Is it legal? Is it ethical? Is it pure? Is it effective? Health care providers should be familiar with common fads and myths that are circulating in the community so that they can approach these individuals and know what to recommend as effective alternatives.

Putting It All Together

Summary

- Many fine muscle fibers and cells, which are triggered by nerve endings, work together to make physical activity possible. Carbohydrate, mainly in the form of complex-carbohydrate foods or starches, is the primary fuel for energy to run this system.
- Carbohydrate metabolism yields circulating blood glucose and stored glycogen in muscles and the liver for fuel. Stored body fat supplies additional fuel as fatty acids, whereas protein provides insignificant energy for exercise. Vitamins and minerals are important parts of coenzymes for the process of energy production.
- Activities of daily living, aerobic exercise, and resistance training have many benefits that increase with practice. Excellent aerobic exercises include sustained fast walking, swimming, jogging, running, and aerobic dancing or similar workouts. Resistance training increases muscle strength, which has a direct influence on metabolic rate and bone density. Weight-bearing exercise is also important for maintaining bone density.
- Exercise increases the need for energy and water. Water is generally the best way to avoid dehydration. Electrolytes that are lost in sweat are replaced during the next meal. The macronutrient needs of athletes do not differ from those of the general population, except that more total calories, protein, and fluids are needed.
- During the week before an athletic event (especially an endurance event), athletes may practice carbohydrate loading to meet the energy demands of competition. However, pregame meals should contain moderate amounts of mainly complex carbohydrates, with little fat, protein, or fiber.

Chapter Review Questions

See answers in Appendix A.

1. Exercise helps maintain healthy blood cholesterol levels by:
   a. Decreasing HDL level.
   b. Increasing LDL level.
   c. Increasing HDL level.
   d. Decreasing dietary cholesterol intake.

2. Jeff is 62 years old and wants to incorporate aerobic exercise into his daily activities. Which activity should he try to incorporate first?
   a. Running a marathon
   b. Walking at a brisk pace
   c. Performing yoga or another stretching exercise
   d. Doing resistance training or weight lifting

3. The type of exercise that primarily uses fat as an energy source is:
   a. High-intensity aerobic exercise.
   b. Low-intensity aerobic exercise.
   c. High-intensity resistance exercise.
   d. Low-intensity resistance exercise.

4. A major source of energy support used during exercise is found in which of the following foods?
   a. Orange juice
   b. Grilled chicken patty
   c. Oatmeal bar
   d. Chocolate bar

5. The most appropriate food choice for a pregame meal would be:
   a. Chicken ravioli, French bread, fresh fruit.
   b. Fried fish, broccoli, yogurt.
   c. Hamburger, fries, low-fat milk.
   d. Grilled steak, onion rings, chocolate cake.

Additional Learning Resources

evolve http://evolve.elsevier.com/Williams/basic/

References and **Further Reading and Resources** in the back of the book provide additional resources for enhancing knowledge.

Nutrition Care

Key Concepts

- Effective health care is centered on the patient and his or her individual needs.
- Comprehensive health care is best provided by a team of health professionals and support staff.
- A personalized health care plan, evaluation, and follow-up care guide actions to promote healing and health.
- Drug-nutrient interactions can create significant medical complications.

People face acute illness or chronic disease and treatment in a variety of settings and locations. Nutrition support is fundamental for the successful treatment of disease, and it is often the primary therapy. To meet individual needs, a broad knowledge of nutrition status, requirements, and ways of meeting the identified needs is essential. Each member of the health care team plays an important role in developing and maintaining a person-centered health care plan.

This chapter focuses on the comprehensive care of the patient's nutrition needs as provided by the registered dietitian nutritionist. Nurses are intimately involved in the care process and often identify nutrition needs within the **nursing diagnosis**. An effective care plan involves all health care team members as well as the patient, the family, and their support system.

THE THERAPEUTIC PROCESS

SETTING AND FOCUS OF CARE

Nutrition support may take place in a variety of settings and in a variety of forms. For example, individuals may seek and receive nutrition support at home, in a private practice, in an outpatient facility, in a hospital, in a long-term care facility, in a rehabilitation center, or in a public health community setting. The ultimate goal of nutrition support is to establish nutritional balance according to specific needs of the individual.

Modern hospitals are a marvel of medical technology, but medical advances sometimes bring confusion to patients, whose illnesses place them in the midst of a complex system of care. Various members of the medical staff come and go, and sometimes the day's schedule does not proceed as planned. Patients need personal advocates. Health care providers such as the

nurse and the dietitian provide essential support and personalized care.

The type of nutrition support may come in many different forms as well, ranging from help with balancing daily meal plans to providing nutrition therapy through intravenous feedings. Nutrition care must be based on individual needs and be person-centered. Figure 17-1 demonstrates the **nutrition care process model,** with the person-centered approach defining the relationship between the patient and the dietetic professional. Needs must constantly be updated with the patient's status. Such personalized care demands great commitment from the health care team. Despite all of the methods, tools, and technologies described in this text and elsewhere, remember this basic fact: the therapeutic use of the self is the most healing tool that a person will ever use. This is a simple yet profound truth, because the human encounter is where health care workers bring themselves and their skills.

HEALTH CARE TEAM

In the area of nutrition care, the registered dietitian nutritionist (RDN), also known as a registered dietitian

---

nursing diagnosis "[a] clinical judgment about individual, family, or community experiences/responses to actual or potential health problems/life processes. Nursing diagnoses provide the basis for selection of nursing interventions to achieve outcomes for which the nurse has accountability," as defined by the North American Nursing Diagnosis Association.

nutrition care process model a systematic approach to providing high-quality individualized nutrition care. The model consists of the following steps: assessment, diagnosis, intervention, and monitoring and evaluation.

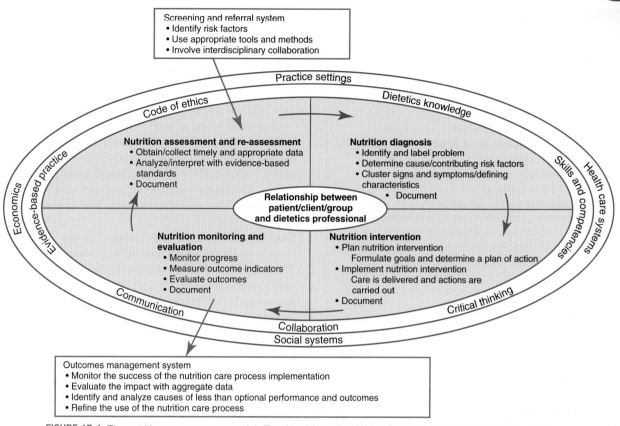

FIGURE 17-1 The nutrition care process model. (Reprinted from the Writing Group of the Nutrition Care Process/ Standardized Language Committee. Nutrition care process and model part I: the 2008 update. *J Am Diet Assoc.* 2008;108(7):1113-1117.)

(RD), carries the major responsibility of medical nutrition therapy. Box 17-1 outlines the qualifications of an RDN. Working closely with the physician, the dietitian determines individual nutrition therapy needs and a plan of care. Team support is essential throughout this process. Nurses are in a unique position to provide additional nutrition support by referring patients to the dietitian when necessary. Of all the health care team members, nurses are in the closest continuous contact with hospitalized patients and their families. Such a relationship is important to ensure the most beneficial health care approach.

Physician and Support Staff
The health care team is headed by the physician and may include several other allied health professionals, depending on the needs of the patient. The team may include some or all of the following members: nurse, dietitian, physical therapist, occupational therapist, speech therapist, respiratory therapist, radiologist, physician assistant, kinesiotherapist, pharmacist, and social worker. When developing this team relationship, all involved parties need each other's expertise for a successful outcome and to best serve the patient's needs.

Roles of the Nurse and the Clinical Dietitian
Successful nutrition care depends on the close collaboration of the dietitian and the nurse. The dietitian determines nutrition needs, plans and manages nutrition therapy, evaluates the plan of care, and documents results. Throughout this entire process, the nurse helps to develop, support, and carry out the plan of care. This teamwork is particularly vital for patients with strict or complicated nutrition requirements. A dietitian may only see a patient once or twice during a

> **medical nutrition therapy** a specific nutrition service and procedure that is used to treat an illness, injury, or condition; it involves an in-depth nutrition assessment of the patient, nutrition diagnosis, nutrition intervention (which includes diet therapy, counseling, and the use of specialized nutrition supplements), and nutrition monitoring and evaluation.
>
> **kinesiotherapist** a health care professional who treats the effects of disease, injury, and congenital disorders through the application of scientifically based exercise principles that have been adapted to enhance the strength, endurance, and mobility of individuals with functional limitations or for those patients who require extended physical conditioning.

Box 17-1   Qualifications of a Registered
Dietitian Nutritionist

WHAT IS A REGISTERED DIETITIAN NUTRITIONIST?

A registered dietitian nutritionist (RDN), also known as a registered dietitian (RD), is a food and nutrition expert who has met academic and professional requirements, including the following:

- Earned a bachelor's degree with course work approved by the Academy of Nutrition and Dietetics Accreditation Council for Education in Nutrition and Dietetics (ACEND); coursework typically includes nutrition sciences, biochemistry, physiology, microbiology, chemistry, sociology and communication, food service systems management, business, economics, and computer science.
- Completed an ACEND-accredited, supervised practice program at a health care facility, community agency, food service corporation or combined with undergraduate or graduate studies. This internship is typically between 6 and 12 months long.
- Passed a national examination administered by the Commission on Dietetic Registration (www.cdrnet.org).
- Completes continuing professional educational requirements to maintain registration.

Approximately 50% of RDNs hold advanced degrees. Some RDNs also hold additional certifications in specialized areas of practice, such as pediatric or renal nutrition, nutrition support, diabetes education, weight management, and sports nutrition.

HOW IS A REGISTERED DIETITIAN NUTRITIONIST DIFFERENT FROM A "NUTRITIONIST"?

- The "RDN" or "RD" (if preferred) credential is a legally protected title that can only be used by practitioners who are authorized by the Commission on Dietetic Registration of the Academy of Nutrition and Dietetics.
- Some RDNs may call themselves "nutritionists," but not all nutritionists are registered dietitians. The definition and requirements for the term *nutritionist* vary. Some states have licensure laws that define the scope of practice for someone who is using the designation, but, in other states, virtually anyone can call himself or herself a "nutritionist," regardless of education or training.

To find out more about what services RDNs provide and what the qualifications are for Dietetic Technician, Registered, please visit www.eatright.org. Go to the *About Us* page.

Source: Academy of Nutrition and Dietetics. www.eatrightpro.org/resources/about-us; accessed February 2015.

hospital stay, whereas the nurse will have constant contact with the patient and will often be the person dealing with immediate nutrition-related questions because of his or her frequent contact.

The nursing process is a specific process by which nurses deliver care to patients and includes the following steps: assessment, diagnosis, outcome/planning, implementation, and evaluation. The nursing diagnosis is the nurse's clinical judgment about a client's response to actual or potential health conditions or needs.[1] A nursing diagnosis may include several issues that are nutrition related, such as diarrhea, malnutrition, failure to thrive, and fluid volume deficit. Although covering the nursing process is not within the scope of this text, an appreciation of the interconnected work of the nurse and the dietitian on the health care team is important.

A skilled nurse is well respected as the thread that ties all of the health care workers together. Nurses are skilled multitaskers, and they carry a heavy load of the overall responsibilities in a clinical setting. When necessary, nurses may also serve as essential coordinators, advocates, interpreters, teachers, and counselors.

Coordinators and advocates. Nurses work more closely with patients than do any other practitioners. They are best able to coordinate the patient's required services and treatments, and they can consult and refer as needed. For example, malnutrition is common in hospital settings and there are many factors involved (e.g., pain or medicine-induced anorexia, surgery, and emotional or psychologic distress). However, sometimes patients have reduced food intake because of conflicts with medical procedures, appointments during meal time, or culture/religious dietary habits that are not being met with the routine hospital diet. The nurse may be able to help resolve such conflicts by coordinating specific meals or meal-delivery times with a consideration of the patient's wishes and scheduled procedures.

Interpreters. The nurse can help to reduce a patient's anxiety with the use of careful, brief, and easily understood explanations about various treatments and plans of care. This may include reinforcement of a prescribed therapeutic diet and the resulting food choices to sustain compliance. These activities may be difficult with uninterested patients, but efforts to understand such patient behaviors are paramount to bridging the gap. A patient's psychologic and emotional status has a strong influence on his or her overall ability to deal with the medical problem at hand and to adhere to the treatment protocol. Patients who are discharged without a proper interpretation of their prognosis or plan of continued care may be noncompliant and experience unnecessary stress, confusion, medical complications, and hospital readmission.

Teachers and counselors. Basic teaching and counseling skills are essential in nursing. Many opportunities exist during daily care for conversations about sound medical and nutrition principles, which will reinforce the care plan with the patient. Learning about health care needs (including nutrition) should begin with the patient's hospital admission or initial contact, carry through the entire period of care, and continue in the home environment, with the support of community resources as needed.

PHASES OF THE CARE PROCESS

The Academy of Nutrition and Dietetics has developed a standardized Nutrition Care Process for RDNs (see the Student Resources section on the Evolve website).[2] The Nutrition Care Process is "a systematic problem-solving method that dietetics professionals use to critically think and make decisions to address nutrition-related problems and provide safe and effective quality nutrition care."[3] It is composed of the following four distinct and interrelated nutrition steps: (1) assessment; (2) diagnosis; (3) intervention; and (4) monitoring and evaluation. The Nutrition Care Process provides a consistent structure and framework for nutrition professionals to use to provide individualized care for patients. This process is used for patients, clients, and groups that have identified nutrition risk factors and that need assistance to achieve or maintain health goals.

NUTRITION ASSESSMENT

To assess nutrition status and provide person-centered care, as much information as possible about the patient's situation is collected. Family and medical history questionnaires are useful methods of gathering pertinent information on admission or during the initial office visit. Appropriate care considers the patient's nutrition status, food habits, and living situation as well as his or her needs, desires, and goals. The patient and his or her family are the primary sources of this information. Other sources include the patient's medical chart, oral or written communication with hospital staff, and related research. Data obtained during the nutrition assessment are organized into five categories. The following table gives examples of information that is gathered within each of the five categories.

Food- and Nutrition-Related History

In most cases, the RDN is responsible for evaluating the diet. Knowledge of the patient's basic eating habits may help to identify possible nutrition deficiencies. The Clinical Applications box entitled "Nutrition

History: Activity-Associated Food Pattern of a Typical Day" shows an example of a general guide for gathering a nutrition history. Sometimes a more specific food history is obtained by using a 3-day food record; this involves the patient recording everything that is consumed, the food items that are used, and the amounts and methods of preparation for 3 full days. A more extended view of the diet may reveal additional information about food habits or problems as they relate to the individual's socioeconomic status, family, living situation, and general support system.

Clinicians should be aware that underreporting energy intake is quite common and that this may affect dietary assessment and recommendations.[4-8] A variety of methods are used to collect dietary intake, all of which have strengths and weaknesses (Table 17-1). Patients often do not volunteer information regarding dietary supplement intake (see the Drug-Nutrient Interaction box, "Dietary Supplement Use"). Thus, direct questions about supplement use (e.g., vitamins, minerals, multivitamin/mineral combinations, herbs) are more likely to yield accurate answers and to provide insight into overall nutrient consumption. Allergies and intolerances should be noted so that alternative recommendations meet nutrition needs without causing negative reactions.

Physical activity logs are similar to dietary intake logs in that all activity is recorded throughout the day in an effort to calculate energy expenditure. Like diet logs, physical activity questionnaires tend to be inaccurate relative to fitness in a portion of the population and overestimate actual energy expenditure when compared to the gold standard of **doubly labeled water method**.[9-11] Thus, the inaccurate estimation of energy

---

doubly labeled water method gold standard for measuring energy expenditure. Participants ingest water labeled with a known concentration of isotopes of hydrogen and oxygen. Elimination of the isotopes is measured to predict the energy expenditure and metabolic rate.

FOOD-/NUTRITION-RELATED HISTORY	ANTHROPOMETRIC MEASUREMENTS	BIOCHEMICAL DATA, MEDICAL TESTS, AND PROCEDURES	NUTRITION-FOCUSED PHYSICAL FINDINGS	CLIENT HISTORY
• Food and nutrient intake • Food and nutrient administration • Medication, complementary/alternative medicine use • Knowledge and beliefs • Availability of food and supplies • Physical activity • Nutrition quality of life	• Height • Weight • Body mass index • Growth pattern indices/percentile ranks • Weight history	• Lab data (e.g., electrolytes, glucose) • Test results (e.g., gastric emptying time, resting metabolic rate)	• Physical appearance • Muscle and fat wasting • Swallow function • Appetite • Affect	• Personal history • Medical, health, and family history • Treatment and complementary or alternative medicine use • Social history

Academy of Nutrition and Dietetics. *Nutrition Care Process SNAPshots.* Cited February 2015; available from www.andeal.org/ncp.

Clinical Applications

Nutrition History: Activity-Associated Food Pattern of a Typical Day

Name: _____ Date: _____

Height: _____ Weight (lb): _____ /(kg): _____ Body mass index: _____

Ideal weight: _____ Usual weight: _____

Referral:

Diagnosis:

Diet order:

Occupation:

Recreation, physical activity:

Present food intake:

TIME/LOCATION	FOOD (AND METHOD OF PREPARATION)	SERVING SIZE	TOLERANCE/COMMENTS
Breakfast			
Snack			
Lunch			
Snack			
Dinner			

Summary: Total servings of foods in each category:

Breads/grains: ____ Vegetables: ____ Fruits: ____ Dairy: ____ Meat: ____ Fat/sugar: ____

Dietary supplements and herbs:

Name of supplement: _____ Dose per day: _____

Drug-Nutrient Interaction

Dietary Supplement Use

Dietary supplements include vitamins, minerals, amino acids, fatty acids, herbs, botanicals, and other substances that have physiologic effects in the body. As noted in the Drug-Nutrient Interaction boxes throughout this textbook, dietary supplements can interact with one another and with medications resulting in either beneficial or detrimental effects on the body. Nutrient intake from food combined with high doses of micronutrients from supplements and from fortified foods and beverages may result in habitual intake above the Upper Tolerable Limit for many vitamins and minerals. This may manifest in gastrointestinal symptoms or overt signs of toxicity.

The use of dietary supplements in the United States has been monitored since the 1970s; 54% of women and 42% of men between the ages of 20 and 69 years old report taking at least one dietary supplement per day.[1] Yet, only half of vitamin/mineral dietary supplement users and 15% of herbal dietary supplement users reported their use to their health care provider.[2] In a study assessing alternative therapies used specifically by cancer patients, 73% of subjects reported using some form of dietary supplement; of those, 47% did *not* disclose supplement use to their medical providers.[3] This oversight may be because patients are unaware of potential interactions with drugs or other therapies or because patients simply forgot about their supplements.

It is evident that patients need more education about the importance of talking to their health care providers about the use of vitamin, mineral, and herbal supplements. Additionally, health care providers may need further training to elicit information about dietary supplement use from their patients. When speaking with patients or clients, be objective about supplement use. Always encourage patients to discuss supplementation with a physician or pharmacist to avoid potential drug-nutrient interactions.

REFERENCES

1. Kennedy ET, Luo H, Houser RF. Dietary supplement use pattern of U.S. adult population in the 2007-2008 National Health and Nutrition Examination Survey (NHANES). *Ecol Food Nutr.* 2013; 52(1):76-84.
2. Shim JM, Schneider J, Curlin FA. Patterns of user disclosure of complementary and alternative medicine (CAM) use. *Med Care.* 2014;52(8):704-708.
3. Rausch SM et al. Complementary and alternative medicine: use and disclosure in radiation oncology community practice. *Support Care Cancer.* 2011;19(4):521-529.

Table 17-1 Strengths and Limitations of Techniques Used to Measure Dietary Intake

TECHNIQUE	BRIEF DESCRIPTION	STRENGTHS	LIMITATIONS
24-hour food recall	A trained interviewer asks the respondent to recall, in detail, all food and drink consumed during the previous 24 hours	Fast, inexpensive, and easy to administer Can provide detailed information about the types of foods consumed Low respondent burden Is not dependent on respondent's level of education, literacy, or writing skills Does not alter respondent's usual intake	One 24-hour recall cannot illustrate typical dietary intake Underreporting and overreporting are common Depends on respondent's memory Accuracy is somewhat dependent upon the skill of the interviewer Omissions of sauces, dressings, and beverages can lead to low estimates of energy intake
Multiple-day food record	The respondent records, at the time of consumption, the identities and amounts of all foods and beverages consumed for 3 to 7 days	Does not rely on memory since the participants record intake immediately following consumption Can provide detailed intake data Multiple-day data are more representative of usual intake Reasonably valid for up to 5 days	Requires high degree of cooperation Client/patient must be literate and able to write Takes more time to obtain data Analysis is labor intensive Act of recording food intake often alters usual intake Underreporting and inaccurately estimating portion sizes are common Respondent burden can result in low response rates
Food frequency questionnaires	The respondent indicates how many times a day, week, month, or year that he or she usually consumes specific foods by using a questionnaire consisting of hundreds of foods or food groups	Can be self-administered Machine readable Relatively inexpensive May be more representative of usual intake over longer periods of time than a few days of diet records Does not alter respondents usual intake	Modest demand on respondent May not represent usual food or portion sizes typically chosen by respondent Cultural/ethnic specific foods are often not included Intake data can be compromised when multiple foods are grouped within single listings Requires literacy and good long-term memory Not effective for monitoring short-term dietary changes
Diet history	A trained nutrition professional interviews the patient about the number of meals eaten per day; his or her appetite and food dislikes; the presence or absence of gastrointestinal distress; the use of dietary supplements; and other lifestyle choices	Assesses usual nutrient intake Can detect seasonal changes Data about all nutrients can be obtained Can correlate well with biochemical measures	Lengthy interview process Requires highly trained interviewers May overestimate nutrient intake Requires the cooperation of a respondent with the ability to recall his or her usual diet Difficult and expensive to code for group analysis

expenditure is another important consideration when providing nutrition recommendations.

Anthropometric Measurements

All providers responsible for taking **anthropometric measurements** should practice taking correct measurements to avoid errors, and maintain proper equipment and careful technique. Height, weight, and body mass index are the most common anthropometric measurements that are used in clinical practice, and they are used to predict basic nutrition risk parameters. In some situations, body composition measurements and waist circumference may be taken as well.

anthropometric measurements the physical measurements of the human body that are used for health assessment, including height, weight, skin fold thickness, and circumference (i.e., of the head, hip, waist, wrist, and mid-arm muscle).

Height. Height should be measured using a wall-mounted measuring tape, if possible, or the moveable measuring rod on a platform clinic scale. Have the person stand as straight as possible, without shoes or a hat. Children who are younger than 2 years old should be measured while they are lying down with a stationary headboard and a movable footboard (Figure 17-2). Alternative measures for nonambulatory patients provide estimates for people who are confined to a bed, who cannot stand up straight, or who have lower-body amputations (Box 17-2).

Weight and body mass index. For accurate results, patients should be weighed at consistent times (e.g., early morning after the bladder is emptied and before breakfast). If the patient is wearing the same clothing each time that he or she is weighed (e.g., an examination gown), a more consistent weight measurement will be obtained. Ask the patient about his or her usual body weight and compare it with standard body mass index tables (see inside back cover of book). Inquire about recent weight loss (e.g., how much over what period of time). Rapid unintentional weight loss

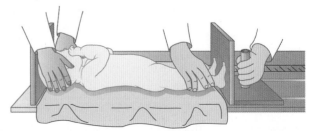

FIGURE 17-2 Measuring height in an infant. (Reprinted from Mahan LK, Escott-Stump S. *Krause's food & nutrition therapy*. 13th ed. Philadelphia: Saunders; 2012.)

Box 17-2   Alternative Measures for Nonambulatory Patients

TOTAL ARM SPAN
- With a flexible metric tape, measure the patient's full arm span from fingertip to fingertip across the front of the clavicles.
- For patients with limited movement in one arm, measure from the fingertip to the midpoint of the sternum on the dominant hand, and then double the measurement.

KNEE HEIGHT[1,2]
- With the client's knees bent at a 90-degree angle, measure the left knee-to-floor height from the outside bony point just under the kneecap (i.e., the fibular head) and down to the floor surface.
- Use the following equations to calculate total body height from knee height:

AGE, GENDER, AND ETHNICITY	EQUATION	STANDARD ERROR FOR AN INDIVIDUAL
Black females		
>60 years old	$89.58 + (1.61 \times KH) - (0.17 \times A)$	3.83 cm
19 to 60 years old	$68.10 + (1.86 \times KH) - (0.06 \times A)$	3.80 cm
6 to 18 years old	$46.59 + (2.02 \times KH)$	4.39 cm
White females		
>60 years old	$82.21 + (1.85 \times KH) - (0.21 \times A)$	3.98 cm
19 to 60 years old	$70.25 + (1.87 \times KH) - (0.06 \times A)$	3.60 cm
6 to 18 years old	$43.21 + (2.15 \times KH)$	3.90 cm
Black males		
>60 years old	$79.69 + (1.85 \times KH) - (0.14 \times A)$	3.81 cm
19 to 60 years old	$73.42 + (1.79 \times KH)$	3.60 cm
6 to 18 years old	$39.60 + (2.18 \times KH)$	4.58 cm
White males		
>60 years old	$78.31 + (1.94 \times KH) - (0.14 \times A)$	3.74 cm
19 to 60 years old	$71.85 + (1.88 \times KH)$	3.97 cm
6 to 18 years old	$40.54 + (2.22 \times KH)$	4.21 cm

KH, Knee height in cm; *A*, age in years.

RECUMBENT BED LENGTH
- Align the body so that the lower extremities, trunk, shoulders, and head are in a straight line.
- Mark on the bed sheet the position of the base of the heels and the top of the crown.
- Measure the distance with a tape measure.

MEASUREMENT WHILE LYING IN THE FETAL POSITION
- Measure four segments of body while the person is lying on his or her side in a "fetal" position: heel (foot flexed) to knee, knee to hip, hip to shoulder, and shoulder to top of head.
- Add the segment measurements together.

REFERENCES
1. Chumlea WC, Guo SS, Steinbaugh ML. Prediction of stature from knee height for black and white adults and children with application to mobility-impaired or handicapped persons. *J Am Diet Assoc.* 1994;94(12):1385-1388, 1391; quiz 1389-1390.
2. Chumlea WC, Guo SS, Wholihan K et al. Stature prediction equations for elderly non-Hispanic white, non-Hispanic black, and Mexican-American persons developed from NHANES III data. *J Am Diet Assoc.* 1998;98(2):137-142.

is significantly associated with increased health risks and mortality, particularly in nursing home patients.[12] Patients who have lost ≥5% of their body weight in 1 month or ≥10% of their body weight over any amount of time for unknown reasons should be referred to an RDN for a thorough evaluation. Recent weight gain should be noted as well. Understanding the patient's general weight history over time (e.g., peaks and lows at what ages) will give a broad view of expected weight fluctuations.

The body mass index is calculated by using both weight and height measurements and it is a helpful assessment tool throughout the life cycle (see Chapter 15).

Body composition. The dietitian may measure various aspects of body size and composition to determine relative levels of lean tissue compared to fat mass. Several methods that are used to measure body composition are covered in Chapter 15. Some methods include a skin fold thickness measurement with calipers, hydrostatic weighing, bioelectrical impedance analysis, dual-energy x-ray absorptiometry, and the BOD POD body composition tracking system (Life Measurement, Inc., Concord, Calif).

Waist circumference. Body mass index and body composition measurements indicate the risk for overweight and obesity (i.e., body fatness), but they do not evaluate where excess fat is stored or relative fitness levels. The location of body fat is an important factor in nutrition assessment, because not all body fat is the same. Individuals who store body fat in the abdominal region have significantly more health risks than their counterparts of the same weight who store fat in the hip and thigh regions. The Expert Panel's National Guidelines for the Management of Overweight and Obesity note that, for a lowered health risk, waist circumference should be <102 cm for men and <88 cm for women.[13] Waist circumference assessment and waist-to-height ratio are important considerations for both overweight and normal-weight individuals, because they indicate the risk for chronic diseases (e.g., type 2 diabetes, cardiovascular disease, hypertension, cancer, overall mortality), even among individuals of normal weight.[14-17]

Biochemical Data, Medical Tests, and Procedures

Laboratory data and radiographic tests are helpful with the nutrition status assessment. Such reports generally are available in the patient's medical chart. Examples of biochemical tests pertinent to nutrition include, but are not limited to, the following:

- *Plasma proteins:* serum albumin and prealbumin evaluate for protein status
- *Liver enzymes:* evaluate liver function
- *Blood urea nitrogen and serum electrolytes:* evaluate renal function
- *Urinary urea nitrogen excretion:* estimate nitrogen balance
- *Creatinine height index:* evaluate protein tissue breakdown
- *Complete blood count:* evaluate for anemia
- *Fasting glucose:* evaluate for hyper- and hypoglycemia
- *Total lymphocyte count:* evaluate immune function

The medical tests that are used for nutrition assessment are generally reliable for people of any age, but some conditions may interfere with test results and should be considered when regarding laboratory values. For example, test results may be altered by hydration status, the presence of chronic diseases, changes in organ function, time from last meal, and certain medications. Depending on the patient, some additional medical tests or procedures may be warranted, such as the following:

Skeletal system integrity. Several tests may be used, especially with older patients, to determine the status of bone integrity and possible osteopenia or osteoporosis. Some tests that are commonly used are x-rays, dual-energy x-ray absorptiometry, and bone scans.

Gastrointestinal function. Medical procedures are also useful to evaluate function, disease, or malfunction along the gastrointestinal tract (e.g., disturbances in gastric emptying time, peptic ulcer disease, inflammatory bowel disease).

Resting metabolic rate. Evaluating a patient's resting metabolic rate helps to establish total energy needs. Both direct and indirect measurement methods are discussed in Chapter 6.

Nutrition-Focused Physical Findings

The careful observation of various areas of the patient's body may reveal signs of poor nutrition. Table 17-2 lists some clinical signs of nutrition status that should be kept in mind when providing general patient care.

Other members of the health care team (e.g., physician, nurse, physical therapist) may also perform physical examinations that are useful for evaluating nutrition status.

Client History

Guided questioning helps clients to identify and remember elements of their histories that may be pertinent. As mentioned previously, dietary supplements such as herbs are often not mentioned unless they are specifically addressed. Other complementary and alternative medicine use should be identified during this stage. Many elements of a client's personal history can affect his or her current nutrition status and help to guide the plan of care; such elements include

Table 17-2   Signs that Suggest Nutrient Imbalance

AREA OF CONCERN	POSSIBLE DEFICIENCY	POSSIBLE EXCESS
Hair		
Dull, dry, and brittle	Pro	
Easily plucked, with no pain	Pro	
Hair loss	Pro, Zn, biotin	Vit A
Flag sign (i.e., loss of hair pigment in strips around the head)	Pro, Cu	
Head and Neck		
Bulging fontanel (in infants)		Vit A
Headache		Vit A, D
Epistaxis (i.e., nosebleed)	Vit K	
Thyroid enlargement	Iodine	
Eyes		
Conjunctival and corneal xerosis (i.e., dryness)	Vit A	
Pale conjunctivae	Fe	
Blue sclerae	Fe	
Corneal vascularization	Vit B_2	
Mouth		
Cheilosis or angular stomatitis (i.e., lesions at the corners of the mouth)	Vit B_2	
Glossitis (i.e., red, sore tongue)	Niacin, folate, vit B_{12}, and other B vit	
Gingivitis (i.e., inflamed gums)	Vit C	
Hypogeusia or dysgeusia (i.e., poor sense of taste or distorted taste)	Zn	
Dental caries	Fluoride	
Mottling of teeth		Fluoride
Atrophy of papillae on tongue	Fe, B vit	
Skin		
Dry or scaly	Vit A, Zn, EFAs	Vit A
Follicular hyperkeratosis (resembles gooseflesh)	Vit A, EFAs, B vit	
Eczematous lesions	Zn	
Petechiae or ecchymoses	Vit C, K	
Nasolabial seborrhea (i.e., greasy, scaly areas between the nose and lip)	Niacin, vit B_{12}, B_6	
Darkening and peeling of skin in areas exposed to sun	Niacin	
Poor wound healing	Pro, Zn, vit C	
Nails		
Spoon shaped	Fe	
Brittle and fragile	Pro	
Heart		
Enlargement, tachycardia, or failure	Vit B_1	
Small heart	Energy	
Sudden failure or death	Se	
Arrhythmia	Mg, K, Se	
Hypertension	Ca, K	Na
Abdomen		
Hepatomegaly	Pro	Vit A
Ascites	Pro	
Musculoskeletal Extremities		
Muscle wasting (especially in the temporal area)	Energy	
Edema	Pro, vit B_1	
Calf tenderness	Vit B_1 or C, biotin, Se	

Table 17-2 Signs that Suggest Nutrient Imbalance—cont'd

AREA OF CONCERN	POSSIBLE DEFICIENCY	POSSIBLE EXCESS
Beading of ribs or "rachitic rosary" in a child	Vit C, D	
Bone and joint tenderness	Vit C, D, Ca, P	
Knock knees, bowed legs, or fragile bones	Vit D, Ca, P, Cu	
Neurologic		
Paresthesias (i.e., pain and tingling or altered sensation in the extremities)	Vit B_1, B_6, B_{12}, biotin	
Weakness	Vit C, B_1, B_6, B_{12}, energy	
Ataxia and decreased position and vibratory senses	Vit B_1, B_{12}	
Tremor	Mg	
Decreased tendon reflexes	Vit B_1	
Confabulation or disorientation	Vit B_1, B_{12}	
Drowsiness and lethargy	Vit B_1	Vit A, D
Depression	Vit B_1, biotin, B_{12}	

Ca, Calcium; *Cu,* copper; *EFAs,* essential fatty acids; *Fe,* iron; *K,* potassium; *Mg,* magnesium; *Na,* sodium; *P,* phosphorus; *Pro,* protein; *Se,* selenium; *Vit,* vitamin(s); *Zn,* zinc.

socioeconomic status, religion, culture, ethnicity, family interactions, living situation, education level, and employment status. Economic needs are paramount for many people in high-risk populations. Health care providers who are cognizant of the personal and cultural needs of their patients will be more effective when helping a patient plan for immediate and long-term nutrition requirements.

Psychologic and emotional problems can weigh heavily on the overall outcome of a patient's prognosis and well-being. For example, geriatric patients in long-term health care facilities often suffer from depression and malnutrition, which are compounding problems when individuals are already in poor health. Although poor nutritional status and unintentional weight loss are associated with depression, it is not always clear if depression is the cause or consequence of poor nutrition.[18] Thus, by inquiring about a patient's psychologic well-being during this step, some of these modifiable factors can be addressed.

At the conclusion of the gathering of nutrition assessment data, health care providers must distinguish relevant from irrelevant data, validate the data, and then determine whether there is a need to obtain additional information.

NUTRITION DIAGNOSIS

A nutrition diagnosis involves the "identification and labeling of an existing nutrition problem that the food and nutrition professional is responsible for treating independently."[2] A careful study of all information that has been gathered thus far reveals basic patient needs. Other needs develop and guide the care plan as the hospitalization or consultation continues. Nutrition diagnoses are organized into the following three categories:

INTAKE	CLINICAL	BEHAVIORAL AND ENVIRONMENTAL
• Too much or too little of a food or nutrient compared with actual or estimated needs	• Nutrition problems that relate to medical or physical conditions	• Knowledge, attitudes, beliefs, physical environment, access to food, and food safety

Academy of Nutrition and Dietetics. *Nutrition Care Process SNAPshots.* Cited February 2015; available from www.andeal.org/ncp.

A nutrition diagnosis statement will have three distinct and concise elements: *Problem, Etiology,* and the *Signs/symptoms.* This is often referred to as a *PES* statement.

Problem

After the careful assessment of nutrition indices, data are analyzed, and a nutrition diagnostic category is assigned. The nutrition diagnostic statement identifies nutrition problems, which may include nutrient deficiencies (e.g., iron-deficiency anemia) or underlying disease that requires a modified diet (e.g., renal disease, liver disease). Such a diagnosis sets realistic and measurable outcome goals. This then allows for the identification of appropriate interventions and a means for tracking the progress toward attaining that specific outcome.

Etiology

The causes or contributing risk factors are identifiable factors that are directly leading to the stated problem. The Academy of Nutrition and Dietetics defines etiology as "a factor gathered during the nutrition assessment that contributes to the existence or the maintenance of pathophysiological, psychosocial, situational, developmental, cultural, and/or environmental problems."[2] Correctly identifying the etiology is the only way to adequately design an intervention plan. Within the nutrition diagnostic PES statement, the etiology should be preceded by the words *related to*.

Signs and Symptoms

Signs and symptoms of nutrition problems are an accumulation of subjective and objective changes in the patient's health status that indicate a nutrition problem and that are the results of the identified etiology. Within a nutrition diagnostic PES statement, the signs and symptoms should be preceded by the words *as evidenced by*.

The nutrition diagnosis will change as the patient's nutrition needs change. The following is an example of a nutrition diagnostic PES statement:

Excessive caloric intake (problem) related to frequent consumption of large portions of high-fat meals (etiology) as evidenced by average daily intake of calories exceeding recommended

amount by 500 kcal and 12-pound weight gain during the past 18 months (signs).[3]

NUTRITION INTERVENTION

After the assessment and diagnosis, dietitians should now be ready to plan and implement the most suitable form of nutrition intervention. Nutrition interventions are "purposefully planned actions designed with the intent of changing a nutrition-related behavior, risk factor, environmental condition, or aspect of health status for an individual, target group, or the community at large."[2] Objectives of the care plan are client-driven, thus focusing attention on personal needs and goals as well as on the identified requirements of medical care for the patient. Suitable and realistic actions then carry out the personal care plan. Such activities ideally include family members and caretakers as well.

The nutrition intervention strategies are organized into four categories:

FOOD AND NUTRIENT DELIVERY	NUTRITION EDUCATION	NUTRITION COUNSELING	COORDINATION OF NUTRITION CARE
• An individualized approach for food and nutrient provision	• A formal process to instruct or train a patient/client in a skill • Impart knowledge to help patients/clients voluntarily manage or modify food, nutrition and physical activity choices, and behavior to maintain or improve health	• A supportive process that is characterized by a collaborative counselor-patient relationship • Sets priorities, establishes goals, and creates individualized action plans that acknowledge and foster responsibility for self-care to treat an existing condition • Promotes health	• Consultation with, referral to, or coordination of nutrition care with other health care providers, institutions, or agencies that can assist with the treatment or management of nutrition-related problems

Academy of Nutrition and Dietetics. *Nutrition Care Process SNAPshots*. Cited February 2015; available from www.andeal.org/ncp.

Food and/or Nutrient Delivery

Personal adaptation. Successful nutrition therapy can occur only when the diet is personalized to meet individual needs. This can be done best by planning with the patient and his or her family. The following four areas must be explored together:

1. *Personal needs:* What personal desires, concerns, goals, or life situation needs must be met?
2. *Disease:* How does the patient's disease or condition affect the body and its normal metabolic functions?
3. *Nutrition therapy:* Prioritize diagnoses on the basis of urgency, impact, and resources. How and why must the diet change to meet the needs created by the patient's particular disease or condition?
4. *Food plan:* How do these necessary nutritional modifications affect daily food choices? Write a nutrition prescription that is focused on the etiology to meet these needs.

Mode of feeding. The primary principle of diet therapy is based on a patient's normal nutrition requirements, and it is only modified as an individual's specific condition requires. Nutrition components of the oral diet may be modified in the following ways:

1. *Energy:* The total energy value of the diet, expressed in kilocalories, may be increased or decreased.
2. *Nutrients:* One or more of the essential nutrients (i.e., protein, carbohydrate, fat, minerals, vitamins, and water) may be modified in amount or form.
3. *Texture:* The texture or seasoning of the diet may be modified (e.g., liquid and low-residue diets).

In the event that nutrient needs cannot be adequately satisfied through oral intake, other methods of nutrient delivery must be considered. When a patient's gastrointestinal tract is functioning but he or she cannot consume food orally, **enteral** feedings are an

enteral a mode of feeding that makes use of the gastrointestinal tract through oral or tube feeding.

option. Enteral feedings are administered by a tube and make use of the digestion and absorption functions of the gastrointestinal tract at some point below the mouth. Feeding tubes are placed within the gastrointestinal tract at the point at which the patient is able to tolerate introduction of food or nutrients. The tube may pass through the nasal cavity down the esophagus to the stomach or small intestine for short-term feedings, or the tube may be surgically placed into the gastrointestinal tract for long-term enteral feedings. Details about when enteral feedings are used, placement of tubes, and types of formula are discussed further in Chapter 22.

If patients are unable to tolerate any nutrient delivery into the gastrointestinal tract, health care providers must consider **parenteral** nutrition therapy. Parenteral nutrition therapy is administered intravenously and thus carries risks associated with its invasive nature. However, it is an effective way of meeting the nutrient needs of a patient whose gastrointestinal tract is not functioning. Chapter 22 also covers parenteral nutrition therapy in greater detail.

Nutrition Education and Counseling

Communicating with a patient about his or her specific nutrition intervention plan is a critical step in the potential success of the treatment. Patients and families who understand the necessary changes to food or nutrient delivery methods are able to appreciate the benefit from such adjustments and are more likely to be compliant. Education may be a one-on-one experience with the dietitian, or it may occur in a group setting. Initial education and counseling interactions during inpatient stays can continue through outpatient appointments, when necessary.

Nutrition intervention plans are generally long-term lifestyle modifications that are meant to promote and improve health. Some patients will have more changes to make than others, and they will need continued nutrition counseling support to reach one goal at a time. Establishing a long-term plan to make such changes takes a commitment to education, counseling, and both professional and personal support. The plan of care will be modified over time as needed and in response to intervention.

Coordination of Nutrition Care

Several health care providers may be involved in a nutrition intervention plan. For example, enteral tube feedings will require the coordination of dietitians, nurses, the prescribing physician, and possibly the clinical pharmacist. Interdisciplinary connections within health care make the coordination of nutrition care possible and more effective. In addition, family, friends, care providers, and other members of the patient's personal support group may be helpful during the coordination of the patient's care. All professional and personal resources and referrals necessary to carry out and maintain the intervention should be identified during this step.

NUTRITION MONITORING AND EVALUATION

Nutrition monitoring and evaluation identifies patient outcomes relevant to the nutrition diagnosis and the intervention plan. This step measures progress toward the patient's goals. The three components of this process are as follows: (1) monitor progress, (2) measure outcomes, and (3) evaluate outcomes.[2]

Outcome measures that are used during this step are organized into the same categories as the nutrition assessment categories, excluding client history, as outlined below.

> **parenteral** a mode of feeding that does not make use of the gastrointestinal tract but that instead provides nutrition support via the intravenous delivery of nutrient solutions.

FOOD-/NUTRITION-RELATED HISTORY OUTCOMES	ANTHROPOMETRIC MEASUREMENT OUTCOMES	BIOCHEMICAL DATA, MEDICAL TESTS, AND PROCEDURE OUTCOMES	NUTRITION-FOCUSED PHYSICAL FINDING OUTCOMES
• Food and nutrient intake • Food and nutrient administration • Medication, complementary/alternative medicine use • Knowledge and beliefs • Availability of food and supplies • Physical activity, nutrition quality of life	• Height • Weight • Body mass index • Growth pattern indices and percentile ranks • Weight history	• Lab data (e.g., electrolytes, glucose) and tests (e.g., gastric emptying time, resting metabolic rate)	• Physical appearance • Muscle and fat wasting • Swallow function • Appetite • Affect

Academy of Nutrition and Dietetics. *Nutrition Care Process SNAPshots*. Cited February 2015; available from www.andeal.org/ncp.

Depending on the care plan, nutrition professionals will collect data that are pertinent to the outcome goals and then compare these data with the patient's previous status to assess progress. Efficacy of the care plan is assessed, and changes are made, if necessary. If changes are not necessary and the patient's goals have been satisfied, the dietitian may discharge the patient from nutrition services at this point.

DIET-DRUG INTERACTIONS

Many negative reactions can occur with polypharmacy, especially among elderly patients, who may also take several dietary supplements and herbal products. Almost half of the U.S. population takes at least one prescription drug per day, 20.6% take three or more, and 10.1% take five or more prescription drugs every day.[19] Patients may respond quite differently from one another, depending on normal dietary habits, the specific disease being treated, compliance, and other medications or supplements that are currently being taken. In addition, there are several different mechanisms in which diet-drug interactions may be classified, each with varying degrees of clinical outcome potentials (Table 17-3).[20] Note that *diet-drug interactions* may be expressed in several different ways, such as drug-diet interactions, food-medication interactions, drug-nutrient interactions, and drug-food interactions. In most cases throughout this text, and elsewhere, the expression *"drug-nutrient interaction"* is used. In this section we are discussing more than single nutrient interactions with medications; thus, the term *diet-drug interactions* is appropriate.

Gathering information about all drug use is essential to the care process; this includes over-the-counter medications, prescribed medications, as well as alcohol and street drugs. Because diet-drug interactions involve medications prescribed by a physician, dispensed by a pharmacist, and food or nutrients consumed by patients, the responsibility for knowledge of such interactions extends to the physician, pharmacist, and dietitian. The nurse must be particularly familiar with diet-drug interactions as well, because it is the nurse who is most commonly administering both items to patients. The bottom line is that all members of the health care team should be aware of potential diet-drug reactions and communicate regularly.

Below is a brief description of the different types of diet-drug interactions. It is not within the scope of this textbook to extensively cover the many possible diet-drug interactions. There are Drug-Nutrient Interaction boxes throughout the text to highlight common interactions of interest within each chapter. Pocket guides such as *Food-Medication Interactions* (www.foodmedinteractions.com) are valuable for onsite reference. Box 17-3 provides a brief list of resources for well-known diet-drug interactions.

DRUG-FOOD INTERACTIONS

Interactions in which food increases or decreases the effect of a drug can adversely influence the health of a patient. Certain foods may affect the absorption, distribution, metabolism, or elimination of a drug, thereby altering the intended dose response. The timing, size, and composition of meals relative to medication administration are all common causes of drug-food

Table 17-3 Classification of Drug-Nutrient Interactions

PRECIPITATING FACTOR	OBJECT OF THE INTERACTION	POTENTIAL CONSEQUENCE	EXAMPLES
Nutrition status	Drug	Treatment failure or drug toxicity	**Obesity** causes lower *ertapenem* concentration following a standard dose, but toxicity of *acyclovir* following a usual dose **Vitamin C** deficiency prolongs *pentobarbital* action
Food or food component	Drug	Treatment failure or drug toxicity	**Enteral nutrition** formula impairs absorption of *ciprofloxacin* **Food** can interfere with *levodopa* and *alendronate* absorption, but improves absorption of *deferasirox* and *gabapentin-enacarbil* **Grapefruit juice** increases *nilotinib* bioavailability and *simvastatin* toxicity
Specific nutrient or other dietary supplement ingredient	Drug	Treatment failure or drug toxicity	**Iron** sulfate reduces *doxycycline* concentration when taken together **Vitamin C** may reduce *fluconazole* activity **Vitamin D** reduces *atorvastatin* concentration **Daidzein** increases bioavailability and reduces clearance of *theophylline*
Drug	Nutrition status	Altered nutrition status	**Capecitabine** may cause *hypertriglyceridemia* Low-dose **quetiqapine** causes significant weight gain **Sorafenib** is associated with sarcopenia
Drug	Specific nutrient	Altered nutrient status	**Carbamazepine** lowers *vitamin D* and *biotin* status **Ezetimibe** reduces *vitamin E* absorption **Isoniazid** impairs vitamin B_6 status **Ribavirin** plus **peginterferon-α2b** impairs *vitamin* B_{12} status

From: Boullata JI and Hudson LM. Drug-nutrient interactions: a broad view with implications for practice. *J Acad Nutr Diet*. 2012;112(4):506-517.

- Avoid Food-Drug Interactions: *A Guide from the National Consumers League and U.S. Food and Drug Administration:* www.fda.gov/downloads/drugs/resourcesforyou/consumers/buyingusingmedicinesafely/ensuringsafeuseofmedicine/generaluseofmedicine/ucm229033.pdf
- Food-Medication Interactions: www.foodmedinteractions.com
- National Center for Biotechnology Information, US National Library of Medicine, National Institutes of Health. PubMed Health: www.ncbi.nlm.nih.gov/pubmedhealth
- Nutrient-Drug Interactions and Food: www.ext.colostate.edu/pubs/foodnut/09361.html

interactions. For example, a high-fat meal increases the absorption of some drugs that are lipophilic (i.e., "fat loving"), whereas a high-fiber meal may bind other drugs and reduce their absorption.

The interaction of grapefruit juice and several medications has been under critical evaluation during recent years. A substance called *furanocoumarin* in grapefruit juice can dramatically alter the bioavailability of certain drugs to a dangerous level.[21] The anticoagulation medication warfarin is a commonly prescribed drug for patients with heart disease, and it is also one of the most highly interactive medications with certain foods, specifically with those that are high in vitamin K, such as green, leafy vegetables.[22] Other examples of drug-food interactions would be as follows: (1) medications that interfere with the appetite as a result of changes in taste or smell sensations (e.g., amitriptyline, metronidazole); and (2) medications that stimulate the appetite (e.g., antihistamines, steroids). Over time, these alterations in appetite may affect nutritional status.

DRUG-NUTRIENT INTERACTIONS

Drug-nutrient interactions are often reactions that occur when medications are taken in combination with over-the-counter vitamin and mineral supplements (see the Clinical Applications box, "Case Study: Drug-Nutrient Interaction"). As mentioned, the patient's use of vitamin and mineral supplements is not always reported to physicians or pharmacists. Patients should be asked what other medications they are taking, with specific questions asked about their vitamin and mineral supplement use. Drug-nutrient interactions may result in the depletion of a nutrient, or the nutrient may induce a change in the rate of metabolism of the drug (see Table 17-3). The Cultural Considerations box entitled "Prescription Medication and Dietary Supplement Use" discusses the prevalence and common demographic traits of patients who are taking both dietary supplements and prescription medications.

Clinical Applications

Case Study: Drug-Nutrient Interaction

Linda, a 24-year-old woman, reported to her doctor with symptoms that included fatigue; headaches; muscle, joint, and bone pain; dry, flaking skin; amenorrhea; hair loss; depression; nausea and vomiting; and weight loss. After a physical examination and laboratory work, Linda was determined to have liver damage. The only prescription medication that Linda takes is isotretinoin (Accutane) for acne. Isotretinoin is known as 13-*cis*-retinoic acid, and it is a vitamin A–related compound. She also reported taking several dietary supplements, including a multivitamin, a vitamin E supplement, and a vitamin D supplement, each of which contains 500% of the Recommended Dietary Allowance of its respective vitamin; an antioxidant liquid mix that contains β-carotene; and an occasional high-antioxidant supplement containing vitamins A, C, and E, zinc, and selenium.

1. Could Linda's dietary supplement use have anything to do with her liver problems? Why?
2. Using resources such as those provided in Box 17-3 or www.drugs.com, research isotretinoin. What foods or nutrients should be avoided when taking isotretinoin?
3. What would you counsel Linda to do regarding her supplement and medication use?
4. Linda also mentions that she is trying to become pregnant. Would you recommend that she change anything with regard to her supplement or medication use?

DRUG-HERB INTERACTIONS

Interactions that involve prescription drugs and herbs are the least well-defined drug interactions. St. John's wort (*Hypericum perforatum*), which is one of the most commonly taken herbs, has been extensively studied for drug interactions. The exact mechanism by which St. John's wort, an antidepressant, interacts with medications varies.[23,24] This herb is thought to have the most drug-herb interactions of the commonly used herbal products, some of which are clinically severe, but not all of which are unfavorable. Medication groups that have documented adverse reactions when taken with St. John's wort include antihistamines; bronchodilators; cardiovascular medications; oral contraceptives; nonsteroidal antiinflammatory medications; corticosteroids; opioids; antimicrobials; anticancer medications; immunosuppressants; hypoglycemic agents; and drugs that act on the gastrointestinal tract.[25]

Other commonly used herbs that are involved in drug interactions include ginkgo (*Ginkgo biloba*), ginger (*Zingiber officinale*), ginseng (*Panax ginseng*), and garlic (*Allium sativum*).[26] Many herbs also have clinically documented medicinal properties and should be evaluated on an individual basis to determine their appropriateness with the patient's current dietary habits and prescribed medications.

🌐 Cultural Considerations

Prescription Medication and Dietary Supplement Use

The concurrent use of prescription medications and dietary supplements is common in the United States. About half of adults report regular use of dietary supplements. If you also include adults who take dietary supplements occasionally or seasonally, the estimates are that 66% of the population uses various forms of vitamin/mineral or herbal dietary supplements.[1] Meanwhile, about half of the adult population is also regularly taking prescription medications.[2]

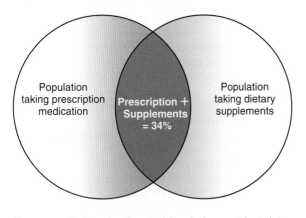

Because of the significant risk of drug-nutrient interactions, nondisclosure of supplement use presents a problem for both health care providers and patients simultaneously taking prescription medications. Although there are always exceptions, some common demographic traits of adults in the United States who take both dietary supplements and prescription medications are as follows[3]:

- Female
- ≥60 years old
- Higher education (college graduate)
- Higher income (≥$75,000)

As discussed in the Drug-Nutrient Interaction box "Dietary Supplement Use," nondisclosure of supplement use is a common problem and a health risk. With one third of the adult population using *both* dietary supplements and prescription medications,[3] it is imperative for health care providers to specifically ask patients about their use of supplements. It is helpful to understand the high use of supplements among certain demographic groups so that extra attention may be given to the matter when working with these patients.

REFERENCES

1. Dickinson A, MacKay D. Health habits and other characteristics of dietary supplement users: a review. *Nutr J.* 2014;13:14.
2. National Center for Health Statistics. *Health, United States, 2014: with special feature of adults aged 55-64.* Hyattsville, Md: U.S. Government Printing Office; 2015.
3. Farina EK, Austin KG, Lieberman HR. Concomitant dietary supplement and prescription medication use is prevalent among US adults with doctor-informed medical conditions. *J Acad Nutr Diet.* 2014;114(11):1784-1790 e2.

Putting It All Together

Summary

- The basis for effective nutrition care begins with the patient's nutrition needs and must involve the patient and his or her family. Such person-centered care requires initial assessment and planning by the dietitian and continuous close teamwork among all team members who are providing primary care.
- The careful assessment of factors that influence nutrition status requires a broad foundation of pertinent information (e.g., physiologic, psychosocial, medical, personal). The patient's medical record is a basic means of communication among health care team members.
- Nutrition therapy is based on the personal and physical needs of the patient. Successful therapy requires a close working relationship among dietetic, medical, and nursing staff in the health care facility. The nurse is in a unique position to reinforce the nutrition principles of the diet with the patient and his or her family.
- Drug interactions with nutrients, foods, or other medications can present complications with patient care. Careful questioning to determine all prescription and over-the-counter supplements and medications that are being taken will help to guide the patient's education needs.

Chapter Review Questions

See answers in Appendix A.

1. A simple measurement that can help indicate risk for chronic disease when used independent of other measurements is:
   a. Waist circumference.
   b. Serum albumin level.
   c. Knee height.
   d. Body weight.

2. A patient has just been diagnosed with type 2 diabetes and needs help to determine a healthy energy intake. The most appropriate member of the health care team to help with this is the:
   a. Registered nurse.
   b. Physician.
   c. Registered dietitian.
   d. Pharmacist.

3. The four steps included in the Nutrition Care Process are:
   a. Planning, intervention, diagnosis, monitoring, and evaluation.
   b. Planning, intervention, monitoring, follow-up, and evaluation.
   c. Assessment, diagnosis, intervention, monitoring, and evaluation.
   d. Assessment, diagnosis, planning, follow-up, and discharge.

4. Warfarin can interact with certain types of foods that are high in:
   a. Vitamin K.
   b. Vitamin B
   c. Potassium.
   d. Iron.

5. With regard to nutrition intervention, the role of the nurse on the health care team for a patient who has just been diagnosed with chronic kidney disease is to:
   a. Assess protein, calorie, and fluid requirements required each day.
   b. Reinforce the nutrition principles of the diet with the patient and family.
   c. Develop a meal plan that will be the most satisfying to the patient.
   d. Determine the most appropriate dietary supplement regimen for the patient.

Additional Learning Resources

evolve Please refer to this text's Evolve website for answers to the Case Study questions.
http://evolve.elsevier.com/Williams/basic/

References and **Further Reading and Resources** in the back of the book provide additional resources for enhancing knowledge.

18 Gastrointestinal and Accessory Organ Problems

Key Concepts

- Diseases of the gastrointestinal (GI) tract and its accessory organs interrupt the body's normal cycle of digestion, absorption, and metabolism.
- Food allergies result from an inappropriate immune response to certain proteins found in food.
- Underlying genetic diseases may cause metabolic defects that block the body's ability to handle specific foods.

The body's highly organized and intricate system for handling food is often taken for granted. However, when something goes wrong with the system, the whole body is affected. The gastrointestinal (GI) tract is a sensitive mirror, both directly and indirectly, of the individual human condition.

This chapter looks at the system that manages food and its nutrients. The digestive process works as a series of cascading events throughout the GI tract and the accessory organs: the pancreas, the liver, and the gallbladder. Nutrition therapy must be based on the functioning of this finely integrated network and on the person whose life it affects.

THE UPPER GASTROINTESTINAL TRACT

Diseases may affect the GI tract anywhere from the mouth to the anus. The most commonly affected areas of the GI tract are discussed in this chapter under the headings that state where the primary problems exist.

MOUTH

Dental Problems

Although the incidence of dental caries has declined somewhat during recent years, tooth decay still plagues children and adults. Some of the decline is attributed to the increased use of fluoridated public water and toothpaste as well as better dental hygiene. Fluoride toothpastes are effective for preventing dental caries at fluoride concentrations of ≥1000 ppm in children and adolescents.[1,2] In elderly people, loss of teeth or the presence of ill-fitting dentures is associated with food avoidance and compromised overall nutrition.[3,4] Specifically, foods such as whole fruits, vegetables, meats, and other high-fiber foods are frequently avoided and excess calories from high-fat and high-sugar foods are consumed. About half of the older adults in the United States have severe tooth loss (i.e.,

0 to 10 teeth remaining) and this prevalence is more pronounced in lower socioeconomic status populations (see the Cultural Considerations box, "Social Disparities and Dental Status").[3,5] Sometimes a **mechanical soft diet** is helpful for individuals who are lacking teeth. For such a diet, all foods are soft cooked, and meats are ground and mixed with sauces or gravies so that less chewing is necessary.

Surgical Procedures

A fractured jaw or other surgeries that involve the mouth and neck pose obvious eating problems. Nutrients must be supplied, usually in the form of high-protein, high-caloric liquids. Table 18-1 provides an example of a simple milkshake. Other prepared commercial formulas are also available and discussed in Chapter 22. As healing progresses, soft foods that require little chewing effort can be added, with the individual progressing to a full diet in accordance with his or her personal tolerance.

Oral Tissue Inflammation

Tissues of the mouth often reflect a person's general nutrition status. Malnutrition—especially severe states—causes the deterioration of the oral tissues, which may result in local infection or injury that brings pain and difficulty with eating. The following conditions of the oral cavity can contribute to malnutrition:

- *Gingivitis:* inflammation of the gums that involves the mucous membrane and its supporting fibrous tissue that circles the base of the teeth (Figure 18-1, *A*)

> **mechanical soft diet** a meal plan that consists of foods that have been chopped, blended, ground, or prepared with extra fluid to make chewing and swallowing easier.

Social Disparities and Dental Status

Large-scale National Health and Nutrition Examination Studies (NHANES) indicate that loss of teeth is highly associated with older age, lower income, and less education in the United States. In addition, black Americans are more prone to tooth loss than other racial segments of the population. However, if income and education are regulated, black people have no greater risk of tooth loss than white people.[1]

As such, there are strong public health implications for which population subgroups to target for education and intervention to decrease tooth loss. Health coverage for dental care is not available to everyone; particularly the elderly population and low-income individuals may not be able to afford such services. Less than half of adults more than 51 years of age in the United States have dental insurance. Although addressing means to overcome poverty and low socioeconomic class is not a typical responsibility of most health care workers, education for oral hygiene is relatively easy and quick to address. Even without twice yearly dental visits, the act of brushing and flossing teeth regularly greatly reduces tooth loss in all ethnic and socioeconomic sects of the population.[2]

Given the health care implications and morbidity associated with the loss of teeth, improving oral hygiene and retention of healthy teeth is a reasonable goal for improving overall health.

REFERENCES

1. Wu B, et al. Social stratification and tooth loss among middle-aged and older Americans from 1988 to 2004. *Commun Dent Oral Epidemiol.* 2014;42(6):495-502.
2. Liang J, et al. Social stratification, oral hygiene, and trajectories of dental caries among old Americans. *J Aging Health.* 2014; 26(6):900-923.

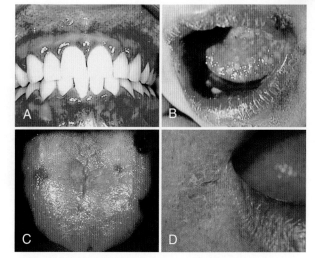

FIGURE 18-1 Tissue inflammation of the mouth. **A,** Gingivitis. **B,** Stomatitis. **C,** Glossitis. **D,** Cheilosis. (**A,** Reprinted from Murray PR, Rosenthal KS, Pfaller MA. *Medical Microbiology.* 2nd ed. St Louis: Mosby; 1994. **B,** Reprinted from Doughty DB, Broadwell-Jackson D. *Gastrointestinal Disorders.* St Louis: Mosby; 1993. **C,** Reprinted from Hoffbrand AV, Pettit JE, eds. *Sandoz Atlas of Clinical Hematology.* London: Gower Medical; 1988. **D,** Reprinted from Lemmi FO, Lemmi CAE. *Physical Assessment Findings* [CD-ROM]. Philadelphia: Saunders; 2000.)

Table 18-1	High-Protein, High-Kilocalorie Formula for Liquid Feedings*†
INGREDIENT	**AMOUNT**
Whole milk, 3.25% milk fat	1 cup
Egg substitute powder	0.35 oz or equivalent of 2 eggs
Ensure Plus	½ cup
Sugar, granulated	2 Tbsp
Ice cream, vanilla	½ cup
Vanilla flavoring	A few drops, as desired

*Approximate food value: 23 g of protein, 22 g of fat, 80 g of carbohydrate, and 618 kcal.
†Prepackaged supplemental feedings are generally used instead of homemade liquid feedings.

- *Stomatitis:* inflammation of the oral mucous lining of the mouth (Figure 18-1, *B*)
- *Glossitis:* inflammation of the tongue (Figure 18-1, *C*)
- *Cheilosis:* a dry, scaling process at the corners of the mouth that affects the lips and the corner angles, thereby making opening the mouth to eat uncomfortable (Figure 18-1, *D*)

Mouth ulcers may develop from three infectious sources: (1) the herpes simplex virus, which causes mouth sores on the inside mucous lining of the cheeks and lips or on the external portion of the lips, where they are commonly called *cold sores* or *fever blisters;* (2) *Candida albicans,* which is a fungus that causes similar sores on the oral mucosa and results in a condition called *candidiasis* or *thrush;* and (3) hemolytic *Streptococcus,* which is a bacteria that causes the mucosal ulcers that are commonly called *canker sores.* Mouth ulcers are usually self-limiting and short lived. Other causes include simple toothbrush abrasions and allergies. Patients with an underlying illness such as cancer or human immunodeficiency virus (HIV)—both of which diminish the body's immune system—often have mouth ulcers. Chemotherapy and radiation treatment to the mouth destroy the fast-replicating cells and can result in painful mouth sores (see Chapter 23).

In these situations, eating may be painful. Progressing from nutritionally dense liquids that are high in protein and calories to soft foods (e.g., nonacidic and bland to avoid irritation) is usually well tolerated. Extremes in temperature are avoided if they cause discomfort. Room-temperature soft or liquid foods are usually better accepted. For a person suffering from mouth pain, a mouthwash that contains a mild topical local anesthetic before meals helps to relieve the irritation that can be caused by eating. In severe cases or cases that last more than 7 to 10 days, a nutrition assessment may be warranted to ensure adequate nutritional needs are being met.

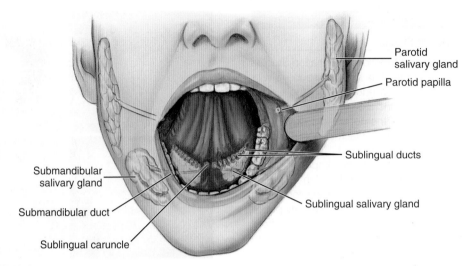

FIGURE 18-2 Location of the salivary glands. (Reprinted from Fehrenbach MJ, Herring SW. *Illustrated Anatomy of the Head and Neck.* 3rd ed. St Louis: Saunders; 2007.)

Salivary Glands

Disorders of the salivary glands in the mouth (Figure 18-2) also affect eating and related nutrition status. Problems may arise from infection, such as the mumps virus that attacks the **parotid gland.** Other problems arise from mucous cysts (i.e., mucoceles) and obstructed salivary ducts, usually on the lower lip or the insides of the cheeks. Both excess salivation and inadequate salivation can interfere with eating and salivary gland function. Excess salivation is seen with numerous disorders that affect the nervous system, local mouth infections, injuries, and drug reactions. Conversely, a dry mouth from a lack of salivation may be temporary and caused by fear, infection, or a drug reaction. Chronic dry mouth, which is called *xerostomia,* sometimes occurs in middle-aged and elderly adults, and it is often associated with rheumatoid arthritis or radiation therapy, or it may occur as a side effect from many drugs that are taken on a long-term basis. Xerostomia causes swallowing and speaking difficulties, taste interference, and tooth decay. The addition of more liquid food items to regular meals such as beverages, soups, stews, juicy fruits, and gravies or sauces may facilitate the eating process. Extreme mouth dryness may be partially relieved by spraying an artificial saliva solution inside the mouth.

Swallowing Disorders

Swallowing is not as simple an act as it may seem. It involves highly integrated actions of the mouth, the **pharynx,** and the esophagus; in addition, after it has been started, swallowing is beyond voluntary control. Swallowing difficulty is a fairly common problem with a variety of causes. It may be only temporary (e.g., as a result of a piece of food lodged in the back of the throat), and the **Heimlich maneuver** may be appropriate first aid. However, **dysphagia** is a more

chronic problem in some patients, and it is particularly common among patients with neurologic disorders such as Alzheimer's disease, Parkinson's disease, and stroke complications. Other common causes of dysphagia are head and neck cancer, tooth loss, xerostomia, and muscular weakness of the larynx. To treat dysphagia effectively, the problem must be identified as either a mechanical obstruction or a neuromuscular disorder, and it is usually diagnosed by a **speech-language pathologist.**

parotid glands the largest of the three pairs of salivary glands; the parotid glands lie, one on each side, above the angle of the jaw and below and in front of the ear; they continually secrete saliva, which passes along the duct of the gland and into the mouth through an opening in the inner cheek that is level with the second upper molar tooth.

pharynx the muscular membranous passage that extends from the mouth to the posterior nasal passages, the larynx, and the esophagus.

Heimlich maneuver (current term is abdominal thrusts) a first-aid maneuver that is used to relieve a person who is choking from the blockage of the breathing passageway by a swallowed foreign object or food particle; to perform the maneuver, when standing behind the choking person, clasp the victim around the waist, place one fist just under the sternum (i.e., the breastbone), grasp the fist with the other hand, and then make a quick, hard, thrusting movement inward and upward to dislodge the object.

dysphagia difficulty swallowing.

speech-language pathologist a specialist in the assessment, diagnosis, treatment, and prevention of speech, language, cognitive communication, voice, swallowing, fluency, and other related disorders.

Subtle symptoms of dysphagia include an unexplained drop in food intake or repeated episodes of pneumonia related to aspiration. Patients with dysphagia have longer hospital stays, compromised nutritional statuses, and increased mortality risks compared with similar patients without dysphagia.[6,7] Watch for warning signs of dysphagia, and report them immediately. These signs may include the reluctance to eat certain food consistencies or any food at all, very slow chewing or eating, fatigue from eating, frequent throat clearing, complaints of food "sticking" in the throat, pockets of food held in the cheeks, painful swallowing, regurgitation, and coughing or choking during attempts to eat.

The problem usually is referred to a team of specialists that includes a physician, a nurse, a dietitian, and a speech-language pathologist. Thin liquids are the most difficult food form to swallow. Thus, the diet is adapted to individual needs in stages of thickened liquids and pureed foods. Pureed foods are generally the consistency of mashed potatoes or pudding. Regular table food can be pureed in a food processor to achieve the desired consistency. Several manufacturers produce pureed foods or food molds that are shaped like various meats or vegetables. Placing pureed food in a food mold to take the shape of the original food (e.g., corn on the cob, a chicken breast) enhances the appeal and appetite of patients who are faced with swallowing disorders, and it has been shown to improve overall nutrition intake.[8]

ESOPHAGUS

Central Tube

The esophagus is a long, muscular tube that extends from the throat to the stomach. It is bound on both ends by circular muscles or sphincters that act as valves to control the passage of food. The upper sphincter muscle remains closed except during swallowing, thereby preventing airflow into the esophagus and the stomach. The sphincter automatically opens when swallowing and then closes immediately afterward. Various disorders along the tube may disrupt normal swallowing, including muscle spasms or uncoordinated contractions as well as the stricture or narrowing of the tube caused by a scar from a previous injury, the ingestion of caustic chemicals, a tumor, or esophagitis. These problems hinder eating and require medical attention through stretching procedures or surgery to widen the tube in addition to drug therapy to heal the inflammation. The diet during such problems ranges from liquid to soft in texture, depending on the extent of the problem and individual tolerance.

Lower Esophageal Sphincter

Defects in the function of the lower esophageal sphincter (LES) may come from changes in the smooth muscle itself or from the nerve, muscle, and hormone control of peristalsis (see Chapter 5). Spasms occur when the LES muscles maintain an excessively high muscle tone, even while resting, thereby failing to open normally when the person swallows. This condition is medically termed achalasia because of its tense muscle state, but it is commonly called *cardiospasm* because of its proximity of the heart (although the condition does not relate to the heart). Symptoms include difficulty swallowing, frequent vomiting, a feeling of fullness in the chest, weight loss, malnutrition, and pulmonary complications and infections caused by the aspiration of food particles, especially during sleep.

Surgical treatment of achalasia involves dilating or cutting (*esophagomyotomy*) the LES muscles. Both procedures can improve the relaxation of the LES, but neither affects the lack of peristalsis. The postoperative nutrition therapy starts with oral liquids and progresses to a regular diet within a few days, depending on tolerance. Patients should avoid very hot or cold foods, citrus juices, and highly spiced foods to prevent irritation. It is also helpful for patients to eat frequent small meals as tolerated, eat slowly, take small bites, and thoroughly chew their food.

Gastroesophageal Reflux Disease

Gastroesophageal reflux disease (GERD) is a serious and difficult problem that has been described as acid "setting up shop" in the esophagus. Unlike the stomach, the esophageal tissue is not protected by mucus from the corrosive acidic content. The constant regurgitation of acidic gastric contents into the lower part of the esophagus results in erosive esophagitis in about half of the patients with this disease (Figure 18-3). Impaired esophageal peristalsis, prolonged LES relaxation, and hiatal hernias are common contributors to chronic GERD.[9,10] Typical symptoms include frequent and severe heartburn within an hour after eating, dysphagia, and excessive belching. The pain sometimes moves into the neck or jaw or down the arms. Long-term complications include stenosis (i.e., a narrowing or stricture of the esophagus), esophageal ulcer, and Barrett's esophagus.

Acid reflux may be attributed to pregnancy, pernicious vomiting, or the extended use of nasogastric tubes. Elderly patients tend to experience more severe cases and complications of GERD compared with younger adults.[11,12] The risk for GERD symptoms and

---

esophagitis inflammation of the esophagus.

achalasia a disorder of the esophagus in which the muscles of the tube fail to relax, thereby inhibiting normal swallowing.

Barrett's esophagus complication of severe gastroesophageal reflux disease in which the squamous cell epithelium of the esophagus changes to resemble the tissue lining the small intestine; increases the risk of esophageal adenocarcinoma.

erosive esophagitis increases with obesity and waist circumference compared with a normal body mass index, thus indicating that overweight patients may respond well to weight-reduction strategies.[13] In addition to weight loss, other conservative measures and dietary goals are outlined in Table 18-2. Proton pump inhibitors (PPIs) are the mainstay of pharmacologic treatment for GERD symptoms and are effective in most patients. **Laparoscopic fundoplication** is a surgical procedure that restores LES function and esophageal peristalsis, thereby treating the condition and not just the symptoms. This procedure is highly successful and

is recommended for patients who cannot be managed with PPI therapy due to complicating side effects from the medication.[14]

Hiatal Hernia

The lower end of the esophagus normally enters the chest cavity through an opening in the diaphragm called the *hiatus*. A hiatal hernia occurs when a portion of the upper stomach also protrudes through this opening, as shown in Figure 18-4. Hiatal hernias are not uncommon, especially in obese adults, for whom weight reduction is essential. Patients with hiatal hernias are advised to eat small amounts of food at a time, to avoid lying down after meals, and to sleep with the head of the bed elevated to prevent the reflux of acidic stomach contents. The frequent use of antacids helps to control the symptoms of heartburn, which is caused by the acid, enzyme, and food mixture irritating the lower esophagus and the upper herniated area of the stomach. Large hiatal hernias or smaller sliding hernias typically require surgical repair.

STOMACH AND DUODENUM: PEPTIC ULCER DISEASE

The mucosal lining of the stomach and duodenum protects the tissue from corrosive gastric acid and enzymatic secretions. If the mucosa is weakened or disturbed and cannot protect against acidic gastric contents, the tissue is damaged. The general term

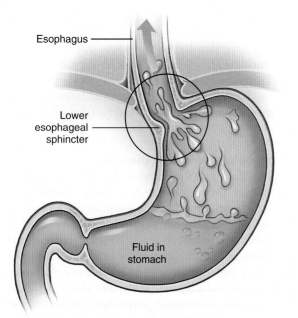

FIGURE 18-3 Reflux of gastric acid up into the esophagus through the lower esophageal sphincter in a patient with gastroesophageal reflux disease. (Reprinted from Thibodeau GA, Patton KT. *Anatomy & Physiology.* 7th ed. St Louis: Mosby; 2010.)

> **laparoscopic fundoplication** a surgery that is used to treat gastroesophageal reflux disease; the upper portion of the stomach (i.e., the fundus) is wrapped around the esophagus and sewn into place so that the esophagus passes through the muscle of the stomach; this strengthens the esophageal sphincter to prevent acid reflux.

Table 18-2 Dietary Care of Gastroesophageal Reflux Disease

GOAL	ACTION
Decrease esophageal irritation	Avoid common irritants such as coffee, strong tea, chocolate, carbonated beverages, tomato and citrus juices, spicy foods, smoking, and alcoholic beverages
Increase lower esophageal sphincter pressure	Ensure adequate intake of lean protein foods Avoid excessive high-fat meals (e.g., fried foods, high-fat meats, cream) Avoid peppermint and spearmint Avoid medications that reduce LES pressure (e.g., anticholinergics, calcium channel blockers, opiates, progesterone)
Decrease reflux frequency and volume	Eat small, frequent meals Sip small amounts of liquid with meals; drink mostly between meals Avoid constipation by consuming adequate fiber and water and avoiding sedentary behaviors; straining increases abdominal pressure reflux Avoid eating at least 3 to 4 hours before going to bed
Clear food materials from the esophagus	Sit upright at the table, and elevate the head of the bed Do not recline for ≥2 hours after eating Wear loose-fitting clothing, especially after a meal

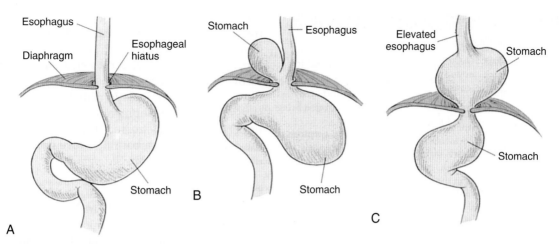

FIGURE 18-4 Hiatal hernia compared with normal stomach placement. **A,** Normal stomach. **B,** Paraesophageal hernia, with the esophagus in its normal position. **C,** Esophageal hiatal hernia, with an elevated esophagus. (Courtesy Bill Ober.)

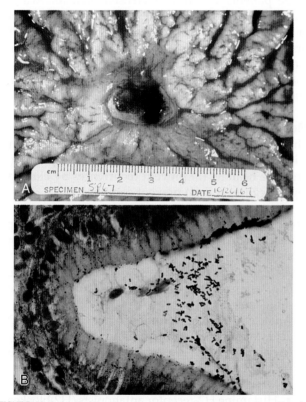

FIGURE 18-5 **A,** Gastric ulcer. **B,** *Helicobacter pylori (black particles)* infecting the stomach mucosa. (Reprinted from Patton KT, Thibodeau GA: *Anatomy & Physiology.* 9th ed. St Louis: Mosby; 2016.)

peptic ulcer refers to an eroded mucosal lesion in the central portion of the GI tract. This lesion can occur in the lower esophagus, the stomach, or the first portion of the duodenum (i.e., the duodenal bulb). Ulcers are common in the duodenal bulb because the gastric contents emptying there are the most concentrated. A peptic ulcer is a crater-like lesion in the wall of the stomach or duodenum that results from the continuous erosion of the tissue through the mucosal layers down to the muscular layers (Figure 18-5, *A*). In extreme cases, the ulcer can perforate.

Etiology

The two most common causes of peptic ulcer disease (PUD) are *H. pylori* infection and the long-term use of nonsteroidal antiinflammatory drugs (NSAIDs).[15] Lesion generally results from an imbalance among some or all of the following three factors: (1) the amount of gastric acid and pepsin secretions; (2) the extent of *Helicobacter pylori* infection; and (3) the degree of tissue resistance and mucosal integrity.

Helicobacter pylori. H. pylori are common, spiraling, rod-shaped bacteria that inhabit the GI area around the pyloric valve (Figure 18-5, *B*). This muscular valve connects the lower part of the stomach with the duodenal bulb. Acidic environments are favorable for *H. pylori* colonization. Infection by *H. pylori* is a major determinant of chronic active gastritis, and it is a critical ingredient, along with gastric acid and pepsin, in the ulcerative process. *H. pylori* infection is common in all areas of the world but not all people with the bacteria will develop an ulcer. As a result of aggressive treatment for *H. pylori* infection, the global incidence rate of PUD has decreased during recent years.[16] The For Further Focus box entitled "Risk for Gastric Ulcer Disease" discusses additional risk factors for PUD and *H. pylori.*

Nonsteroidal antiinflammatory drugs. NSAIDs are widely used medications. This drug class includes ibuprofen (Advil, Motrin) and aspirin (acetylsalicylic acid). Prolonged or excessive use of NSAIDs irritates the gastric mucosa, decreases the mucosal integrity, and may result in erosion, ulceration, and bleeding. The NSAIDs, including at least a dozen antiinflammatory drugs, are so named to distinguish them from steroid drugs, which are synthetic variants of natural adrenal hormones.

Psychologic factors. The influence of psychologic factors in the development of PUD varies. No distinct

Risk for Gastric Ulcer Disease

Before the bacteria *Helicobacter pylori* was shown in 1982 to be the causative organism of peptic ulcer disease, the disease was thought to be the result of excess stress, acid, and spicy food. Although these factors may still exacerbate the disease, infection with *H. pylori* is now known to cause the majority of duodenal and gastric ulcers; the long-term use of nonsteroidal anti-inflammatory drugs is responsible for most of the other cases.

INFECTION WITH *HELICOBACTER PYLORI*

H. pylori infection affects more than ½ of the adult population world-wide. The vast majority of gastric cancer cases are thought to be attributed to *H. pylori*. Thus, there is an especially high prevalence of infection in countries that also have a high rate of gastric cancer (e.g., Korea, Japan, Chili).[1] In the United States, older adults, African Americans, and Hispanics have the highest prevalence of infection. In addition, individuals of a lower socioeconomic status have a higher risk of *H. pylori* infection compared with individuals of a higher socioeconomic status.[2] The mechanism by which *H. pylori* infection is transmitted is not yet known; however, it is believed to be spread through the fecal-oral or oral-oral routes.

ACTIVE *HELICOBACTER PYLORI* ULCERS

Peptic ulcer disease in the United States resulting from *H. pylori* infections have decreased about 20% in the last decade. The rates of *H. pylori* ulcers and hospitalizations due to ulcers remain significantly higher in men than women.[3] The risks for developing an ulcer are not easily defined by genetics, gender, ethnicity, or environment; a combination of all of these factors seems to lead to ulceration. Researchers believe that genetics are less important than environment with regard to determining the risk for ulceration, but both physiologic and psychologic factors are involved in the overall environmental risk.

Physiologic trauma and emotional stress can lead to excess acid secretions in the stomach. For individuals who are already infected with *H. pylori* bacteria, that may be the missing link for creating a perfect environment for rapid growth and inflammation that ultimately results in an ulcer. Therefore, the treatment of peptic ulcers must focus on eliminating the cause (i.e., bacteria or drugs) and focus on the environmental cues that are involved in the promotion of excessive acidic secretions.

REFERENCES

1. Peleteiro B, et al. Prevalence of *Helicobacter pylori* infection worldwide: a systematic review of studies with national coverage. *Dig Dis Sci.* 2014;59(8):1698-1709.
2. Krueger WS, et al. Environmental risk factors associated with *Helicobacter pylori* seroprevalence in the United States: a cross-sectional analysis of NHANES data. *Epidemiol Infect.* 2015:1-12.
3. Feinstein LB, et al. Trends in hospitalizations for peptic ulcer disease, United States, 1998-2005. *Emerg Infect Dis.* 2010;16(9):1410-1418.

personality type is free from the disease. However, a recent study of 3379 adults in Denmark found that those individuals with highly stressful lives were significantly more likely to develop an ulcer, independent of other known risk factors such as *H. pylori* infection or the use of NSAIDs.[17] Several neurologic and physiologic changes that result from severe or long-term stress have negative effects on the GI tract. Such changes include alterations in gut motility, gastric secretions, mucosal permeability, and barrier function; changes in visceral sensitivity; compromised recovery from injured mucosa; and reduction in blood flow.[18] Although the relationship between psychologic stress and the development of PUD is not completely understood, such stressed-induced GI changes and lifestyles may exacerbate the development of gastric ulcer disease in susceptible persons.

Clinical Symptoms

General symptoms of PUD include increased gastric muscle tone and painful contractions when the stomach is empty. With duodenal ulcers, the amount and concentration of hydrochloric acid secretions are increased; with gastric ulcers, the secretions may be normal. Some patients will have increased pain following a meal while others experience relief from the presence of food in the GI tract. Hemorrhage may be one of the first signs. Low plasma protein levels, anemia, and weight loss reveal nutrition deficiencies. Diagnosis is confirmed by radiographs and by visualization with **gastroscopy**.

Medical Management

There are four basic goals for the treatment of patients with PUD: (1) alleviate or minimize the symptoms; (2) promote healing; (3) prevent recurrences by eliminating the cause; and (4) prevent complications.

Drug therapy. Advances in knowledge and therapy have provided physicians with the following four types of drugs for the management of PUD:

1. Antibiotics, which address the *H. pylori* infection (e.g., amoxicillin, clarithromycin, tetracycline, metronidazole).
2. Antacids, which counteract or neutralize the acid. Magnesium and aluminum compounds (e.g., Mylanta, Maalox) are the typical antacids of choice for the treatment of PUD.
3. Hydrochloric acid secretion controllers:
   - Histamine H2-receptor antagonists (H2-blockers) reduce hydrochloric acid production and secretion. These medications are available over-the-counter and include cimetidine (Tagamet), ranitidine (Zantac), famotidine (Pepcid), and nizatidine (Axid).
   - Proton pump inhibitors reduce hydrochloric acid production by inhibiting the hydrogen ion secretion that is needed to produce hydrochloric

gastroscopy an examination of the upper intestinal tract using a flexible tube with a small camera on the end; the tube is approximately 9 mm in diameter, and it takes color pictures as well as biopsy samples, if necessary.

Box 18-1 Risk Factors for Recurring Peptic Ulcer

HIGH RISK

Medical/Physical
- *Helicobacter pylori* infection
- Previous recurrences of peptic ulcer with complications
- Hypersecretion of gastric acid
- Family history of peptic ulcer disease among close relatives
- Use of bisphosphonates to prevent osteoporosis

Emotional
- Continuous and unrelieved emotional stress

Behavioral
- Poor dietary habits
- Failure to maintain prescribed diet and drug therapy
- Smoking
- Frequent use of aspirin and other nonsteroidal antiinflammatory drugs

MODERATE RISK

Medical/Physical
- Age of 50 years old or older

Emotional
- Emotionally stressful environment

Behavioral
- Large, irregular meals
- Distilled alcohol consumption

---

acid. These drugs include lansoprazole (Prevacid), omeprazole (Prilosec), esomeprazole (Nexium), pantoprazole (Protonix), and rabeprazole (AcipHex).

4. Mucosal protectors, which deactivate pepsin and produce a gel-like substance to cover the ulcer and to protect it from acid and pepsin while it heals itself (e.g., bismuth subsalicylate, sucralfate [Carafate]).

Maintenance drug therapy is imperative to stabilize the growth rate of bacteria. A continuous low-dose drug therapy follows initial treatment, with intermittent full-dose treatment or symptomatic self-care with the same agents that are used to heal the initial ulcer infection. Success rates depend on the relative risk factors that influence recurrence (Box 18-1).

See the Drug-Nutrient Interaction boxes titled "Tetracycline and Mineral Absorption" and "Proton Pump Inhibitors and Micronutrient Absorption" for more information about potential nutrient interactions with these commonly prescribed medications.

Lifestyle factors. Adequate rest, relaxation, and sleep have long been the foundation of general care to enhance the body's natural healing process. Incorporating positive coping and relaxation skills into daily life may help patients to better deal with personal psychosocial stress factors. Habits that contribute to ulcer development (e.g., smoking, alcohol use) should be eliminated, and irritating drugs (e.g.,

Drug-Nutrient Interaction

Tetracycline and Mineral Absorption

SARA HARCOURT, MS, RD

Tetracycline is a broad-spectrum antibiotic that is used to treat conditions such as respiratory tract infections, acne, infections of the skin, and stomach ulcers. Minerals with a 2^+ charge—including magnesium, calcium, and iron—bond with tetracycline to form a new compound that the body can no longer absorb. Thus, tetracycline is less effective, and mineral absorption is poor.

To ensure optimal absorption, avoid the following foods or medications 1 hour before and 2 hours after taking tetracycline:
- Foods that contain high amounts of calcium (e.g., milk)
- Calcium supplements
- Antacids
- Laxatives that contain magnesium
- Iron supplements (these should be taken at least 2 hours before or 3 hours after tetracycline)

Drug-Nutrient Interaction

Proton Pump Inhibitors and Micronutrient Absorption

Proton pump inhibitors are routinely prescribed for peptic ulcer disease. The long-term use of proton pump inhibitors (e.g., Zantac, Prilosec) is associated with the decreased absorption of some nutrients. This effect is largely as a result of the reduced acidity of the gastric environment. Gastric acid is required to separate bound nutrients in foods and to stabilize them for absorption. For example, vitamin B_{12} is naturally bound to protein in food. When acid production is reduced, vitamin B_{12} remains bound to protein carriers, and it is thus unavailable for absorption in the intestine.

Malabsorption is more likely to be a problem among elderly patients who may also experience other age-related conditions such as atrophic gastritis. Supplemental vitamin B_{12} is indicated for elderly patients who are receiving long-term proton pump inhibitor therapy. Reduced stomach acid may also affect the absorption of nonheme iron and vitamin C, which can lead to deficiencies of these nutrients. The effect on iron and vitamin C status is more marked when the patient is infected with *Helicobacter pylori*; thus, the supplementation of these nutrients may be indicated.[1]

REFERENCE
1. McColl KE. Effect of proton pump inhibitors on vitamins and iron. *Am J Gastroenterol.* 2009;104(suppl 2):S5-S9.

NSAIDs) should be avoided. Sometimes sedatives are prescribed to aid rest.

Nutrition Intervention

In the past, a highly restrictive and bland diet was used for the care of patients with PUD. A bland diet has long since proved to be ineffective and lacking in adequate nutrition support for the healing process. Such a restrictive diet is unnecessary today, because more effective medication regimens are available to control acid secretions and to assist with healing. Thus, current diet therapy is based on a liberal personalized approach that is guided by individual responses to food in an effort to maintain or improve nutritional status. As part of the nutrition support for medical management, two basic goals guide food habits.

Eating a well-balanced and healthy diet. Supply a well-balanced, regular, healthy diet to help with tissue healing and maintenance. A hearty intake of dietary antioxidants and avoidance of foods/supplements known to increase oxidative stress (e.g., trans fats, excessive supplementation with iron or copper, high alcohol intake) help to restore gastrointestinal well-being.[19] Nutrient needs are outlined in the current Dietary Reference Intakes (see Appendix B) and expressed in the simple food choices of the MyPlate .gov guidelines (see Figure 1-3). Further focus is provided by the goals of the *Dietary Guidelines for Americans* (see Figure 1-4).

Avoiding acid stimulation. Avoid stimulating excess gastric acid secretion, which irritates the gastric mucosa. Only the following few food-related habits are thought to affect acid secretion:

- *Food quantity:* To avoid stomach distention, do not eat large quantities at meals. Avoid eating immediately before going to bed, because food intake stimulates acid output.
- *Irritants:* Individual tolerance is the rule, but some food seasonings such as hot chili peppers, black pepper, and chili powder may irritate an already weakened mucosal layer. Caffeine, chocolate, and alcohol may increase acid secretions or prevent healing in some patients. Patients will need to independently determine which foods are tolerated and which foods worsen symptoms.
- *Smoking:* Complete smoking cessation is best, because smoking provokes GI mucosal injury and hinders ulcer healing in several biochemical and physiologic pathways.[20,21] It also affects gastric acid secretion and hinders the effectiveness of drug therapy.

LOWER GASTROINTESTINAL TRACT

SMALL INTESTINE DISEASES

Diseases within the small intestine generally result in malabsorption as a result of the impaired function of the organ. Malabsorption syndromes are characterized by a defect in the absorption of one or more of the essential nutrients. Malabsorption results from a disturbance in the normal digestive process or absorptive pathway, and the defect may include any of the following processes:

- *Digestion of macronutrients:* Carbohydrates, proteins, and fats are broken down in the small intestines into their basic building blocks (i.e., monosaccharides and disaccharides, amino acids, and fatty acids and glycerol, respectively) with the help of salivary and pancreatic enzymes, hydrochloric acid, and bile acid.
- *Terminal digestion at the brush border mucosa:* Disaccharides and peptides are hydrolyzed by disaccharidases and peptidases for the final step of digestion.
- *Absorption:* The end products of macronutrient digestion, micronutrients (i.e., vitamins, minerals, and electrolytes) and water are absorbed across the epithelium of the small intestine into the general or lymphatic circulation.

Several organ systems and functions are affected by malabsorption disorders. Chronic deficiencies of vitamins, minerals, and macronutrients can lead to several forms of anemia (e.g., iron, pyridoxine, folate, vitamin B_{12}); osteopenia and tetany from calcium; vitamin D and magnesium deficiency; and other musculoskeletal, endocrine, and nervous system abnormalities. The most common symptoms of malabsorption disorders are chronic diarrhea and **steatorrhea**.

Two specific conditions triggering malabsorption—cystic fibrosis (CF) and inflammatory bowel disease (IBD)—are reviewed in this section. Other malabsorption syndromes are listed in Table 18-3. Diarrhea is usually a symptom of a disease or disorder rather than a disease itself. However, it will be discussed in this section as diarrhea pertains to most malabsorption disorders.

Cystic Fibrosis

Disease process. CF is the most common fatal genetic disease in North America for white people; it occurs in approximately 1 in 3300 live Caucasian births and 1 in 15,300 African-American births.[22] Although the disease is characterized as a pulmonary disease, it is a multisystem disorder that has a profound GI tract impact. Because pulmonary diseases are outside of the scope of this text, only the nutrition implications of CF are discussed.

CF is a generalized genetic disease of childhood that is inherited as an autosomal recessive trait that can include multiple defects. Previously, children with CF lived to approximately the age of 10 years, dying from complications such as damaged airways and lung infections as well as fibrous pancreas and malnutrition. However, the discovery of the CF gene and the underlying metabolic defect has improved the management of the disease and helped push the life expectancy of these individuals into adulthood. Despite medical advances, minorities and individuals in the

---

steatorrhea fatty diarrhea; excessive amount of fat in the feces, which is often caused by malabsorption diseases.

Table 18-3 Major Malabsorption Syndromes

SYMPTOMS	ETIOLOGY
Defective Intraluminal Digestion	
Defective digestion of fats and proteins	Pancreatic insufficiency from pancreatitis or cystic fibrosis Zollinger-Ellison syndrome,* with inactivation of pancreatic enzymes by excess gastric acid secretion
Solubilization of fat as a result of defective bile secretion	Ileal dysfunction or resection with decreased bile salt uptake Cessation of bile flow from obstruction or hepatic dysfunction
Nutrient preabsorption or modification	Bacterial overgrowth
Primary Mucosal Cell Abnormalities	
Defective terminal digestion	Disaccharidase deficiency (e.g., lactose intolerance) Bacterial overgrowth with brush border damage
Defective epithelial transport	Abetalipoproteinemia (an inherited disorder of fat metabolism from the inability to synthesize β lipoproteins) Primary bile acid malabsorption that results from mutations in the ileal bile acid transporter
Reduced small intestinal surface area	Gluten-sensitive enteropathy (celiac disease) Crohn's disease
Lymphatic obstruction	Lymphoma Tuberculosis and tuberculous lymphadenitis
Infection	Acute infectious enteritis Parasitic infestation Whipple's disease (bacterial infection)
General malabsorption that results from surgery	Partial or total gastrectomy Short gut syndrome after extensive surgical resection Distal ileal resection or bypass

From the National Institute of Diabetes and Digestive and Kidney Diseases. *Zollinger-Ellison syndrome* (website): <www.niddk.nih.gov/health-information/health-topics/digestive-diseases/zollinger-ellison-syndrome/Pages/facts.aspx>. Accessed March 15, 2015. Modified from Kumar V, Fausto N, Abbas A. *Robbins & Cotran Pathologic Basis of Disease.* 7th ed. Philadelphia: Saunders; 2005.
*This is a rare disorder that causes tumors in the pancreas and duodenum and ulcers in the stomach and duodenum. The tumors secrete a hormone called gastrin that causes the stomach to produce too much hydrochloric acid, which in turn causes stomach and duodenal ulcers.

lowest socioeconomic status have a higher risk of complications, disease severity, and mortality, and they report a lower health-related quality of life compared with patients in the highest income category.[23,24] Identifying and addressing differences among socioeconomic classes with regard to disease self-management, environmental pollutants (e.g., cigarette smoke), and psychologic stress are important to improve the life of all patients with CF.

The metabolic defect of CF inhibits the normal movement of chloride and sodium ions in body tissue fluids (see Chapter 9). These ions become trapped in cells, and this causes thick mucus to form and clog ducts and passageways. Involved organ tissues are damaged so that they no longer function normally. The typical CF symptoms include the following:

- *Thick mucus in the lungs:* causes damaged airways, more difficult breathing, persistent coughing, and pulmonary infections (e.g., bronchitis, pneumonia)
- *Pancreatic insufficiency:* leads to a lack of normal pancreatic enzymes (see Chapter 5) to digest macronutrients and a progressive loss of insulin-producing β cells and eventual diabetes mellitus in approximately 15% of adult patients (see Chapter 20)

- *Malabsorption:* food is left undigested and unabsorbed, with consequential malnutrition, stunted growth, delayed puberty, and infertility
- *Liver and gallbladder disease:* clogged bile ducts lead to a progressive degeneration of functional liver tissue
- *Inflammatory complications:* including arthritis, finger clubbing, and **vasculitis**
- *Increased salt concentration:* in body perspiration, thereby leading to salt depletion

Nutrition management. Nutrition therapy is a critical component of the treatment regimen for CF, and it can have a significant impact on successful growth. Patients who are able to maintain an age-appropriate body mass index percentile have better overall health outcomes.[25] Treatment is augmented with the following: (1) increased knowledge of the disease process; (2) early newborn screening and diagnosis; and (3) improved pancreatic enzyme replacement products.

vasculitis the inflammation of the walls of blood vessels.

Enzyme-replacement products (e.g., pancrelipase [Pancrease]) contain the normal pancreatic enzymes for each energy nutrient (i.e., lipase for fat digestion; amylase for starch digestion; and the proteases trypsin, chymotrypsin, and carboxypeptidase [see Chapter 5]). These enzymes are processed into very small enteric-coated beads that are encased in capsules that have been designed not to open or dissolve until they reach the alkaline medium of the intestine. Generous doses of these enzyme-replacement capsules, which vary with a patient's age, weight, and symptoms, are divided among the day's meals; they are usually taken just before eating. Adequate enzyme replacement is the foundation that makes aggressive diet therapy a possibility for meeting growth needs.[26]

Patients with CF who are older than 2 years of age may require significantly more nutrients than the Dietary Recommended Intakes (DRIs) for their age (110% to 200%), depending on the severity of the disease.[25] Accurately determining energy needs is the first step in designing an appropriate diet to meet nutritional needs. A high-energy, nutritionally adequate diet is required and may include oral or enteral nutritional supplementation to maintain weight and prevent malnutrition[25,27] Routine care is based on regular nutrition assessment, diet counseling, food plans, enzyme and salt replacement, vitamin supplements (especially fat-soluble vitamins), nutrition education, and the exploration of individual emotional and psychologic problems. Box 18-2 outlines the current standards of nutritional care for the management of CF. Try applying these principles of care while completing the Clinical Applications box titled "Case Study: Paul's Adaptation to Cystic Fibrosis."

Clinical Applications

Case Study: Paul's Adaptation to Cystic Fibrosis

Paul is a 12-year-old boy with cystic fibrosis. He is hospitalized with pneumonia, and he has difficulty breathing. Paul is a thin child with little muscle development who tires easily, although he has a large appetite. His stools are large and frequent, and they contain undigested food material.

QUESTIONS FOR ANALYSIS

1. What is cystic fibrosis? Account for the clinical effects of the disease as evidenced by Paul's appearance and symptoms.
2. What are the basic goals of the treatment of cystic fibrosis? Why is vigorous nutrition therapy a primary part of treatment?
3. Describe the role of enzyme replacement therapy in this aggressive nutrition support.
4. Why does Paul require therapeutic doses of multivitamins, including fat-soluble vitamins?

Box 18-2 Nutrition Care for Cystic Fibrosis

EVIDENCE-BASED RECOMMENDATIONS[1]:

1. Energy intake is increased to 110% to 200% of the standards for the healthy population.
2. Optimal ranges of weight-for-age and stature-for-age for children and of body mass index (BMI) for adults are indicated to support better lung function.
   Optimal ranges:
   - Children up to the age of 20 years: ≥50th percentile recommended
   - Women: body mass index of ≥22
   - Men: body mass index of ≥23
3. Pancreatic enzyme preparations are required to ensure efficacy when treating cystic fibrosis–related pancreatic insufficiency.

NUTRITION INTERVENTION DURING CYSTIC FIBROSIS SHOULD FOCUS ON THE FOLLOWING[2]:

1. Increased calorie and fat intake
2. Maintenance of lean body mass

GENERAL DIETARY PRINCIPLES FOR PATIENTS WITH CYSTIC FIBROSIS[2]:

1. Provide three meals and two to three snacks per day.
2. Provide pancreatic enzyme and vitamin supplementation.
3. Provide an unrestricted diet that includes high-fat foods and additives.
4. Encourage a variety of whole grains, nuts, fruits, and vegetables to maintain adequate vitamin and mineral intake.
5. Assess vitamin and mineral intake, including those that are received from supplements.
6. Provide counseling to discuss ideas for calorie boosters, on the basis of the patient's usual intake, to meet energy needs.
7. Know that extra salt will be needed to replace the excess salt that is excreted in sweat, especially during hot weather, when exercising, or when febrile.
8. Ensure adequate calcium, vitamin D, and vitamin K intake to promote optimal bone health.

WHEN ORAL INTAKE IS INADEQUATE AND NOT EXPECTED TO IMPROVE[2]:

1. Enteral nutrition should be considered for patients with a BMI <19 and when weight gain is not achieved after initial attempts at intervention.
2. Enteral nutrition support can provide a safe means of nutritional intake, maintain gut integrity, and possibly improve the patient's outcome.
3. Nocturnal feedings through gastrostomy tubes allow the patients to eat meals during the day and supplement with additional nutrients throughout the night.

REFERENCES

1. Stallings VA, et al. Evidence-based practice recommendations for nutrition-related management of children and adults with cystic fibrosis and pancreatic insufficiency: results of a systematic review. *J Am Diet Assoc.* 2008;108(5):832-839.
2. Academy of Nutrition and Dietetics. *Nutrition Care Manual.* Chicago, Ill: 2015.

Inflammatory Bowel Disease

Inflammatory bowel disease (IBD) is a general term that is used to describe chronic inflammation of the GI tract and the persistent activation of the mucosal immune system against the normal healthy gut flora. Chronic inflammation disrupts the protective epithelial barrier until ulceration of the mucosal surface destroys segments of the GI tract. As a result of lesions, portions of the GI tract are not functional, which causes malabsorption. The related condition of short-bowel syndrome may result if the repeated surgical removal of parts of the small intestine is necessary as the disease progresses.

IBD is more common in northern Europe, the United Kingdom, and North America than in other areas of the world. However, incidence rates are increasing worldwide, particularly in industrialized countries, suggesting environmental risk factors.[28] In North America, the prevalence of IBD ranges from 26 to 246 cases per 100,000 persons and there is a genetic risk factor associated with it.[29] Crohn's disease and ulcerative colitis are the two most common forms of inflammatory bowel disease; both of these are **idiopathic** diseases. These diseases share many symptoms and management strategies, but they differ with regard to their clinical manifestations (Table 18-4).

Crohn's disease. Crohn's disease may affect any portion of the GI tract from the esophagus to the anus, but it is most commonly localized to the ileum and the colon. Risk factors include a family history of the disease, Jewish ancestry, and smoking. Inflammation may skip sections of the GI tract and affect more than one section at a time (Figure 18-6). Symptoms will vary for patients, depending on the location of the inflammation, but they most commonly include the following: abdominal pain, fever, fatigue, anorexia, weight loss, painful and urgent defecation, and diarrhea. Patients may experience long asymptomatic periods between flare-ups, or they may experience continuous and progressive attacks.

Malnutrition and micronutrient deficiencies are common with Crohn's disease as a result of malabsorption, poor food intake, and drug-nutrient

---

idiopathic of unknown cause.

Table 18-4   **Clinical Manifestations of Crohn's Disease and Ulcerative Colitis**

MANIFESTATION	COMMON TO BOTH INFLAMMATORY BOWEL DISEASES	
Etiology	Unknown	
Genetics	15% of patients with inflammatory bowel disease have first-degree relatives with the condition	
Gut flora	Intestinal gut flora plays a role, but there is no specific microbe that is the underlying causative factor	
Immune response	Linked to inappropriate T-cell activation or too little control by regulatory T lymphocytes	
Symptoms	Abdominal pain, diarrhea, and weight loss	
Complications	Malnutrition, osteoporosis, dermatitis, ocular symptoms, liver and gallbladder complications, and kidney stones	
	SPECIFIC TO TYPE OF INFLAMMATORY BOWEL DISEASE	
	CROHN'S DISEASE	*ULCERATIVE COLITIS*
Incidence*	3.1 to 14.6 per 100,000 person-years	2.2 to 14.3 per 100,000 person-years
Additional risk factors	Jewish ancestry and smoking	Former smokers are at higher risk than people who have never smoked
Bowel region affected	Ileum and colon	Colon only
Distribution	Skip lesions	Continuous from rectum
Inflammation	Mucosa and all underlying tissue layers	Mucosa and submucosal layers only
Ulceration	Deep, linear ulcerative lesions	Superficial ulcers
Fat-soluble vitamin malabsorption	If lesions are in ileum	No
Response to surgery	Poor to fair	Good
Long-term complications	Fibrosing strictures, fistulas to other organs, cancer, malabsorption (of vitamin B_{12} and bile salts, thereby causing pernicious anemia and steatorrhea), bowel obstruction, polyarthritis, sacroiliitis, ankylosing spondylitis, erythema nodosum, and clubbing of the fingertips	Perforation and toxic megacolon; these patients also have a high risk for cancer

*The frequency of new cases over a certain time interval. The norm in the IBD literature is cases per 100,000 person-years.

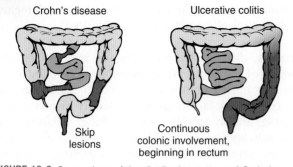

Crohn's disease   Ulcerative colitis

Skip
lesions

Continuous
colonic involvement,
beginning in rectum

FIGURE 18-6 Comparison of the distribution pattern of Crohn's disease and ulcerative colitis. (Reprinted from Kumar V, Fausto N, Abbas A. *Robbins & Cotran Pathologic Basis of Disease.* 7th ed. Philadelphia: Saunders; 2005.)

interactions. Specifically, vitamins A and D, iron, zinc, and protein-energy malnutrition are frequently observed. Iron-deficiency anemia is particularly of concern among patients with Crohn's disease due to the additional issue of blood loss. Protein-energy deficiency is also problematic because the protein needs are higher than normal to allow for tissue healing. Nutrient interactions with necessary medications result in additional complications. For example, long-term corticosteroid use increases the risk for osteoporosis. Surgical removal of portions of the GI tract further exacerbates malabsorption. Malnutrition decreases quality of life, and it can have long-term negative consequences; thus, screening, early detection, and treatment are important parts of the management of this disease.

Ulcerative colitis. Ulcerative colitis (UC) is an inflammatory disease that is limited to the colon. However, it is discussed along with Crohn's disease under the section of Small Intestine Diseases because both diseases are inflammatory bowel diseases with similar manifestations. Symptoms include urgent diarrhea with blood and mucus, abdominal pain, weight loss, fever, and rectal pain. The inflammation does not skip sections of the bowel; rather, it is progressive from the anus (see Figure 18-6).

With the exception of iron-deficiency anemia, UC is not associated with as many micronutrient deficiencies as Crohn's disease because of the location of the inflammation.[30] Dehydration and electrolyte imbalances are more common in UC. However, as pain increases, food intake decreases, or inflammation extends beyond the colon, the same deficiencies as are seen with Crohn's disease may occur. All inflammatory bowel conditions can have severe and often devastating nutrition results as more and more of the absorbing surface area becomes involved or surgical removal is required. Malnutrition can exacerbate an attack and hinder the healing process. Restoring positive nutrition is a basic requirement for tissue healing and health. Enteral nutrition support of either **polymeric formula** or

elemental formula is helpful for many patients to restore nutritional balance and induce remission (see Chapters 17 and 22).[31]

Nutrition therapy. Current studies and clinical practice indicate the benefit of a regular nourishing diet that reflects individual tolerances and disease status for IBD patients. A close working relationship among the physician, the dietitian, and the nurse is essential. The patient's appetite often is poor, but adequate nutrition intake is imperative. A range of feeding modes, including enteral and parenteral nutrition support as needed, is explored to achieve the vigorous nutrition care that is necessary for these individuals. Principles of continuing dietary management of IBD include the following[32]:

During periods of inflammation:
- Use enteral or parenteral nutrition feedings, if necessary.
- Progress to low-fat, high-protein, high-kilocalorie, small, frequent meals when returning to a normal diet as tolerated.
- The diet should be low in fiber only during acute attacks or with strictures. Otherwise, fiber should be increased gradually.
- Vitamin and mineral supplementation should include vitamin D, zinc, calcium, magnesium, folate, vitamin B_{12}, and iron.

During periods of remission:
- Meet energy and protein needs that are specific for weight, and replenish nutrient stores.
- Avoid foods that are high in oxalates for patients with Crohn's disease.
- Increase antioxidant intake, and consider supplementation with omega-3 fatty acids and glutamine.
- Consider the use of **probiotics** and **prebiotics.**

Diarrhea

Diarrhea typically is not a disease of the small intestine but rather a symptom or result of another underlying condition. In some cases, diarrhea may result from intolerance to specific foods or nutrients, such

polymeric formula a nutrition support formula that is composed of complete protein, polysaccharides, and fat as medium-chain fatty acids.
elemental formula a nutrition support formula that is composed of simple elemental nutrient components that require no further digestive breakdown and are thus readily absorbed; these formulas include protein as free amino acids and carbohydrate as the simple sugar glucose.
probiotic a food that contains live microbials, which are thought to benefit the consumer by improving intestinal microbial balance (e.g., lactobacilli in yogurt).
prebiotic nondigestible foods that promote the growth of beneficial microorganisms within the gut.

as in lactose intolerance (see Chapter 2) or acute food poisoning from a specific food-borne organism or toxin (see Chapter 13). A variety of parasites (e.g., *Giardia lamblia, Cryptosporidium parvum, Cyclospora cayetanensis, Entamoeba histolytica*), bacteria (e.g., *Campylobacter, Clostridium difficile, Escherichia coli, Listeria monocytogenes, Salmonella enteritidis, Shigella*), and viral infections (rotavirus, norovirus) are known causes of diarrhea. Traveler's diarrhea, which is often attributed to irregular meals, unfamiliar foods, and travel tensions, is also a well-known GI disturbance; *E. coli*, norovirus, and rotavirus are its most common cause.[33]

Chronic diarrhea (i.e., diarrhea that lasts for more than 2 weeks) can be a life-threatening illness, especially for young children or individuals with compromised immune systems. Diarrheal disease is the fourth leading cause of death globally. Acute infectious diarrhea is the second most common cause of death among children in developing countries.[34] Intravenous fluid and electrolyte replacement may be necessary, or oral rehydration solutions such as Pedialyte, Resol, Ricelyte, CeraLyte, and Rehydralyte may be used. As soon as it is tolerated, a regular refeeding schedule is needed to avoid malnutrition. Nutrition therapy will depend on the underlying causative agent. Determining and treating the cause of diarrhea is paramount to restoring nutritional parameters.

For severely malnourished patients, the resumption of nutrient intake should be carefully monitored. **Refeeding syndrome** is a potentially fatal metabolic disturbance that involves fluid and electrolyte imbalances and that can result in cardiac failure. When malnourished patients are started on a feeding schedule that is too aggressive, sudden shifts in electrolytes leave low serum levels of phosphate, potassium, magnesium, glucose, and thiamine. Malnourished patients require a measured reintroduction to nutrients and close monitoring.

LARGE INTESTINE DISEASES

Diverticular Disease

Diverticulosis is a multifactorial disease that is characterized by the formation of many small pouches or diverticula along the mucosal lining in the colon (Figure 18-7). Segmental circular muscle contractions move waste down the colon to form feces for elimination. When pressures become sufficiently high in a segment with weakened bowel walls, small diverticula may develop. As the diverticula become infected, a condition called **diverticulitis,** the affected area becomes painful.

The commonly used collective term that covers diverticulosis and diverticulitis is *diverticular disease*. Epidemiologic studies have not found one specific cause for diverticular disease. It most often occurs among older people in Western societies, where

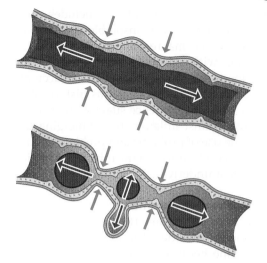

FIGURE 18-7 Mechanism by which low-fiber, low-bulk diets might generate diverticula. When the colon contents are bulky *(top)*, muscular contractions exert pressure longitudinally. If the lumen is small in diameter *(bottom)*, contractions can produce occlusions and exert pressure against the colon wall, which may produce a diverticular "blowout." (Reprinted from Mahan LK, Escott-Stump S. *Krause's Food & Nutrition Therapy.* 13th ed. Philadelphia: Saunders; 2012.)

it is estimated that 70% of the people who are older than 80 years of age will develop diverticulosis, while only 5% of individuals will experience acute diverticulitis.[35] There is evidence that the underlying age-related pathogenesis develops in response to chronic low-grade inflammation, **microbiome** shifts, visceral hypersensitivity, and abnormal gut motility.[36]

As the inflammatory process advances, increased pain and tenderness are localized in the lower left side of the abdomen, and it is accompanied by nausea, vomiting, distention, diarrhea, intestinal spasm, and fever. Perforation sometimes occurs, and surgery is indicated. Underlying malnutrition may also be present. In acute cases of diverticulitis with bloody diarrhea, patients may be restricted to *nothing by mouth* or clear liquids until they can progress slowly to a normal, nutritionally adequate diet. The dietary

refeeding syndrome a potentially lethal condition that occurs when severely malnourished individuals are fed high-carbohydrate diets too aggressively; a sudden shift in electrolytes and fluid retention and a drastic drop in serum phosphorus levels cause a series of complications that involve several organs.

diverticulitis the inflammation of pockets of tissue (i.e., diverticula) in the lining of the mucous membrane of the colon.

microbiome microorganisms living in a specific environment.

Diagnostics. There have been significant improvements in the diagnostic testing for CD in recent years. Serologic testing for IgA anti-tissue transglutaminase antibody can identify CD but diagnosis must be confirmed by duodenal mucosal biopsy while the patient is on a gluten-containing diet.[48] Previously used IgA and IgG anti-gliadin antibody (AGA) tests are no longer recommended. About 40% of the population in the Western world has the genetic polymorphism that leads to CD, but only 1% of people with this genetic predisposition will develop CD, thereby signifying the influence of environmental factors and potentially other genetic factors as well.[49]

Disease process. The pathology of CD is an autoimmune response to a specific sequence of amino acids found in wheat, barley, and rye proteins. The CD-activating proteins are collectively known as *gluten.* However, gluten protein is only found in wheat products. The proteins in barley and rye that cause an adverse reaction are hordein and secalin, respectively. For simplicity, all dietary proteins involved in disease pathogenesis are referred to as *gluten* in this text in keeping with the general public's understanding. Oat products are not problematic for all individuals with CD. However, oats often are processed in facilities that process wheat products, which can result in cross-contamination.

In reaction to the ingestion of a CD-activating protein, the mucosal surface of the small intestine is damaged; this leaves villi that are malformed and with few remaining functional microvilli (Figure 18-8). This injured mucosa effectively reduces the surface area for micronutrient and macronutrient absorption. In addition, the decreased release of peptide hormones, bile, and pancreatic secretions intensifies malabsorption.

Symptoms can vary greatly depending on the extent of the intestinal damage. The major symptoms of diarrhea, steatorrhea, unintended weight loss, and progressive malnutrition are secondary effects of the immunologic response to gluten.

Nutrition management. The goal of nutrition management is to avoid all dietary sources of gluten and to prevent malnutrition through healthy meal alternatives. Wheat, rye, and barley are eliminated from the diet, and a variety of other grains are used instead (Table 18-5). Some individuals with CD are sensitive to oats and also must eliminate oat-containing products. Careful label reading is important for parents and children, because many commercial products use gluten-containing grains as thickeners or fillers. Some commercial products have a gluten-free symbol on their labels to assist with the identification of acceptable foods (Figure 18-9). With the increasing number of processed foods and ethnic dishes available in the marketplace, detecting all food sources of gluten is difficult. Home test kits for gluten are

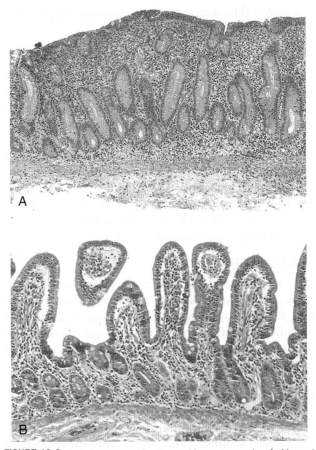

FIGURE 18-8 Celiac disease, gluten-sensitive enteropathy. **A,** Normal mucosal biopsy. **B,** A peroral jejunal biopsy specimen of diseased mucosa shows severe atrophy and the blunting of villi with a chronic inflammatory infiltrate of the lamina propria. (Reprinted from Kumar V, Fausto N, Abbas A. *Robbins & Cotran Pathologic Basis of Disease.* 7th ed. Philadelphia: Saunders; 2005.)

available and may be beneficial for individuals who consume foods without standard ingredient lists. Adhering to a gluten-free diet is the only effective treatment for maintaining a healthy mucosa, and it must be followed for life.

Because of the nature of the malabsorption disorder, patients with CD should be monitored for potential vitamin and mineral deficiencies and partake in supplementation as necessary during flare-ups. In addition, interference with medication absorption and action must be considered with any form of malabsorption disorder.

GASTROINTESTINAL ACCESSORY ORGANS

Three major accessory organs—the liver, the gallbladder, and the pancreas—produce important digestive agents that enter the intestine and help with the digestion and absorption of food (see Figure 5-3). A good understanding of the anatomy and physiology of the accessory organs is paramount to understanding how various diseases of these organs will subsequently affect the GI tract and nutrient metabolism.

Table 18-5 Gluten-Free Diet for Individuals with Celiac Disease*

GRAINS AND PLANT FOODS ALLOWED	GRAINS NOT ALLOWED
Amaranth	Wheat
Arrowroot	Barley
Buckwheat	Rye
Cassava	Malt
Corn	Oats† (unless they are packaged in a
Flax	gluten-free environment)
Indian rice grass	
Job's tears	
Legumes	
Millet	
Finger millet	
Nuts	
Potatoes	
Quinoa	
Rice	
Sago	
Seeds	
Sorghum	
Soy	
Tapioca	
Teff	
Wild rice	
Yucca	

From Academy of Nutrition and Dietetics. *Nutrition Care Manual.* Chicago, Ill: 2015.

*Dietary principles to be addressed include the following: (1) Choose whole-grain, gluten-free products; (2) choose enriched, gluten-free products instead of refined, unenriched products; (3) eat more foods made with alternative plant foods, such as amaranth, quinoa, and buckwheat for good sources of fiber, iron, and B vitamins; (4) eat plenty of nongrain sources of food to meet all of the body's nutrient needs (e.g., lean meats, poultry, pork, fish, dairy products, legumes, seeds, nuts, vegetables, fruit); (5) consider taking a gluten-free multivitamin and mineral supplement.

†Oats and oat products are tolerated by some individuals and do not need to be avoided.

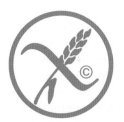

FIGURE 18-9 Gluten-free symbol. (Copyright Coeliac UK, Bucks, UK, 2004.)

LIVER DISEASE

The liver plays several critical roles in basic metabolism and the regulation of body functions (see Box 5-1). Diseases of the liver have the potential to disrupt any of these functions. That being said, the liver is an incredibly regenerative organ. In the event that liver disease is diagnosed early enough, and the causative factor can be removed, the liver is capable of regenerating itself. This regenerative capacity is what allows live-donor liver transplants. One study noted that after healthy live-donors have a **lobectomy** for donation,

their organs had already increased in volume by 73% within 7 days post-surgery.[50] For this amount of organ regeneration to be successful, adequate nutrition is essential to supply the body with the necessary building blocks.

Fatty Liver Disease

Fatty liver disease is the excess accumulation of fat in the liver. It is estimated that up to one third of the U.S. population has some level of **steatosis**.[51] If the disease is a result of alcohol abuse, it is referred to as alcoholic liver disease (ALD). If alcohol is not the cause, it is nonalcoholic fatty liver disease (NAFLD). As the condition progresses, inflammation within the liver ensues. Fat accumulation ("steato") plus inflammation in the liver ("hepatitis") is known as *steatohepatitis*. There are two primary types of steatohepatitis: alcoholic steatohepatitis (ASH) and nonalcoholic steatohepatitis (NASH).

Fat accumulates in the liver in response to high levels of fatty acids in the circulation, exaggerated lipogenesis, and impaired lipolysis. In other words, more fat is made and stored in the liver than is burned or oxidized by the liver. Alcohol-induced disturbances in the liver are multifactorial, progressing from toxicity, steatosis, and mass inflammation to ultimately resulting in organ failure.[52] Disease progression of steatohepatitis may advance to cirrhosis if it is left untreated. Genetic and environmental factors such as chronic inflammation, oxidative stress, insulin resistance, polycystic ovarian syndrome, and obesity increase the risk for the development of NASH.[51,53] Some researchers argue that nonalcoholic fatty liver disease is a precursor to metabolic syndrome, as opposed to a result of the condition.[54]

Basic nutrition guidelines for fatty liver disease and steatohepatitis include a balanced diet, avoidance of alcohol (if indicated), weight loss (if indicated), consideration of antioxidant supplementation, and tight blood glucose level control. Malnutrition is typical in patients with ASH, and enteral nutrition therapy is recommended for such patients as a means for reestablishing adequate nutrient intake.[55]

Hepatitis

Acute hepatitis is an inflammatory condition that is caused by bacteria, viruses, parasites, or toxins (e.g., chloroform, alcohol, drugs). Viral infections and alcohol abuse are the most common forms of hepatitis. Viral infections are often transmitted via the oral-fecal route (i.e., hepatitis A), which is common for many epidemic diseases that involve contaminated food or water. In other cases, the virus may be transmitted by

lobectomy surgical removal of a lobe of an organ.
steatosis accumulation of fat in the liver cells.

transfusions of infected blood or by contaminated syringes or needles (i.e., hepatitis B). Symptoms of hepatitis include anorexia and jaundice with underlying malnutrition.

Treatment focuses on bed rest and nutrition therapy to support the healing and regeneration of the liver tissue (see the Clinical Applications box, "Case Study: Bill's Bout with Infectious Hepatitis"). Dietary restrictions are not usually necessary during acute hepatitis, but they may be required for chronic cases. The following requirements govern the goals of nutrition therapy[32]:

- Avoid substances that are hepatotoxic (e.g., alcohol, drugs, toxins).
- Consume a diet that is adequate in energy, macronutrients, and micronutrients.
- Consume 4 to 6 small meals per day. Most patients will tolerate oral feedings, but enteral feedings may be warranted.
- *Protein:* Protein is essential for regenerating new liver cells and preventing damage from fatty infiltration in liver tissue. The diet should supply 1.0 to 1.2 g/kg of body weight of high-quality protein daily if no complications are present.
- *Carbohydrates:* Available glucose restores protective glycogen reserves in the liver. It also helps to meet the energy demands of the disease process and prevents the breakdown of protein for energy, thus ensuring its use for tissue regeneration. The diet should supply about half of the total kilocalories as carbohydrates. Glucose intolerance and

hypoglycemia are sometimes problematic in patients with liver disease. Therefore, the amount of carbohydrates in the diet depends on individual needs and any co-morbidity (e.g., diabetes).
- *Fat:* In cases of steatorrhea, the diet should not exceed 30% of total kilocalories from fat.
- Sodium is limited to 2000 mg per day to avoid fluid retention.
- As a patient's appetite and food tolerance improve, a full diet is acceptable while observing his or her likes and dislikes and planning ways to encourage optimal food intake.

Cirrhosis

Cirrhosis is a chronic state of liver disease in which the liver is damaged beyond repair with scar tissue and fatty infiltration (Figure 18-10). Progressive cirrhosis and end-stage liver disease is one of the top seven leading causes of death from chronic disease in the United States,[56] and about half of all cases are the result of hepatitis C and alcoholism. Other causes include chronic hepatitis type B; autoimmune hepatitis; NASH; inherited diseases such as Wilson's disease, hemochromatosis (see Chapter 8), and galactosemia (see Chapter 5); blocked bile ducts; and drugs, toxins, and infections.

One of the main functions of the liver is to remove ammonia—and hence nitrogen (see Chapter 5)—from the blood by converting it to urea (via the urea cycle) for urinary excretion. However, with steatohepatitis, the accompanying fatty infiltration kills liver cells and leaves only nonfunctioning fibrous scar tissue. When fibrous scar tissue replaces functional liver tissue, the blood can no longer circulate throughout the liver, which leads to **portal hypertension**. The blood, which is carrying its ammonia load, cannot get to the liver for the normal removal of ammonia and nitrogen. Instead, it must follow the vessels that bypass the liver and proceed to the brain, thereby producing ammonia intoxication and **hepatic encephalopathy**. As a result of portal hypertension, the small blood vessels that surround the esophagus become distended with high pressure, which eventually leads to the development of **esophageal varices**. The rupture of these

portal hypertension high blood pressure in the portal vein.
hepatic encephalopathy a condition in which toxins in the blood lead to alterations in brain homeostasis as a result of liver disease; this results in apathy, confusion, inappropriate behavior, altered consciousness, and eventually coma.
esophageal varices the pathologic dilation of the blood vessels within the wall of the esophagus as a result of liver cirrhosis; these vessels can continue to expand to the point of rupturing.

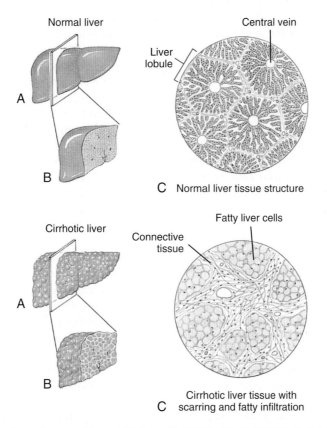

Normal liver

Central vein

Liver lobule

A

B

C   Normal liver tissue structure

Cirrhotic liver

Fatty liver cells

Connective tissue

A

B

C   Cirrhotic liver tissue with scarring and fatty infiltration

FIGURE 18-10 Comparison of a normal liver and a liver with cirrhotic tissue changes. **A,** Anterior view of the organ. **B,** Cross-sectional view. **C,** Tissue structure. (Copyright Medical and Scientific Illustration.)

enlarged veins with massive hemorrhage can result in death.

The liver is responsible for processing and metabolizing medications. Thus, in the case of cirrhosis, medical treatment is limited to removing excess sources of ammonia within the GI tract and nutrition therapy. The most common medications used are lactulose and antibiotics such as neomycin. Lactulose is an unabsorbable sugar that pulls water and ammonia into the colon for elimination. Neomycin works by destroying ammonia-producing bacteria in the gut.

Protein-energy malnutrition and vitamin/mineral deficiencies are a significant issue in patients with cirrhosis.[57] Low plasma protein levels contribute to **ascites.** Nutrition therapy focuses on as much healing support as possible, as follows[32]:

- Avoid substances that are hepatotoxic (e.g., alcohol, drugs, toxins).
- Consume 4 to 6 small meals per day, including nutritional solution products.
- Consume a diet that is adequate in energy, macronutrients, and micronutrients. Vitamin and mineral supplementation and/or enteral or parenteral

nutrition support may be necessary to meet these needs. Of particular consideration are supplemental forms of the B vitamins, zinc, magnesium, and selenium. Cirrhosis patients are also commonly deficient in vitamins A, D, and E as well. Supplementation of the fat soluble vitamins must be handled with care in order to avoid toxicity.[57]

- *Energy:* Total energy intake should equal basal energy needs plus approximately 20%. Practitioners must carefully distinguish body weight from fluid weight, because needs are based on dry weight. Adjustments are made for cases of hypermetabolism or if weight loss is indicated.
- *Carbohydrates:* Approximately half of the total kilocalories in the diet should come from carbohydrates. The total energy provided by carbohydrates depends on individual needs and any co-morbidity (e.g., diabetes, obesity).
- *Protein:* Dietary protein should equal 0.8 to 1.2 g/kg of dry or appropriate body weight in the absence of impending protein-sensitive hepatic encephalopathy. Sufficient protein is needed to correct severe malnutrition, to heal liver tissue, and to restore plasma proteins.
- *Fat:* In the presence of steatorrhea, the dietary intake of fat should not exceed 30% of total kilocalories.

ascites fluid accumulation in the abdominal cavity.

- Sodium is limited to 2000 mg per day to avoid ascites.
- Fluid restrictions are indicated for those with hyponatremia or ascites.
- Reinforce the benefits of daily physical activity.

GALLBLADDER DISEASE

The basic function of the gallbladder is to concentrate and store bile and then release the concentrated bile into the small intestine when fat is present there. Bile emulsifies fat in the intestine to prepare it for digestion and then helps carry it into the mucosal cells of the intestinal wall for preparation to enter the lymphatic circulation (see Chapter 3).

Cholecystitis and Cholelithiasis

Disease process. Inflammation of the gallbladder (cholecystitis) usually results from a low-grade chronic infection or obstruction. Gallstone formation (cholelithiasis) is attributed to impaired metabolism of cholesterol, bile acid, phospholipids, and bilirubin. The risk for cholelithiasis increases with age and is three to four times more likely to develop in women than men during the reproductive years. Other risk factors for cholelithiasis include genetics, overweight/obesity, rapid weight loss, diabetes, certain medications (e.g., corticosteroids, oral contraceptives), pancreatic disease, and liver disease.[58] As the prevalence of obesity and type 2 diabetes increases in the United States, so does the occurrence of cholelithiasis, even in young children.[59]

Gallstones are composed primarily of cholesterol, bilirubin, and fatty acids; and they are classified as either cholesterol stones, pigment stones, or mixed stones.[58] The vast majority of gallstones are cholesterol-containing gallstones. The non–water-soluble cholesterol in bile is normally kept in solution. If the amount of cholesterol is too concentrated, cholesterol may separate out and crystallize to form gallstones. Most gallstones are asymptomatic, but some gallstone carriers experience episodes of intense pain. The typical treatment in such painful and chronic cases is cholecystectomy, which is the surgical removal of the gallbladder. Other medical treatments include litholytic therapy to chemically dissolve the stone and shock wave lithotripsy to shatter the stone.

Nutrition management. As fat enters the intestine, the hormone cholecystokinin triggers gallbladder contractions to release bile. In patients with cholecystitis or cholelithiasis, the normal contraction of the gallbladder often causes pain. Diet therapy centers on controlling fat intake (i.e., less than 30% of calories from fat) and eating small, frequent meals.[32] Table 18-6 outlines a general low-fat diet guide, but the degree of its application depends on individual needs, acuity, and treatment plan.

Following cholecystectomy, the liver continues to produce bile and release it directly into the duodenum to assist with fat digestion. Therefore, most patients will adjust to a normal diet within a few months after surgery. Without a reservoir of stored

Table 18-6   Low-Fat Diet*

FOODS	FOODS ALLOWED	FOODS LIMITED OR AVOIDED
Beverages	Skim milk, coffee, tea, carbonated beverages, and fruit juices	Whole milk, cream, and evaporated and condensed milk
Bread and cereals	Most all	Rich rolls or breads, waffles, and pancakes
Desserts	Gelatin, sherbet, water ices, fruit whips made without cream, angel food cake, and rice and tapioca puddings made with skim milk	Pastries, pies, rich cakes and cookies, and ice cream
Fruits	All fruits as tolerated	Avocado
Eggs	Three allowed per week, cooked any way except fried	Fried eggs
Fats	3 tsp butter or margarine daily	Salad and cooking oils and mayonnaise
Meats	Lean meat such as beef, veal, lamb, liver, lean fish, and fowl that has been baked, broiled, or roasted without added fat	Fried meats, bacon, ham, pork, goose, duck, fatty fish, fish canned in oil, and cold cuts
Cheese	Dry or fat-free cottage cheese	All other cheeses
Potato or substitute	Potatoes, rice, macaroni, noodles, and spaghetti prepared without added fat	Fried potatoes and potato chips
Soups	Bouillon or broth without fat and soups made with skim milk	Cream soups
Sweets	Jam, jelly, and sugar candies without nuts or chocolate	Chocolate, nuts, and peanut butter
Vegetables	All vegetables as tolerated	

*Such dietary restraints on fat are usually only needed during acute or unresolved cases.

bile in the gallbladder, meals that are exceptionally heavy in fat may be uncomfortable for patients after cholecystectomy.

PANCREATIC DISEASE

The pancreas is a key organ in normal digestion and metabolism, and it acts as both an exocrine gland and an endocrine gland. Digestive enzymes and bicarbonate, which are necessary for the breakdown of the macronutrients, are excreted by the pancreas under hormonal control during digestion. The endocrine functions of the pancreas are primarily related to blood glucose level regulation by glucagon and insulin. The endocrine functions of the pancreas will be covered in Chapter 20.

Pancreatitis

Disease process. Inflammation of the pancreas, which is known as *pancreatitis,* inhibits normal exocrine pancreatic function, including the secretion of digestive enzymes. Subsequently, digestion and absorption are severely affected. Mild or moderate episodes may completely subside, but the condition tends to recur, which can lead to chronic pancreatitis. Patients with pancreatitis present with severe abdominal pain and may experience nausea, vomiting, and steatorrhea.

Excessive alcohol consumption is the major causative factor of pancreatitis in the United States. Other causes of chronic pancreatitis include a blocked pancreatic duct due to gallstones, heredity, cystic fibrosis, autoimmune disorders, and other unknown causes.

Nutrition management. Without adequate pancreatic enzymes, the inability to digest food leads to malnutrition. Thus, supplementing with pancreatic enzymes with each meal is a cornerstone of treatment and important for the overall outcome of the patient.[60] Nutrition therapy for cases of mild to moderate pancreatitis includes the following measures[32]:

- *Nothing by mouth* with hydration support during acute phases. This allows for pancreatic rest while providing fluids and correcting for electrolyte and acid-base disturbances.
- Advance to liquid or solid foods as tolerated. For patients with severe acute pancreatitis, a continuous infusion of enteral nutrition is indicated. For patients who cannot tolerate oral or enteral feedings, parenteral nutrition must be considered (see Chapter 22).
- Provide adequate energy and nutrient needs when acute symptoms subside. Energy needs should be based on patient requirements to prevent weight loss. Assess the need for vitamin and mineral supplementation, especially during periods when oral intake is insufficient to meet basic needs.
- The diet should be relatively high in protein and low in fat.
- Avoid alcohol and smoking.

Putting It All Together

Summary

- The nutrition management of GI diseases is based on the degree of interference in the normal processes of ingestion, digestion, absorption, and metabolism that the disease causes.
- Problems in the upper GI tract relate to conditions that hinder chewing, swallowing, or transporting the food mass down the esophagus into the stomach. Esophageal problems such as muscle constriction, acid reflux, esophagitis, and hiatal hernias interfere with the passage of food into the stomach. PUD involves the acidic erosion of the mucosal lining of the stomach or the duodenal bulb. Nutrition therapy is liberal and individual, with the goal of correcting malnutrition and supporting the healing process.
- Problems of the lower GI tract include common functional disorders such as malabsorption and diarrhea, for which symptomatic and personalized treatment is indicated. CD and CF require extensive individualized nutrition support. The inflammatory bowel diseases (e.g., Crohn's disease, ulcerative colitis) involve widespread tissue damage that occasionally requires surgical resection and that results in decreased absorbing surface area. Large intestine problems (e.g., diverticular disease, IBS, constipation) are often multifactorial and may be difficult to resolve. Nutrition therapy is specific to each condition and generally warrants the assistance of a dietitian.
- Diseases of the GI accessory organs also contribute to nutrition problems. Common liver disorders include hepatitis and cirrhosis. Uncontrolled cirrhosis leads to hepatic encephalopathy and eventual liver failure and death. Nutrient and energy levels of the necessary diet therapy vary with the progression of the disease process. Gallbladder disease, infection, and stones involve some acute limitation to fat tolerance, which is modified in accordance with individual need. The treatment for gallstones is the surgical removal of the gallbladder followed by the moderate use of dietary fat. Pancreatitis is a serious condition that requires immediate measures to counter the symptoms of severe pain followed by restorative nutrition support.

Chapter Review Questions

See answers in Appendix A.

1. The best way to prevent constipation is to:
   a. Use stool softeners as needed.
   b. Consume plenty of soluble fiber and fluids.
   c. Use a laxative once a week.
   d. Use a daily multivitamin/multimineral supplement.

2. The meal that is most appropriate for a patient with GERD is:
   a. Coffee, orange juice, sausage patty, and biscuit.
   b. Skim milk, scrambled egg, and whole-wheat toast.
   c. Tomato juice, country fried steak, and hash brown casserole.
   d. Skim milk, peppermint tea, fried chicken, and fried potatoes.

3. A patient with cirrhosis of the liver can help avoid development of hepatic encephalopathy by avoiding excessive intake of:
   a. Fat.
   b. Calories.
   c. Protein.
   d. Thiamin.

4. Pancreatitis is most frequently caused by:
   a. Excessive protein intake.
   b. Protein-energy malnutrition.
   c. Chronic food allergies.
   d. Excessive alcohol intake.

5. A person with celiac disease should avoid:
   a. Barley and vegetable soup.
   b. Grilled chicken and rice.
   c. Rice cakes with strawberries.
   d. Fresh grilled shrimp and baked potato.

Additional Learning Resources

evolve   Please refer to this text's Evolve website for answers to the Case Study questions.
http://evolve.elsevier.com/Williams/basic/

References and **Further Reading and Resources** in the back of the book provide additional resources for enhancing knowledge.

Coronary Heart Disease and Hypertension

Key Concepts

- Cardiovascular disease is the leading cause of death in the United States.
- Several risk factors contribute to the development of coronary heart disease and hypertension, many of which are preventable by improved diet and lifestyle behaviors.
- Other risk factors are nonmodifiable, such as age, sex, family history, and race.

- Hypertension (i.e., chronically elevated blood pressure) may be classified as primary or secondary hypertension.
- Hypertension damages the endothelium of the blood vessels.
- Early education is critical for the prevention of cardiovascular disease.

Cardiovascular disease (CVD) is the leading cause of death in the United States, and it accounts for more than 611,000 deaths each year (Figure 19-1).[1] A similar situation exists in most other developed Western societies. Every day, thousands of people have heart attacks and strokes, and more than 1 million others continue to live with various forms of rheumatic and congestive heart disease.

This chapter discusses the primary underlying disease processes of **atherosclerosis** and hypertension as well as the various risk factors involved. In addition, we will explore ways to use nutrition therapy to reduce risk factors and to help prevent disease.

CORONARY HEART DISEASE

The major arteries and their many branches that serve the heart are called *coronary arteries*, because they lie across the brow of the heart and resemble a crown. Thus, the overall disease process is identified as **coronary heart disease**.

ATHEROSCLEROSIS

Disease Process

The major cause of CVD and the underlying pathologic process in coronary heart disease is atherosclerosis. This process is characterized by fatty **plaques**, which are largely composed of cholesterol, on the inside lining of major blood vessels. Although the exact mechanisms and all of the contributing factors involved are not known, it is believed that the plaques begin as a result of an initial injury to the endothelial lining of the artery and inflammation ensues. Atherosclerotic plaque may begin as early as childhood in susceptible individuals. When tissue is examined, cholesterol can be seen with the unaided eye in the debris of advanced lesions. This fatty plaque

gradually thickens over time to a fibrous plaque that narrows the interior of the vessel. The thickening of the artery or the development of a blood clot may eventually cut off blood flow (Figure 19-2).

Cells die when they are deprived of their normal blood supply. The local area of dying or dead tissue is called an *infarct*. If the affected blood vessel is a major artery that supplies vital nutrients and oxygen to the heart muscle (i.e., the myocardium), then the event is called a **myocardial infarction (MI)** or *heart attack*. A common symptom of its presence is **angina pectoris** or chest pain that typically radiates down the left arm

atherosclerosis the underlying pathology of coronary heart disease; a common form of arteriosclerosis that is characterized by the formation of fatty streaks that contain cholesterol and that develop into hardened plaques in the inner lining of major blood vessels such as the coronary arteries.

coronary heart disease the overall medical problem that results from the underlying disease of atherosclerosis in the coronary arteries, which serve the heart muscle with blood, oxygen, and nutrients.

plaque thick wax-like coating forming inside artery walls; primarily composed of cholesterol, fatty substances, cellular debris, calcium, and fibrin.

myocardial infarction (MI) a heart attack; a myocardial infarction is caused by the failure of the heart muscle to maintain normal blood circulation as a result of the blockage of the coronary arteries with fatty cholesterol plaques that cut off the delivery of oxygen to the affected part of the heart muscle.

angina pectoris a spasmodic, choking chest pain caused by a lack of oxygen to the heart; this is a symptom of a heart attack, and it also may be caused by severe effort or excitement.

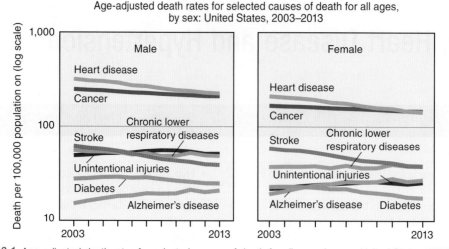

Age-adjusted death rates for selected causes of death for all ages, by sex: United States, 2003–2013

FIGURE 19-1 Age-adjusted death rates for selected causes of death for all ages, by sex: United States, 2003-2013. (National Center for Health Statistics. *Health, United States, 2014: with special feature of adults aged 55-64.* Hyattsville, Md: U.S. Government Printing Office; 2015.)

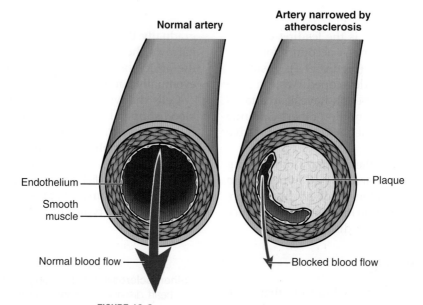

FIGURE 19-2 An atherosclerotic plaque in an artery.

and that is sometimes elicited by excitement or physical effort. If the affected vessel is a major artery that supplies the brain, then it causes a **cerebrovascular accident** or *stroke.*

Relation to Fat Metabolism

See Chapter 3 for details on the dietary lipids involved in the atherogenic disease process. Three of these substances are specifically relevant to CVD and are briefly discussed again here.

Total cholesterol. Although cholesterol is an essential compound in the body, excess total blood levels increase the risk of heart disease in predisposed individuals. High blood cholesterol levels increase the risk for the deposition of cholesterol, fats, fibrous tissue, and macrophages in arteries throughout the body,

which is the beginning of atherosclerosis. The Centers for Disease Control and Prevention reports that 27.8% of American adults ≥20 years old have high total blood cholesterol levels of >240 mg/dL, or are taking cholesterol-lowering medications.[1] Many patients with **hypercholesterolemia** have the related problems of obesity and hypertension; these require

cerebrovascular accident a stroke; a stroke is caused by arteriosclerosis within the blood vessels of the brain that cuts off oxygen supply to the affected portion of brain tissue, thereby paralyzing the actions that are controlled by the affected area.

hypercholesterolemia high cholesterol levels in the blood.

medical counseling and intervention, with nutrition therapy as the primary intervention.

Lipoproteins. Because fat is not soluble in water, it is carried in the bloodstream in small packages wrapped with protein called *lipoproteins.* These compounds are produced (1) in the intestinal mucosal cells after a meal that contains fat and (2) in the liver as part of the ongoing process of fat metabolism. Lipoproteins carry fat and cholesterol to tissues for cell metabolism and then back to the liver for breakdown and excretion as needed. Lipoproteins are grouped and named in accordance with their protein, fat, and cholesterol content (i.e., their density). Those with the highest protein content have the highest density and vice versa. The following lipoproteins are significant in relation to heart disease risk as follows:

1. *Chylomicrons:* These are made predominantly from dietary triglycerides after digestion and absorption from the gastrointestinal tract. Chylomicrons are lipoprotein particles that transport absorbed dietary (i.e., exogenous) triglycerides to plasma and tissues (Figure 19-3, *A*).
2. *Very low-density lipoproteins (VLDLs):* VLDLs are formed in the liver from endogenous fat. VLDLs carry a relatively large load of triglycerides to cells throughout the body, and they also contain approximately 12% cholesterol (Figure 19-3, *B*). They have a very low density of protein.

3. *Intermediate-density lipoproteins (IDLs):* Degradation of VLDLs leaves IDLs in circulation. And like VLDLs, IDLs continue delivering endogenous triglycerides to cells and tissue throughout the body.
4. *Low-density lipoproteins (LDLs):* LDLs carry, in addition to other lipids, at least two thirds of the total plasma cholesterol to body tissues. LDLs are formed endogenously in the liver and in serum from the catabolism of VLDLs and IDLs. Because LDLs deliver cholesterol to the tissue, they are considered the "bad cholesterol." With regard to cardiovascular health, LDL-cholesterol is the major lipoprotein of concern[2] (Figure 19-3, *C*). Sometimes all of the non–high-density lipoprotein fractions (i.e., VLDLs, IDLs, LDLs) are grouped together as a marker for CVD risk. LDLs have a low density of protein.
5. *High-density lipoproteins (HDLs):* HDLs carry less total fat and more protein than the other lipoproteins (Figure 19-3, *D*). They transport cholesterol from the tissues and arteries back to the liver for catabolism. HDLs are endogenously produced in the liver. Compared with LDL-cholesterol, HDL is the "good cholesterol," and higher serum levels are protective against CVD. There are both

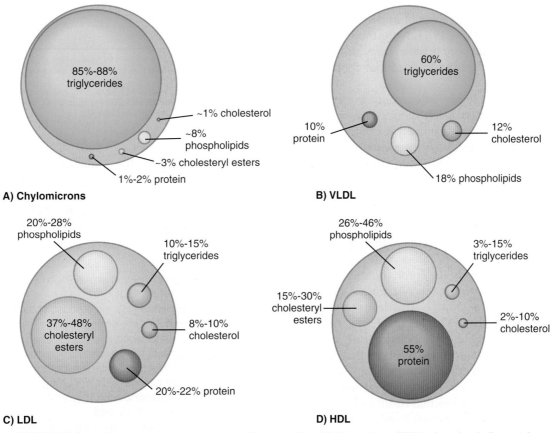

FIGURE 19-3 Serum lipoprotein factions showing lipid composition. **(A)** Chylomicron. **(B)** Very low-density lipoprotein. **(C)** Low-density lipoprotein. **(D)** High-density lipoprotein.

pharmacologic interventions and lifestyle modifications that influence HDL metabolism. Exercise increases metabolic kinetics within the liver, skeletal muscle, and adipose tissue, all of which are cardio-protective and favor HDL production.[3] HDLs have a high density of protein.

We do not consume VLDLs, IDLs, LDLs, or HDLs in our food. Thus, **dyslipidemia** is not nutritionally addressed by "eating less LDL-cholesterol" or "eating more HDL-cholesterol." There are other dietary modifications that can improve lipid profiles, but it is not via a direct consumption or avoidance of these lipoprotein fractions.

Triglycerides. Simple fats, whether in the body or in food, are triglycerides. Cardiovascular disease screenings will test for the levels of total triglycerides circulating in the blood. **Hypertriglyceridemia** is commonly associated with low HDL-cholesterol, both of which are independent risk factors for CVD.[4]

Table 19-1 outlines the standard blood lipid classifications. The current guidelines for starting cholesterol-lowering medications are not based exclusively on these classifications. The algorithm for determining drug therapy needs to take into account many factors, including age, race, sex, family history, blood pressure measurements, co-morbidities, and lifestyle factors.[2]

Risk Factors

The underlying disease process of atherosclerosis has multiple risk factors (Box 19-1). Note the modifiable risk factors over which people have some control compared with those that individuals cannot control (i.e., nonmodifiable):

- *Sex:* CVD occurs more often among men than women until women reach menopause, at which time the relative risks are similar for both sexes.
- *Age:* General risk for CVD increases with age. It is greater for men who are older than 45 and for women who are older than 55.
- *Family history:* A positive family history is defined as a history of premature CVD (see Box 19-1). Early screening for children and adolescents with a high-risk family history is important so that appropriate diet and lifestyle modifications may begin before fatty streaks develop in the coronary arteries.
- *Heredity:* Certain groups (i.e., African Americans, Mexican Americans, Native Americans, and some Asian Americans) have a higher incidence of CVD.[5,6] Some of this heightened incidence rate may be related to ethnicity-associated lifestyles that increase the CVD risk in certain groups (e.g., smoking, obesity), and may not be exclusively genetic factors at play. Genetic anomalies that result in abnormally high serum lipid levels include **familial hypercholesterolemia** and **familial hypertriglyceridemia**.[7] Both

Table 19-1 Cholesterol and Lipoprotein Profile Classification*

CHOLESTEROL READING	CLASSIFICATION
Total Cholesterol (mg/dL)	
<180	Optimal
<200	Near-optimal
200 to 239	Borderline high
≥240	High
Low-Density Lipoprotein Cholesterol (mg/dL)	
<100	Optimal
100 to 129	Near-optimal
130 to 159	Borderline high
160 to 189	High
≥190	Very high
High-Density Lipoprotein Cholesterol (mg/dL)	
≥60	Optimal
40 to 59	Borderline/normal
<40	A major risk factor for heart disease
Total Cholesterol/HDL ratio†	
≤3.5:1	Optimal
<5:1	Near-optimal
>5:1	A major risk factor for heart disease
Triglycerides (mg/dL)	
<150	Optimal
150 to 199	Borderline high
200 to 499	High
≥500	Very high

*NOTE: The 2013 updated guidelines for treating high cholesterol take into account all risk factors. Treatment initiation is not exclusively based on these parameters.
†Divide total cholesterol level by HDL-cholesterol level to determine the ratio. Example: If total cholesterol level is 200 mg/dL and HDL level is 50 mg/dL: 200/50 = 4. Therefore, the ratio would be 4:1.

conditions require the initiation of diet and drug therapy during the second or third decade of life.

- *Blood cholesterol profile:* High total cholesterol and LDL-cholesterol and low HDL-cholesterol are major

dyslipidemia abnormal lipid profile (high cholesterol, LDL, or TG; and/or low HDL).
hypertriglyceridemia high triglycerides in the blood.
familial hypercholesterolemia a genetic disorder that results in elevated blood cholesterol levels despite lifestyle modifications; this condition is caused by absent or nonfunctional low-density lipoprotein receptors, and it requires drug therapy.
familial hypertriglyceridemia a genetic disorder that results in elevated blood triglyceride levels despite lifestyle modifications; it requires drug therapy.

Box 19-1 Risk Factors for Cardiovascular Disease

LIPID RISK FACTORS

- Elevated levels of low-density lipoprotein cholesterol
- Low levels of high-density lipoprotein cholesterol (<40 mg/dL)*
- Elevated total cholesterol levels
- Elevated levels of triglycerides
- Atherogenic dyslipidemia[†]
- High total cholesterol/HDL-cholesterol ratio

NONLIPID RISK FACTORS

Nonmodifiable

- Sex (males have greater risk than females)
- Age (men ≥45 years, women ≥55 years)
- Heredity (including race)
- Family history of premature cardiovascular disease (i.e., myocardial infarction or sudden death at 55 years of age or less in a male first-degree relative or at 65 years of age or less in a female first-degree relative)
- Estimated glomerular filtration rate of <60 mL/min or microalbuminuria
- Type 1 diabetes mellitus

Modifiable

- Poor diet quality: This is the leading risk factor for death and disability in the United States
- Cigarette smoking: approximately one third of all coronary heart disease deaths are attributable to smoking and exposure to second-hand smoke
- Hypertension (blood pressure >140/90 mm Hg or taking antihypertensive medication)
- Physical inactivity
- Obesity (body mass index of >30 kg/m²) and overweight (body mass index of 25 to 29.9 kg/m²)
- Impaired fasting glucose level and type 2 diabetes mellitus
- Metabolic syndrome
- Inflammatory markers (e.g., C-reactive protein)

Sources: National Cholesterol Education Program. *Third report of the NCEP Export Panel on Detection, Evaluation, and Treatment of High Blood Cholesterol in Adults (Adult Treatment Panel III)*. Washington, DC: National Institutes of Health; 2002; Stone NJ et al. 2013 ACC/AHA guideline on the treatment of blood cholesterol to reduce atherosclerotic cardiovascular risk in adults: a report of the American College of Cardiology/American Heart Association Task Force on Practice Guidelines. *J Am Coll Cardiol.* 2014;63(25 Pt B):2889-2934; Mozaffarian D et al. Heart disease and stroke statistics—2015 update: a report from the American Heart Association. *Circulation.* 2015;131(4):e29-322.
*High-density lipoprotein level of >60 mg/dL is cardioprotective.
[†]Atherogenic dyslipidemia is a disorder with four components: borderline high-risk low-density lipoprotein cholesterol level (i.e., 130 to 159 mg/dL), moderately raised (often high normal) triglyceride level, small low-density lipoprotein particles, and low high-density lipoprotein cholesterol level.

Table 19-2 Diagnostic Criteria for Metabolic Syndrome

MEASURE*	CATEGORIC CUT POINTS
Increased waist circumference[†,‡]	≥102 cm (≥40 inches) in men, ≥88 cm (≥35 inches) in women
Elevated level of triglycerides	≥150 mg/dL (1.7 mmol/L) or drug treatment for elevated triglycerides[§]
Reduced HDL-cholesterol level	<40 mg/dL (1.03 mmol/L) in men <50 mg/dL (1.3 mmol/L) in women or drug treatment for reduced HDL-cholesterol[§]
Elevated blood pressure	≥130 mm Hg systolic or ≥85 mm Hg diastolic or drug treatment for hypertension
Elevated fasting glucose level	≥100 mg/dL or drug treatment for elevated glucose

From Grundy SM, Cleeman JI, Daniels SR et al. American Heart Association; National Heart, Lung, and Blood Institute. Diagnosis and management of metabolic syndrome: an American Heart Association/National Heart, Lung, and Blood Institute Scientific Statement. *Circulation.* 2005;112:2735-2752.
*Any three of these five criteria constitute a diagnosis of metabolic syndrome.
[†]To measure waist circumference, locate the top of the right iliac crest. Place a measuring tape in a horizontal plane around the abdomen at the level of the iliac crest. Before reading the tape measure, ensure that the tape is snug but that it does not compress the skin, and be sure that it is parallel to the floor. The measurement is made at the end of a normal expiration.
[‡]Some U.S. adults of non-Asian origin (e.g., Caucasian, African American, Hispanic) with marginally increased waist circumferences (e.g., 94 to 101 cm [37 to 39 inches] in men and 80 to 87 cm [31 to 34 inches] in women) may have a strong genetic contribution to insulin resistance and should benefit from changes in lifestyle habits; this is similar for men with categoric increases in waist circumference. A lower waist circumference cut point (e.g., 90 cm [35 inches] in men and 80 cm [31 inches] in women) appears to be appropriate for Asian Americans.
[§]Fibrates and nicotinic acid are the most commonly used drugs for elevated triglycerides and reduced HDL-cholesterol. Patients who are taking one of these drugs are presumed to have a high triglyceride level and a low HDL-cholesterol level.

risk factors for the disease process, which is worsened by obesity, physical inactivity, diets that are high in trans fat and saturated fat, stress, and smoking. The American Heart Association Task Force recommends cholesterol screening every 4 to 6 years for adults without existing risk factors and more often for those with higher risks.[2]

- *Compounding conditions:* Co-morbidities associated with obesity such as type 2 diabetes, hypertension, and **metabolic syndrome** (Table 19-2) increase the

risk for the development of CVD. Population groups of low socioeconomic status have a higher prevalence of cardiovascular disease.[8]

Dietary Recommendations to Reduce Risk

The American Heart Association notes that poor diet quality is the number 1 risk factor for death and disability in the United States; and poor diet quality seems to be more the rule than the exception.[9] Less than 1% of all children and adults regularly consume a diet that meets at least 4 out of 5 dietary recommendations for a healthy diet (defined as ≥4.5 cups/day of fruits and vegetables, ≥2 servings/week of fish, ≥3 servings/day of whole grains, <36 oz/week of sugar-sweetened beverages, and ≤1500 mg/day of sodium).[9] See the For Further Focus box "Modifiable Risk Factors for Heart

metabolic syndrome a combination of disorders that, when they occur together, increases the risk of cardiovascular disease and diabetes; it is also known as syndrome X and insulin resistance syndrome.

Modifiable Risk Factors for Heart Disease

The American Heart Association uses a seven-metric system for evaluating overall cardiovascular health, which includes: smoking status, weight status, physical activity, diet, total blood cholesterol level, blood pressure, and fasting blood glucose level. Each measurement is a modifiable risk factor that can be addressed with diet and lifestyle adjustments. Of all of the health behaviors, poor dietary habits of American adults are the single largest risk factor contributing to cardiovascular disease.[1] Not incidentally, poor dietary habits negatively influence most of the other measurements in turn (e.g., body mass index, total blood cholesterol, blood pressure, and fasting blood glucose).

IDEAL CARDIOVASCULAR GOALS ARE AS FOLLOWS FOR ADULTS:

- Never smoked or quit >1 year ago
- At least 150 min of moderate or 75 min of vigorous physical activity each week
- Body mass index between 18.5 and 25 kg/m² (see inside back cover of textbook)

- Achieve at least 4 of the 5 following key components of a healthy diet:
  - Fruits and vegetables: consume >4.5 cups per day
  - Fish: consume more than two, 3.5-oz servings per week (preferably oily fish)
  - Fiber-rich whole grains (>1.1 g of fiber per 10 g of carbohydrates): consume three 1-oz-equivalent servings per day
  - Sodium: limit to <1500 mg per day
  - Sugar-sweetened beverages: limit to <450 kcal (36 oz) total per week
- Blood pressure: <120/<80 mm Hg
- Fasting blood glucose: <100 mg/dL
- Cholesterol: <200 mg/dL

REFERENCE

1. Mozaffarian D, et al. Heart disease and stroke statistics—2015 update: a report from the American Heart Association. *Circulation.* 2015;131(4):e29-e322.

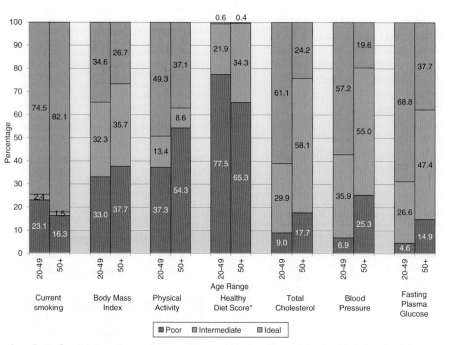

Prevalence (unadjusted) estimates of poor, intermediate, and ideal cardiovascular health for each of the seven metrics of cardiovascular health in the American Heart Association 2020 goals among US adults aged 20 to 49 years and ≥50 years, National Health and Nutrition Examination Survey (NHANES) 2011 to 2012.

*Healthy diet score data reflect 2009 to 2010 NHANES data.

Disease" for additional measures of cardiovascular health behaviors in the United States.

Dietary guidelines. The *Dietary Guidelines for Americans* (see Chapter 1) and the American Heart Association recommend the dietary restriction of certain types of fat and cholesterol to reduce the risk for heart disease

(Box 19-2). However, more importantly is the consideration of the whole diet. Changing one nutrient within an otherwise unhealthy diet will not likely make a significant difference in overall health risk. On the other hand, a shift to a more balanced, well-rounded diet and lifestyle is the primary focus of the *Joint American College of Cardiology (ACC) and the American*

Box 19-2 American Heart Association Dietary Guidelines

WEIGHT AND PHYSICAL ACTIVITY
- Burn at least as many calories as consumed.
- Aim for at least 30 minutes of physical activity on most, if not all, days. To lose weight, do enough activity to burn more calories than eaten every day.

FOODS TO FOCUS ON
- Eat a variety of nutritious foods from all food groups.
- Choose foods like vegetables, fruits, whole-grain products, nuts, and fat-free or low-fat dairy products most often.
- Choose lean meats such as poultry and prepare them without added saturated and trans fats.
- Eat fish at least twice a week.

FOODS TO LIMIT OR CONSUME IN MODERATION
- Limit the amount of saturated fat to 5% to 6% of total calories.
- Avoid trans fat.
- Limit sodium to a maximum of 2400 mg/day (<1500 mg/day reduces blood pressure even more).
- Limit red meat.
- Eat less of the nutrient-poor foods, such as beverages and foods with added sugars.
- Drink alcohol in moderation, if at all. That means one drink per day for women and two drinks per day for men.

GENERAL RECOMMENDATIONS
- Follow the American Heart Association recommendations when eating out, and keep an eye on portion sizes.
- Do not smoke tobacco, and stay away from tobacco smoke.

Source: American Heart Association, Inc. Modified from the American Heart Association. *Diet and lifestyle recommendations* (website): www.heart.org/HEARTORG/GettingHealthy/NutritionCenter/HealthyEating/The-American-Heart-Associations-Diet-and-Lifestyle-Recommendations_UCM_305855_Article.jsp. Accessed March 2015.

Heart Association (AHA) Task Force on Practice Guidelines to Reduce Cardiovascular Disease Risk.[10]

Adult treatment panel guidelines. The National Heart, Lung, and Blood Institute's National Cholesterol Education Program (NCEP) began a campaign against high blood cholesterol in 1988 with the release of its *Report of the Expert Panel on Detection, Evaluation, and Treatment of High Blood Cholesterol in Adults, Adult Treatment Panel (ATP)*. The NCEP designed the Step I and Step II diets, which were also endorsed by the American Heart Association, to lessen the risk of CVD by reducing high blood cholesterol levels. Since the inception of the Step I and Step II diets, the NCEP has released two follow-up reports. In the last NCEP report (ATP III), the organization moved toward an intensive lifestyle habit intervention that focuses on appropriate weight, diet, physical activity, and other controllable risk factors.[11] This approach is referred to as the

Therapeutic Lifestyle Changes (TLC) diet. The most recent Task Force recommendations, however, are broader and are discussed next.

Lifestyle management guideline recommendations. The *ACC/AHA Task Force on Practice Guidelines to Reduce Cardiovascular Disease Risk,* in collaboration with the National Heart, Lung, and Blood Institute, has recently released *Lifestyle Management Guidelines* that are to take the place of the previously used TLC diet. Essential components of the Lifestyle Management approach for all adults, regardless of risk, are as follows[10,12]:

- Consume a dietary pattern that emphasizes intake of vegetables, fruits, and whole grains; includes low-fat dairy products, poultry, fish, legumes, non-tropical vegetable oils and nuts; and limits intake of sodium, sweets, sugar-sweetened beverages, and red meats.
- Adapt this dietary pattern to appropriate calorie requirements, personal and cultural food preferences, and nutrition therapy for other medical conditions (e.g., diabetes mellitus, obesity). This diet should allow for the achievement and maintenance of a healthy weight.
- Achieve this pattern by following plans such as the *Dietary Approaches to Stop Hypertension (DASH)* dietary pattern (discussed later in this chapter), the *Dietary Guidelines for Americans,* or the *American Heart Association Dietary Guidelines* (see Box 19-2).
- Engage in 2 hours and 30 minutes per week of moderate-intensity aerobic physical activity or 1 hour and 15 minutes (75 minutes) per week of vigorous-intensity aerobic physical activity, or an equivalent combination of moderate- and vigorous-intensity aerobic physical activity. Aerobic activity should be performed in episodes of at least 10 minutes, preferably spread throughout the week.

For patients who would specifically benefit from lowering their LDL-cholesterol, the Task Force makes the following additional recommendations:
- Reduce total percent of calories from saturated fat. Aim for a dietary pattern that limits calories from saturated fat to no more than 5% to 6%.
- Reduce percentage of calories from trans fats.
- Engage in three to four sessions of aerobic physical activity, lasting an average of 40 minutes each session, and involving moderate- to vigorous-intensity physical activity.

Therapeutic Lifestyle Changes (TLC) an intensive lifestyle intervention that is focused on appropriate weight, diet, physical activity, and other controllable risk factors to reduce cholesterol levels and to prevent other complications of heart disease.

A diet that is rich in vegetables, fruits, and whole grains; is low in saturated and trans fatty acids; and includes the moderate use of polyunsaturated and monounsaturated food fats (i.e., mostly olive oil, corn oil, and other vegetable oils and products) is the basic guideline. Low-fat and fat-free dairy products as well as lean meat, fish, and poultry are used instead of their high-fat alternatives. These guidelines differ from the TLC guidelines in that specific calorie amounts from each of the macronutrients are not defined.

When the risk factor of obesity is present, weight loss via negative energy balance is encouraged. Interestingly, studies show that weight-loss attempts are largely unsuccessful among patients with CVD; however, when a physician officially diagnoses a patient as overweight, weight-loss attempts are more successful.[13,14] Negative energy balance should be achieved through reduced energy intake and increased energy expenditure from regular physical activity (see Chapter 15). A treadmill exercise tolerance test is ideal to determine the exercise limit for individuals who are older, who are obese, or who have a history of CVD or hypertension before they start an exercise program (Figure 19-4).

Drug Therapy

In the event that the LDL-cholesterol level is above the goal range or multiple risk factors for cardiovascular disease are present, the *ACC/AHH Guidelines on the Treatment of Blood Cholesterol* provide an algorithm for determining the appropriate statin therapy regimen.[2] As the number and severity of risk factors increase, the point at which drug therapy should begin is hastened. For example, a person with few or no risk factors associated with CVD may wait to initiate drug therapy until LDL-cholesterol levels exceed

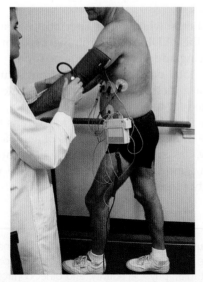

FIGURE 19-4 A patient with a history of cardiac disease is evaluated for exercise tolerance with a treadmill stress test. (Copyright PhotoDisc.)

190 mg/dL, whereas an individual with significant risk for CVD should consider drug therapy when LDL-cholesterol levels rise to more than 100 mg/dL. The guidelines recommend statin therapy for the following groups[2]:

- People without cardiovascular disease who are 40 to 75 years old and have a 7.5% or greater risk for having a heart attack or stroke within 10 years (according to the National Heart, Lung, and Blood Institute's risk assessment tool for estimating 10-year risk of having a heart attack: http://cvdrisk.nhlbi.nih.gov)
- People with a history of a cardiovascular event
- People 21 years old and older who have a very high level of LDL-cholesterol (≥190 mg/dL)
- People with type 1 or type 2 diabetes who are 40 to 75 years old

At any level of drug therapy, the *ACC/AHA Lifestyle Management Guidelines* including nutrition and physical activity should be continued as adjunct therapy.

ACUTE CARDIOVASCULAR DISEASE

When CVD progresses to the point of cutting off the blood supply to major coronary arteries, a critical vascular event (i.e., MI) may occur. During the initial acute phase of the attack, diet modifications may be warranted for healing.

Objective: Cardiac Rest

The term *infarction* means tissue death from a lack of oxygen. Blood tests reveal enzymes and proteins that are released from the damaged heart muscle after infarction; these cardiac markers are one of the tests used for diagnosis. During the care immediately after an MI, patients may be treated with the MONA protocol and given analgesics (e.g., *M*orphine, supplemental *O*xygen, intravenous *N*itroglycerin, and *A*spirin). The individual aspects of the MONA protocol are administered only when indicated, with the exception of aspirin, which is almost always given. For example, if a patient is not in pain, morphine is not necessary. All care, including the diet, is directed toward ensuring cardiac rest so that the damaged heart may be restored to normal functioning.

Principles of Medical Nutrition Therapy

Medical nutrition therapy goals for patients after MI are as follows: (1) promote recovery and strength; and (2) lower LDL-cholesterol and other known risk factors to prevent the progression of CVD.[15] Patients who have experienced an MI are encouraged to follow the *ACC/AHA Lifestyle Management Guidelines* (if they are not already doing so) to reduce further risk factors associated with CVD.

Initially, the diet may be modified with regard to energy value and texture (see the Clinical Applications box, "Case Study: The Patient with a Myocardial Infarction"). After the initial acute phase, dietary

Clinical Applications

Case Study: The Patient with a Myocardial Infarction

Charles Carter is a 56-year-old businessman who works long hours and who carries the major responsibilities of his struggling small business. At his last physical checkup, the physician cautioned him about his pace, because he was already showing mild hypertension. His blood cholesterol level was elevated, and he was overweight, with a body mass index of 28.5 kg/m^2. At his desk job, he gets little exercise, and he finds himself smoking more and eating irregularly as a result of the stress of his increasing financial pressures.

One day while commuting in heavy freeway traffic, Charles felt a pain in his chest, and he became increasingly apprehensive. When he arrived home, the pain increased. He broke out into a cold sweat, and he felt nauseated. When he became more ill after trying to eat dinner, his wife called their physician, and Charles was admitted to the hospital.

After emergency care and tests, the physician placed Charles in the coronary care unit at the hospital. His test results showed elevated total cholesterol, LDL-cholesterol, and triglyceride levels and a low HDL-cholesterol level. The electrocardiogram revealed an infarction of the posterior myocardium wall.

When Charles was first able to take oral nourishment, he could only consume a liquid diet. As his condition stabilized, his diet was increased to 1200 kcal (soft diet) with low saturated fat and low sodium. By the end of the first week, his diet was increased to 1600 kcal (full diet), with low saturated fat,

≤25% of the kilocalories from fat, and a polyunsaturated fat to saturated fat ratio of 1:1.

Charles gradually improved over the next few days and was able to go home. The physician, the nurse, and the dietitian discussed with Charles and his wife the need for care at home during a period of convalescence. They explained that Charles had an underlying lipid disorder and that he needed to continue his weight loss and follow the *ACC/AHA Lifestyle Management Guidelines.*

QUESTIONS FOR ANALYSIS

1. Identify factors in this patient's personal and medical history that place him at high risk for coronary heart disease. Give reasons why each factor contributes to heart disease.
2. Why did Charles receive only a liquid diet at first? What is the reason for each modification in his first diet of solid food?
3. What occurs during the underlying disease process that causes a heart attack? What relationship does dietary fat have to this underlying process?
4. What needs might Charles have when he goes home? How would you help him to prepare to go home? Name some community resources that you might use to help him understand his illness and plan self-care.

---

modifications will depend on the underlying cause and other co-morbidities (e.g., hypertension, atherosclerosis, obesity, diabetes).

Energy. A brief period of reduced energy intake during the first day after the heart attack reduces the metabolic workload on the damaged heart. The metabolic demands for the digestion, absorption, and metabolism of food require a generous cardiac output. Thus, to decrease the level of metabolic activity that the weakened heart can handle, small feedings are spread over the day when an oral diet is started. The patient progresses to eating more as healing occurs. During the recovery period, caloric intake is adjusted to meet the energy needs of the person's ideal body weight.

Texture. Early feedings may include foods that are relatively soft in texture or easily digested to avoid excess effort during eating or the discomfort of gas formation. Some patients benefit from assistance during the feeding process for a short period, especially those with poor appetite or weakness or who become short of breath from the exertion of eating. Smaller and more frequent meals may provide needed nourishment without undue strain or pressure. Depending on the patient's condition, gas-forming

foods, caffeine-containing beverages, and hot or cold temperature extremes in foods in both solids and liquids should be avoided.

Long-Term Dietary Modifications

In order to reduce the risk for additional myocardial infarctions, patients are encouraged to following the *ACC/AHA Lifestyle Management Guidelines.* Many patients will benefit from a very specific daily menu guide to get them started on a healthier eating plan. Research supports the adoption of a Mediterranean diet or the DASH diet (covered later in this chapter) for patients with cardiovascular disease who have had an MI.

Mediterranean diet. Scientific studies evaluating the benefits of the Mediterranean diet are difficult to carry out and difficult to interpret because the definition of the Mediterranean diet is subjective. When patients are told to "eat more fruits and vegetables and replace saturated fat with olive oil," it is often not enough to invoke measureable changes in the otherwise typical Western diet. However, studies in areas of the world where the Mediterranean diet is the standard fair (i.e., Spain), or in studies where participants were specifically given meal plans or provided with food, research findings are more encouraging.

Adherence to a well-defined Mediterranean diet reduces risk factors for CVD, reduces inflammatory markers after an MI, and increases the life span.[16-21] The basic components of a Mediterranean diet are plant-based foods; nuts; whole grains; fish and poultry at least twice a week, with limited red meat; moderate amounts of dairy products and eggs; olive oil as the primary source of fat; the use of herbs and spices in place of salt; moderate red wine intake with meals; fresh fruit as dessert; and minimal intake of processed foods. Mediterranean lifestyles also include regular physical activity and exercise (see Figure 14-5).

Sodium. General attention to reduced sodium content in food selection is important as well (Box 19-3). If the patient has hypertension, sodium restriction to approximately 2400 mg/day may be indicated to control edema.[15] This restriction can be achieved by using little or no salt in cooking, adding no salt when eating, and avoiding salty processed foods. Box 19-4 provides options for salt-free seasoning that patients may find helpful for flavoring their food while cooking in lieu of salt. Nutrition Facts labels provide specific information about the sodium content per serving of any food and may be used as an ideal tool for selectively choosing appropriate foods to include in the diet on an individual basis (see Chapter 13).

Box 19-3	Sodium-Restricted Diet Recommendations*

- Choose low- or reduced-sodium or no-salt-added versions of foods and condiments, when available.
- Choose fresh, frozen, or canned low-sodium or no-salt-added vegetables.
- Cook without salt, and avoid adding salt to prepared meals.
- Avoid salt-preserved foods such as salted or smoked meat (e.g., bacon, bacon fat, bologna, dried or chipped beef, corned beef, frankfurters, ham, kosher meats, luncheon meats, salt pork, sausage), salted or smoked fish (e.g., anchovies, caviar, salted and dried cod, herring, sardines), sauerkraut, and olives. Use fresh poultry, fish, and lean meats instead.
- Avoid highly salted foods such as crackers, pretzels, potato chips, corn chips, salted nuts, and salted popcorn. Choose products that are lower in sodium.
- Limit spices and condiments such as bouillon cubes, ketchup, chili sauce, celery salt, garlic salt, onion salt, monosodium glutamate, meat sauces, meat tenderizers, pickles, prepared mustard, relishes, Worcestershire sauce, and soy sauce.†
- Limit processed foods and convenience foods (e.g., cheese, peanut butter, flavored rice and pasta, frozen dinners, canned soups) that are usually high in salt, or choose reduced-sodium versions.†

*These restrictions are for a mild, low-sodium diet (i.e., 2 to 4 g/day).
†Low-sodium brands may be used.

HEART FAILURE

Congestive heart failure is a form of chronic heart disease. The progressively weakened heart muscle is unable to maintain an adequate cardiac output to sustain normal blood circulation. The resulting fluid imbalances make basic functions of living (e.g., breathing, eating, walking, sleeping) difficult to perform. The most common causes of heart failure are coronary artery disease, MI, and chronic hypertension.

Control of Pulmonary Edema

The goals of diet therapy for a patient with congestive heart failure are to manage shortness of breath and fatigue, and to control the fluid imbalance that results in **pulmonary edema**. The primary causes of fluid accumulation are altered fluid shift mechanisms and inappropriate hormonal responses.

Fluid shift mechanism. With decreased heart function, blood accumulates in the vascular system. This buildup offsets the delicate balance of filtration pressures and causes fluid to collect within intracellular spaces instead of flowing among fluid compartments.

Hormonal alterations. Kidney nephrons sense decreased renal blood flow, which is normally an indication of dehydration and hypovolemia, and they respond by triggering the vasopressin and renin-angiotensin-aldosterone systems to increase blood pressure (see Chapter 9). Unlike dehydration, reduced blood flow in this situation is caused by the inadequate pumping of the heart rather than by hypovolemia. Vasopressin from the pituitary gland, which is also known as *antidiuretic hormone,* stimulates the resorption of water in the kidneys. In addition, aldosterone, which is secreted by the adrenal glands, causes the resorption of sodium (and thus water) in the kidneys. Consequently, fluid retention is increased, and edema is exacerbated.

Principles of Medical Nutrition Therapy

Medical nutrition therapy focuses on achieving nutritional adequacy of the diet while limiting sodium and fluid intake to control edema.[15]

The main source of dietary sodium is common table salt or sodium chloride. The taste for salt is acquired. Some people heavily salt their food out of habit without tasting it first, thereby habituating their taste to high salt levels. Others acquire a taste for less salt by

congestive heart failure a chronic condition of gradually weakening heart muscle; the muscle is unable to pump normal blood through the heart-lung circulation, which results in the congestion of fluids in the lungs.
pulmonary edema an accumulation of fluid in the lung tissues.

Box 19-4   Suggestions for Salt-Free Seasoning

FISH

Breaded, battered fillets
　Dry mustard, onion, oregano, basil, garlic, thyme
Broiled steaks or fillets
　Chili or curry powder, tarragon
Fillets in butter sauce
　Thyme, chervil, dill, fennel
Fish cakes
　Tarragon, savory, dry mustard, white pepper, red
　　pepper, oregano

BEEF

Swiss steak
　Rosemary, black pepper, bay leaf, thyme, clove
Roast beef
　Basil, oregano, bay leaf, nutmeg, tarragon, marjoram
Beef stew
　Chili powder, bay leaf, tarragon, caraway, marjoram
Meatballs
　Garlic, thyme, basil, oregano, onion, black pepper, dry
　　mustard
Beef stroganoff
　Red pepper, onion, garlic, nutmeg, curry powder

POULTRY AND VEAL

Fried chicken
　Basil, oregano, garlic, onion, dill, sesame seed, nutmeg
Roast chicken or turkey
　Ginger, garlic, onion, thyme, tarragon
Chicken croquettes
　Dill, curry, chili, cumin, tarragon, oregano
Veal patties
　Italian seasoning, tarragon, dill, onion, sesame seeds
Barbecue chicken
　Garlic, dry mustard, clove, allspice, basil, oregano

GRAVIES AND SAUCES

Barbecue
　Bay leaf, thyme, red pepper, cinnamon, ginger, allspice,
　　dry mustard, chili powder
Brown
　Chervil, onion, bay leaf, thyme, nutmeg, tarragon
Chicken
　Dry mustard, ginger, garlic, marjoram, thyme, bay leaf
Cream
　White pepper, dry mustard, curry powder, dill, onion,
　　paprika, tarragon, thyme

SOUPS

Chicken
　Thyme, savory, ginger, clove, white pepper, allspice
Clam chowder
　Basil, oregano, nutmeg, white pepper, thyme, garlic
　　powder

Mushroom
　Ginger, oregano, thyme, tarragon, bay leaf, black
　　pepper, chili powder
Onion
　Curry, caraway, marjoram, garlic, cloves
Tomato
　Bay leaf, thyme, Italian seasoning, oregano, onion,
　　nutmeg
Vegetable
　Italian seasoning, paprika, caraway, rosemary, thyme,
　　fennel

SALADS

Chicken
　Curry or chili powder, Italian seasoning, thyme, tarragon
Coleslaw
　Dill, caraway, poppy seeds, dry mustard, ginger
Fish or seafood
　Dill, tarragon, ginger, dry mustard, red pepper, onion,
　　garlic
Macaroni
　Dill, basil, thyme, oregano, dry mustard, garlic
Potato
　Chili powder, curry, dry mustard, onion

PASTA, BEANS, AND RICE

Baked beans
　Dry mustard, chili powder, clove, onion, ginger
Rice and vegetables
　Curry, thyme, onion, paprika, rosemary, garlic, ginger
Spanish rice
　Cumin, oregano, basil, Italian seasoning
Spaghetti
　Italian seasoning, nutmeg, oregano, basil, red pepper,
　　tarragon
Rice pilaf
　Dill, thyme, savory, black pepper

VEGETABLES

Asparagus
　Ginger, sesame seeds, basil, onion
Broccoli
　Italian seasoning, marjoram, basil, nutmeg, onion,
　　sesame seeds
Cabbage
　Caraway, onion, nutmeg, allspice, clove
Carrots
　Ginger, nutmeg, onion, dill
Cauliflower
　Dry mustard, basil, paprika, onion
Tomatoes
　Oregano, chili powder, dill, onion
Spinach
　Savory, thyme, nutmeg, garlic, onion

gradually using smaller and smaller amounts. The Adequate Intake for sodium is 1500 mg per day for adults up to the age of 50 years, and then it declines slightly.[22] Daily adult intakes of sodium range widely in the typical American diet; men consume an average of 4218 mg/day, and women consume an average of 2997 mg/day.[23] Other than the salt that is used in cooking or added at the table, a large amount is used as a preservative in processed food. Remaining sources of sodium include that found as a naturally occurring mineral in certain foods.

Nutrition therapy focuses on the following[15]:

- *Sodium restriction (2 g per day):* For patients with moderate to severe heart failure. No salt is served with meals. Fresh foods are encouraged and should include sodium-free flavorings such as herbs. Salty processed foods are avoided (e.g., pickles, olives, bacon, ham, corn chips, potato chips).
- *Fluid restriction:* Fluid is limited to 2 L per day for patients with serum sodium levels less than 130 mEq/L.
- *Dietary supplements:* Thiamin and potassium supplements may be needed to overcome losses from diuretics. Ensure DRIs are met for folate, vitamin B$_{12}$, and magnesium through diet and/or supplements.
- *Alcohol:* Alcohol intake is limited to one drink per day for women and two drinks per day for men in patients who regularly consume alcohol. Alcohol must be completely avoided by patients in whom alcohol contributed to their heart disease.

Patients may tolerate soft foods better if eating is laborious or uncomfortable. Frequent small meals (e.g., five to six per day) are better suited than large meals to prevent fatigue from eating. Care should be taken to ensure that diet restrictions do not result in nutrient inadequacies in the diet.

ESSENTIAL HYPERTENSION

INCIDENCE AND NATURE

Hypertension or high blood pressure is one of the most common vascular diseases worldwide. Thirty percent of American adults who are older than 20 years have hypertension. Of the adults with hypertension, 55% of them have uncontrolled high blood pressure (Figure 19-5). The incidence of hypertension is highest among African-American women, with a 44.2% prevalence rate.[1] When speaking of the chronic condition of elevated blood pressure, the term *hypertension* is more appropriate than *high blood pressure,* because blood pressure may occasionally be elevated during situations that involve overexertion or stress. With **essential (or primary) hypertension,** the specific etiology is unknown, although some possible dynamics include genetics, congenital defects, lifestyle factors, oxidative stress, and renal abnormalities causing problems with the antidiuretic system, renin-angiotensin-aldosterone system, or sodium imbalance (see Chapter 9).[24,25] More than 90% of cases are

> **essential (or primary) hypertension** an inherent form of high blood pressure with no specific identifiable cause; it is considered to be familial.

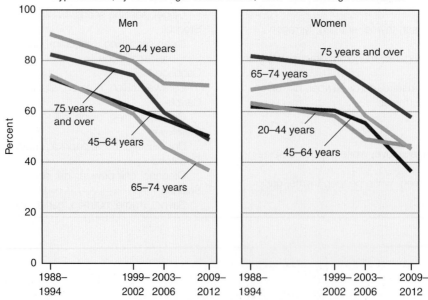

Uncontrolled high blood pressure among adults aged 20 and over with hypertension, by sex and age: United States, 1988–1994 through 2009–2012

FIGURE 19-5 Uncontrolled high blood pressure among adults aged 20 years and older with hypertension, by sex and age: United States, 1988-1994 through 2009-2012. (National Center for Health Statistics. *Health, United States, 2014: with special feature of adults aged 55-64.* Hyattsville, Md: U.S. Government Printing Office; 2015.)

considered to be essential hypertension. **Secondary hypertension** is the result of a known cause; it is a symptom or side effect of another primary condition. For example, individuals with kidney disease often have secondary hypertension.

Hypertension has been called "the silent killer," because no signs indicate its presence. It can have serious effects if it is not detected, treated, and controlled. There are significant indications that many genetic variants play a role in the heritability of hypertension and the individual differences to medication treatment.[26-28] A family history of hypertension quadruples one's risk of developing hypertension. Children of hypertensive parents are twice as likely to develop hypertension; and hypertension during childhood is strongly associated with pervasive hypertension throughout life.[29,30] Obesity worsens the condition through a multitude of pathways, including inflammation, renal damage, endothelial damage, oxidative stress, and hyperinsulinemia.[31] Smoking also increases blood pressure, because nicotine constricts the small vessels. Other risk factors include increasing age, ethnicity, physical inactivity, alcohol consumption, sodium intake, and chronic stress.

> **secondary hypertension** an elevated blood pressure for which the cause can be identified and that is a symptom or side effect of another primary condition.

HYPERTENSIVE BLOOD PRESSURE LEVELS

Common blood pressure measurements indicate the pressure of the blood surge in the arteries of the upper arm with each heartbeat. The power of each surge is measured in millimeters of mercury (mm Hg). Two forces are counted and represented by separate numbers. The numerator of the fraction measures the force of the blood surge when the heart contracts, which is known as the *systolic pressure*. The denominator of the fraction measures the pressure that remains in the arteries when the heart relaxes between beats; this is known as the *diastolic pressure*. Adult blood pressure is considered normal if it is less than 120/80 mm Hg. Current hypertension screening and treatment paradigms identify people with hypertension according to the degree of severity of these pressures and existing co-morbidities (Table 19-3).[32] Specific care is then determined after consideration for all variables.

Prehypertension

Prehypertension is identified by blood pressure measurements that are above normal but are not so high as to meet the diagnostic criteria for hypertension. It is similar in this regard to *prediabetes*. The assumption is that without intervention, the patient will likely progress to stage 1 hypertension.

The initial focus of hypertension treatment is on lifestyle modifications. Lifestyle choices that are encouraged include the following: (1) weight loss, if indicated; (2) increased fruit, vegetable, and low-fat

Table 19-3 Classification of Blood Pressure for Adults*

BLOOD PRESSURE CLASSIFICATION	SYSTOLIC BLOOD PRESSURE (mm Hg)	DIASTOLIC BLOOD PRESSURE (mm Hg)	LIFESTYLE MODIFICATION	INITIAL DRUG THERAPY
Normal	<120	and <80	Encourage	
Prehypertension[†]	120 to 139	or 80 to 89	Yes	No antihypertensive drug indicated
Stage 1 hypertension				There is moderate evidence to support initiating drug treatment with an angiotensin-converting enzyme inhibitor, angiotensin receptor blocker, calcium channel blocker, or thiazide-type diuretic in the nonblack hypertensive population, including those with diabetes. In the black hypertensive population, including those with diabetes, a calcium channel blocker or thiazide-type diuretic is recommended as initial therapy. There is moderate evidence to support initial or add-on antihypertensive therapy with an angiotensin-converting enzyme inhibitor or angiotensin receptor blocker in persons with chronic kidney disease to improve kidney outcomes.
Age 18-59 years old	140 to 159	or 90 to 99	Yes	
Age ≥60 years old	≥150	or 90 to 99	Yes	
Stage 2 hypertension	≥160	or ≥100	Yes	

Modified from James PA et al. 2014 evidence-based guideline for the management of high blood pressure in adults: report from the panel members appointed to the Eighth Joint National Committee (JNC 8). *JAMA.* 2014;311(5):507-520.
*Information for adults 18 years old and older. Treatment is determined by the highest blood pressure category.
†*Prehypertension* means that the blood pressure is above optimal levels but not high enough to be diagnosed with hypertension.

Table **19-4**   Lifestyle Modifications to Prevent and Manage Hypertension*

MODIFICATION	RECOMMENDATION	APPROXIMATE SYSTOLIC BLOOD PRESSURE REDUCTION[†]
Weight reduction	Maintain a healthy body weight (i.e., body mass index of 18.5 to 24.9 kg/m^2)	5 to 20 mm Hg/10 kg
Adopt the DASH eating plan[‡]	Consume a diet that is rich in fruits, vegetables, and low-fat dairy products with a reduced content of saturated and total fat	8 to 14 mm Hg
Lower sodium intake	Consume no more than 2400 mg of sodium/d; further reduction of sodium intake to 1500 mg/d is desirable because it is associated with a greater reduction in blood pressure; reduce sodium intake by at least 1000 mg/d since that will lower blood pressure, even if the desired daily sodium intake is not achieved	2 to 8 mm Hg
Physical activity	Engage in regular aerobic physical activity such as brisk walking at least 30 minutes per day most days of the week	4 to 9 mm Hg
Moderation of alcohol consumption	Limit alcohol consumption to no more than two drinks per day for most men and to no more than one drink per day for women and lighter-weight men[§]	2 to 4 mm Hg

Modified from Go AS et al. An effective approach to high blood pressure control: a science advisory from the American Heart Association, the American College of Cardiology, and the Centers for Disease Control and Prevention. *Hypertension.* 2014;63(4):878-885.
*For overall cardiovascular risk reduction, stop smoking.
[†]The effects of implementing these modifications are dependent on dose and time and could be greater for some individuals.
[‡]Dietary Approaches to Stop Hypertension (DASH) eating plan is discussed later in this chapter.
[§]One drink is defined as 12 oz of beer, 5 oz of wine, 1.5 oz of 80-proof whiskey.

dairy consumption; (3) reduced sodium, total fat, and saturated fat intake; (4) moderation of alcohol use; (5) regular aerobic physical fitness; and (6) cessation of smoking, if indicated.[33,34] Such lifestyle changes are able to reduce the risk of chronic disease and improve blood pressure (Table 19-4).

Stage 1 Hypertension

In addition to the lifestyle modifications encouraged for prehypertension, blood pressure lowering medications are used according to need and usually include a diuretic for patients with stage 1 hypertension. Table 19-3 provides the guidelines' summary for initiating drug therapy in response to hypertensive stage. The continuous use of some diuretic drugs may cause a loss of potassium along with the increased loss of water from the body. Because potassium is necessary for maintaining normal heart muscle action, depletion could become dangerous. Potassium replacement is sometimes necessary. Dietary replacement with the increased use of potassium-rich foods (e.g., fruits, especially bananas and orange juice; vegetables; legumes; nuts; whole grains) is an important part of therapy. The sodium and potassium values of various foods can be found in Appendix C.

Stage 2 Hypertension

In addition to the diet for stage 1 hypertension, vigorous drug therapy is necessary for stage 2 hypertension. The 8th Joint National Committee Guidelines provide practitioners with a detailed algorithm for initiating and evaluating drug therapy for hypertension management.[32] See the Drug-Nutrient Interaction box titled "Grapefruit Juice and Drug Metabolism" for more

information about potential interactions with the medications that are often used for hypertension. Nutrition therapy is important for all types of hypertension, along with other nondrug therapies such as physical activity and stress reduction.

PRINCIPLES OF MEDICAL NUTRITION THERAPY

Regardless of hypertensive stage, lifestyle modifications such as diet and exercise are the foundation for treatment. The *Lifestyle Management Guideline Recommendations* from the ACC/AHA Task Force to reduce the risk for CVD (provided on p. 333) are recommended for all adults.[10] In addition, the following recommendations are specifically encouraged for adults who would benefit from lowering their blood pressure.

Weight Management

In accordance with individual need, weight management requires losing excess body fat and maintaining a healthy weight for one's stature. A sound approach to managing weight loss is discussed in Chapter 15, and guidance for increasing physical activity is provided in Chapter 16. Because excess weight is closely associated with hypertension risk factors, a wisely planned personal program of weight reduction and physical activity is the cornerstone of therapy. In overweight patients, their systolic blood pressure will decrease by 5 to 20 mm Hg, on average, for every 10 kg of weight loss.[34]

Physical Activity

Participating in regular physical activity is important throughout all life-cycle stages for general health and

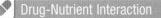

Drug-Nutrient Interaction

Grapefruit Juice and Drug Metabolism

KELLI BOI

A common pathway for drug metabolism makes use of the enzyme CYP3A. This enzyme oxidizes lipid-soluble drugs, thereby making them more water soluble in preparation for urinary excretion. As more of the drug is oxidized, less is absorbed. This system is anticipated when standard dosages of drugs are determined. It is expected that only a percentage of the therapeutic agent will actually reach the circulation.

Compounds in grapefruit juice known as *furanocoumarins* inhibit CYP3A, thereby increasing the amount of the associated drug that enters the circulation. As little as 8 oz of grapefruit juice can increase the absorption of certain drugs for up to 72 hours after consumption. The increased absorption of these medications may cause adverse events and can, in some cases, be fatal. Patients essentially experience drug toxicity from their prescribed dose as a result of the drastic increase in absorption of the active ingredient.

Several cardiovascular drugs make use of the CYP3A pathway for metabolism. The table below shows some of the cardiovascular agents that are influenced by grapefruit's inhibition of CYP3A and their side effects. Hospitals and inpatient facilities do not serve grapefruit juice, and patients who are taking drugs that use the CYP3A pathway for metabolism should avoid drinking grapefruit juice at home.

DRUG NAME	DRUG CLASS	DRUG ACTION	SIDE EFFECTS	ADDITIONAL COMMENTS
Amiodarone (Cordarone)	Antiarrhythmic	Broad-spectrum antiarrhythmic, vasodilator	Anorexia, nausea, vomiting, constipation	High levels may cause fatal pulmonary toxicity
Amlodipine (Norvasc) Nifedipine (Procardia) Nisoldipine	Calcium channel blockers	Antihypertensive	Nausea, dyspepsia, constipation, peripheral edema, muscle cramps, flushing	Alternative calcium channel blockers (e.g., verapamil) are available that do not interact with grapefruit juice
Atorvastatin (Lipitor) Lovastatin (Mevacor) Simvastatin (Zocor)	3-hydroxy-3-methylglutaryl coenzyme A inhibitors/statins	Antihyperlipidemic	Nausea, dyspepsia, abdominal pain, constipation, diarrhea, possible myopathy	Alternative medications in this class are available that do not have significant interactions with grapefruit juice (e.g., fluvastatin, pravastatin, rosuvastatin)

fitness. Participating in at least 30 minutes of aerobic physical activity on most days of the week can lower systolic blood pressure by 4 to 9 mm Hg.[34] The ACC/AHA Task Force recommends patients engage in moderate- to vigorous-intensity aerobic activity 3 to 4 times per week, lasting on average 40 minutes per session to lower blood pressure.[10] For some patients, the combined benefits of weight loss and physical activity are enough to correct for chronically elevated blood pressure and allow them to discontinue medication.

The DASH Diet

The DASH diet is the result of the successful Dietary Approaches to Stop Hypertension landmark study, which was able to lower blood pressure significantly by diet alone within a 2-week period. The diet recommends eating 4 to 6 servings of fruits, 4 to 6 servings of vegetables, and 2 to 3 servings of low-fat dairy foods per day in addition to lean meats, nuts, seeds, dried beans, and high-fiber grains. Studies have found that individuals who follow the diet have an average decrease in systolic blood pressure of 6 to 11 mm Hg.[35]

When combining the DASH diet with a low-sodium diet, the blood–pressure-lowering effects are even greater.[36] Combining the DASH diet with exercise and weight loss also produces a reduction in total cholesterol and LDL-cholesterol levels, a reduced risk for coronary heart disease and heart failure, and improvements in insulin sensitivity.[37-40]

The ACC/AHA Task Force endorses the DASH diet as one method in which the lifestyle modifications can be achieved. The DASH diet is recommended for individuals with high blood pressure, blood pressure in the prehypertension range, and a family history of high blood pressure; it is also recommended for those who are trying to eliminate the use of blood–pressure-lowering medications. The first step in following the DASH diet is to determine the appropriate energy level (in kilocalories) on the basis of the desired weight and activity level (see Chapter 6). The appropriate number of servings per day of each food group should then be based on the total energy need. Table 19-5 outlines the DASH diet and its associated serving sizes; Box 19-5 provides a 1-day sample menu that is based on a 2000-calorie diet.

Table **19-5**   The DASH Eating Plan

CALORIES PER DAY	GRAINS*	VEGETABLES	FRUITS	FAT-FREE OR LOW-FAT MILK AND MILK PRODUCTS	LEAN MEATS, POULTRY, AND FISH	NUTS, SEEDS, AND LEGUMES	FATS AND OILS†	SWEETS AND ADDED SUGARS
1600	6	3 to 4	4	2 to 3	3 to 6	3 per week	2	0
2000	6 to 8	4 to 5	4 to 5	2 to 3	≤6	4 to 5 per week	2 to 3	≤5 per week
2600	10 to 11	5 to 6	5 to 6	3	6	1	3	≤2
3100	12 to 13	6	6	3 to 4	6 to 9	1	4	≤2
Serving sizes	1 slice bread; 1 oz dry cereal‡; ½ cup cooked rice, pasta, or cereal	1 cup raw leafy vegetables, ½ cup cut-up raw or cooked vegetables, ½ cup vegetable juice	1 medium fruit; ¼ cup dried fruit; ½ cup fresh, frozen, or canned fruit; ½ cup fruit juice	1 cup milk or yogurt, 1½ oz cheese	1 oz cooked meat, poultry, or fish; 1 egg§	⅓ cup or 1½ oz nuts, 2 Tbsp peanut butter, 2 Tbsp or ½ oz seeds, ½ cup cooked legumes (dry beans and peas)	1 tsp soft margarine, 1 tsp vegetable oil, 1 Tbsp mayonnaise, 2 Tbsp salad dressing	1 Tbsp sugar, 1 Tbsp jelly or jam, ½ cup sorbet, gelatin; 1 cup lemonade

SERVINGS PER DAY (UNLESS OTHERWISE SPECIFIED)

Modified from the National Institutes of Health; National Heart, Lung, and Blood Institute. *Your guide to lowering your blood pressure with DASH, NIH Publication No. 06-4082.* Washington, DC: U.S. Department of Health and Human Services; 2006.
*Whole grains are recommended for most grain servings as a good source of fiber and nutrients.
†Fat content changes the serving amount for fats and oils. For example, 1 Tbsp of regular salad dressing equals one serving, whereas 1 Tbsp of a low-fat dressing equals a half serving and 1 Tbsp of a fat-free dressing equals zero servings.
‡Serving sizes vary between ½ cup and 1¼ cups, depending on the cereal type. Check the product's Nutrition Facts label.
§Because eggs are high in cholesterol, limit egg yolk intake to no more than four per week; two egg whites have the same protein content as 1 oz of meat.

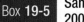

Box 19-5 Sample 1-Day Menu on the Dash Diet, 2000 Calories

BREAKFAST
- ¾ cup bran flakes cereal
- 1 medium banana
- 1 cup low-fat milk
- 1 slice whole-wheat bread
- 1 tsp unsalted soft (tub) margarine
- 1 cup orange juice

LUNCH
- ¾ cup chicken salad
- 2 slices whole-wheat bread
- 1 Tbsp Dijon mustard
- Salad with the following:
  - ½ cup fresh cucumber slices
  - ½ cup tomato wedges
  - 1 Tbsp sunflower seeds
  - 1 tsp Italian dressing, low calorie
- ½ cup fruit cocktail, juice packed

DINNER
- 3 oz beef, eye of round
- 2 Tbsp beef gravy, fat free
- 1 cup green beans, sautéed with ½ tsp canola oil
- 1 small baked potato with the following:
  - 1 Tbsp sour cream, fat free
  - 1 Tbsp grated natural cheddar cheese, reduced fat
  - 1 Tbsp chopped scallions
- 1 small whole-wheat roll
- 1 tsp unsalted soft (tub) margarine
- 1 small apple
- 1 cup low-fat milk

SNACKS
- ⅓ cup almonds, unsalted
- ¼ cup raisins
- ½ cup fruit yogurt, fat free, no sugar added

Modified from the National Institutes of Health; National Heart, Lung, and Blood Institute. *Your guide to lowering your blood pressure with DASH, NIH Publication No. 06-4082.* Washington, DC: U.S. Department of Health and Human Services; 2006.

Sodium Control

About half of the American population with hypertension is salt sensitive, which means that their blood pressure is significantly affected by dietary sodium intake. There is a direct correlation between sodium intake and blood pressure (i.e., high sodium intake leads to high blood pressure), even in patients with **resistant hypertension**.[41-43] However, achieving a palatable diet with sodium restrictions set at <2 g/day may be difficult for patients who rely heavily on processed foods. A dietary restriction of sodium between 1500 and 2400 mg/day is advised.[33] Keep in mind that 2.4 g of sodium is equivalent to approximately 6 g of sodium

chloride (i.e., table salt). See Box 19-3 for ideas on ways to limit sodium intake.

Other Nutrients

The ACC/AHA Task Force concluded that there is insufficient evidence available at this time to determine the specific and independent relationship between hypertension and dietary intake of nutrients such as potassium, magnesium, or calcium.[10]

ADDITIONAL LIFESTYLE FACTORS

The National High Blood Pressure Education Program recommends limiting alcohol intake to no more than two drinks per day for men and one drink per day for most women and smaller men. One alcoholic drink is equal to 12 oz of regular beer, 5 oz of wine, or 1.5 oz of 80-proof whiskey. Moderation of alcohol intake is associated with a reduction of systolic blood pressure by 2 to 4 mm Hg.[34]

Additional lifestyle factors that are associated with hypertension include smoking and chronic stress. Smoking almost doubles the risk of death from hypertensive heart disease.[44] Psychosocial stress, mental stress, and emotional stress are typical aspects of adult life. However, chronic stress takes a toll on the body and leads to elevated blood pressure in many susceptible people.[45] Thus, both smoking cessation and stress-management techniques are lifestyle modifications that can help reduce the burden of hypertension.

EDUCATION AND PREVENTION

Education and disease prevention are concepts that are extremely important in our ever-aging population. Many diseases covered in this text are preventable through modified diet and lifestyle behaviors. As such, the topics covered in this section are applicable for all preventable chronic diseases, not just CVD. Because CVD is the number 1 cause of death in the United States, the topic is presented in this chapter.

PRACTICAL FOOD GUIDES

Food Planning and Purchasing

The *2015-2020 Dietary Guidelines for Americans* (see Figure 1-4), provides a basic outline to guide sound food habits.[46] The food exchange list, which is described in Chapter 20, demonstrates the food groups and includes similar nutrient modifications discussed in this chapter. The food exchange lists also provide a guide for controlling energy intake to help with weight-management planning.

An important part of purchasing food is carefully reading food labels. The Nutrition Facts labels provide basic nutrition information in a standard format that is easily recognized and clearly expressed. All food products that make health claims must follow the strict guidelines provided by the U.S. Food and Drug Administration. A good general guide is to primarily

---

resistant hypertension the presence of high blood pressure despite treatment with three antihypertensive medications.

use fresh, whole foods, with a limited selection of processed foods when necessary. See Chapter 13 for background material regarding food supply and Nutrition Facts labels.

Food Preparation

The public is more aware than ever before of the need to prepare foods with less saturated fat, trans fat, and salt. Consequently, the cookbook industry has responded by providing an abundance of guides and recipes for various age groups and customs. Many seasonings (e.g., herbs, spices, lemon, wine, onion, garlic, nonfat milk and yogurt, fat-free/low-sodium broth) can help to train taste preferences for less sodium. Less animal products overall, and in leaner and smaller portions, can be combined with more complex carbohydrate foods (e.g., potatoes, winter squash, rice, bulgur, and legumes) to make more healthful main dishes. Whole-grain breads and cereals provide needed fiber, and an increased use of fish can add healthier forms of fat in smaller quantities. A variety of vegetables may be used (e.g., in salads or steamed and lightly seasoned), and fruits add interest, taste appeal, and nourishment to meals. The American Heart Association publishes several cookbooks that are excellent guides to lighter, more tasteful, and healthier food preparation (www.shopheart.org).

Person-Centered Approach

The individual adaptation of diet principles is important in all nutrition teaching and counseling. Special attention must be given to personal desires, ethnic diets, economic restrictions, and food habits (see Chapter 14). Effective diet planning must meet both personal and health needs. Lifestyle changes that are the most successful are the ones that include the whole family and last a lifetime.

EDUCATION PRINCIPLES

Starting Early

The prevention of hypertension and heart disease begins during childhood, especially with children from high-risk families. National data indicate that non-HDL lipid levels are already too high in 10.7% of children between the ages of 6 and 19.[47] Preventive measures in family food habits relate to healthy weight maintenance and the limited use of foods that are high in salt, saturated fats, and trans fats. For adults with heart disease and hypertension, learning should be an integral part of all therapy. If a heart attack occurs, education should begin early during convalescence (rather than at hospital discharge) to give patients and their families clear and practical knowledge regarding positive diet and lifestyle needs; and to allow time for questions and guidance on additional outpatient resources.

Focusing on High-Risk Groups

Education about heart disease and hypertension should be particularly directed toward individuals and families with one or more high-risk factors (see Box 19-1). For example, the prevalence of premature cardiovascular mortality is significantly higher in certain high-risk groups, including African Americans and Native Americans.[5] See the Cultural Considerations box, "Influence of Ethnicity and Sociodemographics on a Person's Risk for Heart Disease" for more information on high-risk groups.

Using a Variety of Resources

As researchers learn more about heart disease and hypertension, the American Heart Association and other health agencies are able to provide many excellent resources. The Academy of Nutrition and Dietetics provides a website (www.eatright.org) for the public as well as for health professionals with helpful client education tools, several of which are applicable to heart disease. As professionals and the public have become more aware of health needs and disease prevention, an increasing number of resources and programs are available in most communities. These include various weight-management programs, registered dietitian nutritionists in private practice or in health care centers that provide nutrition counseling, and practical food-preparation materials found in a number of "light cuisine" cooking classes and cookbooks. Bookstores and public libraries as well as health education libraries in health centers and clinics provide an abundance of materials that address health promotion and self-care.

🌐 Cultural Considerations

Influence of Ethnicity and Sociodemographics on a Person's Risk for Heart Disease

Although the death rate from heart disease has declined since the 1960s, it is still the leading cause of death in the United States. The major conditions of heart disease, hypertension, and high blood cholesterol are more prevalent among certain ethnic and sociodemographic groups than others within the United States. Unlike weight and dietary habits, certain aspects constitute nonmodifiable risk factors for cardiovascular disease (e.g., race, sex) as shown in the following graph.[1]

Distinguishing between environmental factors and the genetics associated with a culture is important to help identify the specifics regarding the cause of disease. Only when those factors have been recognized can prevention and treatment programs be directed on an individual basis. A complex

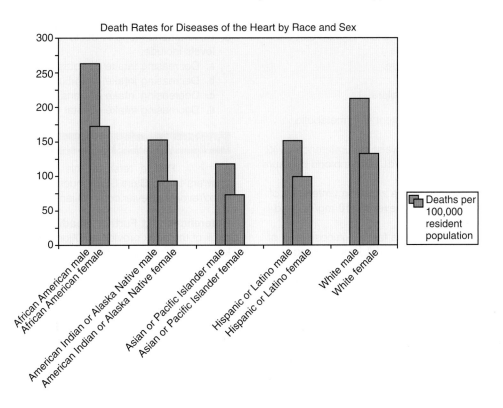

Death Rates for Diseases of the Heart by Race and Sex

combination of sociodemographic risk factors such as education level, annual household income, and employment status may contribute to an individual's risk for death from cardiovascular disease. By acknowledging the risks associated with such factors, health care providers may detect warning signs earlier.

REFERENCE

1. National Center for Health Statistics. *Health, United States, 2014: With Special Feature of Adults Aged 55-64*. Hyattsville, Md: U.S. Government Printing Office; 2015.

Putting It All Together

Summary

- Coronary heart disease is the leading cause of death in the United States. Atherosclerosis is the underlying blood vessel disease. If fatty buildup on the interior surfaces of the blood vessels becomes severe, it cuts off the supply of oxygen and nutrients to the cells, which in turn die. When this occurs in a major coronary artery, the result is an MI.
- The risk for atherosclerosis increases with the amount and type of blood lipids and lipoproteins in circulation. An elevated serum cholesterol level is a primary risk factor for the development of atherosclerosis.
- Current recommendations to help prevent coronary heart disease involve inclusion of a healthy and balanced diet, weight management, and increased physical activity.
- Dietary recommendations for acute CVD include measures to ensure cardiac rest. People with chronic heart disease involving congestive heart failure benefit from a low-sodium diet to control pulmonary edema.

- People with hypertension may improve their condition with weight control, exercise, sodium restriction, and a diet that is rich in fruits, vegetables, whole grains, lean meats, and low-fat dairy products.

Chapter Review Questions

See answers in Appendix A.

1. A high serum level of which of the following lipoproteins is considered protective against CVD?
   a. LDL
   b. VLDL
   c. TG
   d. HDL

2. The best sandwich choice for a patient on a diet with sodium restriction is:
   a. Lean ham.
   b. Pastrami.
   c. Grilled chicken.
   d. Hard salami.

3. Combining the DASH diet with a low-sodium diet can:
   a. Decrease blood pressure.
   b. Decrease risk of liver disease.
   c. Help prevent depression.
   d. Reverse congestive heart failure.

4. An example of a profile consistent with metabolic syndrome is:
   a. A 45-year-old male with a waist circumference of 42 inches, TG level of 225 mg/dL, and a blood pressure of 166/84 mm Hg.
   b. A 32-year-old woman with a waist circumference of 24 inches, fasting glucose level of 110 mg/dL, and HDL level of 63 mg/dL.
   c. A 48-year-old woman with a fasting glucose level of 83 mg/dL, HDL level of 58 mg/dL, and a blood pressure of 124/76 mm Hg.
   d. A 34-year-old male with a waist circumference of 34 inches, TG level of 134 mg/dL, and a blood pressure of 123/68 mm Hg.

5. Recommendations to decrease high LDL-cholesterol levels include:
   a. Decreasing intake of potassium.
   b. Decreasing intake of sodium.
   c. Decreasing intake of trans fats.
   d. Decreasing intake of total fat.

Additional Learning Resources

evolve Please refer to this text's Evolve website for answers to the Case Study questions. http://evolve.elsevier.com/Williams/basic/

References and **Further Reading and Resources** in the back of the book provide additional resources for enhancing knowledge.

Diabetes Mellitus

Key Concepts

- Diabetes mellitus is a metabolic disorder of glucose metabolism that has many causes and forms.
- A consistent and sound diet is a major keystone of diabetes care and control.
- Daily self-care skills enable a person with diabetes to remain healthy and reduce risks for complications.

- Blood glucose monitoring is a critical practice for effective **glycemic control**.
- A personalized care plan that balances food intake, exercise, and insulin regulation is essential to successful diabetes management.

The National Center for Health Statistics reported that 11.7% of the American adult population has diabetes; this includes a significant amount of people (3.3% of the population) that have diabetes but remain undiagnosed. Diabetes is currently the seventh leading cause of death in the United States.[1]

Historically, diabetes mellitus claimed the lives of its victims at a young age. Greater knowledge of the disease and proper self-care practices have enabled people with diabetes to live long and fulfilling lives. However, there is not yet a cure for diabetes, and individuals without health care and access to proper medication continue to die early in life. With professional guidance and support, individuals with diabetes can remain in a state of good health and reduce the risk of long-term complications by consistently practicing sound diet and lifestyle habits.

This chapter examines the nature of diabetes and explains why daily self-care is essential for good health.

THE NATURE OF DIABETES

DEFINING FACTOR

Glucose is the primary and preferred source of energy for the body. As discussed in Chapter 2, carbohydrate foods break down during digestion in the gastrointestinal tract, and they are absorbed into the bloodstream mainly as glucose. Glucose is then circulated throughout the body. For glucose to be used as energy by the cells in the body, it first has to be taken out of the blood and transported into the cells. For this process to happen in most cells, the hormone **insulin** must be present. Insulin is produced by the β cells of the pancreas (see the For Further Focus box, "The History and Discovery of Insulin"). Individuals with diabetes either do not produce insulin or cannot effectively use the

insulin that is produced. Without insulin, glucose accumulates in the bloodstream. The American Diabetes Association defines diabetes as a group of metabolic diseases that are characterized by **hyperglycemia** that results from defects in insulin secretion, insulin action, or both.[2]

CLASSIFICATION OF DIABETES MELLITUS AND GLUCOSE INTOLERANCE

Various types of diabetes mellitus are classified according to the pathogenic process of the disease.

Type 1 Diabetes Mellitus

Type 1 diabetes mellitus accounts for 5% to 10% of all cases of diabetes. It develops rapidly, and it tends to be more severe and unstable than other forms of diabetes. Type 1 diabetes is caused by the autoimmune destruction of the β cells in the pancreas. At least five autoantibodies have been identified as the cause of this destruction in the vast majority of patients: islet cell autoantibodies, autoantibodies to insulin, autoantibodies to glutamic acid decarboxylase, autoantibodies to the tyrosine phosphatases IA-2 and IA-2β, and autoantibodies to zinc transporter protein.[2,3] Patients with type 1 diabetes are also at risk for other forms of autoimmune diseases such as: Graves' disease, Hashimoto's thyroiditis, Addison's disease, celiac disease, autoimmune hepatitis, and autoimmune

---

glycemic control management of appropriate blood glucose levels.

insulin a hormone that is produced by the pancreas, attaches to insulin receptors on cell membranes, and allows the absorption of glucose into the cell.

hyperglycemia an elevated blood glucose level.

The History and Discovery of Insulin

EARLY HISTORY AND NAME

The symptoms of diabetes were first described on an Egyptian papyrus, the Ebers Papyrus, which dates to approximately 1500 BC. During the first century, the Greek physician Areatus wrote of a malady in which the body "ate its own flesh" and gave off large quantities of urine. He named it *diabetes,* from the Greek word meaning "to siphon" or "to pass through." During the seventeenth century, the word *mellitus* from the Latin word meaning "honey" was added because of the sweetness of the urine. The addition of *mellitus* distinguished the disorder from another disorder, *diabetes insipidus,* in which large urine output also was observed. However, diabetes insipidus is a rare and quite different disease that is caused by a lack of the pituitary antidiuretic hormone. Today, the term *diabetes* is almost always in reference to diabetes mellitus.

DIABETIC DARK AGES

Throughout the Middle Ages and the dawning of the scientific era, many early scientists and physicians continued to puzzle over the mystery of diabetes, but the cause remained obscure. For physicians and their patients, these years could be called the "Diabetic Dark Ages." Patients had short life spans and were maintained on a variety of semistarvation and high-fat diets.

DISCOVERY OF INSULIN

The first breakthrough came from a clue that pointed to the involvement of the pancreas in the disease process. This clue was provided by a young German medical student, Paul Langerhans (1847-1888), who found special clusters of cells scattered throughout the pancreas forming little islands of cells. Although he did not yet understand their function, Langerhans could see that these cells were different from the rest of the tissue and assumed that they must be important. When his suspicions later proved true, these clusters of cells were named the *islets of Langerhans* for their young discoverer. In 1922, with the use of this important clue, two Canadian scientists—Frederick Banting and his assistant Charles Best, together with two other research team members, physiologists J.B. Collip and J.J.R. Macleod—extracted the first insulin from animals. It proved to be a hormone that regulates the oxidation of blood glucose and that helps to convert it to heat and energy. They called the hormone *insulin* from the Latin word *insula,* meaning "island." Insulin did prove to be the effective agent for the treatment of diabetes. Leonard Thompson was the first child to be treated with insulin, in January 1922. He lived to adulthood, but he died at the age of 27 years—not from his diabetes but from coronary heart disease caused by the diabetic diet of the day, which obtained 70% of its total kilocalories from fat. Unsurprisingly, his autopsy showed marked atherosclerosis.

SUCCESSFUL USE OF DIET AND INSULIN

The insulin discovery team was more successful on their third try with a young girl who was diagnosed with diabetes at the age of 11 years. She initially had been put on a starvation diet, and her weight fell from 75 to 45 pounds (34 to 21 kg) over a 3-year period. However, the medical research team fortunately had learned the importance of a well-balanced diet for normal growth and health. Thus, with a good diet and the new insulin therapy, this child, Elizabeth Hughes, gained weight and vigor and lived a normal life. She married, had three children, took insulin for 58 years, and died of heart failure at the age of 73 years.

---

enteropathy.[2,4] Several genetic factors are also involved in the complex etiology of type 1 diabetes, the exact mechanisms of which are still under investigation.[4]

The rate of destruction determines the onset of diabetes. The initial onset of type 1 diabetes occurs rapidly among children and adolescents (hence its former name *juvenile-onset diabetes*), but it can occur at any age. For some individuals, the rate of destruction is slower, and symptoms may not appear until adulthood. Individuals with this type of diabetes rely on **exogenous** insulin for survival (hence its other former name *insulin-dependent diabetes*). At the time of diagnosis, individuals with type 1 diabetes have often experienced a recent unexplained weight loss and are at higher risk for acidosis.

Type 2 Diabetes Mellitus

Approximately 90% to 95% of individuals with diabetes have type 2 diabetes. This form is most closely associated with lifestyle and environmental factors that lead to excess body fat, particularly in the abdominal region, and lack of physical activity.[2] Genome-wide association studies have identified several genetic risk factors for the development of both obesity and type 2 diabetes. While many specific genetic loci (90 to date) have been definitively linked to type 2 diabetes risk, these variants do not account for all cases.[5] Box 20-1 lists additional risk factors for the development of type 2 diabetes.

Unlike type 1 diabetes, type 2 diabetes is not caused by an autoimmune response. This form of diabetes results from an insulin resistance or insulin defect: either the body is not producing enough insulin or the insulin that it is being produced cannot be used. These individuals usually do not need exogenous insulin for survival; rather, they rely on diet, exercise, and oral medications for disease management. This form of diabetes, which was previously called *adult-onset diabetes* or *non–insulin-dependent diabetes*, has an onset primarily in adults who are older than 40 years. However, as children get heavier, the prevalence of type 2 diabetes among young people is on the rise. More than 43% of

---

exogenous originating from outside the body.

Box 20-1 Risk Factors for Type 2 Diabetes Mellitus

Overweight (i.e., a body mass index ≥25 kg/m²)

Not physically active on a regular basis

A first-degree relative with diabetes

High-risk race/ethnicity (e.g., African American, Latino, Native American, Asian American, and Pacific Islander)

Women with a history of gestational diabetes or who have delivered an infant weighing ≥9 pounds

Hypertension (≥140/90 mm Hg or on therapy for hypertension)

HDL-cholesterol level <35 mg/dL and/or triglyceride level >250 mg/dL

Woman with polycystic ovarian syndrome

HgA₁c ≥5.7%

Previously identified as having impaired glucose tolerance or prediabetes

History of cardiovascular disease

Other clinical conditions associated with insulin resistance (e.g., severe obesity, acanthosis nigricans)

Age ≥45 years

From American Diabetes Association. Standards of medical care in diabetes—2014. *Diabetes Care.* 2014;37(Suppl 1):S14-S80.

diabetic adolescents in the United States have type 2 diabetes and an estimated 40,000 cases remain undiagnosed and untreated.[6] The Cultural Considerations box entitled "Prevalence of Type 2 Diabetes" discusses this issue in more depth. Many adults and children with type 2 diabetes can improve their symptoms with weight loss, thus requiring diet therapy and balanced exercise programs only.

Table 20-1 summarizes the chief differences between type 1 and type 2 diabetes mellitus.

Gestational Diabetes

Gestational diabetes mellitus (GDM) is a form of diabetes that occurs during pregnancy, with normal blood glucose control usually recovered after delivery. Women who have type 1 or type 2 diabetes before conception do not fall into this category during pregnancy. GDM can present complications for both the mother and the fetus if it is not carefully monitored and controlled. Persistent hyperglycemia is associated with an increased risk of intrauterine fetal death and **macrosomia**.

GDM develops in approximately 7% of all pregnant women.[2] Risk factors for GDM are the same as those for type 2 diabetes (see Box 20-1). Pregnant women who are at high risk for diabetes should be screened with a fasting plasma glucose and glycosylated hemoglobin A₁c test during the first prenatal visit. Women

macrosomia excessive fetal growth that results in an abnormally large infant; this condition carries a high risk for perinatal death.

Cultural Considerations

Prevalence of Type 2 Diabetes

Type 2 diabetes was known for years as *adult-onset diabetes,* because it rarely affected anyone younger than 40 years old. However, this form of diabetes has rapidly become a health care concern among children and adolescents as well. As with the occurrence of type 2 diabetes in adults, it has been reported in all races and ethnic populations, with a disproportionate burden on minority groups. Diabetes, impaired glucose tolerance, obesity, and even cardiovascular disease are beginning to plague the children of America in a similar fashion as they do adults.

CHILDREN

In an effort to define the contributing factors responsible for the increased prevalence of type 2 diabetes in children, researchers have investigated fetal exposure to maternal diabetes and obesity and found such exposures to be strong contributing factors among diverse ethnic groups.[1] Ethnic groups with pronounced risks for type 2 diabetes are African Americans, Hispanic and Latino Americans, and American Indians/Alaska Natives. The estimated number of new cases of type 2 diabetes in children younger than 20 years old is more than 5000 annually,[2] of which about 80% are obese and 10% are overweight at the time of diagnosis.[3]

ADULTS

The Centers for Disease Control and Prevention reported the number of people diagnosed with diabetes from 2010 to 2012 who were ≥20 years old to have the following prevalence by race and ethnicity.[2]

Age-adjusted* percentage of people aged 20 years or older with diagnosed diabetes, by race/ethnicity, United States, 2010–2012

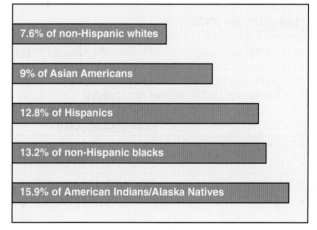

7.6% of non-Hispanic whites

9% of Asian Americans

12.8% of Hispanics

13.2% of non-Hispanic blacks

15.9% of American Indians/Alaska Natives

REFERENCES

1. Dabelea D, et al. Association of intrauterine exposure to maternal diabetes and obesity with type 2 diabetes in youth: the SEARCH Case-Control Study. *Diabetes Care.* 2008;31(7):1422-1426.
2. Centers for Disease Control and Prevention. *National Diabetes Statistics Report: Estimates of Diabetes and Its Burden in The United States, 2014.* Atlanta, Ga: U.S. Department of Health and Human Services; 2014.
3. Liu LL, et al. Prevalence of overweight and obesity in youth with diabetes in USA: the SEARCH for Diabetes in Youth study. *Pediatr Diabetes.* 2010;11(1):4-11.

Table 20-1	Differentiating Type 1 and Type 2 Diabetes Mellitus	
FACTOR	**TYPE 1**	**TYPE 2**
Ethnicity	Increased rates among persons with Northern European heritage	Highest rates are found in those with Native American, Hispanic, African-American, Asian, Pacific Islander, and Mediterranean heritages
Age of onset	Generally younger than 30 years of age, with the peak onset before puberty	Generally older than 40 years of age, although genetic predisposition and obesity may cause onset to occur at younger ages
Weight	Usually normal or underweight; unintentional weight loss often precedes diagnosis	Usually overweight
Treatment	Insulin injections are necessary for life; food and exercise must be balanced with insulin	Weight loss is usually the first goal; oral hypoglycemic agents, insulin, or both may be necessary for good blood glucose management, but they are not necessary to prevent imminent death; diet management and exercise are important
β-cell functioning	No insulin is produced after the "honeymoon period" (a period of about 1 year after diagnosis in which residual insulin is produced)	Excess insulin production is usually evident (i.e., hyperinsulinemia), but insulin resistance occurs at the cellular level; insulin production may also be normal or below normal

Modified from Peckenpaugh NJ. *Nutrition Essentials and Diet Therapy.* 11th ed. Philadelphia: Saunders; 2010.

Box 20-2	Screening and Diagnosis of GDM

"ONE-STEP" (IADPSG CONSENSUS)

Perform a 75-g OGTT, with plasma glucose measurement fasting and at 1 and 2 h, at 24 to 28 weeks of gestation in women not previously diagnosed with overt diabetes. The OGTT should be performed in the morning after an overnight fast of at least 8 hours.

The diagnosis of GDM is made when any of the following plasma glucose values are exceeded:
- Fasting: >92 mg/dL (5.1 mmol/L)
- 1 h: >180 mg/dL (10.0 mmol/L)
- 2 h: >153 mg/dL (8.5 mmol/L)

"TWO-STEP" (NIH CONSENSUS)

Perform a 50-g GLT (nonfasting), with plasma glucose measurement at 1 h (Step 1), at 24-28 weeks of gestation in women not previously diagnosed with overt diabetes. If the plasma glucose level measured 1 h after the load is ≥140 mg/dL* (7.8 mmol/L), proceed to 100-g OGTT (Step 2). The 100-g OGTT should be performed when the patient is fasting.

The diagnosis of GDM is made when at least two of the following four plasma glucose levels (measured fasting, 1 h, 2 h, 3 h after the OGTT) are met or exceeded:

	CARPENTER/COUSTAN	OR	NDDG
• Fasting	95 mg/dL (5.3 mmol/L)		105 mg/dL (5.8 mmol/L)
• 1 h	180 mg/dL (10.0 mmol/L)		190 mg/dL (10.6 mmol/L)
• 2 h	155 mg/dL (8.6 mmol/L)		165 mg/dL (9.2 mmol/L)
• 3 h	140 mg/dL(7.8 mmol/L)		145 mg/dL (8.0 mmol/L)

GLT, Glucose load test; NDDG, National Diabetes Data Group; NIH, National Institutes of Health; OGTT, oral glucose tolerance test.
From American Diabetes Association. Standards of medical care in diabetes—2014. *Diabetes Care.* 2014;37(Suppl 1):S14-S80.
*The American College of Obstetricians and Gynecologists (ACOG) recommends a lower threshold of 135 mg/dL (7.5 mmol/L) in high-risk ethnic minorities with higher prevalence of GDM; some experts also recommend 130 mg/dL (7.2 mmol/L).

who are diagnosed with diabetes at that time are considered to have overt diabetes (usually type 2) rather than gestational diabetes. All women who are not otherwise known to have diabetes or who are at high risk should be screened with a glucose tolerance test between 24 and 28 weeks' gestation.[2] The screening protocol for GDM is provided in Box 20-2.

Women with GDM have their blood glucose levels carefully monitored and are taught to follow a tightly managed program of diet and exercise and to self-test measurements of blood glucose, blood pressure, and urinary protein. For women who are unable to maintain blood glucose levels within an acceptable range (i.e., ≤95 mg/dL fasting, ≤180 mg/dL 1 hour postprandial, or ≤155 mg/dL 2 hours postprandial), insulin therapy is recommended. Oral hypoglycemic agents were not used for GDM in the past for fear of teratogenic effects. However, recent years have seen a large increase in the use of selective oral hypoglycemic agents in this population. Studies indicate that the maternal and fetal outcomes are inferior to those of insulin but that these medications may be appropriate when exogenous insulin is not an option.[7-9]

Complications of GDM for mother and baby are greatly reduced (if not eliminated) by the tight control of blood glucose levels. Women with GDM are also advised to maintain a balanced diet, a regular exercise schedule, and a healthy body mass index and to attend all follow-up visits with their physicians. Women with GDM are at significant risk for having subsequent pregnancies that are complicated by diabetes and for developing type 2 diabetes later in life. However, strict adherence to the recommended lifestyle modifications can prevent or delay the progression to type 2 diabetes.[10-12]

Other Types of Diabetes

Secondary diabetes may be caused by a number of conditions or agents that affect the pancreas, including the following:

- *Genetic defects:* Defects in the β cells or insulin action may result in several forms of diabetes. These forms are not characteristic of the autoimmune destruction found in patients with type 1 diabetes. Mutations on at least six genetic loci have been identified, and these result in impaired insulin secretion (although not the action of the insulin). Other less common defects in the action of insulin (but not in the amount secreted) also result in hyperglycemia and diabetes. Two such syndromes that have been identified in the pediatric population are leprechaunism and Rabson-Mendenhall syndrome.[2]
- *Pancreatic conditions or diseases:* Any condition that causes damage to the pancreatic cells can result in diabetes. Such conditions include tumors that affect the islet cells; acute viral infection by a number of agents, such as the mumps virus; acute pancreatitis from biliary disease, gallstones, or alcoholism; chronic pancreatic insufficiency, such as that which occurs with cystic fibrosis; pancreatic surgery; and severe traumatic abdominal injury.
- *Endocrinopathies:* Insulin works in conjunction with several other hormones in the body. Hormones such as growth hormone, cortisol, glucagon, and epinephrine are all antagonistic to the functions of insulin. Therefore, for patients with disorders in which excessive amounts of antagonistic hormones are produced, the action of insulin is hindered, and hyperglycemia ensues. **Cushing's syndrome**, glucagonoma, **pheochromocytoma**, hyperthyroidism, and **aldosteronoma** are examples of endocrinopathies that ultimately cause symptoms of diabetes. When

the primary disorder (i.e., excessive antagonistic hormone secretion) is removed, the resulting hyperglycemia is usually resolved.

- *Drug- or chemical-induced diabetes:* Certain drugs and toxins can impair insulin secretion or insulin action. The following drugs and toxins have been linked to impaired glucose tolerance and diabetes in susceptible individuals: Vacor (rat poison), pentamidine, nicotinic acid, glucocorticoids, thyroid hormone, thiazides, diazoxide, phenytoin (Dilantin), β-adrenergic agonists, and α-interferon.[2]

Impaired Glucose Tolerance

Individuals whose fasting blood glucose level is higher than normal (>100 mg/dL) but less than the level for the clinical diagnosis of diabetes (≥126 mg/dL) are defined as impaired glucose tolerance (IGT), which is also known as *prediabetes*.[2] IGT is a strong risk factor for the future development of type 2 diabetes. Dietary and lifestyle treatment guidelines follow those that are designed for patients with type 2 diabetes, and can help to prevent or prolong the progression into full-blown diabetes.[13] Overweight individuals with IGT can significantly reduce their risk for developing diabetes by increasing physical activity and by losing 5% to 10% of body weight. Aerobic exercise and resistance training are particularly important aspects of treatment because they increase insulin sensitivity and glucose utilization in skeletal muscles.[14-16]

Individuals with IGT often have a complicated assortment of underlying conditions (e.g., dyslipidemia, obesity, hypertension, chronic inflammation) that build on one another to create the condition known as *metabolic syndrome* (see Table 19-2 for the diagnostic criteria for metabolic syndrome). Lifestyle modifications designed for modest weight loss (i.e., 4% of body weight) over a 1-year period in patients with IGT have been shown to significantly improve cardiac function in addition to insulin sensitivity.[17] This is particularly important for patients with

---

postprandial after eating.

Cushing's syndrome the excess secretion of glucocorticoids from the adrenal cortex; symptoms and complications include protein loss, obesity, fatigue, osteoporosis, edema, excess hair growth, diabetes, and skin discoloration.

pheochromocytoma a tumor of the adrenal medulla or the sympathetic nervous system in which the affected cells secrete excess epinephrine or norepinephrine and cause headache, hypertension, and nausea.

aldosteronoma the excess secretion of aldosterone from the adrenal cortex; symptoms and complications include sodium retention, potassium wasting, alkalosis, weakness, paralysis, polyuria, polydipsia, hypertension, and cardiac arrhythmias.

metabolic syndrome and indicates that slow and modest improvements over time can help reduce risk factors for many chronic diseases of adulthood, including diabetes, cardiovascular disease, and metabolic syndrome.

SYMPTOMS OF DIABETES

Initial Signs

Early signs of diabetes include three primary symptoms: (1) increased thirst (polydipsia); (2) increased urination (polyuria); and (3) increased hunger (polyphagia). Unintentional weight loss often occurs with type 1 diabetes. Additional signs include blurred vision, dehydration, skin irritation or infection, and general weakness and loss of strength. Patients with type 2 diabetes often do not recognize the signs because the symptoms develop gradually over many years. It is not uncommon for some of the long-term complications of diabetes to already be present at the time of diagnosis of type 2 diabetes in older individuals.

Laboratory Tests

Laboratory tests will show hyperglycemia, abnormal glucose tolerance tests, elevated glycosylated hemoglobin A_{1c}, and glucosuria (i.e., glucose in the urine). Although the urinary excretion of glucose is correlated with increasing levels of blood glucose, it is not as sensitive in patients with type 2 diabetes as it is with type 1 diabetes.[18] Glycosylated hemoglobin A_{1c}, which is usually abbreviated as HbA_{1c} or A_{1c}, represents blood glucose levels over a 3-month period. Individuals with a HbA_{1c} test within the range of 5.7% to 6.4% have IGT and are at very high risk for progressing to diabetes.[2] HbA_{1c} levels of 6.5% or more are indicative of diabetes mellitus. Box 20-3 outlines the criteria for the diagnosis of diabetes mellitus, and Table 20-2 gives the correlation between HbA_{1c} values and plasma glucose levels.

Progressive Results

If the disease is left uncontrolled, chronic hyperglycemia causes progressive deterioration throughout the body. These results may include water and electrolyte imbalance, **ketoacidosis**, and coma.

THE METABOLIC PATTERN OF DIABETES

ENERGY SUPPLY AND CONTROL OF BLOOD GLUCOSE

Energy Supply

Diabetes has been called a disease of carbohydrate metabolism, but it is a general metabolic disorder that

---

ketoacidosis the excess production of ketones; a form of metabolic acidosis that occurs with uncontrolled diabetes or starvation from burning body fat for energy fuel; a continuing uncontrolled state can result in coma and death.

Box 20-3	Criteria for the Diagnosis of Diabetes Mellitus

- HbA_{1c} ≥6.5%. The test should be performed in a laboratory using a method that is National Glycohemoglobin Standardization Program (NGSP) certified and standardized to the Diabetes Control and Complications Trial (DCCT) assay*
  or
- Fasting plasma glucose level of ≥126 mg/dL (7.0 mmol/L)
  Fasting is defined as no caloric intake for at least 8 hours*
  or
- A 2-hour plasma glucose level of ≥200 mg/dL (11.1 mmol/L) during an oral glucose tolerance test
    The oral glucose tolerance test should be performed as described by the World Health Organization with the use of a glucose load that contains the equivalent of 75 g of anhydrous glucose dissolved in water*
  or
- In a patient with classic symptoms of hyperglycemia or hyperglycemic crisis, a random plasma glucose level of ≥200 mg/dL (11.1 mmol/L)

Modified from American Diabetes Association. Diagnosis and classification of diabetes mellitus. *Diabetes Care.* 2014;37(Suppl 1):S81-S90.
*In the absence of unequivocal hyperglycemia, results should be confirmed by repeat testing.

Table 20-2	Correlation Between Glycosylated Hemoglobin A_{1c} and Plasma Glucose Levels

	MEAN PLASMA GLUCOSE LEVEL	
HbA_{1c}	mg/dL	mmol/L
6	126	7.0
7	154	8.6
8	183	10.2
9	212	11.8
10	240	13.4
11	269	14.9
12	298	16.5

From American Diabetes Association. Standards of medical care in diabetes—2014. *Diabetes Care.* 2014;37(Suppl 1):S14-S80.

involves all three of the energy-yielding nutrients: carbohydrate, fat, and protein. Diabetes is especially related to the metabolism of the two main fuels, carbohydrate and fat, in the body's overall energy system. The three basic stages of normal glucose metabolism are as follows:

1. Initial interchange with glycogen (glycogenolysis) and reduction to a smaller central compound (glycolysis pathway)
2. Joining with the other two energy-yielding nutrients, fat and protein (pyruvate link)
3. Final common energy production (citric acid cycle and electron transport chain)

Blood Glucose Control

The control of blood glucose level within its normal range is important for general health. Normal control mechanisms ensure sufficient circulating blood glucose to meet the constant energy needs (even the basal metabolic energy needs during sleep), because glucose is the body's preferred fuel. Figure 20-1 shows the balanced sources and uses of glucose at various levels of blood glucose concentrations.

Sources of blood glucose. To ensure a constant supply of the body's main fuel, the following two sources provide the body with glucose:

- *Dietary intake:* the energy-yielding nutrients in food (i.e., carbohydrates and the carbon backbones of fat and protein, as needed; see Chapters 2-6)
- *Glycogen:* the backup source from the constant turnover of stored glycogen in the liver and muscles (i.e., glycogenolysis; see Chapters 2, 5, and 6)

Uses of blood glucose. The body uses glucose as needed in the following actions:

- Burning it during cell oxidation for immediate energy needs (i.e., glycolysis)

- Changing it to glycogen (i.e., glycogenesis), which is briefly stored in the muscles and liver and then withdrawn and changed back to glucose for short-term energy needs
- Converting it to fat, which is stored for longer periods in adipose tissue (i.e., lipogenesis)

Figure 20-2 summarizes the pathways that are involved in glucose metabolism.

Pancreatic Hormonal Control

The specialized cells of the islets of Langerhans in the pancreas provide three hormones that work together to regulate blood glucose levels: insulin, glucagon, and somatostatin. Insulin is produced in the β cells of the islets, which fill its central zone and make up about 60% of each islet gland. The specific arrangement of human islet cells is illustrated in Figure 20-3.

Insulin. Insulin is the major hormone that controls the level of blood glucose. It accomplishes this through the following metabolic actions:

- Helping to transport circulating glucose into cells
- Stimulating glycogenesis
- Stimulating lipogenesis
- Inhibiting lipolysis and protein degradation

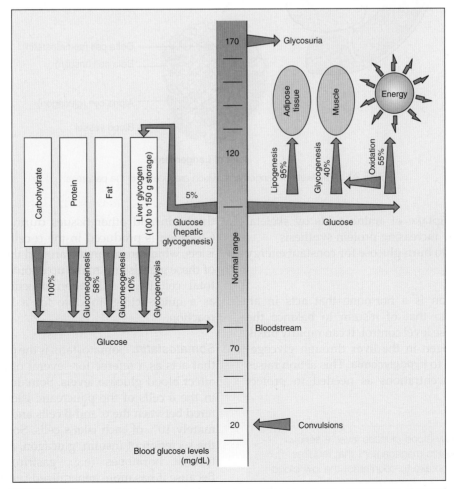

FIGURE 20-1 Sources of blood glucose (e.g., food, stored glycogen) and normal routes of control.

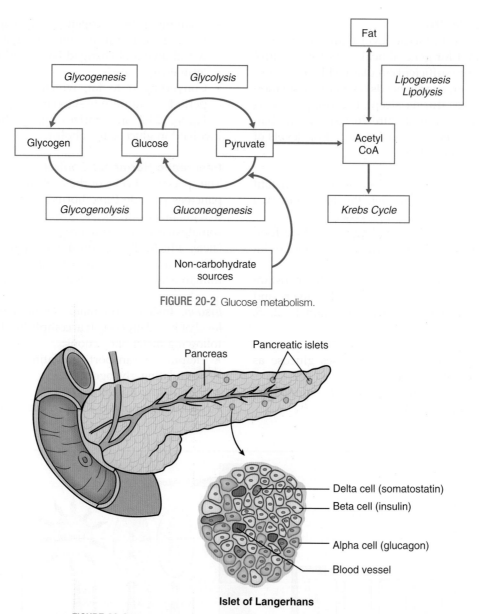

FIGURE 20-2 Glucose metabolism.

Islet of Langerhans

FIGURE 20-3 The islets of Langerhans, which are located in the pancreas.

- Promoting the uptake of amino acids by skeletal muscles, thereby increasing protein synthesis
- Permitting cells to burn glucose for constant energy as needed

Glucagon. Glucagon is a hormone that acts in an opposite manner to that of insulin to balance the overall blood glucose level control. It can rapidly break down stored glycogen in the liver through glycogenolysis in response to **hypoglycemia**. This action raises blood glucose concentrations as needed to protect the brain and other tissues during sleep or fasting. Glucagon is produced in the α cells of the pancreatic islets, which are arranged around the outer rim of each of these glands and make up about 30% of the gland's total cell mass. Glucagon injections may be used as a quick-acting antidote for a low blood glucose reaction.

Somatostatin. Somatostatin is the pancreatic hormone that acts as a referee for several other hormones that affect blood glucose levels. Somatostatin is produced in the δ cells of the pancreatic islets, which are scattered between the α and β cells and make up approximately 10% of each islet's cells. Somatostatin inhibits the secretion of insulin, glucagon, and other gastrointestinal hormones (e.g., gastrin, cholecystokinin). Because it has more generalized functions in the regulation of circulating blood glucose levels, somatostatin

---

hypoglycemia a low blood glucose level; a serious condition in diabetes management that requires immediate sugar intake to counteract the low blood glucose level.

also is produced in other parts of the body (e.g., the hypothalamus).

ABNORMAL METABOLISM IN UNCONTROLLED DIABETES

When insulin action is insufficient, abnormal metabolic changes and imbalances occur among the three macronutrients.

Glucose

Unlike other areas of the body, insulin is not needed for glucose transport into the pancreatic cells. Normally what happens following a meal or snack is that glucose is absorbed into the pancreatic cells and triggers the secretion of insulin into the bloodstream. Insulin is then circulated throughout the blood, attaching to insulin receptor sites on cell membranes throughout the body. Once bound, a signaling cascade begins that phosphorylates **GLUT4** vesicles (within the cell) and results in the migration of GLUT4 vesicles to the cell membrane. Ultimately, GLUT4 transporters allow for the uptake of glucose into the cell (Figure 20-4). Without adequate insulin this process cannot happen. Therefore, cells are essentially starved for glucose as the glucose remains in the blood.

Fat

Insulin promotes lipogenesis and inhibits lipolysis. In essence, when adequate blood glucose is available and insulin is functioning properly, the body uses its preferred energy source (glucose) and stores extra energy for later use as triglycerides in adipose tissue. In the absence of functioning insulin, lipolysis in the adipose tissue increases in an effort to burn fatty acids for energy. This release of fatty acids into the blood results in elevated triglyceride levels. In addition, ketogenesis ensues in the liver. The intermediate products of fat metabolism, called **ketones**, accumulate in the body. Ketones are acids, and their excess accumulation leads to diabetic ketoacidosis (DKA). The appearance of the ketone **acetone** in the urine is one indicator of poor glycemic control as well as of the adverse development of ketoacidosis.

Protein

In the absence of insulin, protein tissues are also broken down in the body's effort to secure energy sources, thereby causing weight loss, muscle weakness, and urinary nitrogen loss.

LONG-TERM COMPLICATIONS

The long-term complications associated with diabetes result from chronic hyperglycemia. These health problems mainly relate to microvascular and macrovascular dysfunction in the vital organs. Individuals with good glycemic control can avoid many such complications.

Retinopathy

Retinopathy involves damage to the small blood vessels in the retina. It often leads to small hemorrhages in the retina that involve yellow, waxy discharge or retinal detachment. Diabetic retinopathy is the leading cause of blindness in adults. The risk for retinopathy significantly increases with incessant hyperglycemia. Retinopathy has few warning signs; however, 28.5% of people with diabetes who are ≥40 years old have diabetic retinopathy.[19] Some treatment

---

GLUT4 an insulin-regulated protein that is responsible for glucose transport into cells.

ketones the chemical name for a class of organic compounds that includes three keto acid bases that occur as intermediate products of fat metabolism.

acetone a major ketone compound that results from fat breakdown for energy in individuals with uncontrolled diabetes; persons with diabetes periodically take urinary acetone tests to monitor the status of ketone production.

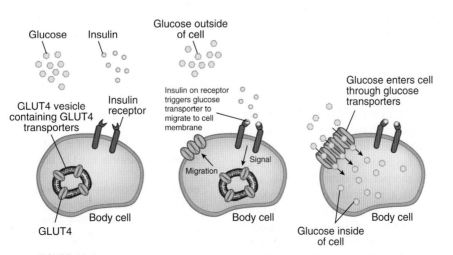

FIGURE 20-4 Insulin allows glucose to enter the cell through the glucose channel.

modalities (e.g., laser photocoagulation therapy) can delay or prevent the onset of this condition; thus, ongoing eye evaluations are an important part of the care plan. The American Diabetes Association recommends that individuals with type 1 diabetes have their first-time eye examination within 5 years after diagnosis and that those with type 2 diabetes have their first eye examination shortly after diagnosis. Examinations with dilation should continue from that point forward every 2 years for patients who have had no evidence of retinopathy and annually for patients with retinopathy.[20] The tight control of the blood glucose level and intensive intervention can reduce retinopathy progression and decrease the development of severe diabetic retinopathy.[21,22]

Retinopathy should not be confused with the blurry vision that sometimes occurs as one of the first signs of diabetes. Blurry vision is caused by the increased glucose concentration in the fluids of the eye, which brings about brief changes in the curved, light-refracting surface of the eye.

Nephropathy

As with retinopathy, hyperglycemia also damages the small vessels within the kidneys. Diabetes is the leading cause of end-stage renal disease in the United States, and it accounts for 44% of all new kidney failure cases.[19] The primary symptom is **microalbuminuria**. Nephropathy and end-stage renal disease cannot be cured, but, with better blood glucose control and antihypertensive therapy, disease progression can be slowed.[21,22] Recommendations for screening are the same as those for retinopathy: within 5 years of diagnosis for type 1 and at diagnosis for type 2, with annual follow-up.[20]

Neuropathy

Diabetes is one of the most common causes of neuropathy. There is also evidence that neuropathy occurs in many patients with impaired glucose tolerance before blood glucose levels are high enough to be diagnostic for diabetes.[23] This indicates the highly sensitive nature of the small nerves throughout the body to chronically elevated blood glucose levels.

Damage to the nerves most commonly involves injury in the peripheral nervous system, especially in the legs and feet. For some patients this causes prickly sensations, increasing pain, and the eventual loss of sensation from damaged nerves. Up to half of the cases of diabetic neuropathy have no symptoms. The loss of nerve sensation can lead to further tissue damage and infection from unfelt foot injuries such as bruises, burns, and deeper **cellulitis**. Patients who are asymptomatic are at a particularly high risk for such complications. Amputations and foot ulcerations are the most common results of severe neuropathy. Approximately 60% of nontraumatic lower-limb amputations in American adults are in patients with diabetes.[19] The risk for neuropathy complications is increased for individuals with peripheral neuropathy and loss of protective sensations, altered biomechanics, increased pressure, bony deformities, peripheral vascular disease, a history of ulcers or amputations, and severe nail pathology.[24] Diabetic neuropathy is also linked to chronic problems such as motor deficits, cardiac ischemia, hypotension, gastroparesis, bladder dysfunction, and sexual dysfunction. Recommendations for screening are the same as those for other microvascular diseases: within 5 years of diagnosis for type 1 and at diagnosis for type 2, with annual follow-up.[20]

Heart Disease

CVD is the major cause of death for people with diabetes, and it occurs about two times more frequently in this population compared with the general population.[19] The standards of medical care for individuals with diabetes include recommendations for the prevention and management of CVD that are specifically aimed at blood lipid levels, blood pressure control, aspirin use, and smoking cessation.[20] Glycemic control is not as strongly related to macrovascular complications (i.e., dyslipidemia and hypertension) as it is to other long-term microvascular complications of diabetes (i.e., retinopathy, nephropathy, and neuropathy). However, the co-morbid conditions of hyperglycemia and dyslipidemia greatly increase the risk of CVD; thus, evaluation and treatment must be part of the overall health care plan for individuals with diabetes.

Dyslipidemia. Elevated triglyceride levels and decreased high-density lipoprotein (HDL) cholesterol levels are characteristic of dyslipidemia in patients with type 2 diabetes. The management of dyslipidemia is prioritized as follows: (1) incorporating lifestyle modifications that focus on the reduction of saturated fats, trans fats, and cholesterol intake; increased intake of omega-3 fatty acids, viscous fiber, and plant stanols/sterols; weight loss, if indicated; and increased physical activity; (2) lowering low-density lipoprotein cholesterol levels; and (3) lowering triglyceride levels.[20] Recommendations for lipid profiles for adults with diabetes are provided in Table 20-3.

---

microalbuminuria low but abnormal levels of albumin in the urine.

cellulitis the diffuse inflammation of soft or connective tissues from injury, bruises, or pressure sores that leads to infection; poor care may result in ulceration and abscess or gangrene.

Table 20-3	Summary of Recommendations for Adults with Diabetes	
PARAMETER	**RECOMMENDATION**	
Glycosylated hemoglobin A_{1c} level	<7.0%	
Preprandial capillary plasma glucose level	70 to 130 mg/dL (3.9 to 7.2 mmol/L)	
Peak postprandial capillary plasma glucose level*	<180 mg/dL (<10.0 mmol/L)	
Blood pressure	<140/80 mm Hg[†]	
Low-density lipoprotein level	<100 mg/dL (<2.6 mmol/L) for individuals without overt cardiovascular disease <70 mg/dL (<1.8 mmol/L) for individuals with overt cardiovascular disease	
Triglyceride level	<150 mg/dL (<1.7 mmol/L)	
High-density lipoprotein level	>40 mg/dL (>1.0 mmol/L) for men >50 mg/dL (>1.3 mmol/L) for women	

- Goals should be individualized on the basis of the following:
  - Duration of diabetes
  - Patient's age and life expectancy
  - Co-morbid conditions
  - Known cardiovascular disease or advanced microvascular complications
  - Hypoglycemia unawareness
  - Individual patient considerations
- More or less stringent glycemic goals may be appropriate for individual patients
- Postprandial glucose may be targeted if HbA_{1c} level goals are not met despite reaching preprandial glucose goals

From American Diabetes Association. Standards of medical care in diabetes—2014. *Diabetes Care*. 2014;37(Suppl 1):S14-S80.
*Postprandial glucose measurements should be made 1 to 2 hours after the beginning of the meal; this is generally when peak levels are seen in patients with diabetes.
[†]Lower systolic pressures of ≤130 mm Hg are an appropriate goal for some younger adults.

Hypertension. Hypertension affects the majority of adults with diabetes (71%), and it is a major risk factor for microvascular complications.[19] CVD mortality is significantly higher for people with both diabetes and hypertension, thereby making blood pressure evaluation and treatment an important part of the health care plan. The recommendation for blood pressure in most adults with diabetes is ≤140/80 mm Hg (see Table 20-3).[20] To achieve such a level of blood pressure, patients are encouraged to adopt lifestyle modifications such as reducing sodium intake; losing weight (if indicated); increasing the consumption of fruits, vegetables, and low-fat dairy products (i.e., following the

DASH diet; see Chapter 19); moderating alcohol intake; and increasing physical activity levels.[20]

GENERAL MANAGEMENT OF DIABETES

EARLY DETECTION AND MONITORING

The guiding principles for the management of diabetes are early detection and the prevention of complications. Community screening programs and annual physical examinations help to identify people with elevated blood glucose levels who may benefit from a glucose tolerance test (e.g., fasting and 2-hour tests with a measured glucose dose) and medical evaluation. The HbA_{1c} assay (normal value <5.7%) provides an effective tool for evaluating the long-term management of diabetes and the degree of control. Because glucose attaches itself to the hemoglobin molecule over the life of the red blood cell, this test reflects the average level of blood glucose over the preceding 3 months. Other tests such as measurement of fructosamine and glycated albumin levels are sometimes used for diagnostic purposes.[25] However, HbA_{1c} is the most commonly used assessment tool for monitoring ongoing blood glucose control and the risk for complications.

BASIC GOALS OF CARE

The health care team may include physicians, nurse practitioners, physician's assistants, nurses, dietitians, pharmacists, and mental health professionals with expertise in diabetes. The team is guided by several objectives when working with patients with diabetes, as follows:

Glycemic Control and Medication

This objective seeks to keep a person relatively free from symptoms of hyperglycemia, **hypoglycemia,** and glycosuria, which indicate poor glycemic control. A number of factors are involved in supporting this goal such as pharmacology (e.g., exogenous insulin injections, oral hypoglycemic agents), diet, exercise, and monitoring. The consistent control of blood glucose levels helps to reduce the risks of chronic complications. Although it is not within the scope of this textbook to extensively cover medications, a summary of basic information follows.

Insulin. There are several types of insulin with different durations of action (Table 20-4), and there are multiple combinations of insulin use (see the For Further Focus box, "Comparative Types of Insulin"). Patients should know how insulin works in the body and how its action relates to the food plan. Learning good insulin injection technique is also an important part of the treatment plan. In addition to the standard injections with needle and syringe or insulin pen, insulin can also be administered with a pump (Figure 20-5).

Table 20-4   **Types of Insulin**

TYPE	EXAMPLES	ONSET OF ACTION	PEAK ACTION	DURATION OF ACTION
Rapid-acting	Apidra (Glulisine) Humalog (Lispro) NovoLog (Aspart)	15 minutes	30 to 90 minutes	3 to 5 hours
Short-acting (regular)	Humulin R Novolin R	30 to 60 minutes	2 to 4 hours	5 to 8 hours
Intermediate-acting	Humulin N (NPH) Novolin N (NPH)	1 to 3 hours	8 hours	12 to 16 hours
Long-acting	Lantus (Glargine) Levemir (Detemir)	1 hour	None	20 to 26 hours
Premixed (intermediate-acting and regular short-acting)	Humulin 70/30 Novolin 70/30 Humulin 50/50	30 to 60 minutes	Varies	10 to 16 hours
Premixed insulin lispro protamine suspension (intermediate-acting) and insulin lispro (rapid-acting)	Humalog Mix 75/25 Humalog Mix 50/50	10 to 15 minutes	Varies	10 to 16 hours
Premixed insulin aspart protamine suspension (intermediate-acting) and insulin aspart (rapid-acting)	NovoLog Mix 70/30	5 to 15 minutes	Varies	10 to 16 hours

From National Diabetes Information Clearinghouse. *Types of Insulin* (website): <http://diabetes.niddk.nih.gov/dm/pubs/medicines_ez/insert_C.aspx>; Accessed April 2015.

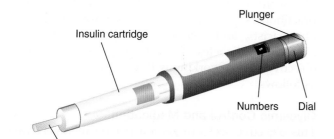

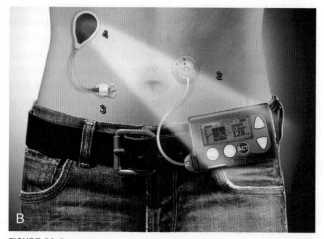

FIGURE 20-5 **(A)** Insulin pen. **(B)** External insulin pump: *(1)* device that delivers insulin; *(2)* where insulin is delivered; *(3)* sensor (beneath the skin) that monitors glucose levels continually; *(4)* transmitter that sends glucose readings to the device via wireless technology. (**B** From Salvo SG: *Mosby's pathology for massage therapists*, ed 2. St Louis, Mosby, 2009.)

Newer forms of insulin-pump therapy continuously deliver insulin to the body in response to a programmed basal rate. Fast-acting insulin can then be delivered in a bolus immediately after a meal based on the number of carbohydrates that the meal contained (as programmed by the user).

Oral hypoglycemic agents. Medications that stimulate insulin activity, comparison of the types and effects of different medications (Table 20-5), and methods that can be used to regulate medication levels are key points that should be well understood by the patient and his or her caretakers. The Drug-Nutrient Interaction box, "Exenatide and Glucose Control," describes the action of one such hypoglycemic medication.

Optimal Nutrition
The second objective is to sustain a high level of nutrition for general health promotion, adequate growth and development, and the maintenance of an appropriate weight. Medical nutrition therapy is an important part of diabetes management throughout the life span and is discussed in detail later in this chapter.

Physical Activity
Current recommendations for adults with diabetes are to perform at least 150 minutes per week of moderate-intensity aerobic physical activity (i.e., 50% to 70% of

For Further Focus

Comparative Types of Insulin

Flexible insulin plans allow patients to use both short-acting and longer-acting types of insulin in a series of several injections per day according to their specific food intake. This requires patients to count their carbohydrates for each meal and snack to calculate the needed fast-acting insulin for each feeding. They will also inject a longer-acting type of insulin once or twice a day to cover basal needs. Experienced patients self-test their blood glucose levels with finger pricks and glucose monitors. These patients are then able to adjust their insulin dosage to their test results; food patterns; work, school, and social activities; and exercise schedules. In some cases, an insulin pump that continuously delivers insulin into the bloodstream may be used to maintain better control over the body's varying insulin needs.

Fixed insulin plans allow patients to cover the day's insulin needs using a premixed insulin dose containing both fast-acting and intermediate-acting insulin combinations. The patient will require fewer injections per day and it is a simple plan. Since the insulin has been injected for the day, patients on this type of plan must make sure to eat meals at about the same time each day, eat about the same amounts of carbohydrates each day, take care not to skip meals or prolong the time between meals, and take their insulin injections at a consistent time each day.

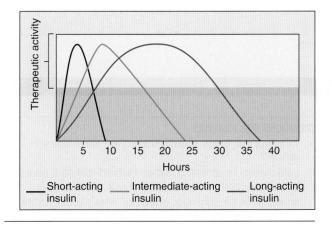

Short-acting insulin — Intermediate-acting insulin — Long-acting insulin

Drug-Nutrient Interaction

Exenatide and Glucose Control

KELLI BOI

Incretins are hormones that are secreted by intestinal cells in response to the presence of food. One of these incretins is known as *glucagon-like peptide 1* (GLP-1). This peptide acts by stimulating glucose-dependent insulin release by the pancreas and inhibiting glucagon secretion when glucose is present. The net effect is an overall reduction in plasma glucose level.

Exenatide (Byetta) is a member of the incretin mimetic class of drugs that is used for the treatment of type 2 diabetes. This drug resembles GLP-1, and it has similar effects when it is injected at meal times. In addition to reducing blood glucose levels, exenatide also slows gastric emptying and nutrient absorption, which enhances satiety and promotes mild weight loss. The most common side effects are nausea, vomiting, indigestion, abdominal pain, and diarrhea.

The powerful interaction between exenatide and glucose is the reason for its effectiveness in the treatment of type 2 diabetes. Exenatide is shown to improve glycemic control and to reduce HbA_{1c} values by 1% to 2%, and it may prolong the time before insulin therapy is needed to control hyperglycemia.[1] Patients who receive higher doses (i.e., 10 mcg twice daily) are at risk for hypoglycemia, primarily when they are using exenatide with sulfonylureas.

REFERENCE

1. Wysham CH, et al. Five-year efficacy and safety data of exenatide once weekly: long-term results from the DURATION-1 randomized clinical trial. *Mayo Clin Proc.* 2015;90(3):356-365.

Diabetes Self-Management Education and Support

Daily self-discipline and informed self-care are necessary for sound diabetes management, because all people with diabetes must ultimately treat themselves, with the support of a good health care team (see the Clinical Applications box, "Case Study: Richard Manages His Diabetes"). Comprehensive diabetes education programs that encourage self-care responsibility are the cornerstone to successful diabetes management.

The objectives of diabetes self-management education are to improve clinical outcomes, health status, and quality of life by supporting informed decision making, self-care behaviors, problem solving, and active collaboration with the health care team.[26] Certified diabetes educators and the American Diabetes Association have developed guidelines for diabetes self-management education that are based on the learning needs, skills, and content areas that are necessary for the self-care of patients with diabetes.

The success of the diabetes education program in any health care facility depends on the sensitivity and training of the staff members who are conducting the program. Continuing education is essential for all professionals and their assistants. Certified diabetes

maximum heart rate). Exercise bouts should be spread over at least 3 days per week with no more than 2 consecutive days without exercise.[20] In addition, people with type 2 diabetes should be encouraged to perform resistance training at least twice per week in the absence of contraindications.[20] Regular moderate-intensity exercise programs help individuals with type 2 diabetes control their blood glucose levels and reduce their risk for cardiovascular disease, hyperlipidemia, hypertension, and obesity. If the patient exhibits long-term complications of diabetes such as retinopathy, neuropathy, or CVD, certain types of exercise may be contraindicated. Health care providers can help make individualized plans for optimal benefits for the patient.

Table 20-5 Oral Hypoglycemic Medications

CATEGORY OF MEDICATION	EXAMPLES	ACTION
α-Glucosidase inhibitor	Acarbose (Precose) Miglitol (Glyset)	Slows breakdown of starches, thereby delaying the rise in blood glucose level that occurs after a meal
Amylin agonists	Pramlintide (Symlin)	Suppresses glucagon production and prevents hyperglycemia following meals
Biguanide	Metformin (Glucophage) Metformin extended release (Glucophage XR)	Suppresses hepatic glucose production
Dipeptidyl peptidase-4 inhibitor	Alogliptin (Nesina) Linagliptin (Tradjenta) Sitagliptin (Januvia) Saxagliptin (Onglyza)	Prevents the breakdown of hormones that increase insulin secretion and suppress glucagon production
Glucagon-like peptide-1 receptor agonists	Exenatide (Byetta) Exenatide Extended Release (Bydureon) Liraglutide (Victoza)	Improves the glucose-dependent secretion of insulin; decreases glucagon secretion after eating; slows gastric emptying and increases satiety
Meglitinide	Nateglinide (Starlix) Repaglinide (Prandin)	Stimulates the release of insulin from β cells
Sodium-glucose transport protein inhibitors	Canagliflozin (Invokana) Dapagliflozin (Farxiga)	Reduces the reabsorption of glucose in the kidneys
Sulfonylurea (second-generation)	Glipizide (Glucotrol, Glucotrol XL) Glyburide (Glynase Prestabs) Glimepiride (Amaryl)	Stimulates the release of insulin from β cells
Thiazolidinedione	Pioglitazone (Actos) Rosiglitazone (Avandia)	Increases insulin sensitivity in muscle and fat

Modified from Academy of Nutrition and Dietetics. *Nutrition Care Manual.* Chicago, Ill: 2015.

Clinical Applications

Case Study: Richard Manages His Diabetes

Richard Smith, who is 21 years old, has type 1 diabetes mellitus. He gives himself two injections per day, and each injection is a combination of medium-acting insulin and regular short-acting insulin. He takes one injection before breakfast and one before dinner, and he usually tests his blood glucose level before each meal and at bedtime. Richard is a college student who is usually active in athletics.

However, this is final examination week, and Richard's schedule is irregular. He is putting in long hours of study, and he is under considerable stress. On the day before a particularly difficult examination, he is reviewing his study materials at home, and he forgets to check his blood glucose level or eat lunch. During the middle of the afternoon, he begins to feel faint. He realizes that his blood glucose level is low and that an insulin reaction is imminent if he does not get a quick source of energy. He looks in the kitchen, but all he can find is orange juice, milk, a loaf of bread, and a jar of peanut butter.

QUESTIONS FOR ANALYSIS

1. Which of the foods should Richard eat immediately? Why?
2. Later, when he is feeling better, Richard makes a peanut butter sandwich, pours a glass of milk, and eats his snack while he continues studying. What carbohydrate food sources of energy are in his snack?
3. Are these carbohydrate sources in a form that the cells can burn for energy? What changes must Richard's body make to these sources to get them into the basic carbohydrate fuel form?
4. What is the complex form of carbohydrate in his snack? Why is this a valuable form of carbohydrate in his diet?
5. If Richard did not take his insulin to provide the necessary control agent for metabolizing the carbohydrate, what would happen to him as the result of improper handling of fat and the accumulation of ketones?

---

educators are the recognized experts in diabetes education for both patient and staff training. Patients and health care providers can locate specialists on their website at www.diabeteseducator.org.

Diabetes educators describe the disease process and treatment options for their patients. In addition, other elements that are involved in a patient's diabetes self-management education program may involve any or all of the following content areas, depending on the specific needs of that individual.[26]

Diet and lifestyle management. People with diabetes should cultivate a lifestyle that involves healthy eating choices that are based on individual nutrition needs, living and working situations, and food habits. Such planning includes understanding how the food plan relates to the maintenance of good glycemic control and the promotion of positive health. Regular physical activity is an important aspect of overall fitness, weight management, and blood glucose control. Patients can work with their health care providers to determine an appropriate activity plan and to discuss how to balance food intake with medications during exercise.

Monitoring. The monitoring of blood glucose levels, urinary acetone levels, weight, and blood pressure is fundamental to diabetes management. This monitoring includes learning accurate self-testing procedures as well as understanding the meaning of the results and knowing what action to take in relation to food, insulin, or exercise. A variety of self-tests are now available for quick blood glucose monitoring. Small glucose testing kits can fit into purses, backpacks, and glove compartments for easy access and convenience. In addition, there are remote blood glucose monitors that allow the user to get real-time feedback from a small sensor that is injected just below the skin to read interstitial blood glucose levels and trends of increasing or decreasing levels (see Figure 20-5, *B*).

Medications. In accordance with their treatment plans, people with diabetes should have a thorough understanding of how their medications work and when to take them. Patients should understand the side effects, efficacy, toxicity, dosage, and effects of missed or delayed doses as well as how to store and travel with their medications.

Problem solving. The prevention, detection, and treatment of acute complications require informed problem-solving skills. Patients and caregivers must recognize the early signs of hypoglycemia and its causes and treatment. This recognition includes the following: (1) knowledge of hypoglycemia's relationship to the interactive balances among insulin, food, and exercise as the basis of the diabetes care plan; (2) daily diabetic care and ways to prevent adverse episodes; (3) the immediate emergency treatment with some form of quick-acting simple carbohydrate to counteract hypoglycemia; and (4) the need to follow the emergency sugar with a snack of complex carbohydrate and protein as soon as possible to sustain a normal blood glucose level.

People living with diabetes should be confident in their ability to deal with illness and other special needs. This knowledge includes how to adjust one's diet and insulin intake and how to plan ahead for events of daily living such as travel, eating out, exercise, and stress.

Reducing risk. Prevention, detection, and a thorough knowledge of treatment options for acute and chronic complications should be well understood by all patients with diabetes. Skills taught in diabetes self-management education programs include the following: blood glucose and blood pressure self-monitoring, smoking cessation, foot care, aspirin use, and the maintenance of personal care records.

Resource awareness. A number of organizations with a wealth of health care tools are available, such as the American Diabetes Association, the Academy of Nutrition and Dietetics, and the American Association of Diabetes Educators. Health care provider resources include certified diabetes educators, hospital and outpatient dietitians, dietitians in private practice, public health nutritionists, and local chapters of the American Diabetes Association. Any resource materials used must be evaluated in terms of individual suitability.

Psychosocial Assessment and Care

Health care providers can help patients address the psychologic and social issues that impede the patient's ability to manage his or her diabetes. Health care providers are encouraged to routinely screen for psychosocial problems such as depression, diabetes-related stress, anxiety, eating disorders, and cognitive impairment.[20] Developing personal strategies to promote health and behavior changes may have significant and long-term effects on a patient's health status and quality of life. Patients should be able to identify appropriate coping mechanisms and support systems.

MEDICAL NUTRITION THERAPY FOR INDIVIDUALS WITH DIABETES

Glycemic control is the primary focus of diabetes management for all patients with diabetes. Medical nutrition therapy (MNT) will be discussed next in terms of recommendations, energy balance, nutrient balance, food distribution, and diet management.

MEDICAL NUTRITION THERAPY

The MNT recommendations and interventions for all people with diabetes or who are at high risk for developing diabetes are as follows[20,27]:

Prediabetes

Overweight and obese adults and children who have one or more additional risk factors should be tested at least once every 3 years to screen for prediabetes and diabetes. For individuals with prediabetes or at risk for type 2 diabetes, decrease the risk of diabetes and CVD by encouraging healthy food choices and at least 150 minutes per week of physical activity to promote and maintain a weight loss of 5% to 10% of body weight. Dietary patterns such as the Mediterranean diet or DASH diet (see Chapter 19) would be an appropriate goal. Other specific recommendations are to limit saturated fat, trans fat, and sugar-sweetened beverage intake.[27] Following the same MNT guidelines as provided for type 2 diabetes is recommended for individuals with prediabetes or impaired glucose tolerance (IGT).

Diabetes

For individuals diagnosed with diabetes, the MNT goals are as follows[28]:

1. Promote and support healthy eating patterns, emphasizing nutrient-dense foods and proper portion sizes.
2. Achieve and maintain blood glucose and lipid profiles as outlined in Table 20-3.
3. Achieve and maintain ideal body weight goals.
4. Prevent or slow the rate of development of the chronic complications of diabetes.
5. Individualize nutrition plans by taking into account personal and cultural preferences, health knowledge and proficiency, access to healthy foods, and willingness to make behavioral change.
6. Maintain the pleasure of eating by only limiting food choices when indicated by scientific evidence.
7. Provide practical tools for day-to-day meal planning rather than only focusing on individual nutrients or single foods.

Additional Considerations

The goals of MNT that apply to specific situations include the following:

1. For youth with type 1 diabetes, youth with type 2 diabetes, and older adults with diabetes, meet the nutrition and psychosocial needs of these unique times of the life cycle.
2. When a woman with diabetes becomes pregnant or when the pregnancy induces GDM, her body metabolism changes to meet the increased physiologic needs of the pregnancy while battling the manifestations of diabetes (see Chapter 10). Careful team monitoring of the mother's diabetes management is essential to ensure her health and the health of her baby. Energy and nutrient intake should be calculated for optimal outcomes.
3. Provide self-management training for the safe conducting of exercise, including the prevention and treatment of hypoglycemia and diabetes treatment during acute illness.

TOTAL ENERGY BALANCE

Type 1 diabetes most commonly begins during childhood; therefore, the normal height/weight charts for children provide a standard for adequate growth and development. During adulthood, maintaining a lean weight continues to be a basic goal. Because type 2 diabetes is associated with excess body fat, a major goal is weight reduction and control.[20]

The total energy value of the diet for a person with diabetes should be sufficient to meet individual needs for normal growth and development, physical activity and exercise, and the maintenance of a desirable lean body weight. Exercise is always an important factor in diabetes control, because it improves the cellular uptake of glucose. Energy intake is adjusted to equal energy output, or a negative energy balance should be achieved if weight loss is the goal. The Dietary Reference Intakes for children and adults (see Appendix B) can serve as guides for total energy needs, with appropriate reductions in kilocalories made for overweight adults (see Chapter 15).

NUTRIENT BALANCE

There is not a specific ratio of calories from each of the macronutrients that is recommended for all individuals with diabetes. The Dietary Reference Intake recommendations for the Acceptable Macronutrient Distribution Range are the basic guide for planning daily food intake: 45% to 65% from carbohydrate, 20% to 35% from fat, and 10% to 35% from protein. The diet for any person with diabetes is always based on the normal nutrition needs of that person for positive health, with a consideration of personal preferences, metabolic goals, and schedule of meals and physical activity.[20] Guidelines for macronutrient, micronutrient, and alcohol intake are based on the recommendations from the American Diabetes Association position statement and outlined in Box 20-4.

Carbohydrate

The primary focus in diabetes care is glycemic control, which involves the regulation of the body's primary fuel: glucose. The quantity and quality of a carbohydrate food consumed will influence the postprandial glycemic response. The American Diabetes Association recommends a diet that includes carbohydrates from fruits, vegetables, whole grains, legumes, and dairy products for good health. Carbohydrate intake should be consistently distributed throughout the day on a day-to-day basis and adjusted in response to blood glucose self-monitoring. Low-carbohydrate diets are not recommended for the management of diabetes.[27]

Starch and sugar. Carbohydrate-containing foods make up a large portion of the food supply. The most obvious of these are breads, cereals, grains, and sugary sweets. Almost all of the calories provided by fruits and vegetables are carbohydrate as well. Individuals with diabetes should not avoid carbohydrate-containing foods, because these represent an important source of energy, vitamins, minerals, and fiber.

Sucrose-containing foods do not have to be eliminated from the diet completely. Eating a sucrose containing food (e.g., piece of cake) will have a similar blood glucose effect as eating another complex carbohydrate containing food of equal caloric value. Generally speaking, sugary foods have less nutritional

Box 20-4 Nutrition Recommendations for the Management of Diabetes

CARBOHYDRATE
- A dietary pattern that includes carbohydrates from fruits, vegetables, whole grains, legumes, and dairy products is encouraged for good health.
- Monitoring carbohydrate levels—whether by carbohydrate counting, exchanges, or experienced-based estimation—remain a key strategy for the achievement of glycemic control.
- The use of low-glycemic load foods in place of higher-glycemic load foods may provide a modest additional benefit over that observed when total carbohydrate is considered alone.
- Sucrose-containing foods can be substituted for other carbohydrates in the meal plan or, if they are added to the meal plan, they must be considered with regard to the dosage of insulin or other glucose-lowering medications. Care should be taken to avoid excess energy intake.
- As for the general population, people with diabetes are encouraged to consume a variety of fiber-containing foods to meet the dietary recommendations.
- Sugar alcohols and nonnutritive sweeteners are safe when they are consumed within the daily intake levels established by the U.S. Food and Drug Administration.
- Fructose from naturally occurring foods such as fruit may result in better glycemic control compared to isocaloric intake of sucrose or starch. Avoid sugar-sweetened beverages (including those made with high-fructose corn syrup).

FAT
- The amount of dietary saturated fat, cholesterol, and trans fat recommendations are the same as those for the general population.
- Increase the selection of foods containing omega-3 fatty acids (EPA and DHA) and omega-3 linolenic acid (ALA).
- Two or more servings of fish per week (with the exception of commercially fried fish filets) provide omega-3 polyunsaturated fatty acids and are recommended.
- For people with type 2 diabetes, a Mediterranean-style, monounsaturated fatty acid–rich eating pattern may benefit glycemic control and CVD risk factors.
- Individuals with diabetes and dyslipidemia may be able to modestly reduce total and LDL-cholesterol by consuming 1.6 to 3 g/day of plant stanols or sterols typically found in enriched foods.

PROTEIN
- For individuals with diabetes and normal renal function, evidence is insufficient to suggest that usual protein intake (i.e., 15% to 20% of energy) should be modified.
- For individuals with type 2 diabetes, ingested protein can increase the insulin response without increasing plasma glucose concentrations. Therefore, carbohydrate foods that are also high in protein should not be used to prevent or treat acute hypoglycemia.

SODIUM
- For individuals with both diabetes and hypertension, a reduction in dietary sodium below the recommendations for the general public (≤2300 mg/day) is advisable.

ALCOHOL
- If adults with diabetes choose to use alcohol, daily intake should be limited to a moderate amount (i.e., one drink per day or less for women and two drinks per day or less for men).
- Be aware that alcohol consumption may place people with diabetes at increased risk for delayed hypoglycemia, especially if taking insulin or insulin secretagogues.

MICRONUTRIENTS
- No clear evidence demonstrates a benefit from vitamin or mineral supplementation in people with diabetes (as compared with the general population) who do not have underlying deficiencies.
- Routine supplementation with antioxidants (e.g., vitamins E and C, carotene), chromium, magnesium, vitamin D, or herbs is not advised because of a lack of evidence of efficacy and, in some cases, concern related to long-term safety.

Adapted from Evert AB et al. Nutrition therapy recommendations for the management of adults with diabetes. *Diabetes Care.* 2013;36(11):3821-3842.

value than other forms of starch and thus consumption should be limited in favor of nutrient-dense complex carbohydrate sources.[28] Sugar-sweetened beverages should be limited or avoided altogether.[20]

Glycemic index. The use of the glycemic index for individuals with diabetes may provide a modest benefit for glycemic control; however, there is conflicting evidence of its effectiveness.[20] For now, personal preference dictates the use of glycemic index values. See the For Further Focus box in Chapter 2 titled "Carbohydrate Complications" for more details about the glycemic index.

Fiber. As for all individuals, the consumption of dietary fiber is encouraged for patients with diabetes. There are no reasons for these individuals to consume greater amounts of fiber than what is recommended for the general public. Current recommendations are to consume approximately 14 g of fiber per 1000 kcal (approximately 25 g/day for women and 38 g/day for men).[29]

Sugar substitutes and sweeteners. Nutritive and nonnutritive sweeteners are safe to consume in moderation and as part of a nutritious and well-balanced diet. Various sugar substitutes are listed in Table 2-4 in Chapter 2. The use of nutritive sweeteners (e.g., sucrose, fructose, sorbitol) must be accounted for in a meal plan. Nonnutritive sweeteners do not influence the blood glucose levels.

Protein

There is no evidence that a specific amount of protein consumption will optimize glycemic control.[28] Patients with normal renal function should be able to adequately meet their protein needs on diets that supply the usual amount of kilocalories as protein.[27] Excessively high protein intake is not recommended because of its unnecessary stress on the kidneys for patients with diabetic nephropathy.

Fat

There is no evidence to support a specific recommendation for dietary fat consumption as a percentage of total calories. Fat quality appears to be more important than fat quantity; thus recommendations for dietary patterns such as the Mediterranean diet (high monounsaturated fats) are favored over low-fat, high-carbohydrate diets.[20] Recommendations for omega-3 fatty acids, saturated fat, dietary cholesterol, and trans fats are the same for individuals with diabetes as they are for the general public. Because diabetes increases the risk for cardiovascular disease, cardioprotective nutrition interventions aimed at normalizing lipid profiles should be addressed in the overall diet plan.

FOOD DISTRIBUTION

Food distribution, including amount and quality of carbohydrate-containing foods, should be coordinated with the patient's daily schedule, exercise plans, and specific type of medications used to control blood glucose levels.

Daily Schedule

Food distribution should be planned ahead when using oral hypoglycemic agents or long-acting insulin, and adjusted according to each day's scheduled activities and blood glucose monitoring to prevent episodes of hypoglycemia. The careful distribution of food and snacks is especially important for children and adolescents with diabetes to balance with insulin during the growth spurts and changing hormone patterns of puberty. Practical consideration should be given to school and work schedules, athletics, social events, and stressful periods. A stressful event caused by any

source (e.g., injury, anxiety, fear, pain) brings an adrenaline (epinephrine) rush. This fight-or-flight effect counteracts insulin activity and can contribute to a glycemic response.

Exercise and Glycemic Control

For people who are using insulin, any exercise or additional physical activity must be covered in the food distribution plan. The energy demands of exercise are discussed separately in Chapter 16. The following guidelines are recommended for regulating the glycemic response to exercise in individuals with diabetes who use insulin[20,28]:

1. Achieve metabolic control before physical activity.
   - In the presence of hyperglycemia: use caution if glucose levels are elevated and if no ketosis is present; avoid vigorous physical activity if ketosis is present.
   - Ingest added carbohydrate if glucose levels are less than 100 mg/dL.
2. Monitor blood glucose levels before and after physical activity.
   - Identify when changes in insulin or food intake are necessary.
   - Learn the glycemic response to different physical activity conditions.
3. Monitor food and fluid intake.
   - Consume added carbohydrate as needed to avoid hypoglycemia (Table 20-6).
   - Carbohydrate-based foods should be readily available during and after physical activity.
   - Ensure adequate fluid intake.

Table 20-6	Meal Planning Guide for Active People with Type 1 Diabetes	
ACTIVITY LEVEL	**EXCHANGE NEEDS**	**SAMPLE FOOD EXCHANGES**
Moderate		
30 minutes	Usually not necessary unless blood glucose is <100 mg/dL	
1 hour	1 carbohydrate serving (15 g of carbohydrate)	1 small apple, ½ banana, 6 saltine crackers, 2 tablespoons raisins, or 1 cup of milk
Strenuous		
1 to 2 hours	2 carbohydrate servings (30 g of carbohydrate)	1⅓ cup plain yogurt, ½ large bagel, 1 cup oatmeal or starchy vegetable, or 1 cup orange juice

Drug Therapy

The food distribution pattern is also influenced by any form of drug therapy (i.e., type, amount, and dose schedule of insulin or oral hypoglycemic agent) that is necessary for glucose control. For example, individuals taking insulin will usually administer a specific dose of insulin relative to the amount of carbohydrate consumed at each meal. If patients are using a pre-mixed insulin plan, injections should be at consistent times every day and meals need to be consumed at a similar time each day. If patients are using a fixed insulin plan, the amount of carbohydrates each day should match the fixed insulin dose.

Individuals taking oral hypoglycemic agents do not change the dose of their medication to reflect each meal consumed; therefore, the daily meal plan should provide a moderate and consistent amount of carbohydrates throughout the day. For patients taking oral hypoglycemic agents, the following food distribution guidelines are applicable: patients using insulin secretagogues should be diligent to include a source of carbohydrates at each meal and snack; patients using biguanides should take their medication with food or 15 minutes after a meal if symptoms persist; patients taking α-glucosidase inhibitors should take their medication at the very beginning of a meal, and patients taking incretin mimetics should inject their medication before the meal.[28] Successful self-care means that the patient can adjust his or her diet, medications, and exercise on the basis of the result of blood glucose monitoring.

DIET MANAGEMENT

The nature of an individual's diabetes, his or her treatment regimen, and his or her health status largely determine the necessary personal diet management. Table 20-7 provides guidelines for dietary strategies for type 1 and type 2 diabetes.

Every person with diabetes is unique, with a particular form and degree of diabetes as well as a different living situation, a different background, and different food habits. All of these personal needs must be considered (as discussed in Chapters 14 and 17) if appropriate and realistic care is to be planned. The nutrition counselor, who usually is the registered dietitian nutritionist or certified diabetes educator, should determine these various needs as part of a careful initial nutrition assessment that includes medical, socioeconomic, and psychosocial needs as well as personal lifestyle characteristics. This information provides the basis for determining the diet prescription.

A major principle of diabetes management is the variety of methods and dietary guidelines that the nutrition team can use when planning for and supporting patients. Of these dietary guides, carbohydrate counting and the food exchange method—when tailored to meet individual needs—remain the two most commonly used approaches. Materials that can be used for planning the diet are available from the American Diabetes Association and the Academy of Nutrition and Dietetics in both English and Spanish.

Carbohydrate Counting

Carbohydrate counting is one way to balance the carbohydrate intake with insulin injections (i.e., the insulin-to-carbohydrate ratio). Patients count the total number of carbohydrates contained within a meal and then inject an appropriate amount of insulin to process the glucose. One carbohydrate serving equals 15 g of carbohydrate. There are multiple resources (e.g., books, online programs, handheld devices, phone applications) available that list grams of carbohydrates for thousands of foods. One benefit of carbohydrate counting is that meal plans are much less stringent and flexibility is more easily accommodated. For this type of meal and insulin planning to work, the patient must be well versed in calculating the total number of carbohydrate grams consumed per meal or snack.

Additional information and tool kits for dietary planning based on carbohydrate counting can be

Table 20-7 Dietary Strategies for Type 1 and Type 2 Diabetes Mellitus

DIETARY STRATEGY	TYPE 1	TYPE 2
Decrease energy intake (kilocalories)	No	Yes, if weight loss is recommended
Increase frequency of feedings	Sometimes	Usually no
Have regular daily intake of kilocalories from carbohydrate, protein, and fat	Very important	Yes
Plan consistent daily ratio of protein, carbohydrate, and fat for each feeding	Desirable	Yes, but not as tightly controlled
Use extra or planned food to treat or prevent hypoglycemia	Very important	Usually not necessary
Plan regular times for meals and snacks	Very important	Yes
Use extra food for unusual exercise	Yes	Usually not necessary
During illness, use small, frequent feedings of carbohydrates to prevent starvation ketoacidosis	Important	Usually not necessary because of resistance to ketoacidosis

found on the American Diabetes Association website (www.diabetes.org) and the Academy of Nutrition and Dietetics website (www.eatright.org).

Food Exchange System

The dietitian uses the food exchange system to calculate a patient's energy and nutrient needs as well as to distribute foods in a balanced meal and snack pattern. The food exchange system is called this because people with diabetes use the system to select a variety of foods from the various food groups in accordance with their personal diet plans.

With this system, commonly used foods are grouped into exchange lists according to roughly equal portions based on macronutrient values. A standard serving of a carbohydrate food (e.g., bread, cereal, legumes, starchy vegetables) has 15 grams of carbohydrates. A serving of fruit or a serving of sweets or desserts would also contain 15 grams of carbohydrates. Dairy products have 12 grams of carbohydrates per serving. Nonstarchy vegetables all have 5 grams of carbohydrates per serving. The exchange list also has defined portions based on macronutrient content for meat and meat substitutes, fats, and alcohol. The exchange system uses lists of all foods (and the serving size) that count as one serving from each of the food groups. The dietitian can help define how many servings the patient needs from each food group per day. Then the patient may choose from any food within those food group lists to personalize their daily diet (see the exchange lists provided on the Evolve website). Thus, a variety of foods may be chosen from these lists to fulfill the food plan while the basic diet prescription of total energy and a balanced ratio of nutrients are maintained. The booklet entitled *Choose Your Foods: Exchange Lists for Diabetes* provides a detailed tutorial on using the exchange lists and is available for purchase from the Academy of Nutrition and Dietetics or the American Diabetes Association. In addition, the National Institutes of Health provides a list of example serving sizes of each of the food groups online (www.nih.gov [search "Exchange list"]). Table 20-8 illustrates a calculated 2200-kcal diet and food pattern example using the exchange system. Box 20-5 outlines a sample menu that is based on this pattern.

Special Concerns

Special concerns arise in daily living and become an important part of ongoing dietary counseling. Some suggestions for these concerns are given in the following sections.

Special diet food items. Little need exists for special "diabetic" foods. People with diabetes should eat the regular, well-balanced diet that is recommended for the general population to promote health and prevent disease. This kind of a healthful diet primarily makes use of regular fresh foods from all of the basic food groups, with the limited use of processed foods and an increased use of flavorful, low-fat seasonings. The simple principles of moderation and variety should guide food choices and amounts.

Alcohol. The occasional use of alcohol in an adult diabetic diet can be planned, but caution must be exercised. Individuals who use insulin or insulin secretagogues and consume alcohol should eat food when they drink and not increase their insulin dose, because the overall effect of alcohol is to lower the blood glucose level. In addition, education concerning the recognition and management of delayed hypoglycemia is warranted.[20] Occasional use is defined as moderate intake: one drink or less per day for women and two drinks or less per day for men. Equivalent portions are 12 oz of regular beer, 5 oz of wine, or 1.5 oz of 80-proof whiskey. The same precautions for the use of alcohol that apply to the general public apply to people with diabetes.

A person with type 1 diabetes should not substitute alcohol for food exchanges in the diet. When a person's blood glucose levels begin to drop, the liver typically responds to the hormone glucagon and releases glucose into the blood to reestablish normal blood glucose levels. However, when alcohol is in the system, the liver's primary role is to detoxify the blood of alcohol, and it will not respond to impending hypoglycemia until the alcohol is cleared. Therefore, alcohol should only be consumed slowly, in moderation, and in conjunction with food. Sugar-free mixes should be used in cocktails and light beer is recommended. Alcohol may be used in cooking as desired because it vaporizes in the cooking process and contributes only its flavor to the finished product.

Hypoglycemia. The brain depends on a constant supply of glucose for metabolism and proper function; a prolonged lack of glucose can lead to brain damage. Hypoglycemia (i.e., a blood glucose level of less than 70 mg/dL) may occur from too much insulin or oral hypoglycemic agents that act by stimulating the islet cells in the pancreas to secrete more insulin. Hypoglycemia can also occur if a person with diabetes delays a meal or snack, does not eat enough carbohydrate, or exercises too much without sufficient food. Table 20-9 lists symptoms of both hyperglycemia and hypoglycemia. Because behavior is often irrational and movements are uncoordinated, patients in this state may be mistaken for being intoxicated. Thus, an identification bracelet or pendant is an ideal means of informing others about the true condition so that proper treatment—glucose replacement in the form of a food or beverage or an injection of glucagon—can be given.

People with type 1 diabetes should always carry a convenient form of sugar (e.g., sugar lumps or glucose

Table 20-8   Calculation of a Diabetic Diet Using the Exchange System (2200 kcal)

FOOD GROUP	TOTAL DAY'S EXCHANGES	CARBOHYDRATES: 275 g (50% kcal)	PROTEIN: 110 g (20% kcal)	FAT: 74 g (30% kcal)	BREAKFAST	LUNCH	DINNER	SNACKS AFTERNOON	SNACKS BEDTIME
Carbohydrates									
Starch	11.5	172	34.5	—	3	3	3	1	1.5
Fruit	3	45	—	—	1	1		1	
Milk									
Fat free	2	24	16	1	1				1
Sweets, Desserts, and Other Carbohydrates	1	15	Varies	Varies			1		
Nonstarchy Vegetables	4	20	8	—		2	2		
Meat and Meat Substitutes									
Very lean	2	—	14	0 to 1				1	1
Lean	3	—	21	9			3		
Medium fat	2	—	14	10	1	1			
Fat	11	—	—	55	3	3	3	1	1
Total grams		276	107.5	75					

Box 20-5   Sample Menu Prescription: 2200 Kilocalories

- 275 g of carbohydrate (50% kcal)
- 110 g of protein (20% kcal)
- 75 g of fat (30% kcal)

BREAKFAST
- 1 medium fresh peach
- 1 bagel (3 oz)
- 1 soft-boiled egg
- 1 Tbsp of butter
- 1 cup of low-fat milk
- Coffee or tea without sweetener

LUNCH
- Vegetable soup with whole-wheat crackers
- Tuna sandwich on whole-wheat bread
  - Tuna (½ cup, drained)
  - Mayonnaise (1 Tbsp)
  - Chopped dill pickle
  - Chopped celery
- 1 fresh pear

DINNER
- Pan-broiled pork chop (well-trimmed)
- 1 cup of brown rice
- ½ cup of green beans
- 1 cup of tossed green salad
- Salad dressing (1 Tbsp)
- ⅓ cup of fat-free frozen yogurt

AFTERNOON SNACK
- ½ pita pocket with 2 Tbsp of peanut butter
- 1 medium orange

EVENING SNACK
- 3 cups of plain popped popcorn
- 1 oz of cheese
- 1 cup of low-fat milk

tablets) with them to take at the first sign of a hypoglycemic attack. Blood glucose level should be retested within 15 to 20 minutes after administering glucose to determine if additional glucose is needed. Blood glucose level should be checked again 60 minutes later to ensure normoglycemia.[27] Patients in a severe hypoglycemic condition may not be conscious enough to swallow without risk of aspirating. In this case, someone else may need to assist by placing glucose gel (or the equivalent) inside the patient's cheek for absorption or by administering a glucagon injection.

Illness. Illnesses can complicate diet management and blood glucose control. As such, it is recommended that individuals with diabetes receive an annual influenza vaccine, along with other preventive vaccines as indicated (e.g., pneumococcal polysaccharide vaccine, hepatitis B vaccines).[20] When general illness occurs, food and insulin should be adjusted accordingly. The texture of the food can be modified to make use of easily digested and absorbed liquid foods. In general, people with diabetes who are experiencing short-term illness (e.g., cold, flu, vomiting, diarrhea) should do the following[27]:

- Monitor the blood glucose level frequently. Fever, infection, or stress hormones can raise blood glucose levels.
- Administer supplemental insulin as indicated by blood glucose level.
- Monitor urine for ketones, a sign of diabetic ketoacidosis (DKA).
- Maintain food and fluid intake. Fluids, carbohydrates, and electrolytes must be replaced. Liquid or soft foods may replace carbohydrate-containing solid foods if necessary.
- Contact a physician if the illness lasts for more than 24 hours, if the fever remains high, or if blood glucose concentration remains ≥250 mg/dL and moderate to large ketone levels are present.

Table 20-9   Symptoms of Hyperglycemia and Hypoglycemia

FACTOR	HYPERGLYCEMIA	HYPOGLYCEMIA
Cause	Too much food, not enough insulin, illness, or stress	Not enough food, too much insulin, too much exercise, or alcohol intake without food
Symptoms	Polydipsia Polyuria Polyphagia Dry or itchy skin Blurred vision Drowsiness Nausea Fatigue Shortness of breath Weakness Confusion Coma	Sudden shaking Nervousness Sweating Anxiety and irritability Dizziness Impaired vision Weakness Headache Hunger Confusion Tingling sensations around the mouth Seizure

Travel. When a trip is planned, clients may benefit from consulting with the dietitian or diabetes educator, particularly for newly diagnosed patients, to make decisions about food choices that reflect what will be available. In general, preparation activities may include the following:

- Review meal-planning skills, the number and type of exchanges at each meal, basic portion sizes, and tips on eating out.
- Learn about foods that will be available (e.g., ordering a "diabetic meal" ahead from an airline).
- Select appropriate snacks to carry, and plan time intervals for their use.
- Plan for time-zone changes with regard to medication, exercise, and diet routines.
- Carry some quick-acting form of carbohydrate (e.g., sugar lumps, glucose tablets) at all times, and tell companions about the signs, symptoms, and treatment of hypoglycemia.
- Wear an identification bracelet or pendant.
- Secure a physician's letter that addresses syringes and insulin prescriptions.

Eating out. In general, people with diabetes should plan ahead so that food that is eaten at home before and after a meal out can be accommodated to maintain the continuing day's balance. Choosing restaurants wisely also makes menu selection easier. Timing insulin doses to food arrival is important, because taking insulin too long before eating will result in hypoglycemia.

Stress. Physiologic or psychosocial stress may affect glycemic control in patients with diabetes because of the hormonal responses that are antagonistic to insulin. In particular, diabetes-specific emotional stress is associated with poor HbA_{1c} control in individuals with type 1 and type 2 diabetes.[30,31] People with diabetes, especially those who use insulin, should learn useful stress-reduction exercises and activities as part of their self-care skills and practices. Stress-reducing activities can vary greatly from one person to the next (e.g., meditation, running, yoga, journaling, playing music). Finding the best coping mechanism may require trial and error.

Putting It All Together

Summary

- Diabetes mellitus is a syndrome with varying forms and degrees that has the common characteristic of hyperglycemia. Its underlying metabolic disorder involves all three of the energy-yielding nutrients and influences energy balance. The major controlling hormone involved is insulin from the pancreas, and people with diabetes have either a lack of insulin or a resistance to its action.
- Type 1 diabetes affects approximately 5% to 10% of all people with diabetes; it most commonly presents itself first during childhood, and it is more severe and unstable. The treatment of type 1 diabetes involves regular meals and snacks that are balanced with insulin and exercise. The self-monitoring of blood glucose levels is a critical part of disease management.
- Type 2 diabetes occurs mostly among adults, especially those who are overweight. Acidosis is rare. Treatment involves weight reduction and maintenance along with regular exercise. Oral hypoglycemic medications or insulin may be needed.
- Diabetes self-management education is a cornerstone of the overall success of patients who are managing their diabetes.

- A significant keystone of care for all forms of diabetes is sound nutrition therapy. The basic food plan should be rich in complex carbohydrates and dietary fiber; low in simple sugars, saturated fats, and cholesterol; and moderate in protein. Food should be distributed throughout the day in fairly regular amounts and at regular times, and it should be tailored to meet individual needs.

Chapter Review Questions

See answers in Appendix A.

1. A risk factor for type 2 diabetes is:
   a. A BMI of 20.
   b. A BMI of 28.
   c. Exercising 60 minutes a day.
   d. A blood pressure of 130/85 mm Hg.

2. A form of metabolic acidosis that occurs in uncontrolled diabetes is called:
   a. Metabolic syndrome.
   b. Ketoacidosis.
   c. Ketoalkalosis.
   d. Hypoglycemia.

3. The hormone responsible for promoting the uptake of amino acids by skeletal muscle is:
   a. Insulin.
   b. Somatostatin.
   c. Glucagon.
   d. Leptin.

4. A dietary strategy that can assist individuals with type 2 diabetes is:
   a. Replace all sugar with noncaloric sweeteners.
   b. Restrict carbohydrate intake to 50 grams or less per day.
   c. Learn appropriate portion sizes for different types of foods.
   d. Focus on choosing foods with a high glycemic index.

5. One serving of sliced bread (1 ounce) from the exchange list provides:
   a. 5 grams of carbohydrate.
   b. 10 grams of carbohydrate.
   c. 15 grams of carbohydrate.
   d. 20 grams of carbohydrate.

Additional Learning Resources

evolve Please refer to this text's Evolve website for answers to the Case Study questions.
http://evolve.elsevier.com/Williams/basic/

References and **Further Reading and Resources** in the back of the book provide additional resources for enhancing knowledge.

Kidney Disease

Key Concepts

- Kidney disease interferes with the normal capacity of nephrons to filter the waste products of metabolism.
- Short-term kidney disease requires basic nutrition support for healing.
- The progressive degeneration of chronic kidney disease requires dialysis treatment and nutrient

modification in accordance with each individual's disease status.
- Current therapy for kidney stones depends more on basic nutrition and health support for medical treatment than on major food and nutrient restrictions.

More than 114,000 Americans are diagnosed with end-stage renal disease (ESRD) annually.[1] And there are many more with compromised kidney function who remain undiagnosed and untreated. The National Health and Nutrition Examination Survey found that 90% of individuals with more than two clinical markers for chronic kidney disease (CKD) are unaware of their condition.[2] These kidney problems are costly as a result of lost productivity, income, leisure time, and overall quality of life.

This chapter reviews the medical nutrition therapy (MNT) for people with various forms of kidney disease. **Dialysis** extends the lives of patients with CKD; however, it does so at an emotional, physical, and financial cost.

BASIC STRUCTURE AND FUNCTION OF THE KIDNEY

Tremendous quantities of fluid (approximately 1.2 L) are filtered through the kidneys every minute. Most of this fluid is reabsorbed back into the vascular system to maintain circulating blood volume. As the blood circulates through the kidneys, these twin organs repeatedly "launder" it to monitor and maintain its quantity and quality. Indeed, the composition of various body fluids is determined not as much by what the mouth takes in as by what the kidneys keep; they are the master chemists of the internal environment.

STRUCTURES

The basic functional unit of the kidney is the **nephron**. Each human kidney is made up of approximately 1 million nephrons, all of which are independently capable of forming urine. Key parts of the nephron include the glomerulus and the tubules (Figure 21-1).

Glomerulus

At the head of each nephron, a cup-shaped membrane referred to as **Bowman's capsule** holds the entering blood capillary and its clump of smaller vessels. Within Bowman's capsule, the afferent arteriole branches into a cluster of capillaries to form the **glomerulus** (see Figure 21-1). Only the larger blood proteins and cells remain behind in the circulating blood as it leaves the glomerulus via the efferent arteriole. The rate at which blood is filtered through the glomerulus, which is

---

dialysis the process of separating crystalloids (i.e., crystal-forming substances) and colloids (i.e., glue-like substances) in solution by the difference in their rates of diffusion through a semipermeable membrane; crystalloids (e.g., blood glucose, other simple metabolites) pass through readily, and colloids (e.g., plasma proteins) pass through slowly or not at all. Dialysis is used to remove waste and excess fluid from the blood when one's kidneys are not functioning.

nephron the functional unit of the kidney that filters and reabsorbs essential blood constituents, secretes hydrogen ions as needed to maintain the acid-base balance, reabsorbs water, and forms and excretes a concentrated urine for the elimination of wastes.

Bowman's capsule the membrane at the head of each nephron; this capsule was named for the English physician Sir William Bowman, who in 1843 first established the basis of plasma filtration and consequent urine secretion in the relationship of the blood-filled glomeruli and the filtration across the enveloping membrane.

glomerulus the first section of the nephron; a cluster of capillary loops that are cupped in the nephron head that serves as an initial filter.

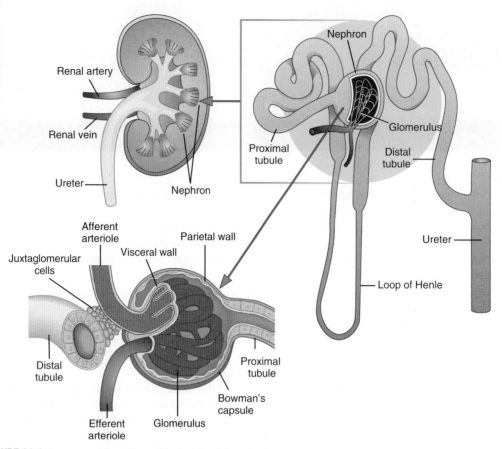

FIGURE 21-1 Anatomy of the kidney. (*Top*, Reprinted from Peckenpaugh NJ. *Nutrition essentials and diet therapy.* 11th ed. St. Louis, Saunders, 2010. *Bottom*, Reprinted from Thibodeau GA, Patton KT. *Anatomy & physiology.* 6th ed. St Louis: Mosby; 2007.)

called the **glomerular filtration rate (GFR)**, is the current method for monitoring kidney function and for defining stages of kidney disease. CKD is defined as a GFR of <60 mL/min (adjusted to a standard body surface area of 1.73 m^2) for 3 or more months or a urinary albumin-to-creatinine ratio of >30 mg/g.[3]

Tubules

From the cupped head of each nephron, a small tubule carries the filtered fluid through its winding pathway and empties into the central area of the kidney medulla. Specific substances are reabsorbed and secreted along the way in each of the four parts of these tubules (Table 21-1).

Proximal tubule. Most of the needed nutrients are reabsorbed in this first part of the tubule and returned to the blood. The surface area of the tubule is greatly increased by a brush border membrane that contains

> **glomerular filtration rate (GFR)** the volume of fluid that is filtered from the renal glomerular capillaries into Bowman's capsule per unit of time; this term is used clinically as a measure of kidney function.

thousands of microvilli. Glucose and amino acids as well as approximately 80% of the water and other substances are usually reabsorbed here. Approximately 20% of the filtered fluid remains to enter the next section of the tube.

Loop of Henle. The tubule's midsection narrows and dips down into the central part of the kidney. Here, the important exchange of sodium, chloride, and water occurs. This fluid environment maintains the necessary osmotic pressure to concentrate the urine as it passes through the distal tubule and ureter on its way to the bladder for elimination.

Distal tubule. The latter part of the tubule winds back up into the outer area of the kidney cortex. Here, the secretion of hydrogen ions occurs as needed to control the acid-base balance. Additional sodium is also reabsorbed as needed under the influence of the adrenal hormone aldosterone (see Chapter 9).

Collecting tubule. In this final section of the tubule, concentrated urine is produced by the following water-reabsorbing actions: (1) the influence of antidiuretic hormone (see Chapter 9); and (2) the osmotic pressure from the more dense surrounding fluid in the central

Table **21-1**	Reabsorption and Secretion In Parts of the Nephron	
PART	**FUNCTION**	**SUBSTANCE MOVED**
Proximal tubule	Reabsorption (active)	Sodium, glucose, amino acids
	Reabsorption (passive)	Chloride, phosphate, urea, water, other solutes
Loop of Henle		
Descending limb	Reabsorption (passive)	Water
	Secretion (passive)	Urea
Ascending limb	Reabsorption (active)	Sodium
	Reabsorption (passive)	Chloride
Distal tubule	Reabsorption (active)	Sodium
	Reabsorption (passive)	Chloride, other anions, water (in the presence of antidiuretic hormone)
	Secretion (passive)	Ammonia
	Secretion (active)	Potassium, hydrogen, some drugs
Collecting duct	Reabsorption (active)	Sodium
	Reabsorption (passive)	Urea, water (in the presence of antidiuretic hormone)
	Secretion (passive)	Ammonia
	Secretion (active)	Potassium, hydrogen, some drugs

From Thibodeau GA, Patton KT. *Anatomy & physiology*. 7th ed. St Louis: Mosby; 2010.

area of the kidney. The urine, which is now concentrated and ready for excretion, only amounts to 0.5% to 1% of the original fluid and materials that have been filtered through the glomerulus.

FUNCTION

Nephron structure is adapted in fine detail to balance the internal fluids that are necessary for life. At birth, each person has far more nephrons than are actually needed, but they are gradually lost with advancing age. Chronic hyperglycemia (i.e., uncontrolled diabetes) and hypertension exacerbate damage to the glomerulus and increase the rate of lost functioning nephrons.

Excretory and Regulatory Functions

The following excretory and regulatory tasks are performed while blood flows through the nephron:

- *Filtration:* Most particles in blood are filtered out, except for the larger components of red blood cells and proteins.
- *Reabsorption:* As the filtrate continues through the winding tubules, substances that the body needs are selectively reabsorbed and returned to the blood to maintain the electrolyte, acid-base, and fluid balances.
- *Secretion:* Along the tubules, additional hydrogen ions are secreted as needed to maintain the acid-base balance.
- *Excretion:* Waste materials are excreted in the now-concentrated urine.

Endocrine Functions

In addition to major functions in the regulation of the blood constituents and the production and elimination of concentrated urine, the kidneys perform several endocrine functions. The endocrine system is composed of glands that secrete hormones directly into the circulatory system. Many of the hormones released from glands throughout the body have a response within the kidney, as follows:

- *Renin secretion:* When the **arteriole** pressure falls, the kidneys activate and secrete renin, which is an enzyme that initiates the renin-angiotensin-aldosterone mechanism to reabsorb sodium and to maintain hormonal control of the body water balance (see Chapter 9).
- *Erythropoietin secretion:* The kidneys are responsible for producing the body's major supply (80% to 90%) of **erythropoietin**.
- *Vitamin D activation:* The kidneys convert an intermediate inactive form of vitamin D into the final active vitamin D hormone in the proximal tubules of the nephrons (see Chapter 7). This action is stimulated by the parathyroid hormone.

DISEASE PROCESS AND DIETARY CONSIDERATIONS

GENERAL CAUSES OF KIDNEY DISEASE

Several disease conditions may interfere with the normal functioning of nephrons and eventually result in kidney disease.

Infection and Obstruction

Symptoms of bacterial urinary tract infection may range from the discomfort of bladder infections to

---

arteriole the smallest branch of an artery that connects with the capillaries.

erythropoietin hormone that stimulates the production of red blood cells in the bone marrow.

more involved chronic disease and obstruction from kidney stones. Obstruction anywhere in the urinary tract blocks drainage and may cause further infection and general tissue damage.

Damage from Other Diseases

Diabetes mellitus is the leading cause of ESRD in the United States (Figure 21-2).[1] Hyperglycemia and hypertension associated with diabetes can damage small renal arteries, thereby leading to glomerulosclerosis (i.e., the loss of functioning nephrons) and eventual CKD. Circulatory disorders such as prolonged and poorly controlled hypertension can cause the degeneration of the small arteries within the kidney and interfere with normal nephron function. More than 84% of all patients with CKD have a history of hypertension.[1] Increased demands on the remaining nephrons may in turn cause further hypertension and additional damage. Other chief causes are glomerulonephritis and cystic kidney disease. Autoimmune diseases such as systemic lupus erythematosus may also lead to compromised kidney function or disease.

Toxins

Various environmental agents (e.g., chemical pesticides, solvents), animal venom, certain plants, heavy metals, and some drugs (e.g., nonsteroidal antiinflammatory drugs, aminoglycoside antibiotics, radiographic contrast dye) are **nephrotoxic** and can cause kidney damage.

Genetic or Congenital Defects

Cystic diseases (e.g., polycystic kidney disease, medullary cystic disease) are genetically linked kidney diseases that may lead to ESRD later in life. Congenital abnormalities of both kidneys can contribute to kidney disease with extensive distortion of kidney structure.

---

nephrotoxic toxic to the kidney.

Individuals with only one kidney do not necessarily have kidney disease or even impaired function. People born with a single kidney are often unaware of the fact and usually lead full lives without compromised kidney function.

Risk Factors

Risks for CKD are higher among individuals who have diabetes, hypertension, or cardiovascular disease (CVD); who are older than 60 years; who are obese; and who have a family history of kidney disease.[1] Malnutrition can intensify the rate of renal tissue destruction and increase susceptibility to infection. The prevalence of CKD is higher in racial and ethnic minority populations; and higher among individuals with low-socioeconomic status due in part to modifiable contributing factors such as smoking, alcohol intake, and limited access to health care.[4] Box 21-1 lists risk factors and common causes of kidney disease.

Box 21-1 | **Risk Factors and Common Causes of Kidney Disease**

SOCIODEMOGRAPHIC FACTORS
- Older age
- Family history of chronic kidney disease
- Hereditary diseases affecting the kidneys (e.g., polycystic kidney disease)

CLINICAL FACTORS
- Poor glycemic control in diabetes
- Hypertension
- Obesity
- Autoimmune disease
- Glomerulonephritis
- Systemic infection
- Repetitive urinary tract infection or kidney stones
- Lower urinary tract obstruction
- History of acute kidney injury
- Reduction in kidney mass or congenital malformations
- Exposure to certain nephrotoxic drugs or environmental conditions

---

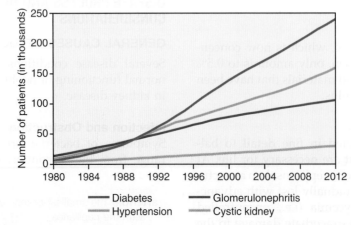

FIGURE 21-2 Prevalence of chronic kidney disease by primary diagnosis. (U.S. Renal Data System. *2014 Annual data report: epidemiology of kidney disease in the United States.* Bethesda, Md: National Institutes of Health, National Institute of Diabetes and Digestive and Kidney Diseases; 2014.)

MEDICAL NUTRITION THERAPY IN KIDNEY DISEASE

During the treatment of kidney disease, appropriate MNT is based on the severity of the disease, the presence of metabolic abnormalities, and the treatment modality (e.g., renal replacement therapy, medications).

Length of Disease

During short-term acute disease that results from infection, drug therapy with antibiotics usually controls the disease. Nutrition therapy is aimed at optimal nutrition support for healing and normal growth. More specific nutrient modifications may be necessary if the patient is a child or if the disease progresses to a chronic state.

Degree of Impaired Kidney Function and Clinical Symptoms

For milder acute disease with few nephrons involved, less interference occurs with general kidney function, because the large number of backup nephrons can meet basic needs. However, with progressive chronic disease, more and more nephrons become involved, which results in CKD. In such cases, extensive MNT is required to help maintain kidney function as long as possible. With continuing disease, nutrient modifications are designed to meet individual needs to address clinical symptoms. Working closely with a registered dietitian nutritionist for personalized nutrition therapy is especially important for patients with advanced kidney disease.

This chapter's discussion focuses primarily on the serious degenerative process of CKD. MNT and clinical practice guidelines are discussed for each type of kidney disease in the following sections.

NEPHRON DISEASES

ACUTE GLOMERULONEPHRITIS OR NEPHRITIC SYNDROME

Disease Process

This inflammatory process affects the glomeruli, which are the small blood vessels in the cupped membrane at the head of the nephron. Glomerulonephritis is the third leading cause of stage 5 CKD, which is also known as *ESRD*.[1]

Clinical Symptoms

Classic symptoms include **hematuria** and **proteinuria** although edema and hypertension also may occur. These patients may experience anorexia in advanced stages, which contributes to feeding problems and malnutrition. If the disease progresses to more kidney involvement, signs of **oliguria** or **anuria** may develop. Table 21-2 outlines the five glomerular syndromes and their respective clinical manifestations.

Table 21-2   Glomerular Syndromes

SYNDROME	CLINICAL MANIFESTATIONS
Acute nephritic syndrome	Hematuria, azotemia, variable proteinuria, oliguria, edema, and hypertension
Rapidly progressive glomerulonephritis	Acute nephritis, proteinuria, and acute kidney failure
Nephrotic syndrome	>3.5 g of proteinuria, hypoalbuminemia, hyperlipidemia, and lipiduria
Chronic kidney failure	Azotemia and uremia that progress for years
Asymptomatic hematuria or proteinuria	Glomerular hematuria and subnephrotic proteinuria

From Kumar V, Fausto N, Abbas A. *Robbins and Cotran pathologic basis of disease.* 7th ed. Philadelphia: Saunders; 2005.

Medical Nutrition Therapy

Nephrologists and dietitians favor overall optimal nutrition support for growth with adequate protein. Diet modifications are not crucial in most patients with acute short-term disease. Fluid intake is adjusted to output and insensible losses.

NEPHROTIC SYNDROME

Disease Process

Nephrotic syndrome or **nephrosis** results from nephron tissue damage to the major filtering membrane of the glomerulus, thereby allowing protein to pass into the tubule. This high protein concentration may cause further damage to the tubule. Both filtration and reabsorption functions of the nephron are disrupted. Nephrosis may be caused by infection, medications, neoplasms, preeclampsia, progressive glomerulonephritis, or diseases such as diabetes and systemic lupus erythematosus.

Clinical Symptoms

Nephrotic syndrome is characterized by a group of symptoms that result from nephron tissue damage and impaired function. The large protein losses (i.e., ≥3 g/day or more in adults) lead to hypoalbuminemia, edema, and ascites. The abdomen becomes distended as fluid accumulates, and the plasma protein level is

hematuria the abnormal presence of blood in the urine.
proteinuria an abnormal excess of serum proteins (e.g., albumin) in the urine.
oliguria the secretion of small amounts of urine in relation to fluid intake (i.e., 0.5 mL/kg per hour or less).
anuria the absence of urine production; anuria indicates kidney shutdown or failure.
nephrosis degenerative lesions of the renal tubules of the nephrons and especially of the thin basement membrane of the glomerulus that helps to support the capillary loops; marked by edema, albuminuria, and a decreased serum albumin level.

greatly reduced because of losses in the urine. As protein loss continues, tissue proteins are broken down, and general malnutrition follows. Severe edema and ascites often mask the extent of body tissue wasting. Other clinical manifestations include hyperlipidemia, **lipiduria**, blood clotting abnormalities, and imbalances in several minerals (e.g., iron, copper, zinc, calcium) due to the loss of key proteins that are necessary for their transport or metabolism.

Medical Nutrition Therapy

Medical nutrition therapy is directed toward controlling major symptoms, replacing the nutrients that are lost in the urine, reducing the progression to CKD, and decreasing the risk of atherosclerosis. Current standards of care are as follows[5]:

- *Protein:* The diet is usually moderate in protein (0.8 to 1.0 g/kg of body weight/day), with an emphasis on protein from high biologic value sources, including soy protein. Total protein intake may be modified on the basis of **blood urea nitrogen** and GFR results. If blood urea nitrogen level is elevated and urine output is decreased, dietary protein may be restricted.
- *Energy:* Total energy intake should be adequate to support nutrition status. Needs may be as high as 35 kcal/kg/day. To provide sufficient energy in kilocalories, complex carbohydrates should be given liberally, which also helps to combat the catabolism of tissue protein and to prevent starvation **ketosis**.
- *Fat:* Total fat intake should not exceed 30% total kcal/day, cholesterol intake should not exceed 200 mg/day, trans fats should be limited, and up to 10% of kilocalories should come from polyunsaturated fats, including fish. Controlling the dietary intake of fat and cholesterol may help to alleviate dyslipidemia and the resulting risk for atherosclerosis.
- *Sodium and potassium:* To reduce symptoms of edema, a sodium restriction of 1 to 2 g/day is advised to maintain the sodium and fluid balance. Sodium overload is difficult to treat because of the characteristic hypoalbuminuria and **hypotension**; therefore, careful monitoring is necessary. The renal clearance of potassium is impaired with oliguria. Thus, potassium intake should be monitored and adjusted in accordance with individual needs.

---

lipiduria lipid droplets found in the urine that are composed mostly of cholesterol esters.

blood urea nitrogen a test of nephron function that measures the ability to filter urea nitrogen, which is a product of protein metabolism, from the blood.

ketosis the accumulation of ketones, which are intermediate products of fat metabolism, in the blood.

hypotension low blood pressure.

- *Calcium and phosphorus:* Some calcium is bound to albumin in the blood. As albumin is lost through the tubule, bound calcium is also lost. In addition, low serum levels of active vitamin D decrease calcium absorption. Thus, the recommendations are to consume 1 to 1.5 g of calcium per day and to limit phosphorus intake to 12 mg/kg/day.
- *Fluid:* Fluid intake may be restricted in response to urine output and insensible losses. If restriction is not indicated, fluids can be consumed as desired.

KIDNEY FAILURE

The two types of kidney failure—acute and chronic—have a number of symptoms that reflect interference with normal nephron functions and nutrient metabolism. Both forms are addressed with similar nutrition therapy, depending on the extent of renal tissue damage and the treatment method used.

ACUTE KIDNEY INJURY

Disease Process

Healthy kidneys may suddenly shut down after metabolic insult or traumatic injury, thereby causing a life-threatening situation. Baseline risk factors for the development of in-hospital acute kidney injury (also known as *acute renal failure*) include older age, diabetes, and underlying renal insufficiency attributable to systemic infection, organ failure, or the use of nephrotoxic medications.[6] This is a medical emergency in which the dietitian and the nurse play important supportive roles. Depending on the underlying cause, acute kidney injury (AKI) is divided into three categories[7]:

1. *Prerenal:* Prerenal injury is the most common form of AKI, accounting for 60% to 70% of cases. It involves inadequate blood flow to the kidneys and a subsequent reduction in GFR. Common causes include renal vasoconstriction or occlusion, nephrotoxic medications (e.g., nonsteroidal antiinflammatory drugs, angiotensin-converting enzyme inhibitors, angiotensin receptor blockers), systemic vasodilation (e.g., sepsis, shock), and severe dehydration and hypotension.
2. *Intrinsic:* Intrinsic AKI results from damage to a specific part of the kidney. Common causes include glomerulonephritis, acute tubular necrosis, acute interstitial nephritis, vascular obstruction, infection, or nephrotoxicity from antibiotics, antimicrobial agents, radiographic contrast agents, chemotherapeutic agents, or other drugs.
3. *Postrenal obstruction:* Postrenal obstruction involves the obstruction of urine flow. Common causes include prostatic hypertrophy with urinary retention, ureteral stones, and other obstructions (e.g., tumors, blood clots).

AKI occurs in as many as one in five hospitalized patients and significantly increases the length of stay in the hospital and the death rate.[8,9] For those patients who do recover, the episode of AKI may last from days to weeks, with normal function returning when the condition that is causing the failure is resolved. Depending on the extent of renal tissue damage, regaining full function may take months. However, some individuals do not regain normal kidney function, and the disease then progresses to CKD. Patients suffering an acute kidney injury and who have a high risk for advancing to CKD are those with significantly reduced GFR (measurement of severity), repetitive and/or long episodes of AKI, endothelial damage, and persistent fibrosis.[10]

Clinical Symptoms

AKI is classified according to the RIFLE classification system, which assesses the severity of **R**isk, **I**njury, **F**ailure, and the outcomes of either **L**oss or **E**SRD and the Acute Kidney Injury Network (AKIN) criteria.[11] The diagnostic criteria for AKI are an increase in serum **creatinine** levels and oliguria, which is caused when cellular debris from the tissue damage blocks the tubules. Diminished urine output may be accompanied by proteinuria or hematuria. Other symptoms include nausea, vomiting, fatigue, muscle weakness, swelling in the lower extremities, itchy skin, confusion, uremia, and malnutrition. Water balance also becomes a crucial factor. **Continuous renal replacement therapy**, which is a type of dialysis, may be needed to support kidney function for critical patients.

Medical Nutrition Therapy

Basic objectives. The major challenge during AKI is to improve or maintain nutrition status while the patient is faced with marked catabolism. Current standards indicate the need for highly individualized therapy that is focused on the following: (1) treating the underlying cause; (2) preventing further kidney damage and complications from nutrient deficiencies; and (3) correcting any fluid, electrolyte, or uremic abnormalities.[5] Loss of appetite is common and enteral nutrition may be required. If enteral nutrition is contraindicated, parenteral nutrition may then be necessary (see Chapter 22).

Principles. Nutrition support in acutely ill patients helps reduce the risks for energy and protein malnutrition. General recommendations for AKI are presented next. Keep in mind that kidney function and treatment modality may vary greatly among patients; thus, MNT should be adjusted accordingly.[5]

- *Protein:* Adequate protein is important for supporting kidney function and for preserving lean tissue. For patients who are not receiving dialysis and who are not experiencing catabolism, a protein intake of 0.8 to 1.2 g/kg is recommended. For patients who are experiencing catabolism or who are on dialysis, 1.2 to 1.5 g/kg of daily protein is recommended to allow for nutrient replenishment and to account for losses.
- *Energy:* Energy intake in the range of 25 to 35 kcal/kg is suggested. This amount needs to be adjusted on an individual basis, depending on metabolic stress and the nutritional status of the patient. If the patient is on dialysis, energy intake from the **dialysate** must be included in the total energy intake.
- *Sodium and potassium:* During a diuretic phase, patients may lose excessive electrolytes. Losses of both sodium and potassium (2 to 3 g/day each) should be replaced during this phase. These levels are further adjusted depending on blood pressure and the presence of edema. During oliguria or anuria phases, electrolytes may need to be restricted because of accumulation in the blood and increased risk for hyperkalemia, a potentially fatal condition (see Chapter 8).
- *Phosphate and calcium:* Dietary phosphorus intake is determined on the basis of body weight, with a range of 8 to 15 mg of phosphorus per kg of body weight. Hyperphosphatemia during anuria phases results in calcium resorption from bones. Phosphate binders taken with meals help prevent phosphate absorption. The MNT goal for calcium is to maintain serum value levels within normal limits and to adjust dietary intake accordingly.
- *Vitamins and minerals:* A patient's diet should be balanced to prevent nutrient deficiencies by meeting the Dietary Reference Intakes for all other vitamins and minerals. If the patient is experiencing catabolism or other complications, nutrient intakes may be modified to meet specific needs.
- *Fluid:* Fluid needs are highly variable with AKI. Treatment modality, hydration, and fluid loss should be considered on an individual basis. Insensible fluid loss may increase as a result of fever, and sensible fluid loss (e.g., urine output, vomitus, diarrhea) will vary considerably among patients.

---

creatinine a nitrogen-carrying product of normal tissue protein breakdown; it is excreted in the urine; serum creatinine levels are an indicator of renal function.

continuous renal replacement therapy (CRRT) a method of blood purification that is used continuously (i.e., 24 hr/day) for critically ill patients in intensive care settings. There are several forms of CRRT that vary according to the vascular access route, presence or absence of dialysate, type of semipermeable membrane used, and the mechanism of solute removal.

dialysate the cleansing solution used in dialysis; contains dextrose and other chemicals similar to those in the body.

A starting point recommendation is 500 mL of fluid plus urine output daily.

CHRONIC KIDNEY DISEASE

Disease Process

CKD is a progressive breakdown of kidney tissue, which impairs all kidney functions. Few functioning nephrons remain and they gradually deteriorate. CKD develops slowly, and no cure exists. Approximately 14% of the U.S. population has CKD with individuals more than 60 years of age having the highest prevalence.[1]

CKD is most commonly a result of the following:

- Metabolic diseases with kidney involvement (e.g., diabetes, hypertension, CVD, metabolic syndrome, obesity)
- Primary glomerular disease
- Inherited diseases (e.g., polycystic kidney disease) or congenital abnormality
- Other causes: immune disease such as lupus, obstructions such as kidney stones, chronic urinary tract infections, and long-term use of nephrotoxic medications

Modifiable risk factors include blood pressure, glycemic control, and addressing dyslipidemia; reducing sodium intake; making necessary dietary adjustments to potassium, phosphorus, and protein intake; increasing physical activity; achieving a healthy body weight; and quitting smoking.[3] CKD is categorized into five stages on the basis of the GFR (Table 21-3). This section will focus on stages 1 through 4 and the following section will discuss stage 5.

Clinical Symptoms

Depending on the nature of the underlying kidney disease, chronic kidney changes may involve extensive scarring of renal tissue, which distorts the kidney structure and causes vascular damage. As nephrons are lost, the remaining nephrons gradually lose their ability to sustain metabolic balance. Long-term complications most commonly include malnutrition, bone and mineral disorders, anemia, and CVD.

Water balance. During the early stages of chronic kidney failure, the kidneys are unable to reabsorb water or to properly concentrate urine. Therefore, large amounts of dilute urine are produced (i.e., polyuria). Dehydration is a risk factor at this point, and it may become critical. As the disease progresses, urine production declines to a point of oliguria and finally anuria. Without the urinary excretion of waste products, dangerous levels of urea accumulate in the blood.

Nitrogen retention. An increasing loss of nephron function results in elevated levels of nitrogenous metabolites such as urea. Elevated blood urea nitrogen, serum creatinine, and serum uric acid levels are reflected in the characteristic laboratory finding of azotemia. Protein-energy malnutrition is a common complication of protein catabolism.

Electrolyte and mineral balance. Several imbalances among electrolytes result from decreasing nephron function. The failing kidney cannot appropriately maintain the vital sodium and potassium balance that guards body water (see Chapter 9). A concentration of materials (e.g., phosphate, sulfate, organic acids) is produced by the metabolism of nutrients. Without appropriate filtering, these materials accumulate in the blood, thereby causing metabolic acidosis. The disturbed metabolism of calcium and phosphorus, the abnormal levels of parathyroid hormone, and the lack of activated vitamin D (a process that occurs in the kidneys) lead to bone pain, abnormal bone metabolism, and chronic kidney disease-mineral and bone disorder (CKD-MBD) or osteodystrophy.

Table 21-3	Stages of Chronic Kidney Disease*

STAGE	DESCRIPTION	GLOMERULAR FILTRATION RATE (ML/MIN/1.73 M²)
1	Kidney damage with normal or elevated GFR	≥90
2	Kidney damage with mild decrease in GFR	60 to 89
3	Mild to moderate decrease in GFR	30 to 59
4	Severely decreased GFR	15 to 29
5	Kidney failure or end-stage renal disease	<15 (or dialysis)

Data from Kidney Disease: Improving Global Outcomes (KDIGO) CKD Work Group. KDIGO 2012 clinical practice guideline for the evaluation and management of chronic kidney disease. *Kidney Int.* 2013;3(Suppl):1-150.
GFR, Glomerular filtration rate.
*Chronic kidney disease is defined as either kidney damage or a glomerular filtration rate of less than 60 mL/min per 1.73 m² for 3 or more months. Kidney damage is defined as pathologic abnormalities or markers of damage, including abnormalities in blood or urine tests or imaging studies.

urea the chief nitrogen-carrying product of dietary protein metabolism; urea appears in the blood, lymph, and urine.
azotemia an excess of urea and other nitrogenous substances in the blood.
chronic kidney disease-mineral and bone disorder a clinical syndrome that develops as a systemic disorder of mineral and bone metabolism in patients with chronic kidney disease; results from abnormalities of calcium, phosphorus, parathyroid hormone, or vitamin D metabolism; causes abnormalities in bone turnover, mineralization, volume, linear growth, strength, and soft-tissue calcification.
osteodystrophy an alteration of bone morphology found in patients with chronic kidney disease.

Anemia. The damaged kidney cannot accomplish its normal initiation of red blood cell production through erythropoietin. Therefore, fewer red blood cells are produced, and those that are produced have a decreased survival time. The Kidney Disease–Improving Global Outcomes Work Group has published clinical guidelines for the monitoring and treatment of anemia in patients with CKD.[12]

Hypertension. When blood flow to the kidney tissues is increasingly impaired, renal hypertension develops. In turn, hypertension causes cardiovascular damage and the further deterioration of the nephrons. The Kidney Disease–Improving Global Outcomes Work Group has also published specific clinical guidelines for the monitoring and treatment of hypertension in patients with CKD.[13]

General Signs and Symptoms

Increasing loss of kidney function causes progressive weakness, shortness of breath, fatigue, anemia, swelling in the extremities, and itchy skin rashes. Anorexia, nausea, and vomiting are common, thus worsening malnutrition and weight loss. Protein-energy wasting (PEW) syndrome is a common occurrence in patients with CKD. PEW is multifactorial, results in a loss of muscle and visceral protein stores, and is associated with high morbidity and mortality.[14,15] Malnutrition lowers resistance to infection, and some patients may experience bone and joint pain. In advanced stages, irregular cyclic breathing (i.e., Kussmaul's breathing) indicates acidosis. Acidosis may cause mouth ulcers, a foul taste, and bad breath in the patient. Nervous system involvement may involve muscular twitching and peripheral neuropathy.

Medical Nutrition Therapy

Basic objectives. Treatment must always be individual and adjusted according to the progression of the illness, the type of treatment, and the patient's response. The nutritional status of patients with CKD should be monitored at regular intervals to identify dietary risk factors and to help prevent malnutrition.[3]

Principles. Nutrition therapy for CKD patients who are not on dialysis involves several nutrient adjustments that should be made in accordance with individual need. The MNT recommendations for patients with CKD are as follows[5,16]:

- *Protein:* The goal is to provide adequate protein to maintain tissue integrity while avoiding excess. Protein is generally limited to 0.6 to 0.8 g/kg/day for individuals who are not on dialysis with a GFR of <30 mL/min per 1.73 m². Protein sources should focus on high biologic value protein (see Chapter 4) to ensure an adequate intake of essential amino acids. Avoid high protein intakes of >1.3 g/kg in adults at risk for further progression of CKD.[3]

- *Energy:* Carbohydrate and fat must provide sufficient nonprotein kilocalories to supply energy and spare protein for tissue synthesis. The recommended energy intake is 23 to 35 kcal/kg/day. Energy needs are less for overweight individuals with both CKD and diabetes to allow for weight loss. Because cardiovascular disease is accelerated in patients with CKD, the remaining calories should support cardiovascular health principles (e.g., substitute monounsaturated and polyunsaturated fats for saturated and trans fats, reduce total cholesterol intake; see Chapter 19). For patients with diabetes, glycemic control is an important part of intervention (see Chapter 20). The recommendation is to achieve an HbA_{1c} value of ≈7%.[3]

- *Sodium and potassium:* The general population recommendations for sodium (<2.4 g/day) and potassium are applicable until complications are present. If hypertension and edema are present, sodium intake is limited to 2 g/day.[3] As CKD advances to stages 3 and 4, potassium is not cleared adequately from the blood. Dietary intake is determined by assessing laboratory values. If blood levels of potassium are elevated and other nondietary causes are eliminated, then a potassium-restricted diet (<2.4 g/day) may be indicated.

- *Phosphorus and calcium:* Inappropriate blood phosphorus and calcium levels negatively affect bone composition. As the kidney loses function, the activation of vitamin D and the control of blood calcium levels are inhibited. This problem is worsened by excess blood phosphorus levels, which results in calcium resorption from the bone to establish a calcium/phosphorus equilibrium in the blood. Thus, moderate dietary phosphorus restriction depends on laboratory values in the patient who is not undergoing dialysis, and it is generally limited to 800 to 1000 mg/day when the serum phosphorus level is 4.6 mg/dL or more or when the parathyroid hormone level is elevated.

- *Vitamins and minerals:* A protein-restricted diet does not contribute the full daily requirement of all essential nutrients (review the Clinical Applications box, "Case Study: A Patient with Chronic Kidney Disease"). Supplemental fat-soluble vitamins A and E are not recommended, because they may accumulate to toxic levels in patients with kidney failure. Excesses of vitamins D and K are contraindicated, because the kidney cannot convert vitamin D to its active form, and vitamin K can adversely affect clotting time. The specific MNT recommendations are to help patients meet their Dietary Reference Intakes for the B-complex vitamins and vitamin C and to determine the patient-specific needs for vitamin D and iron.

- *Fluid:* Fluid intake should be sufficient to maintain adequate urine volume in patients who are not undergoing dialysis. Intake usually is balanced with output, and it is not otherwise restricted.

Case Study: a Patient with Chronic Kidney Disease

Gary is 49 years old and is an active man who works at a large manufacturing plant. Recently he has begun to tire more easily, has little appetite, has lost 5% of his normal body weight, and generally feels ill most of the time. He recently noticed some ankle swelling and blood in his urine. At his family's insistence, he finally decided to see his physician.

After a complete workup, the physician's findings included the following:

- No prior illness except a case of the flu with a throat infection during his overseas service in the Army
- Laboratory tests: presence of albumin, red blood cells, and white blood cells in the urine; high blood potassium, phosphorus, creatinine, and urea levels; and severely decreased glomerular filtration rate of 20 mL/min per 1.73 m^2
- Other symptoms: hypertension, edema in the lower legs, headache, occasional blurry vision, and low-grade fever

The physician discussed the findings and the serious prognosis of stage 4 chronic kidney disease with Gary and his wife. Together with the renal dietitian, they explored his immediate medical and nutrition needs. They also discussed the ultimate need for medical management with dialysis or transplantation. The physician prescribed medications to control Gary's growing symptoms and discomfort.

Over the next 10 months, Gary's symptoms worsened. He lost more weight, became anemic, and had increased bone and joint pain. Nausea increased, and he had occasional muscle twitching and spasms. Small mouth ulcers made eating a painful effort. Gary and his wife made an appointment with their dietitian to learn how to manage his present predialysis diet at home.

QUESTIONS FOR ANALYSIS

1. What metabolic imbalances in chronic kidney disease do you think account for Gary's symptoms?
2. Of these metabolic imbalances, what is contributing to his edema?
3. What are the objectives of the treatment of chronic kidney disease?
4. What are the basic principles of Gary's predialysis diet? Describe this type of diet. Plan a 1-day menu for Gary with the use of the dietary analysis program that is included with this text.
5. How does a predialysis diet differ from a diet prescribed for patients on hemodialysis?

END-STAGE RENAL DISEASE

Disease Process

When CKD advances to its end stage, life-support decisions face the patient, the family, and the physician. ESRD is diagnosed when the patient's GFR decreases to less than 15 mL/min per 1.73 m^2. This decrease in GFR indicates irreversible damage to a majority of the kidneys' nephrons. At this point, the patient has two options: long-term kidney dialysis or kidney transplant. The lives of an estimated 630,000 people in the United States are prolonged by dialysis and kidney transplants annually.[1] Dialysis is the principal treatment for ESRD.

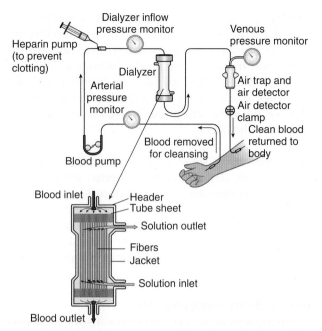

FIGURE 21-3 Hemodialysis cleans and filters blood with a special filter called a *dialyzer* that functions as an artificial kidney. Blood travels through tubes into the dialyzer, which filters wastes and extra water, and then the cleaned blood flows through another set of tubes and back into the body. (From National Institute of Diabetes and Digestive and Kidney Diseases. *Treatment methods for hemodialysis*. National Institutes of Health Publication No. 07-4666. Bethesda, Md: National Institutes of Health; 2006.)

Two forms of dialysis are used: hemodialysis and peritoneal dialysis. For a thorough understanding of the treatment options that are available for ESRD, please refer to the article by Burkhalter and colleagues listed in the "Further Reading and Resources" for Chapter 21 at the back of this textbook.

Treatment Options and Respective Medical Nutrition Therapy

Hemodialysis. Hemodialysis is the use of an "artificial kidney machine" to remove toxic substances from the blood and to restore nutrients and metabolites to normal blood levels (Figure 21-3). To prepare a patient for hemodialysis therapy, vascular access must be established. This procedure ideally takes place 4 to 16 weeks before treatments begin to allow for adequate healing. The three basic kinds of vascular access for hemodialysis are arteriovenous fistula, arteriovenous graft, and a venous catheter (Figure 21-4). An arteriovenous fistula is the most commonly used access for long-term dialysis,[1] and it is made by joining an artery and a vein on the forearm just beneath the skin. After the fistula has healed, a cannula (i.e., a large-bore needle) is inserted through the tissue and connected by tubes to the dialysis machine.

A patient on hemodialysis usually receives three treatments per week, each of which lasts 3 to 4 hours. However, studies indicate that patients receiving hemodialysis up to six times per week with shorter sessions (i.e., about 2 hours per session) experience health

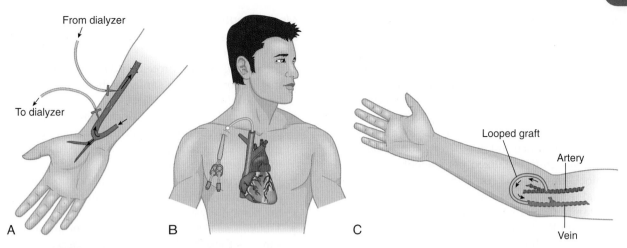

FIGURE 21-4 Types of access for hemodialysis. **A,** Forearm arteriovenous fistula. **B,** Venous catheter for temporary hemodialysis access. **C,** Artificial loop graft. (From National Institute of Diabetes and Digestive and Kidney Diseases. *Kidney failure: choosing a treatment that's right for you.* National Institutes of Health Publication No. 00-2412. Bethesda, Md: National Institutes of Health; 2007.)

benefits such as improved self-reported physical health, physical function, and mental health with no reported loss in quality of life.[17,18] However, patients who receive frequent hemodialysis do have a tendency to require more interventions related to vascular access.[19]

During each treatment, the patient's blood makes several complete cycles through the dialyzer, which removes excess waste to maintain normal blood levels of life-sustaining substances, a function the patient's own kidneys can no longer accomplish. Two compartments in the machine are separated by a selective semipermeable membrane. One compartment contains blood from the patient with all of the excess fluids and waste; the other contains the dialysate, which is a type of "cleaning fluid." As during normal capillary filtration, the blood cells are too large to pass through the pores in the membrane. However, the remaining smaller molecules in the blood pass through the membrane and are carried away by the dialysate. If the patient's blood is deficient in certain nutrients, they may be added to the dialysate. These nutrients will cross the membrane via osmosis or diffusion to establish equilibrium between the dialysate and the blood.

Medical nutrition therapy for hemodialysis. The diet of a patient who is undergoing hemodialysis is an important aspect of maintaining biochemical balance. PEW syndrome remains a significant concern for patients on hemodialysis. The loss of muscle mass through progressive protein catabolism is associated with mortality.[20] Registered dietitian nutritionists who specialize in renal care are heavily involved with meal planning and diet education. The goal of the MNT during hemodialysis is to maintain optimal nutrition while preventing the accumulation of excess waste products between treatments. In most cases, MNT can be planned with more liberal nutrient allowances than for nondialysis patients, as follows[5,16]:

- *Protein:* Protein-energy malnutrition, as indicated by dietary intake and the biomarkers of protein status, is a major concern for patients on dialysis, and it is considered one of the most significant predictors of overall malnutrition and adverse outcomes.[21-23] For most adult patients on dialysis, a protein allowance of 1.1 to 1.5 g/kg is ideal to prevent protein malnutrition. This amount provides nutrition needs, maintains positive nitrogen balance, does not produce excessive nitrogenous waste, and replaces the amino acids that are lost during each dialysis treatment. At least 50% of this daily allowance should consist of protein foods of high biologic value (e.g., eggs, meat, fish, poultry).
- *Energy:* MNT recommendations for energy intake are 25 to 35 kcal/kg/day to achieve and maintain goal body weight. Interestingly, the death rate decreases as the body mass index increases above normal ranges (i.e., ≥ 25 kg/m^2), purportedly as the result of a complex association between malnutrition and clinical outcomes.[24,25] The unfortunate combination is that decreased appetite is common in ESRD when the GFR falls below 60 mL/min per 1.73 m^2. A generous amount of carbohydrates with some fat continues to supply needed kilocalories for energy and protein sparing.
- *Sodium and potassium:* To control body fluid retention and hypertension, sodium is limited to 2 to 3 g/day. Sodium intake is not as stringently regulated for patients on dialysis as it is for those with CKD and not yet on dialysis, because the dialysis process rids the body of excess sodium. To prevent potassium accumulation, which can cause cardiac problems, intake is restricted to 2 to 4 g/day, with adjustments based on serum potassium levels as indicated.
- *Phosphorus and calcium:* With careful monitoring to control for co-morbid bone conditions, the dietary intake of phosphorus is limited to 800 to 1000 mg/

day or 10 to 12 mg of phosphorus per gram of protein when serum phosphorus levels exceed 5.5 mg/dL or when parathyroid hormone level is elevated. Calcium intake should not exceed 2 g/day, including the amount received through food, dietary supplements, and medications such as binders.

- *Vitamins and minerals:* The general recommendation for all water-soluble vitamins is to achieve the Dietary Reference Intakes. Iron and vitamin D intakes are individualized per patient on the basis of biochemical markers. Other micronutrients of special interest are as follows:
  - Vitamin C: 60 to 100 mg/day
  - Vitamin B_6: 2 mg/day
  - Folate: 1 to 5 mg/day
  - Vitamin B_{12}: 3 mcg/day
  - Vitamin E: 15 IU/day
  - Zinc: 15 mg/day
- *Fluid:* Fluid intake is limited to 1000 mL/day plus an amount equal to urine output.

Peritoneal dialysis. An alternative form of treatment is peritoneal dialysis, which has the convenience of mobility. Approximately 9% of patients with ESRD who are on dialysis use this form of dialysis.[1] During this process, the patient introduces the dialysate solution directly into the **peritoneal cavity**, where the peritoneal membrane serves as the filter in which metabolic waste products can pass into the dialysate for removal from the body. Because this form of dialysis is continuous within the body, the process is called *continuous ambulatory peritoneal dialysis.* An automated device may be used to provide several solution exchanges during sleep hours and one continuous exchange during the day for a technique that is called *continuous cyclic peritoneal dialysis.*

First, the patient is prepared by surgically inserting a permanent catheter into the peritoneal cavity. Treatments are then carried out by doing the following: (1) attaching a disposable bag that contains the dialysate solution to the abdominal catheter, which leads into the peritoneal cavity; (2) emptying the dialysate into the peritoneal cavity and allowing 4 to 6 hours for the solution exchange, known as dwell time; (3) lowering the bag to allow gravity to pull the waste-containing fluid back out of the peritoneal cavity; and (4) repeating the procedure (Figure 21-5). Patients on peritoneal dialysis can move about in their normal daily activities throughout the dwell times but must remain stationary during the exchange of the dialysate and waste solution into and out of the bags. The use of self-administered peritoneal dialysis at home gives the patient a sense of control, independence, and improved satisfaction with care. However, the treatment is a daily intensive therapy and some patients experience more symptoms of depression and poorer self-reported physical health than patients treated with hemodialysis.[26,27]

Medical nutrition therapy for peritoneal dialysis. A slightly more liberal diet may be used with peritoneal dialysis, as follows[5,16]:

- *Protein and energy:* Protein and energy intake recommendations are the same as those for patients on hemodialysis (see p. 381).
- *Sodium and potassium:* Sodium intake is limited to 2 to 4 g/day, contingent on fluid balance. Potassium intake recommendations are 3 to 4 g/day, depending on serum levels.
- *Phosphorus and calcium:* Recommendations for phosphorus and calcium intake remain the same as those for hemodialysis.
- *Vitamins and minerals:* All recommendations are the same as those for hemodialysis, as described previously, with the following exception: patients may need 1.5 to 2 mg/day of thiamin (vitamin B_1) as a result of losses that occur during dialysis.
- *Fluid:* Fluid intake is limited to 1000 mL/day plus an amount equal to urine output.

Transplantation. Kidney transplantation, which is another treatment modality, improves affected individuals' quality of life and survival rates, and it is more cost-effective than maintenance dialysis.[1,28] Current advances in surgical techniques, immunosuppressive drugs to prevent rejection, and antibiotics to control infection have helped to ensure successful outcomes (see the Drug-Nutrient Interaction box, "Immunosuppressive Therapies after Kidney Transplantation"). Patients who have undergone kidney transplantation have significantly lower rates of CVD progression and CVD mortality than patients who remain on dialysis, despite the continuous use of immunosuppressive therapy.[1]

The difficulty with transplantation is that waiting lists can be long and donor matches difficult to find, even when using **expanded-criteria donors** (matches with more liberal criteria). See the Cultural Considerations box entitled "Cultural Disparities in Kidney Transplant Availability and Success in Certain Ethnic and Racial Groups" for more details. Survival rates are significantly improved for recipients of living donor transplants over those of deceased donors.[1]

---

peritoneal cavity a serous membrane that lines the abdominal and pelvic walls and the undersurface of the diaphragm to form a sac that encloses the body's vital visceral organs.

expanded-criteria donors any brain-dead donor who is older than 60 years old or a donor who is older than 50 years old with two of the following conditions: history of hypertension, a terminal serum creatinine level of at least 1.5 mg/dL, or death from a cerebrovascular accident.

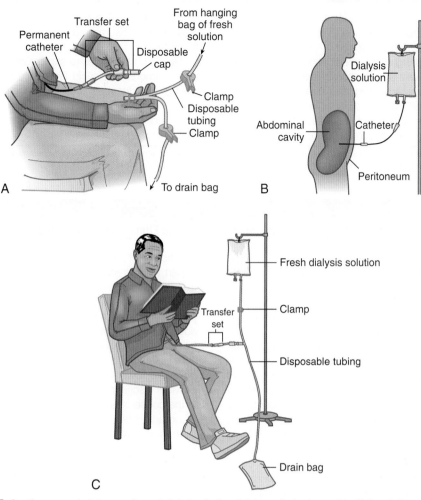

FIGURE 21-5 Continuous ambulatory peritoneal dialysis. **A,** A soft tube catheter is used to fill the abdomen with a cleansing dialysis solution. **B,** The walls of the abdominal cavity are lined with a peritoneal membrane that allows waste products and extra fluid to pass from the blood into the dialysis solution. **C,** Waste and fluid then leave the body when the dialysis solution is drained. The time during which the dialysis solution remains in the abdominal cavity (i.e., dwell time) ranges from 4 to 6 hours, and the patient can be mobile during this time. An exchange takes approximately 30 to 40 minutes, and a typical schedule requires four to five exchanges every day. (From National Institute of Diabetes and Digestive and Kidney Diseases. *Treatment methods for kidney failure: peritoneal dialysis.* National Institutes of Health Publication No. 06-4688. Bethesda, Md: National Institutes of Health; 2006.)

Drug-Nutrient Interaction

Immunosuppressive Therapies after Kidney Transplantation

KELLI BOI

The kidney is the most common solid organ that is transplanted worldwide, and the need for kidney transplantation has grown over the past decade. Survival after kidney transplant is largely dependent on a successful immunosuppressive regimen. Several antirejection medications are used after an organ transplant. Most kidney transplant recipients undergo multidrug immunosuppressive therapy that includes corticosteroids to reduce the risk of acute rejection. Over time, the patient may be weaned from steroid use but continue on long-term maintenance regimens that include other antirejection medications. The use of corticosteroids is associated with a number of adverse side effects that specifically affect overall nutritional status, such as the following:

- Gastrointestinal irritation: esophagitis, dyspepsia, peptic ulcer disease

- Increased appetite and weight gain
- Hyperglycemia
- Protein catabolism and negative nitrogen balance
- Fluid retention
- Growth retardation (in children)
- Bone disease
- Cardiovascular disease and mortality

Corticosteroids also increase the excretion of several nutrients. Additional consumption of vitamins A, B$_6$, B$_{12}$, and C; folate; potassium; phosphorus; magnesium; zinc; and protein may be needed in the diet or provided as a dietary supplement. Supplemental calcium and vitamin D are recommended with long-term corticosteroid use. Other antirejection medications are often used concomitantly with corticosteroids, and these may also interact with nutrient bioavailability. For example, cyclosporine and tacrolimus (Prograf) are calcineurin inhibitors.

These immunosuppressants may cause hyperkalemia; thus, high potassium intake from food or supplements should be avoided when these drugs are included in the drug regimen. When the patient is taking these medications, serum drug levels and electrolyte levels are monitored and the dosage is adjusted for optimal therapeutic benefit. Azathioprine (Imuran) and mycophenolate (CellCept) are other antirejection medications that do not have significant nutrient interactions, but they can cause nausea, vomiting, abdominal pain, and diarrhea in some patients. This can become a concern if the patient is unable to consume adequate nutrition and is at risk for malnutrition.

Research continues to explore alternative immunosuppressive regimens that avoid or reduce long-term steroid use. In the last two decades, the prevalence of steroid-free transplant regimens has increased but long-term survival rates have not improved. Further research is needed before new protocols can be accepted.

References and recommended readings: Steiner RW. Steroid-free chronic immunosuppression in renal transplantation. *Curr Opin Nephrol Hypertens*. 2012;21(6):567-573; Adesina S et al. Steroid withdrawal in kidney allograft recipients. *Expert Rev Clin Immunol*. 2014;10(9):1229-1239.

🌐 Cultural Considerations

Cultural Disparities in Kidney Transplant Availability and Success in Certain Ethnic and Racial Groups

JENNIFER E. SCHMIDT

Kidney transplantation is generally considered the optimal treatment for patients with end-stage renal disease. More than 17,000 kidney transplants are performed in the United States annually, of which approximately 11,500 of the donated kidneys are from deceased donors and 5500 are from living donors. Almost half of the organ transplants go to Caucasian recipients; however, Caucasians only make up 36.6% of those on the waiting list to receive a transplant.[1] Advances in both medical technology and immunosuppressive therapies have led to longer lives for transplant recipients among all racial groups over the past several decades. Despite this increase in survival rates, African-American kidney transplant recipients continue to have a higher incidence of the transplant failing within 10 years as well as a higher rate of death among transplant recipients compared with their white counterparts. Hispanic and Asian transplant recipients are reported to have the best outcomes.[2]

Several theories exist to explain these disparities in transplantation rates and survival among various groups. Racial variation with regard to transplant success can be attributed in part to differences in immunologic function among different racial groups. There are also social factors that affect the disparity of transplantation (see figure). Minorities are less likely to pursue live donor kidney transplants as a result of lack of knowledge, discomfort with talking to family members or individuals from other social networks about the procedure, difficulty with finding suitable donors, insufficient education from health care providers, lower availability of health insurance, and health care provider discrimination.[3] Provider inequity is related to variations in the consensus regarding the appropriate and just allocation of organs. Many providers believe that an organ should go to the recipient who is likely to receive the greatest benefit or live the longest as a result of the transplant. Factors such as African-American race, lower socioeconomic status, co-morbid diseases, and limited access to health care all decrease survival rate and length of life despite transplantation. To compound this issue, the longer that a recipient is on dialysis while waiting for a transplant, the lower the success rate of the transplant.[4]

To decrease these disparities, many interventions have been suggested. Immunosuppression regimens should be modified for different racial groups. Education methods and materials should also be culturally sensitive and consider the patients' cultural beliefs, values, language, socioeconomic status, and social context.[2] In addition, dialysis providers should be educated regarding kidney transplantation so that they can supply quality education to both potential transplant patients and potential live donors. Education about live donor kidney transplant should be offered to families of patients with end-stage renal disease to increase the donor pool and thus ease the matching process for donors for these groups. Research indicates that education that is provided early during the course of treatment and frequently throughout treatment leads to an increase across all ethnic groups with regard to patients' pursuit of transplantation.[3,4]

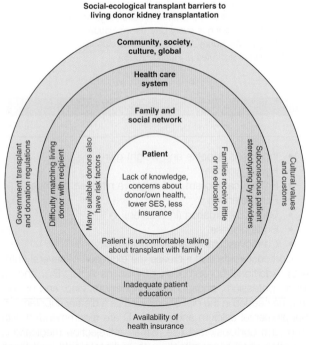

Social-ecological transplant barriers to living donor kidney transplantation

Community, society, culture, global

Health care system

Family and social network

Patient

Lack of knowledge, concerns about donor/own health, lower SES, less insurance

Government transplant and donation regulations

Difficulty matching living donor with recipient

Many suitable donors also have risk factors

Families receive little or no education

Subconscious patient stereotyping by providers

Cultural values and customs

Patient is uncomfortable talking about transplant with family

Inadequate patient education

Availability of health insurance

SES, Socioeconomic status. From Waterman AD, Rodrigue JR, Purnell TS, et al. Addressing racial/ethnic disparities in live donor kidney transplantation: priorities for research and intervention. *Semin Nephrol.* 2010;30(1):90-98.

REFERENCES

1. Organ Procurement and Transplantation Network. *Transplants in the U.S. by Recipient Ethnicity: U.S. Transplants Performed January 1, 1988-January 31, 2015.* Washington, DC: U.S. Department of Health and Human Services; 2015.
2. Gordon EJ, et al. Disparities in kidney transplant outcomes: a review. *Semin Nephrol.* 2010;30(1):81-89.
3. Waterman AD, et al. Addressing racial and ethnic disparities in live donor kidney transplantation: priorities for research and intervention. *Semin Nephrol.* 2010;30(1):90-98.
4. Courtney AE, Maxwell AP. The challenge of doing what is right in renal transplantation: balancing equity and utility. *Nephron Clin Pract.* 2009;111(1):c62-c67, discussion c68.

Recommended reading: Williams AW. Health policy, disparities, and the kidney. *Adv Chronic Kidney Dis.* 2015;22(1):54-59.

MNT for patients who choose kidney transplantation will be highly individualized and must take into consideration any co-morbidities and level of kidney function following surgery. Table 21-4 summarizes the nutrition guidelines for various levels of kidney disease and treatments.

Complications

Long-term complications of ESRD and dialysis include bone disorders, malnutrition, anemia, hormonal and blood pressure imbalances, depression, and diminished quality of life as a result of constant dependence on treatments. Several of these conditions have been addressed earlier in the chapter. Additional complications of chronic kidney disease that are found in patients with ESRD include the following:

Enteral or parenteral nutrition support. There are special considerations for patients on dialysis who are in medical need of nutrition support via enteral or

Table 21-4 Recommended Nutrition Guidelines for Adults with Chronic Kidney Disease

NUTRIENT	CKD STAGES 3 TO 5 WITHOUT RRT (GFR CATEGORIES 3 TO 5)	CKD STAGE 5 WITH RRT (KIDNEY FAILURE)	POSTTRANSPLANTATION (GUIDED BY CKD STAGE/CATEGORY OF KIDNEY FUNCTION)
Protein	0.6 to 0.8 g/kg of BW/day with at least 50% HBV to potentially slow disease progression (particularly in patients with diabetes) and achieve/maintain adequate serum albumin	1.1 to 1.5 g/kg of BW/day (HD with at least 50% HBV to achieve/maintain adequate serum albumin levels in conjunction with sufficient protein-sparing caloric intake)	0.8 to 1.0 g/kg of BW/day with 50% coming from HBV sources
Energy	25 to 35 kcal/kg of BW/day to achieve or maintain goal body weight	25 to 35 kcal/kg of BW/day to achieve or maintain goal body weight; include estimated caloric absorption from PD fluid as applicable	25 to 35 kcal/kg of BW/day to achieve or maintain goal body weight
Fat	General population recommendation of <30% of total calories from fat; emphasis on healthy fat sources	Focus on type of fat and carbohydrate to manage dyslipidemia, if present	Focus on type of fat and carbohydrate to reduce cardiovascular risk or manage immunosuppressant medication adverse effect (e.g., dyslipidemia, glucose intolerance)
Saturated fat	Same as for general population; <7% of total fat	Reduce and substitute saturated fat sources with healthier fat sources	Reduce and substitute saturated fat sources with healthier fat sources
Sodium	General population recommendation of 2.4 g/day	2.0 to 3.0 g/day (HD) to control interdialytic fluid gain; 2.0 to 4.0 g/day (PD) to control hydration status	General population recommendation of 2.4 g/day
Potassium	Typically not restricted until hyperkalemia is present, then individualized	2.0 to 4.0 g/day or 40 mg/kg of BW/day in HD or individualized in PD to achieve normal serum levels	No restriction unless hyperkalemia is present, then individualized
Calcium	No restriction	2 g elemental/day from dietary and medication sources	Individualized to kidney function
Phosphorus	Typically not restricted until hyperphosphatemia is present, then individualized to maintain normal serum levels by diet and/or phosphate binders	800 to 1000 mg/day to achieve goal serum level of 3.5 to 5.5 mg/dL or below; coordinate with oral phosphate binder prescription	Individualized to stage of kidney function
Fiber	Same as general population; 25 to 35 g/day	Same as general population; 25 to 35 g/day	Same as general population; 25 to 35 g/day
Fluid	No restriction	1000 mL/day (+ urine output if present) in HD; greater in PD; individualized to fluid status	No restriction; matched to urine output if appropriate

From Beto JA, Ramirez WE, Bansal VK. Medical nutrition therapy in adults with chronic kidney disease: integrating evidence and consensus into practice for the generalist registered dietitian nutritionist. *J Acad Nutr Diet.* 2014;114(7):1077-1087.
BW, Body weight; *CKD,* chronic kidney disease; *GFR,* glomerular filtration rate; *HBV,* high biologic value; *HD,* hemodialysis; *PD,* peritoneal dialysis; *RRT,* renal replacement therapy (hemodialysis, peritoneal dialysis).

parenteral feedings. A medical necessity of nutrition support usually means that the patient is experiencing severe malnutrition, inflammation, and anorexia. The type of and tolerance of dialysis must be considered when choosing an appropriate nutrition support modality, and the current GFR, metabolic state, stress, and nitrogen balance must also be considered. The American Society for Parenteral and Enteral Nutrition has published clinical guidelines for administering and evaluating nutrition support specifically for patients with CKD.[29]

Osteodystrophy. Bone disease and disorders are prevalent in CKD, and they are a leading cause of morbidity. Several factors contribute to renal osteodystrophy and CKD-MBD. The decreased activation of vitamin D has a cascading effect that results in elevated levels of parathyroid hormone, reduced calcium absorption from the gastrointestinal tract, and low serum calcium levels. Patients also have elevated serum phosphorus levels as a result of the inability of the kidney to excrete phosphorus. This combination causes abnormal changes in bone structure and function. Hyperphosphatemia is associated with increased mortality risk; thus, phosphate binders are an important management aspect of CKD. Patients with a GFR <45 mL/min per 1.73 m^2 should be evaluated for bone disease and disorders of calcium and phosphorus metabolism. Treatment strategies for bone disorders require a highly individualized management plan and continue to evolve in the light of new research.[30]

Neuropathy. In the absence of functioning kidneys, toxic substances accumulate in the blood, resulting in a uremic state. These toxic substances damage nerve tissues and lead to painful neuropathies in the majority of individuals with ESRD. Central and peripheral neurologic disturbances may be present at the initiation of dialysis, particularly for patients with diabetes. Symptoms of neuropathy are more common when the GFR falls to less than 20 mL/min per 1.73 m^2 and when serum creatinine levels rise. Patients should be periodically assessed for neuropathy irrespective of symptoms because some cases are asymptomatic. Addressing pain management is an important aspect of health care to maintain quality of life in patients with ESRD.

KIDNEY STONE DISEASE

In the United States, approximately 7.1% of women and 10.6% of men form kidney stones at some point during their lives.[31] The etiology of **nephrolithiasis** is unknown, but many factors that relate to the nature of the urine itself (e.g., pH, concentration) or to conditions of the urinary tract environment contribute to **supersaturation** and stone formation. Co-morbidities

such as obesity, diabetes, gout, and hyperparathyroidism increase the risk for stone formation.[31-33] The most common types of kidney stones are calcium, struvite, and uric acid. Figure 21-6 illustrates various types of stones. Box 21-2 lists additional risk factors that are associated with kidney stone development.

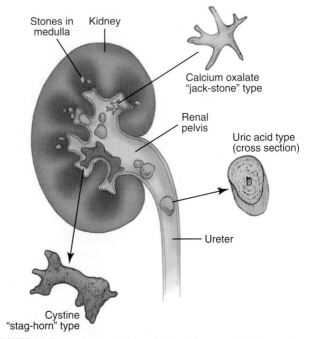

FIGURE 21-6 Renal calculi: stones in the kidney, renal pelvis, and ureter.

Box 21-2	Risk Factors for the Development of Kidney Stones

- Dietary
  - Inadequate fluid intake
  - Low calcium intake
  - High animal protein intake
  - High sodium intake
- Diseases or disorders
  - Eating disorders, multiple food restrictions, or food intolerances or allergies
  - Chronic diarrhea from malabsorption disorders or bowel disease
  - Obesity, type 2 diabetes, gout, hyperparathyroidism, metabolic syndrome
  - Chronic urinary tract infections
- Familial
  - Personal history or family history of urolithiasis
  - Genetic predisposition for stone formation
  - Congenital disorders of the kidneys

nephrolithiasis the formation of a kidney stone.
supersaturation (pertaining to urine) excess concentration of solutes.

DISEASE PROCESS

Calcium Stones

Calcium oxalate and calcium phosphate stones are the most common types, and they account for approximately 80% of all kidney stones. The supersaturation of kidney stone materials in the urine may result from the following[32]:

- Excess calcium in the blood (hypercalcemia) or urine (hypercalciuria)
- Excess oxalate (hyperoxaluria) or uric acid in the urine (hyperuricosuria)
- Low levels of citrate in the urine (hypocitraturia)

High levels of urinary oxalate increase the risk of an individual forming a calcium oxalate stone. Oxalates are derived from endogenous synthesis (relative to lean body mass) and dietary sources (Box 21-3). A small percentage of the population are "hyperabsorbers" of dietary oxalate and thus are at higher risk of forming stones. Oxalic acid is a metabolite of ascorbic acid. Therefore, the long-term supplementation of vitamin C in excess of the tolerable upper intake (2000 mg/day) may pose a potential health risk for kidney stone formation.[34,35]

Adequate dietary calcium intake from all sources (i.e., dairy foods, nondairy foods, and supplements) is inversely associated with calcium oxalate stone formation.[36,37] Essentially, individuals with a low dietary intake of calcium are at a *higher* risk for calcium oxalate stone formation than those who consume the DRI for calcium. Dietary calcium binds oxalates in the intestines, preventing absorption and thus concentration of oxalates in the urine. Historically, it was a common misunderstanding to restrict the calcium intake of those patients who form calcium oxalate stones.

Struvite Stones

Struvite stones, which account for approximately 10% of all stones, are composed of magnesium ammonium phosphate and carbonate apatite. They often are called *infection stones* because they are primarily caused by urinary tract infections and because they are not associated with any specific nutrient. Thus, no particular diet therapy is involved. Struvite stones are usually large "staghorn" stones that are surgically removed.

Uric Acid Stones

Approximately 9% of kidney stones are uric acid stones. The primary risk factors for uric acid stone formation are overly acidic urine, excess urinary excretion of uric acid, and low urine volume.[38] Hyperuricosuria may result from an impairment that involves the metabolism of purine, which is a nitrogen end product of protein metabolism from which uric acid is formed. This impairment occurs with diseases such as gout, and it can also occur with rapid tissue breakdown during wasting disease. Other conditions that are associated with persistently acidic urine and uric acid stone formation are diarrheal illness (e.g., short-gut syndrome, inflammatory bowel disease), type 2 diabetes, obesity, and metabolic syndrome.[38,39]

Other Stones

Other rare forms of kidney stones are often reflective of inherited disorders or complications of medications. For example, cystine stones are caused by a genetic defect in the renal reabsorption of the amino acid cystine (as well as other dibasic amino acids), thereby causing an accumulation in the urine (cystinuria). Cystine is not soluble and thus a high concentration may result in stone formation.

Clinical Symptoms

The main symptom of kidney stones is severe pain. Many other urinary symptoms may result from the presence of the stones, and general weakness and sometimes fever are present. Laboratory examination of the urine and of any passed stones helps to determine treatment.

Box 21-3	High-Oxalate Foods and Drinks

DRINKS
Chocolate drink mixes, soymilk, Ovaltine, instant iced tea, fruit juices of fruits listed in this table

FRUITS
Apricots (dried), red currants, figs, kiwi, rhubarb

VEGETABLES
Beans (wax, dried), beets and beet greens, chives, collard greens, eggplant, escarole, dark greens of all kinds, kale, leeks, okra, parsley, green peppers, potatoes, rutabagas, spinach, Swiss chard, tomato paste, watercress, zucchini

BREADS, CEREALS, AND GRAINS
Amaranth, barley, white corn flour, fried potatoes, fruit cake, grits, soybean products, sweet potatoes, wheat germ and bran, buckwheat flour, All-Bran cereal, graham crackers, pretzels, whole-wheat bread

MEAT, MEAT REPLACEMENTS, FISH, AND POULTRY
Dried beans, peanut butter, soy burgers, miso

DESSERTS AND SWEETS
Carob, chocolate, marmalades

FATS AND OILS
Nuts (peanuts, almonds, pecans, cashews, hazelnuts), nut butters, sesame seeds, tahini (a paste made from sesame seeds)

OTHER FOODS
Poppy seeds

From American Dietetic Association. *ADA nutrition care manual.* Chicago, Ill: 2010.

MEDICAL NUTRITION THERAPY

General Objectives

MNT may include several aspects, and it will vary depending on the type of stone. General MNT recommendations are as follows[5,40]:

- *Energy:* Overweight and obesity increase the risk for several chronic diseases as well as for kidney stone formation. Total energy intake should be customized to achieve an ideal body weight. Diets such as the DASH diet or Mediterranean diet are ideal (see Chapter 19). High-protein, low-carbohydrate diets are specifically discouraged for individuals at risk for stone formation.[41]
- *Protein:* Excessive protein intake from animal sources is a risk factor for stone formation. Thus, patients should normalize their intake to healthy population standard recommendations of 0.8 to 1.0 g/kg/day.
- *Calcium:* Low dietary calcium intake is a risk for calcium oxalate stone formation. Thus, patients should be encouraged to normalize calcium intake to 800 mg/day for men and 1200 mg/day for women and balance intake throughout the day.
- *Sodium and potassium:* High sodium intake increases the amount of calcium excretion in the urine, thereby precipitating hypercalciuria, and it is associated with an increased risk of stone formation. All stone formers should be counseled on a low-sodium diet (<2300 mg/day). Citrate and potassium are helpful in solubilizing calcium salts and preventing calcium oxalate stone formation. The diet should be rich in fruits (particularly citrus fruits) and vegetables to provide a potassium intake of >4.7 g/day.
- *Oxalates:* Limiting dietary oxalates reduces urinary oxalate excretion and the risk of calcium oxalate stone formation.[42] Thus, avoiding foods that are high in oxalates is advised. Intake should be <200 mg/day (see Box 21-3).
- *Vitamins and minerals:* Vitamin C should be limited to the Dietary Reference Intake, and all other vitamin and mineral intakes should meet the Dietary Reference Intake standards.
- *Fluid:* A large fluid intake of ≥2 to 3 L/day helps to produce more dilute urine and thus to prevent the accumulation of materials that form stones. Exact fluid intake needs vary by patient, but enough fluids—preferably water—should be ingested to produce at least 2 to 2.5 L of clear urine daily. For patients who consume soft drinks, reducing soft-drink intake may lower the risk of recurrent stone formation.

Objectives Specific to Type of Stone

The nutrition care plan may be further individualized relative to the nature of the specific stone formed. A variety of medications are useful for the treatment of kidney stones in combination with diet therapy. For medications to be most effective, the specific type of stone must be identified. This is not always possible and therefore limits drug therapy in some individuals.

Dietary recommendations relative to specific type of stone formation are summarized in Table 21-5.

Calcium stones. In some cases, dietary control of the stone constituents may help to reduce the recurrence of such stone formation. If a stone is made of calcium oxalate, then avoiding foods that are high in oxalate (see Box 21-3) may be beneficial. If a stone is made of calcium phosphate, additional sources of phosphorus (e.g., meats, legumes, nuts) should be controlled.

Table 21-5　Summary of Dietary Principles In Kidney Stone Disease

STONE TYPE	CALCIUM	OXALATE	SODIUM*	POTASSIUM†	ANIMAL PROTEIN	CITRATE	FRUCTOSE	FLUIDS
Calcium								
• Idiopathic calcium oxalate	800-1200 mg	Avoid oxalate-rich foods	Reduce to <2300 mg	Increase to >120 mEq	Reduce to <1.2 g/kg	Increase	Reduce	Increase
• Calcium phosphate	800-1200 mg		Reduce to <2300 mg	?	Reduce to <1.2 g/kg	?		Increase
Uric acid				Increase	Reduce (also purines)	Increase		Increase
Cystine			Reduce to <2300 mg	Increase	Reduce to <1.2 g/kg	Increase		Increase
Struvite	800-1200 mg		Reduce to <2300 mg					Increase

Source: Heilberg IP, Goldfarb DS. Optimum nutrition for kidney stone disease. *Adv Chronic Kidney Dis.* 2013;20(2):165-174. Empty boxes indicate that nutrient intake is not considered relevant; question marks indicate unclear if dietary modification is beneficial or adverse.
*2300 mg Na corresponds to about 6 g of NaCl.
†120 mEq K corresponds to 4.7 g of K.

In addition to the recommendations listed previously, fiber intake should be considered in the case of calcium stones. Materials that bind potential stone elements in the intestine can prevent their absorption and remove them from the body. For example, phytate can bind calcium and thus help to prevent the crystallization of oxalate calcium salts. Phytates are found in high-fiber plant foods such as whole wheat, bran, and soybeans.

Uric acid stones. Dietary attempts to alter urinary pH with **alkaline diets** low in purines are helpful to prevent an increase of the concentration of uric acid and stone

> **alkaline diet** diet that is low in animal protein and high in fruits and vegetables.

formation within the kidneys. Acidic urine favors the kidneys' reuptake of uric acid whereas alkaline urine favors the excretion of uric acid.[43] Potassium citrate treatments may also be used to raise the urinary pH, which decreases the supersaturation of uric acid.[44] The primary goals of therapy are to establish and maintain a healthy weight and alkalization of the urine through a vegetarian-type diet with limited animal protein (including red meat, fish, and poultry).[40,45]

Cystine stones. Dietary modifications are geared toward reducing urinary cystine concentrations by decreasing intake of animal foods high in cystine and methionine; reducing sodium intake; increasing the intake of vegetables high in organic anions; and diluting the urine.[45] Diluting the urine requires the intake of copious amounts of water daily in order to void at least 4 L of urine per day.[44]

Putting It All Together

Summary

- The nephrons are the functional units of the kidneys. Through these unique structures, the kidney maintains homeostasis in the blood of the materials that are required for life and health. The nephrons accomplish their tremendous task by constantly cleaning the blood, returning necessary elements to the blood, and eliminating the remainder in concentrated urine.
- Various diseases that interfere with the vital function of nephrons can cause kidney disease. Kidney diseases have predisposing factors, such as diabetes, recurrent urinary tract infections that may lead to renal calculi, and progressive glomerulonephritis that may lead to chronic nephrotic syndrome and kidney failure.
- At its end stage, CKD is treated by dialysis or kidney transplantation. Patients who are undergoing dialysis require close monitoring for protein, water, and electrolyte balance.
- Kidney stones may be formed from a variety of substances. For some patients, a change in the dietary intake of the identified substance (e.g., sodium, oxalate, purine) and an increase in fluid intake may decrease stone formation.

Chapter Review Questions

See answers in Appendix A.

1. The hormone that acts on the distal nephron tubule to stimulate reabsorption of sodium is:
   a. Insulin.
   b. Aldosterone.
   c. Antidiuretic hormone.
   d. Erythropoietin.

2. Which of the following do the kidneys convert from an intermediate inactive form to its active form?
   a. Vitamin E
   b. Vitamin D
   c. Hemoglobin
   d. Nitrogen

3. A patient with nephrotic syndrome is likely to have:
   a. Low serum albumin levels.
   b. High serum albumin levels.
   c. Low plasma glucose levels.
   d. High plasma glucose levels.

4. Medical nutrition therapy for a patient with stage 3 CKD includes:
   a. Energy intake limited to 20 kcal/kg body weight.
   b. Fluid intake limited to 500 mL per day.
   c. Sodium intake limited to 4 g per day.
   d. Protein intake limited to 0.6 to 0.8 g/kg body weight.

5. A protein source that is of high biologic value is:
   a. Grilled chicken.
   b. Baked beans.
   c. Oatmeal.
   d. Spinach.

Additional Learning Resources

evolve Please refer to this text's Evolve website for answers to the Case Study questions. http://evolve.elsevier.com/Williams/basic/

References and **Further Reading and Resources** in the back of the book provide additional resources for enhancing knowledge.

22

Surgery and Nutrition Support

Key Concepts

- Surgical procedures may require nutrition support for tissue healing and recovery.
- Gastrointestinal (GI) surgery may necessitate diet modifications if the surgery alters the normal digestion or passage of food.
- To ensure optimal nutrition for postsurgical or critically ill patients, diet management may involve **enteral** or **parenteral** nutrition support.

Malnutrition contributes to morbidity, mortality, extended length of stay in the hospital, and significant additional treatment costs. Approximately 3.2% of all hospitalized patients in the United States are diagnosed with malnutrition before discharge.[1] Effective nutrition support should reverse malnutrition, improve prognosis, and speed recovery in a cost-effective manner. The surgical process also places physiologic and psychologic stress on the patient, which may lead to further nutrition demands and increases the risk for clinical problems.

This chapter looks at the nutrition needs of surgical and burn patients and the enteral and parenteral feeding methods of providing nutrition support. Careful attention to both preoperative and postoperative nutrition support can reduce complications and provide essential resources for healing and health.

NUTRITION NEEDS OF GENERAL SURGERY PATIENTS

A patient who is undergoing surgery often faces significant physical and psychologic stress. As a result, nutrition demands are increased during this period, and deficiencies can develop that manifest as malnutrition and subsequent clinical complications. Therefore, careful attention must be given to a patient's nutrition status in preparation for surgery as well as to the individual nutrition needs that follow to address wound healing and recovery. Poor nutrition status and the following clinical problems are well documented[1-5]:

- Impaired wound healing and increased risk of infection
- Increased necessity of enteral or parenteral nutrition support
- Longer hospital stay and increased medical cost
- Increased morbidity and mortality rate
- Reduced quality of life

The diagnosis of malnutrition includes the following general characteristics: insufficient energy intake; weight loss; loss of muscle mass; loss of subcutaneous fat; localized or generalized fluid accumulation; and diminished functional status as measured by strength of hand grip.[6] A diagnosis can be made when two or more of those criteria are met. Table 22-1 provides the clinical diagnostic criteria for malnutrition.

PREOPERATIVE NUTRITION CARE: NUTRIENT RESERVES

When the surgery is elective (i.e., not emergent), body nutrient stores can be built up to fortify a patient for the demands of the surgery and the period that immediately follows, when food intake may be limited. Particular needs center on protein, energy, vitamins, and minerals.

Protein

Protein deficiencies among pediatric and geriatric hospital patients are not uncommon, particularly among the critically ill patients.[5,7,8] Every patient facing surgery must be equipped with adequate body protein to counteract blood losses that occur during surgery and to prevent tissue catabolism during the immediate postoperative period (see the For Further Focus box, "Protein-Energy Malnutrition after Surgery"). For example, extensive bone healing may be involved in orthopedic surgery. Protein, in addition to other vital nutrients such as calcium, is essential for establishing healthy bone mineral density.[9,10] Establishing

---

enteral a mode of feeding that makes use of the gastrointestinal tract through oral or tube feedings.

parenteral a mode of feeding that does not involve the gastrointestinal tract but that instead provides nutrition support via the intravenous delivery of nutrient solutions.

Table 22-1   Clinical Diagnostic Criteria for Malnutrition

Characteristics to Diagnose Severe Malnutrition

Characteristic	Acute Illness or Injury Related Malnutrition	Chronic Disease Related Malnutrition	Social or Environmental Related Malnutrition
Weight loss	>2%/1 week >5%/1 month >7.5%/3 months	>5%/1 month >7.5%/3 months >10%/6 months > 20%/1 year	>5%/1 month >7.5%/3 months >10%/6 months > 20%/1 year
Energy intake	≤50% for ≥5 days	≤75% for ≥1 month	≤50% for ≥1 month
Body fat	Moderate depletion	Severe depletion	Severe depletion
Muscle mass	Moderate depletion	Severe depletion	Severe depletion
Fluid accumulation	Moderate → severe	Severe	Severe
Grip strength	Not recommended in intensive care unit	Reduced for age/gender	Reduced for age/gender

Characteristics to Diagnose Moderate Malnutrition

Characteristic	Acute Illness or Injury Related Malnutrition	Chronic Disease Related Malnutrition	Social or Environmental Related Malnutrition
Weight loss	1%–2%/1 week 5%/1 month 7.5%/3 months	5%/1 month 7.5%/3 months 10%/6 months 20%/1 year	5%/1 month 7.5%/3 months 10%/6 months 20%/1 year
Energy intake	<75% for >7 days	<75% for ≥1 month	<75% for ≥3 months
Body fat	Mild depletion	Mild depletion	Mild depletion
Muscle mass	Mild depletion	Mild depletion	Mild depletion
Fluid accumulation	Mild	Mild	Mild
Grip strength	Not applicable	Not applicable	Not applicable

From: Malone A, Hamilton C. *The Academy of Nutrition and Dietetics/the American Society for Parenteral and Enteral Nutrition consensus malnutrition characteristics: application in practice.* Nutr Clin Pract. 2013;28(6):639-650.

For Further Focus

Protein-Energy Malnutrition after Surgery

Protein-energy malnutrition (PEM) compromises quality of life and the ability to recover from surgery and injury. As general health declines with age and the risk for unplanned surgery increases, so does the prevalence of PEM. Actively evaluating the nutritional status of older people in the home, the hospital, or the nursing home may provide valuable information about the preoperative needs of these individuals. Use of oral supplements or enteral feedings for malnourished elderly patients before surgery is a cost-effective way to improve outcome, reduce hospital stay, and reduce the risk of complications associated with surgery.

Even without a formal nutrition assessment, PEM can be identified by monitoring unintended weight loss. Unplanned weight loss is indicative of PEM as well as of the inability to deal with physiologic stress. Unintentional weight loss of up to 5% over a 1-month period or of 10% over a 6-month period is considered a *significant loss*. Unintentional weight loss of more than 5% in 1 month or 10% in 6 months is classified as *severe*. Identifying and treating those individuals who are at risk for PEM may also prevent poor outcomes in the event of injury or emergency surgery.

and maintaining good bone mineral density throughout life are especially relevant for the growing U.S. population of elderly individuals and their risk for debilitating bone fractures (see Chapter 12). The adequate dietary consumption of high-quality complete proteins (i.e., those that contain all of the essential amino acids) is associated with the maintenance of lean tissue, bone mineral density, and bone mineral content.[11,12]

Energy

Sufficient energy must be provided when increased protein is necessary for tissue building. The increased source of kilocalories supports the added energy demands and spares protein for its tissue-building function. For example, carbohydrate intake should be adequate to maintain optimal glycogen stores in the liver as a necessary resource for immediate energy, thereby directing protein to its tissue synthesis task. If a person is underweight, extra energy may be required to increase weight to an ideal maintenance level before surgery. If a person is overweight and the surgery is elective, some weight reduction before the procedure may help to reduce surgical complications.

Table 22-2   **Fiber-Restricted Diet***

FOOD TYPE	FOODS ALLOWED	FOODS NOT ALLOWED
Dairy	Buttermilk and kefir Fat-free and low-fat milk and milk-substitute products (e.g., soy, rice, almond milk) Yogurt and mild cheese Lactose-free dairy products	Whole milk Half-and-half Cream and sour cream Dairy products with nuts or fruit
Grains	Grains with <2 g of fiber per serving Grain products made with white or refined flour	Grains made with whole wheat or whole grains Grains made with seeds or nuts Popcorn
Fruit	Canned, soft, or well-cooked fruit without skin, seeds, or membranes Fruit juice without pulp	Raw fruits Fruit with skin Dried fruit Fruit juice with pulp Prune juice
Vegetables	Canned, soft, or well-cooked vegetables without skin, seeds, or hulls Mashed potatoes Vegetable juice without skin	Raw or undercooked vegetables High-fiber vegetables Gas-forming vegetables
Fats and oils	Limit to less than 8 tsp daily	Coconut Avocado

Source: Academy of Nutrition and Dietetics. *Nutrition Care Manual.* Chicago, Ill: 2015.
*Presurgical fiber-restricted diet: This diet includes foods that are low in fiber, seeds, and skins and with a minimal amount of residue. The diet should be adequate in protein and energy, but may be inadequate in micronutrients. If patients are to continue this diet for a long period, supplementary vitamins and minerals should be administered. Postsurgical fiber-restricted diet: This diet is slightly higher in fiber, but it has greater variety. The average daily menu contains slightly more protein, energy, vitamins, and minerals compared with the presurgical diet.

Vitamins and Minerals

When increased protein and energy are necessary, the appropriate intake of vitamins and minerals involved in protein and energy metabolism (e.g., B-complex vitamins) must also be supplied. Any specifically identified deficiency states (e.g., iron-deficiency anemia) should be corrected. In addition, electrolyte and water balance is necessary to prevent dehydration.

Immediate Preoperative Period

The usual preparation for surgery requires nothing to be taken orally for at least 8 hours before the procedure. This protocol is to ensure that the stomach retains no food during surgery. The presence of food may cause complications, such as the aspiration of food particles during anesthesia or in the course of recovery from anesthesia if the patient vomits. In addition, any food present in the stomach may interfere with the surgical procedure or increase the risk for postoperative gastric retention and expansion. Before GI surgery, a fiber-restricted diet may be followed for several days to clear the surgical site of any food residue (Table 22-2). Commercial nonresidue **elemental formulas** can provide a complete diet in liquid form. These formulas can be administered by tube or made more palatable for oral use with various flavorings.

elemental formula a nutrition support formula composed of simple elemental nutrient components that require no further digestive breakdown and are thus readily absorbed (e.g., glucose, amino acids, medium-chain triglycerides).

Emergency Surgery

If the surgery is urgent, no time is available for building up ideal nutrition reserves, which is another reason to maintain good nutrition status through a healthy diet at all times. If optimal nutrition is maintained, then reserves are available to meet needs during times of stress and risks associated with malnutrition are minimized.

POSTOPERATIVE NUTRITION CARE: NUTRIENT NEEDS FOR HEALING

Adequate nutrition support is necessary to help with recovery from surgery when nutrient losses are great. At the same time, food intake may be diminished or even absent for a period. If a patient is not able to resume adequate oral intake within a few days, an alternative form of nutrition support such as enteral or parenteral routes must be considered. Several nutrients require particular attention during this time.

Protein

Optimal protein intake during the postoperative recovery period is important for all patients. Protein is needed to replace losses that occur during surgery and to meet the increased demands of the healing process. During the period immediately following major surgery, body tissues may undergo considerable catabolism, which means that the process of tissue breakdown and loss exceeds the process of tissue buildup. Weight loss and malnutrition are common among patients who are experiencing catabolic stress but the maintenance of lean body mass improves the survival of some catabolic patients.[13]

In addition to protein losses from tissue breakdown, other losses of protein from the body may occur. These losses include plasma protein loss from hemorrhage, blood loss, and various body fluid losses or exudates. The increased loss of plasma protein from extensive tissue destruction, inflammation, infection, and trauma should be monitored. If any degree of prior malnutrition or chronic infection existed, a patient's protein deficiency could present significant complications. Several reasons exist for this increased protein demand, and these will be detailed in the following paragraphs.

Building tissue. The process of wound healing requires building a great deal of new body tissue, which depends on an adequate amount of essential amino acids. Necessary amino acids must come from dietary protein (either oral or tube feedings) or from parenteral nutrition if a patient cannot eat or tolerate enteral feedings for an extended period. Dietary protein recommendations may increase above normal needs to restore lost protein and to build new tissues at the wound site.

Controlling edema. A sufficient supply of plasma protein—mainly albumin—is necessary to maintain blood volume. If the plasma albumin level drops, pressure to keep tissue fluid circulating between the capillaries and cells is insufficient. Without adequate pressure, water leaves the capillaries, and it cannot be drawn back into circulation; this results in edema (see Chapter 9). Edema is characterized by puffiness or swelling of the tissue from the excess fluid being held there instead of returning to circulation. Generalized edema may adversely affect heart and lung function. Local edema at the wound site also interferes with the closure of the wound, hindering the healing process.

Controlling shock. Excessive loss of blood out of the body or out of circulation (as a result of low albumin level and subsequent edema) may lead to symptoms of shock as the body attempts to restore euvolemia.

Healing bone. Protein and mineral matter are essential to the foundation of bone tissue for proper formation and healing. Protein provides a matrix for calcium and phosphorus, and these are required for strong bones.

Resisting infection. Protein is the major component of the body's immune system, which provides the body's defense against infection. The immune system's defensive agents include specialized white cells called *lymphocytes* as well as antibodies and various other blood cells, hormones, and enzymes. Tissue strength is a major defense barrier against infection at all times.

Transporting lipids. Fat is also an important component of tissue structure. It forms the lipid bilayer of cell membranes, and it participates in many other necessary metabolic activities. Protein is necessary to transport fat via the bloodstream to all tissues and to the liver for metabolism (e.g., lipoproteins).

Because protein has many important functions during recovery from surgery, protein deficiency at this time can lead to many clinical complications. Such problems include poor wound healing, the rupture of the suture lines (i.e., dehiscence), the delayed healing of fractures, depressed heart and lung function, anemia, the failure of GI stomas, a reduced resistance to infection, liver damage, extensive weight loss, muscle wasting, and an increased mortality risk.

Energy

As always, when increased protein is demanded for tissue building, enough nonprotein kilocalories must be provided to spare protein for its vital tissue-building function. Therefore, the fuel sources (i.e., carbohydrate and fat) must be sufficient in the diet. In situations of acute metabolic stress (e.g., with extensive surgery or burns), energy needs may increase to as much as 1.2 to 2 kcal/kg of body weight/day over basal energy requirements. Energy requirements can be estimated by first calculating the individual's basal metabolic rate (BMR) with the Mifflin-St. Jeor equation (see Chapter 6) and then multiplying by an injury factor (1.0 to 2, depending on the patient's status) to meet the added energy needs of stress and sepsis:

$$Male = [(10 \times Weight\ in\ kg) + (6.25 \times Height\ in\ cm)$$
$$- (5 \times Age\ in\ years) + 5] \times injury\ factor$$
$$Female = [(10 \times Weight\ in\ kg) + (6.25 \times Height\ in\ cm)$$
$$- (5 \times Age\ in\ years) - 161] \times injury\ factor$$

Carbohydrates spare protein for tissue building and help to avoid liver damage by maintaining glycogen reserves in the liver. Adipose tissue heals poorly and is more susceptible to infection. Therefore, overfeeding should be avoided to prevent the accumulation of extra fat tissue during recovery.

exudate various materials such as cells, cellular debris, and fluids that have escaped from the blood vessels and that are deposited in or on the surface tissues, usually as a result of inflammation; the protein content of exudate is high.
euvolemia normal blood volume.
dehiscence a splitting open; the separation of the layers of a surgical wound that may be partial, superficial, or complete and that involves total disruption and resuturing.
stoma the opening that is established in the abdominal wall that connects with the ileum or the colon for the elimination of intestinal wastes after the surgical removal of nonfunctional portions of the intestines.

Water

Surgery induces altered fluid distribution in the patient. Sufficient fluid replacement is necessary to prevent dehydration, to maintain circulation, and to prevent complications. The specific fluid therapy goals for each patient during and after surgery must be individualized to maximize support and outcome for the patient.[14] Elderly patients, whose thirst mechanisms may be depressed, warrant special attention to total fluid intake and hydration status. During the postoperative period, large water losses may also occur from vomiting, hemorrhage, fever, infection, or **diuresis**. A variety of solutions are available for intravenous administration, depending on the patient's needs. Intravenous fluids after surgery supply some initial hydration needs, but oral intake should begin as soon as possible and be sufficiently maintained.

Vitamins

Several vitamins require particular attention during wound healing. Vitamin C is vital for building connective tissue and capillary walls during the healing process, but levels are often low in critically ill patients. Studies demonstrate that the parenteral administration of vitamin C protects microvascular functions, decreases length of stay in the hospital for post cardiac-surgery patients,[15] decreases the risk for morbidity, and may be particularly beneficial for critically ill patients with sepsis.[16,17] If extensive tissue building is necessary, as much as 1 to 3 g/day of vitamin C may be beneficial during the postoperative period for critically ill patients.[18,19] (Long-term supplementation at this level is not recommended.) Antioxidant supplementation with vitamins C and E and with *n*-3 fatty acids may also be helpful in preventing postsurgical complications such as arrhythmias, oxidative stress, and inflammation.[20] As energy and protein intake are increased, the B-complex vitamins that have important coenzyme roles in protein and energy metabolism (e.g., thiamin, riboflavin, niacin) must be increased. Other B-complex vitamins (e.g., folate, B_{12}, pyridoxine, and pantothenic acid) play important roles in building hemoglobin and thus must meet the demands of an increased blood supply and general metabolic stress. Vitamin K, which is essential for blood clotting, is usually present in a sufficient amount because it is synthesized by intestinal bacteria. However, patients who are treated with long-term antibiotics may have decreased gut flora and vitamin K synthesis.

Minerals

Although there is no universally accepted list of minerals or doses that should be supplemented in postsurgical or critically ill patients, attention to mineral deficiencies is important and supplementation may prove advantageous.[21] Tissue catabolism results in cell potassium and phosphorus loss. Electrolyte imbalances of sodium and chloride also result from fluid imbalances. Iron-deficiency anemia may develop from blood loss or inadequate iron absorption (see the Drug-Nutrient Interaction box, "Aspirin and Iron Absorption"). Patients with critical illness or sepsis have low levels of zinc and selenium in response to the inflammatory response, increasing their risk for added oxidative stress and inflammation.[22,23] Zinc is also important for wound healing. Adequate protein-rich food consumption usually meets this need, because most dietary zinc is found in protein foods of animal origin. However, even if patients have adequate dietary intake of zinc, surgical trauma and infection may lead to reduced serum zinc status and elevated needs.

GENERAL DIETARY MANAGEMENT

The nutrition support needed for the hospitalized patient can vary greatly between individuals. The necessary medical nutrition therapy (MNT) will depend on the patient's nutritional status upon arrival, the metabolic results of the patient's condition, the patient's ability to consume food, and the patient's advance directive, or living will, regarding nutrition support.

INITIAL INTRAVENOUS FLUID AND ELECTROLYTES

Routine intravenous fluids (IV fluids) are used to supply hydration needs and electrolytes; they cannot sustain energy and nutrient balance. For example, a 5% dextrose solution with normal saline (i.e., 0.9%

💊 Drug-Nutrient Interaction

Aspirin and Iron Absorption

SARA HARCOURT

Aspirin is one of the most common analgesics used in the United States. Its use is implicated in the presence of other conditions as well, such as transient ischemic attacks (i.e., mini strokes), myocardial infarctions, arthritis and other inflammatory diseases, blood-clotting disorders, and insomnia.

Long-term aspirin use may lead to poor iron absorption. The acetylsalicylic acid found in aspirin can irritate the stomach lining and prevent or slow the normal excretion of gastric acid. Gastric acid is needed to keep iron in its Fe^{3+} state until absorption can occur in the duodenum. When gastric acid levels are low, the bioavailability of iron is compromised.

Aspirin should be taken on an empty stomach with a large glass of water. This dilutes the acetylsalicylic acid, thereby preventing the erosion of the stomach lining and the disruption of gastric acid secretion. Aspirin may be taken with other liquids but never with alcohol; it increases the bioavailability of alcohol and thus increases the risk for adverse side effects.

---

diuresis the increased excretion of urine.

sodium chloride solution) contains only 5 g of dextrose/dL or approximately 170 kcal/L (dextrose provides 3.4 kcal/g), although the patient's total energy need is typically more than 10 times that amount. For a patient only receiving IV fluids, a return to regular eating should be encouraged and maintained as soon as tolerated.

METHODS OF NUTRITION SUPPORT

The method of nutrition support used in the nutrition care plan depends on the patient's condition. Many patients experience malnutrition during hospital stays, and the risk for malnutrition increases with advanced age, disease status, and length of hospital stay.[1,24] The appropriate and timely administration of nutrition support is an important predictor of overall health outcomes and quality of life.[25,26] The physician, the dietitian, and the nurse work together to manage the diet by using oral, enteral, or parenteral feeding as necessary:

- *Oral:* nourishment through the regular GI route by oral feedings; may include a variety of diet plans, textures, and meal replacement liquid supplements
- *Enteral:* technically refers to nourishment through the regular GI route either by regular oral feedings or by tube feedings; however, in medical nutrition therapy, enteral feedings imply *tube feedings*
- *Parenteral:* nourishment through the veins (either small peripheral veins or a large central vein) bypassing the GI tract

When a patient is capable of meeting his or her nutrient needs by oral feedings and when feedings are well tolerated, that is the feeding method of choice. Table 22-3 lists conditions that often require nutrition support by tube feeding or parenteral nutrition. General criteria for selecting the most appropriate nutrition support method are listed in Box 22-1. In addition, the algorithm for determining the route for nutrition support administration is provided in Figure 22-1.

Oral Feedings

When the GI tract can be used, it is the preferred route of feeding: orally if possible and by feeding tube if not. Most general surgical patients can and should receive oral feedings as soon as feasible to provide adequate

Table 22-3 | Conditions that Often Require Nutrition Support

RECOMMENDED ROUTE OF FEEDING	CONDITION	EXAMPLES
Enteral nutrition	Impaired nutrient ingestion	Neurologic disorders Facial, oral, or esophageal trauma or surgery Congenital anomalies Respiratory failure Cystic fibrosis Traumatic brain injury Anorexia and wasting with severe eating disorders
	Inability to consume adequate nutrition orally	Hyperemesis gravidarum Hypermetabolic states (e.g., burns) Comatose states Anorexia with congestive heart failure, cancer, chronic obstructive pulmonary disease, and eating disorders Congenital heart disease Severe dysphagia Premature birth without suck reflex Spinal cord injury
	Impaired digestion, absorption, and metabolism	Severe gastroparesis Inborn errors of metabolism Crohn's disease Obstruction in the upper gastrointestinal tract Short-bowel syndrome with minimal resection
	Severe wasting or depressed growth	Cystic fibrosis Failure to thrive Cancer, HIV/AIDS Sepsis Cerebral palsy Myasthenia gravis
Parenteral nutrition	Gastrointestinal incompetence	Nothing by mouth before surgery for more than 7 days Obstruction in the lower gastrointestinal tract Intestinal infarction Short-bowel syndrome or major resection

Continued

Table 22-3	Conditions that Often Require Nutrition Support—cont'd	

RECOMMENDED ROUTE OF FEEDING	CONDITION	EXAMPLES
		Severe acute pancreatitis Severe inflammatory bowel disease Small-bowel ischemia Intestinal atresia Severe liver failure Major gastrointestinal surgery
	Critical illness with poor enteral tolerance or accessibility	Multiorgan system failure Major trauma or burns Bone marrow transplantation Acute respiratory failure with ventilator dependency and gastrointestinal malfunction Severe wasting with renal failure and dialysis Small-bowel transplantation, immediately after surgery

Adapted from Mahan LK, Escott-Stump S. *Krause's Food & Nutrition Therapy*. 13th ed. St Louis: Saunders; 2012.

Box 22-1	Criteria for Selecting a Nutrition Support Method

The physician and dietitian will decide the most appropriate method of medical nutrition therapy for the patient with the use of the following criteria. Either the pharmacist or the registered dietitian nutritionist will make the calculations for the enteral formula or parenteral nutrition solution that will be used.

ENTERAL NUTRITION SUPPORT

Is indicated for patients with the following characteristics:
- They have enough functional gastrointestinal tract to allow adequate digestion and absorption.
- They cannot eat enough to meet their nutrient needs orally.
- They are at risk for malnutrition without nutrition support.

PARENTERAL NUTRITION SUPPORT

Is indicated for patients with the following characteristics:
- They do not have sufficient gastrointestinal tract function and they need long-term nutrition support.
- They are unable to meet nutrient needs after 7 to 10 days of enteral nutrition.
- There is a need for bowel rest (e.g., enteral fistulas, acute inflammatory bowel disease).
- They do not have access for feeding tube placement and need nutrition support.
- They repeatedly pull out their feeding tubes.
    The decision is then made for which form of parenteral nutrition support:
    Peripheral Parenteral Nutrition
    - Length of therapy of ≤10 to 14 days
    - Not hypermetabolic
    - No fluid restriction
    Central Parenteral Nutrition
    - Long-term therapy needed
    - Hypermetabolic
    - Fluid restriction
    - Poor peripheral access or central access already in place

nutrition. Oral feedings provide needed nutrients and help to stimulate the normal action of the GI tract. Early initiation of oral feedings (i.e., within 24 hours after injury, surgery, or hospital admission) is associated with reduced complications and infections, and, in some cases, reduced hospital stays.[27-29] When oral feedings begin, the patient may begin with clear or full liquids and then progress to a soft or regular diet as indicated. Individual tolerance and needs are always the guide, but encouragement and help should be supplied as part of the general care of postsurgical patients to facilitate eating as soon as possible. If inadequate caloric intake is a concern, the energy value of foods in the regular diet may also be increased with added sauces, dried protein powder, and dressings. Alternatively, a general food supplement formula such as Boost or Ensure may be added orally with or between meals. More frequent, less bulky, and concentrated small meals may be helpful to make every bite count.

Routine house diets. A schedule of routine "house" diets that is based on a cyclic menu is typically followed in most hospitals. The basic modification is in texture, and this ranges from clear liquid (no milk) to full liquid (including milk) and from soft food to a full regular diet. Mechanically altered soft diets are designed for patients with chewing or swallowing problems. Small amounts of liquid may be added to regular foods to achieve an appropriate consistency when puréed. These diets may be further modified, depending on the patient's needs. For example, low-sodium, low-fat, or high-protein requirements can still be met with mechanically altered diets. Therapeutic soft diets are used to transition between liquid and regular diets. Whole foods that are low in fiber and limited seasonings are included as

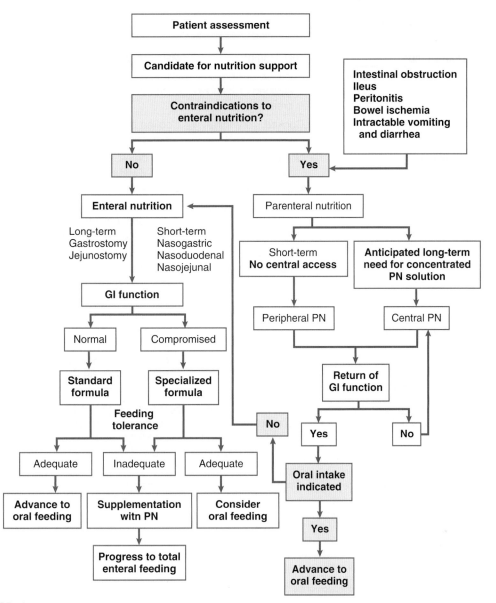

FIGURE 22-1 Route of administration algorithm for nutrition support. (Reprinted from Ukleja A, et al. Standards for nutrition support: adult hospitalized patients. *Nutr Clin Pract*. 2010;25[4]:403-414.) *PN,* Parenteral nutrition.

tolerated. Table 22-4 summarizes the basic details of routine hospital diets.

Assisted oral feeding. In accordance with the patient's condition, assistance with eating may be needed. Patients should maintain independence as much as possible and health care providers should encourage them to do so with whatever degree of assistance that is necessary. Plate guards or special utensils to facilitate independence are usually welcomed by both the patient and the staff. The staff should try to learn each patient's needs and limitations so that little things (e.g., having the meat precut or the bread buttered before bringing the tray to the bedside) can be done without making the patient feel inadequate or dependent. Box 22-2 provides guidelines for personnel when assistance is needed at meal times.

Assisted feeding times provide a special opportunity for nutrition counseling and support. Important observations can be made during this time. The assistant can closely observe the patient's physical appearance and responses to the foods served, the patient's appetite and tolerance for certain foods, and the meaning of food to the person. These observations help the nurse and the dietitian to adapt the patient's diet to meet any particular individual needs. Helping patients learn more about their own nutrition needs is an important part of personal care. People who understand the role of good food in health (e.g., that it helps them to regain strength and recover from illness) are more likely to accept the diet prescription. Patients also feel more encouraged to maintain sound eating habits after discharge from the hospital as well as to improve their eating habits in general.

Table 22-4   Routine Hospital Diets

FOOD	CLEAR LIQUID*	FULL LIQUID†	MECHANICAL SOFT‡	REGULAR HOUSE DIET
Soup	Clear, fat-free broth; bouillon	Same as clear, plus strained or blended cream soups	Same as clear and full, plus all cream soups	All
Cereal	Not included	Cooked, very-thin, refined cereal	Cooked cereal, corn flakes, rice, noodles, macaroni, and spaghetti	All
Bread	Not included	Not included	White bread, crackers, Melba toast, and Zwieback	All
Protein foods	Not included	Milk, cream, milk drinks, and yogurt	Same as full, plus eggs (not fried), mild cheeses, cottage and cream cheeses, poultry, fish, tender beef, veal, lamb, and liver	All
Vegetables	Not included	Vegetable juices or puréed vegetables	Potatoes: baked, mashed, creamed, steamed, or scalloped; tender, cooked, whole, bland vegetables; fresh lettuce, and tomatoes	All
Fruit and fruit juices	Strained fruit juices as tolerated and flavored fruit drinks	Fruit juices	Same as full, plus cooked fruit: peaches, pears, apple sauce, peeled apricots, and white cherries; ripe peaches, pears, and bananas; orange and grapefruit sections without membrane	All
Desserts and gelatin	Fruit-flavored gelatin, fruit ices, and popsicles	Same as clear, plus sherbet, ice cream, puddings, custard, and frozen yogurt	Same as full, plus plain sponge cakes, plain cookies, plain cake, puddings, and pies made with allowed foods	All
Miscellaneous	Soft drinks as tolerated, coffee, tea, sugar, honey, salt, hard candy, Polycose (Abbott Nutrition, Columbus, Ohio), and residue-free supplements	Same as clear, plus margarine and all supplements	Same as full, plus mild salad dressings	All

*Clear liquids are liquid at room temperature and require minimal digestion. Should be limited to 24 to 48 hours.
†Full liquid diets are usually a stepping stone to a diet with solid food.
‡Mechanically altered diets can vary depending on the condition of the patient. This may include puréed foods, mechanically soft foods, or mechanically advanced diets that focus on foods with high moisture.

Box 22-2   Assisted Oral Feeding Guidelines

- Have the tray securely placed within the patient's sight.
- Sit down beside the bed if this is more comfortable, and make simple conversation or remain silent as the patient's condition indicates. Do not carry on a conversation with another patient or co-worker or engage in any form of mobile phone use; this will make the patient feel excluded.
- Offer small amounts, and do not rush the feeding.
- Allow ample time for a patient to chew and swallow or to rest between mouthfuls.
- Offer liquids between the solids, with a drinking straw if necessary.
- Wipe the patient's mouth with a napkin during and after each meal; or offer a napkin to the patient if he or she is capable of doing this on his or her own.

- Let the patient hold his or her bread if desired and able to do so.
- When feeding a patient who is blind or who has eye dressings, describe the food on the tray so that a mental image helps create a desire to eat. Sometimes the analogy of the face of a clock helps a patient to visualize the position of certain foods on the plate (e.g., indicate that the meat is at 12 o'clock, the potatoes are at 3 o'clock, and so on).
- Warn the patient that soup feels particularly hot when it is taken through a straw.
- Identify each food that is being served beforehand and allow about three bites of each food before moving on to another food.

Enteral Feedings

When a patient cannot tolerate eating food orally but the remaining portions of the GI tract can be used, an alternate form of enteral nutrition (EN) that accesses the GI tract by tube further down provides nutrition support. Enteral tube feedings preserve gut function, they are less invasive, and they are less expensive than parenteral nutrition. Even when patients can only tolerate small feedings enterally, every effort should be made to provide some portion of the day's nutrient needs through the GI tract. Maintaining some level of gut function helps to prevent atrophy of the GI tract. As with all parts of the body, if you do not use it, you lose it.

The most common route of EN is the nasogastric tube, which is inserted through the patient's nasal cavity and down to the stomach. For patients who are at risk for aspiration, reflux, or continual vomiting, a nasoduodenal or nasojejunal tube may be more appropriate (Figure 22-2, A). In both cases, a tube is first inserted through the nose and then passed down the esophagus and into the stomach. It is then passed through the stomach and into the appropriate portion of the small intestine by peristaltic activity or endoscopic or fluoroscopic guidance. Correct placement of the tube is verified by radiography, **auscultation,** or gastric content aspiration. Modern small-bore nasoenteric feeding tubes are made of soft and flexible polyurethane and silicone materials. These feeding tubes

> **auscultation** listening to the sounds of the gastrointestinal tract with a stethoscope.

are relatively comfortable for the patient, and they easily carry the variety of nutrient materials that are available in EN support formulas.

Routes. The patient's disease state, estimated length of enteral therapy, GI anatomy and function, and ability to safely access the GI tract are all important aspects to consider when determining the most appropriate access point for EN. The nasoenteric route is indicated for short-term therapy of 6 weeks or less in many clinical situations. For long-term feedings, however, an enterostomy (i.e., the surgical placement of the tube at progressive points along the GI tract) provides a more comfortable route, as follows (Figure 22-2, B):

- *Esophagostomy:* A cervical esophagostomy is placed at the level of the cervical spine to the side of the neck after head and neck surgeries or traumatic injury. This placement removes the discomfort of the nasal route and enables the entry point to be easily concealed under clothing.
- *Percutaneous endoscopic gastrostomy:* A gastrostomy tube may be surgically placed through the abdominal wall into the stomach if the patient is not at risk for aspiration.
- *Percutaneous endoscopic jejunostomy:* A jejunostomy tube is surgically placed through the abdominal wall and passed through the duodenum into the jejunum. This procedure is indicated for patients with gastroparesis, gastric obstructions, or a history of reflux or aspiration or for those who otherwise cannot tolerate gastric feedings.

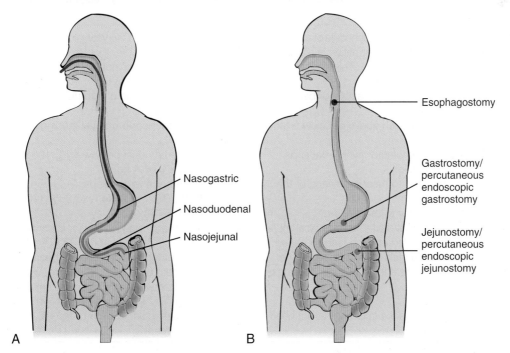

FIGURE 22-2 Types of enteral feeding. **A,** Nonsurgical routes accessed through the nasal cavity. **B,** Surgically placed feeding routes. (Copyright Rolin Graphics.)

Formula. The EN formula is generally prescribed by the physician and the clinical dietitian in accordance with the patient's nutrition needs and tolerance. In addition to the immediate needs of the patient, other considerations include preexisting conditions, co-morbidities, food allergies, food intolerances, and other aspects of nutrient needs that are specific to the patient. Several varieties of commercial formulas are available and designed to meet particular needs. These products may be made from intact nutrients (polymeric formulas) for use with a fully functioning GI system that is capable of digestion and absorption. Others may be made from hydrolyzed elemental or semi-elemental nutrients that are readily absorbed with only minimal residue. Still others may be formulated with single-nutrient modules of protein, carbohydrate, and fat mixed together as calculated by the dietitian to meet a patient's specific needs.

Commercial formulas provide a sterile, homogenized solution that is suitable for small-bore feeding tubes and that ensures a fixed profile of nutrients. With the development of improved formulas and feeding equipment, the question of using blender-mixed formulas of regular foods seldom arises. The use of puréed table food for tube feedings may present the following problems:

- *Physical form:* Foods that are broken down and mixed in a blender yield a sticky, larger-particle mixture that does not pass through the small feeding tubes easily and thus requires the use of the more uncomfortable large-bore tubing.

- *Safety:* Blender-mixed formulas carry problems of bacterial growth and infection as well as inconsistent nutrient composition because the solid components settle out.

- *Digestion and absorption:* Puréed food requires a fully functioning GI system to digest the food and absorb its released nutrients. Many patients have GI deficits that require nutrients with varying degrees of hydrolysis or smaller molecular structure.

Formulas are available in varying caloric densities (e.g., 1 kcal/mL, 1.5 kcal/mL, 2 kcal/mL) to meet a patient's energy needs in a given volume of fluid. Carbohydrates are provided as sucrose, maltodextrins, or corn syrup; protein is provided as casein or whey protein; and fat is usually from soy, canola, corn, or safflower oil, or medium-chain triglycerides as indicated. All formulas are enriched with essential vitamins and minerals. In addition to the standard formulas, there are also "specialty formulas" that are intended to meet the needs of patients with unique requirements. Some examples of specialty formulas include those that are designed for patients with trauma, cancer, human immunodeficiency virus (HIV), renal conditions, and pediatric conditions.

Rate. For any form of EN, the amount of formula and the rate at which it is given must be monitored and regulated. See the Clinical Applications box entitled "Calculating a Tube Feeding" for details about setting the rate of administration for a tube feeding.

Clinical Applications

Calculating a Tube Feeding*

To calculate the nutrient needs and feeding schedule of a patient receiving enteral nutrition, the following information is required:
1. Ideal body weight in kilograms (lb ÷ 2.2). This can be estimated by using the HAMWI formula:
   - Female: 100 lb ± 5 lb for every inch above or below 5 feet
   - Male: 106 lb ± 6 lb for every inch above or below 5 feet
2. Energy needs
   - Basal metabolic rate[†] × Injury factor (which depends on the condition of the patient)
3. The type of formula to be used to meet the needs of the patient
4. Total formula needed for the day to meet energy requirements (energy needs [kcal/day] ÷ formula [kcal/mL])
5. Amount of formula to be provided at each feeding based on the prescribed feeding schedule (total formula for the day ÷ number of feedings or hours for continuous feedings)

CRITICAL THINKING
How many milliliters of formula does the following patient need at each feeding?

- Our patient is a 37-year-old woman who is 5 feet and 7 inches tall.
- She is under considerable catabolic stress, with an injury factor of 1.8.
- The energy value of formula that she will be provided is 1.5 kcal/mL.
- She is to receive 6 equal feedings per day.

Steps:
1. Determine her ideal body weight: 100 lb + (7 in. × 5 lb) = 135 lb/2.2 = 61.4 kg
2. Calculate her energy needs:
   - BMR[†]: (10 × 61.4 kg) + (6.25 × 170.2 cm) − (5 × 37) − 161 = 1332 kcal/day
   - Total energy needs (BMR × injury factor): 1332 kcal/day × 1.8 (injury factor) = 2398 kcal/day
3. The type of formula has already been decided for us and will provide 1.5 kcal/mL. Therefore, we need to calculate the total formula needed to meet her energy needs: 2398 kcal/day ÷ 1.5 kcal/mL = 1599 mL/day
4. Feeding schedule: 1599 mL/day ÷ 6 feedings/day = 266.5 mL/feeding

---

*These equations require the weight in kilograms, the height in centimeters, and the age in years.
[†]As calculated by the Mifflin-St. Jeor equation: female basal metabolic rate = (10 × Weight) + (6.25 × Height) − (5 × Age) − 161; male basal metabolic rate = (10 × Weight) + (6.25 × Height) − (5 × Age) + 5.

Adults who are receiving **bolus feedings** that are introduced into the stomach generally tolerate full-strength formulas from the beginning if they are provided as three to eight feedings per day. The amount given is increased by 60 to 120 mL every 8 to 12 hours until the goal volume for nutrient needs is met. Intermittent feedings may be administered by gravity or with a pump. Typically, intermittent feedings provide 240 to 720 mL of formula infused over a 20-minute to 60-minute period, 4 to 6 times daily. Pump-assisted feedings are used for small-bowel feedings and for critically ill patients to allow for the slower administration of **continuous feedings.** Critically ill patients or those who have not been fed enterally for some time will not be able to tolerate large feedings at initiation and should start with slow rates (10 to 40 mL/hr), with gradual increases to the goal rate (e.g., increase by 10 to 20 mL/hr every 8 to 12 hours).[30] Feeding rates may also be set to administer the formula over a shorter continuous period of time (e.g., 12-hour infusion or 8-hour nocturnal infusion). In the absence of metabolic or systemic complications, the current recommendations are to advance to goal rate within 24 to 48 hours.[27]

Monitoring for complications. Patients given EN require continuous monitoring for appropriate feeding schedules, tolerance, and potential complications. For patients who are fed by tube, diarrhea is the most frequently reported GI complication. A number of factors may contribute to diarrhea in tube-fed patients, such as medications, bacterial overgrowth, infections, or conditions that predispose the patient to diarrhea.[27] Medications and *Clostridium difficile* enterocolitis are common culprits and should be ruled out before further changes are made to the enteral feeding protocol. If the enteral feeding regimen is suspected, some modifications to the type of formula, the rate of infusion, the volume, or the addition of guar gum fiber may improve bowel function and help to reduce the incidence of diarrhea. However, fiber-supplemented formulas are contraindicated for patients with impaired gastric emptying.

No matter what type of feeding tube or formula is used to meet a patient's physiologic needs, this feeding method may contribute to a patient's psychologic stress. Support for a patient's quality of life is an important part of the planning of patient care. Box 22-3 provides guidelines for an ideal monitoring schedule,

---

Box 22-3	Monitoring the Patient Who is Receiving Enteral Nutrition

ANTHROPOMETRICS
- Weight (daily for 3 to 4 days until stable and then at least three times per week)
- Length or height in pediatric patients (monthly)

PHYSICAL ASSESSMENT
- Signs and symptoms of edema (daily)
- Fluid balance (daily)
- Adequacy of enteral intake (at least two times per week)
- GI motility (every 2 to 4 hours during initiation of feedings, every 8 hours when stable)
  - Abdominal distention and discomfort
  - Nausea and vomiting; risk for aspiration
  - Gastric residuals
  - Stool output and consistency
- Tube placement: make sure that the tube is in the desired location (daily for the short term or as needed if there are indications of migration)

BIOCHEMICAL MEASURES
- Glucose (three times daily until stable, then two to three times per week)
- Serum electrolytes (daily until stable, then two to three times per week)
- Blood urea nitrogen (one to two times per week)
- Serum calcium, magnesium, and phosphorus (one to two times per week)
- Complete blood count and transferrin or prealbumin (once a week)

Adapted from Moore MC. *Nutrition Assessment and Care.* 6th ed. St Louis: Mosby; 2009; and Bankhead R, Boullata J, Brantley S, et al. A.S.P.E.N. Board of Directors. Enteral nutrition practice recommendations. *JPEN J Parenter Enteral Nutr.* 2009;33(2):122-167.

---

and Table 22-5 gives problem-solving suggestions for common issues that may be encountered with EN.

Parenteral Feedings

If a patient cannot tolerate or absorb food or formula in the GI tract, alternative methods of nutrition support are necessary. The term *parenteral nutrition* refers to any feeding method other than one that involves the GI route. In current medical terminology, parenteral nutrition (PN) specifically refers to the feeding of nutrients directly into the blood circulation through certain veins (e.g., a peripheral vein in the arm or the subclavian vein) when the GI tract cannot be used. Compared with EN, parenteral feedings are more invasive and expensive, and they introduce more risk. However, for patients in whom part or all of the gastrointestinal system is not functioning, it is necessary. Table 22-3 outlines indications for PN. Depending on the nutrition support necessary, the following two routes are available:
- Peripheral PN is used when a solution of <900 mOsm/L is sufficient to provide nutrient needs and when feeding is necessary for only a brief

---

bolus feeding a volume of feeding from 250 to 500 mL administered by a syringe over a short period of time (usually 10 to 15 minutes) that is given in several feedings per day.

continuous feeding an enteral feeding schedule with which the formula is infused via a pump over a 24-hour period.

Table 22-5	Problem-Solving Tips for Patients Who Are Receiving Enteral Nutrition

PROBLEM	SUGGESTED SOLUTIONS
Thirst and oral dryness	Lubricate the lips
	Chew sugarless gum
	Brush the teeth
	Rinse the mouth frequently
Tube discomfort	Gargle with a mixture of warm water and mouthwash
	Gently blow the nose
	Clean the tube regularly with water or a water-soluble lubricant
	If persistent, gently pull out the tube, clean it, and reinsert it
	Request a smaller tube
Tension and fullness	Relax and breathe deeply after each feeding
Reflux or aspiration	Lift the head of the bed to 30 to 45 degrees
Constipation	Use a fiber-containing formula
	Assess for adequate fluid intake
Diarrhea	Take antidiarrheal medications if bacterial infections have been ruled out
	Avoid excess sorbitol and hypertonic solutions
	Use continuous feedings instead of bolus feedings
	Evaluate for lactose intolerance and intestinal mucosal atrophy
Gustatory Distress*	
General dissatisfaction with feeding	Warm or chill feedings *Caution:* Feedings that are too cold may cause diarrhea
	Serve favorite foods that have been liquefied
Persistent hunger	Chew gum
	Suck hard candy
Inability to drink	Rinse the mouth frequently with water and other liquids

*This refers to the frustration that is experienced when the sense of taste is not satisfied.

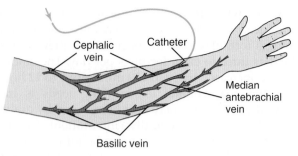

FIGURE 22-3 Peripheral parenteral nutrition feeding into the small veins of the arm.

is needed for longer periods. A large central vein (usually the subclavian vein that leads directly into the rapid flow of the superior vena cava to the heart) is used for the surgical placement of the catheter. The catheter may access the superior vena cava by direct access (Figure 22-4, *A*); a peripherally inserted central catheter (Figure 22-4, *B*); or a tunneled catheter (Figure 22-4, *C*). Nutrition support solutions of high osmolality are tolerated by the central veins.

PN is used in cases of major surgery or complications, especially those that involve the GI tract or when the patient is unable to obtain sufficient nourishment enterally. PN provides crucial nutrition support from solutions that contain glucose, amino acids, electrolytes, vitamins, and minerals. Fat in the form of lipid emulsions from soybean or safflower oil is also used to supply needed energy and the essential fatty acids. A basic PN solution may contain between 3% and 20% crystalline amino acids, 2.5% to 70% dextrose, and 10% to 30% fat emulsions, with additional micronutrients that are specific to patient needs. Each constituent of the parenteral solution contributes to the overall osmolality. Because the peripheral access point has a limited capacity for high osmolality, this must be considered when choosing an appropriate site for access.

A team of specialists including physicians, dietitians, pharmacists, and nurses works closely together during the administration of PN. The physician and the clinical dietitian on the nutrition support team determine the individual formula that is needed on the basis of a detailed individual nutrition assessment and concurrent medication use (see the Drug-Nutrient Interaction box, "Propofol and Lipids in Nutrition Support"). The pharmacist on the nutrition support team mixes the PN solutions in accordance with the prescription. The administration of the solution is an important nursing responsibility (Box 22-4).

The use of either PN or EN must first be discussed with the patient or the patient's family. The use of assisted medical technology in feeding is not always welcomed and may be against the will of the patient for ethical, cultural, religious, or personal reasons. See the Cultural Considerations box entitled "Cultural Differences in Advanced Care Planning" for more information.

period of 10 to 14 days or less or as a supplement to enteral feedings. The osmolality (i.e., mOsm/L) of a solution depends on the concentration of its total particles, including dextrose, protein, and electrolytes. Small peripheral veins, usually in the arm, are used to deliver the less-concentrated solutions (Figure 22-3). Some catheters allow for an extended feeding period in a peripheral vein for individuals with large veins who can tolerate the extended dwell catheter.

- Central PN is used when the energy and nutrient requirement is large or when full nutrition support

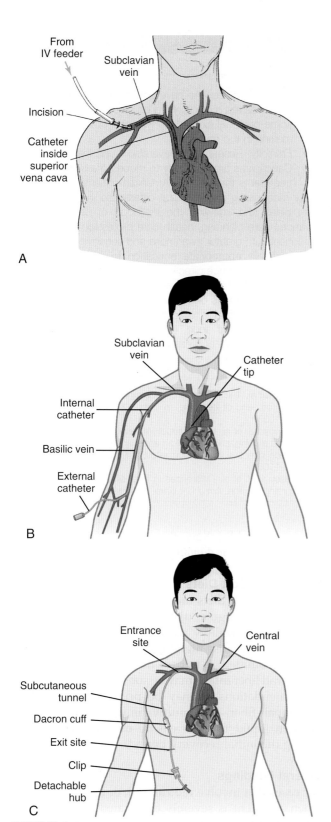

FIGURE 22-4 Catheter placement for parenteral nutrition. **A,** A direct line via the subclavian vein to the superior vena cava. **B,** A peripherally inserted central catheter line. **C,** A tunneled catheter.

Box 22-4	The Administration of Parenteral Nutrition Formulas

The careful administration of parenteral nutrition formulas is essential. The physician will make the decision regarding the most appropriate access point for parenteral nutrition for the patient. Specific protocols will vary but generally include the following points:

- *Ensure proper access.* Make sure that the proper route for access is in place and has been verified.
- *Start slowly.* Optimize fluid and electrolyte status and glycemic control before beginning infusion. Allow time for the patient to adapt to the increased glucose concentration and osmolality of the solution.
- *Schedule carefully and increase volume gradually.* The goal rate of administration should be reached within 72 to 96 hours of initiating parenteral nutrition.
- *Monitor closely.* Note the metabolic effects of glucose and electrolytes. Both hyperglycemia and hypoglycemia present complications. The blood glucose goal for critically ill adult patients is between 140 and 180 mg/dL.
- *Make changes cautiously.* Watch for the effect of all changes, and proceed slowly.
- *Maintain a constant rate.* Keep the correct hourly infusion rate, with no "catch up" or "slow down" efforts made to meet the original volume order.
- *Discontinue slowly.* Take the patient off of the parenteral nutrition feeding by reducing the rate and daily volume gradually. Patients may be given dextrose 10% to help them adjust to lower glucose levels or may be started on enteral feedings simultaneously.

Drug-Nutrient Interaction

Propofol and Lipids in Nutrition Support

KELLI BOI

Propofol is a drug that is often used for sedation and anesthesia during surgery or to maintain sedation in mechanically ventilated patients in the intensive care unit. The drug is fat soluble, and it is emulsified in an oil and water solution for intravenous administration. During long-term sedation, patients often receive nutrition support in the form of enteral or parenteral nutrition. One important consideration for the nutrition support team is the concurrent administration of propofol because the lipid emulsion contributes 1.1 kcal/mL. Therefore, enteral or parenteral nutrition solutions must provide reduced calories from fat to compensate for those that are provided with the propofol.

Propofol and other intravenous lipid emulsions are designed like chylomicrons. They are cleared from the bloodstream by the same enzyme/lipoprotein lipase ratio. Elevated serum triglyceride levels may result if the infusion rate of propofol exceeds the clearance rate. This is more likely to occur with long-term use of propofol when other risk factors are present (e.g., advanced age, cardiovascular disease, renal failure) or when the overall amount of lipids provided exceeds the patient's needs. Serum triglyceride levels should be monitored during propofol infusion to prevent hypertriglyceridemia.

Cultural Differences in Advanced Care Planning

JENNIFER E. SCHMIDT

Advanced care planning is the process by which the future treatment of a patient is determined before it is needed. Advance directives and living wills are examples of documents that are recognized in the United States by all health care institutions. The Patient Self-Determination Act of 1991 was intended to promote the use of advanced care procedures and to strengthen the rights of patients during end-of-life medical procedures. Such documents are the best way that the treatment preferences of the patient can be carried out during times of unconsciousness or when there is otherwise an inability to communicate.

Some consider enteral and parenteral nutrition support to be a life-sustaining intervention that is not welcomed. Studies suggest that significant differences exist among various racial and ethnic patients and their caregivers with regard to advanced care planning and end-of-life decisions. When demographic values are examined, several factors are related to the completion of a living will, a do-not-resuscitate order, or orders that address the removal of life support. These values include the following[1-3]:

- *Gender:* Females are more likely than males to complete advance directives.
- *Education:* Individuals with at least a high school education are more likely to have completed an advance directive.
- *Religion:* Individuals with a religious affiliation are more likely to have end-of-life preferences or a living will.

- *Age:* Individuals who have completed advance directives are more likely to be older and have had some personal experience with end-of-life decision making in the past.
- *Ethnicity:* Researchers have also found that Caucasians are less likely to request life-supportive treatments than African-American patients.

By recognizing such cultural differences in desired treatment plans and knowing the likelihood of patients having advanced care planning, health care professionals can assist the patient with greater awareness and sensitivity and provide more culturally appropriate education to patients and their families about advance directives, living wills, and all methods of life support that may be available. Even if the patient has verbally expressed his or her wishes to the family, sometimes family members find it difficult to follow through with the patient's wishes. Advanced care planning can alleviate the burden on the family and ensure that the patient's wishes are known and honored.

REFERENCES

1. Muni S, et al. The influence of race/ethnicity and socioeconomic status on end-of-life care in the ICU. *Chest.* 2011;139(5): 1025-1033.
2. Van Scoy LJ, et al. Family structure, experiences with end-of-life decision making, and who asked about advance directives impacts advance directive completion rates. *J Palliat Med.* 2014;17(10): 1099-1106.
3. Johnson RW, et al. Differences in level of care at the end of life according to race. *Am J Crit Care.* 2010;19(4):335-343, quiz 344.

SPECIAL NUTRITION NEEDS AFTER GASTROINTESTINAL SURGERY

Because the GI system is uniquely designed to handle food, a surgical procedure on any part of this system requires special dietary attention and possibly nutrient modification.

MOUTH, THROAT, AND NECK SURGERY

Surgery that involves the mouth, jaw, throat, or neck may require modification with regard to the mode of eating. These patients usually cannot chew or swallow normally, so accommodations must be made to address individual limitations. The ultimate goals are to promote healing, prevent nutrient deficiencies, and minimize complications such as malabsorption, maldigestion, and dysphagia.[27]

Oral Liquid Feedings

If patients are able to drink and swallow without complication or undue stress, a concentrated liquid formula may be provided to ensure that adequate nutrition is supplied. An enriched commercial formula can be used several times a day to supply needed nourishment. For patients who have had an esophagectomy, they may be at risk for dumping syndrome, in which case liquid feedings are not recommended. These

patients should follow the same recommendations covered below for *dumping syndrome*.

Mechanical Soft Diets

Mechanical soft diets are used to transition between full-liquid and regular diets. Whole foods that are easy to chew and swallow are included as tolerated (see Table 22-4). Because high-fiber foods (e.g., vegetables) are often omitted as part of the mechanical soft diet, the overall fiber intake may be substantially lower than recommendations. It may be prudent to provide a functional fiber and multivitamin/mineral supplement in liquid form to ensure micronutrient intake during the initial recovery period.

Enteral Feedings

For cases that involve radical neck or facial surgery or when a patient is severely debilitated, tube feedings may be indicated. For long-term needs, improved equipment and standardized commercial formulas have made continued home EN through tube feeding possible for many patients. A nasogastric tube is often used, but an obstruction of the esophagus or other complications may require the surgeon to make a gastrostomy access point. As with any patient in need of EN, the earliest functioning point of access to the GI tract should be used to maintain gut integrity from that point onward. In other words, if the esophagus and stomach are working properly, it is contraindicated to bypass these parts of the GI tract and access the small intestine instead.

GASTRIC SURGERY
Nutrition Problems
Because the stomach is the first major food reservoir in the GI tract, gastric surgery poses special problems for the maintenance of adequate nutrition. Some of these problems may develop immediately after the surgery, depending on the type of surgical procedure and the individual patient's response. Other physical or malabsorption complications may occur later, when the person begins to eat a regular diet. Refer back to Chapter 5 to review the digestive processes that take place in the stomach. The goals of nutrition therapy are to promote healing, to prevent dumping syndrome and nutrient deficiency, and to minimize complications such as malabsorption and maldigestion. Multivitamin/mineral supplements in liquid form, vitamin B_{12} injections, and functional fiber may be warranted to maintain nutrient balance.[27]

Gastrectomy
Serious nutritional deficits may occur after a gastrectomy. Increased gastric fullness and distention may result if the gastric resection also involved a **vagotomy**. Because it lacks the normal nerve stimulus, the stomach becomes **atonic** and empties poorly. Food fermentation occurs, and this produces discomfort, gas, and diarrhea. Weight loss is common after extensive gastric surgery.

To cover the immediate postoperative nutrition needs after a gastrectomy procedure, surgeons may prepare a jejunostomy through which the patient can be fed an elemental formula. Frequent small oral feedings are resumed in accordance with the patient's tolerance. A typical pattern of simple dietary progression may cover several weeks. The basic principles of such diet therapy for the immediate postgastrectomy period involve both the size of the meals (which should be small and frequent) and the nature of the meals (which are generally simple, easily digested, bland, and low in bulk).

Dumping Syndrome
Dumping syndrome is the most frequently encountered complication subsequent to extensive gastric resection. After the initial recovery from surgery, when the patient begins to feel better and eats a regular diet in greater volume and variety, discomfort may occur

vagotomy the cutting of the vagus nerve, which supplies a major stimulus for gastric secretions.
atonic without normal muscle tone.

10 to 20 minutes after meals with *early-onset dumping syndrome*. A cramping and full feeling develops, the pulse rate becomes rapid, and a wave of weakness, cold sweating, and dizziness may follow. Abdominal pain and diarrhea terminate the event. For patients with *intermediate dumping syndrome*, symptoms begin within 20 to 30 minutes after eating; and for patients experiencing *late-onset dumping syndrome*, the symptoms begin 1 to 3 hours following a meal.

This multifaceted condition constitutes a shock syndrome that results when a meal containing a large proportion of readily soluble carbohydrates rapidly enters or "dumps" into the small intestine. When the stomach is bypassed, food quickly passes from the esophagus into the small intestine. This rapidly entering food mass is a concentrated solution with a higher osmolality compared with the surrounding circulation of blood. To achieve osmotic balance (i.e., a state of equal concentrations of fluids within the small intestine and the surrounding blood circulation), water is drawn from the circulatory system into the intestine. This water shift rapidly shrinks the vascular fluid volume, thereby causing shock. Blood pressure drops, and signs of rapid heart rate to rebuild the blood volume appear; these include a rapid pulse rate, sweating, weakness, and tremors.

If the meal consisted of simple carbohydrates, late dumping may occur approximately 2 hours after eating. The initial concentrated solution of simple carbohydrate has been rapidly absorbed, which results in a rapid rise in blood glucose level and stimulates an overproduction of insulin. Blood sugar level eventually drops below normal, with symptoms of hypoglycemia (e.g., weakness, shaky, sweating, confusion). These distressing reactions to food increase anxiety. As a result, less and less food is eaten. Weight loss and general malnutrition may follow.

Careful adherence to the postoperative diet allows dramatic relief from these distressing symptoms. Patients may also find that eating slowly, eliminating fluids during meals, and lying down for 15 to 30 minutes after eating help to decrease the rate of gastric emptying (see the Clinical Applications box "Case Study: John Has a Gastrectomy").

BARIATRIC SURGERY
Special considerations must be made after bariatric surgery; because patients are at high risk for deficiencies in several micronutrients for an extended period (see the For Further Focus box "Nutrient Deficiencies after Bariatric Surgery"). After gastric bypass, patients progress slowly from a clear liquid diet to a regular diet at approximately 6 weeks after surgery, but they are generally limited to approximately 1 cup of food per meal from that point forward, and they are subject to dumping syndrome.[31] Patients should avoid using a straw to reduce air swallowing, which can cause

Clinical Applications

Case Study: John Has a Gastrectomy

After a long experience with persistent peptic ulcer disease that involved more and more gastric tissue, John and his physician decided that surgery was needed. John then entered the hospital for a total gastrectomy. John weathered the surgery well and received some initial nutrition support from an elemental formula fed through a tube that the surgeon had placed into his jejunum. After a few days, the tube was removed. Over the next 2-week period, John was gradually able to tolerate a soft diet in small oral feedings. He soon recovered enough to go home, and he gradually felt his strength returning. He was relieved to be free of his former ulcer pain, and he began to resume more and more of his usual activities, including eating a regular diet of increasing volume and variety.

However, as time went by, John began having more discomfort after meals. He felt a cramping sensation, an increased heartbeat, and then a wave of weakness with sweating and dizziness. John would often become nauseated and have diarrhea. As his anxiety increased, he began to eat less and less, and his weight began to drop. He was soon in a state of general malnutrition.

John finally sought medical help. The physician and the clinical dietitian outlined necessary changes in his eating habits, and a specialized food plan was developed for him. John followed the new diet plan faithfully because he had felt so ill. To his surprise, he soon found that his previous symptoms after eating had almost completely disappeared. His weight gradually returned to normal, and his state of nutrition markedly improved. John found that he always felt better if he would nibble on food items throughout the day rather than consume large meals as he did in the past.

QUESTIONS FOR ANALYSIS

1. What were John's nutrition needs immediately after surgery and for the next 2 weeks?
2. Why did his feedings need to be resumed cautiously?
3. Why is emphasis given to postsurgical protein sources? How should this nutrient be provided?
4. After John recovered from surgery and resumed eating, why did he become ill? Describe why his symptoms developed.
5. Using the principles of diet management for dumping syndrome, plan a day's meal and snack pattern for John that includes basic instructions and suggestions that you would discuss with him.

For Further Focus

Nutrient Deficiencies after Bariatric Surgery

Bariatric surgery for obese patients is becoming more common around the world. Bariatric surgery is effective for weight loss and maintenance, but it is not without drawbacks. Restrictive eating patterns, dumping syndrome, and nutrient deficiencies from malabsorption are common complications after bariatric surgery. The quality-of-life cost-benefit ratio of surgery is difficult to assess. While obesity increases the morbidity and mortality rates, the complications of surgery can introduce a new set of risks.

The Roux-en-Y gastric bypass procedure (see Chapter 15), in which the amount of bowel that is capable of absorbing nutrients is reduced, is the surgery of choice for obesity in the United States. Obese patients are at risk for complications during surgery from co-morbid conditions such as diseases of the cardiovascular, endocrine, renal, pulmonary, gastrointestinal, and musculoskeletal systems. Therefore, special care must be taken to prepare the patient for surgery.

Bariatric surgery that induces malabsorption (e.g., gastric bypass, biliopancreatic diversion) presents particular nutritional problems. Protein-energy malnutrition is a significant risk for many patients, and it may result in hospitalization and the necessity of nutrition support in severe cases. In addition, micronutrient deficiencies from limited intake and malabsorption warrant multivitamin/mineral supplementation postoperatively for life. The nutrients at risk for deficiency are highly dependent upon the form of bariatric surgery performed. Specific nutrients of concern include the following[1,2]:

- Vitamins: A, B_1, B_6, B_{12}, C, D, E, K, and folate
- Minerals: calcium, copper, iron, selenium, and zinc

Patients who have undergone bariatric procedures should have follow-up appointments with a registered dietitian nutritionist to be screened for dietary adequacy. It is recommended that bariatric patients take the following supplements daily following surgery: 2 multivitamin/mineral supplements with iron; calcium citrate (1200 to 1500 mg/day); and vitamin D (3000 IU/day). These supplements should be in chewable or liquid form for the first couple of months following surgery. In addition, patients should take a sublingual vitamin B_{12} supplement (350 to 500 mcg/day) or receive a monthly injection of 1000 mcg.[3]

REFERENCES

1. Fujioka K, DiBaise JK, Martindale RG. Nutrition and metabolic complications after bariatric surgery and their treatment. *JPEN J Parenter Enteral Nutr.* 2011;35(5 suppl):52S-59S.
2. Strohmayer E, Via MA, Yanagisawa R. Metabolic management following bariatric surgery. *Mt Sinai J Med.* 2010;77(5):431-445.
3. Mechanick JI, et al. Clinical practice guidelines for the perioperative nutritional, metabolic, and nonsurgical support of the bariatric surgery patient—2013 update: cosponsored by American Association of Clinical Endocrinologists, the Obesity Society, and American Society for Metabolic & Bariatric Surgery. *Surg Obes Relat Dis.* 2013;9(2):159-191.

discomfort. The combination of severely reduced intake coupled with dumping syndrome dramatically reduces nutrient availability.[32] The specific guidelines for dietary advancement after bariatric surgery are individualized to the type of surgery performed.

As with other forms of gastric surgeries, adherence to the postoperative diet should provide relief from difficult symptoms as well as the gradual stabilization of weight. The careful reintroduction of milk in small amounts may later be used to test tolerance. Various forms of bariatric surgery are discussed further in Chapter 15.

GALLBLADDER SURGERY

For patients with acute gallbladder inflammation (i.e., cholecystitis) or gallstones (i.e., cholelithiasis) (Figure 22-5), the treatment is usually cholecystectomy (see Chapter 18). The modern procedure for this removal, called *laparoscopic cholecystectomy,* requires only minimal surgery that involves small skin punctures; the previous surgery required a transverse right upper quadrant incision. Through these small openings, the surgeon can insert needed instruments and a laparoscope fitted with a miniature camera and bright fiber-optic lighting.

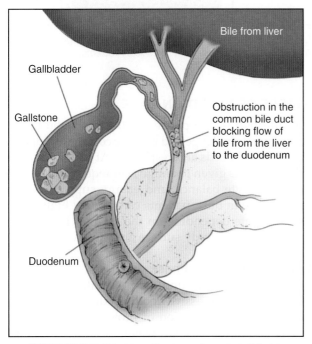

FIGURE 22-5 Gallbladder with stones (i.e., cholelithiasis).

Because the function of the gallbladder is to concentrate and store bile, which helps with the digestion and absorption of fat, some moderation in dietary fat intake is usually indicated. After surgery, the control of fat in the diet (e.g., less than 30% of total energy intake as fat) facilitates wound healing and comfort,[27] because the hormonal stimulus for bile secretion still functions in the surgical area, thereby causing pain with the high intake of fatty foods. The body also needs a period to adjust to the more dilute supply of bile that is available to assist with fat digestion and absorption directly from the liver; see the low-fat diet guide given for gallbladder disease in Table 18-6.

INTESTINAL SURGERY

Intestinal disease that involves tumors, lesions, or obstructions may require the surgical resection of the affected intestinal area. For complicated cases that require the removal of large sections of the small intestine, the use of EN support may be difficult at first. In such cases, PN is used for nutrition support, with a small allowance of oral feeding for personal food desires when tolerated. After general resection for less severe cases, a diet that is relatively low in dietary fiber may be beneficial in the beginning to allow for healing and comfort.

Intestinal surgery involving the latter portions of the GI tract sometimes requires making an opening in the abdominal wall to the intestine, called a *stoma,* for the elimination of fecal waste. If the opening is in the area of the ileum, which is the last section of the small intestine, it is called an *ileostomy* (Figure 22-6, *A*). The food mass is still fairly liquid at this point in the GI tract, and more problems are encountered with management. If the opening is farther along in the large intestine, it is called a *colostomy* (Figure 22-6, *B*). In the large intestine, the water is predominantly reabsorbed and the remaining feces are more solid, thereby making management easier. Patients with an ostomy begin a

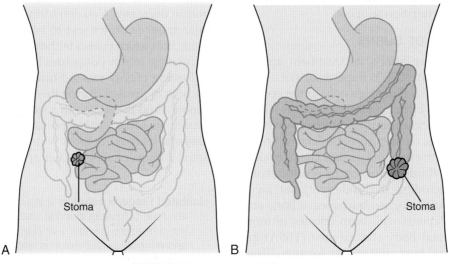

FIGURE 22-6 A, Ileostomy. **B,** Colostomy.

clear liquid diet during the immediate postoperative period. Patients progress toward small, frequent feedings of meals that are relatively low in dietary fiber, as tolerated.[27] Encouraging patients to limit fluids with meals and instead drink adequate fluids between meals may help to reduce diarrhea. Lactose intolerance and fat malabsorption are common complications in patients with ileostomies and should be monitored, with dietary adjustments made as indicated.

Patients need support and practical help with learning about self-care for an ostomy. Eliminating gas-producing foods, odor-causing foods, and foods that may cause an obstruction will help to facilitate maintenance. The goal is to advance to an individualized diet that is acceptable to the patient as soon as tolerated. Progression to a regular diet is important for nutritional value and emotional support. Regular food provides psychologic comfort, and dietary adjustments to individual preferences for specific foods can be made.

RECTAL SURGERY

For a brief period after rectal surgery or hemorrhoidectomy, a clear fluid or fiber-restricted diet (see Table 22-2) may be indicated to reduce painful elimination and to allow for healing. In some cases, a nonresidue commercial elemental formula may be used to delay bowel movements until the surgical area has healed. Return to a regular diet is usually rapid.

SPECIAL NUTRITION NEEDS FOR PATIENTS WITH BURNS

In the United States, there are approximately 450,000 visits to emergency departments and 3400 deaths per year as a result of burn injuries.[33] The treatment of severe burns presents a tremendous nutrition challenge. The location and severity of the burn will greatly affect the prognosis and plan of care for the patient. Co-morbidities and other injuries complicate care, but they must be considered when deciding when, where, and how to initiate nutrition support.

TYPE AND EXTENT OF BURNS

The depth of the burn affects its treatment and its healing process (Figure 22-7). Superficial (i.e., first-degree) burns involve cell damage only to the epidermis. Second-degree burns are classified as either superficial partial-thickness burns, which involve cell damage to the dermis, or deep partial-thickness burns, which involve both the first and second layers of skin. Full-thickness (i.e., third-degree) burns result in complete skin loss, including the underlying fat layer. Subdermal (i.e., fourth-degree) burns leave bone and tendon exposed. Patients with burn injuries of more than 10% of the total body surface area (TBSA) are referred to a regional burn unit facility for specialized burn team care that includes nutrition support.

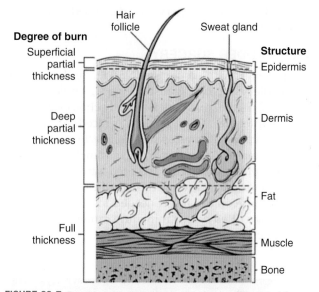

FIGURE 22-7 Depth of skin area involved in burns. (Reprinted from Lewis SM, Heitkemper MM, Dirksen SR. *Medical-Surgical Nursing: Assessment and Management of Clinical Problems*. 7th ed. St Louis: Mosby; 2007.)

STAGES OF NUTRITION CARE

The nutrition care of patients with massive burns presents a great challenge and must be constantly adjusted to individual needs and responses. At each stage, critical attention is given to amino acid requirements, fluid and electrolyte balance, and energy support. Energy expenditure in burn patients can be very high, and it will fluctuate depending on the stage of healing and the extent of the body surface area involved.

Burn Shock or Ebb Phase

From the first hours until approximately the second day after a burn, massive flooding edema occurs at the burn site. The destruction of protective skin leads to immediate losses of heat, water, electrolytes (mainly sodium), and protein. As water is drawn from surrounding blood to replace the losses, general loss continues, blood volume and pressure drop, and urine output decreases. Cell dehydration follows as intracellular water is drawn out to balance the loss of tissue fluid. Potassium is also withdrawn from the cells, and circulating serum potassium levels rise.

Resting energy expenditure and body temperature are both depressed during this phase. Immediate intravenous fluid therapy with a salt solution (e.g., 6% hetastarch in saline, balanced salt solution) or **lactated Ringer's solution** replaces water and electrolytes and helps to prevent shock. After approximately 12 hours,

---

lactated Ringer's solution a sterile solution of calcium chloride, potassium chloride, sodium chloride, and sodium lactate in water that is given to replenish fluid and electrolytes; this solution was developed by the English physiologist Sidney Ringer (1835-1910).

when vascular permeability returns to normal and losses begin to decrease at the burn site, albumin solutions or plasma can be used to help restore blood volume. The stability of the patient and his or her resuscitation needs are great during this phase and must be established before nutrition efforts are considered. However, metabolic needs should be addressed and ideally nutrition support would be initiated within 12 hours of injury, preferably by the enteral route. The motility of the gut is reduced in some severely burned patients. In such cases, introducing enteral feedings into the small intestine is indicated.[34]

Acute or Flow Phase

After approximately 48 to 72 hours, tissue fluids and electrolytes are gradually reabsorbed, and the pattern of massive tissue loss is stabilized. A sudden diuresis occurs, and this indicates successful initial therapy. Constant attention to fluid intake and output with evaluation for any signs of dehydration or overhydration is essential. Toward the end of the first week after the injury, adequate bowel function usually returns. This flow phase of hypermetabolism may last weeks to months. The following three major reasons exist for these increased nutrient and energy demands:

1. Tissue destruction brings large losses of protein and electrolytes that must be replaced.
2. Tissue catabolism follows the injury and involves a further loss of lean body mass and nitrogen.
3. Increased metabolism brings added nutrition needs to cover the energy costs of infection, fever, and the increased protein metabolism of tissue replacement and skin grafting.

Medical Nutrition Therapy

Most patients with burns of less than 20% of the TBSA are able to consume an oral meal plan that is adequate in nutrient needs, unless the burn site hinders eating. Successful nutrition therapy during this critical feeding period is based on vigorous protein and energy intake as follows[27,34]:

- *High energy:* Individual energy needs will vary greatly among patients and should be calculated with the most precise method available, ideally indirect calorimetry (see Chapter 6). If indirect calorimetry is not available, energy needs should be calculated according to the equations provided in Table 22-6.
- High energy needs are necessary to spare the protein that is essential for tissue rebuilding and to supply the greatly increased metabolic demands of the whole body. Approximately 55% to 60% of the total kilocalories should come from carbohydrates along with a moderate amount of fat (<35% of kcal). Overfeeding increases metabolic stress and should be avoided. The frequent recalculation of energy needs may be necessary if the patient is gaining or losing weight. One goal of MNT is for patients to

Table 22-6	Estimated Energy Needs for Burn Patients	
	EQUATION	**FORMULA**
Adults	Toronto	kcal/day = −4343 + 10.5 × %TBSA + 0.23 × previous 24 hours' caloric intake + 0.84 × Harris-Benedict equation + 114 × previous 24 hours' maximal temperature − 4.5 × days post-burn injury
Girls 3-10 yr	Shofield	kcal/day = (16.97 × weight in kg) + (1.618 × height in cm) + 371.2
Boys 3-10 yr	Shofield	kcal/day = (19.6 × weight in kg) + (1.033 × height in cm) + 414.9
Girls 10-18 yr	Shofield	kcal/day = (8.365 × weight in kg) + (4.65 × height in cm) + 200
Boys 10-18 yr	Shofield	kcal/day = (16.25 × weight in kg) + (1.372 × height in cm) + 515.5

Reference: Rousseau AF, et al. ESPEN endorsed recommendations: nutritional therapy in major burns. *Clin Nutr.* 2013;32(4):497-502.

not lose more than 10% of their body weight from the point of admission.
- *High protein:* The aggressive supplementation of protein is crucial to promote early wound healing and to support immune function. Depending on the extent of the burn and the associated catabolic losses, individual protein needs vary from 1.5 to 2 g/kg/day in adults and from 1.5 to 3 g/kg/day in children. This level of protein will equal 20% to 25% of energy intake. For obese individuals or patients with burns that cover less than 10% of the TBSA, protein intake is calculated at 1.2 g/kg.
- *High vitamin, high mineral:* Increased vitamin C (500 mg/day) may be needed as a partner with amino acids for tissue rebuilding. Vitamin A (10,000 IU/day) and zinc are specifically important for optimal immune function, and they are often supplemented. Increased thiamin, riboflavin, and niacin are necessary for increased energy and protein metabolism. Special attention to electrolyte imbalances and to calcium to phosphorus ratios in the blood are warranted during this period. Patients are given a daily multivitamin supplement.

Dietary management. With any method, a careful dietary intake record must be maintained to measure progress toward the increased nutrition goals. Oral feedings are preferred if they are well tolerated and if they allow nutrition needs to be met. Concentrated liquids with added protein or amino acids and commercial formulas such as Ensure may be used as added interval nourishment. Solid foods given on the basis of individual preferences are usually tolerated by the second week. However, hypermetabolic states, pain, and poor appetite make oral feedings difficult for patients with major burns.

Either enteral or parenteral methods of feeding may be used to meet crucial nutrient demands when oral intake is inadequate, which is defined as less than 75% of goal intake for more than 3 days. When enteral feedings are impossible because of associated injuries or complications, parenteral feeding can provide essential nutrition support. Studies evaluating early versus delayed EN support indicate that initiating nutrition support soon after the burn injury (e.g., as early as 6 to 12 hours after injury) is effective and safe, stimulates protein retention, and reduces the hypermetabolic response, stress hormones, risk of infection, and length of hospital stay.[34-37]

Follow-up reconstruction. Continued nutrition support is essential to maintain tissue strength for successful skin grafting or reconstructive plastic surgery. Patients need the physical rebuilding of body resources that surgery requires as well as personal support to rebuild their will and spirit, because disfigurement and disability are quite possible. Optimal physical stamina that is gained through persistent and supportive medical, nutrition, and nursing care helps patients to rebuild the personal resources that they need to cope.

Putting It All Together

Summary

- Before surgery, the goals are to correct any existing deficiencies and to build nutrition reserves to meet surgical demands. After surgery, the goals are to replace losses and to support recovery. The additional task of encouraging eating is often necessary during this period of healing.
- Postsurgical feedings are given in a variety of ways, and the oral route is always preferred. However, the inability to eat or damage to the intestinal tract may require enteral tube feedings or parenteral feedings. Special formulas are used for such alternate means of nourishment, and these are designed to meet individual needs.
- For patients who are undergoing surgery of the GI tract, special diets are modified in accordance with the surgical procedure being performed.
- For patients with severe burns, increased nutrition support is necessary in successive stages in response to the burn injury and to the continuing requirements of tissue rebuilding.

Chapter Review Questions

See answers in Appendix A.

1. Edema may indicate inadequate intake of:
   a. Sodium.
   b. Potassium.
   c. Dietary fiber.
   d. Protein.

2. Parenteral nutrition support is most appropriate for a patient with:
   a. Short-bowel syndrome.
   b. Failure to thrive.
   c. Facial trauma.
   d. Comatose state.

3. Patients receiving tube feedings who have a fully functioning GI system may have improved bowel function and less diarrhea if they are given an enteral formula that is:
   a. Fiber-supplemented.
   b. High in protein.
   c. Hydrolyzed elemental.
   d. Semi-elemental.

4. If patients have undergone gastric resection for treatment of gastric cancer, they would be most likely to experience dumping syndrome if they ate:
   a. String cheese.
   b. Peanuts.
   c. Cupcakes.
   d. Bacon.

5. Medical nutrition therapy during the acute or flow phase of recovering from a large burn for a patient consists of feedings that are:
   a. High protein, high calorie.
   b. High protein, low carbohydrate.
   c. High protein, low calorie.
   d. Low protein, high calorie.

Additional Learning Resources

evolve Please refer to this text's Evolve website for answers to the Case Study Questions.
http://evolve.elsevier.com/Williams/basic/

References and **Further Reading and Resources** in the back of the book provide additional resources for enhancing knowledge.

Nutrition Support in Cancer and HIV

Key Concepts

- Environmental agents, genetic factors, and weaknesses in the body's immune system can contribute to the development of cancer.
- The strength of the body's immune system is influenced by its overall nutritional status.
- Nutrition problems affect the nature of the disease process and the medical treatment methods for

patients with cancer or human immunodeficiency virus (HIV).
- The progressive effects of HIV to the final stage of acquired immunodeficiency syndrome (AIDS) have many nutrition implications and often require aggressive medical nutrition therapy.

Cancer continues to be a prevalent cause for morbidity and mortality in the United States. Because cancer is generally associated with aging, increases in life expectancy contribute to this growing incidence. Although cancer and HIV/AIDS share a direct relationship with the body's immune system and basic nutrition needs, their courses and outcomes are distinct.

This chapter looks at nutrition support in relation to both cancer and HIV/AIDS. Both diseases have important nutrition connections for prevention and therapy.

SECTION I CANCER

PROCESS OF CANCER DEVELOPMENT

THE NATURE OF CANCER

One of the difficulties with the study and treatment of cancer is that it is not a single problem: it has a highly variable nature, and it expresses itself in multiple forms. Cancer is the second leading cause of death in the United States. It is responsible for 23% of all deaths, whereas cardiovascular disease causes 24% of all deaths in the United States.[1] The general term *cancer* is used to designate a malignant tumor or **neoplasm.** The many forms of cancer vary in prevalence worldwide and change as populations migrate to different environments. The Cultural Considerations box entitled "Types and Incidence of Cancer in American Populations" outlines the prevalence of cancer in the United States relative to race/ethnicity and socioeconomic characteristics.

The continuous process of cell division is guided by the genetic code that is contained in the deoxyribonucleic acid (DNA) of the cell nucleus. This orderly process can be lost as the result of a **mutation,** particularly when the mutation occurs in a regulatory

gene. Growth of a mutated cell may form a malignant tumor when normal gene control is lost. Thus, the misguided cell and its tumor tissue represent normal cell growth that has gone wrong. Malignancies are identified by their primary site of origin, their stage or tumor size, the presence of **metastasis,** and their grade (i.e., how aggressive the tumor is).

Carcinogenesis is often described as having three phases: initiation, promotion, and progression. *Initiation* is the point at which a mutagen causes irreversible damage to the DNA. *Promotion* is caused by an agent that triggers the mutated cell to grow and reproduce. *Progression* is the phase during which the cancer cells advance and become a malignant tumor that is capable of metastasizing.

CAUSES OF CANCER CELL DEVELOPMENT

The underlying cause of cancer is the fundamental loss of cell control over normal cell reproduction. Several factors may contribute to this loss and change a normal cell into a cancer cell, including chemical carcinogens, radiation, oncogenic viruses, epidemiologic factors (e.g., race, region, age, heredity, occupation), psychologic stress, and dietary factors. As such, many aspects of cancer are outside of the scope of this text and will not be addressed in detail here. The discussion here will focus on the nutritional aspects of cancer development and treatment.

---

neoplasm any new or abnormal cellular growth, specifically one that is uncontrolled and aggressive.
mutation a permanent transmissible change in a gene.
metastasis the spread to other tissue.
carcinogenesis the development of cancer.

Cultural Considerations

Types and Incidence of Cancer in American Populations

The prevalence of cancer at any given time has many variables. The National Center for Health Statistics has reported the prevalence of cancer by race/ethnicity and family income as such[1]:

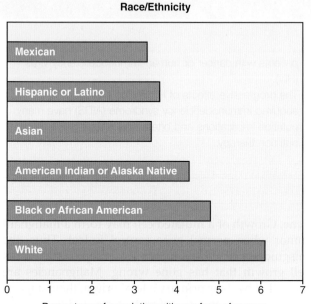

Race/Ethnicity

Mexican
Hispanic or Latino
Asian
American Indian or Alaska Native
Black or African American
White

Percentage of population with any form of cancer, aged 18 years old and older

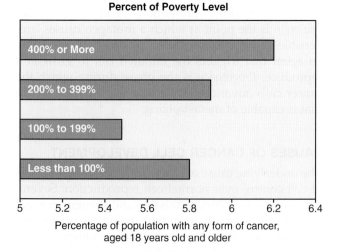

Percent of Poverty Level

400% or More
200% to 399%
100% to 199%
Less than 100%

Percentage of population with any form of cancer, aged 18 years old and older

The confounding factors associated with cancer risk are complicated and multifactorial. A health care trend toward the prevention of cancer is a goal of the *Healthy People 2020* national objectives. With a continued dedication to research, ideally prevention instead of treatment will become the norm. Identifying high-risk patients and encouraging regular physical examinations are important aspects of general health care as well as valuable prevention tools.

REFERENCE

1. National Center for Health Statistics. *Health, United States, 2014: With Special Feature of Adults Aged 55-64.* Hyattsville, Md: U.S. Government Printing Office; 2015.

Dietary Factors

Nutrition and cancer care focus on the following two fundamental areas:

- *Prevention,* in relation to the environment and the body's natural defense system
- *Therapy,* in relation to nutrition support for medical treatment and rehabilitation

The association between diet and cancer is complex. Although it has been the subject of much research, many questions are still unanswered. Foods naturally contain both carcinogenic and anticarcinogenic compounds. Research indicates that there is an increase in cancer risk for individuals who consume diets high in trans fat, and alcohol.[2,3] But there are conflicting results regarding the protective role of specific micronutrients as well as total fruit and vegetable consumption.[4] Some studies show no significant protective role of fruit and vegetable intake with cancer risk[5]; some studies show that fruit intake is more protective than vegetable intake[6]; and some studies show that vegetable intake is more protective against cancer than fruit intake.[7] A general consensus links adequate vitamin and mineral intake (through either food or dietary supplement) with a decreased risk of DNA damage and cancer incidence.[8,9] Thus, a well-balanced diet that includes an ample intake of fruits, vegetables, whole grains, and fiber and limits excess fat and alcohol is the general recommendation for health promotion and disease prevention. Because obesity is associated with several types of cancer,[10,11] diet and lifestyle behaviors should also support and maintain an ideal body weight.

THE BODY'S DEFENSE SYSTEM

The body's defense system is remarkably efficient and complex. Special cells protect the body from external invaders such as bacteria and viruses and from internal aliens such as cancer cells.

Defensive Cells of the Immune System

Two major cell populations provide the immune system's primary "search and destroy" defense for detecting and killing non-self substances that propagate potential disease. These two populations of lymphocytes, which are special types of white blood cells, develop early during life from a common stem cell in the bone marrow. The two types are T cells, which are derived from thymus cells, and B cells, which are derived from bursal intestinal cells (Figure 23-1). A major function of T cells is to activate the phagocytes, which are the cells that destroy invaders and kill disease-carrying **antigens.** A major function

antigen any foreign or non-self substance (e.g., toxins, viruses, bacteria, foreign proteins) that triggers the production of antibodies that are specifically designed to counteract their activity.

of B cells is to produce **antibodies,** which also kill antigens.

Relation of Nutrition to Immunity and Healing

Immunity. Balanced nutrition is necessary to maintain the integrity of the human immune system. Severe malnutrition compromises the capacity of the immune system because of **atrophy** of the organs and tissues that are involved in immunity (e.g., liver, bowel wall, bone marrow, spleen, lymphoid tissue). Nutrition is also fundamental for combating sustained attacks of diseases such as cancer. The core of the immune system is made up of the internally derived antibodies. A direct and simple example of the important role of nutrition in immunity is the link between protein-energy malnutrition and the subsequent suppression of immune function.

Healing. The strength of any body tissue is maintained through the constant building and rebuilding of tissue protein. Strong tissue is a front line of the body's defense. This process of tissue building and healing requires optimal nutrition intake. Specific nutrients that include protein, essential fatty acids, and key vitamins and minerals must be constantly supplied in the diet. The wise and early use of medical nutrition therapy (MNT) for patients with cancer speeds the recovery of nutritional status after surgery; this includes **immunocompetence,** which improves a patient's response to therapy as well as his or her prognosis.[12-14]

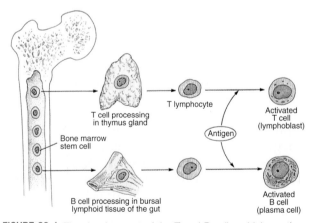

FIGURE 23-1 The development of the T and B cells, which are the lymphocyte components of the body's immune system. (Courtesy Eileen Draper.)

antibodies any of numerous protein molecules produced by B cells as a primary immune defense for attaching to specific related antigens.
atrophy tissue wasting.
immunocompetence the ability or capacity to develop an immune response (i.e., antibody production or cell-mediated immunity) after exposure to an antigen.

NUTRITION COMPLICATIONS OF CANCER TREATMENT

Three major forms of therapy are used today as medical treatment for cancer: surgery, radiation, and chemotherapy. Each requires nutrition support. Drug-nutrient interactions are also a complication that may happen with any form of treatment.

SURGERY

Any surgery requires nutrition support for the healing process (see Chapter 22). This requirement is particularly true for patients with cancer, because their general condition is often weakened by the disease process and its drain on the body's resources. With early diagnosis and sound nutrition support both before and after surgery, many tumors can be successfully removed. Nutrition support has specifically been shown to improve postoperative outcomes and to reduce the complications of patients with cancer of the gastrointestinal tract.[14,15] MNT also includes any needed modifications in food texture or specific nutrients, depending on the site of the surgery or the function of the organ involved. Various methods of nutrition support following surgery are covered in Chapter 22.

RADIATION

Radiation therapy is often used by itself or in conjunction with other treatments. This type of therapy involves treatment with high-energy radiography that is targeted to the cancer site to kill or shrink tumors. Radiation may be administered to the body by an external machine (Figure 23-2) or by implanted radioactive materials at the cancer site. Although the goal is for only the cancer cells to die, other cells within close proximity to the target site and rapidly growing cells often die as well.

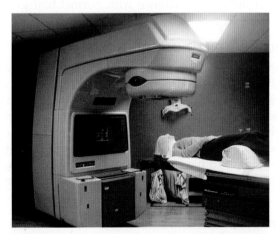

FIGURE 23-2 A radiation treatment machine. (Courtesy Jormain Cady, Virginia Mason Medical Center, Seattle, Wash. In: Lewis SM, Heitkemper MM, Dirksen SR, et al, eds. *Medical-Surgical Nursing: Assessment and Management of Clinical Problems.* 7th ed. St Louis: Mosby; 2007.)

The site and intensity of the radiation treatment determine the nature of the nutrition-related problems that the patient may encounter. For example, radiation of the head, neck, or esophagus affects the oral mucosa and salivary secretions, thereby affecting taste sensations and sensitivity to food texture and temperature. Means of enhancing the appetite through food appearance and aroma as well as texture must be explored. Similarly, radiation to the abdominal area affects the intestinal mucosa, causing a loss of villi and possibly nutrient malabsorption. Ulcers, inflammation, obstructions, or **fistulas** may also develop as a result of tissue breakdown, and these conditions interfere with the normal functioning of the involved tissue. General malabsorption within the gastrointestinal (GI) tract may be further compounded by a lack of food intake as a result of anorexia and nausea.

CHEMOTHERAPY

Chemotherapeutic agents destroy rapidly growing cancer cells. Unlike radiation therapy, chemotherapy is administered via general blood circulation throughout the body. Because chemotherapeutic medications are highly toxic, they also affect normal, healthy cells. This accounts for their side effects on rapidly growing tissues (e.g., bone marrow, GI tract, hair follicles) as well as the problems that they cause for nutrition management. General complications include the following:

- *Bone marrow:* Interference with the production of specific blood factors causes a reduced red blood cell count and anemia, a reduced white blood cell count and lowered resistance to infections, and a reduced blood platelet level that may prevent the formation of blood clots when needed to stop bleeding.
- *GI tract:* Numerous problems may develop that interfere with food tolerance, such as nausea and vomiting, a loss of normal taste sensations, anorexia, diarrhea, ulcers, malabsorption, and **mucositis.**
- *Hair follicle:* Interference with normal hair growth results in general hair loss.

DRUG-NUTRIENT INTERACTIONS

Many medications used in cancer treatment have a high potential for drug-nutrient interactions. Several antineoplastic drugs have known drug-nutrient interactions that should be addressed with patients on an individual basis (Table 23-1). In addition, many patients experiment with dietary supplements and herbs that are thought to have a protective role in cancer treatment or prevention. Some of the more commonly used

---

Table 23-1 Drug-Nutrient Interactions with Commonly Used Medications in Patients with Cancer

ANTINEOPLASTIC DRUGS	POSSIBLE INTERACTIONS
Bexarotene (Targretin)	Grapefruit juice may increase drug concentration and toxicities
Methotrexate (Folex, Rheumatrex)	Alcohol may increase hepatotoxicity
Plicamycin (Mithracin)	Supplements that contain calcium and vitamin D may decrease effectiveness
Procarbazine (Matulane)	A mild monoamine oxidase inhibitor; a low-tyramine diet should be followed
Temozolomide (Temodar)	Food may decrease drug rate and absorption

Source: National Cancer Institute. *Nutrition in cancer care: other nutrition issues.* Website: <www.cancer.gov>. Accessed May 2015.

---

herbs have well-known food-drug interactions that may adversely affect the patient or their treatment regimen (see the *Complementary and Alternative Medicine* information at www.cancer.gov). Careful questioning will reveal dietary supplement and herb use, and any potential interactions should be discussed.

MEDICAL NUTRITION THERAPY IN THE PATIENT WITH CANCER

NUTRITION PROBLEMS RELATED TO THE DISEASE PROCESS

Individual nutrition problems throughout the continuum of care for cancer patients will vary greatly. Not all patients with cancer will need MNT. For example, basal cell carcinoma is the most common type of skin cancer and in most cases, excision of the lesion is the only intervention required. In such circumstances, nutrition intervention is usually not necessary. However, general nutrition obstacles may pose a challenge for patients with advanced stages of cancer, for patients undergoing surgery or radiation therapy affecting the gastrointestinal system, and for patients receiving chemotherapy. These problems relate to the overall systemic effects of cancer as well as to the specific individual responses to the treatment involved.

General Systemic Effects

Cancer generally causes the following three basic systemic effects with regard to nutrition status:

- *Anorexia,* or loss of appetite, which results in poor food intake
- *Increased metabolism,* which results in increased nutrient and energy needs
- *Negative nitrogen balance,* which results in lean tissue catabolism

---

fistulas from the Latin word for "pipe," an abnormal opening or passageway within the body or to the outside.
mucositis an inflammation of the tissues around the mouth or other orifices of the body.

Unfortunately, this creates a snowball effect: cancer causes poor nutritional status and poor nutritional status is associated with an increased rate of hospital admission rates for oncology patients and poor overall outcome.[16] The extent of these effects may vary widely from a mild response, to malnutrition, or to an extreme form of debilitating cachexia. Extreme weight loss and weakness are caused by an inability to ingest or use nutrients, which results in the patient's body feeding off of its own tissue. Although the prevalence of cachexia varies with the type of cancer, approximately half of all patients with advanced cancer experience some level of cachexia-associated weight loss. Cachexia greatly increases morbidity, mortality, length of hospital stays, medical costs, and contributes to poor quality of life.[17] The 1-year mortality rate of cancer cachexia is estimated to be between 20% and 80%.[18] An involuntary weight loss of >5% of the premorbid weight within a 1-month period or >10% in the previous 6 months is indicative of cachexia. The best way to treat cancer-related cachexia is to alleviate the cancer and the metabolic abnormalities associated with it. However, because this is not always a possibility, aggressive MNT is indicated.

Effects Specific to the Type of Cancer

In addition to the primary nutrition problems that are caused by the disease process itself, secondary problems with eating or nutrient metabolism result from tumors that cause obstructions or lesions in the GI tract, accessory organs, or the surrounding tissue. Such conditions limit food intake and digestion as well as nutrient absorption. Patients with forms of cancer that involve hormone or steroid therapy (e.g., breast and prostate cancer) are at risk for significant weight gain. Their MNT should focus on diet and lifestyle modifications that help to avoid unintentional weight gain. Depending on the nature and location of the cancer and the mode of treatment, MNT must always be individualized to help overcome these difficulties.

BASIC OBJECTIVES OF THE NUTRITION PLAN

The fundamental principles of identifying needs and planning care on the basis of those needs underlie all sound patient care (see Chapter 17).

Nutrition Screening and Assessment

Assessing and monitoring the nutritional status of each patient is the primary responsibility of the registered dietitian nutritionist. Various members of the health care team may take part in anthropometric measurements and the calculations of body composition,

laboratory tests and the interpretation of their results, physical examination and clinical observations, and dietary analysis. Weight can change rapidly in some patients; therefore, accurate measurements must be taken instead of relying on self-reported or estimated values. All cancer patients should be evaluated for malnutrition. There are several validated and reliable assessment tools available to screen for malnutrition, such as the Patient-Generated Subjective Global Assessment (PG-SGA), Malnutrition Screening Tool (MST), Malnutrition Screening Tool for Cancer Patients (MSTC), and the Malnutrition Universal Screening Tool (MUST).[19] Malnutrition or severe alterations in weight indicate complications that may change medication dosages, alter the treatment plan, or otherwise require medical intervention.

Nutrition Intervention

The basic objectives of the nutrition intervention plan for patients with cancer are as follows[19]:
- Prevent weight loss, even among overweight patients
- Maintain lean body mass
- Prevent unintentional weight gain, particularly in certain groups of patients (e.g., those with hormone-related cancers such as prostate or breast cancer, those taking long-term high-dose steroids)
- Identify and manage treatment-related side effects

Nutrient specifics of the plan are outlined in the Medical Nutrition Therapy section later in this chapter.

Prevention of catabolism. Every effort is made to meet the increased metabolic demands of the disease process in an effort to prevent extensive catabolic effects and tissue breakdown. Maintaining nutrition from the beginning is far more efficient than rebuilding the body after extensive wasting. The nutrition intervention recommendations for patients with or at risk for cancer-related cachexia are to maximize the oral intake of nutrient-dense foods while liberalizing any diet restrictions and encouraging small, frequent meals. Dietary supplements and nutrient-dense nourishments (e.g., Ensure, Boost, Carnation Breakfast Essentials) may benefit the patient and help him or her to meet nutrient needs. If patients are taking dietary supplements containing antioxidants, they should be advised not to take more than the Upper Tolerable Intake according to the Dietary Reference Intakes.[19]

A variety of drugs are currently in use to increase appetite, decrease nausea, spare protein degradation, and improve caloric intake. Some examples include megestrol acetate, corticosteroids, ghrelin, glucocorticoids, branched-chain amino acids, eicosapentaenoic acid, cyproheptadine, and cannabinoids, all of which have limitations.[20] See the For Further Focus box entitled "Cannabis as a Treatment for Anorexia" for information about the use of cannabis for combating unintended weight loss in patients who suffer from

---

cachexia a specific profound syndrome that is characterized by wasting, reduced food intake, and systemic inflammation.

cancer-related cachexia. For patients who are unable to meet their metabolic needs orally, enteral or parenteral nutrition should be considered.

Relief of symptoms. The symptoms of cancer and the side effects of treatment can be devastating for a patient. Stress management, pain management, relaxation techniques, psychologic support, and physical activity (as tolerated) are important aspects of overall patient care, and they can improve a patient's quality of life.

Although the dietitian and the physician have the primary responsibility for planning and managing the MNT plan, a tremendous contribution is made by the nursing staff and other health care personnel with regard to day-to-day support and counseling to help patients meet their nutrient requirements. This kind of constant care and support is the difference between personnel who are going through the motions of daily duties versus those who are ensuring the comfort and well-being of their patients in a successful relationship.

Nutrition Monitoring and Evaluation

On the basis of detailed information that is gathered about each patient, including his or her living situation

For Further Focus

Cannabis as a Treatment for Anorexia

SARA HARCOURT

Both sides of the debate for the legalization of cannabis (medical marijuana) have genuine concerns. Proponents argue in favor of the effectiveness that marijuana has on relieving the nausea caused by cancer treatment, the wasting effects of HIV, and the pain of glaucoma. Critics cite studies that indicate the addictiveness of marijuana and that link it to cancer and lung damage.

Dronabinol, which is sold under the brand name Marinol, is a capsule form of marijuana that has been approved by the U.S. Food and Drug Administration. It contains tetrahydrocannabinol, which is the active ingredient found in the marijuana plant; thus, the drug has similar side effects:

Dizziness	Stomach pain
Anxiety	Nausea/vomiting
Paranoid reaction	Memory loss
Somnolence (sleepiness)	Hallucinations
Weakness	Strange or unusual thoughts

Dronabinol is indicated for the treatment of anorexia associated with unintentional weight loss in patients with HIV and for the nausea and vomiting associated with cancer chemotherapy in patients who have not adequately responded to conventional antiemetic treatments.

The dosage should be strictly regulated by the physician because each patient responds to dronabinol differently. Because this drug can be habit-forming, the lowest dose needed to produce the desired result is recommended.

and other personal and social needs, the dietitian develops a personal MNT plan for each patient. This plan should be evaluated for efficacy on a regular basis with the patient and his or her family or care providers. The plan should be updated as needed to meet the nutrition demands of the patient's condition as well as his or her individual desires and tolerances.

MEDICAL NUTRITION THERAPY

Guidelines for MNT will vary depending on the cancer site, the stage of disease, the treatment modality, and the current nutritional status of the patient. Guidelines for MNT must meet specific nutrient needs and goals related to the accelerated metabolism and protein-tissue synthesis.

Energy

An adult patient with good nutritional status needs approximately 25 to 30 kcal/kg of body weight for maintenance requirements. More kilocalories may be needed in accordance with the degree of metabolic stress, the amount of tissue synthesis that is taking place, and physical activity levels. A malnourished patient may require significantly more energy, depending on the degree of malnutrition, the extent of tissue injury, or the amount of anabolism taking place. Patients receiving chemotherapy or radiation, hypermetabolic patients, and severely stressed patients have energy needs up to 35 kcal/kg.[19] Symptoms and side effects of the cancer or of the cancer treatment also have significant impacts on energy needs and oral intake. Anorexia, diarrhea, cachexia, nausea, malabsorption, fever, xerostomia, pain, infection, and early satiety are all examples of complications that will alter a patient's energy needs and consumption. Indirect calorimetry is the gold standard for determining exact energy needs if calculated estimates are not maintaining weight.

Protein

Essential amino acids and nitrogen are necessary for tissue building and healing and to offset the tissue breakdown that is caused by the disease or the treatment. Efficient protein use depends on an optimal protein-to-energy ratio to prevent catabolism. An adult nonstressed cancer patient with good nutritional status needs from 1.0 to 1.2 g/kg/day of protein to meet maintenance requirements, with an emphasis on high-quality protein sources. A malnourished patient needs additional protein to replenish deficits and to restore a positive nitrogen balance. The recommendations are that patients undergoing treatment should aim for 1.2 to 1.5 g/kg, stem cell transplant patients should aim for 1.5 to 2.0 g/kg, and patients with protein-losing enteropathies or wasting may need up to 2.5 g/kg of protein per day.[19]

Vitamins and Minerals

Key vitamins and minerals help to control protein and energy metabolism through their coenzyme roles in specific cell enzyme pathways, and they also play important roles in building and maintaining strong tissue (see Chapters 7 and 8). Therefore, an optimal intake of vitamins and minerals (at least to the Dietary Reference Intake standards) is ideal. Vitamin and mineral supplements are often indicated to ensure dietary intake (see the Drug-Nutrient Interaction box "Antiestrogens and Breast Cancer"). However, the unsubstantiated megadosing of dietary supplements (specifically those that contain antioxidants) may be counterproductive to the health of the patient (see the Drug-Nutrient Interaction box "Antioxidants and Chemotherapy").

The Academy of Nutrition and Dietetics *Nutrition Care Manual* notes a potential benefit from the supplementation of the following nutrients for patients with specific types of cancer[19]:

- *Vitamin E:* patients with breast cancer who are receiving radiation; patients with head and neck cancer
- *Omega-3 fatty acid supplements:* patients with pancreatic cancer
- *Arginine:* patients with breast cancer; patients with head and neck cancer
- *Eicosapentaenoic acid:* patients with oral and laryngeal cancer
- *Honey:* patients who are receiving radiation on the head or neck

- *Glutamine:* patients undergoing hematopoietic cell transplantation
- *Antioxidants at levels higher than the Tolerable Upper Intake Level:* patients with non–small-cell lung cancer who are receiving chemotherapy

Drug-Nutrient Interaction

Antioxidants and Chemotherapy

Complementary and alternative medicine (CAM) is best described as diverse health care systems, products, and practices that are not generally considered part of conventional medicine. This type of treatment includes dietary supplement use, acupuncture, massage, herbal medicines, and mind-body techniques. The use of CAM—and most notably dietary supplement use—is highly prevalent in patients with cancer.

Antioxidant supplements, particularly vitamin C, are often used by cancer patients in an effort to boost their immune system or to improve general health. This practice may not be helpful, and it can in fact be harmful for patients who are being treated for certain types of cancer. Tumor cells are characterized by their rapid rate of division, but normal, healthy cells such as skin cells and the cells that line the digestive tract divide quickly as well. Antineoplastic drugs target the rapidly dividing cells and produce free radicals that cause oxidative damage. Although vitamin C supplementation may help to alleviate the unpleasant side effects of chemotherapy, it may also reduce the effectiveness of the anticancer treatment. Even at typical supplemental doses of 500 mg per day, vitamin C has been shown to prevent the cytotoxic effects of antineoplastic agents from killing tumor cells, not just healthy cells.[1] In other words, the vitamin C *protects the cancer cells*.[2] To date, the efficacy of large dose intravenous administration of vitamin C for cancer patients is lacking, despite its popularity.[3,4]

Resveratrol is another dietary supplement commonly used as an adjunct to cancer treatment. It is a phytochemical that has been found to have anticancer as well as antioxidant activity. Resveratrol shows promise in increasing tumor cell response to the effects of chemotherapeutic agents and increasing apoptosis (programmed cell death) of breast cancer cells.[5] This research is still in its infancy, and general recommendations cannot yet be made regarding dietary supplements of resveratrol during cancer treatment. To ensure safety during chemotherapy, patients should carefully discuss their use of supplemental vitamin C or other potent dietary antioxidants with their health care providers.

Drug-Nutrient Interaction

Antiestrogens and Breast Cancer

SARA HARCOURT

Tamoxifen citrate is an antiestrogenic drug that is used to treat breast cancer. Some common symptoms of interactions with this drug that are related to nutrition include the following:

Nausea	Stomach cramps
Increased bone or tumor pain	Constipation
Fluid retention	Excessive tiredness
Weight loss	Loss of appetite

Estrogen is needed for bone formation along with vitamin D, calcium, and magnesium. With low levels of estrogen, calcium is taken from the bone, and bone resorption may result. Calcium and magnesium supplements can help to reduce resorption, but they should be taken separately from the tamoxifen citrate by at least 2 hours. Grapefruit juice should be avoided, because it can interfere with absorption, as can soy supplements and soy-based foods because of their estrogenic effect. Soy products do not contain estrogen, but they do contain compounds that are similar in structure to estrogen. Because of the similarity, these estrogen-like compounds may fit into the active site of the drug and therefore act as decoys to the true estrogen target.

REFERENCES

1. Heaney ML, et al. Vitamin C antagonizes the cytotoxic effects of antineoplastic drugs. *Cancer Res.* 2008;68(19):8031-8038.
2. Subramani T, et al. Vitamin C suppresses cell death in MCF-7 human breast cancer cells induced by tamoxifen. *J Cell Mol Med.* 2014;18(2):305-313.
3. Jacobs C, et al. Is there a role for oral or intravenous ascorbate (vitamin C) in treating patients with cancer? A systematic review. *Oncologist.* 2015;20(2):210-223.
4. Fritz H, et al. Intravenous vitamin C and cancer: a systematic review. *Integr Cancer Ther.* 2014;13(4):280-300.
5. Diaz-Chavez J, et al. Proteomic profiling reveals that resveratrol inhibits HSP27 expression and sensitizes breast cancer cells to doxorubicin therapy. *PLoS ONE.* 2013;8(5):e64378.

Fluid

Adequate fluid intake must be ensured for the following reasons:

- To replace GI losses from fever, infection, vomiting, or diarrhea
- To help the kidneys dispose of metabolic breakdown products from destroyed cancer cells and from the drugs that are used in chemotherapy

Some chemotherapeutic drugs (e.g., cyclophosphamide [Cytoxan]) require hyperhydration by forced fluids daily to prevent hemorrhagic cystitis.

NUTRITION MANAGEMENT

Achieving these nutrition objectives and needs in the face of frequent food intolerance, anorexia, or the inability to eat presents a great challenge for the patient and the nutrition support team. The specific method of feeding depends on the patient's condition. The dietitian and the physician may manage a patient's nutrition care with the use of high-calorie nutritional supplements (e.g., Ensure, Boost) or with enteral or parenteral nutrition support (see Chapter 22).

Oral Diet with Nutrient Supplementation

An oral diet with supplementation (if indicated) is the most desired form of feeding when tolerated. A personal food plan must include adjustments in food texture and temperature, food choices, and tolerances, and it should provide as much energy and nutrient density as possible in smaller volumes of food. Special attention is given to eating problems that are caused by a loss of appetite, oral complications, GI problems, and pain. Table 23-2 provides strategies for improving food intake in patients with cancer or HIV.

Loss of appetite. Anorexia is a major problem in patients with cancer, and it curtails food intake when it is needed most. Anorexia often sets up a vicious cycle that can lead to the gross malnutrition of

Table 23-2	Dietary Modifications for Nutrition-Related Side Effects of Cancer, Human Immunodeficiency Virus, and Acquired Immunodeficiency Syndrome
SYMPTOM	**SUGGESTIONS**
Anorexia	Plan a menu in advance that involves small, frequent, high-calorie meals (every 2 hours)
	Add extra protein and calories to food
	Consume one third of the daily protein and calorie requirements at breakfast
	Prepare and store small portions of favorite foods
	Snack between meals
	Choose foods that appeal to the sense of smell
	Be creative with desserts
	Experiment with different foods
	Arrange for help with purchasing and preparing food and meals
	Perform frequent mouth care to relieve symptoms and to decrease aftertastes
Nausea and vomiting	Avoid spicy foods, greasy foods, and foods with strong odors
	Eat dry, bland, soft, and easy-to-digest foods such as crackers, breadsticks, and toast throughout the day
	Avoid heavy meals
	Remain upright for at least 1 hour after eating
	Avoid eating in areas with strong cooking odors or that are too warm
	Consume liquids between meals
	Rinse out the mouth before and after eating
	Suck on hard candies (e.g., peppermints, lemon drops) if there is a bad taste in the mouth
Taste and smell alterations	Try new foods when feeling best
	Use plastic utensils if foods taste metallic
	Use sugar-free lemon drops, gum, or mints when experiencing a bitter taste in the mouth
	Substitute poultry, fish, eggs, and cheese for red meat
	Eat small, frequent meals and healthy snacks
	Be flexible: eat meals when hungry rather than at set meal times
	Plan meals that include favorite foods
	Plan to eat with family and friends
	Have others prepare the meal
	A vegetarian or Chinese cookbook can provide useful meatless, high-protein recipes
	Add spices, herbs, seasonings, and sauces to foods
	Eat meat with something sweet, such as cranberry sauce, jelly, or applesauce

Table 23-2	Dietary Modifications for Nutrition-Related Side Effects of Cancer, Human Immunodeficiency Virus, and Acquired Immunodeficiency Syndrome—cont'd

SYMPTOM	SUGGESTIONS
Xerostomia	Drink plenty of fluids (25-30 mL/kg per day) Eat moist foods with extra sauces and gravies Keep water handy at all times to moisten the mouth Perform oral hygiene at least four times per day, but avoid rinses that contain alcohol Brush dentures after each meal Consume very sweet or tart foods and beverages, which may stimulate saliva production Drink fruit nectar instead of juice Use hard candy, frozen desserts, chewing gum, and ice pops between meals to moisten the mouth
Diarrhea	Avoid greasy foods, hot and cold liquids, and caffeine Drink at least 1 cup of liquid after each loose bowel movement Limit gas-forming foods and beverages such as soda, cruciferous vegetables, legumes and lentils, chewing gum, and milk (if not well tolerated) Limit the use of sorbitol Drink plenty of fluids throughout the day; room-temperature fluids may be better tolerated
Constipation	Gradually increase fiber consumption to 25 to 35 g/day Drink 8 to 10 cups of fluid each day Maintain regular physical activity
Mucositis and stomatitis	Eat foods that are soft, easy to chew and swallow Moisten foods with gravy, broth, or sauces Avoid known irritants such as acidic, spicy, salty, and coarse-textured foods Cook foods until they are soft and tender, or cut foods into small bites Eat foods at room temperature Use a straw to drink liquids Supplement meals with high-calorie, high-protein drinks Maintain good oral hygiene Numb the mouth with ice chips or flavored ice pops
Neutropenia*	Check expiration dates on food; do not buy or use if the food is out of date Do not buy or use food in cans that are swollen, dented, or damaged Thaw foods in the refrigerator or microwave; never thaw foods at room temperature Cook foods immediately after thawing Refrigerate all leftovers within 2 hours of cooking, and eat them within 24 hours Keep hot foods hot and cold foods cold Avoid old, moldy, or damaged fruits and vegetables Avoid tofu in open bins or containers Cook all meat, poultry, and fish thoroughly; avoid raw eggs and fish Buy individually packaged foods Avoid salad bars and buffets when eating out Limit exposure to large groups of people and people with infections Practice good hygiene, and wash hands often
Dehydration	Drink 8 to 12 cups of liquids a day, regardless of thirst Add soup, flavored ice pops, and other sources of fluid to the diet Limit caffeine Drink most fluids between meals Use antiemetics for relief from nausea and vomiting

Modified from National Cancer Institute. *Nutrition in cancer care: nutrition implications of cancer therapies* (website): <www.cancer.gov/about-cancer/treatment/side-effects/appetite-loss/nutrition-hp-pdq#link/_120_toc>. Accessed May 2015.
*Neutropenia involves a low white blood cell count and an increased risk of infection.

cancer-related cachexia, as discussed previously. A vigorous program of eating that does not depend on appetite for stimulus must be planned with the patient and his or her support system. The overall goal is to provide food with as much nutrient density as possible so that every bite counts.

Oral complications. Various problems that contribute to eating difficulties may stem from a sore mouth, mucositis, or altered taste and smell acuity. Decreased saliva and sore mouth often result from radiation to the head and neck area or from chemotherapy. Spraying the mouth with artificial saliva or an oral numbing solution may be helpful. Good oral care habits are important to avoid infection and to prevent dental caries, both of which could further impede healthy eating. Basic mouth care includes the following:

- Visiting the dentist before treatment begins
- Examining the mouth daily for sores or irritation
- Brushing and flossing regularly with a soft-bristled toothbrush
- Ensuring that dentures fit correctly
- Using mouthwash that does not contain alcohol, which dries out the mouth

Frequent small snacks are often better accepted than traditional meals. The treatment may alter the tongue's taste buds, thereby causing taste distortion, taste blindness, and the inability to distinguish sweet, sour, salt, or bitter, thereby resulting in more food aversions. Strong food seasonings (for those who can tolerate them) and high-protein liquid drinks may be helpful. Because the treatment may also alter salivary secretions, foods with a high liquid content are favored. Solid foods may be swallowed more easily with the use of sauces, gravies, broth, yogurt, or salad dressings. A food processor or blender can turn foods into semisolid or liquid forms for easier swallowing. Any dental problems should be corrected to help with chewing.

Gastrointestinal problems. Chemotherapy often causes nausea and vomiting, which require special individual attention (see Table 23-2). Food that is hot, sweet, fatty, or spicy sometimes exacerbates nausea and should be avoided in accordance with individual tolerances. Small and frequent feedings of soft or liquid cold or room-temperature foods that are eaten slowly with rests in between may be helpful. The use of anti-nausea drugs (e.g., prochlorperazine [Compazine, Zofran, Kytril]) may help with food tolerances. Surgical treatment that involves the GI tract requires related dietary modifications as covered in Chapter 22. Chemotherapy and radiation treatment can affect the mucosal cells that secrete lactase and thus induce lactose intolerance. In such cases, soy-based dairy substitutes or nutrient supplements (e.g., Ensure [Ross Products, Columbus, Ohio]) may be helpful.

Loss of lean tissue. Dietary supplements containing fish oil may be effective at preserving or improving lean body mass in adult oncology patients experiencing unintentional weight loss. Therefore, the dietitian may recommend a dietary supplement containing 0.26 to 6.0 g/day of eicosapentaenoic acid (EPA) or a medical food supplement containing fish oil with 1.1 to 2.2 g of EPA daily as a nutrition intervention for patients who continue to lose weight and lean body mass.[16]

Pain and discomfort. Patients are more able to eat if severe pain is controlled and if they are positioned as comfortably as possible. The current medical consensus is to administer pain-controlling medication as needed in close consultation with the patient and his or her care providers or family and then to carefully monitor patient responses. This is especially important for children with cancer who are undergoing painful treatments. Constipation is a common side effect of several pain medications. Preventive therapy to avoid additional discomfort from constipation should focus on adequate fluids, soluble fiber, and regular physical activity (even short walks can help).

Enteral and Parenteral Nutrition Support

When the GI tract can still be used but the patient is unable to eat and requires more assistance to achieve essential intake goals, tube feeding may be indicated. When the GI tract cannot be used and nutrition support is vital, parenteral feedings must be initiated. See Box 22-1 for indications requiring enteral and parenteral nutrition support. Details of enteral and parenteral methods of feeding are covered in Chapter 22.

CANCER PREVENTION

Based on the most current information about cancer research and prevention, the American Cancer Society has issued guidelines to encourage healthy lifestyle choices to reduce the risk of cancer.[21] The World Cancer Research Fund and the American Institute for Cancer Research published the second report regarding the global perspective of food, nutrition, and physical activity as they are related to cancer prevention in 2008.[22] The combined recommendations from these two reports are outlined in the next section of this chapter. In addition, the U.S. Food and Drug Administration (FDA) has defined specific food-labeling guidelines for associating certain foods and nutrients to the decreased risk of cancer.[23] A variety of other government and privately funded research studies are ongoing in the hopes of identifying a more specific cause of and cure for cancer.

AMERICAN CANCER SOCIETY, WORLD CANCER RESEARCH FUND, AND THE AMERICAN INSTITUTE FOR CANCER RESEARCH: GUIDELINES FOR CANCER PREVENTION

The most recent expert panel publications recommend the following lifestyle factors to reduce the risk of cancer[21,22]:

1. Be as lean as possible within the normal range of body weight throughout life.
   - Balance caloric intake with physical activity.

- Avoid excessive weight gain at all ages. For overweight or obese individuals, losing even a small amount of weight is helpful.
2. Adopt a physically active lifestyle.
   - Children and adolescents: participate in at least 60 minutes every day of moderate to vigorous physical activity, with vigorous intensity activity included at least 3 days per week.
   - Adults: engage in at least 150 minutes of moderate intensity or 75 minutes of vigorous physical activity each week; preferably spread throughout the week.
   - Examples of moderate activity include walking, skating, yoga, softball or baseball, downhill skiing, gardening, and lawn care. Examples of vigorous activities include running, aerobics, fast bicycling, circuit weight training, soccer, singles tennis, basketball, cross-country skiing, and heavy manual labor.
   - Limit sedentary behaviors.
3. Consume a healthy diet that has an emphasis on plant sources.
   - Become familiar with standard serving sizes and read food labels to become more aware of actual servings consumed. Choose foods that will help achieve and maintain a healthy body weight.
   - Limit the consumption of salty foods and foods that are processed with sodium.
   - Limit the consumption of energy-dense foods, particularly processed foods that are high in added sugar, low in fiber, or high in fat. Avoid sugary drinks.
   - Eat at least 2.5 cups of vegetables and fruits every day.
   - Choose whole grains instead of processed (refined) grains and sugars. Avoid moldy grains and legumes.
   - Choose fish, poultry, and beans as alternatives to beef, pork, and lamb. Select lean cuts and small portions, and prepare the meat by baking, broiling, or poaching rather than frying. Avoid processed meats.
4. If alcoholic beverages are consumed, limit their intake. Limit alcohol intake to two drinks per day for men and one drink per day for women. One drink is defined as 12 oz of beer, 5 oz of wine, or 1.5 oz of 80-proof distilled spirits.
5. Aim to meet nutritional needs through diet alone; do not rely on supplements.
6. Aim to breastfeed infants exclusively for 6 months and continue to breastfeed while offering complementary food after 6 months.

Dietary choices and physical activity are the most modifiable risk factors for cancer prevention. In a study of more than 475,000 participants followed for 10+ years, adherence to the preceding guidelines significantly reduced the incidence of cancer and cancer mortality for both men and women.[24] The reduction in risk varies between sex and type of cancer with a risk reduction ranging from 15% (lung cancer in men) to 65% (gallbladder cancer in both sexes). Adopting a healthy lifestyle and avoiding tobacco have tremendous health benefits and reduce the risk of several other forms of chronic disease as well.

U.S. Food and Drug Administration Health Claims

Health claims approved for use on food labels are regulated by the FDA (see Chapter 13). The qualified health claims about cancer risk for use on food labels in the United States link the following nutrients with reduced risk[23]:

- *Dietary fat (lipids) and cancer.* An example claim approved for use: "Eating a healthful diet low in fat may help reduce the risk of some types of cancers. Development of cancer is associated with many factors, including a family history of the disease, cigarette smoking, and what you eat."
- *Fiber-containing grain products, fruits, vegetables, and cancer.* An example claim approved for use: "Development of cancer depends on many factors. Eating a diet low in fat and high in grain products, fruits, and vegetables that contain dietary fiber may reduce your risk of some cancers."
- *Fruits and vegetables and cancer.* An example claim approved for use on broccoli: "Low fat diets rich in fruits and vegetables (foods that are low in fat and may contain dietary fiber, vitamin A, and vitamin C) may reduce the risk of some types of cancer, a disease associated with many factors. Broccoli is high in vitamins A and C, and it is a good source of dietary fiber."

On the basis of these associations, the Centers for Disease Control and Prevention (CDC) encourages Americans to eat several servings of fruits and vegetables every day, which is one of the nation's *Healthy People 2020* objectives.[25] The personalized serving recommendation is based on age, gender, and activity level (www.cdc.gov/nutrition/everyone/fruitsvegetables). Most people need a total of about 5 servings of fruits and vegetables per day. In addition, the CDC works closely with the Association of State and Public Health Nutritionists (www.asphn.org), which is comprised of nutrition coordinators involved in food and nutrition policy, programs, and services at the state and national level.

Ongoing Cancer Research

Research that links specific elements of the diet with the risk for cancer is difficult to do and complicated to interpret. Some studies have shown that diets that are low in fat and high in fiber, fruits, and vegetables, which are major sources of micronutrients and phytochemicals, are associated with decreased incidences and mortality rates for various cancers. The exact mechanisms by which such diets are protective against cancer are not yet clearly defined for each association and are still under investigation. Some examples of recent findings include the following:

- *Breast cancer:* Overweight/obesity increases the risk for breast cancer through several metabolic and inflammatory pathways.[26] Women following the World Cancer Research Fund and the American Institute for Cancer Research Guidelines significantly reduce their risk for breast cancer.[27] The dietary factors with the strongest protective association are avoiding high energy-dense foods and excess alcohol and consuming predominantly plant-based foods.

- *Gastric cancer:* A diet rich in fruits and vegetables such as the Mediterranean diet appears to be protective against gastric cancer compared with the typical Western diet that is rich in starchy foods, sweets, meat, and fat.[28] Specifically, the intake of carotenoids, retinol, α-tocopherol, and cereal fiber is protective. The intake of total meat, red meat, and processed meat are risk factors.[29]

- *Colorectal cancer:* It has been estimated that 70% to 90% of colorectal cancer is due to dietary factors. Diets rich in vitamin D, calcium, folate, polyphenols, and fish appear to be protective against colorectal cancer. Red meat and processed meat intake, abdominal obesity, high body mass index, and alcohol consumption are risk factors for colorectal cancer.[29,30]

Many other associations have been investigated, with some controversy. The article by Kabat and colleagues[24] provides detailed information about the dietary factors and lifestyle choices that are associated with a reduced risk of specific types of cancer (see the references for Chapter 23 listed at the back of this textbook).

The CDC hosts many programs that are aimed at preventing and controlling cancers as well as researching cause-and-effect relationships, including the National Comprehensive Cancer Control Program; the National Breast and Cervical Cancer Early Detection Program; the National Program of Cancer Registries; and the Colorectal Cancer Control Program. In addition to these programs, there are several initiatives that focus on education and awareness campaigns and research activities that are aimed at lung, skin, prostate, and gynecologic cancers and cancer survivorship.[31] Many of these programs have nutrition-related objectives.

DIETS AND SUPPLEMENTS PROMOTED AS "CANCER CURES"

Diets and dietary supplements promoting the ability to cure cancer have been around for many decades, the vast majority of which have been proven inconsequential, some of which are downright dangerous, and some of which are currently undergoing clinical trial.

The Academy of Nutrition and Dietetics *Nutrition Care Manual* reports on the following diets and supplements that are commonly associated with cancer: Gerson Diet, Gonzalez Diet, Livingston-Wheeler Diet, high-dose vitamin C supplements, hydrazine sulfate, laetrile, shark cartilage, juice therapies, and mega-antioxidant supplement therapies.[19] Some of these that have been tested and failed to produce any positive or cancer-protective results include the Gerson Diet, Livingston-Wheeler Diet, high-dose vitamin C, laetrile, and hydrazine sulfate diets. Macrobiotic diets have also been hyped for cancer prevention but they are discouraged because of the restrictive nature of the diet and the risk for multiple nutrient deficiencies.

Complementary and alternative medicine (CAM) is commonly used by patients with cancer,[32-34] but less than half of those patients, on average, disclosed that information to their doctors.[35] Health care practitioners should always be open to the needs of their patients and respectful of their desires. The most important thing to ensure is that all alternative practices are discussed with the health care team to determine any potential interactions, dangers, or risks. Alternative practices that may have nutritional or drug-nutrient interaction potentials include specific diets, supplements, herbs, infusions, injections, and enemas, for example. As a health care provider, be sure to ask about the use of any of these practices. Some dietary supplements can have dangerous interactions with chemotherapeutic agents or other treatment regimens. If patients are made to feel uncomfortable about discussing their CAM practices with their health care provider, they are much less likely to disclose the use of CAM and serious consequences may result.

SECTION 2   HUMAN IMMUNODEFICIENCY VIRUS

PROGRESSION OF HUMAN IMMUNODEFICIENCY VIRUS

This section looks at HIV and compares its relationship to the body's immune system and course of development with that of cancer. According to the CDC, about 50,000 people are infected with HIV every year in the United States alone, ≈80% of which are male.[36] See the Cultural Considerations box "Types and Incidence of Human Immunodeficiency Virus and Acquired Immunodeficiency Syndrome in American Populations" for more information on the incidence of HIV in the United States.

EVOLUTION OF HUMAN IMMUNODEFICIENCY VIRUS

The earliest known case of AIDS was identified in a blood sample collected in 1959 from a Bantu man

Types and Incidence of Human Immunodeficiency Virus and Acquired Immunodeficiency Syndrome in American Populations

More than 1.2 million people in the United States are currently living with HIV and 14% of them are unaware of their infection. The largest percentage of new HIV infections each year occurs as a result of male-to-male sexual contact. High-risk heterosexual activity and injection drug use are the next most common causes of HIV transmission. Acquired immunodeficiency syndrome (AIDS) is the ninth leading cause of death among Americans between the ages of 25 and 44 years.[1]

The percentage of new HIV infections according to race is disproportionate to the total U.S. population. For example, African Americans make up approximately 12% of the total U.S. population, but 44% of new HIV infection cases occur among African Americans. Efforts to increase education, awareness, and prevention are important for the specific populations most affected.

The Centers for Disease Control and Prevention has reported the race and ethnicity of people with HIV/AIDS who were diagnosed during 2013 as follows[2]:

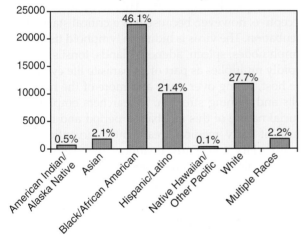

Estimated Number of Diagnoses of HIV Infection by Race or Ethnicity, 2013

Because no cures or vaccines for HIV are currently available, prevention is the only means of protection, regardless of race or gender.

REFERENCES

1. National Center for Health Statistics. *Health, United States, 2014: With Special Feature of Adults Aged 55-64*. Hyattsville, Md: U.S. Government Printing Office; 2015.
2. Centers for Disease Control and Prevention. *HIV surveillance report, 2013*. 2015. <www.cdc.gov/hiv/library/reports/surveillance/>.

living in what is currently the Democratic Republic of Congo, an area from which the current world epidemic is believed to have originated.[37] Early during the 1960s in the African country of Uganda, strange deaths began to occur from simple common infections such as pneumonia that did not respond to the usual antibiotic drugs. By the late 1970s and early 1980s, the same peculiar deaths were occurring in Europe and America. Similar reports of unexplained immune system failure increased rapidly in various parts of the world, and the **pandemic** spread. These early cases came from people with diverse social and medical backgrounds, including heterosexual and homosexual men, intravenous drug users, and recipients of transfused blood and blood products (e.g., patients with hemophilia, medical and surgical patients). After feverish research, the underlying infectious agent was finally discovered in May 1983. The French scientist Luc Montagnier, a leading pioneer in AIDS research, reported that he and his team at the Pasteur Institute in Paris had isolated the viral cause, which is now known as *HIV*.

PARASITIC NATURE OF THE VIRUS

No virus can have a life of its own. As a result of their structure and reproductive nature, viruses are the ultimate **parasites**. They are mere shreds of genetic material, a small packet of genetic information encased in a protein coat. Viruses only contain a small chromosome of nucleic acids (RNA or DNA), usually with fewer than five genes. They can live only through a host that they invade and infect, and they hijack the host's cell machinery to make a multitude of copies of themselves. Scientists agree that HIV, which is genetically similar to a virus found in African primates (simian immunodeficiency virus), was probably transmitted to human beings as hunters accidentally cut themselves while butchering their kills for food. The deadly strength of HIV results from its aggressive growth within an increasing number of hosts. Worldwide, 35 million people are living with HIV/AIDS; the majority of these individuals are in sub-Saharan Africa.[38]

Transmission and Stages of Disease Progression

HIV is transmitted from an infected person to another person through sexual contact (i.e., oral, anal, or vaginal), through the sharing of needles or syringes, or through mother-to-child transmission. Blood, tissue, and organ donations are now very closely screened for HIV antibodies in most countries, thereby reducing this form of transmission. The primary mode of HIV transmission is sexual contact, which accounts for the vast majority of new cases (Figure 23-3).

pandemic a widespread epidemic distributed throughout a region, a continent, or the world.
parasite an organism that lives in or on an organism of another species, known as the *host*, from whom all nourishment is obtained.

The individual clinical course of HIV infection varies substantially, but the following three distinct stages mark the progression of the disease:

- Primary HIV infection and extended latent period of viral incubation
- HIV-related diseases
- AIDS

There are two classification systems that are used for staging HIV: the CDC Classification System and the World Health Organization Clinical Staging and Disease Classification System. The CDC Classification System assesses HIV stages on the basis of the lowest documented helper T white blood cell count (i.e., CD4 cell count stages 0, 1, 2, 3, and unknown) and the presence of specific HIV-related conditions (i.e., clinical categories A, B, and C).[39] The World Health Organization Staging System is generally used in areas where laboratory values of CD4 cell counts are unavailable. This system relies on clinical manifestations to stage the severity of HIV. The CDC Classification System is used in the United States and will be discussed here.

CDC Classification System for HIV

Table 23-3 provides the CDC Classification System for HIV-infected adults and adolescents ≥6 years of age. In addition to stages 1 to 3, there are also *stages 0* and *unknown* as follows:

- *Stage 0:* Early HIV infection, inferred from a negative or indeterminate HIV test result within 6 months of a confirmed positive test
- *Stage unknown:* HIV test positive but no CD4+ T-lymphocyte count available

After the patient has been staged by their CD4+ T-lymphocyte count, the patient's clinical category is determined on the basis of symptomatic conditions.

Category A: asymptomatic or acute HIV. Approximately 2 to 4 weeks after initial exposure and infection, a mild flu-like episode may occur. This brief (i.e., days to weeks) and mild response reflects the initial development of antibodies to the viral infection. Any subsequent HIV testing is positive. For a number of years, the person typically feels well. This long well period is deceptive, however, because it is a critical stage of viral incubation. The virus is hiding in lymphoid tissues (e.g., lymph nodes, spleen, adenoid glands, tonsils), where it rapidly multiplies as part of its parasite life cycle within the host, taking over more and more of the host's CD4 cells and gaining strength. Researchers emphasize the crucial nature of this incubation period and the importance of early medical treatment intervention after a positive HIV test. Early treatment may slow the viral strengthening time while drugs and vaccines are developed to combat its steady progression.

Category B: symptomatic conditions. After the asymptomatic HIV-positive stage, associated infectious illnesses begin to invade the body. This period of opportunistic illnesses is so named because, at this point, the HIV infection has killed enough host-protective T lymphocytes to damage the immune system severely and to lower the body's normal disease

Estimated Number of Male Diagnosis of HIV by Transmission, 2013

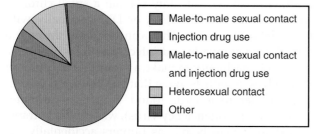

- Male-to-male sexual contact
- Injection drug use
- Male-to-male sexual contact and injection drug use
- Heterosexual contact
- Other

Estimated Number of Female Diagnosis of HIV by Transmission, 2013

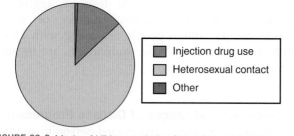

- Injection drug use
- Heterosexual contact
- Other

FIGURE 23-3 Mode of HIV transmission for males and females. (Source: Centers for Disease Control and Prevention. *HIV surveillance report, 2013.* 2015: <www.cdc.gov/hiv/library/reports/surveillance/>.)

Table 23-3 CDC Classification System for HIV

	CLINICAL CATEGORIES		
CD4+ T-LYMPHOCYTE COUNT	**A** ASYMPTOMATIC, ACUTE HIV, OR PGL	**B** SYMPTOMATIC CONDITIONS	**C*** AIDS-INDICATOR CONDITIONS
Stage 1: ≥500 cells/μL	A1	B1	C1
Stage 2: 200-499 cells/μL	A2	B2	C2
Stage 3: >200 cells/μL*	A3	B3	C3

PGL, Persistent generalized lymphadenopathy.
*Patients in any stage 3 CD4+ lymphocyte count or clinical category C are considered to have AIDS. Shaded in gray in the table.

Box 23-1	Common Types of Opportunistic Infections in Patients Infected with Human Immunodeficiency Virus: Category B

EXAMPLES OF CATEGORY B OPPORTUNISTIC ILLNESSES

- Bacillary angiomatosis
- Candidiasis, oropharyngeal (thrush)
- Candidiasis, vulvovaginal; persistent, frequent, or poorly responsive to therapy
- Cervical dysplasia (moderate or severe), cervical carcinoma in situ
- Constitutional symptoms, such as fever (38.5° C/101.3° F) or diarrhea lasting longer than 1 month
- Hairy leukoplakia, oral
- Herpes zoster (shingles) involving two or more distinct episodes or at least one dermatome
- Idiopathic thrombocytopenic purpura
- Pelvic inflammatory disease, particularly if complicated by tuboovarian abscess
- Peripheral neuropathy

Box 23-2	Common Types of Opportunistic Infections in Patients Infected with Human Immunodeficiency Virus: Category C

CATEGORY C DEFINING OPPORTUNISTIC ILLNESSES

- Bacterial infections, multiple or recurrent[*]
- Candidiasis of the bronchi, trachea, or lungs
- Candidiasis, esophageal
- Cervical cancer, invasive[†]
- Coccidioidomycosis, disseminated or extrapulmonary
- Cryptococcosis, extrapulmonary
- Cryptosporidiosis, chronic intestinal (>1 month in duration)
- Cytomegalovirus disease (other than liver, spleen, or nodes), onset at age >1 month
- Cytomegalovirus retinitis with loss of vision
- Encephalopathy, related to HIV
- Herpes simplex: chronic ulcers (>1 month in duration); bronchitis, pneumonitis, or esophagitis
- Histoplasmosis, disseminated or extrapulmonary
- Isosporiasis, chronic intestinal (>1 month in duration)
- Kaposi's sarcoma
- Lymphoma, Burkitt's, immunoblastic (or equivalent term)
- Lymphoma, primary, of brain
- *Mycobacterium avium* complex or *Mycobacterium kansasii*, disseminated or extrapulmonary
- *Mycobacterium tuberculosis*, of any site, pulmonary,[†] disseminated or extrapulmonary
- *Mycobacterium*, other species or unidentified species, disseminated or extrapulmonary
- *Pneumocystis jiroveci* pneumonia
- Pneumonia, recurrent[†]
- Progressive multifocal leukoencephalopathy
- *Salmonella* septicemia, recurrent
- Toxoplasmosis of brain, onset at age >1 month
- Wasting syndrome attributed to HIV

From the Centers for Disease Control and Prevention. Revised surveillance case definition for HIV infection—United States, 2014. *MMWR Recomm Rep.* 2014;63(RR-03):1-10.
*Only among children aged <6 years.
†Only among adults, adolescents, and children aged ≥6 years.

resistance so that even the most common everyday infections have an opportunity to take root and grow (Box 23-1). Common symptoms during this period include persistent fatigue, diarrhea and fever, mouth sores from thrush (i.e., oral *Candida albicans*), night sweats, unintentional weight loss, remarkable headaches, shingles, cervical dysplasia or carcinoma, new or unusual cough, unusual bruises or skin discoloration, and peripheral neuropathy.

Category C: AIDS-indicator conditions. The terminal stage of HIV infection, which is designated as *AIDS*, is marked by rapidly declining T-lymphocyte counts and the presence of opportunistic illnesses (Box 23-2). Kaposi's sarcoma is the most common AIDS-associated cancer, and it is characterized by malignant and rapidly growing tumors of the skin and mucous linings of the GI and respiratory tracts; these tumors may cause severe internal bleeding. Low-dose radiation therapy or anticancer drugs may be used to slow the spread of tumors.

During severe immunodeficiency, protozoan parasites (i.e., primitive single-celled organisms) appear and infect a number of body organs. At lymphocyte counts of less than $50/mm^3$, cytomegalovirus (i.e., a herpes virus that causes lesions on the mucous linings of body organs) and lymphoma (i.e., any cancer of the lymphoid tissue) can flourish. This series of HIV effects on the body brings marked changes in body weight in both men and women (i.e., wasting syndrome), with women losing disproportionately more body fat. Other common conditions include infection with *Mycobacterium tuberculosis*, *Pneumocystis jiroveci* pneumonia, AIDS dementia complex, and progressive multifocal leukoencephalopathy.

When the virus kills enough white cells to overwhelm the immune system's weakened resistance to the disease complications, death follows.

MEDICAL MANAGEMENT OF THE PATIENT WITH HIV/AIDS

INITIAL EVALUATION AND GOALS

The initial medical evaluation of a person who has been newly diagnosed with HIV is critical to provide guidelines for ongoing comprehensive care by the HIV/AIDS team. This professional team includes medical, nutrition, nursing, and psychosocial health care specialists. Box 23-3 outlines an initial evaluation guide that emphasizes special coordinated medical care and the importance of allied health care support.

From U.S. Department of Health and Human Services, Agency for Healthcare Research and Quality. *National Guideline Clearinghouse: guideline summary: primary care approach to the HIV-infected patient* (website): <www.guideline.gov/content.aspx?id=34268>. Accessed May 2015.

Box 23-3 — Initial Evaluation of Patients Who Have Been Newly Diagnosed with Human Immunodeficiency Virus

- General history
  - History of present illness and past hospitalizations
  - Current prescription and nonprescription medicines
  - Vaccination history
  - Partner information for disclosure of human immunodeficiency virus (HIV) status
  - Occupational history
  - Allergies
  - Reproductive history
- HIV treatment and staging
  - HIV exposure history
  - Most recent viral load and CD4 count
  - Current and previous antiretroviral regimens
  - Previous adverse antiretroviral drug reactions
  - Opportunistic infections
- Mental health and substance use history
- Sexual history
- Review of systems (including questions about common symptoms related to HIV infection)
- Comprehensive physical examination
  - Vital signs and pain assessment
  - Ophthalmologic assessment
  - Oral examination
  - Head, ears, nose, and throat examination
  - Dermatologic examination
  - Lymph node examination
  - Endocrinologic examination
  - Pulmonary and cardiac examination
  - Abdominal examination
  - Genital examination
  - Rectal examination
  - Musculoskeletal examination
  - Neuropsychologic examination
- Diagnostic and laboratory assessment
  - Immunologic and virologic assessment
  - Tuberculosis evaluation
  - Screening for sexually transmitted infections
  - Cytologic screening
  - Hematologic assessment
  - Renal and hepatic assessment
  - Metabolic assessment

The medical management of HIV infection is constantly evolving as a result of intensive medical research. Basic current goals are to achieve the following:

- Delay the progression of the infection and boost the immune system.
- Prevent opportunistic illnesses.
- Recognize the infection early and provide rapid treatment for complications, including infections and cancer.

DRUG THERAPY

Developing effective drugs is difficult because of the highly evolved nature of the virus. One of the earliest findings in the drug research for HIV has been a group of compounds called *nucleoside/nucleotide reverse transcriptase inhibitors* (NRTIs) that inhibit the virus's necessary enzyme for copying itself, thereby effectively preventing viral increase. Multiple toxic side effects have been reported (Table 23-4), but some of these (e.g., nausea) may be helped by dietary modifications or antinausea medications. Other types of antiretroviral drugs approved by the FDA and currently in use in the United States are non-NRTIs (NNRTIs), protease inhibitors, fusion inhibitors, entry inhibitors, and HIV integrase strand-transfer inhibitors.[40] NNRTIs prevent the reproduction of the viral cells by inhibiting reverse transcriptase. Protease inhibitors help to stop HIV by inhibiting the basic enzyme protease, which is essential to HIV's development. Unfortunately, the virus is capable of mutation in response to some drugs (specifically protease inhibitors) and thus becomes resistant to treatment. Fusion inhibitors prevent the infection of healthy cells by binding to HIV. A combination of these medications, which is referred to as *highly active antiretroviral therapy* (HAART), is the primary drug treatment regimen that is used to slow the progression of HIV.

In addition to these antiretroviral drugs, many other drugs have been approved by the FDA to prevent or treat AIDS-related illnesses. Full descriptions and current approved therapies for the treatment of HIV/AIDS complications can be found on the FDA's website at www.fda.gov.

Vaccine Development

A successful HIV vaccine would train the body's immune system to identify and destroy the virus. The development and testing of vaccines takes several years. After a potential vaccine is identified, it must go through the following three phases of testing and be deemed effective before the FDA can approve it for public use:

- *Phase I:* The vaccine is tested in small groups of healthy, low-risk participants. This phase typically lasts 12 to 18 months.
- *Phase II:* The vaccine is tested in hundreds of high-risk and low-risk participants. This phase can last up to 2 years.
- *Phase III:* Thousands of high-risk participants are tested for both the safety and the effectiveness of the vaccine. This phase usually lasts an additional 3 to 4 years.

Thailand became the first country to begin a phase III HIV vaccine trial. The two-vaccine combination was considered safe and somewhat effective for the prevention of HIV infection (the vaccine efficacy was 31% one year after vaccination).[41] The CDC and the National

Table 23-4 Antiretroviral Therapy and Toxic Effects and Cautions

DRUG	MAJOR TOXIC EFFECTS AND CAUTIONS
Nucleoside Reverse Transcriptase Inhibitors	
Abacavir/Ziagen	Hypersensitivity reactions (human leukocyte antigen screening should be performed before initiation)
Didanosine/Videx EC	Pancreatitis Peripheral neuropathy Retinal changes Lactic acidosis with hepatic steatosis Nausea and vomiting Insulin resistance/diabetes mellitus Potential association with noncirrhotic portal hypertension
Emtricitabine/Emtriva	Severe acute exacerbation of hepatitis may occur in HBV-coinfected patients stopping treatment Hyperpigmentation/skin discoloration
Lamivudine/Epivir	Severe acute exacerbation of hepatitis may occur in HBV-coinfected patients stopping treatment
Stavudine/Zerit	Peripheral neuropathy Lipoatrophy Pancreatitis Lactic acidosis or severe hepatomegaly with hepatic steatosis Hyperlipidemia Insulin resistance/diabetes mellitus Rapidly progressive ascending neuromuscular weakness (rare)
Tenofovir disoproxil fumarate/Viread	Renal insufficiency Osteomalacia Severe acute exacerbation of hepatitis Weakness, headache, diarrhea, nausea, vomiting, and flatulence
Zidovudine/Retrovir	Headache, nausea, and insomnia Bone marrow suppression: macrocytic anemia or neutropenia Lipoatrophy Lactic acidosis or severe hepatomegaly with hepatic steatosis Hyperlipidemia Insulin resistance/diabetes mellitus Myopathy
Non-Nucleoside Reverse Transcriptase Inhibitors	
Efavirenz/Sustiva	Rash Neuropsychiatric symptoms Increased transaminase levels Hyperlipidemia Potentially teratogenic during the first trimester of pregnancy
Etravirine/Intelence	Rash, including Stevens-Johnson syndrome Hypersensitivity reactions Nausea
Nevirapine/Viramune	Rash, including Stevens-Johnson syndrome Symptomatic hepatitis, including fatal hepatic necrosis, has been reported
Rilpivirine/Edurant	Rash Depression, insomnia, headache Hepatoxicity
Protease Inhibitors	
Atazanavir/Reyataz, Evotaz	Indirect hyperbilirubinemia Hyperglycemia Fat maldistribution Cholelithiasis Nephrolithiasis Renal insufficiency Skin rash Serum transaminase elevations Hyperlipidemia Increase in serum creatinine level

Continued

Table 23-4   Antiretroviral Therapy and Toxic Effects and Cautions—cont'd

DRUG	MAJOR TOXIC EFFECTS AND CAUTIONS
Darunavir/Prezista, Prezcobix	Skin rash Hepatotoxicity Diarrhea, nausea, and headache Hyperlipidemia Serum transaminase elevation Hyperglycemia Fat maldistribution Increase in serum creatinine level
Fosamprenavir/ Lexiva	Skin rash Diarrhea, nausea, and vomiting Headache Hyperlipidemia Serum transaminase level elevation Hyperglycemia Fat maldistribution Possible increased bleeding in hemophiliac patients Nephrolithiasis
Indinavir/Crixivan	Gastrointestinal intolerance and nausea Nephrolithiasis Hepatitis Indirect hyperbilirubinemia Hyperlipidemia Headache, weakness, blurred vision, dizziness, rash, metallic taste, thrombocytopenia, alopecia, and hemolytic anemia Hyperglycemia Fat maldistribution Possible increased bleeding in hemophiliac patients
Lopinavir + ritonavir/ Kaletra	Gastrointestinal intolerance, nausea, vomiting, and diarrhea Pancreatitis Weakness Hyperlipidemia Serum transaminase level elevation Hyperglycemia Insulin resistance/diabetes mellitus Fat maldistribution Possible increased bleeding in hemophiliac patients
Nelfinavir/Viracept	Diarrhea Hyperlipidemia Hyperglycemia Fat maldistribution Possible increased bleeding in hemophiliac patients Serum transaminase elevation
Ritonavir/Norvir	Gastrointestinal intolerance, nausea, and vomiting Paresthesias (circumoral and extremities) Hyperlipidemia Hepatitis Weakness Altered taste Hyperglycemia Fat maldistribution Possible increased bleeding in hemophiliac patients
Saquinavir/Invirase	Gastrointestinal intolerance, nausea, and diarrhea Headache Serum transaminase elevation Hyperlipidemia Hyperglycemia Fat maldistribution Possible increased bleeding in hemophiliac patients

Table 23-4   Antiretroviral Therapy and Toxic Effects and Cautions—cont'd

DRUG	MAJOR TOXIC EFFECTS AND CAUTIONS
Tipranavir/Aptivus	Hepatotoxicity Skin rash Intracranial hemorrhage (rare) Hyperlipidemia Hyperglycemia Fat maldistribution Possible increased bleeding in hemophiliac patients
Integrase Inhibitor	
Dolutegravir/Tivicay, Triumeq	Rash and organ dysfunction Insomnia Headache
Elvitegravir/Vitekta	Nausea Diarrhea
Stribild	Nausea Diarrhea New onset or worsening renal impairment Potential decrease in bone mineral density Severe acute exacerbation of hepatitis
Raltegravir/Isentress	Rash, including Stevens-Johnson syndrome, hypersensitivity reaction, and toxic epidermal necrolysis Nausea Headache Diarrhea Pyrexia Creatine phosphokinase elevation, muscle weakness, and rhabdomyolysis Insomnia
Fusion Inhibitor	
Enfuvirtide/Fuzeon	Injection site reaction Increased bacterial pneumonia Hypersensitivity reaction
CCR5 Antagonist	
Maraviroc/Selzentry	Abdominal pain Cough Dizziness Musculoskeletal symptoms Pyrexia Rash Upper respiratory tract infections Hepatotoxicity Orthostatic hypotension
Integrase Inhibitors	
Dolutegravir/Tivicay	Hypersensitivity reaction Insomnia Headache
Elvitegravir/Vitekta	Nausea and diarrhea
Stribild	Nausea and diarrhea New onset or worsening renal impairment Potential decrease in bone mineral density Severe acute exacerbation of hepatitis may occur in HBV-coinfected patients stopping treatment
Raltegravir/Isentress	Rash, including Stevens-Johnson syndrome, hypersensitivity reaction, and toxic epidermal necrolysis Nausea Headache Diarrhea Pyrexia Creatine phosphokinase elevation, muscle weakness, and rhabdomyolysis Insomnia

Modified from Panel on Antiretroviral Guidelines for Adults and Adolescents—A Working Group of the Office of AIDS Research, Advisory Council. *Guidelines for the Use of Antiretroviral Agents in HIV-1-Infected Adults and Adolescents.* Department of Health and Human Services; 2015. Available at <www.aidsinfo.nih.gov/ContentFiles/AdultandAdolescentGL.pdf>. Accessed May 2015.

Institutes of Health are involved in coordinating vaccine research in the United States, and they are working in conjunction with other agencies worldwide to expedite the development of a more effective vaccine. A combination medication consisting of 300 mg of tenofovir disoproxil fumarate and 200 mg of emtricitabine, known as Truvada, has been approved for use as a preexposure prophylaxis in high-risk individuals in the United States.[42] The medication is taken daily in tablet form and appears to reduce the risk of HIV infection by 44% to 75% in high-risk individuals.[43] Research regarding the safety of long-term use of this preexposure prophylaxis in healthy adults is currently underway. Challenges to the development of an effective vaccine include the degree of diversity of the virus, the ability of the virus to evade the host's immunity, the cross-reactivity and incorrect presentation of the vaccine antigen, nonresponders, and several more.[44] More information about preventive and therapeutic vaccines can be found at https://aidsinfo.nih.gov.

MEDICAL NUTRITION THERAPY

ASSESSMENT

A comprehensive nutrition assessment provides the baseline information that is necessary for starting and continuing nutrition care. The registered dietitian nutritionist on the multidisciplinary team conducts this assessment. The assessment should include the typical ABCD nutrition evaluations: *a*nthropometric, *b*iochemical, *c*linical, and *d*ietary parameters (see Chapter 17).[45] Further person-centered nutrition care for HIV-infected patients may be indicated, as discussed in the Clinical Applications box, "The ABCDEFs of Nutrition Assessment for Patients with HIV/AIDS."

INTERVENTION

This portion of the nutrition care process includes planning, implementing, and documenting appropriate patient-specific interventions. There are no specific macronutrient or micronutrient recommendations for the patient with HIV, other than meeting his or her general needs. The key MNT objective is to reduce or eliminate malnutrition and to correct nutrition problems that are identified in the nutrition assessment.[19] Suggestions for nutrition-related symptom management are outlined in Table 23-2.

Dietitians can help to plan a patient-specific diet so that energy, protein, fluid, and micronutrient needs are met while not interfering with medication schedules. Food and water safety are important for all patients with compromised immunity, especially patients with HIV. Thus, the prevention of food-borne illness through appropriate cooking and storing food methods should be discussed during nutrition

---

Clinical Applications

The ABCDEFs of Nutrition Assessment for Patients with HIV/AIDS

The initial nutrition assessment visit with a patient infected with HIV is a vital encounter serving both informational and relational functions. It provides the necessary baseline information for planning practical, individual nutrition support. More importantly, however, the initial visit establishes the essential provider/patient relationship, which is the human context in which continuing nutrition care and support are provided. The basic ABCDs of nutrition assessment (*a*nthropometry, *b*iochemical tests, *c*linical observations, and *d*ietary evaluations) provide a practical guide (see Chapter 17), with two more points added for HIV-infected patients.

*E*nvironmental, behavioral, and psychologic assessment
- Living situation, personal support
- Food environment, types of meals, eating assistance needed

*F*inancial assessment
- Medical insurance
- Income, financial support through caregivers
- Ability to afford food, enteral supplements, additional vitamins or minerals

---

counseling. Complications from medications and co-morbidities should also be addressed. Common co-morbidities include cardiovascular disease, impaired renal function, diabetes, cancer, liver disease, and malnutrition.

WASTING EFFECTS OF HIV ON NUTRITIONAL STATUS

Malnutrition and Weight Loss

Patients with advanced stages of HIV regularly have a decreased appetite and an insufficient energy intake coupled with an elevated resting energy expenditure. Some of the energy imbalance is due to the nature of the disease and the rest is attributable to the side effects of medications. Significant weight loss follows and eventually leads to cachexia that is similar to what is seen in patients with cancer. Malnutrition suppresses cellular immune function, thereby perpetuating the onset of opportunistic infections, which is the ultimate cause of death in patients with AIDS. The chronic and relentless body wasting of AIDS is so striking that in Africa it is called the "slim disease." This wasting process plays a major role in the patient's debilitating weakness and fatigue, decreased quality of life, and the progression of the disease.

Causes of Body Wasting

The characteristic body wasting of HIV infection may result from any of the following processes, either alone or in combination:
- *Inadequate food intake:* An important factor in the profound weight loss seen in HIV/AIDS patients is

anorexia. This state is related to the patient's life-changing situation as well as the body's physiologic response to the disease and to drug-nutrient interactions. In addition to anorexia, food insecurity complicates the lives of many individuals who are living with HIV, especially in developing countries. Incorporating nutrition support and adding programs to provide food security have become recognized as important aspects within the treatment regimen for individuals with HIV worldwide.[46,47]

- *Malabsorption of nutrients:* Diarrhea and malabsorption are common symptoms that are related to drug-diet interactions and to the progressive effects of HIV infection. The viral infection causes the blunting of the intestinal villi and the secretion of abnormal intestinal enzymes. During the later stages of AIDS, the damaged intestinal tissues are open to opportunistic organisms, which results in severe diarrhea and malabsorption. Probiotics and prebiotics may be beneficial for preserving gut function and reducing inflammation in some patients.[48]

- *Disordered metabolism:* During the final stage of weight loss in patients with AIDS, changes in metabolism (e.g., hypermetabolism, altered energy metabolism) occur. The progressive depletion of lean body mass and an increased resting energy expenditure also result.[49]

- *Lean tissue wasting:* A decreased level of physical activity and exercise is to be expected among terminally ill patients who are undergoing extensive medical therapy with a multitude of negative side effects. Disuse coupled with systemic inflammation exacerbate muscle wasting and increase mortality. Resistance training, appropriate nutrition, and the administration of hormone replacement therapy may be effective for preventing lean tissue losses in some conditions of muscle wasting. Providing a lipid-based nutritional supplement with soy or whey protein early in antiretroviral therapy (ART) treatment has been shown to help maintain lean body mass and strength for some patients.[50]

Lipodystrophy

Lipodystrophy is not well-defined or objectively diagnosed; however, it is described as a disproportionate gaining of fat mass in the neck and abdomen with a concurrent loss of body fat in the face, buttocks, arms, and legs. Patients with lipodystrophy continue to lose lean tissue while unbalanced changes in fat mass are taking place. The combined effects add to the abnormal body composition seen in patients with AIDS and contribute to the development of cardiometabolic co-morbidities (e.g., hypertriglyceridemia, low HDL cholesterol, and insulin resistance).

The most well understood causative factor for lipodystrophy is treatment with antiretroviral therapy (see the For Further Focus box "Highly Active Antiretroviral Therapy and Lipodystrophy"). Other possible

For Further Focus

Highly Active Antiretroviral Therapy and Lipodystrophy

Lipodystrophy in patients with HIV involves lipoatrophy (i.e., body fat reduction) in the limbs and face and lipohypertrophy (i.e., increased fat mass) around the abdomen and the back of the neck. This redistribution of fat is associated with metabolic abnormalities and an increased risk for chronic conditions such as dyslipidemia, hypertension, and insulin resistance.

The introduction of antiretroviral drugs was an important step in the treatment of HIV. Since that time, mortality and morbidity from HIV have significantly declined. Although the natural process of aging over time and the HIV infection can lead to lipodystrophy, other body fat changes are attributed to the side effects of antiretroviral drugs. Nucleoside reverse transcriptase inhibitors and protease inhibitors are associated with lipoatrophy, and protease inhibitors may be associated with lipohypertrophy.

There is no cure for lipodystrophy; however, diet and exercise are key interventions to manage hyperlipidemia, insulin resistance, and central adiposity related to HIV-associated lipodystrophy. The dietary management of these patients is similar to that of patients without HIV who have cardiovascular risk factors. A diet that is low in saturated and trans fats; rich in fruits, vegetables, and whole grains; and adequate in protein, in combination with daily exercise, can reduce cardiovascular risk.

Recommended reading: da Cunha J, et al. Impact of antiretroviral therapy on lipid metabolism of human immunodeficiency virus-infected patients: old and new drugs. *World J Virol*. 2015;4(2):56-77.

risk factors include age, sex, body mass index, ethnicity, genetic factors, CD4 count, viral load, and duration of HIV infection.[51] To date, effective interventions to mitigate the burden of lipodystrophy in ART-treated individuals have not been identified. The dietary recommendations are to follow a well-balanced diet that is particularly heart-healthy, such as those discussed in Chapter 19 (e.g., DASH diet, Mediterranean diet, Lifestyle Management Guidelines from the American College of Cardiology and the American Heart Association Task Force).

NUTRITION COUNSELING, EDUCATION, AND SUPPORTIVE CARE

Education and counseling are important factors of MNT and should focus on the following:
- Adequate food intake to maintain appropriate body composition and nutritional status
- A review of nutritional strategies and additional therapies for symptom management to reduce the effects of disease progression, co-morbidities, and medication intolerance
- Potential drug-nutrient interactions
- Benefits and risks of dietary supplements

The basic goal of nutrition counseling is to make the least amount of changes necessary in a person's lifestyle and food patterns to promote optimal nutritional status while providing maximal comfort and quality of life. In this person-centered care process, the following counseling principles are particularly important:

- *Motivation:* Changes in behavior in any area require the motivation, desire, and ability to achieve one's goals. HIV/AIDS is no exception. Until a patient perceives food patterns and behaviors as appropriate goals, wait for a better time, and start with establishing a general supportive climate in which to continue working together. Specific obstacles that are raised by the patient (e.g., time, physical limitations, money, anxiety) can be met with related suggestions to consider, while also respecting the patients apprehensions.

- *Rationale:* Any diet or food behavior change with possible benefits or risks must be clearly explained to the patient. Patients with HIV/AIDS may be particularly vulnerable to the lure of unproven therapies.

- *Provider-patient agreement:* When the patient is ready, any change must involve an agreement, and it must fit daily routines and include caregivers and resource support as needed.

- *Manageable steps:* All information and actions should proceed in manageable steps that are as small as necessary and in order of complexity and difficulty. Do the simple and easy things first; information overload can discourage anyone. Clinicians should also keep in mind any cognitive or central nervous system decline in the patient. Such decline may contribute to memory loss and the inability to follow nutrition advice. Include individuals from the patient's support group in consultations and provide the patient with written instructions.

PERSONAL FOOD MANAGEMENT SKILLS

The patient's living situation and general practical skills with regard to planning, purchasing, and preparing food must be considered. The need for information and guidance when developing these skills or locating sources of help should be addressed. It is the responsibility of the registered dietitian nutritionist to establish patient-specific dietary plans that support the patient's medication regimens; this may include individualized plans for meal timing, macronutrient and micronutrient modulations, and symptom management.[45]

Community Programs

Information about available community food programs (e.g., Meals on Wheels for the delivery of prepared meals when the patient is too ill to shop for food or prepare it) may be needed. Information about food-assistance programs (e.g., the Supplemental Nutrition Assistance Program [SNAP] or food commodities [see Chapter 13]), for which lower-income patients may qualify, may be warranted. As mentioned earlier, nutrition support is a recognized important aspect of the care plan. Health care providers should ensure that a patient is economically, physically, and mentally capable of meeting his or her daily food needs or refer the patient to a social worker to assist in finding available programs within a patient's community to help secure the patient's access to food.

Psychosocial Support

Every aspect of health care provided should be given in a form and manner that provides genuine psychosocial support. All health care providers who work with patients with HIV/AIDS must be particularly sensitive to the psychologic and social issues that confront their patients. Major stress areas include issues related to autonomy and dependency, a sense of uncertainty and fear of the unknown, grief, change and loss, fear of symptoms and abandonment, spirituality, and quality of life. Common emotions are hostility, denial, withdrawal, depression, anxiety, guilt, and confusion. Health care providers must always be aware of how the patient and his or her caregivers relate to the disease and utilize the assistance of social workers and clinical psychologists as needed. Stress-reduction groups and activities—including exercise training—are helpful, as they are for other chronic conditions.

Health care workers must also examine their own stresses, values, and fears about sexual orientation, lifestyle behaviors, intravenous drug use, and fear of HIV transmission. Preconceived judgments are easily sensed by patients and threaten the provider-patient relationship. Before they can be effective with patients, all health care workers must first deal with their own fears and prejudices and learn to let go of judgmental behavior and support the needs of the patient.

Putting It All Together

Summary

- The general term *cancer* is given to various abnormal malignant tumors in different tissue sites. The cancer cell is derived from a normal cell that loses control over its growth and reproduction. Cancer cell development occurs as a result of the mutation of regulatory genes, and it is influenced by environmental chemical carcinogens, radiation, and viruses. Other lifestyle factors associated with an increased risk for cancer include poor diet, excessive alcohol use, and smoking.

- Cell integrity is mediated by the body's immune system, primarily through its two types of white blood cells: T cells that kill invading agents that cause disease and B cells that make specific antibodies to attack these agents.

- Cancer treatment primarily consists of surgery, radiation, and chemotherapy. Supportive nutrition care must be highly individualized in accordance with the patient's responses to the disease and its treatment.
- The nutrition care of patients with HIV/AIDS must be built on knowledge and compassion, with a sensitivity and concern for individual patient needs.
- The overall disease progression of HIV follows the three distinct stages: (1) HIV infection; (2) symptomatic disease with opportunistic infection and illnesses; and (3) symptomatic AIDS with complicating diseases that lead to death.
- The medical management of HIV infection involves the supportive treatment of associated illnesses and diseases. During the terminal AIDS stage, the virus eventually gains enough strength to destroy the host's immune system.
- Nutrition management centers on providing individual nutrition support to counteract the body wasting and malnutrition that are characteristic of HIV. The process of nutrition care involves a comprehensive nutrition assessment, the evaluation of personal needs, the planning of care with patient and caregivers, and the meeting of food needs.

Chapter Review Questions

See answers in Appendix A.
1. Cells that activate phagocytes are called:
   a. Antigens.
   b. Antibodies.
   c. T cells.
   d. B cells.

2. Appropriately planned medical nutrition therapy has been shown to be advantageous in patients with cancer by preventing extensive:
   a. Anabolism.
   b. Catabolism
   c. Pain.
   d. Depression.

3. A patient who is having difficulty eating because of mucositis would most likely tolerate which of the following food items?
   a. Flavored yogurt
   b. Hot chili with beans
   c. Cheese and crackers
   d. Chips and salsa

4. A disproportionate gaining of fat mass is referred to as:
   a. Cellulite.
   b. Cellulitis.
   c. Lipodystrophy.
   d. Hyperlipidemia.

5. Strategies to help prevent development of cancer include:
   a. Focusing on energy-dense meals and snacks.
   b. Eating standard serving sizes and emphasizing plant-based foods.
   c. Avoiding any consumption of alcoholic beverages.
   d. Using vitamin and mineral supplements to ensure adequate intake.

Additional Learning Resources

evolve http://evolve.elsevier.com/Williams/basic/

References and Further Reading and Resources in the back of the book provide additional resources for enhancing knowledge.

References

CHAPTER 1

1. U.S. Department of Health and Human Services. *Healthy People 2020*. Washington, DC: U.S. Government Printing Office; 2010.
2. National Center for Health Statistics. *Health, United States, 2014: with Special Feature Of Adults Aged 55-64*. Hyattsville, MD: U.S. Government Printing Office; 2015.
3. Sebastian RS, Wilkinson Enns C, Goldman JD. *MyPyramid Intakes and Snacking Patterns of U.S. Adults: What We Eat in America, NHANES 2007-2008*. Food Surveys Research Group Dietary Data Brief; 2011 Available from: <http://ars.usda.gov/Services/docs.htm?docid=19476>.
4. U.S. Department of Agriculture, Agricultural Research Service. *Nutrient intakes from food: mean amounts consumed per individual, by gender and age, what we eat in America, NHANES 2009-2010*. 2012.
5. Calder PC. Feeding the immune system. *Proc Nutr Soc*. 2013;72(3):299-309.
6. Kirkland LL, et al. Nutrition in the hospitalized patient. *J Hosp Med*. 2013;8(1):52-58.
7. Food and Nutrition Board, Institute of Medicine. *Dietary Reference Intakes for Calcium, Phosphorus, Magnesium, Vitamin D, and Fluoride*. Washington, DC: National Academies Press; 1997.
8. Food and Nutrition Board, Institute of Medicine. *Dietary Reference Intakes for Thiamin, Riboflavin, Niacin, Vitamin B$_6$, Folate, Vitamin B$_{12}$, Pantothenic Acid, Biotin, and Choline*. Washington, DC: National Academies Press; 1998.
9. Food and Nutrition Board, Institute of Medicine. *Dietary Reference Intakes for Vitamin C, Vitamin E, Selenium, and Carotenoids*. Washington, DC: National Academies Press; 2000.
10. Food and Nutrition Board, Institute of Medicine. *Dietary Reference Intakes for Vitamin A, Vitamin K, Arsenic, Boron, Chromium, Copper, Iodine, Iron, Manganese, Molybdenum, Nickel, Silicon, Vanadium, and Zinc*. Washington, DC: National Academies Press; 2001.
11. Food and Nutrition Board, Institute of Medicine. *Dietary Reference Intakes for Energy, Carbohydrate, Fiber, Fat, Fatty Acids, Cholesterol, Protein, and Amino Acids*. Washington, DC: National Academies Press; 2002.
12. Food and Nutrition Board, Institute of Medicine. *Dietary Reference Intakes for Water, Potassium, Sodium, Chloride, and Sulfate*. Washington, DC: National Academies Press; 2004.
13. Food and Nutrition Board, Institutes of Health. *Dietary Reference Intakes for Calcium and Vitamin D*. Washington, DC: National Academy of Sciences; 2010.
14. U.S. Department of Agriculture. Center for Nutrition Policy and Promotion. *USDA's MyPlate home page (website)*. Available from: <www.choosemyplate.gov>; Accessed June 6, 2015.
15. U.S. Department of Health and Human Services and U.S. Department of Agriculture. *2015-2020 Dietary Guidelines for Americans*. 8th ed. December 2015. Available at <http://health.gov/dietaryguidelines/2015/guidelines/>.

CHAPTER 2

1. U.S. Department of Agriculture. *2007-10 National Health and Nutrition Examination Survey (NHANES), two-day averages*. Available from: <www.ers.usda.gov/data-products/food-consumption-and-nutrient-intakes/documentation.aspx#.U7BiY3awXG4>; 2014 Accessed June 6, 2015.
2. U.S. Department of Health and Human Services and U.S. Department of Agriculture. *2015-2020 Dietary Guidelines for Americans*. 8th ed. December 2015. Available at <http://health.gov/dietaryguidelines/2015/guidelines/>.
3. U.S. Department of Agriculture, Economic Research Service. *Food availability (per capita) data system, sugar and sweeteners (added)*. Available from: <www.ers.usda.gov/data-products/food-availability-%28per-capita%29-data-system/.aspx#.U7BpG3awXG4>; 2014 Accessed June 6, 2015.
4. Food and Nutrition Board, Institute of Medicine. *Dietary Reference Intakes for Energy, Carbohydrate, Fiber, Fat, Fatty Acids, Cholesterol, Protein, and Amino Acids*. Washington, DC: National Academies Press; 2002.
5. Ross AB, et al. A whole-grain cereal-rich diet increases plasma betaine, and tends to decrease total and LDL-cholesterol compared with a refined-grain diet in healthy subjects. *Br J Nutr*. 2011;105(10):1492-1502.
6. Tighe P, et al. Effect of increased consumption of whole-grain foods on blood pressure and other cardiovascular risk markers in healthy middle-aged persons: a randomized controlled trial. *Am J Clin Nutr*. 2010;92(4):733-740.
7. Slavin JL, Lloyd B. Health benefits of fruits and vegetables. *Adv Nutr*. 2012;3(4):506-516.
8. Bijkerk CJ, et al. Soluble or insoluble fibre in irritable bowel syndrome in primary care? Randomised placebo controlled trial. *BMJ*. 2009;339:b3154.
9. Burger KN, et al. Dietary fiber, carbohydrate quality and quantity, and mortality risk of individuals with diabetes mellitus. *PLoS ONE*. 2012;7(8):e43127.
10. Ye EQ, et al. Greater whole-grain intake is associated with lower risk of type 2 diabetes, cardiovascular disease, and weight gain. *J Nutr*. 2012;142(7):1304-1313.
11. Othman RA, Moghadasian MH, Jones PJ. Cholesterol-lowering effects of oat beta-glucan. *Nutr Rev*. 2011;69(6):299-309.
12. Guenther PM, et al. Most Americans eat much less than recommended amounts of fruits and vegetables. *J Am Diet Assoc*. 2006;106(9):1371-1379.
13. O'Neil CE, et al. Whole-grain consumption is associated with diet quality and nutrient intake in adults: the National Health and Nutrition Examination Survey, 1999-2004. *J Am Diet Assoc*. 2010;110(10):1461-1468.
14. U.S. Department of Agriculture, Agricultural Research Service. Nutrient intakes from food: mean amounts consumed per individual, by gender and age, what we eat in America. *NHANES 2009-2010*, 2012.
15. Fitch C, et al. Position of the Academy of Nutrition and Dietetics: use of nutritive and nonnutritive sweeteners. *J Acad Nutr Diet*. 2012;112(5):739-758.
16. U.S. Department of Agriculture, Center for Nutrition Policy and Promotion. *USDA's MyPlate home page (website)*. Available from: <www.choosemyplate.gov>; Accessed June 6, 2015.

CHAPTER 3

1. Kiage JN, et al. Intake of trans fat and incidence of stroke in the REasons for Geographic And Racial Differences in Stroke (REGARDS) cohort. *Am J Clin Nutr.* 2014;99(5):1071-1076.

2. Vannice G, Rasmussen H. Position of the Academy of Nutrition and Dietetics: dietary fatty acids for healthy adults. *J Acad Nutr Diet.* 2014;114(1):136-153.

3. Chien KL, et al. Comparison of predictive performance of various fatty acids for the risk of cardiovascular disease events and all-cause deaths in a community-based cohort. *Atherosclerosis.* 2013;230(1):140-147.

4. Food and Nutrition Board, Institute of Medicine. *Dietary Reference Intakes for Energy, Carbohydrate, Fiber, Fat, Fatty Acids, Cholesterol, Protein, and Amino Acids.* Washington, DC: National Academies Press; 2013.

5. U.S. Department of Health and Human Services and U.S. Department of Agriculture. *2015-2020 Dietary Guidelines for Americans.* 8th ed. December 2015. Available at <http://health.gov/dietaryguidelines/2015/guidelines/>.

6. Fernandez ML. Rethinking dietary cholesterol. *Curr Opin Clin Nutr Metab Care.* 2012;15(2):117-121.

7. U.S. Department of Agriculture, Center for Nutrition Policy and Promotion. *Nutrient content of the U.S. food supply, 1909-2010,* 2014.

8. Beauchesne-Rondeau E, et al. Plasma lipids and lipoproteins in hypercholesterolemic men fed a lipid-lowering diet containing lean beef, lean fish, or poultry. *Am J Clin Nutr.* 2003;77(3):587-593.

9. Roussell MA, et al. Beef in an optimal lean diet study: effects on lipids, lipoproteins, and apolipoproteins. *Am J Clin Nutr.* 2012;95(1):9-16.

10. Binkoski AE, et al. Balance of unsaturated fatty acids is important to a cholesterol-lowering diet: comparison of mid-oleic sunflower oil and olive oil on cardiovascular disease risk factors. *J Am Diet Assoc.* 2005;105(7):1080-1086.

11. Iggman D, et al. Replacing dairy fat with rapeseed oil causes rapid improvement of hyperlipidaemia: a randomized controlled study. *J Intern Med.* 2011;270(4):356-364.

12. Astrup A, et al. The role of reducing intakes of saturated fat in the prevention of cardiovascular disease: where does the evidence stand in 2010? *Am J Clin Nutr.* 2011;93(4):684-688.

13. Lawrence GD. Dietary fats and health: dietary recommendations in the context of scientific evidence. *Adv Nutr.* 2013;4(3):294-302.

14. Ravnskov U, et al. The questionable benefits of exchanging saturated fat with polyunsaturated fat. *Mayo Clin Proc.* 2014;89(4):451-453.

15. Ramsden CE, et al. n-6 fatty acid-specific and mixed polyunsaturated dietary interventions have different effects on CHD risk: a meta-analysis of randomised controlled trials. *Br J Nutr.* 2010;104(11):1586-1600.

16. U.S. Food and Drug Administration. *Health claims meeting significant scientific agreement (SSA).* Available from: <www.fda.gov/Food/IngredientsPackagingLabeling/LabelingNutrition/ucm2006876.htm#Approved_Health_Claims>; Accessed July 17, 2014.

17. U.S. Department of Agriculture. *2007-10 National Health and Nutrition Examination Survey (NHANES), two-day averages.* 2014 June 29, 2014. Available from: <www.ers.usda.gov/data-products/food-consumption-and-nutrient-intakes/documentation.aspx#.U7BiY3awXG4>.

18. Bastien M, et al. Overview of epidemiology and contribution of obesity to cardiovascular disease. *Prog Cardiovasc Dis.* 2014;56(4):369-381.

19. Flegal KM, et al. Association of all-cause mortality with overweight and obesity using standard body mass index categories: a systematic review and meta-analysis. *JAMA.* 2013;309(1):71-82.

20. Jenkins DJ, et al. Adding monounsaturated fatty acids to a dietary portfolio of cholesterol-lowering foods in hypercholesterolemia. *CMAJ.* 2010;182(18):1961-1967.

21. Yang J, et al. Modified Mediterranean diet score and cardiovascular risk in a North American working population. *PLoS ONE.* 2014;9(2):e87539.

22. Casas R, et al. The effects of the Mediterranean diet on biomarkers of vascular wall inflammation and plaque vulnerability in subjects with high risk for cardiovascular disease. A randomized trial. *PLoS ONE.* 2014;9(6):e100084.

23. Mozaffarian D, Aro A, Willett WC. Health effects of trans-fatty acids: experimental and observational evidence. *Eur J Clin Nutr.* 2009;63(suppl 2):S5-S21.

24. Food and Drug Administration *Final determination regarding partially hydrogenated oil, Food and Drug Administration,* 2015, *Federal Register.*

25. Centers for Disease Control and Prevention. Prevalence of abnormal lipid levels among youths—United States, 1999-2006. *MMWR Morb Mortal Wkly Rep.* 2010;59(2):29.

26. Simopoulos AP. The importance of the omega-6/omega-3 fatty acid ratio in cardiovascular disease and other chronic diseases. *Exp Biol Med (Maywood).* 2008;233(6):674-688.

27. U.S. Department of Agriculture, Center for Nutrition Policy and Promotion. *USDA's myplate home page (website).* Available from: <www.choosemyplate.gov>; Accessed June 16, 2014.

CHAPTER 4

1. Food and Nutrition Board, Institute of Medicine. *Dietary Reference Intakes for Energy, Carbohydrate, Fiber, Fat, Fatty Acids, Cholesterol, Protein, and Amino Acids.* Washington, DC: National Academies Press; 2002.

2. Craig WJ, Mangels AR. American Dietetic. Position of the American Dietetic Association: vegetarian diets. *J Am Diet Assoc.* 2009;109(7):1266-1282.

3. Stahler C. *How often do Americans eat vegetarian meals? And how many adults in the US are vegetarian, 2012?* Available from: <www.vrg.org/journal/vj2011issue4/vj2011issue4poll.php>; Accessed June 11, 2015.

4. Fraser GE. Vegetarian diets: what do we know of their effects on common chronic diseases? *Am J Clin Nutr.* 2009;89(5):1607S-1612S.

5. Yokoyama Y, et al. Vegetarian diets and blood pressure: a meta-analysis. *JAMA Intern Med.* 2014;174(4):577-587.

6. Mishra S, et al. A multicenter randomized controlled trial of a plant-based nutrition program to reduce body weight and cardiovascular risk in the corporate setting: the GEICO study. *Eur J Clin Nutr.* 2013;67(7):718-724.

7. Clarys P, et al. Dietary pattern analysis: a comparison between matched vegetarian and omnivorous subjects. *Nutr J.* 2013;12:82.

8. Ley SH, et al. Prevention and management of type 2 diabetes: dietary components and nutritional strategies. *Lancet.* 2014;383(9933):1999-2007.

9. Kahleova H, et al. Vegetarian diet improves insulin resistance and oxidative stress markers more than conventional diet in subjects with Type 2 diabetes. *Diabet Med.* 2011;28(5):549-559.

10. Crowe FL, et al. Risk of hospitalization or death from ischemic heart disease among British vegetarians and nonvegetarians: results from the EPIC-Oxford cohort study. *Am J Clin Nutr.* 2013;97(3):597-603.

11. Tantamango-Bartley Y, et al. Vegetarian diets and the incidence of cancer in a low-risk population. *Cancer Epidemiol Biomarkers Prev.* 2013;22(2):286-294.

12. Segasothy M, Phillips PA. Vegetarian diet: panacea for modern lifestyle diseases? *QJM.* 1999;92(9):531-544.

13. Craig WJ. Nutrition concerns and health effects of vegetarian diets. *Nutr Clin Pract.* 2010;25(6):613-620.

14. Madry E, et al. The impact of vegan diet on B-12 status in healthy omnivores: five-year prospective study. *Acta Sci Pol Technol Aliment*. 2012;11(2):209-212.

15. Rizzo NS, et al. Nutrient profiles of vegetarian and nonvegetarian dietary patterns. *J Acad Nutr Diet*. 2013;113(12): 1610-1619.

16. Wallace TC, Reider C, Fulgoni VL 3rd. Calcium and vitamin D disparities are related to gender, age, race, household income level, and weight classification but not vegetarian status in the United States: analysis of the NHANES 2001-2008 data set. *J Am Coll Nutr*. 2013;32(5):321-330.

17. Millward DJ, et al. Protein quality assessment: impact of expanding understanding of protein and amino acid needs for optimal health. *Am J Clin Nutr*. 2008;87(5):1576S-1581S.

18. Millward DJ. Amino acid scoring patterns for protein quality assessment. *Br J Nutr*. 2012;108(suppl 2):S31-S43.

19. Tome D. Criteria and markers for protein quality assessment – a review. *Br J Nutr*. 2012;108(suppl 2):S222-S229.

20. Ahmed T, Rahman S, Cravioto A. Oedematous malnutrition. *Indian J Med Res*. 2009;130(5):651-654.

21. Meek RL, et al. Glomerular cell death and inflammation with high-protein diet and diabetes. *Nephrol Dial Transplant*. 2013;28(7):1711-1720.

22. U.S. Department of Agriculture, Agricultural Research Service. *Nutrient intakes from food: mean amounts consumed per individual, by gender and age, what we eat in America, NHANES 2009-2010*. 2012.

23. U.S. Department of Health and Human Services and U.S. Department of Agriculture. *2015-2020 Dietary Guidelines for Americans*. 8th ed. December 2015. Available at <http://health.gov/dietaryguidelines/2015/guidelines/>.

24. U.S. Department of Agriculture, Center for Nutrition Policy and Promotion. *USDA's MyPlate home page (website)*. Available from: <www.choosemyplate.gov>; Accessed June 6, 2015.

CHAPTER 5

1. Food and Nutrition Board, Institute of Medicine. *Dietary Reference Intakes for Calcium, Phosphorus, Magnesium, Vitamin D, and Fluoride*. Washington, DC: National Academies Press; 1997.

2. Food and Nutrition Board, Institute of Medicine. *Dietary Reference Intakes for Thiamin, Riboflavin, Niacin, Vitamin B6, Folate, Vitamin B12, Pantothenic Acid, Biotin, and Choline*. Washington, DC: National Academies Press; 2000.

3. Food and Nutrition Board, Institute of Medicine. *Dietary Reference Intakes for Vitamin C, Vitamin E, Selenium, and Carotenoids*. Washington, DC: National Academies Press; 2000.

4. Food and Nutrition Board, Institute of Medicine. *Dietary Reference Intakes for Vitamin A, Vitamin K, Arsenic, Boron, Chromium, Copper, Iodine, Iron, Manganese, Molybdenum, Nickel, Silicon, Vanadium, and Zinc*. Washington, DC: National Academies Press; 2001.

5. Food and Nutrition Board, Institute of Medicine. *Dietary Reference Intakes for Energy, Carbohydrate, Fiber, Fat, Fatty Acids, Cholesterol, Protein, and Amino Acids*. Washington, DC: National Academies Press; 2002.

6. Food and Nutrition Board, Institute of Medicine. *Dietary Reference Intakes for Water, Potassium, Sodium, Chloride, and Sulfate*. Washington, DC: National Academies Press; 2004.

7. Cerreto M, et al. Reversal of metabolic and neurological symptoms of phenylketonuric mice treated with a PAH containing helper-dependent adenoviral vector. *Curr Gene Ther*. 2012;12(1):48-56.

8. Harding C. Progress toward cell-directed therapy for phenylketonuria. *Clin Genet*. 2008;74(2):97-104.

9. Yagi H, et al. Recovery of neurogenic amines in phenylketonuria mice after liver-targeted gene therapy. *Neuroreport*. 2012;23(1):30-34.

10. Longo N, et al. Single-dose, subcutaneous recombinant phenylalanine ammonia lyase conjugated with polyethylene glycol in adult patients with phenylketonuria: an open-label, multicentre, phase 1 dose-escalation trial. *Lancet*. 2014; 384(9937):37-44.

11. Jahja R, et al. Neurocognitive evidence for revision of treatment targets and guidelines for phenylketonuria. *J Pediatr*. 2014;164(4):895-899, e2.

12. Berry GT. Classic galactosemia and clinical variant galactosemia. In: Pagon RA, Adam MP, Ardinger HH, et al., eds. *GeneReviews(R)*. Seattle: Wash; 2014.

13. Karadag N, et al. Literature review and outcome of classic galactosemia diagnosed in the neonatal period. *Clin Lab*. 2013;59(9-10):1139-1146.

14. Jumbo-Lucioni PP, et al. Diversity of approaches to classic galactosemia around the world: a comparison of diagnosis, intervention, and outcomes. *J Inherit Metab Dis*. 2012;35(6): 1037-1049.

15. Mayatepek E, Hoffmann B, Meissner T. Inborn errors of carbohydrate metabolism. *Best Pract Res Clin Gastroenterol*. 2010;24(5):607-618.

CHAPTER 6

1. Food and Nutrition Board, Institute of Medicine. *Dietary Reference Intakes for Energy, Carbohydrate, Fiber, Fat, Fatty Acids, Cholesterol, Protein, and Amino Acids*. Washington, DC: National Academies Press; 2002.

2. Psota T, Chen KY. Measuring energy expenditure in clinical populations: rewards and challenges. *Eur J Clin Nutr*. 2013;67(5):436-442.

3. Bosy-Westphal A, et al. Effect of organ and tissue masses on resting energy expenditure in underweight, normal weight and obese adults. *Int J Obes Relat Metab Disord*. 2004;28(1): 72-79.

4. Javed F, et al. Brain and high metabolic rate organ mass: contributions to resting energy expenditure beyond fat-free mass. *Am J Clin Nutr*. 2010;91(4):907-912.

5. Gallagher D, et al. Organ-tissue mass measurement allows modeling of REE and metabolically active tissue mass. *Am J Physiol*. 1998;275(2 Pt 1):E249-E258.

6. Heymsfield SB, et al. Evolving concepts on adjusting human resting energy expenditure measurements for body size. *Obes Rev*. 2012;13(11):1001-1014.

7. McClave SA, Martindale RG, Kiraly L. The use of indirect calorimetry in the intensive care unit. *Curr Opin Clin Nutr Metab Care*. 2013;16(2):202-208.

8. Cooney RN, Frankenfield DC. Determining energy needs in critically ill patients: equations or indirect calorimeters. *Curr Opin Crit Care*. 2012;18(2):174-177.

9. Hipskind P, et al. Do handheld calorimeters have a role in assessment of nutrition needs in hospitalized patients? A systematic review of literature. *Nutr Clin Pract*. 2011;26(4): 426-433.

10. McDoniel SO. Systematic review on use of a handheld indirect calorimeter to assess energy needs in adults and children. *Int J Sport Nutr Exerc Metab*. 2007;17(5):491-500.

11. Nieman DC, et al. Validation of a new handheld device for measuring resting metabolic rate and oxygen consumption in children. *Int J Sport Nutr Exerc Metab*. 2005;15(2): 186-194.

12. Frankenfield D, Roth-Yousey L, Compher C. Comparison of predictive equations for resting metabolic rate in healthy nonobese and obese adults: a systematic review. *J Am Diet Assoc*. 2005;105(5):775-789.

13. Ravussin E, et al. Determinants of 24-hour energy expenditure in man. Methods and results using a respiratory chamber. *J Clin Invest*. 1986;78(6):1568-1578.

14. Astrup A, et al. Prediction of 24-h energy expenditure and its components from physical characteristics and body

composition in normal-weight humans. *Am J Clin Nutr.* 1990;52(5):777-783.

15. Krems C, et al. Lower resting metabolic rate in the elderly may not be entirely due to changes in body composition. *Eur J Clin Nutr.* 2005;59(2):255-262.

16. Luhrmann PM, Edelmann-Schafer B, Neuhauser-Berthold M. Changes in resting metabolic rate in an elderly German population: cross-sectional and longitudinal data. *J Nutr Health Aging.* 2010;14(3):232-236.

17. St-Onge MP, Gallagher D. Body composition changes with aging: the cause or the result of alterations in metabolic rate and macronutrient oxidation? *Nutrition.* 2010;26(2): 152-155.

18. Butte NF, King JC. Energy requirements during pregnancy and lactation. *Public Health Nutr.* 2005;8(7A):1010-1027.

19. Landsberg L. Core temperature: a forgotten variable in energy expenditure and obesity? *Obes Rev.* 2012;13(suppl 2): 97-104.

20. Kreitschmann-Andermahr I, et al. GH/IGF-I regulation in obesity—mechanisms and practical consequences in children and adults. *Horm Res Paediatr.* 2010;73(3):153-160.

21. Vallance JK, et al. Physical activity and health-related quality of life among older men: an examination of current physical activity recommendations. *Prev Med.* 2012;54(3-4): 234-236.

22. Moilanen JM, et al. Physical activity and change in quality of life during menopause—an 8-year follow-up study. *Health Qual Life Outcomes.* 2012;10:8.

23. Messier V, et al. Menopause and sarcopenia: a potential role for sex hormones. *Maturitas.* 2011;68(4):331-336.

24. Toth MJ, et al. Menopause-related changes in body fat distribution. *Ann N Y Acad Sci.* 2000;904:502-506.

25. Maltais ML, Desroches J, Dionne IJ. Changes in muscle mass and strength after menopause. *J Musculoskelet Neuronal Interact.* 2009;9(4):186-197.

26. U.S. Department of Health and Human Services and U.S. Department of Agriculture. *2015-2020 Dietary Guidelines for Americans.* 8th ed. December 2015. Available at <http://health.gov/dietaryguidelines/2015/guidelines/>.

27. U.S. Department of Agriculture, Center for Nutrition Policy and Promotion. *USDA's myplate home page (website).* Available from: <www.choosemyplate.gov>; Accessed June 16, 2014.

CHAPTER 7

1. Lind J. *A Treatise of the Scurvy.* Edinburgh, Scotland: Sands, Murray & Cochran; 1753.

2. Hopkins FG. Feeding experiments illustrating the importance of accessory factors in normal dietaries. *J Physiol.* 1912;44(5-6):425-460.

3. Funk C. The etiology of the deficiency diseases. Beri-beri, polyneuritis in birds, epidemic dropsy, scurvy, experimental scurvy in animals, infantile scurvy, ship beri-beri, pellagra. *J State Med.* 1912;20:341.

4. Age-Related Eye Disease Study 2 Research Group, et al. Secondary analyses of the effects of lutein/zeaxanthin on age-related macular degeneration progression: AREDS2 report No. 3. *JAMA Ophthalmol.* 2014;132(2):142-149.

5. World Health Organization. *Global Prevalence of Vitamin A Deficiency in Populations at Risk 1995-2005.* Geneva, Switzerland: World Health Organization; 2009.

6. Food and Nutrition Board, Institute of Medicine. *Dietary Reference Intakes for Vitamin A, Vitamin K, Arsenic, Boron, Chromium, Copper, Iodine, Iron, Manganese, Molybdenum, Nickel, Silicon, Vanadium, and Zinc.* Washington, DC: National Academies Press; 2001.

7. Reboul E. Absorption of vitamin A and carotenoids by the enterocyte: focus on transport proteins. *Nutrients.* 2013;5(9): 3563-3581.

8. Castenmiller JJ, West CE. Bioavailability and bioconversion of carotenoids. *Annu Rev Nutr.* 1998;18:19-38.

9. McCollum EV, Simmonds N, Becker JE, Shipley PG. Studies on experimental rickets. XXI. An experimental demonstration of the existence of a vitamin which promotes calcium deposition. *J Biol Chem.* 1922;53:293-312.

10. Hiligsmann M, et al. Cost-effectiveness of vitamin D and calcium supplementation in the treatment of elderly women and men with osteoporosis. *Eur J Public Health.* 2014;25(1): 20-25.

11. de Jong A, et al. Vitamin D insufficiency in osteoporotic hip fracture patients: rapid substitution therapy with high dose oral cholecalciferol (vitamin D3). *Acta Orthop Belg.* 2013; 79(5):578-586.

12. Holick MF. Optimal vitamin D status for the prevention and treatment of osteoporosis. *Drugs Aging.* 2007;24(12): 1017-1029.

13. Troesch B, et al. Dietary surveys indicate vitamin intakes below recommendations are common in representative Western countries. *Br J Nutr.* 2012;108(4):692-698.

14. Holick MF, Chen TC. Vitamin D deficiency: a worldwide problem with health consequences. *Am J Clin Nutr.* 2008; 87(4):1080S-1086S.

15. Bendik I, et al. Vitamin D: a critical and essential micronutrient for human health. *Front Physiol.* 2014;5:248.

16. Wagner CL, et al. Prevention of rickets and vitamin D deficiency in infants, children, and adolescents. *Pediatrics.* 2008; 122(5):1142-1152.

17. Gutierrez OM, et al. Racial differences in the relationship between vitamin D, bone mineral density, and parathyroid hormone in the National Health and Nutrition Examination Survey. *Osteoporos Int.* 2011;22(6):1745-1753.

18. Powe CE, et al. Vitamin D-binding protein and vitamin D status of black Americans and white Americans. *N Engl J Med.* 2013;369(21):1991-2000.

19. Food and Nutrition Board, Institute of Medicine. *Dietary Reference Intakes for Calcium and Vitamin D.* Washington, DC: National Academies Press; 2011.

20. Evans HM, Bishop KS. On the existence of a hitherto unrecognized dietary factor essential for reproduction. *Science.* 1922;56(1458):650-651.

21. Food and Nutrition Board, Institute of Medicine. *Dietary Reference Intakes for Vitamin C, Vitamin E, Selenium, and Carotenoids.* Washington, DC: National Academies Press; 2000.

22. Rimbach G, et al. Gene-regulatory activity of alpha-tocopherol. *Molecules.* 2010;15(3):1746-1761.

23. Yu AL, Moriniere J, Welge-Lussen U. Vitamin E reduces TGF-beta2-induced changes in human trabecular meshwork cells. *Curr Eye Res.* 2013;38(9):952-958.

24. Traber MG. Vitamin E and K interactions—a 50-year-old problem. *Nutr Rev.* 2008;66(11):624-629.

25. Dam H. The antihaemorrhagic vitamin of the chick. *Biochem J.* 1935;29(6):1273-1285.

26. Bugel S. Vitamin K and bone health in adult humans. *Vitam Horm.* 2008;78:393-416.

27. Bollet AJ. Politics and pellagra: the epidemic of pellagra in the U.S. in the early twentieth century. *Yale J Biol Med.* 1992;65(3):211-221.

28. Food and Nutrition Board, Institute of Medicine. *Dietary Reference Intakes for Thiamin, Riboflavin, Niacin, Vitamin B6, Folate, Vitamin B12, Pantothenic Acid, Biotin, and Choline.* Washington, DC: National Academies Press; 1998.

29. Clarke R, et al. Effects of lowering homocysteine levels with B vitamins on cardiovascular disease, cancer, and cause-specific mortality: meta-analysis of 8 randomized trials involving 37485 individuals. *Arch Intern Med.* 2010;170(18): 1622-1631.

30. Ohrvik VE, Witthoft CM. Human folate bioavailability. *Nutrients.* 2011;3(4):475-490.

31. Copp AJ, Greene ND. Neural tube defects—disorders of neurulation and related embryonic processes. *Wiley Interdiscip Rev Dev Biol.* 2013;2(2):213-227.

32. Centers for Disease Control and Prevention. Racial/ethnic differences in the birth prevalence of spina bifida—United States, 1995-2005. *MMWR Morb Mortal Wkly Rep.* 2009; 57(53):1409-1413.

33. Youngblood ME, et al. 2012 Update on global prevention of folic acid-preventable spina bifida and anencephaly. *Birth Defects Res A Clin Mol Teratol.* 2013;97(10):658-663.

34. Langan RC, Zawistoski KJ. Update on vitamin B12 deficiency. *Am Fam Physician.* 2011;83(12):1425-1430.

35. Wolf B. Biotinidase deficiency: "if you have to have an inherited metabolic disease, this is the one to have". *Genet Med.* 2012;14(6):565-575.

36. Buchman AL, et al. Choline deficiency causes reversible hepatic abnormalities in patients receiving parenteral nutrition: proof of a human choline requirement: a placebo-controlled trial. *JPEN J Parenter Enteral Nutr.* 2001;25(5): 260-268.

37. Hollenbeck CB. The importance of being choline. *J Am Diet Assoc.* 2010;110(8):1162-1165.

38. Liu RH. Health-promoting components of fruits and vegetables in the diet. *Adv Nutr.* 2013;4(3):384S-392S.

39. de Kok TM, van Breda SG, Manson MM. Mechanisms of combined action of different chemopreventive dietary compounds: a review. *Eur J Nutr.* 2008;47(suppl 2):51-59.

40. Centers for Disease Control and Prevention. *What counts as a cup?* September 2014. Available from: <www.cdc.gov/nutrition/everyone/fruitsvegetables/cup.html>.

41. Wang X, et al. Fruit and vegetable consumption and mortality from all causes, cardiovascular disease, and cancer: systematic review and dose-response meta-analysis of prospective cohort studies. *BMJ.* 2014;349:4490.

42. McGuire S. State Indicator Report on Fruits and Vegetables, 2013, Centers for Disease Control and Prevention, Atlanta, Ga. *Adv Nutr.* 2013;4(6):665-666.

43. Krebs-Smith SM, et al. Americans do not meet federal dietary recommendations. *J Nutr.* 2010;140(10):1832-1838.

44. Office of Dietary Supplements. *Mission statement.* September 2014. Available from: <http://ods.od.nih.gov/About/MissionOriginMandate.aspx>.

45. Marra MV, Boyar AP. Position of the American Dietetic Association: nutrient supplementation. *J Am Diet Assoc.* 2009;109(12):2073-2085.

46. Schleicher RL, et al. Serum vitamin C and the prevalence of vitamin C deficiency in the United States: 2003-2004 National Health and Nutrition Examination Survey (NHANES). *Am J Clin Nutr.* 2009;90(5):1252-1263.

47. Ramanathan VS, et al. Hypervitaminosis A inducing intrahepatic cholestasis—a rare case report. *Exp Mol Pathol.* 2010;88(2):324-325.

48. Khasru MR, et al. Acute hypervitaminosis A in a young lady. *Mymensingh Med J.* 2010;19(2):294-298.

49. Hayman RM, Dalziel SR. Acute vitamin A toxicity: a report of three paediatric cases. *J Paediatr Child Health.* 2012;48(3): E98-E100.

50. Crowe KM, et al. Position of the Academy of Nutrition and Dietetics: functional foods. *J Acad Nutr Diet.* 2013;113(8): 1096-1103.

CHAPTER 8

1. Khosla S. Update in male osteoporosis. *J Clin Endocrinol Metab.* 2010;95(1):3-10.

2. Banu J. Causes, consequences, and treatment of osteoporosis in men. *Drug Des Devel Ther.* 2013;7:849-860.

3. Becker DJ, Kilgore ML, Morrisey MA. The societal burden of osteoporosis. *Curr Rheumatol Rep.* 2010;12(3):186-191.

4. Budhia S, et al. Osteoporotic fractures: a systematic review of U.S. healthcare costs and resource utilization. *Pharmacoeconomics.* 2012;30(2):147-170.

5. Cauley JA, et al. Objective measures of physical activity, fractures and falls: the osteoporotic fractures in men study. *J Am Geriatr Soc.* 2013;61(7):1080-1088.

6. Balasubramanian A, et al. Declining rates of osteoporosis management following fragility fractures in the U.S., 2000 through 2009. *J Bone Joint Surg Am.* 2014;96(7):e52.

7. U.S. Department of Agriculture, Agricultural Research Service. *Nutrient intakes from food and beverages: mean amounts consumed per individual, by gender and age, what we eat in America, NHANES 2011-2012.* 2014.

8. Peters BS, Martini LA. Nutritional aspects of the prevention and treatment of osteoporosis. *Arq Bras Endocrinol Metabol.* 2010;54(2):179-185.

9. Caroli A, et al. Invited review: dairy intake and bone health: a viewpoint from the state of the art. *J Dairy Sci.* 2011; 94(11):5249-5262.

10. Radimer K, et al. Dietary supplement use by US adults: data from the National Health and Nutrition Examination Survey, 1999-2000. *Am J Epidemiol.* 2004;160(4):339-349.

11. Pivnick EK, et al. Rickets secondary to phosphate depletion. A sequela of antacid use in infancy. *Clin Pediatr (Phila).* 1995;34(2):73-78.

12. Neumann L, Jensen BG. Osteomalacia from Al and Mg antacids. Report of a case of bilateral hip fracture. *Acta Orthop Scand.* 1989;60(3):361-362.

13. Chines A, Pacifici R. Antacid and sucralfate-induced hypophosphatemic osteomalacia: a case report and review of the literature. *Calcif Tissue Int.* 1990;47(5):291-295.

14. Food and Nutrition Board, Institute of Medicine. *Dietary Reference Intakes for Calcium, Phosphorus, Magnesium, Vitamin D, and Fluoride.* Washington, DC: National Academies Press; 1997.

15. Savica V, Bellinghieri G, Kopple JD. The effect of nutrition on blood pressure. *Annu Rev Nutr.* 2010;30:365-401.

16. Food and Nutrition Board, Institute of Medicine. *Dietary Reference Intakes for Water, Potassium, Sodium, Chloride, and Sulfate.* Washington, DC: National Academies Press; 2004.

17. U.S. Department of Health and Human Services and U.S. Department of Agriculture. *2015-2020 Dietary Guidelines for Americans.* 8th ed. December 2015. Available at <http://health.gov/dietaryguidelines/2015/guidelines/>.

18. Musso CG. Magnesium metabolism in health and disease. *Int Urol Nephrol.* 2009;41(2):357-362.

19. Assadi F. Hypomagnesemia: an evidence-based approach to clinical cases. *Iran J Kidney Dis.* 2010;4(1):13-19.

20. Food and Nutrition Board, Institute of Medicine. *Dietary Reference Intakes for Vitamin A, Vitamin K, Arsenic, Boron, Chromium, Copper, Iodine, Iron, Manganese, Molybdenum, Nickel, Silicon, Vanadium, and Zinc.* Washington, DC: National Academies Press; 2001.

21. McLean E, et al. Worldwide prevalence of anaemia, WHO Vitamin and Mineral Nutrition Information System, 1993-2005. *Public Health Nutr.* 2009;12(4):444-454.

22. Chang TP, Rangan C. Iron poisoning: a literature-based review of epidemiology, diagnosis, and management. *Pediatr Emerg Care.* 2011;27(10):978-985.

23. Madiwale T, Liebelt E. Iron: not a benign therapeutic drug. *Curr Opin Pediatr.* 2006;18(2):174-179.

24. Crownover BK, Covey CJ. Hereditary hemochromatosis. *Am Fam Physician.* 2013;87(3):183-190.

25. World Health Organization. *Assessment of Iodine Deficiency Disorders and Monitoring Their Elimination.* Geneva: WHO; 2008.

26. Pearce EN, Andersson M, Zimmermann MB. Global iodine nutrition: where do we stand in 2013? *Thyroid.* 2013;23(5): 523-528.

27. Hynes KL, et al. Mild iodine deficiency during pregnancy is associated with reduced educational outcomes in the offspring: 9-year follow-up of the gestational iodine cohort. *J Clin Endocrinol Metab.* 2013;98(5):1954-1962.

28. Markou KB, et al. Treating iodine deficiency: long-term effects of iodine repletion on growth and pubertal development in school-age children. *Thyroid*. 2008;18(4):449-454.

29. Almandoz JP, Gharib H. Hypothyroidism: etiology, diagnosis, and management. *Med Clin North Am*. 2012;96(2):203-221.

30. Stanbury JB, et al. Iodine-induced hyperthyroidism: occurrence and epidemiology. *Thyroid*. 1998;8(1):83-100.

31. Haase H, Rink L. Multiple impacts of zinc on immune function. *Metallomics*. 2014;6(7):1175-1180.

32. Gibson RS, et al. Does zinc deficiency play a role in stunting among primary school children in NE Thailand? *Br J Nutr*. 2007;97(1):167-175.

33. Prasad AS. Zinc in human health: effect of zinc on immune cells. *Mol Med*. 2008;14(5-6):353-357.

34. Plum LM, Rink L, Haase H. The essential toxin: impact of zinc on human health. *Int J Environ Res Public Health*. 2010;7(4):1342-1365.

35. Craig WJ, Mangels AR. Position of the American Dietetic Association: vegetarian diets. *J Am Diet Assoc*. 2009;109(7):1266-1282.

36. MacFarquhar JK, et al. Acute selenium toxicity associated with a dietary supplement. *Arch Intern Med*. 2010;170(3):256-261.

37. Food and Nutrition Board, Institute of Medicine. *Dietary Reference Intakes for Vitamin C, Vitamin E, Selenium, and Carotenoids*. Washington, DC: National Academies Press; 2000.

38. U.S. Department of Agriculture, Agricultural Research Service, *Nutrient Data Laboratory. USDA nutrient database for standard reference 2014 October 11*, 2014. Available from: <http://ndb.nal.usda.gov/>.

39. Tumer Z, Moller LB. Menkes disease. *Eur J Hum Genet*. 2010;18(5):511-518.

40. Gouider-Khouja N. Wilson's disease. *Parkinsonism Relat Disord*. 2009;15(suppl 3):S126-S129.

41. Hardy G. Manganese in parenteral nutrition: who, when, and why should we supplement? *Gastroenterology*. 2009;137(5 suppl):S29-S35.

42. Gunton JE, et al. Chromium supplementation does not improve glucose tolerance, insulin sensitivity, or lipid profile: a randomized, placebo-controlled, double-blind trial of supplementation in subjects with impaired glucose tolerance. *Diabetes Care*. 2005;28(3):712-713.

43. Di Bona KR, et al. Chromium is not an essential trace element for mammals: effects of a "low-chromium" diet. *J Biol Inorg Chem*. 2011;16(3):381-390.

44. Vincent JB. Chromium: celebrating 50 years as an essential element? *Dalton Trans*. 2010;39(16):3787-3794.

45. Vincent JB, Love ST. The need for combined inorganic, biochemical, and nutritional studies of chromium(III). *Chem Biodivers*. 2012;9(9):1923-1941.

46. Food and Nutrition Board, Institute of Health. *Dietary Reference Intakes for Calcium and Vitamin D*. Washington, DC: National Academy of Sciences; 2011.

47. Golden NH, et al. Optimizing bone health in children and adolescents. *Pediatrics*. 2014;134(4):e1229-e1243.

48. Prentice RL, et al. Health risks and benefits from calcium and vitamin D supplementation: Women's Health Initiative clinical trial and cohort study. *Osteoporos Int*. 2013;24(2):567-580.

49. Reid R, et al. Managing menopause. *J Obstet Gynaecol Can*. 2014;36(9):830-833.

CHAPTER 9

1. Cannon WB. *The Wisdom of The Body*. New York: W.W. Norton; 1932. xv p., 1 l., 19-312 p.

2. Food and Nutrition Board, Institute of Medicine. *Dietary Reference Intakes for Water, Potassium, Sodium, Chloride, and Sulfate*. Washington, DC: National Academies Press; 2004.

3. Maughan RJ, Shirreffs SM. Nutrition for sports performance: issues and opportunities. *Proc Nutr Soc*. 2012;71(1):112-119.

4. Rodriguez NR, DiMarco NM, Langley S. Position of the American Dietetic Association, Dietitians of Canada, and the American College of Sports Medicine: nutrition and athletic performance. *J Am Diet Assoc*. 2009;109(3):509-527.

5. Maughan RJ, Griffin J. Caffeine ingestion and fluid balance: a review. *J Hum Nutr Diet*. 2003;16(6):411-420.

6. Zhang Y, et al. Caffeine and diuresis during rest and exercise: a meta-analysis. *J Sci Med Sport*. 2014;18(5):569-574.

7. Manz F. Hydration and disease. *J Am Coll Nutr*. 2007;26(5 suppl):535s-541s.

8. Masento NA, et al. Effects of hydration status on cognitive performance and mood. *Br J Nutr*. 2014;111(10):1841-1852.

9. Kenney WL, Chiu P. Influence of age on thirst and fluid intake. *Med Sci Sports Exerc*. 2001;33(9):1524-1532.

10. Farrell MJ, et al. Effect of aging on regional cerebral blood flow responses associated with osmotic thirst and its satiation by water drinking: a PET study. *Proc Natl Acad Sci U S A*. 2008;105(1):382-387.

11. Farrell DJ, Bower L. Fatal water intoxication. *J Clin Pathol*. 2003;56(10):803-804.

12. Guggenheimer J, Moore PA. Xerostomia: etiology, recognition and treatment. *J Am Dent Assoc*. 2003;134(1):61-69.

13. World Health Organization. *Diarrhoeal disease*, 2013. Available from: <www.who.int/mediacentre/factsheets/fs330/en/>; Cited November 1, 2014.

CHAPTER 10

1. Simpson JW, Lawless RW, Mitchell AC. Responsibility of the obstetrician to the fetus. II. Influence of prepregnancy weight and pregnancy weight gain on birthweight. *Obstet Gynecol*. 1975;45(5):481-487.

2. Food and Nutrition Board, Institute of Medicine. *Dietary Reference Intakes for Calcium and Vitamin D*. Washington, DC: National Academies Press; 2011.

3. Food and Nutrition Board, Institute of Medicine. *Dietary Reference Intakes for Thiamin, Riboflavin, Niacin, Vitamin B6, Folate, Vitamin B12, Pantothenic Acid, Biotin, and Choline*. Washington, DC: National Academies Press; 1998.

4. Food and Nutrition Board, Institute of Medicine. *Dietary Reference Intakes for Vitamin C, Vitamin E, Selenium, and Carotenoids*. Washington, DC: National Academies Press; 2000.

5. Food and Nutrition Board, Institute of Medicine. *Dietary Reference Intakes for Vitamin A, Vitamin K, Arsenic, Boron, Chromium, Copper, Iodine, Iron, Manganese, Molybdenum, Nickel, Silicon, Vanadium, and Zinc*. Washington, DC: National Academies Press; 2001.

6. Food and Nutrition Board, Institute of Medicine. *Dietary Reference Intakes for Energy, Carbohydrate, Fiber, Fat, Fatty Acids, Cholesterol, Protein, and Amino Acids*. Washington, DC: National Academies Press; 2002.

7. Food and Nutrition Board, Institute of Medicine. *Dietary Reference Intakes for Water, Potassium, Sodium, Chloride, and Sulfate*. Washington, DC: National Academies Press; 2004.

8. U.S. Department of Health and Human Services and U.S. Department of Agriculture. *2015-2020 Dietary Guidelines for Americans*. 8th ed. December 2015. Available at <http://health.gov/dietaryguidelines/2015/guidelines/>.

9. Oken E, Gillman MW. Fetal origins of obesity. *Obes Res*. 2003;11(4):496-506.

10. Han Z, et al. Low gestational weight gain and the risk of preterm birth and low birthweight: a systematic review and meta-analyses. *Acta Obstet Gynecol Scand*. 2011;90(9):935-954.

11. U.S. Department of Agriculture, Agriculture Research Service. *Nutrient intakes from food and beverages: mean amounts consumed per individual, by gender and age, what we eat in America, NHANES 2011-2012*. 2014.

12. Procter SB, Campbell CG. Position of the Academy of Nutrition and Dietetics: nutrition and lifestyle for a healthy pregnancy outcome. *J Acad Nutr Diet.* 2014;114(7):1099-1103.

13. King JC. Physiology of pregnancy and nutrient metabolism. *Am J Clin Nutr.* 2000;71(5 suppl):1218S-1225S.

14. Milman N, et al. Iron prophylaxis during pregnancy—how much iron is needed? A randomized dose-response study of 20-80 mg ferrous iron daily in pregnant women. *Acta Obstet Gynecol Scand.* 2005;84(3):238-247.

15. Picciano MF, McGuire MK. Use of dietary supplements by pregnant and lactating women in North America. *Am J Clin Nutr.* 2009;89(2):663S-667S.

16. Copp AJ, Stanier P, Greene ND. Neural tube defects: recent advances, unsolved questions, and controversies. *Lancet Neurol.* 2013;12(8):799-810.

17. Racial/ethnic differences in the birth prevalence of spina bifida—United States, 1995-2005. *MMWR Morb Mortal Wkly Rep.* 2009;57(53):1409-1413.

18. Blencowe H, et al. Folic acid to reduce neonatal mortality from neural tube disorders. *Int J Epidemiol.* 2010;39(suppl 1):i110-i121.

19. Grundmann M, von Versen-Hoynck F. Vitamin D—roles in women's reproductive health? *Reprod Biol Endocrinol.* 2011;9:146.

20. Urrutia RP, Thorp JM. Vitamin D in pregnancy: current concepts. *Curr Opin Obstet Gynecol.* 2012;24(2):57-64.

21. Rasmussen KM, Yaktine AL, eds. *Weight Gain During Pregnancy: Reexamining the Guidelines.* Washington, DC: National Academies Press; 2009.

22. Einarson TR, Piwko C, Koren G. Prevalence of nausea and vomiting of pregnancy in the USA: a meta analysis. *J Popul Ther Clin Pharmacol.* 2013;20(2):e163-e170.

23. Lacroix R, Eason E, Melzack R. Nausea and vomiting during pregnancy: a prospective study of its frequency, intensity, and patterns of change. *Am J Obstet Gynecol.* 2000;182(4):931-937.

24. Matthews A, et al. Interventions for nausea and vomiting in early pregnancy. *Cochrane Database Syst Rev.* 2014;(3):CD007575.

25. Viljoen E, et al. A systematic review and meta-analysis of the effect and safety of ginger in the treatment of pregnancy-associated nausea and vomiting. *Nutr J.* 2014;13:20.

26. Ding M, Leach M, Bradley H. The effectiveness and safety of ginger for pregnancy-induced nausea and vomiting: a systematic review. *Women Birth.* 2013;26(1):e26-e30.

27. Herrell HE. Nausea and vomiting of pregnancy. *Am Fam Physician.* 2014;89(12):965-970.

28. Niebyl JR. Clinical practice. Nausea and vomiting in pregnancy. *N Engl J Med.* 2010;363(16):1544-1550.

29. Trogstad LI, et al. Recurrence risk in hyperemesis gravidarum. *BJOG.* 2005;112(12):1641-1645.

30. Creanga AA, et al. Pregnancy-related mortality in the United States, 2006-2010. *Obstet Gynecol.* 2015;125(1):5-12.

31. Hamilton BE, Osterman MJK, Curtin SC. Births: preliminary data for 2013. *Natl Vital Stat Rep.* 2014;(2):63.

32. Curtin SC, Abma JC, Ventura SJ, Henshaw SK. *Pregnancy Rates for U.S. Women Continue to Drop. NCHS Data Brief, No 136.* Hyattsville, Md: National Center for Health Statistics; 2013.

33. Johnson JA, et al. Delayed child-bearing. *J Obstet Gynaecol Can.* 2012;34(1):80-93.

34. Khalil A, et al. Maternal age and adverse pregnancy outcome: a cohort study. *Ultrasound Obstet Gynecol.* 2013;42(6):634-643.

35. Karabulut A, et al. Perinatal outcomes and risk factors in adolescent and advanced age pregnancies: comparison with normal reproductive age women. *J Obstet Gynaecol.* 2013;33(4):346-350.

36. Aliyu MH, et al. Extreme parity and the risk of stillbirth. *Obstet Gynecol.* 2005;106(3):446-453.

37. Aliyu MH, et al. High parity and fetal morbidity outcomes. *Obstet Gynecol.* 2005;105(5 Pt 1):1045-1051.

38. Hinkle SN, et al. Excess gestational weight gain is associated with child adiposity among mothers with normal and overweight prepregnancy weight status. *J Nutr.* 2012;142(10):1851-1858.

39. May PA, et al. Prevalence and epidemiologic characteristics of FASD from various research methods with an emphasis on recent in-school studies. *Dev Disabil Res Rev.* 2009;15(3):176-192.

40. Tong VT, et al. Trends in smoking before, during, and after pregnancy—Pregnancy Risk Assessment Monitoring System, United States, 40 sites, 2000-2010. *MMWR Surveill Summ.* 2013;62(6):1-19.

41. Salmasi G, et al. Environmental tobacco smoke exposure and perinatal outcomes: a systematic review and meta-analyses. *Acta Obstet Gynecol Scand.* 2010;89(4):423-441.

42. Einarson A, Riordan S. Smoking in pregnancy and lactation: a review of risks and cessation strategies. *Eur J Clin Pharmacol.* 2009;65(4):325-330.

43. Kawashima A, et al. Effects of maternal smoking on the placental expression of genes related to angiogenesis and apoptosis during the first trimester. *PLoS ONE.* 2014;9(8):e106140.

44. Lavezzi AM, et al. Possible role of the alpha7 nicotinic receptors in mediating nicotine's effect on developing lung – implications in unexplained human perinatal death. *BMC Pulm Med.* 2014;14:11.

45. Murphy DJ, et al. Population-based study of smoking behaviour throughout pregnancy and adverse perinatal outcomes. *Int J Environ Res Public Health.* 2013;10(9):3855-3867.

46. Kocherlakota P. Neonatal abstinence syndrome. *Pediatrics.* 2014;134(2):e547-e561.

47. Dai WS, LaBraico JM, Stern RS. Epidemiology of isotretinoin exposure during pregnancy. *J Am Acad Dermatol.* 1992;26(4):599-606.

48. Brent RL, Christian MS, Diener RM. Evaluation of the reproductive and developmental risks of caffeine. *Birth Defects Res B Dev Reprod Toxicol.* 2011;92(2):152-158.

49. Peck JD, Leviton A, Cowan LD. A review of the epidemiologic evidence concerning the reproductive health effects of caffeine consumption: a 2000-2009 update. *Food Chem Toxicol.* 2010;48(10):2549-2576.

50. Leviton A, Cowan L. A review of the literature relating caffeine consumption by women to their risk of reproductive hazards. *Food Chem Toxicol.* 2002;40(9):1271-1310.

51. Young SL, et al. Association of pica with anemia and gastrointestinal distress among pregnant women in Zanzibar, Tanzania. *Am J Trop Med Hyg.* 2010;83(1):144-151.

52. Young SL. Pica in pregnancy: new ideas about an old condition. *Annu Rev Nutr.* 2010;30:403-422.

53. Miao D, Young SL, Golden CD. A meta-analysis of pica and micronutrient status. *Am J Hum Biol.* 2015;27(1):84-93.

54. Haider BA, et al. Anaemia, prenatal iron use, and risk of adverse pregnancy outcomes: systematic review and meta-analysis. *BMJ.* 2013;346:f3443.

55. McLean E, et al. *Worldwide Prevalence of Anaemia 1993-2005 WHO Global Database on Anaemia.* Spain: World Health Organization; 2008.

56. McLean E, et al. Worldwide prevalence of anaemia, WHO Vitamin and Mineral Nutrition Information System, 1993-2005. *Public Health Nutr.* 2009;12(4):444-454.

57. World Health Organization. *Guideline: Intermittent Iron and Folic Acid Supplementation in Menstruating Women.* Geneva: 2011.

58. Mook-Kanamori DO, et al. Risk factors and outcomes associated with first-trimester fetal growth restriction. *JAMA*. 2010;303(6):527-534.

59. Class QA, et al. Birth weight, physical morbidity, and mortality: a population-based sibling-comparison study. *Am J Epidemiol*. 2014;179(5):550-558.

60. Vest AR, Cho LS. Hypertension in pregnancy. *Cardiol Clin*. 2012;30(3):407-423.

61. Magee LA, et al. Diagnosis, evaluation, and management of the hypertensive disorders of pregnancy: executive summary. *J Obstet Gynaecol Can*. 2014;36(5):416-441.

62. American Diabetes Association. Diagnosis and classification of diabetes mellitus. *Diabetes Care*. 2014;37(suppl 1): S81-S90.

63. Bellamy L, et al. Type 2 diabetes mellitus after gestational diabetes: a systematic review and meta-analysis. *Lancet*. 2009;373(9677):1773-1779.

64. World Health Organization. *Global Strategy for Infant and Young Child Feeding*. Geneva: 2003.

65. Centers for Disease Control and Prevention. *Breastfeeding among U.S. children born 2001–2011, CDC National Immunization Survey*, 2011. Available from: <www.cdc.gov/breastfeeding/data/NIS_data>; Cited November 14, 2014.

66. World Health Organization. *Comprehensive Implementation Plan on Maternal, Infant and Young Child Nutrition*. Geneva: 2014.

67. National Center for Health Statistics. *Health, United States, 2014: with Special Feature of Adults Aged 55-64*. Hyattsville, Md: U.S. Government Printing Office; 2015.

68. U.S. Department of Health and Human Services. *Healthy People 2020*. Washington, DC: U.S. Government Printing Office; 2010.

69. Bergmann RL, et al. Breastfeeding is natural but not always easy: intervention for common medical problems of breastfeeding mothers—a review of the scientific evidence. *J Perinat Med*. 2014;42(1):9-18.

70. Li R, et al. Why mothers stop breastfeeding: mothers' self-reported reasons for stopping during the first year. *Pediatrics*. 2008;122(suppl 2):S69-S76.

71. O'Brien M, et al. Exploring the influence of psychological factors on breastfeeding duration, phase 1: perceptions of mothers and clinicians. *J Hum Lact*. 2009;25(1):55-63.

72. McNiel ME, Labbok MH, Abrahams SW. What are the risks associated with formula feeding? A re-analysis and review. *Birth*. 2010;37(1):50-58.

73. Kramer MS, et al. Breastfeeding and child cognitive development: new evidence from a large randomized trial. *Arch Gen Psychiatry*. 2008;65(5):578-584.

74. Horta BL, Victora CG. *Long-Term Effects of Breastfeeing: a Systematic Review*. Geneva: World Health Organization; 2013.

75. American Academy of Pediatrics Committee on Nutrition. Breastfeeding and the use of human milk. *Pediatrics*. 2012; 129(3):e827-e841.

76. James DC, Lessen R. Position of the American Dietetic Association: promoting and supporting breastfeeding. *J Am Diet Assoc*. 2009;109(11):1926-1942.

CHAPTER 11

1. Grummer-Strawn LM, et al. Use of World Health Organization and CDC growth charts for children aged 0-59 months in the United States. *MMWR Recomm Rep*. 2010; 59(RR-9):1-15.

2. Food and Nutrition Board, Institute of Medicine. *Dietary Reference Intakes for Energy, Carbohydrate, Fiber, Fat, Fatty Acids, Cholesterol, Protein, and Amino Acids*. Washington, DC: National Academies Press; 2002.

3. Su BH. Optimizing nutrition in preterm infants. *Pediatr Neonatol*. 2014;55(1):5-13.

4. Agostoni C, et al. Enteral nutrient supply for preterm infants: commentary from the European Society of Paediatric Gastroenterology, Hepatology and Nutrition Committee on Nutrition. *J Pediatr Gastroenterol Nutr*. 2010;50(1):85-91.

5. Specker B. Nutrition influences bone development from infancy through toddler years. *J Nutr*. 2004;134(3):691S-695S.

6. Rizzoli R, et al. Maximizing bone mineral mass gain during growth for the prevention of fractures in the adolescents and the elderly. *Bone*. 2010;46(2):294-305.

7. Pitukcheewanont P, Punyasavatsut N, Feuille M. Physical activity and bone health in children and adolescents. *Pediatr Endocrinol Rev*. 2010;7(3):275-282.

8. Braun M, et al. Racial differences in skeletal calcium retention in adolescent girls with varied controlled calcium intakes. *Am J Clin Nutr*. 2007;85(6):1657-1663.

9. Congdon EL, et al. Iron deficiency in infancy is associated with altered neural correlates of recognition memory at 10 years. *J Pediatr*. 2012;160(6):1027-1033.

10. Riggins T, et al. Consequences of low neonatal iron status due to maternal diabetes mellitus on explicit memory performance in childhood. *Dev Neuropsychol*. 2009;34(6): 762-779.

11. Food and Nutrition Board, Institute of Medicine. *Dietary Reference Intakes for Vitamin A, Vitamin K, Arsenic, Boron, Chromium, Copper, Iodine, Iron, Manganese, Molybdenum, Nickel, Silicon, Vanadium, and Zinc*. Washington, DC: National Academies Press; 2001.

12. American Academy of Pediatrics Committee on Nutrition. Breastfeeding and the use of human milk. *Pediatrics*. 2012;129(3):e827-e841.

13. Wagner CL, et al. Prevention of rickets and vitamin D deficiency in infants, children, and adolescents. *Pediatrics*. 2008;122(5):1142-1152.

14. Thiele DK, Senti JL, Anderson CM. Maternal vitamin D supplementation to meet the needs of the breastfed infant: a systematic review. *J Hum Lact*. 2013;29(2):163-170.

15. Bauer J, Gerss J. Longitudinal analysis of macronutrients and minerals in human milk produced by mothers of preterm infants. *Clin Nutr*. 2011;30(2):215-220.

16. James DC, Lessen R. Position of the American Dietetic Association: promoting and supporting breastfeeding. *J Am Diet Assoc*. 2009;109(11):1926-1942.

17. Turck D. Safety aspects in preparation and handling of infant food. *Ann Nutr Metab*. 2012;60(3):211-214.

18. Labiner-Wolfe J, Fein SB, Shealy KR. Infant formula-handling education and safety. *Pediatrics*. 2008;122(suppl 2):S85-S90.

19. Grimshaw KE, et al. Introduction of complementary foods and the relationship to food allergy. *Pediatrics*. 2013;132(6): e1529-e1538.

20. Fleischer DM, et al. Primary prevention of allergic disease through nutritional interventions. *J Allergy Clin Immunol Pract*. 2013;1(1):29-36.

21. Moyer VA, U.S. Preventive Services Task Force. Prevention of dental caries in children from birth through age 5 years: US Preventive Services Task Force recommendation statement. *Pediatrics*. 2014;133(6):1102-1111.

22. Scaglioni S, et al. Determinants of children's eating behavior. *Am J Clin Nutr*. 2011;94(6 suppl):2006S-2011S.

23. Harris JL, Bargh JA. Television viewing and unhealthy diet: implications for children and media interventions. *Health Commun*. 2009;24(7):660-673.

24. Lissner L, et al. Television habits in relation to overweight, diet and taste preferences in European children: the IDEFICS study. *Eur J Epidemiol*. 2012;27(9):705-715.

25. Falbe J, et al. Longitudinal relations of television, electronic games, and digital versatile discs with changes in diet in adolescents. *Am J Clin Nutr*. 2014;100(4):1173-1181.

26. McCann JC, Ames BN. An overview of evidence for a causal relation between iron deficiency during development and

deficits in cognitive or behavioral function. *Am J Clin Nutr.* 2007;85(4):931-945.

27. Schwimmer JB, Burwinkle TM, Varni JW. Health-related quality of life of severely obese children and adolescents. *JAMA.* 2003;289(14):1813-1819.

28. Spiotta RT, Luma GB. Evaluating obesity and cardiovascular risk factors in children and adolescents. *Am Fam Physician.* 2008;78(9):1052-1058.

29. Toschke AM, et al. Adjusted population attributable fractions and preventable potential of risk factors for childhood obesity. *Public Health Nutr.* 2007;10(9):902-906.

30. Harris HR, Willett WC, Michels KB. Parental smoking during pregnancy and risk of overweight and obesity in the daughter. *Int J Obes (Lond).* 2013;37(10):1356-1363.

31. Olstad DL, McCargar L. Prevention of overweight and obesity in children under the age of 6 years. *Appl Physiol Nutr Metab.* 2009;34(4):551-570.

32. Scaglioni S, Salvioni M, Galimberti C. Influence of parental attitudes in the development of children eating behaviour. *Br J Nutr.* 2008;99(suppl 1):S22-S25.

33. Centers for Disease Control and Prevention. Blood lead levels in children aged 1-5 years – United States, 1999-2010. *MMWR Morb Mortal Wkly Rep.* 2013;62(13):245-248.

34. United States Department of Health and Human Services. *Healthy People 2020.* Washington, DC: U.S. Government Printing Office; 2010.

35. Ahmed ML, Ong KK, Dunger DB. Childhood obesity and the timing of puberty. *Trends Endocrinol Metab.* 2009;20(5): 237-242.

36. Widen E, et al. Pubertal timing and growth influences cardiometabolic risk factors in adult males and females. *Diabetes Care.* 2012;35(4):850-856.

37. Golub MS, et al. Public health implications of altered puberty timing. *Pediatrics.* 2008;121(suppl 3):S218-S230.

38. Prentice P, Viner RM. Pubertal timing and adult obesity and cardiometabolic risk in women and men: a systematic review and meta-analysis. *Int J Obes (Lond).* 2013;37(8): 1036-1043.

39. Stensland SO, et al. Interpersonal violence and overweight in adolescents: The HUNT Study. *Scand J Public Health.* 2014;43(1):18-26.

40. Matkovic V, et al. Timing of peak bone mass in Caucasian females and its implication for the prevention of osteoporosis. Inference from a cross-sectional model. *J Clin Invest.* 1994;93(2):799-808.

41. Matkovic V, et al. Nutrition influences skeletal development from childhood to adulthood: a study of hip, spine, and forearm in adolescent females. *J Nutr.* 2004;134(3): 701S-705S.

42. Pedersen TP, et al. Meal frequencies in early adolescence predict meal frequencies in late adolescence and early adulthood. *BMC Public Health.* 2013;13:445.

CHAPTER 12

1. U.S. Department of Health and Human Services. *Healthy People 2020.* Washington, DC: U.S. Government Printing Office; 2010.

2. U.S. Census Bureau, Population Division. *Projections of the Population and Components of Change for the United States: 2010 to 2050.* Washington, DC: U.S. Government Printing Office; 2014.

3. U.S. Census Bureau, Population Division. *Projections of the Population by Selected Age Groups and Sex for the United States: 2015 to 2060.* Washington, DC: U.S. Government Printing Office; 2014.

4. U.S. Census Bureau, Population Division. *Projected Life Expectancy at Birth by Sex, Race, and Hispanic Origin for the United States: 2015 to 2060.* Washington, DC: U.S. Government Printing Office; 2014.

5. Singh GK, Siahpush M. Widening rural-urban disparities in life expectancy, U.S., 1969-2009. *Am J Prev Med.* 2014;46(2): e19-e29.

6. Mykletun A, et al. Levels of anxiety and depression as predictors of mortality: the HUNT study. *Br J Psychiatry.* 2009;195(2):118-125.

7. Schoevers RA, et al. Depression and excess mortality: evidence for a dose response relation in community living elderly. *Int J Geriatr Psychiatry.* 2009;24(2):169-176.

8. Borg C, Hallberg IR, Blomqvist K. Life satisfaction among older people (65+) with reduced self-care capacity: the relationship to social, health and financial aspects. *J Clin Nurs.* 2006;15(5):607-618.

9. National Center for Health Statistics. *Health, United States, 2014: with Special Feature of Adults Aged 55-64.* Hyattsville, Md: U.S. Government Printing Office; 2015.

10. McMinn J, Steel C, Bowman A. Investigation and management of unintentional weight loss in older adults. *BMJ.* 2011;342:d1732.

11. Robertson RG, Montagnini M. Geriatric failure to thrive. *Am Fam Physician.* 2004;70(2):343-350.

12. St-Onge MP, Gallagher D. Body composition changes with aging: the cause or the result of alterations in metabolic rate and macronutrient oxidation? *Nutrition.* 2010;26(2): 152-155.

13. Javed F, et al. Brain and high metabolic rate organ mass: contributions to resting energy expenditure beyond fat-free mass. *Am J Clin Nutr.* 2010;91(4):907-912.

14. Wall BT, Cermak NM, van Loon LJ. Dietary protein considerations to support active aging. *Sports Med.* 2014;44(suppl 2):185-194.

15. Centers for Disease Control and Prevention. *State Indicator Report on Physical Activity, 2014.* Atlanta, Ga: U.S. Department of Health and Human Services; 2014.

16. U.S. Department of Health and Human Services. *2008 Physical Activity Guidelines for Americans.* Washington, DC: U.S. Department of Health and Human Services; 2008.

17. Food and Nutrition Board, Institute of Medicine. *Dietary Reference Intakes for Energy, Carbohydrate, Fiber, Fat, Fatty Acids, Cholesterol, Protein, and Amino Acids.* Washington, DC: National Academies Press; 2002.

18. Rillamas-Sun E, et al. Obesity and late-age survival without major disease or disability in older women. *JAMA Intern Med.* 2014;174(1):98-106.

19. U.S. Department of Agriculture, Agricultural Research Service. *Nutrient intakes from food: mean amounts consumed per individual, by gender and age, what we eat in America, NHANES 2009-2010.* 2012.

20. Deutz NE, et al. Protein intake and exercise for optimal muscle function with aging: recommendations from the ESPEN Expert Group. *Clin Nutr.* 2014;33(6):929-936.

21. Food and Nutrition Board, Institute of Medicine. *Dietary Reference Intakes for Thiamin, Riboflavin, Niacin, Vitamin B6, Folate, Vitamin B12, Pantothenic Acid, Biotin, and Choline.* Washington, DC: National Academies Press; 1998.

22. Norman AW, Bouillon R. Vitamin D nutritional policy needs a vision for the future. *Exp Biol Med (Maywood).* 2010; 235(9):1034-1045.

23. LeFevre ML. Screening for vitamin D deficiency in adults: U.S. Preventive Services Task Force Recommendation Statement. *Ann Intern Med.* 2015;162(2):133-140.

24. Food and Nutrition Board, Institute of Medicine. *Dietary Reference Intakes for Calcium and Vitamin D.* Washington, DC: National Academies Press; 2011.

25. LeBlanc ES, et al. Screening for vitamin D deficiency: a systematic review for the U.S. Preventive Services Task Force. *Ann Intern Med.* 2015;162(2):109-122.

26. Wallace TC, McBurney M, Fulgoni VL 3rd. Multivitamin/mineral supplement contribution to micronutrient intakes

in the United States, 2007-2010. *J Am Coll Nutr.* 2014;33(2): 94-102.

27. Diekmann R, et al. Screening for malnutrition among nursing home residents – a comparative analysis of the mini nutritional assessment, the nutritional risk screening, and the malnutrition universal screening tool. *J Nutr Health Aging.* 2013;17(4):326-331.

28. Young AM, et al. Malnutrition screening tools: comparison against two validated nutrition assessment methods in older medical inpatients. *Nutrition.* 2013;29(1):101-106.

29. Gil-Montoya JA, et al. Association of the oral health impact profile with malnutrition risk in Spanish elders. *Arch Gerontol Geriatr.* 2013;57(3):398-402.

30. Kenney WL, Chiu P. Influence of age on thirst and fluid intake. *Med Sci Sports Exerc.* 2001;33(9):1524-1532.

31. Farrell MJ, et al. Effect of aging on regional cerebral blood flow responses associated with osmotic thirst and its satiation by water drinking: a PET study. *Proc Natl Acad Sci U S A.* 2008;105(1):382-387.

32. Ogden CL, et al. Prevalence of childhood and adult obesity in the United States, 2011-2012. *JAMA.* 2014;311(8):806-814.

33. Bauer J, et al. Evidence-based recommendations for optimal dietary protein intake in older people: a position paper from the PROT-AGE Study Group. *J Am Med Dir Assoc.* 2013; 14(8):542-559.

34. Herman KM, et al. Physical activity, body mass index, and health-related quality of life in Canadian adults. *Med Sci Sports Exerc.* 2012;44(4):625-636.

35. U.S. Department of Health and Human Services and U.S. Department of Agriculture. *2015-2020 Dietary Guidelines for Americans.* 8th ed. December 2015. Available at <http://health.gov/dietaryguidelines/2015/guidelines/>.

36. Aguiar EJ, et al. Efficacy of interventions that include diet, aerobic and resistance training components for type 2 diabetes prevention: a systematic review with meta-analysis. *Int J Behav Nutr Phys Act.* 2014;11:2.

37. Douen AG, et al. Exercise induces recruitment of the "insulin-responsive glucose transporter". Evidence for distinct intracellular insulin- and exercise-recruitable transporter pools in skeletal muscle. *J Biol Chem.* 1990;265(23): 13427-13430.

38. Centers for Disease Control and Prevention. *The Power of Prevention: Chronic Disease … the Public Health Challenge of the 21st Century.* Atlanta, Ga: National Center for Chronic Disease Prevention and Health Promotion, CDC; 2009.

39. Eslami E. *Trends in Supplemental Nutrition Assistance Program Participation Rates: Fiscal Year 2010 to Fiscal Year 2012.* Alexandria, Va: United States Department of Agriculture; 2014.

40. Dorner B, et al. Position of the American Dietetic Association: individualized nutrition approaches for older adults in health care communities. *J Am Diet Assoc.* 2010;110(10): 1549-1553.

41. Desai J, et al. Changes in type of foodservice and dining room environment preferentially benefit institutionalized seniors with low body mass indexes. *J Am Diet Assoc.* 2007;107(5):808-814.

CHAPTER 13

1. Ollberding NJ, Wolf RL, Contento I. Food label use and its relation to dietary intake among US adults. *J Am Diet Assoc.* 2010;110(8):1233-1237.

2. Temple NJ, Fraser J. Food labels: a critical assessment. *Nutrition.* 2014;30(3):257-260.

3. U.S. Department of Health and Human Services. *Food Labeling: Revision of the Nutrition and Supplement Facts Labels.* Rockville, Md: Federal Registry, FDA; 2014.

4. U.S. Department of Health and Human Services. *A Food Labeling Guide: Guidance for Industry.* College Park, Md:

Center for Food Safety and Applied Nutrition, FDA; 2013.

5. Roberto CA, et al. Evaluation of consumer understanding of different front-of-package nutrition labels, 2010-2011. *Prev Chronic Dis.* 2012;9:E149.

6. Hawley KL, et al. The science on front-of-package food labels. *Public Health Nutr.* 2013;16(3):430-439.

7. Alkerwi A. Diet quality concept. *Nutrition.* 2014;30(6): 613-618.

8. Nestle M, Ludwig DS. Front-of-package food labels: public health or propaganda? *JAMA.* 2010;303(8):771-772.

9. U.S. Department of Agriculture. *National Organic Program.* Washington, DC: U.S. Department of Agriculture, U.S. Government Publishing Office, Electronic Code of Federal Regulations; 2014.

10. Smith-Spangler C, et al. Are organic foods safer or healthier than conventional alternatives? A systematic review. *Ann Intern Med.* 2012;157(5):348-366.

11. Meier MS, et al. Environmental impacts of organic and conventional agricultural products – Are the differences captured by life cycle assessment? *J Environ Manage.* 2015;149C: 193-208.

12. U.S. Department of Agriculture, Economic Research Service. *Adoption of Genetically Engineered Crops in the U.S.* Washington, DC: National Agricultural Statistics Service, U.S. Department of Agriculture; 2014.

13. Hoff M, et al. Serum testing of genetically modified soybeans with special emphasis on potential allergenicity of the heterologous protein CP4 EPSPS. *Mol Nutr Food Res.* 2007;51(8):946-955.

14. National Center for Emerging and Zoonotic Infection Diseases. *Irradiation of food.* Available from: <www.cdc.gov/nczved/divisions/dfbmd/diseases/irradiation_food/#what>; Cited January 2015.

15. Crim SM, et al. Preliminary incidence and trends of infection with pathogens transmitted commonly through food – Foodborne Diseases Active Surveillance Network, 10 U.S. sites, 2006-2014. *MMWR Morb Mortal Wkly Rep.* 2015;64(18): 495-499.

16. Centers for Disease Control and Prevention (CDC). *Surveillance for Foodborne Disease Outbreaks, United States, 2013, Annual Report.* Atlanta, Ga: 2015.

17. Centers for Disease Control and Prevention, National Center for Emerging and Zoonotic Infectious Diseases. *Salmonellosis.* Available from: <www.cdc.gov/nczved/divisions/dfbmd/diseases/salmonellosis/>; Cited January 2015.

18. Centers for Disease Control and Prevention, National Center for Emerging and Zoonotic Infectious Diseases. *Shigellosis.* Available from: <www.cdc.gov/shigella/general-information.html>; Cited January 2015.

19. Centers for Disease Control and Prevention, National Center for Emerging and Zoonotic Infectious Diseases. *Listeriosis.* Available from: <www.cdc.gov/listeria/definition.html>; Cited January 2015.

20. Centers for Disease Control and Prevention, National Center for Emerging and Zoonotic Infectious Diseases. *E. coli (Escherichia coli).* Available from: <www.cdc.gov/ecoli/general/index.html>; Cited January 2015.

21. Centers for Disease Control and Prevention, National Center for Emerging and Zoonotic Infectious Diseases. *Vibrio illness (vibriosis).* Available from: <www.cdc.gov/vibrio/index.html>; Cited January 2015.

22. Centers for Disease Control and Prevention. *Staphylococcal food poisoning.* Available from: <www.cdc.gov/ncidod/dbmd/diseaseinfo/staphylococcus_food_g.htm>; Cited January 2015.

23. Raymond J, et al. Lead screening and prevalence of blood lead levels in children aged 1-2 years—Child Blood Lead Surveillance System, United States, 2002-2010 and National

Health and Nutrition Examination Survey, United States, 1999-2010. *MMWR Surveill Summ.* 2014;63(suppl 2):36-42.

24. Centers for Disease Control and Prevention. Blood lead levels in children aged 1-5 years—United States, 1999-2010. *MMWR Morb Mortal Wkly Rep.* 2013;62(13):245-248.

25. U.S. Department of Health and Human Services. *Healthy People 2020.* Washington, DC: U.S. Government Printing Office; 2010.

26. Dixon SL, et al. Exposure of U.S. children to residential dust lead, 1999-2004: II. The contribution of lead-contaminated dust to children's blood lead levels. *Environ Health Perspect.* 2009;117(3):468-474.

27. Jusko TA, et al. Blood lead concentrations <10 microg/dL and child intelligence at 6 years of age. *Environ Health Perspect.* 2008;116(2):243-248.

28. Liu J, et al. Impact of low blood lead concentrations on IQ and school performance in Chinese children. *PLoS ONE.* 2013;8(5):e65230.

29. Wright RO, et al. Association between iron deficiency and blood lead level in a longitudinal analysis of children followed in an urban primary care clinic. *J Pediatr.* 2003;142(1):9-14.

30. Skoet J, Stamoulis K. *The State of Food Insecurity in the World: 2006.* Rome, Italy: Food and Agriculture Organization of the United Nations; 2006.

31. Food and Agriculture Organization of the United Nations. *Strategic Framework for FAO: 2000-2015.* Rome, Italy: Food and Agriculture Organization of the United Nations; 2009.

32. Coleman-Jensen A, Gregory C, Singh A. *Household Food Security in the United States in 2013, ERR-173.* Washington, DC: U.S. Department of Agriculture, Economic Research Service; 2014.

33. Food and Nutrition Services. *Commodity supplemental food program fact sheet.* Available from: <www.fns.usda.gov/sites/default/files/pfs-csfp.pdf>; 2014 Cited January 2015.

34. Food and Nutrition Services. *Supplemental Nutrition Assistance Program Participation and Costs.* Washington, DC: U.S. Department of Agriculture; 2016.

35. Food and Nutrition Services. *WIC Program Participation and Costs.* Washington, DC: U.S. Department of Agriculture; 2016.

36. Johnson B, Thorn B, McGill B, et al. *WIC Participant and Program Characteristics 2012.* Prepared by Insight Policy Research under Contract No. AG-3198-C-11-0010. Alexandria, Va: U.S. Department of Agriculture, Food and Nutrition Service; 2013.

37. Bergman EA, Gordon RW. Position of the American Dietetic Association: local support for nutrition integrity in schools. *J Am Diet Assoc.* 2010;110(8):1244-1254.

38. Food and Nutrition Services. *Nutrition Standards in the National School Lunch and School Breakfast Programs, 2012.* Washington, DC: U.S. Department of Agriculture, Federal Register; 2012:4088.

39. Center for Nutrition Policy and Promotion, U.S. Department of Agriculture. *Official USDA Food Plans: Cost of Food at Home at Four Levels, U.S. Average, May 2015.* Alexandria, Va: U.S. Department of Agriculture; 2015.

CHAPTER 14

1. Roberto CA, et al. Influence of licensed characters on children's taste and snack preferences. *Pediatrics.* 2010;126(1):88-93.

2. Kotler JA, Schiffman JM, Hanson KG. The influence of media characters on children's food choices. *J Health Commun.* 2012;17(8):886-898.

3. Powell LM, Schermbeck RM, Chaloupka FJ. Nutritional content of food and beverage products in television advertisements seen on children's programming. *Child Obes.* 2013;9(6):524-531.

4. Mink M, et al. Nutritional imbalance endorsed by televised food advertisements. *J Am Diet Assoc.* 2010;110(6):904-910.

5. DeNavas-Walt C, Proctor BD. *U.S. Census Bureau, Current Population Reports, P60-252, Income and Poverty in the United States: 2015.* Washington, DC: U.S. Government Printing Office; 2015.

6. Powell LM, Han E, Chaloupka FJ. Economic contextual factors, food consumption, and obesity among U.S. adolescents. *J Nutr.* 2010;140(6):1175-1180.

7. Powell LM, et al. Assessing the potential effectiveness of food and beverage taxes and subsidies for improving public health: a systematic review of prices, demand and body weight outcomes. *Obes Rev.* 2013;14(2):110-128.

8. Glickman D, et al. *Accelerating Progress in Obesity Prevention: Solving the Weight of the Nation.* Washington, DC; 2012.

9. Painter J, Rah JH, Lee YK. Comparison of international food guide pictorial representations. *J Am Diet Assoc.* 2002;102(4):483-489.

10. Washburn KK. *Indian Entities Recognized and Eligible to Receive Services from the United States Bureau of Indian Affairs.* Bureau of Indian Affairs, Department of the Interior; 2015:1943-1948 Federal Register.

11. Rastogi S, Johnson TD, Hoeffel EM, Drewery MP. *The Black Population, 2010 Census Briefs.* Washington, DC: U.S. Department of Commerce, Economics and Statistics Administration, U.S. Census Bureau; 2011.

12. The Gilder Lehrman Institute of American History. *Facts about the slave trade and slavery.* Available from: <www.gilderlehrman.org/>; Cited January 2015. New York City, NY.

13. U.S. Bureau of Labor Statistics. *Women in the labor force: a databook, 2014.* U.S. Department of Labor, BLS Reports 1049; 2014.

14. Smith LP, Ng SW, Popkin BM. Trends in US home food preparation and consumption: analysis of national nutrition surveys and time use studies from 1965-1966 to 2007-2008. *Nutr J.* 2013;12:45.

15. Eisenberg ME, et al. Family meals and substance use: is there a long-term protective association? *J Adolesc Health.* 2008;43(2):151-156.

16. Skeer MR, Ballard EL. Are family meals as good for youth as we think they are? A review of the literature on family meals as they pertain to adolescent risk prevention. *J Youth Adolesc.* 2013;42(7):943-963.

17. Powell LM, Nguyen BT. Fast-food and full-service restaurant consumption among children and adolescents: effect on energy, beverage, and nutrient intake. *JAMA Pediatr.* 2013;167(1):14-20.

18. Ello-Martin JA, Ledikwe JW, Rolls BJ. The influence of food portion size and energy density on energy intake: implications for weight management. *Am J Clin Nutr.* 2005;82(1 suppl):236S-241S.

19. Piernas C, Popkin BM. Increased portion sizes from energy-dense foods affect total energy intake at eating occasions in US children and adolescents: patterns and trends by age group and sociodemographic characteristics, 1977-2006. *Am J Clin Nutr.* 2011;94(5):1324-1332.

20. Almiron-Roig E, et al. Large portion sizes increase bite size and eating rate in overweight women. *Physiol Behav.* 2015;139C:297-302.

21. Johnson SL, et al. Portion sizes for children are predicted by parental characteristics and the amounts parents serve themselves. *Am J Clin Nutr.* 2014;99(4):763-770.

22. Young LR, Nestle M. Expanding portion sizes in the US marketplace: implications for nutrition counseling. *J Am Diet Assoc.* 2003;103(2):231-234.

23. Bauer KW, et al. Energy content of U.S. fast-food restaurant offerings: 14-year trends. *Am J Prev Med.* 2012;43(5):490-497.

24. Freeland-Graves JH, et al. Position of the academy of nutrition and dietetics: total diet approach to healthy eating. *J Acad Nutr Diet*. 2013;113(2):307-317.

CHAPTER 15

1. Ogden CL, et al. Prevalence of childhood and adult obesity in the United States, 2011-2012. *JAMA*. 2014;311(8):806-814.
2. National Center for Health Statistics. *Health, United States, 2014: With Special Feature of Adults Aged 55-64*. Hyattsville, Md: U.S. Government Printing Office; 2015.
3. Vogelezang S, et al. Adult adiposity susceptibility loci, early growth and general and abdominal fatness in childhood. The Generation R Study. *Int J Obes (Lond)*. 2015;39(6):1001-1009.
4. Kaminsky LA, American College of Sports Medicine. *ACSMs Health-Related Physical Fitness Assessment Manual*, Vol 14. 4th ed. Philadelphia: Wolters Kluwer Health/Lippincott Williams & Wilkins; 2014:174.
5. Wan CS, et al. Bioelectrical impedance analysis to estimate body composition, and change in adiposity, in overweight and obese adolescents: comparison with dual-energy x-ray absorptiometry. *BMC Pediatr*. 2014;14:249.
6. Bedogni G, et al. Comparison of dual-energy x-ray absorptiometry, air displacement plethysmography and bioelectrical impedance analysis for the assessment of body composition in morbidly obese women. *Eur J Clin Nutr*. 2013;67(11):1129-1132.
7. Velazquez-Alva Mdel C, et al. A comparison of dual energy x-ray absorptiometry and two bioelectrical impedance analyzers to measure body fat percentage and fat-free mass index in a group of Mexican young women. *Nutr Hosp*. 2014;29(5):1038-1046.
8. Holmes JC, et al. Body-density measurement in children: the BOD POD versus hydrodensitometry. *Int J Sport Nutr Exerc Metab*. 2011;21(3):240-247.
9. Lowry DW, Tomiyama AJ. *Air* displacement plethysmography versus dual-energy x-ray absorptiometry in underweight, normal-weight, and overweight/obese individuals. *PLoS ONE*. 2015;10(1):e0115086.
10. Hames KC, et al. Body composition analysis by air displacement plethysmography in normal weight to extremely obese adults. *Obesity (Silver Spring)*. 2014;22(4):1078-1084.
11. Bertoli S, et al. Evaluation of air-displacement plethysmography and bioelectrical impedance analysis vs dual-energy x-ray absorptiometry for the assessment of fat-free mass in elderly subjects. *Eur J Clin Nutr*. 2008;62(11):1282-1286.
12. Toombs RJ, et al. The impact of recent technological advances on the trueness and precision of DXA to assess body composition. *Obesity (Silver Spring)*. 2012;20(1):30-39.
13. Li C, et al. Estimates of body composition with dual-energy x-ray absorptiometry in adults. *Am J Clin Nutr*. 2009;90(6):1457-1465.
14. Patel AV, Hildebrand JS, Gapstur SM. Body mass index and all-cause mortality in a large prospective cohort of white and black U.S. Adults. *PLoS ONE*. 2014;9(10):e109153.
15. Miller KK. Endocrine dysregulation in anorexia nervosa update. *J Clin Endocrinol Metab*. 2011;96(10):2939-2949.
16. Dunford M. *Nutrition for Sport and Exercise*. 3rd ed. Stamford, Conn: Cengage Learning; 2014.
17. Guh DP, et al. The incidence of co-morbidities related to obesity and overweight: a systematic review and meta-analysis. *BMC Public Health*. 2009;9:88.
18. Dombrowski SU, Avenell A, Sniehott FF. Behavioural interventions for obese adults with additional risk factors for morbidity: systematic review of effects on behaviour, weight and disease risk factors. *Obes Facts*. 2010;3(6):377-396.
19. Kramer CK. Weight loss is a useful therapeutic objective. *Can J Cardiol*. 2015;31(2):211-215.
20. Tudor-Locke C, et al. A step-defined sedentary lifestyle index: <5000 steps/day. *Appl Physiol Nutr Metab*. 2013;38(2):100-114.
21. Zhang Y, et al. Positional cloning of the mouse obese gene and its human homologue. *Nature*. 1994;372(6505):425-432.
22. Farooqi IS, O'Rahilly S. 20 years of leptin: human disorders of leptin action. *J Endocrinol*. 2014;223(1):T63-T70.
23. Kalra SP. Central leptin insufficiency syndrome: an interactive etiology for obesity, metabolic and neural diseases and for designing new therapeutic interventions. *Peptides*. 2008;29(1):127-138.
24. Patterson M, Bloom SR, Gardiner JV. Ghrelin and appetite control in humans—potential application in the treatment of obesity. *Peptides*. 2011;32(11):2290-2294.
25. Pradhan G, Samson SL, Sun Y. Ghrelin: much more than a hunger hormone. *Curr Opin Clin Nutr Metab Care*. 2013;16(6):619-624.
26. Schwenk RW, Vogel H, Schurmann A. Genetic and epigenetic control of metabolic health. *Mol Metab*. 2013;2(4):337-347.
27. Hoelscher DM, et al. Position of the Academy of Nutrition and Dietetics: interventions for the prevention and treatment of pediatric overweight and obesity. *J Acad Nutr Diet*. 2013;113(10):1375-1394.
28. Dulloo AG, Jacquet J, Montani JP. How dieting makes some fatter: from a perspective of human body composition autoregulation. *Proc Nutr Soc*. 2012;71(3):379-389.
29. Sachdev M, et al. Effect of fenfluramine-derivative diet pills on cardiac valves: a meta-analysis of observational studies. *Am Heart J*. 2002;144(6):1065-1073.
30. Ioannides-Demos LL, Piccenna L, McNeil JJ. Pharmacotherapies for obesity: past, current, and future therapies. *J Obes*. 2011;2011:179674.
31. Colquitt JL, et al. Surgery for weight loss in adults. *Cochrane Database Syst Rev*. 2014;(8):CD003641.
32. Sundbom M. Laparoscopic revolution in bariatric surgery. *World J Gastroenterol*. 2014;20(41):15135-15143.
33. Kulick D, Hark L, Deen D. The bariatric surgery patient: a growing role for registered dietitians. *J Am Diet Assoc*. 2010;110(4):59593-59599.
34. Seagle HM, et al. Position of the American Dietetic Association: weight management. *J Am Diet Assoc*. 2009;109(2):330-346.
35. Karl JP, et al. Independent and combined effects of eating rate and energy density on energy intake, appetite, and gut hormones. *Obesity (Silver Spring)*. 2013;21(3):E244-E252.
36. U.S. Department of Health and Human Services and U.S. Department of Agriculture. *2015-2020 Dietary Guidelines for Americans*. 8th ed. December 2015. Available at <http://health.gov/dietaryguidelines/2015/guidelines/>.
37. Ozier AD, Henry BW, American Dietetic Association. Position of the American Dietetic Association: nutrition intervention in the treatment of eating disorders. *J Am Diet Assoc*. 2011;111(8):1236-1241.
38. Franko DL, et al. A longitudinal investigation of mortality in anorexia nervosa and bulimia nervosa. *Am J Psychiatry*. 2013;170(8):917-925.
39. Matthews-Ewald MR, Zullig KJ, Ward RM. Sexual orientation and disordered eating behaviors among self-identified male and female college students. *Eat Behav*. 2014;15(3):441-444.
40. Culbert KM, Racine SE, Klump KL. Research Review: what we have learned about the causes of eating disorders—a synthesis of sociocultural, psychological, and biological research. *J Child Psychol Psychiatry*. 2015;56(11):1141-1164.
41. Hudson JI, et al. The prevalence and correlates of eating disorders in the National Comorbidity Survey Replication. *Biol Psychiatry*. 2007;61(3):348-358.
42. American Dietetic Association. Position of the American Dietetic Association: nutrition intervention in the treatment

of anorexia nervosa, bulimia nervosa, and other eating disorders. *J Am Diet Assoc.* 2006;106(12):2073-2082.

CHAPTER 16

1. National Center for Health Statistics. *Health, United States, 2014: with Special Feature on Adults Aged 55-64.* Hyattsville, Md: U.S. Government Printing Office; 2015.
2. Koh HK. A 2020 vision for healthy people. *N Engl J Med.* 2010;362(18):1653-1656.
3. United States Department of Health and Human Services. *2008 Physical Activity Guidelines for Americans: Be Active, Healthy, and Happy!* Office of Disease Prevention and Health Promotion publication. Washington, DC: 2008;9:61.
4. Powell KE, Paluch AE, Blair SN. Physical activity for health: What kind? How much? How intense? On top of what? *Annu Rev Public Health.* 2011;32:349-365.
5. Taylor D. Physical activity is medicine for older adults. *Postgrad Med J.* 2014;90(1059):26-32.
6. Mann S, Beedie C, Jimenez A. Differential effects of aerobic exercise, resistance training and combined exercise modalities on cholesterol and the lipid profile: review, synthesis and recommendations. *Sports Med.* 2014;44(2):211-221.
7. Go AS, et al. Heart disease and stroke statistics—2013 update: a report from the American Heart Association. *Circulation.* 2013;127(1):e6-e245.
8. Brook RD, et al. Beyond medications and diet: alternative approaches to lowering blood pressure: a scientific statement from the American Heart Association. *Hypertension.* 2013;61(6):1360-1383.
9. Thent ZC, Das S, Henry LJ. Role of exercise in the management of diabetes mellitus: the global scenario. *PLoS ONE.* 2013;8(11):e80436.
10. Kilbride L, et al. Managing blood glucose during and after exercise in Type 1 diabetes: reproducibility of glucose response and a trial of a structured algorithm adjusting insulin and carbohydrate intake. *J Clin Nurs.* 2011;20(23-24):3423-3429.
11. Deslandes A. The biological clock keeps ticking, but exercise may turn it back. *Arq Neuropsiquiatr.* 2013;71(2):113-118.
12. Zschucke E, Gaudlitz K, Strohle A. Exercise and physical activity in mental disorders: clinical and experimental evidence. *J Prev Med Public Health.* 2013;46(suppl 1):S12-S21.
13. Garber CE, et al. American College of Sports Medicine position stand. Quantity and quality of exercise for developing and maintaining cardiorespiratory, musculoskeletal, and neuromotor fitness in apparently healthy adults: guidance for prescribing exercise. *Med Sci Sports Exerc.* 2011;43(7):1334-1359.
14. Hulston CJ, et al. Training with low muscle glycogen enhances fat metabolism in well-trained cyclists. *Med Sci Sports Exerc.* 2010;42(11):2046-2055.
15. Sawka MN, Cheuvront SN, Kenefick RK. High skin temperature and hypohydration impair aerobic performance. *Exp Physiol.* 2012;97(3):327-332.
16. Merry TL, Ainslie PN, Cotter JD. Effects of aerobic fitness on hypohydration-induced physiological strain and exercise impairment. *Acta Physiol (Oxf).* 2010;198(2):179-190.
17. Jeukendrup AE. Nutrition for endurance sports: marathon, triathlon, and road cycling. *J Sports Sci.* 2011;29(suppl 1):S91-S99.
18. Ortenblad N, Westerblad H, Nielsen J. Muscle glycogen stores and fatigue. *J Physiol.* 2013;591(Pt 18):4405-4413.
19. Vandenbogaerde TJ, Hopkins WG. Effects of acute carbohydrate supplementation on endurance performance: a meta-analysis. *Sports Med.* 2011;41(9):773-792.
20. Correia-Oliveira CR, et al. Strategies of dietary carbohydrate manipulation and their effects on performance in cycling time trials. *Sports Med.* 2013;43(8):707-719.
21. Phillips SM. Dietary protein requirements and adaptive advantages in athletes. *Br J Nutr.* 2012;108(suppl 2):S158-S167.
22. Bonci LJ. Eating for performance: bringing science to the training table. *Clin Sports Med.* 2011;30(3):661-670.
23. Gleeson M. Nutritional support to maintain proper immune status during intense training. *Nestle Nutr Inst Workshop Ser.* 2013;75:85-97.
24. Walsh NP, et al. Position statement. Part two: Maintaining immune health. *Exerc Immunol Rev.* 2011;17:64-103.
25. Manore MM. Weight management in the performance athlete. *Nestle Nutr Inst Workshop Ser.* 2013;75:123-133.
26. Cunningham JJ. A reanalysis of the factors influencing basal metabolic rate in normal adults. *Am J Clin Nutr.* 1980;33:2372-2374.
27. Burke LM. Fueling strategies to optimize performance: training high or training low? *Scand J Med Sci Sports.* 2010;20(suppl 2):48-58.
28. U.S. Department of Agriculture Agricultural Research Service. *Table 5. Energy Intakes: Percentages of Energy from Protein, Carbohydrate, Fat, and Alcohol, by Gender and Age, in What We Eat in America, NHANES 2009-2010.* 2012.
29. Burke LM, et al. Carbohydrates for training and competition. *J Sports Sci.* 2011;29(suppl 1):S17-S27.
30. Zoorob R, et al. Sports nutrition needs: before, during, and after exercise. *Prim Care.* 2013;40(2):475-486.
31. Beelen M, et al. Nutritional strategies to promote postexercise recovery. *Int J Sport Nutr Exerc Metab.* 2010;20(6):515-532.

CHAPTER 17

1. Herdman TH, Kamitsuru S. *Nursing Diagnoses 2015-2017: Definitions and Classification.* 10th ed. Oxford: Wiley Blackwell; 2014.
2. Nutrition care process and model part I: the 2008 update. *J Am Diet Assoc.* 2008;108(7):1113-1117.
3. Lacey K, Pritchett E. Nutrition care process and model: ADA adopts road map to quality care and outcomes management. *J Am Diet Assoc.* 2003;103(8):1061-1072.
4. Tooze JA, et al. Psychosocial predictors of energy underreporting in a large doubly labeled water study. *Am J Clin Nutr.* 2004;79(5):795-804.
5. Scagliusi FB, et al. Characteristics of women who frequently under report their energy intake: a doubly labelled water study. *Eur J Clin Nutr.* 2009;63(10):1192-1199.
6. Bailey RL, et al. Assessing the effect of underreporting energy intake on dietary patterns and weight status. *J Am Diet Assoc.* 2007;107(1):64-71.
7. Freedman LS, et al. Pooled results from 5 validation studies of dietary self-report instruments using recovery biomarkers for energy and protein intake. *Am J Epidemiol.* 2014;180(2):172-188.
8. Poslusna K, et al. Misreporting of energy and micronutrient intake estimated by food records and 24 hour recalls, control and adjustment methods in practice. *Br J Nutr.* 2009;101(suppl 2):S73-S85.
9. Csizmadi I, et al. The Sedentary Time and Activity Reporting Questionnaire (STAR-Q): reliability and validity against doubly labeled water and 7-day activity diaries. *Am J Epidemiol.* 2014;180(4):424-435.
10. Neilson HK, et al. Estimating activity energy expenditure: how valid are physical activity questionnaires? *Am J Clin Nutr.* 2008;87(2):279-291.
11. Foley LS, et al. Doubly labeled water validation of a computerized use-of-time recall in active young people. *Metabolism.* 2013;62(1):163-169.
12. Bell CL, et al. Prevalence and measures of nutritional compromise among nursing home patients: weight loss, low body mass index, malnutrition, and feeding dependency, a

systematic review of the literature. *J Am Med Dir Assoc.* 2013;14(2):94-100.

13. Jensen MD, et al. 2013 AHA/ACC/TOS guideline for the management of overweight and obesity in adults: a report of the American College of Cardiology/American Heart Association Task Force on Practice Guidelines and The Obesity Society. *J Am Coll Cardiol.* 2014;(25 Pt B).

14. Feller S, Boeing H, Pischon T. Body mass index, waist circumference, and the risk of type 2 diabetes mellitus: implications for routine clinical practice. *Dtsch Arztebl Int.* 2010; 107(26):470-476.

15. Sabah KM, et al. Body mass index and waist/height ratio for prediction of severity of coronary artery disease. *BMC Res Notes.* 2014;7:246.

16. Jacobs EJ, et al. Waist circumference and all-cause mortality in a large US cohort. *Arch Intern Med.* 2010;170(15):1293-1301.

17. de Hollander EL, et al. The association between waist circumference and risk of mortality considering body mass index in 65- to 74-year-olds: a meta-analysis of 29 cohorts involving more than 58 000 elderly persons. *Int J Epidemiol.* 2012;41(3):805-817.

18. Tamura BK, et al. Factors associated with weight loss, low BMI, and malnutrition among nursing home patients: a systematic review of the literature. *J Am Med Dir Assoc.* 2013;14(9):649-655.

19. National Center for Health Statistics. *Health, United States, 2014: with Special Feature of Adults Aged 55-64.* Hyattsville, Md: U.S. Government Printing Office; 2015.

20. Chan LN. Drug-nutrient interactions. *JPEN J Parenter Enteral Nutr.* 2013;37(4):450-459.

21. Paine MF, et al. A furanocoumarin-free grapefruit juice establishes furanocoumarins as the mediators of the grapefruit juice-felodipine interaction. *Am J Clin Nutr.* 2006; 83(5):1097-1105.

22. Holbrook AM, et al. Systematic overview of warfarin and its drug and food interactions. *Arch Intern Med.* 2005;165(10): 1095-1106.

23. Meng Q, Liu K. Pharmacokinetic interactions between herbal medicines and prescribed drugs: focus on drug metabolic enzymes and transporters. *Curr Drug Metab.* 2014; 15(8):791-807.

24. Rahimi R, Abdollahi M. An update on the ability of St. John's wort to affect the metabolism of other drugs. *Expert Opin Drug Metab Toxicol.* 2012;8(6):691-708.

25. Russo E, et al. *Hypericum perforatum:* pharmacokinetic, mechanism of action, tolerability, and clinical drug-drug interactions. *Phytother Res.* 2014;28(5):643-655.

26. Chen XW, et al. Herb-drug interactions and mechanistic and clinical considerations. *Curr Drug Metab.* 2012;13(5): 640-651.

CHAPTER 18

1. Cury JA, Tenuta LM. Evidence-based recommendation on toothpaste use. *Braz Oral Res.* 2014;28(Spec):1-7.

2. Wong MC, et al. Cochrane reviews on the benefits/risks of fluoride toothpastes. *J Dent Res.* 2011;90(5):573-579.

3. Savoca MR, et al. Severe tooth loss in older adults as a key indicator of compromised dietary quality. *Public Health Nutr.* 2010;13(4):466-474.

4. Savoca MR, et al. Impact of denture usage patterns on dietary quality and food avoidance among older adults. *J Nutr Gerontol Geriatr.* 2011;30(1):86-102.

5. Wu B, et al. Social stratification and tooth loss among middle-aged and older Americans from 1988 to 2004. *Commun Dent Oral Epidemiol.* 2014;42(6):495-502.

6. Cichero JA, Altman KW. Definition, prevalence and burden of oropharyngeal dysphagia: a serious problem among older adults worldwide and the impact on prognosis and hospital resources. *Nestle Nutr Inst Workshop Ser.* 2012;72:1-11.

7. Altman KW, Yu GP, Schaefer SD. Consequence of dysphagia in the hospitalized patient: impact on prognosis and hospital resources. *Arch Otolaryngol Head Neck Surg.* 2010;136(8): 784-789.

8. Germain I, Dufresne T, Gray-Donald K. A novel dysphagia diet improves the nutrient intake of institutionalized elders. *J Am Diet Assoc.* 2006;106(10):1614-1623.

9. Boeckxstaens GE, Rohof WO. Pathophysiology of gastroesophageal reflux disease. *Gastroenterol Clin North Am.* 2014; 43(1):15-25.

10. Lee YY, McColl KE. Pathophysiology of gastroesophageal reflux disease. *Best Pract Res Clin Gastroenterol.* 2013;27(3): 339-351.

11. Achem SR, DeVault KR. Gastroesophageal reflux disease and the elderly. *Gastroenterol Clin North Am.* 2014;43(1): 147-160.

12. Soumekh A, Schnoll-Sussman FH, Katz PO. Reflux and acid peptic diseases in the elderly. *Clin Geriatr Med.* 2014;30(1): 29-41.

13. Wu YW, et al. Association of esophageal inflammation, obesity and gastroesophageal reflux disease: from FDG PET/CT perspective. *PLoS ONE.* 2014;9(3):e92001.

14. Frazzoni M, et al. Laparoscopic fundoplication for gastroesophageal reflux disease. *World J Gastroenterol.* 2014;20(39): 14272-14279.

15. Yeomans ND. The ulcer sleuths: the search for the cause of peptic ulcers. *J Gastroenterol Hepatol.* 2011;26(suppl 1): 35-41.

16. Sung JJ, Kuipers EJ, El-Serag HB. Systematic review: the global incidence and prevalence of peptic ulcer disease. *Aliment Pharmacol Ther.* 2009;29(9):938-946.

17. Levenstein S, et al. Psychological stress increases risk for peptic ulcer, regardless of *Helicobacter pylori* infection or use of nonsteroidal anti-inflammatory drugs. *Clin Gastroenterol Hepatol.* 2015;13(3):498-506, e1.

18. Konturek PC, Brzozowski T, Konturek SJ. Stress and the gut: pathophysiology, clinical consequences, diagnostic approach and treatment options. *J Physiol Pharmacol.* 2011; 62(6):591-599.

19. Bhattacharyya A, et al. Oxidative stress: an essential factor in the pathogenesis of gastrointestinal mucosal diseases. *Physiol Rev.* 2014;94(2):329-354.

20. Zhang L, et al. Effects of cigarette smoke and its active components on ulcer formation and healing in the gastrointestinal mucosa. *Curr Med Chem.* 2012;19(1):63-69.

21. Li LF, et al. Cigarette smoking and gastrointestinal diseases: the causal relationship and underlying molecular mechanisms (review). *Int J Mol Med.* 2014;34(2):372-380.

22. Merck and Co, Inc. *The Merck Manual for Healthcare Professionals.* Whitehouse Station, NJ: 2015.

23. Quittner AL, et al. Impact of socioeconomic status, race, and ethnicity on quality of life in patients with cystic fibrosis in the United States. *Chest.* 2010;137(3):642-650.

24. Schechter MS, et al. Association of socioeconomic status with the use of chronic therapies and healthcare utilization in children with cystic fibrosis. *J Pediatr.* 2009;155(5):634-639, e1-4.

25. Stallings VA, et al. Evidence-based practice recommendations for nutrition-related management of children and adults with cystic fibrosis and pancreatic insufficiency: results of a systematic review. *J Am Diet Assoc.* 2008;108(5): 832-839.

26. Haupt ME, et al. Pancreatic enzyme replacement therapy dosing and nutritional outcomes in children with cystic fibrosis. *J Pediatr.* 2014;164(5):1110-1115, e1.

27. Culhane S, et al. Malnutrition in cystic fibrosis: a review. *Nutr Clin Pract.* 2013;28(6):676-683.

28. Burisch J, Munkholm P. The epidemiology of inflammatory bowel disease. *Scand J Gastroenterol.* 2015;50(8):942-951.

29. Loftus EV Jr. Clinical epidemiology of inflammatory bowel disease: incidence, prevalence, and environmental influences. *Gastroenterology*. 2004;126(6):1504-1517.

30. Antunes CV, et al. Anemia in inflammatory bowel disease outpatients: prevalence, risk factors, and etiology. *Biomed Res Int*. 2015;2015:728925.

31. Lee D, et al. Diet in the pathogenesis and treatment of inflammatory bowel diseases. *Gastroenterology*. 2015;148(6):1087-1106.

32. Academy of Nutrition and Dietetics. *Nutrition Care Manual*. Chicago, Ill: 2015.

33. Steffen R, Hill DR, DuPont HL. Traveler's diarrhea: a clinical review. *JAMA*. 2015;313(1):71-80.

34. GBD 2013 Mortality Causes of Death, Collaborators. Global, regional, and national age-sex specific all-cause and cause-specific mortality for 240 causes of death, 1990-2013: a systematic analysis for the Global Burden of Disease Study 2013. *Lancet*. 2015;385(9963):117-171.

35. Everhart JE, Ruhl CE. Burden of digestive diseases in the United States part II: lower gastrointestinal diseases. *Gastroenterology*. 2009;136(3):741-754.

36. Strate LL, et al. Diverticular disease as a chronic illness: evolving epidemiologic and clinical insights. *Am J Gastroenterol*. 2012;107(10):1486-1493.

37. Choung RS, Locke GR 3rd. Epidemiology of IBS. *Gastroenterol Clin North Am*. 2011;40(1):1-10.

38. Quigley EM, et al. A global perspective on irritable bowel syndrome: a consensus statement of the World Gastroenterology Organisation Summit Task Force on irritable bowel syndrome. *J Clin Gastroenterol*. 2012;46(5):356-366.

39. World Gastroenterology Organization. *WGO practice guideline—irritable bowel syndrome: a global perspective*, 2009 March 11, 2015. Available from: <www.worldgastroenterology.org/irritable-bowel-syndrome.html>.

40. Chey WD, Kurlander J, Eswaran S. Irritable bowel syndrome: a clinical review. *JAMA*. 2015;313(9):949-958.

41. Jones M, et al. Pathways connecting cognitive behavioral therapy and change in bowel symptoms of IBS. *J Psychosom Res*. 2011;70(3):278-285.

42. Canadian Agency for Drugs and Technologies in Health. *Treatments for Constipation: A Review of Systematic Reviews*. Ottawa, Ontario: 2014.

43. Suares NC, Ford AC. Systematic review: the effects of fibre in the management of chronic idiopathic constipation. *Aliment Pharmacol Ther*. 2011;33(8):895-901.

44. Leung J, Crowe SE. Food allergy and food intolerance. *World Rev Nutr Diet*. 2015;111:76-81.

45. Boyce JA, et al. Guidelines for the diagnosis and management of food allergy in the United States: summary of the NIAID-sponsored expert panel report. *Nutr Res*. 2011;31(1):61-75.

46. Sicherer SH, Sampson HA. Food allergy: epidemiology, pathogenesis, diagnosis, and treatment. *J Allergy Clin Immunol*. 2014;133(2):291-307, quiz 308.

47. Choung RS, et al. Trends and racial/ethnic disparities in gluten-sensitive problems in the United States: findings from the national health and nutrition examination surveys from 1988 to 2012. *Am J Gastroenterol*. 2015;110(3):455-461.

48. Armstrong C. ACG releases guideline on diagnosis and management of celiac disease. *Am Fam Physician*. 2014;89(6):485-487.

49. Koning F. Pathophysiology of celiac disease. *J Pediatr Gastroenterol Nutr*. 2014;59(suppl 1):S1-S4.

50. Ju MK, et al. Difference of regeneration potential between healthy and diseased liver. *Transplant Proc*. 2012;44(2):338-340.

51. Vernon G, Baranova A, Younossi ZM. Systematic review: the epidemiology and natural history of non-alcoholic fatty liver disease and non-alcoholic steatohepatitis in adults. *Aliment Pharmacol Ther*. 2011;34(3):274-285.

52. Neuman MG, et al. Alcoholic and non-alcoholic steatohepatitis. *Exp Mol Pathol*. 2014;97(3):492-510.

53. Cusi K. Role of obesity and lipotoxicity in the development of nonalcoholic steatohepatitis: pathophysiology and clinical implications. *Gastroenterology*. 2012;142(4):711-725, e6.

54. Lonardo A, et al. Nonalcoholic fatty liver disease: a precursor of the metabolic syndrome. *Dig Liver Dis*. 2015;47(3):181-190.

55. Plauth M, et al. ESPEN guidelines on enteral nutrition: liver disease. *Clin Nutr*. 2006;25(2):285-294.

56. National Center for Health Statistics. *Health, United States, 2014: with Special Feature of Adults Aged 55-64*. Hyattsville, Md: U.S. Government Printing Office; 2015.

57. Bemeur C, Butterworth RF. Nutrition in the management of cirrhosis and its neurological complications. *J Clin Exp Hepatol*. 2014;4(2):141-150.

58. Reshetnyak VI. Concept of the pathogenesis and treatment of cholelithiasis. *World J Hepatol*. 2012;4(2):18-34.

59. Fradin K, Racine AD, Belamarich PF. Obesity and symptomatic cholelithiasis in childhood: epidemiologic and case-control evidence for a strong relation. *J Pediatr Gastroenterol Nutr*. 2014;58(1):102-106.

60. Lindkvist B. Diagnosis and treatment of pancreatic exocrine insufficiency. *World J Gastroenterol*. 2013;19(42):7258-7266.

CHAPTER 19

1. National Center for Health Statistics. *Health, United States, 2014: with Special Feature of Adults Aged 55-64*. Hyattsville, Md: U.S. Government Printing Office; 2015.

2. Stone NJ, et al. 2013 ACC/AHA guideline on the treatment of blood cholesterol to reduce atherosclerotic cardiovascular risk in adults: a report of the American College of Cardiology/American Heart Association Task Force on Practice Guidelines. *J Am Coll Cardiol*. 2014;63(25 Pt B):2889-2934.

3. Zhang B, et al. Therapeutic approaches to the regulation of metabolism of high-density lipoprotein. Novel HDL-directed pharmacological intervention and exercise. *Circ J*. 2013;77(11):2651-2663.

4. Tenenbaum A, Klempfner R, Fisman EZ. Hypertriglyceridemia: a too long unfairly neglected major cardiovascular risk factor. *Cardiovasc Diabetol*. 2014;13(1):159.

5. Graham G. Population-based approaches to understanding disparities in cardiovascular disease risk in the United States. *Int J Gen Med*. 2014;7:393-400.

6. Liao Y, et al. Surveillance of health status in minority communities—Racial and ethnic approaches to community health across the U.S. (REACH U.S.) Risk Factor Survey, United States, 2009. *MMWR Surveill Summ*. 2011;60(6):1-44.

7. Lewis GF, Xiao C, Hegele RA. Hypertriglyceridemia in the genomic era: a new paradigm. *Endocr Rev*. 2015;36(1):131-147.

8. Karlamangla AS, et al. Socioeconomic and ethnic disparities in cardiovascular risk in the United States, 2001-2006. *Ann Epidemiol*. 2010;20(8):617-628.

9. Mozaffarian D, et al. Heart disease and stroke statistics—2015 update: a report from the American Heart Association. *Circulation*. 2015;131(4):29-322.

10. Eckel RH, et al. 2013 AHA/ACC guideline on lifestyle management to reduce cardiovascular risk: a report of the American College of Cardiology/American Heart Association Task Force on Practice Guidelines. *J Am Coll Cardiol*. 2014;63(25 Pt B):2960-2984.

11. Third Report of the National Cholesterol Education Program (NCEP) Expert Panel on Detection, Evaluation, and Treatment of High Blood Cholesterol in Adults (Adult Treatment Panel III) final report. *Circulation*. 2002;106(25):3143-3421.

12. Millen BE, et al. 2013 American Heart Association/American College of Cardiology Guideline on Lifestyle Management to Reduce Cardiovascular Risk: practice opportunities for

registered dietitian nutritionists. *J Acad Nutr Diet.* 2014; 114(11):1723-1729.

13. Pool AC, et al. The impact of physician weight discussion on weight loss in US adults. *Obes Res Clin Pract.* 2014; 8(2):e131-e139.

14. Singh S, et al. Physician diagnosis of overweight status predicts attempted and successful weight loss in patients with cardiovascular disease and central obesity. *Am Heart J.* 2010;160(5):934-942.

15. Academy of Nutrition and Dietetics. *Nutrition Care Manual.* Chicago, Ill: 2015.

16. Martinez-Gonzalez MA, Bes-Rastrollo M. Dietary patterns, Mediterranean diet, and cardiovascular disease. *Curr Opin Lipidol.* 2014;25(1):20-26.

17. Casas R, et al. The effects of the Mediterranean diet on biomarkers of vascular wall inflammation and plaque vulnerability in subjects with high risk for cardiovascular disease. A randomized trial. *PLoS ONE.* 2014;9(6):e100084.

18. Panagiotakos DB, et al. Mediterranean diet and inflammatory response in myocardial infarction survivors. *Int J Epidemiol.* 2009;38(3):856-866.

19. Perez-Lopez FR, et al. Effects of the Mediterranean diet on longevity and age-related morbid conditions. *Maturitas.* 2009;64(2):67-79.

20. Guallar-Castillon P, et al. Major dietary patterns and risk of coronary heart disease in middle-aged persons from a Mediterranean country: the EPIC-Spain cohort study. *Nutr Metab Cardiovasc Dis.* 2012;22(3):192-199.

21. Prinelli F, et al. Mediterranean diet and other lifestyle factors in relation to 20-year all-cause mortality: a cohort study in an Italian population. *Br J Nutr.* 2015;1-9.

22. Food and Nutrition Board, Institute of Medicine. *Dietary Reference Intakes for Water, Potassium, Sodium, Chloride, and Sulfate.* Washington, DC: National Academies Press; 2004.

23. U.S. Department of Agriculture, Agriculture Research Service. *Nutrient intakes from food and beverages: mean amounts consumed per individual, by gender and age, what we eat in America, NHANES 2011-2012.* 2014.

24. Johnson RJ, et al. The discovery of hypertension: evolving views on the role of the kidneys, and current hot topics. *Am J Physiol Renal Physiol.* 2015;308(3):F167-F178.

25. Gonzalez J, et al. Essential hypertension and oxidative stress: new insights. *World J Cardiol.* 2014;6(6):353-366.

26. Padmanabhan S, Newton-Cheh C, Dominiczak AF. Genetic basis of blood pressure and hypertension. *Trends Genet.* 2012;28(8):397-408.

27. Ehret GB, Caulfield MF. Genes for blood pressure: an opportunity to understand hypertension. *Eur Heart J.* 2013;34(13): 951-961.

28. Lind JM, Chiu CL. Genetic discoveries in hypertension: steps on the road to therapeutic translation. *Heart.* 2013;99(22):1645-1651.

29. Bloetzer C, et al. Performance of parental history for the targeted screening of hypertension in children. *J Hypertens.* 2015;33(6):1167-1173.

30. Chen X, Wang Y. Tracking of blood pressure from childhood to adulthood: a systematic review and meta-regression analysis. *Circulation.* 2008;117(25):3171-3180.

31. Vaneckova I, et al. Obesity-related hypertension: possible pathophysiological mechanisms. *J Endocrinol.* 2014;223(3): R63-R78.

32. James PA, et al. 2014 evidence-based guideline for the management of high blood pressure in adults: report from the panel members appointed to the Eighth Joint National Committee (JNC 8). *JAMA.* 2014;311(5):507-520.

33. Go AS, et al. An effective approach to high blood pressure control: a science advisory from the American Heart Association, the American College of Cardiology, and the Centers for Disease Control and Prevention. *Hypertension.* 2014;63(4):878-885.

34. National Institutes of Health, National Heart, Lung, and Blood Institute, and National High Blood Pressure Education Program. *The Seventh Report of the Joint National Committee on Prevention, Detection, Evaluation, and Treatment of High Blood Pressure.* Bethesda, Md: National Institutes of Health; 2004.

35. Appel LJ, et al. A clinical trial of the effects of dietary patterns on blood pressure. DASH Collaborative Research Group. *N Engl J Med.* 1997;336(16):1117-1124.

36. Sacks FM, et al. Effects on blood pressure of reduced dietary sodium and the Dietary Approaches to Stop Hypertension (DASH) diet. DASH-Sodium Collaborative Research Group. *N Engl J Med.* 2001;344(1):3-10.

37. Chen ST, Maruthur NM, Appel LJ. The effect of dietary patterns on estimated coronary heart disease risk: results from the Dietary Approaches to Stop Hypertension (DASH) trial. *Circ Cardiovasc Qual Outcomes.* 2010;3(5):484-489.

38. Harsha DW, et al. Effect of dietary sodium intake on blood lipids: results from the DASH-sodium trial. *Hypertension.* 2004;43(2):393-398.

39. Blumenthal JA, et al. Effects of the dietary approaches to stop hypertension diet alone and in combination with exercise and caloric restriction on insulin sensitivity and lipids. *Hypertension.* 2010;55(5):1199-1205.

40. Levitan EB, Wolk A, Mittleman MA. Consistency with the DASH diet and incidence of heart failure. *Arch Intern Med.* 2009;169(9):851-857.

41. He FJ, Li J, Macgregor GA. Effect of longer term modest salt reduction on blood pressure: Cochrane systematic review and meta-analysis of randomised trials. *BMJ.* 2013;346: f1325.

42. Pimenta E, et al. Effects of dietary sodium reduction on blood pressure in subjects with resistant hypertension: results from a randomized trial. *Hypertension.* 2009;54(3): 475-481.

43. Kanbay M, et al. Mechanisms and consequences of salt sensitivity and dietary salt intake. *Curr Opin Nephrol Hypertens.* 2011;20(1):37-43.

44. Carter BD, et al. Smoking and mortality—beyond established causes. *N Engl J Med.* 2015;372(7):631-640.

45. Spruill TM. Chronic psychosocial stress and hypertension. *Curr Hypertens Rep.* 2010;12(1):10-16.

46. U.S. Department of Health and Human Services and U.S. Department of Agriculture. *2015-2020 Dietary Guidelines for Americans.* 8th ed. December 2015. Available at <http://health.gov/dietaryguidelines/2015/guidelines/>.

47. Dai S, et al. Non-high-density lipoprotein cholesterol: distribution and prevalence of high serum levels in children and adolescents: United States National Health and Nutrition Examination Surveys, 2005-2010. *J Pediatr.* 2014;164(2): 247-253.

CHAPTER 20

1. National Center for Health Statistics. *Health, United States, 2014: with Special Feature of Adults Aged 55-64.* Hyattsville, Md: U.S. Government Printing Office; 2015.

2. American Diabetes Association. Diagnosis and classification of diabetes mellitus. *Diabetes Care.* 2014;37(suppl 1): S81-S90.

3. Chiang JL, et al. Type 1 diabetes through the life span: a position statement of the American Diabetes Association. *Diabetes Care.* 2014;37(7):2034-2054.

4. Morran MP, et al. Immunogenetics of type 1 diabetes mellitus. *Mol Aspects Med.* 2015;42:42-60.

5. Grarup N, et al. Genetic susceptibility to type 2 diabetes and obesity: from genome-wide association studies to rare variants and beyond. *Diabetologia.* 2014;57(8):1528-1541.

6. Mohamadi A, Cooke DW. Type 2 diabetes mellitus in children and adolescents. *Adolesc Med State Art Rev.* 2010;21(1): 103-119, x.

7. Balsells M, et al. Glibenclamide, metformin, and insulin for the treatment of gestational diabetes: a systematic review and meta-analysis. *BMJ*. 2015;350:h102.

8. Buschur E, Brown F, Wyckoff J. Using oral agents to manage gestational diabetes: what have we learned? *Curr Diab Rep*. 2015;15(2):570.

9. Holt RI, Lambert KD. The use of oral hypoglycaemic agents in pregnancy. *Diabet Med*. 2014;31(3):282-291.

10. Morton S, Kirkwood S, Thangaratinam S. Interventions to modify the progression to type 2 diabetes mellitus in women with gestational diabetes: a systematic review of literature. *Curr Opin Obstet Gynecol*. 2014;26(6):476-486.

11. Ratner RE, et al. Prevention of diabetes in women with a history of gestational diabetes: effects of metformin and lifestyle interventions. *J Clin Endocrinol Metab*. 2008;93(12):4774-4779.

12. Knowler WC, et al. Reduction in the incidence of type 2 diabetes with lifestyle intervention or metformin. *N Engl J Med*. 2002;346(6):393-403.

13. Djousse L, et al. Association between modifiable lifestyle factors and residual lifetime risk of diabetes. *Nutr Metab Cardiovasc Dis*. 2013;23(1):17-22.

14. Prior SJ, et al. Increased skeletal muscle capillarization after aerobic exercise training and weight loss improves insulin sensitivity in adults with IGT. *Diabetes Care*. 2014;37(5):1469-1475.

15. Ryan AS, et al. Aerobic exercise + weight loss decreases skeletal muscle myostatin expression and improves insulin sensitivity in older adults. *Obesity (Silver Spring)*. 2013;21(7):1350-1356.

16. Aguiar EJ, et al. Efficacy of interventions that include diet, aerobic and resistance training components for type 2 diabetes prevention: a systematic review with meta-analysis. *Int J Behav Nutr Phys Act*. 2014;11:2.

17. Labbe SM, et al. Improved cardiac function and dietary fatty acid metabolism after modest weight loss in subjects with impaired glucose tolerance. *Am J Physiol Endocrinol Metab*. 2014;306(12):E1388-E1396.

18. Wilding JP. The role of the kidneys in glucose homeostasis in type 2 diabetes: clinical implications and therapeutic significance through sodium glucose co-transporter 2 inhibitors. *Metabolism*. 2014;63(10):1228-1237.

19. Centers for Disease Control and Prevention. *National Diabetes Statistics Report: Estimates of Diabetes and Its Burden in the United States, 2014*. Atlanta, Ga: U.S. Department of Health and Human Services; 2014.

20. American Diabetes Association. Standards of medical care in diabetes–2014. *Diabetes Care*. 2014;37(suppl 1):S14-S80.

21. Mattila TK, de Boer A. Influence of intensive versus conventional glucose control on microvascular and macrovascular complications in type 1 and 2 diabetes mellitus. *Drugs*. 2010;70(17):2229-2245.

22. Fullerton B, et al. Intensive glucose control versus conventional glucose control for type 1 diabetes mellitus. *Cochrane Database Syst Rev*. 2014;(2):CD009122.

23. Rajabally YA. Neuropathy and impaired glucose tolerance: an updated review of the evidence. *Acta Neurol Scand*. 2011;124(1):1-8.

24. Mayfield JA, et al. Preventive foot care in diabetes. *Diabetes Care*. 2004;27(suppl 1):S63-S64.

25. Danese E, et al. Advantages and pitfalls of fructosamine and glycated albumin in the diagnosis and treatment of diabetes. *J Diabetes Sci Technol*. 2015;9(2):169-176.

26. Haas L, et al. National standards for diabetes self-management education and support. *Diabetes Care*. 2012;35(11):2393-2401.

27. Academy of Nutrition and Dietetics. *Nutrition Care Manual*. Chicago, Ill: 2015.

28. Evert AB, et al. Nutrition therapy recommendations for the management of adults with diabetes. *Diabetes Care*. 2013;36(11):3821-3842.

29. Food and Nutrition Board, Institute of Medicine. *Dietary Reference Intakes for Energy, Carbohydrate, Fiber, Fat, Fatty Acids, Cholesterol, Protein, and Amino Acids*. Washington, DC: National Academies Press; 2002.

30. Strandberg RB, et al. Relationships of diabetes-specific emotional distress, depression, anxiety, and overall well-being with HbA1c in adult persons with type 1 diabetes. *J Psychosom Res*. 2014;77(3):174-179.

31. Fisher L, Glasgow RE, Strycker LA. The relationship between diabetes distress and clinical depression with glycemic control among patients with type 2 diabetes. *Diabetes Care*. 2010;33(5):1034-1036.

CHAPTER 21

1. U.S. Renal Data System. *2014 Annual Data Report: Epidemiology of Kidney Disease in the United States. National Institutes of Health, National Institute of Diabetes and Digestive and Kidney Diseases*. Bethesda, Md: National Institute of Diabetes and Digestive and Kidney Diseases; 2014.

2. Tuot DS, et al. Chronic kidney disease awareness among individuals with clinical markers of kidney dysfunction. *Clin J Am Soc Nephrol*. 2011;6(8):1838-1844.

3. Kidney Disease; Improving Global Outcomes (KDIGO) CKD Work Group. KDIGO 2012 clinical practice guideline for the evaluation and management of chronic kidney disease. *Kidney Int Suppl*. 2013;3:1-150.

4. Vart P, et al. Mediators of the association between low socioeconomic status and chronic kidney disease in the United States. *Am J Epidemiol*. 2015;181(6):385-396.

5. Academy of Nutrition and Dietetics. *Nutrition Care Manual*. Chicago, Ill: 2015.

6. Leblanc M, et al. Risk factors for acute renal failure: inherent and modifiable risks. *Curr Opin Crit Care*. 2005;11(6):533-536.

7. Rahman M, Shad F, Smith MC. Acute kidney injury: a guide to diagnosis and management. *Am Fam Physician*. 2012;86(7):631-639.

8. Wang HE, et al. Acute kidney injury and mortality in hospitalized patients. *Am J Nephrol*. 2012;35(4):349-355.

9. Zeng X, et al. Incidence, outcomes, and comparisons across definitions of AKI in hospitalized individuals. *Clin J Am Soc Nephrol*. 2014;9(1):12-20.

10. Chawla LS, et al. Acute kidney injury and chronic kidney disease as interconnected syndromes. *N Engl J Med*. 2014;371(1):58-66.

11. Kidney Disease: Improving Global Outcomes (KDIGO) Acute Kidney Injury Work Group. KDIGO Clinical Practice Guideline for Acute Kidney Injury. *Kidney Int Suppl*. 2013;2:1-138.

12. Kidney Disease: Improving Global Outcomes (KDIGO) Anemia Work Group. KDIGO Clinical Practice Guideline for Anemia in Chronic Kidney Disease. *Kidney Int Suppl*. 2012;2:279-335.

13. Kidney Disease: Improving Global Outcomes (KDIGO) Blood Pressure Work Group. KDIGO Clinical Practice Guideline for the Management of Blood Pressure in Chronic Kidney Disease. *Kidney Int Suppl*. 2012;2:337-414.

14. Carrero JJ, et al. Etiology of the protein-energy wasting syndrome in chronic kidney disease: a consensus statement from the International Society of Renal Nutrition and Metabolism (ISRNM). *J Ren Nutr*. 2013;23(2):77-90.

15. Gracia-Iguacel C, et al. Defining protein-energy wasting syndrome in chronic kidney disease: prevalence and clinical implications. *Nefrologia*. 2014;34(4):507-519.

16. Beto JA, Ramirez WE, Bansal VK. Medical nutrition therapy in adults with chronic kidney disease: integrating evidence

and consensus into practice for the generalist registered dietitian nutritionist. *J Acad Nutr Diet*. 2014;114(7): 1077-1087.

17. Hall YN, et al. Effects of six versus three times per week hemodialysis on physical performance, health, and functioning: Frequent Hemodialysis Network (FHN) randomized trials. *Clin J Am Soc Nephrol*. 2012;7(5):782-794.

18. Unruh ML, et al. Effects of 6-times-weekly versus 3-times-weekly hemodialysis on depressive symptoms and self-reported mental health: Frequent Hemodialysis Network (FHN) Trials. *Am J Kidney Dis*. 2013;61(5):748-758.

19. Chertow GM, et al. In-center hemodialysis six times per week versus three times per week. *N Engl J Med*. 2010; 363(24):2287-2300.

20. Gracia-Iguacel C, et al. Prevalence of protein-energy wasting syndrome and its association with mortality in haemodialysis patients in a centre in Spain. *Nefrologia*. 2013;33(4): 495-505.

21. Nafzger S, et al. Detection of malnutrition in patients undergoing maintenance haemodialysis: a quantitative data analysis on 12 parameters. *J Ren Care*. 2015;41(3):168-176.

22. Edalat-Nejad M, et al. Geriatric nutritional risk index: a mortality predictor in hemodialysis patients. *Saudi J Kidney Dis Transpl*. 2015;26(2):302-308.

23. Herselman M, et al. Relationship between serum protein and mortality in adults on long-term hemodialysis: exhaustive review and meta-analysis. *Nutrition*. 2010;26(1): 10-32.

24. Herselman M, et al. Relationship between body mass index and mortality in adults on maintenance hemodialysis: a systematic review. *J Ren Nutr*. 2010;20(5):281-292, 7 p following 292.

25. Vashistha T, et al. Effect of age and dialysis vintage on obesity paradox in long-term hemodialysis patients. *Am J Kidney Dis*. 2014;63(4):612-622.

26. Griva K, et al. Quality of life and emotional distress between patients on peritoneal dialysis versus community-based hemodialysis. *Qual Life Res*. 2014;23(1):57-66.

27. Turkmen K, et al. Health-related quality of life, sleep quality, and depression in peritoneal dialysis and hemodialysis patients. *Hemodial Int*. 2012;16(2):198-206.

28. U.S. Renal Data System. *USRDS 2013 Annual Data Report: Atlas of Chronic Kidney Disease and End-Stage Renal Disease in the United States*. Bethesda, Md: National Institutes of Health, National Institute of Diabetes and Digestive and Kidney Diseases; 2013.

29. Brown RO, Compher C. ASPEN clinical guidelines: nutrition support in adult acute and chronic renal failure. *JPEN J Parenter Enteral Nutr*. 2010;34(4):366-377.

30. Kidney Disease: Improving Global Outcomes (KDIGO). Chronic Kidney Disease-Mineral and Bone Disorder Work Group. KDIGO clinical practice guideline for the diagnosis, evaluation, prevention, and treatment of Chronic Kidney Disease-Mineral and Bone Disorder (CKD-MBD). *Kidney Int Suppl*. 2009;113:S1-S130.

31. Scales CD Jr, et al. Prevalence of kidney stones in the United States. *Eur Urol*. 2012;62(1):160-165.

32. Dawson CH, Tomson CR. Kidney stone disease: pathophysiology, investigation and medical treatment. *Clin Med*. 2012; 12(5):467-471.

33. Evan AP. Physiopathology and etiology of stone formation in the kidney and the urinary tract. *Pediatr Nephrol*. 2010;25(5):831-841.

34. Thomas LD, et al. Ascorbic acid supplements and kidney stone incidence among men: a prospective study. *JAMA Intern Med*. 2013;173(5):386-388.

35. Massey LK, Liebman M, Kynast-Gales SA. Ascorbate increases human oxaluria and kidney stone risk. *J Nutr*. 2005;135(7):1673-1677.

36. Sorensen MD, et al. Impact of nutritional factors on incident kidney stone formation: a report from the WHI OS. *J Urol*. 2012;187(5):1645-1649.

37. Taylor EN, Curhan GC. Dietary calcium from dairy and nondairy sources, and risk of symptomatic kidney stones. *J Urol*. 2013;190(4):1255-1259.

38. Wiederkehr MR, Moe OW. Uric acid nephrolithiasis: a systemic metabolic disorder. *Clin Rev Bone Miner Metab*. 2011;9(3-4):207-217.

39. Sakhaee K. Epidemiology and clinical pathophysiology of uric acid kidney stones. *J Nephrol*. 2014;27(3):241-245.

40. Tracy CR, et al. Animal protein and the risk of kidney stones: a comparative metabolic study of animal protein sources. *J Urol*. 2014;192(1):137-141.

41. Reddy ST, et al. Effect of low-carbohydrate high-protein diets on acid-base balance, stone-forming propensity, and calcium metabolism. *Am J Kidney Dis*. 2002;40(2):265-274.

42. Lieske JC, et al. Diet, but not oral probiotics, effectively reduces urinary oxalate excretion and calcium oxalate supersaturation. *Kidney Int*. 2010;78(11):1178-1185.

43. Kanbara A, et al. Effect of urine pH changed by dietary intervention on uric acid clearance mechanism of pH-dependent excretion of urinary uric acid. *Nutr J*. 2012;11:39.

44. Xu H, et al. Kidney stones: an update on current pharmacological management and future directions. *Expert Opin Pharmacother*. 2013;14(4):435-447.

45. Heilberg IP, Goldfarb DS. Optimum nutrition for kidney stone disease. *Adv Chronic Kidney Dis*. 2013;20(2):165-174.

CHAPTER 22

1. Corkins MR, et al. Malnutrition diagnoses in hospitalized patients: United States, 2010. *JPEN J Parenter Enteral Nutr*. 2014;38(2):186-195.

2. Harris CL, Fraser C. Malnutrition in the institutionalized elderly: the effects on wound healing. *Ostomy Wound Manage*. 2004;50(10):54-63.

3. Calder PC, et al. Inflammatory disease processes and interactions with nutrition. *Br J Nutr*. 2009;101(suppl 1): S1-S45.

4. Rasheed S, Woods RT. Malnutrition and quality of life in older people: a systematic review and meta-analysis. *Ageing Res Rev*. 2013;12(2):561-566.

5. Robinson MK, et al. The relationship among obesity, nutritional status, and mortality in the critically ill. *Crit Care Med*. 2015;43(1):87-100.

6. Malone A, Hamilton C. The Academy of Nutrition and Dietetics/the American Society for Parenteral and Enteral Nutrition consensus malnutrition characteristics: application in practice. *Nutr Clin Pract*. 2013;28(6):639-650.

7. Mehta NM, et al. Nutritional practices and their relationship to clinical outcomes in critically ill children—an international multicenter cohort study. *Crit Care Med*. 2012;40(7): 2204-2211.

8. Drevet S, et al. Prevalence of protein-energy malnutrition in hospital patients over 75 years of age admitted for hip fracture. *Orthop Traumatol Surg Res*. 2014;100(6):669-674.

9. Jesudason D, Clifton P. The interaction between dietary protein and bone health. *J Bone Miner Metab*. 2011;29(1): 1-14.

10. Mangano KM, Sahni S, Kerstetter JE. Dietary protein is beneficial to bone health under conditions of adequate calcium intake: an update on clinical research. *Curr Opin Clin Nutr Metab Care*. 2014;17(1):69-74.

11. Wolfe RR. The role of dietary protein in optimizing muscle mass, function and health outcomes in older individuals. *Br J Nutr*. 2012;108(suppl 2):S88-S93.

12. Loenneke JP, et al. Short report: relationship between quality protein, lean mass and bone health. *Ann Nutr Metab*. 2010;57(3-4):219-220.

13. Huang JW, et al. Lean body mass predicts long-term survival in Chinese patients on peritoneal dialysis. *PLoS ONE*. 2013;8(1):e54976.

14. Navarro LH, et al. Perioperative fluid therapy: a statement from the international Fluid Optimization Group. *Perioper Med (Lond)*. 2015;4:3.

15. Sadeghpour A, et al. Impact of vitamin C supplementation on post-cardiac surgery ICU and hospital length of stay. *Anesth Pain Med*. 2015;5(1):e25337.

16. Wilson JX. Evaluation of vitamin C for adjuvant sepsis therapy. *Antioxid Redox Signal*. 2013;19(17):2129-2140.

17. Wilson JX. Mechanism of action of vitamin C in sepsis: ascorbate modulates redox signaling in endothelium. *Biofactors*. 2009;35(1):5-13.

18. Rumelin A, et al. Metabolic clearance of the antioxidant ascorbic acid in surgical patients. *J Surg Res*. 2005;129(1):46-51.

19. Long CL, et al. Ascorbic acid dynamics in the seriously ill and injured. *J Surg Res*. 2003;109(2):144-148.

20. Rodrigo R, et al. A randomized controlled trial to prevent post-operative atrial fibrillation by antioxidant reinforcement. *J Am Coll Cardiol*. 2013;62(16):1457-1465.

21. Rech M, et al. Heavy metal in the intensive care unit: a review of current literature on trace element supplementation in critically ill patients. *Nutr Clin Pract*. 2014;29(1):78-89.

22. Mertens K, et al. Low zinc and selenium concentrations in sepsis are associated with oxidative damage and inflammation. *Br J Anaesth*. 2015;114(6):990-999.

23. Stefanowicz F, et al. Assessment of plasma and red cell trace element concentrations, disease severity, and outcome in patients with critical illness. *J Crit Care*. 2014;29(2):214-218.

24. Leandro-Merhi VA, de Aquino JL. Determinants of malnutrition and post-operative complications in hospitalized surgical patients. *J Health Popul Nutr*. 2014;32(3):400-410.

25. Ha L, et al. Individual, nutritional support prevents undernutrition, increases muscle strength and improves QoL among elderly at nutritional risk hospitalized for acute stroke: a randomized, controlled trial. *Clin Nutr*. 2010;29(5):567-573.

26. Vashi PG, et al. A longitudinal study investigating quality of life and nutritional outcomes in advanced cancer patients receiving home parenteral nutrition. *BMC Cancer*. 2014;14:593.

27. Academy of Nutrition and Dietetics. *Nutrition Care Manual*. Chicago, Ill: 2015.

28. Pragatheeswarane M, et al. Early oral feeding vs. traditional feeding in patients undergoing elective open bowel surgery—a randomized controlled trial. *J Gastrointest Surg*. 2014;18(5):1017-1023.

29. Zhuang CL, et al. Early versus traditional postoperative oral feeding in patients undergoing elective colorectal surgery: a meta-analysis of randomized clinical trials. *Dig Surg*. 2013;30(3):225-232.

30. Bankhead R, et al. Enteral nutrition practice recommendations. *JPEN J Parenter Enteral Nutr*. 2009;33(2):122-167.

31. Jastrzebska-Mierzynska M, et al. Dietetic recommendations after bariatric procedures in the light of the new guidelines regarding metabolic and bariatric surgery. *Rocz Panstw Zakl Hig*. 2015;66(1):13-19.

32. Fujioka K, DiBaise JK, Martindale RG. Nutrition and metabolic complications after bariatric surgery and their treatment. *JPEN J Parenter Enteral Nutr*. 2011;35(5 suppl):52S-59S.

33. American Burn Association. *Burn incidence and treatment in the United States: 2013 Fact Sheet 2013*. Available from: <www.ameriburn.org/resources_factsheet.php>; Cited May 2015.

34. Rousseau AF, et al. ESPEN endorsed recommendations: nutritional therapy in major burns. *Clin Nutr*. 2013;32(4):497-502.

35. Lu G, et al. Influence of early post-burn enteral nutrition on clinical outcomes of patients with extensive burns. *J Clin Biochem Nutr*. 2011;48(3):222-225.

36. Vicic VK, Radman M, Kovacic V. Early initiation of enteral nutrition improves outcomes in burn disease. *Asia Pac J Clin Nutr*. 2013;22(4):543-547.

37. Khorasani EN, Mansouri F. Effect of early enteral nutrition on morbidity and mortality in children with burns. *Burns*. 2010;36(7):1067-1071.

CHAPTER 23

1. National Center for Health Statistics. *Health, United States, 2014: with Special Feature of Adults Aged 55-64*. Hyattsville, Md: U.S. Government Printing Office; 2015.

2. Laake I, et al. Intake of trans fatty acids from partially hydrogenated vegetable and fish oils and ruminant fat in relation to cancer risk. *Int J Cancer*. 2013;132(6):1389-1403.

3. Bagnardi V, et al. Alcohol consumption and site-specific cancer risk: a comprehensive dose-response meta-analysis. *Br J Cancer*. 2015;112(3):580-593.

4. Key TJ. Fruit and vegetables and cancer risk. *Br J Cancer*. 2011;104(1):6-11.

5. Wang X, et al. Fruit and vegetable consumption and mortality from all causes, cardiovascular disease, and cancer: systematic review and dose-response meta-analysis of prospective cohort studies. *BMJ*. 2014;349:4490.

6. Bradbury KE, Appleby PN, Key TJ. Fruit, vegetable, and fiber intake in relation to cancer risk: findings from the European Prospective Investigation into Cancer and Nutrition (EPIC). *Am J Clin Nutr*. 2014;100(suppl 1):394S-398S.

7. Oyebode O, et al. Fruit and vegetable consumption and all-cause, cancer and CVD mortality: analysis of Health Survey for England data. *J Epidemiol Community Health*. 2014;68(9):856-862.

8. Gaziano JM, et al. Multivitamins in the prevention of cancer in men: the Physicians' Health Study II randomized controlled trial. *JAMA*. 2012;308(18):1871-1880.

9. Ames BN, Wakimoto P. Are vitamin and mineral deficiencies a major cancer risk? *Nat Rev Cancer*. 2002;2(9):694-704.

10. Boeing H. Obesity and cancer—the update 2013. *Best Pract Res Clin Endocrinol Metab*. 2013;27(2):219-227.

11. De Pergola G, Silvestris F. Obesity as a major risk factor for cancer. *J Obes*. 2013;2013:291546.

12. Chen Y, et al. Nutrition support in surgical patients with colorectal cancer. *World J Gastroenterol*. 2011;17(13):1779-1786.

13. Vashi PG, et al. The relationship between baseline nutritional status with subsequent parenteral nutrition and clinical outcomes in cancer patients undergoing hyperthermic intraperitoneal chemotherapy. *Nutr J*. 2013;12:118.

14. Qiu M, et al. Nutrition support can bring survival benefit to high nutrition risk gastric cancer patients who received chemotherapy. *Support Care Cancer*. 2015;23(7):1933-1939.

15. Wang X, et al. Enteral nutrition improves clinical outcome and shortens hospital stay after cancer surgery. *J Invest Surg*. 2010;23(6):309-313.

16. Academy of Nutrition and Dietetics: Oncology Work Group. Oncology evidence-based nutrition practice guidelines. In: *Evidence Analysis Library*. Chicago, Ill: 2013.

17. Arthur ST, et al. One-year prevalence, comorbidities and cost of cachexia-related inpatient admissions in the USA. *Drugs Context*. 2014;3:212265.

18. von Haehling S, Anker SD. Prevalence, incidence and clinical impact of cachexia: facts and numbers-update 2014. *J Cachexia Sarcopenia Muscle*. 2014;5(4):261-263.

19. Academy of Nutrition and Dietetics. *Nutrition Care Manual.* Chicago, Ill: 2015.

20. Suzuki H, et al. Cancer cachexia—pathophysiology and management. *J Gastroenterol.* 2013;48(5):574-594.

21. Kushi LH, et al. American Cancer Society Guidelines on nutrition and physical activity for cancer prevention: reducing the risk of cancer with healthy food choices and physical activity. *CA Cancer J Clin.* 2012;62(1):30-67.

22. Wiseman M. The second World Cancer Research Fund/ American Institute for Cancer Research expert report. Food, nutrition, physical activity, and the prevention of cancer: a global perspective. *Proc Nutr Soc.* 2008;67(3):253-256.

23. U.S. Food and Drug Administration. *Health claims meeting significant scientific agreement (SSA).* Available from: <www.fda.gov/Food/IngredientsPackagingLabeling/ LabelingNutrition/ucm2006876.htm#Approved_Health_ Claims>; Accessed May 2015.

24. Kabat GC, et al. Adherence to cancer prevention guidelines and cancer incidence, cancer mortality, and total mortality: a prospective cohort study. *Am J Clin Nutr.* 2015;101(3): 558-569.

25. U.S. Department of Health and Human Services. *Healthy People 2020.* Washington DC: U.S. Government Printing Office; 2010.

26. Patterson RE, et al. Metabolism and breast cancer risk: frontiers in research and practice. *J Acad Nutr Diet.* 2013;113(2): 288-296.

27. Castello A, et al. Lower breast cancer risk among women following the World Cancer Research Fund and American Institute for Cancer Research Lifestyle Recommendations: EpiGEICAM case-control study. *PLoS ONE.* 2015;10(5): e0126096.

28. Bertuccio P, et al. Dietary patterns and gastric cancer risk: a systematic review and meta-analysis. *Ann Oncol.* 2013;24(6): 1450-1458.

29. Gonzalez CA, Riboli E. Diet and cancer prevention: contributions from the European Prospective Investigation into Cancer and Nutrition (EPIC) study. *Eur J Cancer.* 2010; 46(14):2555-2562.

30. Pericleous M, Mandair D, Caplin ME. Diet and supplements and their impact on colorectal cancer. *J Gastrointest Oncol.* 2013;4(4):409-423.

31. Centers for Disease Control and Prevention. *Cancer prevention and control, 2015.* Available from: <www.cdc.gov/ cancer/>; Cited May 2015.

32. Wilkinson JM, Stevens MJ. Use of complementary and alternative medical therapies (CAM) by patients attending a regional comprehensive cancer care centre. *J Complement Integr Med.* 2014;11(2):139-145.

33. Rossi E, et al. Complementary and alternative medicine for cancer patients: results of the EPAAC survey on integrative oncology centres in Europe. *Support Care Cancer.* 2015;23(6): 1795-1806.

34. Saydah SH, Eberhardt MS. Use of complementary and alternative medicine among adults with chronic diseases: United States 2002. *J Altern Complement Med.* 2006;12(8):805-812.

35. Davis EL, et al. Cancer patient disclosure and patient-doctor communication of complementary and alternative medicine use: a systematic review. *Oncologist.* 2012;17(11): 1475-1481.

36. Centers for Disease Control and Prevention. *HIV surveillance report, 2013.* Accessed 2015 from: <www.cdc.gov/hiv/ library/reports/surveillance/>.

37. Zhu T, et al. An African HIV-1 sequence from 1959 and implications for the origin of the epidemic. *Nature.* 1998; 391(6667):594-597.

38. UNAIDS. *Fact sheet 2014: global statistics, 2014.* Available from: <www.unaids.org/sites/default/files/en/media/ unaids/contentassets/documents/factsheet/2014/ 20140716_FactSheet_en.pdf>.

39. Centers for Disease Control and Prevention. Revised surveillance case definition for HIV infection—United States, 2014. *MMWR Recomm Rep.* 2014;63(RR–03):1-10.

40. U.S. Food and Drug Administration. *Antiretroviral drugs used in the treatment of HIV infection.* September 2014. Available from: <www.fda.gov/forpatients/illness/ hivaids/treatment/ucm118915.htm>; Cited May 2015.

41. Rerks-Ngarm S, et al. Vaccination with ALVAC and AIDSVAX to prevent HIV-1 infection in Thailand. *N Engl J Med.* 2009;361(23):2209-2220.

42. Centers for Disease Control and Prevention. *Preexposure Prophylaxis for the Prevention of HIV Infection in the United States–2014 Clinical Practice Guideline.* Atlanta, Ga: U.S. Public Health Service, Centers for Disease Control and Prevention; 2014.

43. Plosker GL. Emtricitabine/tenofovir disoproxil fumarate: a review of its use in HIV-1 pre-exposure prophylaxis. *Drugs.* 2013;73(3):279-291.

44. Schiffner T, Sattentau QJ, Dorrell L. Development of prophylactic vaccines against HIV-1. *Retrovirology.* 2013;10: 72.

45. Fields-Gardner C, Campa A. Position of the American Dietetic Association: nutrition intervention and human immunodeficiency virus infection. *J Am Diet Assoc.* 2010; 110(7):1105-1119.

46. Aberman NL, et al. Food security and nutrition interventions in response to the AIDS epidemic: assessing global action and evidence. *AIDS Behav.* 2014;18(suppl 5): S554-S565.

47. Nagata JM, et al. Descriptive characteristics and health outcomes of the food by prescription nutrition supplementation program for adults living with HIV in Nyanza Province, Kenya. *PLoS ONE.* 2014;9(3):e91403.

48. Gonzalez-Hernandez LA, et al. Synbiotic therapy decreases microbial translocation and inflammation and improves immunological status in HIV-infected patients: a double-blind randomized controlled pilot trial. *Nutr J.* 2012; 11:90.

49. Kosmiski L. Energy expenditure in HIV infection. *Am J Clin Nutr.* 2011;94(6):1677S-1682S.

50. Olsen MF, et al. Effects of nutritional supplementation for HIV patients starting antiretroviral treatment: randomised controlled trial in Ethiopia. *BMJ.* 2014;348:g3187.

51. Domingo P, et al. Fat redistribution syndromes associated with HIV-1 infection and combination antiretroviral therapy. *AIDS Rev.* 2012;14(2):112-123.

Further Reading and Resources

CHAPTER 1

The following organizations are key sources of up-to-date information and research regarding nutrition. Each site has a unique focus and may be helpful for keeping abreast of current topics.

- Academy of Nutrition and Dietetics. www.eatright.org
- American Society for Nutrition. www.nutrition.org
- Dietary Guidelines for Americans. www.health.gov/dietaryguidelines
- Food and Agriculture Organization of the United Nations. www.fao.org
- Healthy People 2020. http://healthypeople.gov/2020/
- Institute of Medicine (Food and Nutrition). www.iom.edu/Global/Topics/Food-Nutrition.aspx
- Society for Nutrition Education and Behavior. www.sneb.org
- USDA Choose MyPlate. www.choosemyplate.gov
- World Health Organization. www.who.int
- Slining MM, Popkin BM. Trends in intakes and sources of solid fats and added sugars among U.S. children and adolescents: 1994-2010. *Pediatr Obes.* 2013;8(4):307-324.
  - *Despite dietary guidelines and healthy recommendations, Americans do not eat appropriate ratios of food from the recommended food groups. This study takes a specific look at the food choices of children and adolescents in the United States.*
- Freeland-Graves JH et al. Position of the academy of nutrition and dietetics: total diet approach to healthy eating. *J Acad Nutr Diet.* 2013;113(2):307-317.
  - *The authors discuss the use of a person-centered approach in applying healthy eating messages such as the Dietary Guidelines, MyPlate, Healthy People 2020, and the Dietary Reference Intakes.*

CHAPTER 2

The following organizations are valuable resources for nutrition and health-related information.

- Centers for Disease Control and Prevention site for *Nutrition Basics—Carbohydrates.* www.cdc.gov/nutrition/everyone/basics/carbs.html
- Women's Health.gov (U.S. Department of Health and Human Services) site for *Nutrition and Fitness—Carbohydrates.* www.womenshealth.gov/fitness-nutrition/nutrition-basics/carbohydrates.html
- Food and Nutrition Information Center (USDA) site for *Carbohydrate information.* http://fnic.nal.usda.gov/food-composition/macronutrients/carbohydrates
- Whole Grains Council. www.wholegrainscouncil.org
- Bray GA. Energy and fructose from beverages sweetened with sugar or high-fructose corn syrup pose a health risk for some people. *Adv Nutr.* 2013;4(2):220-225.
- Johnson RJ et al. Sugar, uric acid, and the etiology of diabetes and obesity. *Diabetes.* 2013;62(10):3307-3315.
  - *The authors explore the health dangers of excess consumption of high-fructose corn syrup.*
- Noto H et al. Low-carbohydrate diets and all-cause mortality: a systematic review and meta-analysis of observational studies. *PLoS One.* 2013;8(1):e55030.
  - *Carbohydrates are the topic of much debate in weight-loss programs. This review examines the long-term effects of a low-carbohydrate diet on all-cause mortality. The authors answer the following question: "Are the short-term benefits worth the long-term risk?"*

CHAPTER 3

- Lipids in Health and Disease. www.lipidworld.com
  - *An online journal of peer-reviewed articles about all aspects of lipids that is open access and free to the public*
- Mayo Clinic. www.mayoclinic.com
  - *A site search for "dietary fat" results in several informative articles*
- USDA Nutrient Data Laboratory. http://ndb.nal.usda.gov/
  - *A useful website for finding the nutrient content of the foods that you most enjoy, including their trans-fat content*
- U.S. Food and Drug Administration. www.fda.gov
  - *A site search for 'trans fat' results in several informative articles regarding the current regulations on the use of partially hydrogenated oils in the food supply*
- Vannice G, Rasmussen H. Position of the Academy of Nutrition and Dietetics: dietary fatty acids for healthy adults. *J Acad Nutr Diet.* 2014;114(1):136-153.
- Walker TB, Parker MJ. Lessons from the war on dietary fat. *J Am Coll Nutr.* 2014;33:1-5.

CHAPTER 4

The following organizations are good sources of information about vegetarian diets.

- Food and Nutrition Information Center. http://fnic.nal.usda.gov

- Medline Plus site for *Vegetarian Diets*. www.nlm .nih.gov/medlineplus/vegetariandiet.html
- North American Vegetarian Society. www.navs -online.org
- Vegetarian Nutrition Dietetic Practice Group. http://vegetariannutrition.net/
- The Vegetarian Resource Group. www.vrg.org
- Tuso PJ et al. Nutritional update for physicians: plant-based diets. *Perm J.* 2013;17(2):61-66.
- Food and Agriculture Organization of the United Nations. *Dietary protein quality evaluation in human nutrition: report of an FAO Expert Consultation,* Rome, 2013, ISBN 978-92-5-107417-6. Available from www.fao.org.

CHAPTER 5

The following organizations provide up-to-date research and reliable information about matters of the GI tract and metabolism.

- The American College of Gastroenterology. www .gi.org
- The American Gastroenterological Association. www.gastro.org
- The American Journal of Gastroenterology. www .amjgastro.com
- Metabolism. www.metabolism.com
- Nutrition & Metabolism. www. nutritionandme tabolism.com
- Rasmussen HH et al. Nutrition in chronic pancreatitis. *World J Gastroenterol.* 2013;19(42):7267-7275.

This article will give the reader insight into the complex issues that result when one accessory organ fails to provide the necessary enzymes for normal digestion.

CHAPTER 6

The following websites provide methods for predicting total energy needs and for evaluating energy expenditure.

- Adult energy needs and body mass index calculator. www.bcm.edu/cnrc/caloriesneed.cfm
- Children's energy needs calculator. www.bcm.edu/ cnrc/healthyeatingcalculator/eatingCal.html
- Mayo Clinic. Site search for *burn calories.* www .mayoclinic.com
- Choose MyPlate.gov Daily Food Plans and Worksheets. www.choosemyplate.gov/supertracker -tools/daily-food-plans.html
- Mullur R, Liu YY, Brent GA. Thyroid hormone regulation of metabolism. *Physiol Rev.* 2014;94(2): 355-382.
- Camps SG, Verhoef SP, Westerterp KR. Weight loss, weight maintenance, and adaptive thermogenesis. *Am J Clin Nutr.* 2013;97(5):990-994.
  - *This study examines the effect of weight loss on adaptive thermogenesis. Since one of the factors that affects resting energy expenditure is body size, it is expected that REE would decline after weight loss because the body is smaller. Researchers in this study found that*

the REE decreased more than expected after weight loss, resulting in a disproportionately lower REE for the given age, gender, and body size.

CHAPTER 7

For more information about the role of folic acid with regard to neural tube defects, see the following websites:

- Centers for Disease Control and Prevention. *Spina Bifida.* www.cdc.gov/ncbddd/spinabifida/ data.html
- Spina Bifida Association of America. www.sbaa .org

The following organizations and articles provide current information and guidelines regarding dietary recommendations for nutrient consumption:

- Center for Science in the Public Interest. www .cspinet.org
- Centers for Disease Control and Prevention. *Nutrition for everyone, fruits and vegetables.* www.cdc.gov/ nutrition/everyone/fruitsvegetables/index.html
- Office of Dietary Supplements. http://ods.od.nih .gov
- Wolf G. The discovery of vitamin D: the contribution of Adolf Windaus. *J Nutr.* 2004;134(6): 1299-1302.
- Public Health Reports, June 26, 1914. The etiology of pellagra. The significance of certain epidemiological observations with respect thereto. *Public Health Rep.* 1975;90(4):373-375.
  - *The articles listed above are two short and remarkable papers on the history of vitamin D discovery and the pellegra epidemic, both in the early 1900s.*
- Liu RH. Dietary bioactive compounds and their health implications. *J Food Sci.* 2013;78(Suppl 1): A18-A25.

CHAPTER 8

The following websites are good sources for information about certain minerals in diets and their role in general health. You can also go to the National Heart, Lung, and Blood Institute website to learn about the relationship between several minerals (sodium, potassium, magnesium, and calcium) and hypertension. Examine the American Dental Association Oral Health Topics for more information about the protective role of fluoride in dental hygiene.

- American Dental Association. www.ada.org/ fluoride.aspx
- National Digestive Diseases Information Clearinghouse, hemochromatosis. http://digestive.niddk .nih.gov/ddiseases/pubs/hemochromatosis/
- National Heart, Lung, and Blood Institute. www .nhlbi.nih.gov/health/health-topics/topics/dash/
- National Osteoporosis Foundation. www.nof.org
- Varacallo MA, Fox EJ. Osteoporosis and its complications. *Med Clin North Am.* 2014;98(4):817-831, xii-xiii.

- Prasad AS. Discovery of human zinc deficiency: its impact on human health and disease. *Adv Nutr.* 2013;4(2):176-190.

CHAPTER 9

The following organizations provide up-to-date recommendations regarding water and electrolyte balance in addition to a plethora of other health information.

- American College of Sports Medicine. www.acsm.org (search for Fluid Requirements)
- Mayo Clinic. www.mayoclinic.org/healthy-lifestyle (see Food and Healthy Eating)
- Maughan RJ. Hydration, morbidity, and mortality in vulnerable populations. *Nutr Rev.* 2012;70(Suppl 2):S152-S155.
- Popkin BM, D'Anci KE, Rosenberg IH. Water, hydration, and health. *Nutr Rev.* 2010;68(8): 439-458

These two review articles address the importance of maintaining adequate hydration.

- Robinson JR. Water, the indispensable nutrient. *Nutr Today.* 1970;5(1):16-23, 28-29.

This classic article by a New Zealand physician who is a world authority in this field clearly describes the processes that are involved in body water balance. This article is filled with excellent charts and diagrams to illustrate key principles.

CHAPTER 10

Each of the following organizations has an earnest interest in the health care of pregnant women and their children. For information about a variety of topics involving pregnancy and lactation, explore their websites.

- American Academy of Pediatrics. www.aap.org
- Birth Defect Research for Children, Inc. www.birthdefects.org
- Canadian Paediatric Society. www.cps.ca
- La Leche League International, Inc. www.llli.org
- March of Dimes Birth Defects Foundation. www.marchofdimes.org
- U.S. Department of Agriculture WIC Program. www.fns.usda.gov/wic
- Herrell HE. Nausea and vomiting of pregnancy. *Am Fam Physician.* 2014;89(12):965-970.
- Kramer MS, Aboud F, Mironova E et al. Breastfeeding and child cognitive development: new evidence from a large randomized trial: Promotion of Breastfeeding Intervention Trial (PROBIT) Study Group. *Arch Gen Psychiatry.* 2008;65(5):578-584.

Researchers outline and discuss one of the largest randomized trials addressing the benefits of breastfeeding for child cognitive development.

- Gibbs BG, Forste R. Breastfeeding, parenting, and early cognitive development. *J Pediatr.* 2014;164(3): 487-493.

Researchers discuss breastfeeding as an indication of overall parenting skills and the link to cognitive development, as opposed to any nutrient element found in breast milk.

CHAPTER 11

- Food and Nutrition Service. School Meals. www.fns.usda.gov/school-meals/child-nutrition-programs
- Kidnetic. www.kidnetic.com
- KidsHealth. www.kidshealth.org
- MyPlate tools for kids (6 to 11 years old). www.choosemyplate.gov/children-over-five.html
- MyPlate tools for preschoolers. www.choosemyplate.gov/preschoolers.html
- National Center for Education in Maternal and Child Health. www.ncemch.org
- World Health Organization child growth standards. www.who.int/childgrowth/en/

These websites are excellent resources for childhood nutrition information. One of the most important parts of working with parents and children on feeding and health issues is to have access to up-to-date information and ideas. Explore these sites to discover current topics that address the health and nutrition issues that face youth today.

- Hancock ME, Brown J. Formula-feeding safety: what nurses need to teach parents who choose to formula-feed. *Nurs Womens Health.* 2010;14(4): 302-309.
- Savona-Ventura C, Savona-Ventura S. The inheritance of obesity. *Best Pract Res Clin Obstet Gynaecol.* 2015;29(3):300-308.

CHAPTER 12

- Administration on Aging. www.aoa.gov
- American Geriatrics Society. www.americangeriatrics.org
- American Society on Aging. www.asaging.org
- Assisted Living Federation of America. www.alfa.org
- CDC site for *Chronic Disease Prevention and Health Promotion:* www.cdc.gov/chronicdisease/overview/index.htm
- Centers for Medicare & Medicaid Services. www.cms.hhs.gov
- The Gerontological Society of America. www.geron.org
- LeadingAge. www.leadingage.org
- National Council on Aging. www.ncoa.org
- National Institute on Aging. www.nia.nih.gov
- National Osteoporosis Foundation. www.nof.org
- U.S. Department of Agriculture, Food and Nutrition Service, Commodity Supplemental Food Program. www.fns.usda.gov/csfp/about-csfp

These organizations are excellent sources of information about nutrition, health, and community services for the elderly.

- Centers for Disease Control and Prevention. *The power of prevention: chronic disease...the public health challenge of the 21st century* (website). Available at www.cdc.gov/chronicdisease/pdf/2009-Power-of-Prevention.pdf.

- van Dijk GM et al. Health issues for menopausal women: the top 11 conditions have common solutions. *Maturitas*. 2015;80(1):24-30.
- Agarwal E et al. Malnutrition in the elderly: a narrative review. *Maturitas*. 2013;76(4):296-302.

CHAPTER 13

Explore these websites for current information and regulations regarding food safety, food-borne illness, and food labeling standards.

- Centers for Disease Control and Prevention. Food-borne illness in the United States. www.cdc.gov/foodborneburden
- Food and Agriculture Organization of the United Nations: www.fao.org/economic
- Food Value Analysis: www.foodvalueanalysis.org/ This site offers "a way to compare a range of values for various forms of processed foods compared to foods prepared from a recipe in the home kitchen."
- U.S. Department of Agriculture: Agricultural Marketing Service, The National Organic Program. www.ams.usda.gov/AMSv1.0/nop
- U.S. Department of Agriculture. Food and nutrition services: nutrition assistance programs. www.fns.usda.gov
- U.S. Food and Drug Administration. Ingredients, Packaging, and Labeling. www.fda.gov/Food/IngredientsPackagingLabeling/default.htm
- U.S. Department of Agriculture. Food Safety Education. www.fsis.usda.gov/wps/portal/fsis/topics/food-safety-education
- U.S. Department of Agriculture: National Institute of Food and Agriculture. www.csrees.usda.gov
- Greene D et al. Peeling lead paint turns into poisonous dust. Guess where it ends up? A media campaign to prevent childhood lead poisoning in New York City. *Health Educ Behav*. 2015;42(3):409-421.
- Caruso ML, Cullen KW. Quality and cost of student lunches brought from home. *JAMA Pediatr*. 2015;169(1):86-90.
- Cullen KW et al. Differential improvements in student fruit and vegetable selection and consumption in response to the new national school lunch program regulations: a pilot study. *J Acad Nutr Diet*. 2015;115(5):743-750.

A look into the effects of the new National School Lunch Program and a comparison of those lunches brought from home.

CHAPTER 14

- Anthropology of Food. http://aof.revues.org
- Association for the Study of Food and Society. www.food-culture.org
- CDC: Racial and Ethnic Minority Populations. www.cdc.gov/minorityhealth/populations/remp.html
- Food and Agricultural Organization of the United Nations. www.fao.org/home/en/

- Kraak VI, Story M. Influence of food companies' brand mascots and entertainment companies' cartoon media characters on children's diet and health: a systematic review and research needs. *Obes Rev*. 2015;16(2):107-126.
- Birch LL, Savage J, Fisher JO. Right sizing prevention: food portion size effects on children's eating and weight. *Appetite*. 2015;88:11-16.

CHAPTER 15

- Academy of Nutrition and Dietetics: Wellness www.eatright.org/resources/health/wellness
- Centers for Disease Control and Prevention: Healthy Weight www.cdc.gov/healthyweight/index.html
- Intuitive Eating www.intuitiveeating.org
- Nutrition.gov www.nutrition.gov click on "Weight Management"
- Office of the Surgeon General. Obesity www.surgeongeneral.gov/topics/obesity/
- Culbert KM, Racine SE, Klump KL. Research Review: what we have learned about the causes of eating disorders – a synthesis of sociocultural, psychological, and biological research. *J Child Psychol Psychiatry*. 2015;56(11):1141-1164.

CHAPTER 16

Review the following websites for information, guidelines, research, and suggestions regarding exercise and physical fitness.

- American College of Sports Medicine. www.acsm.org
- Sports, Cardiovascular, and Wellness Nutrition. www.scandpg.org
- Nancy Clark's Sports Nutrition Guidebook. www.nancyclarkrd.com
- National Coalition for Promoting Physical Activity. www.ncppa.org
- National Institutes of Health, Office of Dietary Supplements. ods.od.nih.gov
- The Surgeon General's Vision for a Healthy and Fit Nation. www.surgeongeneral.gov/initiatives/healthy-fit-nation/obesityvision2010.pdf
- Denison HJ et al. Prevention and optimal management of sarcopenia: a review of combined exercise and nutrition interventions to improve muscle outcomes in older people. *Clin Interv Aging*. 2015;10:859-869.
- Brocklebank LA et al. Accelerometer-measured sedentary time and cardiometabolic biomarkers: a systematic review. *Prev Med*. 2015;76:92-102.

CHAPTER 17

- Academy of Nutrition and Dietetics, *Nutrition Care Process*. www.eatrightpro.org/resources/practice/nutrition-care-process
- American Society for Parenteral and Enteral Nutrition. www.nutritioncare.org

This association provides education, publications, conferences, and resources about clinical nutrition therapy for health care professionals. The association is made up of physicians, dietitians, nurses, pharmacists, scientists, and other allied health care professionals.

- NANDA International, *Diagnosis Development*. www.nanda.org/nanda-international-diagnosis-development.html
- Bell CL, Lee AS, Tamura BK. Malnutrition in the nursing home. *Curr Opin Clin Nutr Metab Care*. 2015;18(1):17-23.
- Boullata JI. Drug and nutrition interactions: not just food for thought. *J Clin Pharm Ther*. 2013;38(4): 269-271.

CHAPTER 18

- American Academy of Allergy, Asthma, & Immunology. www.aaaai.org
- Asthma and Allergy Foundation of America. www.aafa.org
- Celiac Support Association. www.csaceliacs.org
- Crohn's and Colitis Foundation of America. www.ccfa.org
- Cystic Fibrosis Foundation. www.cff.org
- Cystic Fibrosis.com. www.cysticfibrosis.com
- Dysphagia Research Society. www.dysphagiaresearch.org
- International Foundation for Functional Gastrointestinal Disorders. www.iffgd.org
- National Digestive Diseases Information Clearinghouse, Irritable Bowel Syndrome. www.niddk.nih.gov
- United Ostomy Associations of America. www.ostomy.org/Home.html

These organizations provide support for individuals who are affected by disorders of the gastrointestinal tract. Health care providers should be familiar with these organizations and their websites to refer patients to organizations that can continue to give them support, understanding, and up-to-date information about their diseases.

- Biesiekierski JR et al. No effects of gluten in patients with self-reported non-celiac gluten sensitivity after dietary reduction of fermentable, poorly absorbed, short-chain carbohydrates. *Gastroenterology*. 2013; 145(2):320-328, e1-3.
- Jones SM, Burks AW, Dupont C. State of the art on food allergen immunotherapy: oral, sublingual, and epicutaneous. *J Allergy Clin Immunol*. 2014;133(2): 318-323.

CHAPTER 19

- American Heart Association. www.heart.org
- Centers for Disease Control and Prevention. Heart disease prevention: What you can do. www.cdc.gov/HeartDisease/prevention.htm
- National Heart, Lung, and Blood Institute. Systematic Evidence Reviews and Clinical Practice Guidelines for Heart Disease. www.nhlbi.nih.gov/health-pro/guidelines

- National Heart, Lung, and Blood Institute. Risk assessment tool for estimating 10-year risk of having a heart attack. http://cvdrisk.nhlbi.nih.gov/
- National Heart, Lung, and Blood Institute. Heart and Vascular Resources. www.nhlbi.nih.gov/health-pro/resources/heart

These organizations are valuable sources of information regarding the most current recommendations for healthy lifestyles to prevent and treat heart disease. The websites also provide educational materials for both health care professionals and the public.

- Ooi EM et al. Dietary fatty acids and lipoprotein metabolism: new insights and updates. *Curr Opin Lipidol*. 2013;24(3):192-197.
- Martinez-Gonzalez MA, Bes-Rastrollo M. Dietary patterns, Mediterranean diet, and cardiovascular disease. *Curr Opin Lipidol*. 2014;25(1):20-26.
- Liese AD et al. The Dietary Patterns Methods Project: Synthesis of Findings across Cohorts and Relevance to Dietary Guidance. *J Nutr*. 2015;145(3): 393-402.

CHAPTER 20

- American Association of Diabetes Educators. www.diabeteseducator.org
- American Diabetes Association. www.diabetes.org
- Juvenile Diabetes Research Foundation International. http://jdrf.org
- National Institute of Diabetes and Digestive and Kidney Diseases. www.niddk.nih.gov
- National Diabetes Information Clearinghouse. www.diabetes.niddk.nih.gov

The preceding organizations are dedicated to providing the most current information about the evaluation, treatment, and prevention of diabetes. These websites are excellent resources for both health care professionals and patients.

- Poomalar GK. Changing trends in management of gestational diabetes mellitus. *World J Diabetes*. 2015;6(2):284-295.

CHAPTER 21

- American Urological Association. www.urologyhealth.org
- End Stage Renal Disease National Coordinating Center. http://esrdncc.org
- National Institute of Diabetes and Digestive and Kidney Diseases. www.niddk.nih.gov
- National Kidney Disease Education Program. http://nkdep.nih.gov
- National Kidney Foundation. www.kidney.org, a site search for "Understanding kidney disease and treatment options" will provide the viewer with an excellent series of short videos on kidney function, disease, and treatment modalities.

These websites provide additional information about various forms of kidney disease. Several national organizations provide free education and support for health care providers, patients, and family members.

Dietary restrictions for patients with kidney disease can sometimes be overwhelming. To fully understand such diets, continuous follow-up and feedback are needed.

- Burkhalter F, Steiger J, Dickenmann M. A road map for patients with imminent end-stage renal disease. *Swiss Med Wkly*. 2012;142:w13713.
- McCarthy MS, Phipps SC. Special nutrition challenges: current approach to acute kidney injury. *Nutr Clin Pract*. 2014;29(1):56-62.
- Obi Y et al. Latest consensus and update on protein-energy wasting in chronic kidney disease. *Curr Opin Clin Nutr Metab Care*. 2015;18(3):254-262.

CHAPTER 22

- American Burn Association. www.ameriburn.org
- American Society for Parenteral and Enteral Nutrition. www.nutritioncare.org
- Burn Foundation. www.burnfoundation.org
- Critical Care Nutrition. www.criticalcarenutrition.com
- Rosenthal MD et al. Evolving paradigms in the nutritional support of critically ill surgical patients. *Curr Probl Surg*. 2015;52(4):147-182.
- Elrazek AE, Elbanna AE, Bilasy SE. Medical management of patients after bariatric surgery: principles and guidelines. *World J Gastrointest Surg*. 2014;6(11):220-228.

CHAPTER 23

- AIDS information, education, and action. www.aids.org
- *AIDS*, the official journal of the International AIDS Society. www.aidsonline.com
- AIDS.gov. www.aids.gov
- American Cancer Society. www.cancer.org
- Centers for Disease Control and Prevention. Cancer prevention and control. www.cdc.gov/cancer
- Centers for Disease Control and Prevention. National Center for HIV/AIDS, Viral Hepatitis, STD, and TB Prevention. www.cdc.gov/nchhstp
- Joint United Nations Program on HIV/AIDS. www.unaids.org
- National Cancer Institute. www.cancer.gov
- The National Institute of Allergy and Infectious Diseases. HIV/AIDS vaccines. www.niaid.nih.gov/topics/hivaids/research/vaccines/Pages/default.aspx
- Argiles JM et al. Cancer cachexia: understanding the molecular basis. *Nat Rev Cancer*. 2014;14(11):754-762.
- Mankal PK, Kotler DP. From wasting to obesity, changes in nutritional concerns in HIV/AIDS. *Endocrinol Metab Clin North Am*. 2014;43(3):647-663.
- Richert L et al. Recent developments in clinical trial designs for HIV vaccine research. *Hum Vaccin Immunother*. 2015;11(4):1022-1029.

Glossary

1α-hydroxylase the enzyme in the kidneys that catalyzes the hydroxylation reaction of 25-hydroxycholecalciferol (i.e., calcidiol) to calcitriol, which is the active form of vitamin D; 1α-hydroxylase activity is increased by parathyroid hormone when blood calcium levels are low.

A

abdominal thrusts (formerly called Heimlich maneuver) a first-aid maneuver that is used to relieve a person who is choking from the blockage of the breathing passageway by a swallowed foreign object or food particle; to perform the maneuver, when standing behind the choking person, clasp the victim around the waist, place one fist just under the sternum (i.e., the breastbone), grasp the fist with the other hand, and then make a quick, hard, thrusting movement inward and upward to dislodge the object.

absorption (in terms of digestion and metabolism) the process by which nutrients are taken into the cells that line the gastrointestinal tract.

acculturation the process of an individual or group of people adopting the behaviors and lifestyle habits of a new culture.

acetone a major ketone compound that results from fat breakdown for energy in individuals with uncontrolled diabetes; persons with diabetes periodically take urinary acetone tests to monitor the status of ketone production.

achalasia a disorder of the esophagus in which the muscles of the tube fail to relax, thereby inhibiting normal swallowing.

acidic or alkaline diets diets based on the theory that diets high in acidic foods (e.g., animal protein, caffeine, simple sugars) will disrupt the body's normal pH balance, which is slightly alkaline.

acidosis a blood pH of less than 7.35; *respiratory acidosis* is caused by an accumulation of carbon dioxide (an acid); *metabolic acidosis* may be caused by a variety of conditions that result in the excess accumulation of acids in the body or by a significant loss of bicarbonate (a base).

adaptive thermogenesis an adjustment to heat production in response to changing environmental influences (e.g., external temperature, diet).

adipocytes fat cells.

adipose fat stored in the cells of adipose (fatty) tissue.

adipose tissue the storage site for excess fat.

aerobic capacity a state in which oxygen is required to proceed; milliliters of oxygen consumed per kilogram of body weight per minute as influenced by body composition.

aldosterone a hormone of the adrenal glands that acts on the distal nephron tubule to stimulate the reabsorption of sodium in an ion exchange with potassium; the aldosterone mechanism is essentially a sodium-conserving mechanism, but it also indirectly conserves water, because water absorption follows sodium resorption.

aldosteronoma the excess secretion of aldosterone from the adrenal cortex; symptoms and complications include sodium retention, potassium wasting, alkalosis, weakness, paralysis, polyuria, polydipsia, hypertension, and cardiac arrhythmias.

alkaline diets diets that are low in animal protein and high in fruits and vegetables.

alkalosis a blood pH of more than 7.45; *respiratory alkalosis* is caused by hyperventilation and an excess loss of carbon dioxide; *metabolic alkalosis* is seen with extensive vomiting in which a significant amount of hydrochloric acid is lost and bicarbonate (a base) is secreted.

allergens proteins that elicit an immune system response or an allergic reaction; symptoms may include itching, swelling, hives, diarrhea, and difficulty breathing as well as anaphylaxis in the worst cases.

allergy a state of hypersensitivity to particular substances in the environment that works on body tissues to produce problems in the functioning of the affected tissues; the agent involved (i.e., the allergen) may be a certain food that is eaten or a substance (e.g., pollen) that is inhaled or touched.

alpha-linolenic acid an essential fatty acid with 18 carbon atoms and 3 double bonds. The first double bond is located at the third carbon from the omega end, making it an omega-3 fatty acid. Found in soybean, canola, and flaxseed oil.

amenorrhea or ammenorrheic the absence of a menstrual period in a woman of reproductive age.

amino acids the nitrogen-bearing compounds that form the structural units of protein; after digestion, amino acids are available for the synthesis of required proteins.

aminopeptidase a specific protein-splitting enzyme secreted by glands in the walls of the small intestine that breaks off the nitrogen-containing amino end (i.e., NH_2) of the peptide chain, thereby producing smaller-chained peptides and free amino acids.

anabolism the metabolic process of building large substances from smaller parts; the opposite of catabolism.

anaerobic a microorganism that can live and grow in an oxygen-free environment.

anaphylactic shock or anaphylaxis a severe and sometimes fatal allergic reaction that results from exposure to a protein that the body perceives as foreign and that elicits a systemic response that involves multiple organs.

anemia a condition that is characterized by a decreased number of circulating red blood cells, decreased hemoglobin level, or both.

anencephaly the congenital absence of the brain that results from the incomplete closure of the upper end of the neural tube.

angina pectoris a spasmodic, choking chest pain caused by a lack of oxygen to the heart; this is a symptom of a heart attack, and it also may be caused by severe effort or excitement.

angiotensin I inactive peptide hormone that is the precursor to angiotensin II.

angiotensin-converting enzyme (ACE) the enzyme found on the capillary walls within the lungs that converts angiotensin I to angiotensin II. ACE is also present to a lesser extent in the endothelial cells and the epithelial cells within the kidneys.

angiotensin II an active hormone that constricts blood vessels and stimulates the release of aldosterone. Both actions lead to an increase in blood pressure.

angiotensinogen an inactive enzyme produced by the liver that circulates within the blood at all times. Angiotensinogen is activated by renin to becomes angiotensin I.

anorexia nervosa an extreme psychophysiologic aversion to food that results in life-threatening weight loss; a psychiatric eating disorder that results from a morbid fear of fatness in which a person's distorted body image is reflected as fat when the body is malnourished and extremely thin as a result of self-starvation.

anthropometric measurements the physical measurements of the human body that are used for health assessment, including height, weight, skin fold thickness, and circumference (i.e., of the head, hip, waist, wrist, and mid-arm muscle).

antibody any of numerous protein molecules produced by B cells as a primary immune defense for attaching to specific related antigens.

antidiuretic hormone a hormone of the pituitary gland that acts on the distal nephron tubule to conserve water by reabsorption; also called *vasopressin.*

antigen any foreign or non-self substance (e.g., toxins, viruses, bacteria, foreign proteins) that triggers the production of antibodies that are specifically designed to counteract their activity.

antioxidant a molecule that prevents the oxidation of cellular structures by free radicals.

anuria the absence of urine production; anuria indicates kidney shutdown or failure.

appetite-regulating network a hormonally controlled system of appetite stimulation and suppression.

arteriole the smallest branch of an artery that connects with the capillaries.

ascites the accumulation of serous fluid (i.e., blood and lymph serum) in the abdominal cavity.

ascorbic acid the chemical name for vitamin C; the vitamin was named after its ability to cure scurvy.

atherosclerosis the underlying pathology of coronary heart disease; a common form of arteriosclerosis that is characterized by the formation of fatty streaks that contain cholesterol and that develop into hardened plaques in the inner lining of major blood vessels such as the coronary arteries.

atonic without normal muscle tone.

atopy patch test a diagnostic test that is used to assess for allergic reactions on the skin.

atrophy tissue wasting.

auscultation listening to the sounds of the gastrointestinal tract with a stethoscope.

azotemia an excess of urea and other nitrogenous substances in the blood.

B

baby bottle tooth decay the decay of the baby teeth as a result of inappropriate feeding practices such as putting an infant to bed with a bottle; also called *nursing bottle caries, bottle mouth,* and *bottle caries.*

Barrett's esophagus complication of severe gastroesophageal reflux disease in which the squamous cell epithelium of the esophagus changes to resemble the tissue lining the small intestine; increases the risk of esophageal adenocarcinoma.

basal energy expenditure (BEE) the amount of energy (in kcal) needed by the body for the maintenance of life when a person is at complete digestive, physical, mental, thermal, and emotional rest (i.e., 10 to 12 hours after eating and 12 to 18 hours after physical activity); measured immediately upon waking. Also referred to as basal metabolic rate (BMR).

beriberi a disease of the peripheral nerves that is caused by a deficiency of thiamin (vitamin B_1) and is characterized by pain (neuritis) and paralysis of legs and arms, cardiovascular changes, and edema.

bile an emulsifying agent produced by the liver and transported to the gallbladder for concentration and storage; it is released into the duodenum with the entry of fat to facilitate enzymatic fat digestion by acting as an emulsifier.

binge-eating disorder a psychiatric eating disorder that is characterized by the occurrence of binge-eating episodes at least twice a week for a 6-month period.

biologic age age of the body relative to physiologic and maturity developmental standards.

blood urea nitrogen a test of nephron function that measures the ability to filter urea nitrogen, which is a product of protein metabolism, from the blood.

body composition the relative sizes of the four body compartments that make up the total body: lean body mass (muscle mass), fat, water, and bone.

body dysmorphic disorder an obsession with a perceived defect of the body.

body mass index the body weight in kilograms divided by the square of the height in meters (kg/m^2); this measurement correlates with body fatness and the health risks associated with obesity.

bolus feeding a volume of feeding from 250 mL to 500 mL administered by a syringe over a short period of time (usually 10 to 15 minutes) that is given in several feedings per day.

Bowman's capsule the membrane at the head of each nephron; this capsule was named for the English physician Sir William Bowman, who in 1843 first established the basis of plasma filtration and consequent urine secretion in the relationship of the blood-filled glomeruli and the filtration across the enveloping membrane.

branched-chain amino acids amino acids with branched side chains; three of the essential amino acids are branched-chain amino acids: leucine, isoleucine, and valine.

breastfed exclusively feeding the infant only breast milk with no supplemental liquids or solid foods, other than necessary medications or nutrient supplements when needed.

brush border the cells that are located on the microvilli within the lining of the intestinal tract; the microvilli are tiny hair-like projections that protrude from the mucosal cells and help to increase the surface area for the digestion and absorption of nutrients.

bulimia nervosa a psychiatric eating disorder related to a person's fear of fatness in which cycles of gorging on large quantities of food are followed by compensatory mechanisms (e.g., self-induced vomiting, the use of diuretics and laxatives) to maintain a "normal" body weight.

C

cachexia a specific profound syndrome that is characterized by wasting, reduced food intake, and systemic inflammation.

Cajun a group of people with an enduring tradition whose French-Catholic ancestors established permanent communities in the southern Louisiana coastal waterways after being expelled from Acadia (now Nova Scotia, Canada) by the reigning English during the late eighteenth century; they developed a unique food pattern from a blend of native French influence and the Creole cooking that was found in the new land.

calcitriol the activated hormone form of vitamin D.

calorie a measure of heat; the energy necessary to do work is measured as the amount of heat produced by the body's work; the energy value of a food is expressed as the number of kilocalories that a specified portion of the food will yield when it is oxidized in the body.

carboxypeptidase a specific protein-splitting enzyme secreted as the inactive zymogen procarboxypeptidase by the pancreas; after it has been activated by trypsin, it acts in the small intestine to break off the acid (i.e., carboxyl) end of the peptide chain, thereby producing smaller-chained peptides and free amino acids.

carcinogenesis the development of cancer.

carotene a group name for three red and yellow pigments (α-, β-, and γ-carotene) that are found in plant foods; β-carotene is most important to human nutrition because the body can convert it to vitamin A, thus making it a primary source of the vitamin.

carotenoids organic pigments that are found in plants; known to have functions such as scavenging free radicals, reducing the risk of certain types of cancer, and helping to prevent age-related eye diseases; more than 600 carotenoids have been identified, with β-carotene being the most well-known.

catabolism the metabolic process of breaking down large substances to yield smaller building blocks.

cellulitis the diffuse inflammation of soft or connective tissues from injury, bruises, or pressure sores that leads to infection; poor care may result in ulceration and abscess or gangrene.

cerebrovascular accident a stroke; a stroke is caused by arteriosclerosis within the blood vessels of the brain that cuts off oxygen supply to the affected portion of brain tissue, thereby paralyzing the actions that are controlled by the affected area.

chelator a ligand that binds to a metal to form a metal complex.

cholecalciferol the chemical name for vitamin D_3 in its inactive form; it is often shortened to *calciferol*.

cholecystectomy the removal of the gallbladder.

cholecystitis acute gallbladder inflammation.

cholecystokinin (CCK) hormone secreted from the mucosal epithelium of the small intestine in response to the presence of fat and certain amino acids in chyme. CCK inhibits gastric motility, increases the release of pancreatic enzymes, and stimulates the gallbladder to secrete bile into the small intestine.

cholelithiasis gallstones.

cholesterol a fat-related compound called a sterol that is synthesized only in animal tissues; a normal constituent of bile and a principal constituent of gallstones; in the body, cholesterol is primarily synthesized in the liver; in the diet, cholesterol is found in animal food sources.

chronic dieting syndrome a cyclic pattern of weight loss by dieting followed by rapid weight gain; this abnormal psychophysiologic food pattern becomes chronic, changing a person's natural body metabolism and relative body composition to the abnormal state of a metabolically obese person of normal weight.

chronic kidney disease-mineral and bone disorder a clinical syndrome that develops as a systemic disorder of mineral and bone metabolism in patients with chronic kidney disease; results from abnormalities of calcium, phosphorus, parathyroid hormone, or vitamin D metabolism; causes abnormalities in bone turnover, mineralization, volume, linear growth, strength, and soft-tissue calcification.

chronologic age amount of time a person has lived.

chylomicron a lipoprotein formed in the intestinal cell that is composed of triglycerides, cholesterol, phospholipids, and protein; chylomicrons allow for the absorption of fat into the lymphatic circulatory system before entering the blood circulation.

chyme the semifluid food mass in the gastrointestinal tract that is present after gastric digestion.

chymotrypsin a protein-splitting enzyme secreted as the inactive zymogen chymotrypsinogen by the pancreas; after it has been activated by trypsin, it acts in the small intestine to continue breaking down proteins into shorter-chain polypeptides and dipeptides.

clinically severe or significant obesity a BMI of 40 or more or a BMI of 35 to 39 with at least one obesity-related disorder; also referred to as extreme obesity and morbid obesity.

cobalamin the chemical name for vitamin B_{12}; this vitamin is found mainly in animal protein food sources; it is closely related to amino acid metabolism and the formation of the heme portion of hemoglobin; the absence of hydrochloric acid and intrinsic factor leads to pernicious anemia and degenerative effects on the nervous system.

colloidal osmotic pressure (COP) the fluid pressure that is produced by protein molecules in the plasma and the cell; because proteins are large molecules, they do not pass through the separating membranes of the capillary walls; thus, they remain in their respective compartments and exert a constant osmotic pull that protects vital plasma and cell fluid volumes in these areas.

colostrum fluid secreted by the mammary glands for the first few days after birth, preceding the mature breast milk. Colostrum contains up to 20% protein, including a large amount of lactalbumin, minerals, and immunoglobulins that represent the antibodies found in maternal blood. It has less lactose and fat than mature milk.

competitive foods any food or beverage that is served outside of a federal meal program in a food-program setting, regardless of nutritional value.

complex carbohydrates large complex molecules of carbohydrates composed of many sugar units (polysaccharides); the complex forms of dietary carbohydrates are starch and dietary fiber.

conditionally indispensable amino acids the six amino acids that are normally considered dispensable amino acids because the body can make them; however, under certain circumstances (e.g., illness), the body cannot make them in high enough quantities, and they become indispensable (cannot do without) in the diet.

congestive heart failure a chronic condition of gradually weakening heart muscle; the muscle is unable to pump normal blood through the heart-lung circulation, which results in the congestion of fluids in the lungs.

continuous feeding an enteral feeding schedule with which the formula is infused via a pump continuously over a 24-hour period.

continuous renal replacement therapy (CRRT) a method of blood purification that is used continuously (i.e., 24 hr/day) for critically ill patients in intensive care settings. There are several forms of CRRT that vary according to the vascular access route, presence or absence of dialysate, type of semipermeable membrane used, and the mechanism of solute removal.

coronary heart disease the overall medical problem that results from the underlying disease of atherosclerosis in the coronary arteries, which serve the heart muscle with blood, oxygen, and nutrients.

crawfish boil traditional Louisiana Cajun festive meal. Typically includes crawfish, crab, shrimp, small ears of corn, new potatoes, onions, garlic and seasonings such as cayenne pepper, hot sauce, salt, lemons, and bay leaf. Smoked sausage links are occasionally added. All ingredients are added to a large pot and boiled. The contents are then spread out on newspaper covered tables for everyone to eat from directly.

creatinine a nitrogen-carrying product of normal tissue protein breakdown; it is excreted in the urine; serum creatinine levels are an indicator of renal function.

Cushing's syndrome the excess secretion of glucocorticoids from the adrenal cortex; symptoms and complications include protein loss, obesity, fatigue, osteoporosis, edema, excess hair growth, diabetes, and skin discoloration.

D

deamination the removal of the nitrogen containing part (amino group) from an amino acid.

dehiscence a splitting open; the separation of the layers of a surgical wound that may be partial, superficial, or complete and that involves total disruption and resuturing.

dialysate the cleansing solution used in dialysis; contains dextrose and other chemicals similar to those in the body.

dialysis the process of separating crystalloids and colloids in solution by the difference in their rates of diffusion through a semipermeable membrane; crystalloids (e.g., blood glucose, other simple metabolites) pass through readily, and colloids (e.g., plasma proteins) pass through slowly or not at all. Dialysis is used to remove waste and excess fluid from the blood when one's kidneys are not functioning.

Dietary Reference Intakes (DRIs) reference values for the nutrient intake needs of healthy individuals for each gender and age group.

dietetics the management of the diet and the use of food; the science concerned with nutrition planning, medical nutrition therapy, and the preparation of foods.

digestion the process by which food is broken down in the gastrointestinal tract to release nutrients in forms that the body can absorb.

dipeptidase the final enzyme in the protein-splitting system that releases free amino acids from dipeptide bonds.

dispensable amino acids the five amino acids that the body can synthesize from other amino acids that are supplied through the diet and thus do not have to be consumed on a daily basis.

diuresis the increased excretion of urine.

diuretic any substance that induces urination and subsequent fluid loss.

diverticulitis the inflammation of pockets of tissue (i.e., diverticula) in the lining of the mucous membrane of the colon.

doubly labeled water method gold standard for measuring energy expenditure. Participants ingest water labeled with a known concentration of isotopes of hydrogen and oxygen. Elimination of the isotopes is measured to predict the energy expenditure and metabolic rate.

dual-energy x-ray absorptiometry radiography that makes use of two beams (i.e., dual) that measure bone density and body composition.

dumping syndrome condition in which there is a quick emptying of the stomach of a hyperosmolar content into the small intestine, causing fluid to shift into the intestinal lumen from the intravascular compartment.

dynamic equilibrium the process of maintaining balance (i.e., equilibrium) through constant change or motion by energy or action (i.e., dynamic).

dysbiosis imbalance of the intestinal microbiome.

dyslipidemia abnormal lipid profile (high cholesterol, LDL, or TG; and/or low HDL).

dysphagia difficulty swallowing.

E

early-onset obesity a genetically associated obesity that occurs during early childhood.

eating disorder not otherwise specified subthreshold disordered eating that is not consistent with the diagnostic criteria for bulimia nervosa or anorexia nervosa.

edema an unusual accumulation of fluid in the interstitial compartments (i.e., the small structural spaces between tissue parts) of the body.

element a single type of atom; a total of 118 elements have been identified, of which 94 occur naturally on Earth; elements cannot be broken down into smaller substances.

elemental formula a nutrition support formula that is composed of simple elemental nutrient components that require no further digestive breakdown and are thus readily absorbed; these formulas include protein as free amino acids and carbohydrate as the simple sugar glucose.

emulsifier an agent that breaks down large fat globules into smaller, uniformly distributed particles; the action is chiefly accomplished in the intestine by bile acids, which lower the surface tension of the fat particles, thereby breaking the fat into many smaller droplets and facilitating contact with the fat-digesting enzymes.

energy-yielding nutrient nutrients that break down to yield energy within the body: including carbohydrates, fat, protein.

enriched a word that is used to describe foods to which vitamins and minerals have been added back to a food after a refining process that caused a loss of some nutrients; for example, iron may be lost during the refining process of a grain, so the final product will be enriched with additional iron.

enteral a mode of feeding that makes use of the gastrointestinal tract through oral or tube feeding.

enterokinase an enzyme produced and secreted in the duodenum in response to food entering the small intestine; it activates trypsinogen to its active form of trypsin.

enzymes the proteins produced in the body that digest or change nutrients in specific chemical reactions without being changed themselves during the process, thus their action is that of a catalyst; digestive enzymes in gastrointestinal secretions act on food substances to break them down into simpler compounds. (An enzyme usually is named after the substance [i.e., substrate] on which it acts, with the common word ending of -ase; for example, sucrase is the specific enzyme for sucrose, which it breaks down into glucose and fructose.)

ergocalciferol the chemical name for vitamin D_2 in its inactive form; it is produced by some organisms (not humans) upon ultraviolet irradiation from the precursor ergosterol.

ergogenic the tendency to increase work output; various substances that increase work or exercise capacity and output.

erythropoietin hormone that stimulates the production of red blood cells in the bone marrow.

esophageal varices the pathologic dilation of the blood vessels within the wall of the esophagus as a result of liver cirrhosis; these vessels can continue to expand to the point of rupturing.

esophagitis inflammation of the esophagus.

essential (or primary) hypertension an inherent form of high blood pressure with no specific identifiable cause; it is considered to be familial.

essential nutrients nutrients a person must obtain from food because the body cannot make them for itself in sufficient quantity to meet physiologic needs.

estrogen hormones sex hormones produced primarily by the ovaries.

euvolemia normal blood volume.

exogenous originating from outside the body.

expanded-criteria donors any brain-dead donor who is older than 60 years old or a donor who is older than 50 years old with two of the following conditions: history of hypertension, a terminal serum creatinine level of at least 1.5 mg/dL, or death from a cerebrovascular accident.

extrusion reflex the normal infant reflex to protrude the tongue outward when it is touched.

exudate various materials such as cells, cellular debris, and fluids that have escaped from the blood vessels and that are deposited in or on the surface tissues, usually as a result of inflammation; the protein content of exudate is high.

F

familial hypercholesterolemia a genetic disorder that results in elevated blood cholesterol levels despite lifestyle modifications; this condition is caused by absent or nonfunctional low-density lipoprotein receptors and it requires drug therapy.

familial hypertriglyceridemia a genetic disorder that results in elevated blood triglyceride levels despite lifestyle modifications; it requires drug therapy.

fatty acids the major structural components of fats.

ferritin the storage form of iron.

fetal alcohol spectrum disorders a group of physical and mental birth defects that are found in infants who are born to mothers who used alcohol during pregnancy; the physical and mental disabilities vary in severity; there is no cure.

fetal alcohol syndrome (FAS) a combination of physical and mental birth defects that are found in infants who are born to mothers who used alcohol during pregnancy; this is the most severe of the fetal alcohol spectrum disorders; there is no cure.

filé powder a substance that is made from ground sassafras leaves; it seasons and thickens the dish into which it is added.

fistulas from the Latin word for "pipe," an abnormal opening or passageway within the body or to the outside.

fluorosis an excess intake of fluoride that causes the yellowing of teeth, white spots on the teeth, and the pitting or mottling of tooth enamel.

food insecurity limited or uncertain availability of nutritionally adequate and safe foods or limited or uncertain ability to acquire acceptable foods in socially acceptable ways.

food jag brief sprees or binges of eating one particular food.

food neophobia the fear of new food.

G

galactosemia an autosomal recessive genetic disorder in which the liver does not produce the enzyme that is needed to metabolize galactose.

gastrin a hormone that helps with gastric motility, that stimulates the secretion of gastric acid by the parietal cells of the stomach, and that stimulates the chief cells to secrete pepsinogen.

gastroscopy an examination of the upper intestinal tract with a flexible tube with a small camera on the end; the tube is approximately 9 mm in diameter, and it takes color pictures as well as biopsy samples, if necessary.

glomerular filtration rate (GFR) the volume of fluid that is filtered from the renal glomerular capillaries into Bowman's capsule per unit of time; this term is used clinically as a measure of kidney function.

glomerulus the first section of the nephron; a cluster of capillary loops that are cupped in the nephron head that serves as an initial filter.

glucagon a hormone secreted by the alpha cells of the pancreatic islets of Langerhans in response to hypoglycemia; it has an effect opposite to that of insulin in that it raises the blood glucose concentration and thus is used as a quick-acting antidote for a low blood glucose reaction; it also counteracts the overnight fast during sleep by breaking down liver glycogen to keep blood glucose levels normal and to maintain an adequate energy supply for normal nerve and brain function.

gluconeogenesis the formation of glucose from noncarbohydrate substances such as amino acids.

GLUT4 an insulin-regulated protein that is responsible for glucose transport into cells.

glycemic control management of appropriate blood glucose levels.

glycemic index a ranking of foods relative to the increase above fasting in the blood glucose level more than 2 hours after the ingestion of a constant amount of that food divided by the response to a reference food.

glycerides the chemical group name for fats; fats are formed from a glycerol base with one, two, or three fatty acids attached to make monoglycerides, diglycerides, and triglycerides, respectively; glycerides are the principal constituents of adipose tissue, and they are found in animal and vegetable fats and oils.

glycogen a polysaccharide; a complex carbohydrate that is the main storage form of carbohydrates found in animal tissue that is composed of many glucose units linked together; stored primarily in the liver and to a lesser extent in muscle tissue.

glycogenesis the anabolic process of creating stored glycogen from glucose.

glycolipid a lipid with a carbohydrate attached.

goiter an enlarged thyroid gland that is usually caused by a lack of iodine to produce the thyroid hormone thyroxine.

gynecomastia the excessive development of the male mammary glands, frequently as a result of increased estrogen levels.

H

Hamwi method a formula for estimating the ideal body weight on the basis of gender and height.

health a state of optimal physical, mental, and social well-being; relative freedom from disease or disability.

health promotion the active engagement in behaviors or programs that advance positive well-being.

hematuria the abnormal presence of blood in the urine.

hemochromatosis genetic disease resulting in iron overload.

hemoglobin a conjugated protein in red blood cells that is composed of a compact, rounded mass of polypeptide chains that forms globin (the protein portion) and that is attached to an iron-containing red pigment called *heme;* hemoglobin carries oxygen in the blood to cells.

hemolytic uremic syndrome a condition that results most often from infection with *Escherichia coli* and that presents with a breaking up of red blood cells (i.e., hemolysis) and kidney failure.

hepatic encephalopathy a condition in which toxins in the blood lead to alterations in brain homeostasis as a result of liver disease; this results in apathy, confusion, inappropriate behavior, altered consciousness, and eventually coma.

hepatitis the inflammation of the liver cells; symptoms of acute hepatitis include flu-like symptoms, muscle and joint aches, fever, nausea, vomiting, diarrhea, headache, dark urine, and yellowing of the eyes and skin; symptoms of chronic hepatitis include jaundice, abdominal swelling and sensitivity, low-grade fever, and ascites.

homeostasis the state of relative dynamic equilibrium within the body's internal environment; a balance that is achieved through the operation of various interrelated physiologic mechanisms.

human milk fortifiers powder or liquid mixed with breast milk to increase the concentration of calories and protein in the milk for premature and low birth weight infants who need more kcals/mL than provided in breast milk.

hydrostatic pressure the force exerted by a fluid pushing against a surface.

hypercalcemia a serum calcium level that is greater than normal.

hypercholesterolemia high cholesterol levels in the blood.

hyperemesis gravidarum a condition that involves prolonged and severe vomiting in pregnant women, with a loss of more than 5% of body weight and the presence of ketonuria, electrolyte disturbances, and dehydration.

hyperglycemia an elevated blood glucose level.

hyperhomocysteinemia the presence of high levels of homocysteine in the blood; associated with cardiovascular disease.

hyperkalemia a serum potassium level that is greater than normal.

hypernatremia a serum sodium level that is greater than normal.

hyperphosphatemia a serum phosphorus level that is greater than normal.

hypertension chronically elevated blood pressure; systolic blood pressure is consistently 140 mm Hg or more or diastolic blood pressure is consistently 90 mm Hg or more.

hypertriglyceridemia high levels of triglycerides in the blood.

hypocalcemia a serum calcium level that is less than normal.

hypogeusia impaired taste.

hypoglycemia an abnormally low blood glucose level that may lead to muscle tremors, cold sweat, headache, and confusion; a serious condition in diabetes management that requires immediate sugar intake to counteract the low blood glucose level.

hypokalemia a serum potassium level that is less than normal.

hypomagnesemia a serum magnesium level that is less than normal.

hyponatremia a serum sodium level that is less than normal.

hypophosphatemia a serum phosphorus level that is less than normal.

hyposmia impaired ability to smell.

hypotension low blood pressure.

hypovolemia low blood volume.

I

idiopathic of unknown cause.

immunocompetence the ability or capacity to develop an immune response (i.e., antibody production or cell-mediated immunity) after exposure to an antigen.

indispensable amino acids the nine amino acids that must be obtained from the diet because the body does not make adequate amounts to support body needs.

insulin a hormone that is produced by the pancreas, attaches to insulin receptors on cell membranes, and allows the absorption of glucose into the cell.

intrauterine growth restriction (IUGR) a condition that occurs when a newborn baby weighs less than 10% of predicted fetal weight for gestational age.

K

ketoacidosis the excess production of ketones; a form of metabolic acidosis that occurs with uncontrolled diabetes or starvation from burning body fat for energy fuel; a continuing uncontrolled state can result in coma and death.

ketones the chemical name for a class of organic compounds that includes three keto acid bases that occur as intermediate products of fat metabolism.

ketosis the accumulation of ketones, which are intermediate products of fat metabolism, in the blood.

kilocalorie the general term *calorie* refers to a unit of heat measure, and it is used alone to designate the small calorie; the calorie that is used in nutrition science and the study of metabolism is the large Calorie or kilocalorie, which avoids the use of large numbers in calculations; a kilocalorie, which is composed of 1000 calories, is the measure of heat that is necessary to raise the temperature of 1000 g (1 L) of water by 1° C.

kinesiotherapist a health care professional who treats the effects of disease, injury, and congenital disorders through the application of scientifically based exercise principles that have been adapted to enhance the strength, endurance, and mobility of individuals with functional limitations or for those patients who require extended physical conditioning.

L

lactated Ringer's solution a sterile solution of calcium chloride, potassium chloride, sodium chloride, and sodium lactate in water that is given to replenish fluid and electrolytes; this solution was developed by the English physiologist Sidney Ringer (1835-1910).

lactation specialist health care professionals with specialized knowledge and clinical expertise in breastfeeding and human lactation. Also known as a lactation consultant.

laparoscopic fundoplication a surgery that is used to treat gastroesophageal reflux disease; the upper portion of the stomach (i.e., the fundus) is wrapped around the esophagus and sewn into place so that the esophagus passes through the muscle of the stomach; this strengthens the esophageal sphincter to prevent acid reflux.

life expectancy the number of years that a person of a given age may expect to live; this is affected by environment, lifestyle, sex, and race.

linoleic acid an essential fatty acid that consists of 18 carbon atoms and 2 double bonds. The first double bond is located at the sixth carbon from the omega end, making it an omega-6 fatty acid. Found in vegetable oils.

lipectomy the surgical removal of subcutaneous fat by suction through a tube that is inserted into a surface incision or by the removal of larger amounts of subcutaneous fat through a major surgical incision.

lipids the chemical group name for organic substances of a fatty nature; the lipids include fats, oils, waxes, and other fat-related compounds such as cholesterol.

lipiduria lipid droplets found in the urine that are composed mostly of cholesterol esters.

lipogenesis the anabolic process of forming fat.

lipoproteins chemical complexes of fat and protein that serve as the major carriers of lipids in the plasma; they vary in density according to the size of the fat load being carried (i.e., the lower the density, the higher the fat load); the combination package with water-soluble protein makes possible the transport of non–water-soluble fatty substances in the water-based blood circulation.

lobectomy surgical removal of a lobe of an organ.

M

macrosomia excessive fetal growth that results in an abnormally large infant; this condition carries a high risk for perinatal death.

major minerals the group of minerals that are required by the body in amounts of more than 100 mg/day.

masculinization a condition marked by the attainment of male characteristics (e.g., facial hair) either physiologically as part of male maturation or pathologically by either sex.

mechanical soft diet a meal plan that consists of foods that have been chopped, blended, ground, or prepared with extra fluid to make chewing and swallowing easier.

medical nutrition therapy a specific nutrition service and procedure that is used to treat an illness, injury, or condition; it involves an in-depth nutrition assessment of the patient, nutrition diagnosis, nutrition intervention (which may include diet therapy, counseling, and the use of specialized nutrition supplements), and nutrition monitoring and evaluation.

melatonin the hormone responsible for regulating body rhythms.

menopause the end of a woman's menstrual activity and capacity to bear children.

metabolic syndrome a combination of disorders that, when they occur together, increases the risk of cardiovascular disease and diabetes; it is also known as syndrome X and insulin resistance syndrome.

metabolism the sum of all chemical changes that take place in the body by which it maintains itself and produces energy for its functioning; products of the various reactions are called *metabolites*.

metastasis the spread to other tissue.

micelles packages of free fatty acids, monoglycerides, and bile salts; the hydrophobic fat particles are found in the middle of the package, whereas the hydrophilic part faces outward and allows for the absorption of fat into intestinal mucosal cells.

microalbuminuria low but abnormal levels of albumin in the urine.

microbiome microorganisms living in a specific environment.

microvilli extremely small, hair-like projections that cover all of the villi on the surface of the small intestine and that greatly increase the total absorbing surface area; they are visible through an electron microscope.

mucosal folds the large, visible folds of the mucous lining of the small intestine that increase the absorbing surface area.

mucositis an inflammation of the tissues around the mouth or other orifices of the body.

mutation a permanent transmissible change in a gene.

myocardial infarction (MI) a heart attack; a myocardial infarction is caused by the failure of the heart muscle to maintain normal blood circulation as a result of the blockage of the coronary arteries with fatty cholesterol plaques that cut off the delivery of oxygen to the affected part of the heart muscle.

MyPlate a visual pattern of the current basic five food groups—grains, vegetables, fruits, dairy, and protein—arranged on a plate to indicate proportionate amounts of daily food choices.

N

negative energy balance more total energy is expended than consumed.

neoplasm any new or abnormal cellular growth, specifically one that is uncontrolled and aggressive.

nephrolithiasis the formation of a kidney stone.

nephron the functional unit of the kidney that filters and reabsorbs essential blood constituents, secretes hydrogen ions as needed to maintain the acid-base balance, reabsorbs water, and forms and excretes a concentrated urine for the elimination of wastes.

nephrosis degenerative lesions of the renal tubules of the nephrons and especially of the thin basement membrane of the glomerulus that helps to support the capillary loops; marked by edema, albuminuria, and a decreased serum albumin level.

nephrotoxic toxic to the kidney.

niacin the chemical name for vitamin B_3; this vitamin was discovered in relation to the deficiency disease pellagra; it is important as a coenzyme factor in many cell reactions related to energy and protein metabolism.

nonessential nutrient a nutrient that can be manufactured in the body by means of other nutrients. Thus, it is not essential to consume regularly in the diet.

nursing diagnosis clinical judgment about individual, family, or community experiences/responses to actual or potential health problems/life processes. Nursing diagnoses provide the basis for selection of nursing interventions to achieve outcomes for which the nurse has accountability.

nursing process the means by which nurses deliver care to patients; it includes the following steps: assessment, diagnosis, planning, implementation, and evaluation.

nutrition the sum of the processes involved with the intake of nutrients as well as assimilating and using them to maintain body tissue and provide energy; a foundation for life and health.

nutrition care process model a systematic approach to providing individualized nutrition care. The model consists of the following steps: assessment, diagnosis, intervention, and monitoring and evaluation.

nutrition integrity a level of performance that ensures all foods and beverages available in schools are consistent with the *Dietary Guidelines for Americans,* and, when combined with nutrition education, physical activity, and a healthful school environment; contributes to enhanced learning and development of lifelong, healthful eating habits.

nutrition science the body of science, developed through controlled research, that relates to the processes involved in nutrition internationally, clinically, and in the community.

O

oliguria the secretion of small amounts of urine in relation to fluid intake (i.e., 0.5 mL/kg per hour or less).

One-Step diagnosis A method for diagnosing diabetes using a 75-gram oral glucose tolerance test. The patient's fasting plasma glucose level is measured, then the patient drinks a solution with 75 mg of glucose and plasma glucose level is measured again at 1 hr and 2 hr post consumption. Diagnostic criteria are based on the levels of plasma glucose at each measurement.

organic farming the use of farming methods that employ natural means of pest control and that meet the standards set by the National Organic Program of the U.S. Department of Agriculture; organic foods are grown or produced without the use of synthetic pesticides or fertilizers, sewage sludge, genetically modified organisms, or ionizing radiation.

osmosis the passage of a solvent (e.g., water) through a membrane that separates solutions of different concentrations and that tends to equalize the concentration pressures of the solutions on either side of the membrane.

osmotic pressure hydrostatic pressure across a semipermeable membrane that is necessary to maintain the normal movement of fluid between the capillaries and the surrounding tissue.

osteoblast cells that are responsible for the mineralization and formation of bone.

osteodystrophy an alteration of bone morphology found in patients with chronic kidney disease.

osteopenia a condition that involves a low bone mass and an increased risk for fracture.

osteoporosis an abnormal thinning of the bone that produces a porous, fragile, lattice-like bone tissue of enlarged spaces that are prone to fracture or deformity.

outbreak of food-borne illness the occurrence of two or more similar illnesses resulting from ingestion of a common food.

oxytocin hormone released from the posterior pituitary gland that stimulates milk let-down.

P

pancreatic amylase a major starch-splitting enzyme that is secreted by the pancreas and that acts in the small intestine.

pancreatic lipase a major fat-splitting enzyme produced by the pancreas and secreted into the small intestine to digest fat.

pandemic a widespread epidemic distributed throughout a region, a continent, or the world.

pantothenic acid a B-complex vitamin that is found widely distributed in nature and that occurs throughout the body tissues; it is an essential constituent of the body's main activating agent, coenzyme A.

parasite an organism that lives in or on an organism of another species, known as the *host,* from whom all nourishment is obtained.

parenteral a mode of feeding that does not make use of the gastrointestinal tract but that instead provides nutrition support via the intravenous delivery of nutrient solutions.

parotid glands the largest of the three pairs of salivary glands; the parotid glands lie, one on each side, above the angle of the jaw and below and in front of the ear; they continually secrete saliva, which passes along the duct of the gland and into the mouth through an opening in the inner cheek that is level with the second upper molar tooth.

pellagra the deficiency disease caused by a lack of dietary niacin and an inadequate amount of protein that contains the amino acid tryptophan, which is a precursor of niacin; pellagra is characterized by skin lesions that are aggravated by sunlight as well as by gastrointestinal, mucosal, neurologic, and mental symptoms.

pepsin the main gastric enzyme specific to proteins; it begins breaking large protein molecules into shorter-chain polypeptides; gastric hydrochloric acid is necessary for its activation.

peritoneal cavity a serous membrane that lines the abdominal and pelvic walls and the undersurface of the diaphragm to form a sac that encloses the body's vital visceral organs.

pernicious anemia a form of megaloblastic anemia that is caused by destroyed gastric parietal cells that produce intrinsic factor; without intrinsic factor, vitamin B_{12} cannot be absorbed.

pharynx the muscular membranous passage that extends from the mouth to the posterior nasal passages, the larynx, and the esophagus.

pheochromocytoma a tumor of the adrenal medulla or the sympathetic nervous system in which the affected cells secrete excess epinephrine or norepinephrine and cause headache, hypertension, and nausea.

photosynthesis the process by which plants that contain chlorophyll are able to manufacture carbohydrate by combining carbon dioxide and water; sunlight is used as energy, and chlorophyll is a catalyst.

phylloquinone a fat-soluble vitamin of the K group that is found primarily in green plants.

plaque thick wax-like coating forming inside artery walls; primarily composed of cholesterol, fatty substances, cellular debris, calcium, and fibrin.

plasma protein any of a number of protein substances that are carried in the circulating blood; a major one is *albumin*, which maintains the fluid volume of the blood through colloidal osmotic pressure.

polarity the interaction between the positively charged end of one molecule and the negative end of another (or the same) molecule.

polydipsia excessive thirst and drinking.

polymeric formula a nutrition support formula that is composed of complete protein, polysaccharides, and fat as medium-chain fatty acids.

polypharmacy the use of multiple medications by the same patient.

polyuria excessive urination.

portal an entrance or gateway; for example, the portal blood circulation designates the entry of blood vessels from the intestines into the liver; it carries nutrients for liver metabolism, and it then drains into the body's main systemic circulation to deliver metabolic products to body cells.

portal hypertension high blood pressure in the portal vein.

postprandial after eating.

prebiotic nondigestible foods that promote the growth of beneficial microorganisms within the gut.

pregnancy-induced hypertension the development of hypertension during pregnancy after the twentieth week of gestation.

primary deficiency deficiency of a nutrient due to inadequate dietary intake. Different from secondary causes where the deficiency is due to malabsorption or other bioavailability hindrances.

probiotic a food that contains live microbials, which are thought to benefit the consumer by improving intestinal microbial balance (e.g., lactobacilli in yogurt).

proenzyme an inactive precursor (i.e., a forerunner substance from which another substance is made) that is converted to the active enzyme by the action of an acid, another enzyme, or other means.

prohormone a precursor substance that the body converts to a hormone; for example, a cholesterol compound in the skin is first irradiated by sunlight and then converted through successive enzyme actions in the liver and kidney into the active vitamin D hormone, which then regulates calcium absorption and bone development.

prolactin hormone released from the anterior pituitary gland that stimulates milk production.

proteinuria an abnormal excess of serum proteins (e.g., albumin) in the urine.

pulmonary edema an accumulation of fluid in the lung tissues.

pyridoxine the chemical name of vitamin B_6; in its activated phosphate form (i.e., B_2PO_4), pyridoxine functions as an important coenzyme factor in many reactions in cell metabolism that are related to amino acids, glucose, and fatty acids.

R

Ramadan the ninth month of the Muslim year, which is a period of daily fasting from sunrise to sunset.

Recommended Dietary Allowances (RDAs) the average daily dietary intake level that is sufficient to meet the nutrient requirement of nearly all healthy individuals in a group.

refeeding syndrome a potentially lethal condition that occurs when severely malnourished individuals are fed high-carbohydrate diets too aggressively; a sudden shift in electrolytes and fluid retention and a drastic drop in serum phosphorus levels cause a series of complications that involves several organs.

registered dietitian (RD) a professional dietitian accredited with an academic degree from an undergraduate or graduate study program who has passed required registration examinations administered by the Commission on Dietetic Registration (CDR). The RD and RDN (registered dietitian nutritionists) credentials are legally protected titles that may only be used by practitioners authorized by the CDR. The term *nutritionist* alone is not a legally protected title in most states and may be used by virtually anyone. See *www.eatright. org* for more details.

renin an enzyme released from the kidney because of hypovolemia; it converts angiotensinogen to angiotensin I.

rennin the milk-curdling enzyme of the gastric juice of human infants and young animals (e.g., calves); rennin should not be confused with renin, which is an important enzyme produced by the kidneys that plays a vital role in the activation of angiotensin.

resistant hypertension the presence of high blood pressure despite treatment with three antihypertensive medications.

resorption the destruction, loss, or dissolution of a tissue or a part of a tissue by biochemical activity (e.g., the loss of bone, the loss of tooth dentin).

resting energy expenditure (REE) the amount of energy (in kcal) needed by the body for the maintenance of life at rest over a 24-hour period; this is often used interchangeably with the term *basal energy expenditure,* but in actuality it is slightly higher because the protocol for measurement does not put the person at complete rest. Also referred to as resting metabolic rate (RMR).

retinol the chemical name of vitamin A; the name is derived from the vitamin's visual functions related to the retina of the eye, which is the back inner lining of the eyeball that catches the light refractions of the lens to form images that are interpreted by the optic nerve and the brain and that makes the necessary light-dark adaptations.

riboflavin the chemical name for vitamin B_2; it has a role as a coenzyme factor in many cell reactions related to energy and protein metabolism.

rickets a disease of childhood that is characterized by the softening of the bones from an inadequate intake of vitamin D and insufficient exposure to sunlight; it is also associated with impaired calcium and phosphorus metabolism.

rooting reflex reflex that occurs when an infant's cheek is stroked or touched. The infant will turn toward the stimuli and make sucking (or rooting) motions in an effort to nurse.

S

saccharide the chemical name for sugar molecules; may occur as single molecules in monosaccharides (glucose, fructose, galactose), two molecules in disaccharides (sucrose, lactose, maltose), or multiple molecules in polysaccharides (starch, dietary fiber, glycogen).

salivary amylase a starch-splitting enzyme that is secreted by the salivary glands in the mouth and that is commonly called *ptyalin* (from the Greek word *ptyalon,* meaning "spittle").

sarcopenia loss of lean tissue mass associated with aging.

saturated the state of being filled; the state of fatty acid components being filled in all their available carbon bonds with hydrogen, thus making the fat harder and more solid at room temperature; such solid food fats are generally from animal sources.

school breakfast and lunch programs federally assisted meal programs that operate in public and nonprofit private schools and residential child-care institutions; these programs provide nutritionally balanced, low-cost, or free meals to children each school day.

screen time time spent in front of any electronic screen— television, computer, phone, DVD players, portable gaming devices, etc.

scurvy a hemorrhagic disease caused by a lack of vitamin C that is characterized by diffuse tissue bleeding, painful limbs and joints, thickened bones, and skin discoloration from bleeding; bones fracture easily, wounds do not heal, gums swell and tend to bleed, and the teeth loosen.

secondary hypertension an elevated blood pressure for which the cause can be identified and which is a symptom or side effect of another primary condition.

secretin hormone that stimulates gastric and pancreatic secretions. Secretin secretion is increased in response to a low pH in the duodenum. Secretin stimulates the pancreatic release of bicarbonate to increase the pH to an alkaline environment. Secretin also stimulates the secretion of pepsinogen from the chief cells of the stomach.

senescence the process or condition of growing old.

simple carbohydrates sugars with a simple structure of one or two single-sugar (saccharide) units; a monosaccharide is composed of one sugar unit, and a disaccharide is composed of two sugar units.

small for gestational age (SGA) infant is smaller than a gender and gestational age matched infant. Birth weight is below the 10th percentile.

sorbitol a sugar alcohol that is often used as a nutritive sugar substitute; it is named for where it was discovered in nature, in ripe berries of the *Sorbus aucuparia* tree; it also occurs naturally in small quantities in various other berries, cherries, plums, and pears.

speech-language pathologist a specialist in the assessment, diagnosis, treatment, and prevention of speech, language, cognitive communication, voice, swallowing, fluency, and other related disorders.

spina bifida a congenital defect in the embryonic fetal closing of the neural tube to form a portion of the lower spine, which leaves the spine unclosed and the spinal cord open to various degrees of exposure and damage.

state land grant universities an institution of higher education that has been designated by the state to receive unique federal support as a result of the Morrill Acts of 1862 and 1890.

steatorrhea fatty diarrhea; excessive amount of fat in the feces, which is often caused by malabsorption diseases.

steatosis accumulation of fat in the liver cells.

stillbirth the death of a fetus after the twentieth week of pregnancy.

stoma the opening that is established in the abdominal wall that connects with the ileum or the colon for the elimination of intestinal wastes after the surgical removal of nonfunctional portions of the intestines.

sugar alcohols nutritive sweeteners that provide 2 to 3 kcal/g; examples include sorbitol, mannitol, and xylitol; these are produced in food-industry laboratories for use as sweeteners in candies, chewing gum, beverages, and other foods.

supersaturation (pertaining to urine) excess concentration of solutes.

T

teratogen a substance or factor resulting in birth defects or miscarriage of an embryo or fetus.

teratogenic causing a birth defect.

Therapeutic Lifestyle Changes (TLC) an intensive lifestyle intervention that is focused on appropriate weight, diet, physical activity, and other controllable risk factors to reduce cholesterol levels and to prevent other complications of heart disease.

thermic effect of food an increase in energy expenditure caused by the activities of digestion, absorption, transport, and metabolism of ingested food; a meal that consists of a usual mixture of carbohydrates, protein, and fat increases the energy expenditure equivalent to approximately 10% of the food's energy content (e.g., a 300-kcal piece of pizza would elicit an energy expenditure of 30 kcal to digest the food).

thiamin the chemical name of vitamin B_1; this vitamin was discovered in relation to the classic deficiency disease beriberi, and it is important in body metabolism as a coenzyme factor in many cell reactions related to energy metabolism.

thyroid-stimulating hormone (TSH) hormone released from the pituitary gland that stimulates the thyroid gland to produce thyroxine (T_4) and triiodothyronine (T_3).

thyrotropin-releasing hormone (TRH) a hormone that is produced by the hypothalamus and that stimulates the release of thyroid-stimulating hormone by the pituitary.

thyroxine (T_4) an iodine-dependent thyroid prohormone; the active hormone form is T_3; it is the major controller of basal metabolic rate.

tocopherol the chemical name for vitamin E, which was named by early investigators because their initial work with rats indicated a reproductive function (Greek translation=child bearing); in people, vitamin E functions as a strong antioxidant that preserves structural membranes such as cell walls.

Total Diet Study FDA program beginning in 1961 that evaluates the levels of nutrients and contaminants in foods.

trace minerals the group of elements that are required by the body in amounts of less than 100 mg/day.

transferrin a protein that binds and transports iron through the blood.

transport (in terms of nutrition and metabolism) the movement of nutrients through the circulatory system from one area of the body to another.

triglycerides the chemical name for fats in the body or in food; three fatty acids attached to a glycerol base.

trypsin a protein-splitting enzyme secreted as the inactive proenzyme trypsinogen by the pancreas and that is activated by enterokinase; works in the small intestine to reduce proteins to shorter-chain polypeptides and dipeptides.

Two-Step diagnosis A method for diagnosing diabetes using a two-step method of oral glucose tolerance test in a non-fasting patient. Step 1: The patient drinks a 50-g glucose solution and plasma glucose is measured at 1 hr post consumption. If the patient's plasma glucose level is ≥140 g/dL then the patient must return for Step 2, which is a fasting 100-g glucose tolerance test.

U

ultrasonography an ultrasound-based diagnostic imaging technique that is used to visualize the muscles and internal organs; also referred to as *sonography.*

unintentional weight loss weight loss of 5% of body weight over a 6- to 12-month period that is not intentional.

urea the chief nitrogen-carrying product of dietary protein metabolism; urea appears in the blood, lymph, and urine.

V

vagotomy the cutting of the vagus nerve, which supplies a major stimulus for gastric secretions.

vasculitis the inflammation of the walls of blood vessels.

vasopressin a hormone of the pituitary gland that acts on the distal nephron tubule to conserve water by reabsorption; also known as *antidiuretic hormone.*

villi small protrusions from the surface of a membrane; finger-like projections that cover the mucosal surfaces of the small intestine and that further increase the absorbing surface area; they are visible through a regular microscope.

VO$_2$max the maximal uptake volume of oxygen during exercise; this is used to measure the intensity and duration of exercise that a person can perform.

W

waist circumference the measurement of the waist at its narrowest point width-wise, just above the navel; waist circumference is a rough measurement of abdominal fat and a predictor of risk factors for cardiovascular disease; this risk factor increases with a waist measurement of more than 40 inches in men and of more than 35 inches in women.

weaning the process of gradually acclimating a young child to food other than the mother's milk or a breast milk substitute as the child's natural need to suckle wanes.

Wilson's disease an autosomal recessive genetic disorder in which copper accumulates in tissue and causes damage to organs.

X

xerostomia the condition of dry mouth that results from a lack of saliva; saliva production can be hindered by certain diseases (e.g., diabetes, Parkinson's disease) and by some prescription and over-the-counter medications.

Z

zymogen an inactive enzyme precursor.

appendix

A

Answers to Chapter Review Questions

Chapter 1: Food, Nutrition, and Health
1. a
2. a
3. b
4. d
5. a

Chapter 2: Carbohydrates
1. a
2. c
3. b
4. c
5. b

Chapter 3: Fats
1. a
2. b
3. b
4. b
5. c

Chapter 4: Proteins
1. d
2. b
3. c
4. a
5. b

Chapter 5: Digestion, Absorption, and Metabolism
1. c
2. a
3. b
4. a
5. c

Chapter 6: Energy Balance
1. d
2. c
3. b
4. b
5. c

Chapter 7: Vitamins
1. b
2. a
3. a
4. a
5. d

Chapter 8: Minerals
1. a
2. c
3. b
4. d
5. a

Chapter 9: Water and Electrolyte Balance
1. c
2. d
3. a
4. b
5. a

Chapter 10: Nutrition during Pregnancy and Lactation
1. a
2. a
3. c
4. b
5. c

Chapter 11: Nutrition during Infancy, Childhood, and Adolescence
1. d
2. b
3. b
4. b
5. c

Chapter 12: Nutrition for Adults: The Early, Middle, and Later Years
1. b
2. d
3. b
4. b
5. c

Chapter 13: Community Food Supply and Health
1. d
2. a
3. a
4. c
5. b

Chapter 14: Food Habits and Cultural Patterns
1. a
2. b
3. a
4. c
5. d

Chapter 15: Weight Management
1. c
2. b
3. a
4. b
5. c

Chapter 16: Nutrition and Physical Fitness
1. c
2. b
3. b
4. c
5. a

Chapter 17: Nutrition Care
1. a
2. c
3. c
4. a
5. b

Chapter 18: Gastrointestinal and Accessory Organ Problems
1. b
2. b
3. c
4. d
5. a

Chapter 19: Coronary Heart Disease and Hypertension
1. d
2. c
3. a
4. a
5. c

Chapter 20: Diabetes Mellitus
1. b
2. b
3. a
4. c
5. c

Chapter 21: Kidney Disease
1. b
2. b
3. a
4. d
5. a

Chapter 22: Surgery and Nutrition Support
1. d
2. a
3. a
4. c
5. a

Chapter 23: Nutrition Support in Cancer and HIV
1. c
2. b
3. a
4. c
5. b

Dietary Reference Intake (DRI)

Dietary Reference Intakes (DRIs): Recommended Dietary Allowances and Adequate Intakes, Vitamins*; Food and Nutrition Board, Institute of Medicine, National Academies

LIFE STAGE GROUP	VITAMIN A (mcg/d)[a]	VITAMIN C (mg/d)	VITAMIN D (IU/d)[b,c]	VITAMIN E (mg/d)[d]	VITAMIN K (mcg/d)	THIAMIN (mg/d)	RIBOFLAVIN (mg/d)	NIACIN (mg/d)[e]	VITAMIN B$_6$ (mg/d)	FOLATE (mcg/d)[f]	VITAMIN B$_{12}$ (mcg/d)	PANTOTHENIC Acid (mg/d)	BIOTIN (mcg/d)	CHOLINE (mg/d)[g]
Infants														
Birth to 6 mo	400*	40*	400	4*	2.0*	0.2*	0.3*	2*	0.1*	65*	0.4*	1.7*	5*	125*
6 to 12 mo	500*	50*	400	5*	2.5*	0.3*	0.4*	4*	0.3*	80*	0.5*	1.8*	6*	150*
Children														
1-3 yr	300	15	600	6	30*	0.5	0.5	6	0.5	150	0.9	2*	8*	200*
4-8 yr	400	25	600	7	55*	0.6	0.6	8	0.6	200	1.2	3*	12*	250*
Males														
9-13 yr	600	45	600	11	60*	0.9	0.9	12	1.0	300	1.8	4*	20*	375*
14-18 yr	900	75	600	15	75*	1.2	1.3	16	1.3	400	2.4	5*	25*	550*
19-30 yr	900	90	600	15	120*	1.2	1.3	16	1.3	400	2.4	5*	30*	550*
31-50 yr	900	90	600	15	120*	1.2	1.3	16	1.3	400	2.4	5*	30*	550*
51-70 yr	900	90	600	15	120*	1.2	1.3	16	1.7	400	2.4[h]	5*	30*	550*
>70 yr	900	90	800	15	120*	1.2	1.3	16	1.7	400	2.4[h]	5*	30*	550*
Females														
9-13 yr	600	45	600	11	60*	0.9	0.9	12	1.0	300	1.8	4*	20*	375*
14-18 yr	700	65	600	15	75*	1.0	1.0	14	1.2	400[i]	2.4	5*	25*	400*
19-30 yr	700	75	600	15	90*	1.1	1.1	14	1.3	400[i]	2.4	5*	30*	425*
31-50 yr	700	75	600	15	90*	1.1	1.1	14	1.3	400[i]	2.4	5*	30*	425*
51-70 yr	700	75	600	15	90*	1.1	1.1	14	1.5	400	2.4[h]	5*	30*	425*
>70 yr	700	75	800	15	90*	1.1	1.1	14	1.5	400	2.4[h]	5*	30*	425*

Life Stage Group													
Pregnancy													
14-18 yr	750	80	600	15	75*	1.4	1.4	18	1.9	600	2.6	6*	30*	450*
19-30 yr	770	85	600	15	90*	1.4	1.4	18	1.9	600	2.6	6*	30*	450*
31-50 yr	770	85	600	15	90*	1.4	1.4	18	1.9	600	2.6	6*	30*	450*
Lactation													
14-18 yr	1200	115	600	19	75*	1.4	1.6	17	2.0	500	2.8	7*	35*	550*
19-30 yr	1300	120	600	19	90*	1.4	1.6	17	2.0	500	2.8	7*	35*	550*
31-50 yr	1300	120	600	19	90*	1.4	1.6	17	2.0	500	2.8	7*	35*	550*

Sources: Dietary Reference Intakes for Calcium, Phosphorus, Magnesium, Vitamin D, and Fluoride (1997); Dietary Reference Intakes for Thiamin, Riboflavin, Niacin, Vitamin B_6, Folate, Vitamin B_{12}, Pantothenic Acid, Biotin, and Choline (1998); Dietary Reference Intakes for Vitamin C, Vitamin E, Selenium, and Carotenoids (2000); Dietary Reference Intakes for Vitamin A, Vitamin K, Arsenic, Boron, Chromium, Copper, Iodine, Iron, Manganese, Molybdenum, Nickel, Silicon, Vanadium, and Zinc (2001); Dietary Reference Intakes for Water, Potassium, Sodium, Chloride, and Sulfate (2005); and Dietary Reference Intakes for Calcium and Vitamin D (2011). These reports may be accessed via www.nap.edu.

NOTE: This table (taken from the DRI reports, see www.nap.edu) presents Recommended Dietary Allowances (RDAs) in **boldface type** and Adequate Intakes (AIs) in lightface type followed by an asterisk (*). An RDA is the average daily dietary intake level; sufficient to meet the nutrient requirements of nearly all (97%-98%) healthy individuals in a group. It is calculated from an Estimated Average Requirement (EAR). If sufficient scientific evidence is not available to establish an EAR, and thus calculate an RDA, an AI is usually developed. For healthy breastfed infants, an AI is the mean intake. The AI for other life stage and gender groups is believed to cover the needs of all healthy individuals in the groups, but lack of data or uncertainty in the data prevent being able to specify with confidence of the percentage of individuals covered by this intake.

aAs retinol activity equivalents (RAEs). 1 RAE = 1 mcg of retinol, 12 mcg of β-carotene, 24 mcg of α-carotene, or 24 mcg of β-cryptoxanthin. The RAE for dietary provitamin A carotenoids is twofold greater than retinol equivalents (REs), whereas the RAE for preformed vitamin A is the same as the RE for vitamin A.

bAs cholecalciferol. 1 mcg of cholecalciferol = 40 IU of vitamin D.

cUnder the assumption of minimal sunlight.

dAs α-Tocopherol. α-Tocopherol includes RRR-α-tocopherol, the only form of α-tocopherol that occurs naturally in foods, and the 2R-stereoisomeric forms of α-tocopherol (RRR-, RSR-, RRS-, and RSS-α-tocopherol) that occur in fortified foods and supplements. It does not include the 2S-stereoisomeric forms of α-tocopherol (SRR-, SSR-, SRS-, and SSS-α-tocopherol), also found in fortified foods and supplements.

eAs niacin equivalents (NEs). 1 mg of niacin = 60 mg of tryptophan; 0-6 months = preformed niacin (not NE).

fAs dietary folate equivalents (DFEs). 1 DFE = 1 mcg of food folate = 0.6 mcg of folic acid from fortified food or as a supplement consumed with food = 0.5 mcg of a supplement taken on an empty stomach.

gAlthough AIs have been established for choline, there are few data to assess whether a dietary supply of choline is needed at all stages of the life cycle, and it may be that the choline requirement can be met by endogenous synthesis at some of these stages.

hBecause 10% to 30% of older people may malabsorb food-bound B_{12}, it is advisable for those older than 50 years to meet their RDA mainly by consuming foods fortified with B_{12} or a supplement containing B_{12}.

iIn view of evidence linking folate intake with neural tube defects in the fetus, it is recommended that all women capable of becoming pregnant consume 400 mcg from supplements or fortified foods in addition to intake of food folate from a varied diet.

jIt is assumed that women will continue consuming 400 mcg from supplements or fortified food until their pregnancy is confirmed and they enter prenatal care, which ordinarily occurs after the end of the periconceptional period—the critical time for formation of the neural tube.

Dietary Reference Intakes (DRIs): Recommended Dietary Allowances and Adequate Intakes, Minerals; Food and Nutrition Board, Institute of Medicine, National Academies

Life Stage Group	Calcium (mg/d)	Chromium (mcg/d)	Copper (mcg/d)	Fluoride (mg/d)	Iodine (mcg/d)	Iron (mg/d)	Magnesium (mg/d)	Manganese (mg/d)	Molybdenum (mcg/d)	Phosphorus (mg/d)	Selenium (mcg/d)	Zinc (mg/d)	Potassium (g/d)	Sodium (g/d)	Chloride (g/d)
Infants															
Birth to 6 mo	200*	0.2*	200*	0.01*	110*	0.27*	30*	0.003*	2*	100*	15*	2*	0.4*	0.12*	0.18*
6 to 12 mo	260*	5.5*	220*	0.5*	130*	11	75*	0.6*	3*	275*	20*	3	0.7*	0.37*	0.57*
Children															
1-3 yr	700	11*	340	0.7*	90	7	80	1.2*	17	460	20	3	3.0*	1.0*	1.5*
4-8 yr	1000	15*	440	1*	90	10	130	1.5*	22	500	30	5	3.8*	1.2*	1.9*
Males															
9-13 yr	1300	25*	700	2*	120	8	240	1.9*	34	1250	40	8	4.5*	1.5*	2.3*
14-18 yr	1300	35*	890	3*	150	11	410	2.2*	43	1250	55	11	4.7*	1.5*	2.3*
19-30 yr	1000	35*	900	4*	150	8	400	2.3*	45	700	55	11	4.7*	1.5*	2.3*
31-50 yr	1000	35*	900	4*	150	8	420	2.3*	45	700	55	11	4.7*	1.5*	2.3*
51-70 yr	1000	30*	900	4*	150	8	420	2.3*	45	700	55	11	4.7*	1.3*	2.0*
>70 yr	1200	30*	900	4*	150	8	420	2.3*	45	700	55	11	4.7*	1.2*	1.8*
Females															
9-13 yr	1300	21*	700	2*	120	8	240	1.6*	34	1250	40	8	4.5*	1.5*	2.3*
14-18 yr	1300	24*	890	3*	150	15	360	1.6*	43	1250	55	9	4.7*	1.5*	2.3*
19-30 yr	1000	25*	900	3*	150	18	310	1.8*	45	700	55	8	4.7*	1.5*	2.3*
31-50 yr	1000	25*	900	3*	150	18	320	1.8*	45	700	55	8	4.7*	1.5*	2.3*
51-70 yr	1200	20*	900	3*	150	8	320	1.8*	45	700	55	8	4.7*	1.3*	2.0*
>70 yr	1200	20*	900	3*	150	8	320	1.8*	45	700	55	8	4.7*	1.2*	1.8*
Pregnancy															
14-18 yr	1300	29*	1000	3*	220	27	400	2.0*	50	1250	60	12	4.7*	1.5*	2.3*
19-30 yr	1000	30*	1000	3*	220	27	350	2.0*	50	700	60	11	4.7*	1.5*	2.3*
31-50 yr	1000	30*	1000	3*	220	27	360	2.0*	50	700	60	11	4.7*	1.5*	2.3*
Lactation															
14-18 yr	1300	44*	1300	3*	290	10	360	2.6*	50	1250	70	13	5.1*	1.5*	2.3*
19-30 yr	1000	45*	1300	3*	290	9	310	2.6*	50	700	70	12	5.1*	1.5*	2.3*
31-50 yr	1000	45*	1300	3*	290	9	320	2.6*	50	700	70	12	5.1*	1.5*	2.3*

Sources: Dietary Reference Intakes for Calcium, Phosphorus, Magnesium, Vitamin D, and Fluoride (1997); Dietary Reference Intakes for Thiamin, Riboflavin, Niacin, Vitamin B₆, Folate, Vitamin B₁₂, Pantothenic Acid, Biotin, and Choline (1998); Dietary Reference Intakes for Vitamin C, Vitamin E, Selenium, and Carotenoids (2000); and Dietary Reference Intakes for Vitamin A, Vitamin K, Arsenic, Boron, Chromium, Copper, Iodine, Iron, Manganese, Molybdenum, Nickel, Silicon, Vanadium, and Zinc (2001); Dietary Reference Intakes for Water, Potassium, Sodium, Chloride, and Sulfate (2005); and Dietary Reference Intakes for Calcium and Vitamin D (2011). These reports may be accessed via www.nap.edu.

NOTE: This table (taken from the DRI reports, see www.nap.edu) presents Recommended Dietary Allowances (RDAs) in **boldface type** and Adequate Intakes (AIs) in lightface type followed by an asterisk (*). An RDA is the average daily dietary intake level; sufficient to meet the nutrient requirements of nearly all (97-98%) healthy individuals in a group. It is calculated from an Estimated Average Requirement (EAR). If sufficient scientific evidence is not available to establish an EAR, and thus calculate an RDA, an AI is usually developed. For healthy breastfed infants, an AI is the mean intake. The AI for other life stage and gender groups is believed to cover the needs of all healthy individuals in the groups, but lack of data or uncertainty in the data prevent being able to specify with confidence of the percentage of individuals covered by this intake.

Dietary Reference Intake of Energy from Birth to 18 Years of Age Per Day*

	AGE	ESTIMATED ENERGY REQUIREMENT
Infants	0 to 3 months	(89 × Weight [kg] − 100) + 175 kcal
	4 to 6 months	(89 × Weight [kg] − 100) + 56 kcal
	7 to 12 months	(89 × Weight [kg] − 100) + 22 kcal
	13 to 36 months	(89 × Weight [kg] − 100) + 20 kcal
Boys	3 to 8 years	88.5 − (61.9 × Age [yr]) + PA × (26.7 × Weight [kg] + 903 × Height [m]) + 20 kcal
	9 to 18 years	88.5 − (61.9 × Age [yr]) + PA × (26.7 × Weight [kg] + 903 × Height [m]) + 25 kcal
Girls	3 to 8 years	135.3 − (30.8 × Age [yr]) + PA × (10.0 × Weight [kg] + 934 × Height [m]) + 20 kcal
	9 to 18 years	135.3 − (30.8 × Age [yr]) + PA × (10.0 × Weight [kg] + 934 × Height [m]) + 25 kcal

*PA, Physical activity level. Data from the Food and Nutrition Board, Institute of Medicine. *Dietary reference intakes for energy, carbohydrate, fiber, fat, fatty acids, cholesterol, protein, and amino acids (macronutrients).* Washington, DC: National Academies Press; 2002.

Dietary Reference Intakes (DRIs): Recommended Dietary Allowances and Adequate Intakes, Total Water, Fiber, Essential Fatty Acids, and Protein;* Food and Nutrition Board, Institute of Medicine, National Academies

LIFE STAGE GROUP	TOTAL WATER[a] (L/d)	TOTAL FIBER (g/d)	LINOLEIC ACID (g/d)	α-LINOLENIC ACID (g/d)	PROTEIN[b] (g/d)
Infants					
Birth to 6 mo	0.7*	ND	4.4*	0.5*	9.1*
6 to 12 mo	0.8*	ND	4.6*	0.5*	**11.0**
Children					
1-3 yr	1.3*	19*	7*	0.7*	**13**
4-8 yr	1.7*	25*	10*	0.9*	**19**
Males					
9-13 yr	2.4*	31*	12*	1.2*	**34**
14-18 yr	3.3*	38*	16*	1.6*	**52**
19-30 yr	3.7*	38*	17*	1.6*	**56**
31-50 yr	3.7*	38*	17*	1.6*	**56**
51-70 yr	3.7*	30*	14*	1.6*	**56**
>70 yr	3.7*	30*	14*	1.6*	**56**
Females					
9-13 yr	2.1*	26*	10*	1.0*	**34**
14-18 yr	2.3*	26*	11*	1.1*	**46**
19-30 yr	2.7*	25*	12*	1.1*	**46**
31-50 yr	2.7*	25*	12*	1.1*	**46**
51-70 yr	2.7*	21*	11*	1.1*	**46**
>70 yr	2.7*	21*	11*	1.1*	**46**
Pregnancy					
14-18 yr	3.0*	28*	13*	1.4*	**71**
19-30 yr	3.0*	28*	13*	1.4*	**71**
31-50 yr	3.0*	28*	13*	1.4*	**71**
Lactation					
14-18 yr	3.8*	29*	13*	1.3*	**71**
19-30 yr	3.8*	29*	13*	1.3*	**71**
31-50 yr	3.8*	29*	13*	1.3*	**71**

Source: *Dietary Reference Intakes for Energy, Carbohydrate, Fiber, Fat, Fatty Acids, Cholesterol, Protein, and Amino Acids* (2002/2005) and *Dietary Reference Intakes for Water, Potassium, Sodium, Chloride, and Sulfate* (2005). The report may be accessed via www.nap.edu.
***NOTE:** This table (taken from the DRI reports, see www.nap.edu) presents Recommended Dietary Allowances (RDA) in **boldface type** and Adequate Intakes (AIs) in ordinary type followed by an asterisk (*). An RDA is the average daily dietary intake level; sufficient to meet the nutrient requirements of nearly all (97%-98%) healthy individuals in a group. It is calculated from an Estimated Average Requirement (EAR).
If sufficient scientific evidence is not available to establish an EAR, and thus calculate an RDA, an AI is usually developed. For healthy breastfed infants, an AI is the mean intake. The AI for other life stage and gender groups is believed to cover the needs of all healthy individuals in the groups, but lack of data or uncertainty in the data prevent being able to specify with confidence the percentage of individuals covered by this intake.
[a]Total water includes all water contained in food, beverages, and drinking water.
[b]Based on grams of protein per kilogram of body weight for the reference body weight (e.g., for adults 0.8 g/kg body weight for the reference body weight).

Dietary Reference Intakes (DRIs): Acceptable Macronutrient Distribution Ranges; Food and Nutrition Board, Institute of Medicine, National Academies

MACRONUTRIENT	RANGE (PERCENT OF ENERGY)		
	CHILDREN, 1-3 yr	CHILDREN, 4-18 yr	ADULTS
Fat	30-40	25-35	20-35
n-6 polyunsaturated fatty acids[a] (linoleic acid)	5-10	5-10	5-10
n-3 polyunsaturated fatty acids[a] (α-linolenic acid)	0.6-1.2	0.6-1.2	0.6-1.2
Carbohydrate	45-65	45-65	45-65
Protein	5-20	10-30	10-35

Source: *Dietary Reference Intakes for Energy, Carbohydrate, Fiber, Fat, Fatty Acids, Cholesterol, Protein, and Amino Acids* (2002/2005). The report may be accessed via www.nap.edu.
[a]Approximately 10% of the total can come from longer-chain n-3 or n-6 fatty acids.

Dietary Reference Intakes (DRIs): Acceptable Macronutrient Distribution Ranges; Food and Nutrition Board, Institute of Medicine, National Academies

MACRONUTRIENT	RECOMMENDATION
Dietary cholesterol	As low as possible while consuming a nutritionally adequate diet
Trans fatty acids	As low as possible while consuming a nutritionally adequate diet
Saturated fatty acids	As low as possible while consuming a nutritionally adequate diet
Added sugars[a]	Limit to no more than 25% of total energy

Source: *Dietary Reference Intakes for Energy, Carbohydrate, Fiber, Fat, Fatty Acids, Cholesterol, Protein, and Amino Acids* (2002/2005). The report may be accessed via www.nap.edu.
[a]Not a recommended intake. A daily intake of added sugars that individuals should aim for to achieve a healthful diet was not set.

Dietary Reference Intakes (DRIs): Tolerable Upper Intake Levels, Vitamins; Food and Nutrition Board, Institute of Medicine, National Academies

LIFE STAGE GROUP	VITAMIN A (mcg/d)[a]	VITAMIN C (mg/d)	VITAMIN D (IU/d)	VITAMIN E (mg/d)[b,c]	NIACIN (mg/d)[c]	VITAMIN B$_6$ (mg/d)	FOLATE (mcg/d)[c]	CHOLINE (g/d)	CAROTENOIDS[d]
Infants									
Birth to 6 mo	600	ND[e]	1000	ND	ND	ND	ND	ND	ND
6 to 12 mo	600	ND	1500	ND	ND	ND	ND	ND	ND
Children									
1-3 yr	600	400	2500	200	10	30	300	1.0	ND
4-8 yr	900	650	3000	300	15	40	400	1.0	ND
Males									
9-13 yr	1700	1200	4000	600	20	60	600	2.0	ND
14-18 yr	2800	1800	4000	800	30	80	800	3.0	ND
19-30 yr	3000	2000	4000	1000	35	100	1000	3.5	ND
31-50 yr	3000	2000	4000	1000	35	100	1000	3.5	ND
51-70 yr	3000	2000	4000	1000	35	100	1000	3.5	ND
>70 yr	3000	2000	4000	1000	35	100	1000	3.5	ND
Females									
9-13 yr	1700	1200	4000	600	20	60	600	2.0	ND
14-18 yr	2800	1800	4000	800	30	80	800	3.0	ND
19-30 yr	3000	2000	4000	1000	35	100	1000	3.5	ND
31-50 yr	3000	2000	4000	1000	35	100	1000	3.5	ND
51-70 yr	3000	2000	4000	1000	35	100	1000	3.5	ND
>70 yr	3000	2000	4000	1000	35	100	1000	3.5	ND
Pregnancy									
14-18 yr	2800	1800	4000	800	30	80	800	3.0	ND
19-30 yr	3000	2000	4000	1000	35	100	1000	3.5	ND
31-50 yr	3000	2000	4000	1000	35	100	1000	3.5	ND
Lactation									
14-18 yr	2800	1800	4000	800	30	80	800	3.0	ND
19-30 yr	3000	2000	4000	1000	35	100	1000	3.5	ND
31-50 yr	3000	2000	4000	1000	35	100	1000	3.5	ND

NOTE: A Tolerable Upper Intake Level (UL) is the highest level of daily nutrient intake that is likely to pose no risk of adverse health effects to almost all individuals in the general population. Unless otherwise specified, the UL represents total intake from food, water, and supplements. Due to a lack of suitable data, ULs could not be established for vitamin K, thiamin, riboflavin, vitamin B$_{12}$, pantothenic acid, biotin, and carotenoids. In the absence of a UL, extra caution may be warranted in consuming levels above recommended intakes. Members of the general population should be advised not to routinely exceed the UL. The UL is not meant to apply to individuals who are treated with the nutrient under medical supervision or to individuals with predisposing conditions that modify their sensitivity to the nutrient.

[a]As preformed vitamin A only.

[b]As α-tocopherol; applies to any form of supplemental α-tocopherol.

[c]The ULs for vitamin E, niacin, and folate apply to synthetic forms obtained from supplements, fortified foods, or a combination of the two.

[d]β-Carotene supplements are advised only to serve as a provitamin A source for individuals at risk of vitamin A deficiency.

[e]ND = Not determinable due to lack of data of adverse effects in this age group and concern with regard to lack of ability to handle excess amounts. Source of intake should be from food only to prevent high levels of intake.

SOURCES: *Dietary Reference Intakes for Calcium, Phosphorus, Magnesium, Vitamin D, and Fluoride* (1997); *Dietary Reference Intakes for Thiamin, Riboflavin, Niacin, Vitamin B$_6$, Folate, Vitamin B$_{12}$, Pantothenic Acid, Biotin, and Choline* (1998); *Dietary Reference Intakes for Vitamin C, Vitamin E, Selenium, and Carotenoids* (2000); *Dietary Reference Intakes for Vitamin A, Vitamin K, Arsenic, Boron, Chromium, Copper, Iodine, Iron, Manganese, Molybdenum, Nickel, Silicon, Vanadium, and Zinc* (2001); and *Dietary Reference Intakes for Calcium and Vitamin D* (2011). These reports may be accessed via www.nap.edu.

Dietary Reference Intakes (DRIs): Tolerable Upper Intake Levels, Minerals; Food and Nutrition Board, Institute of Medicine, National Academies

LIFE STAGE GROUP	ARSENIC[a]	BORON (mg/d)	CALCIUM (mg/d)	COPPER (mcg/d)	FLUORIDE (mg/d)	IODINE (mcg/d)	IRON (mg/d)	MAGNESIUM (mg/d)[b]
Infants								
0 to 6 mo	ND[e]	ND	1000	ND	0.7	ND	40	ND
6 to 12 mo	ND	ND	1500	ND	0.9	ND	40	ND
Children								
1-3 yr	ND	3	2500	1000	1.3	200	40	65
4-8 yr	ND	6	2500	3000	2.2	300	40	110
Males								
9-13 yr	ND	11	3000	5000	10	600	40	350
14-18 yr	ND	17	3000	8000	10	900	45	350
19-30 yr	ND	20	2500	10000	10	1100	45	350
31-50 yr	ND	20	2500	10000	10	1100	45	350
51-70 yr	ND	20	2000	10000	10	1100	45	350
>70 yr	ND	20	2000	10000	10	1100	45	350
Females								
9-13 yr	ND	11	3000	5000	10	600	40	350
14-18 yr	ND	17	3000	8000	10	900	45	350
19-30 yr	ND	20	2500	10000	10	1100	45	350
31-50 yr	ND	20	2500	10000	10	1100	45	350
51-70 yr	ND	20	2000	10000	10	1100	45	350
>70 yr	ND	20	2000	10000	10	1100	45	350
Pregnancy								
14-18 yr	ND	17	3000	8000	10	900	45	350
19-30 yr	ND	20	2500	10000	10	1100	45	350
61-50 yr	ND	20	2500	10000	10	1100	45	350
Lactation								
14-18 yr	ND	17	3000	8000	10	900	45	350
19-30 yr	ND	20	2500	10000	10	1100	45	350
31-50 yr	ND	20	2500	10000	10	1100	45	350

NOTE: A Tolerable Upper Intake Level (UL) is the highest level of daily nutrient intake that is likely to pose no risk of adverse health effects to almost all individuals in the general population. Unless otherwise specified, the UL represents total intake from food, water, and supplements. Due to a lack of suitable data, ULs could not be established for all minerals. In the absence of a UL, extra caution may be warranted in consuming levels above recommended intakes. Members of the general population should be advised not to routinely exceed the UL. The UL is not meant to apply to individuals who are treated with the nutrient under medical supervision or to individuals with predisposing conditions that modify their sensitivity to the nutrient.

[a]Although the UL was not determined for arsenic, there is no justification for adding arsenic to food or supplements.

[b]The ULs for magnesium represent intake from a pharmacologic agent only and do not include intake from food and water.

[c]Although silicon has not been shown to cause adverse effects in humans, there is no justification for adding silicon to supplements.

[d]Although vanadium in food has not been shown to cause adverse effects in humans, there is no justification for adding vanadium to food and vanadium supplements should be used with caution. The UL is based on adverse effects in laboratory animals and this data could be used to set a UL for adults but not children and adolescents.

[e]ND = Not determinable due to lack of data of adverse effects in this age group and concern with regard to lack of ability to handle excess amounts. Source of intake should be from food only to prevent high levels of intake.

SOURCES: *Dietary Reference Intakes for Calcium, Phosphorus, Magnesium, Vitamin D, and Fluoride* (1997); *Dietary Reference Intakes for Thiamin, Riboflavin, Niacin, Vitamin B$_6$, Folate, Vitamin B$_{12}$, Pantothenic Acid, Biotin, and Choline* (1998); *Dietary Reference Intakes for Vitamin C, Vitamin E, Selenium, and Carotenoids* (2000); *Dietary Reference Intakes for Vitamin A, Vitamin K, Arsenic, Boron, Chromium, Copper, Iodine, Iron, Manganese, Molybdenum, Nickel, Silicon, Vanadium, and Zinc* (2001); and *Dietary Reference Intakes for Calcium and Vitamin D* (2011). These reports may be accessed via www.nap.edu.

MANGANESE (mg/d)	MOLYBDENUM (mcg/d)	NICKEL (mg/d)	PHOSPHORUS (g/d)	SELENIUM (mcg/d)	SILICON[c]	VANADIUM (mg/d)[d]	ZINC (mg/d)	SODIUM (g/d)	CHLORIDE (g/d)
ND	ND	ND	ND	45	ND	ND	4	ND	ND
ND	ND	ND	ND	60	ND	ND	5	ND	ND
2	300	0.2	3	90	ND	ND	7	1.5	2.3
3	600	0.3	3	150	ND	ND	12	1.9	2.9
6	1100	0.6	4	280	ND	ND	23	2.2	3.4
9	1700	1.0	4	400	ND	ND	34	2.3	3.6
11	2000	1.0	4	400	ND	1.8	40	2.3	3.6
11	2000	1.0	4	400	ND	1.8	40	2.3	3.6
11	2000	1.0	4	400	ND	1.8	40	2.3	3.6
11	2000	1.0	3	400	ND	1.8	40	2.3	3.6
6	1100	0.6	4	280	ND	ND	23	2.2	3.4
9	1700	1.0	4	400	ND	ND	34	2.3	3.6
11	2000	1.0	4	400	ND	1.8	40	2.3	3.6
11	2000	1.0	4	400	ND	1.8	40	2.3	3.6
11	2000	1.0	4	400	ND	1.8	40	2.3	3.6
11	2000	1.0	3	400	ND	1.8	40	2.3	3.6
9	1700	1.0	3.5	400	ND	ND	34	2.3	3.6
11	2000	1.0	3.5	400	ND	ND	40	2.3	3.6
11	2000	1.0	3.5	400	ND	ND	40	2.3	3.6
9	1700	1.0	4	400	ND	ND	34	2.3	3.6
11	2000	1.0	4	400	ND	ND	40	2.3	3.6
11	2000	1.0	4	400	ND	ND	40	2.3	3.6

FOOD AND DESCRIPTION	SODIUM (mg)	POTASSIUM (mg)
Almonds		
Dried	4	773
Roasted and salted	198	773
Apple Brown Betty	153	100
Apple butter	2	252
Apple juice, canned or bottled	1	101
Apples		
Raw, pared	1	110
Frozen, sliced, sweetened	14	68
Applesauce, canned, sweetened	2	65
Apricot nectar, canned (approximately 40% fruit)	Trace	151
Apricots		
Raw	1	281
Canned, syrup pack, light	1	239
Dried, sulfured, cooked, fruit and liquid	8	318
Asparagus		
Cooked spears, boiled, drained	1	183
Canned spears, green		
Regular pack, solids and liquid	236*	166
Special dietary pack (low sodium), solids and liquid	3	166
Frozen		
Cuts and tips, cooked, boiled, drained	1	220
Spears, cooked, boiled, drained	1	238
Avocados, raw, all commercial varieties	4	604
Bacon, cured, cooked, broiled or fried, drained	1021	236
Bacon, Canadian, cooked, broiled or fried, drained	2555	432
Banana, raw, common	1	370
Barbecue sauce	815	174
Bass, black sea, raw	68	256
Beans, common, mature seeds, dry		
White, cooked	7	416
White, canned, solids and liquid, with pork and tomato sauce	463	210
Red, cooked	3	340
Beans, lima		
Immature seeds		
Cooked, boiled, drained	1	442
Canned		
Regular pack, solids and liquid	236*	222
Special dietary pack (low sodium), solids and liquid	4	222
Frozen, thin-seeded types, commonly called *baby limas*		
Cooked, boiled, drained	129	394
Mature seeds, dry, cooked	2	612

FOOD AND DESCRIPTION	SODIUM (mg)	POTASSIUM (mg)
Beans, mung, sprouted seeds, cooked, boiled, drained	4	156
Beans, snap		
Green		
Cooked, boiled, drained	4	151
Canned		
Regular pack, solids and liquid	236*	95
Special dietary pack (low sodium), solids and liquid	2	95
Frozen, cut, cooked, boiled, drained	1	152
Yellow or wax		
Cooked, boiled, drained	3	151
Canned		
Regular pack, solids and liquid	236*	95
Special dietary pack (low sodium), solids and liquid	2	95
Frozen, cut, cooked, boiled, drained	1	164
Beans and frankfurters, canned	539	262
Beef		
Retail cuts, trimmed to retail level		
Round	60	370
Rump	60	370
Hamburger, regular ground, cooked	47	450
Heart, lean, cooked, braised	104	232
Liver, cooked, fried	184	380
Tongue, medium fat, cooked, braised	61	164
Beef and vegetable stew, canned	411	174
Beef, corned, boneless		
Cooked, medium fat	1740	150
Canned corned beef hash (with potato)	540	200
Beef, dried, cooked, creamed	716	153
Beef potpie, commercial, frozen, unheated	366	93
Beet greens, common, canned, cooked, boiled, drained		
Regular pack, solids and liquid	236*	167
Special dietary pack (low sodium), solids and liquid	46	167
Biscuit dough, commercial, frozen	910	86
Biscuit mix, with enriched flour, and biscuits baked from mix		
Dry form	1300	80
Made with milk	973	116
Biscuits, baking powder, made with enriched flour	626	117
Blackberries, including dewberries, boysenberries, and youngberries, raw	1	170
Blackberries, canned, solids and liquid		
Water pack, with or without artificial sweetener	1	115
Syrup pack, heavy	1	109
Blueberries		
Raw	1	81
Frozen, not thawed, sweetened	1	66
Bluefish, cooked		
Baked or broiled	104	—
Fried	146	—
Bouillon cubes or powder	24,000	100
Boysenberries, frozen, not thawed, sweetened	1	105
Bran, added sugar and malt extract	1060	1070
Bran flakes (40% bran), added thiamin	925	—
Bran flakes with raisins, added thiamin	800	—
Brazil nuts	1	715
Bread crumbs, dry, grated	736	152
Bread stuffing mix and stuffing prepared from mix, dry form	1331	172

FOOD AND DESCRIPTION	SODIUM (mg)	POTASSIUM (mg)
Breads		
Boston brown bread	251	292
Cracked wheat	529	134
French or Vienna, enriched	580	90
Italian, enriched	585	74
Raisin	365	233
Rye	660	166
White enriched, made with 3% to 4% nonfat dry milk	507	105
Whole wheat, made with 2% nonfat dry milk	527	273
Broccoli		
Cooked, spears, boiled, drained	10	267
Frozen, spears, cooked, boiled, drained	12	220
Brussels sprouts, frozen, cooked, boiled, drained	14	295
Buffalo fish, raw	52	293
Bulgur (parboiled wheat), canned, made from hard red winter wheat		
Unseasoned[†]	599	87
Seasoned[‡]	460	112
Butter[§]	987	23
Buttermilk, liquid, cultured (made from skim milk)	130	140
Cabbage		
Common varieties (Danish, domestic, and pointed types)		
Raw	20	233
Cooked, boiled until tender, drained, shredded, cooked in small amount of water	14	163
Red, raw	26	268
Cabbage, Chinese (also called *celery cabbage* or *pe-tsai*)	23	253
Cakes		
Homemade		
Angel food	283	88
Fruit cake, made with enriched flour, dark	158	496
Gingerbread, made with enriched flour	237	454
Plain cake or cupcake, without icing	300	79
Pound, modified	178	78
Frozen, commercial, devil's food, with chocolate icing	420	119
Candy		
Caramels, plain or chocolate	226	192
Chocolate, sweet	33	269
Chocolate coated, chocolate fudge	228	193
Gum drops, starch jelly pieces	35	5
Hard	32	4
Marshmallows	39	6
Peanut bars	10	448
Carp, raw	50	286
Carrots		
Raw	47	341
Canned		
Regular pack, solids and liquid	236*	120
Special dietary pack (low sodium), solids and liquid	39	120
Cashews	15[‖]	464
Catfish, freshwater, raw	60	330
Cauliflower		
Cooked, boiled, drained	9	206
Frozen, cooked, boiled, drained	10	207
Caviar, sturgeon, granular	2200	180
Celery, all, including green and yellow varieties		
Raw	126	341
Cooked, boiled, drained	88	239

FOOD AND DESCRIPTION	SODIUM (mg)	POTASSIUM (mg)
Chard, Swiss, cooked, boiled, drained	86	321
Cheese straws	721	63
Cheeses		
Natural cheeses		
Cheddar (domestic type)	700	82
Cottage (large or small curd)		
Creamed	229	85
Uncreamed	290	72
Cream	250	74
Parmesan	734	149
Swiss (domestic)	710	104
Pasteurized processed cheese, American	1136¶	80
Pasteurized processed cheese spread, American	1625¶	240
Cherries		
Raw, sweet	2	191
Canned		
Sour, red, solids and liquid, water pack	2	130
Sweet, solids and liquid, syrup pack, light	1	128
Frozen, not thawed, sweetened	2	130
Chicken, all classes		
Light meat without skin, cooked, roasted	64	411
Dark meat without skin, cooked, roasted	86	321
Gizzard, chicken, all classes, cooked, simmered	57	211
Chicken potpie, commercial, frozen, unheated	411	153
Chicory, witloof (also called *French* or *Belgian endive*), bleached head (forced), raw	7	182
Chili con carne, canned, with beans	531	233
Chocolate, bitter or baking	4	830
Chocolate syrup, fudge type	89	284
Chop suey, with meat, canned	551	138
Chow mein, chicken (without noodles), canned	290	167
Citron, candied	290	120
Clams, raw		
Soft meat only	36	235
Hard or round meat only	205	311
Clams, canned, including hard, soft, razor, and unspecified solids and liquid	—	140
Cocoa and chocolate-flavored beverage powders		
Cocoa powder with nonfat dry milk	525	800
Mix for hot chocolate	382	605
Cocoa, dry powder, high fat or breakfast		
Plain	6	1522
Processed with alkali	717	651
Coconut cream (liquid expressed from grated coconut meat)	4	324
Coconut meat, fresh	23	256
Cod		
Cooked, broiled	110	407
Dehydrated, lightly salted	8100	160
Coffee, instant, water-soluble solids		
Beverage	1	36
Collards, cooked, boiled, drained, leaves (including stems) cooked in small amount of water	25	234
Cookie dough, plain, chilled in roll, baked	548	48

FOOD AND DESCRIPTION	SODIUM (mg)	POTASSIUM (mg)
Cookies		
Assorted, packaged, commercial	365	67
Butter, thin, rich	418	60
Gingersnaps	571	462
Molasses	386	138
Oatmeal with raisins	162	370
Sandwich type	483	38
Vanilla wafer	252	72
Corn, sweet		
Cooked, boiled, drained, white and yellow, kernels, cut off cob before cooking	Trace	165
Canned		
Regular pack, cream style, white and yellow, solids and liquid	236*	(97)
Special dietary pack (low sodium), cream style, white and yellow, solids and liquid	2	(97)
Frozen, kernels cut off cob, cooked, boiled, drained	1	184
Corn fritters	477	133
Corn grits, degermed, enriched, dry form	1	80
Corn products used mainly as ready-to-eat breakfast cereals		
Corn flakes, added nutrients	1005	120
Corn, puffed, added nutrients	1060	—
Corn, rice and wheat flakes, mixed, added nutrients	950	—
Cornbread mix and cornbread baked from mix, made with egg and milk	744	127
Cornmeal, white or yellow, degermed, enriched, dry form	1	120
Cowpeas, including black-eyed peas		
Immature seeds, canned, solids and liquid	236*	352
Young pods, with seeds, cooked, boiled, drained	3	196
Crab, canned	1000	110
Crackers		
Butter	1092	113
Graham, plain	670	384
Saltines	1072	154
Sandwich type, peanut butter or cheese	992	226
Cranberries, raw	2	82
Cranberry juice cocktail, bottled (approximately 33% cranberry juice)	1	10
Cranberry sauce, sweetened, canned, strained	1	30
Cream, liquid, light, coffee or table, 20% fat	43	122
Cream substitutes, dried, containing cream, skim milk (calcium reduced), and lactose	575	—
Cream puffs with custard filling	83	121
Cress, garden, raw	14	606
Croaker, Atlantic, cooked, baked	120	323
Cucumbers, raw, pared	6	160
Custard, baked	79	146
Dates, domestic, natural and dry	1	648
Doughnuts, cake type	501	90
Duck, domesticated, raw, flesh only	74	285
Eggplant, cooked, boiled, drained	1	150
Eggs, chicken		
Raw		
Whole, fresh and frozen	122	129
Whites, fresh and frozen	146	139
Yolks, fresh	52	98
Endive (curly endive and escarole), raw	14	294

FOOD AND DESCRIPTION	SODIUM (mg)	POTASSIUM (mg)
Farina		
Enriched		
Regular	2	83
Dry form	144	9
Cooked		
Quick cooking, cooked	165	10
Instant cooking, cooked	188	13
Nonenriched, regular, dry form	2	83
Figs, canned, solids and liquid, syrup pack, light	2	152
Flat fish (flounder, sole, sand dabs), raw	78	342
Fruit, cocktail, canned, solids and liquid, water pack, with or without artificial sweetener	5	168
Garlic, cloves, raw	19	529
Ginger root, fresh	6	264
Goose, domesticated, flesh only, cooked, roasted	124	605
Gooseberries, canned, solids and liquid, syrup pack, heavy	1	98
Grapefruit		
Raw, pulp, pink, red, white, all varieties	1	135
Canned, juice, sweetened	1	162
Grapefruit juice and orange juice, blended, canned, sweetened	1	184
Grapes, raw, American type (slip skin), such as Concord, Delaware, Niagara, Catawba, and Scuppernong	3	158
Grape juice, canned or bottled	2	116
Guava, whole, raw, common	4	289
Haddock, cooked, fried	177	348
Hake, including Pacific hake, squirrel hake, and silver hake or whiting, raw	74	363
Halibut, Atlantic and Pacific, cooked, broiled	134	525
Ham croquette	342	83
Herring		
Raw, Pacific	74	420
Smoked, hard	6231	157
Honey, strained or extracted	5	51
Horseradish, prepared	96	290
Ice cream and frozen custard, regular (approximately 17% fat)	63**	181
Ice cream cones	232	244
Ice milk	68**	195
Jams and preserves	12	88
Kale, cooked, boiled, drained, leaves including stems	43	221
Lake herring (cisco), raw	83	250
Lamb, retail cuts	70	290
Lemon juice, canned or bottled, unsweetened	1	141
Lettuce, raw crisphead varieties such as iceberg, New York, and Great Lakes	9	175
Lime juice, canned or bottled, unsweetened	1	104
Lobster, northern, canned or cooked	210	180
Loganberries, canned, solids and liquid, syrup pack, light	1	111
Macadamia nuts	—	164
Macaroni, unenriched, dry form	2	197
Macaroni and cheese	802	423
Margarine††	987	23
Mayonnaise	597	34

FOOD AND DESCRIPTION	SODIUM (mg)	POTASSIUM (mg)
Milk, cow		
Liquid (pasteurized and raw)		
Whole, 3.7% fat	50	144
Skim	52	145
Canned, evaporated (unsweetened)	118	303
Dry, skim (nonfat solids), regular	532	1745
Malted		
Dry powder	440	720
Beverage	91	200
Chocolate drink, liquid, commercial		
Made with skim milk	46	142
Made with whole (3.5% fat) milk	47	146
Molasses, cane		
First extraction or light	15	917
Third extraction or blackstrap	96	2927
Muffin mixes, corn, and muffins baked from mixes		
Made with egg and milk	479	110
Made with egg and water	346	104
Mushrooms		
Raw	15	414
Canned, solids and liquid	400	197
Muskmelon, raw, cantaloupe and other netted varieties	12	251
Mussels, Atlantic and Pacific, raw, meat only	289	315
Mustard greens, cooked, boiled, drained	18	220
Mustard, prepared		
Brown	1307	130
Yellow	1252	130
Nectarines, raw	6	294
Noodles, egg, enriched, cooked	2	44
Oat products used mainly as hot breakfast cereals, oatmeal, or rolled oats		
Dry form	2	352
Cooked	218	61
Oat products used mainly as ready-to-eat breakfast cereals, with or without corn, puffed, added nutrients	1267	—
Ocean perch, Atlantic (redfish)		
Raw	79	269
Cooked, fried	153	284
Ocean perch, Pacific, raw	63	390
Oils, salad or cooking	0	0
Okra		
Raw	3	249
Cooked, boiled, drained	2	174
Olives, pickled, canned or bottled		
Green	2400	55
Ripe, Ascolano (extra large, mammoth, giant jumbo)	813	34
Ripe, salt cured, oil coated, Greek style	3288	—
Onions, mature (dry), raw	10	157
Onions, young, green (bunching varieties), raw, bulb and entire top	5	231
Orange, raw, peeled, all commercial varieties	1	200
Orange juice		
Raw, all commercial varieties	1	200
Canned, unsweetened	1	199
Frozen concentrate, unsweetened, diluted with three parts water, by volume	1	186

FOOD AND DESCRIPTION	SODIUM (mg)	POTASSIUM (mg)
Oysters		
Raw, meat only, eastern	73	121
Cooked, fried	206	203
Frozen, solids and liquid	380	210
Oyster stew, commercial, frozen, prepared with equal volume of milk	366	176
Pancake and waffle mixes, baked, plain and buttermilk, made with egg and milk	564	154
Parsnips, cooked, boiled, drained	8	379
Peaches		
Raw	1	202
Canned, solids and liquid, water pack, with or without artificial sweetener	2	137
Frozen, sliced, sweetened, not thawed	2	124
Peanut butters made with small amounts of added fat and salt	607	670
Peanuts		
Roasted with skins	5	701
Roasted and salted	418	674
Pears		
Raw, including skin	2	130
Canned, solids and liquid, syrup pack, light	1	85
Peas, green, immature		
Cooked, boiled, drained, canned, Alaska (early or June peas)		
Regular pack, solids and liquid	236*	96
Special dietary pack (low sodium), solids and liquid	3	96
Frozen, cooked, boiled, drained	115	135
Peas, mature seeds, dry, whole, raw	35	1005
Peas and carrots, frozen, cooked, boiled, drained	84	157
Pecans	Trace	603
Peppers, hot, chili, mature, red, raw, pods excluding seeds	25	564
Peppers, sweet, garden varieties, immature, green, raw	13	213
Perch, yellow, raw	68	230
Pickles, cucumber, dill	1428	200
Pie crust or plain pastry, made with enriched flour, baked	611	50
Pies, baked, pie crust made with unenriched flour		
Apple	301	80
Cherry	304	105
Mincemeat	448	178
Pumpkin	214	160
Pike, walleye, raw	51	319
Pineapple		
Raw	1	146
Frozen chunks, sweetened, not thawed	2	100
Pizza, homemade, baked		
With cheese topping only	702	130
With sausage and cheese topping	729	168
Plate dinners, frozen, commercial, unheated		
Beef pot roast, whole oven-browned potatoes, peas, and corn	259	244
Fried chicken, mashed potatoes, and mixed vegetables (carrots, peas, corn, beans)	344	112
Meat loaf with tomato sauce, mashed potatoes, and peas	393	115
Sliced turkey, mashed potatoes, and peas	400	176
Plums		
Raw, damson	2	299
Canned, solids and liquid, purple (Italian prunes), syrup pack, light	1	145
Popcorn, popped		
Plain	(3)	—
Oil and salt added	1940	—

FOOD AND DESCRIPTION	SODIUM (mg)	POTASSIUM (mg)
Pork, fresh, retail cuts, trimmed to retail level, loin	65	390
Pork, lightly cured, commercial, ham, medium-fat class, separable, lean, cooked, roasted	930	326
Pork, cured, canned ham, contents of can	(1100)	(340)
Potatoes		
Cooked, boiled in skin	3‡‡	407
Dehydrated, mashed, flakes, without milk		
Dry form	89	1600
Prepared, with water, milk, and table fat added	231	286
Pretzels	1680§§	130
Prunes, dried, softened, cooked (fruit and liquid), with added sugar	3	262
Pudding mixes and puddings made from mixes, with starch base		
With milk, cooked	129	136
With milk, uncooked	124	129
Pumpkin, canned	2	240
Radishes, raw, common	18	322
Raisins, natural (unbleached), cooked, fruit and liquid, added sugar	13	355
Raspberries		
Canned, solids and liquid, water pack, with or without artificial sweetener, red	1	114
Frozen, red, sweetened, not thawed	1	100
Rhubarb, cooked	2	203
Rice		
Brown		
Raw	9	214
Cooked	282	70
White (fully milled or polished), enriched, common commercial varieties, all types		
Raw	5	92
Cooked	374	28
Wild, raw	7	220
Rice products used mainly as ready-to-eat breakfast cereals		
Rice flakes, added nutrients	987	180
Rice, puffed, added nutrients, without salt	2	100
Rice, puffed or open popped, presweetened, honey and added nutrients	706	—
Rockfish, including black, canary, yellowtail, rasphead, and bocaccio, cooked, oven steamed	68	446
Roe, cooked, baked or broiled, cod and shad‖‖	73	132
Rolls and buns, commercial, ready to serve		
Danish pastry	366	112
Hard rolls, enriched	625	97
Plain (pan rolls), enriched	506	95
Sweet rolls	389	124
Rusk	246	161
Rutabagas, cooked, boiled, drained	4	167
Rye wafers, whole grain	882	600

FOOD AND DESCRIPTION	SODIUM (mg)	POTASSIUM (mg)
Salad dressings, commercial[¶¶]		
Bleu and Roquefort cheese		
Regular	1094	37
Special dietary (low calorie), low fat (approximately 5 kcal/tsp)	1108	34
French		
Regular	1370	79
Special dietary (low calorie), low fat (approximately 5 kcal/tsp)	787	79
Thousand Island		
Regular	700	113
Special dietary (low calorie, approximately 10 kcal/tsp)	700	113
Salmon, Coho (sliver)		
Raw	48[***]	421
Canned, solids and liquid	351[†††]	339
Salt pork, raw	1212	42
Sandwich spread (with chopped pickle)		
Regular	626	92
Special dietary (low calorie, approximately 5 kcal/tsp)	626	92
Sardines, Atlantic, canned in oil, drained solids	823	590
Sardines, Pacific, in tomato sauce, solids and liquid	400	320
Sauerkraut, canned, solids and liquid	747[‡‡‡]	140
Sausage, cold cuts, and luncheon meats		
Bologna, all samples	1300	230
Frankfurters, raw, all samples	1100	220
Luncheon meat, pork, cured ham or shoulder, chopped, spiced or unspiced, canned	1234	222
Pork sausage, links or bulk, cooked	958	269
Scallops, bay and sea, cooked, steamed	265	476
Soups, commercial, canned		
Beef broth, bouillon, and consommé, prepared with an equal volume of water	326	54
Chicken noodle, prepared with an equal volume of water	408	23
Tomato		
Prepared with an equal volume of water	396	94
Prepared with an equal volume of milk	422	167
Vegetable beef, prepared with an equal volume of water	427	66
Soy sauce	7325	366
Spaghetti, enriched, cooked, tender stage	1	61
Spaghetti, in tomato sauce with cheese, canned	382	121
Spinach		
Cooked, boiled, drained	50	324
Canned		
Regular pack, drained solids	236[*]	250
Special dietary pack (low sodium), solids and liquid	34	250
Frozen, chopped, cooked, boiled, drained	52	333
New Zealand spinach, cooked, boiled, drained	92	463
Squash, summer, all varieties, cooked, boiled, drained	1	141
Squash, frozen		
Summer, yellow crookneck, cooked, boiled, drained	3	167
Winter, heated	1	207

FOOD AND DESCRIPTION	SODIUM (mg)	POTASSIUM (mg)
Strawberries		
Raw	1	164
Frozen, sweetened, not thawed, sliced	1	112
Sturgeon, cooked, steamed	108	235
Succotash (corn and lima beans), frozen, cooked, boiled, drained	38	246
Sugars, beet or cane, brown	30	344
Sweet potatoes		
Cooked, all, baked in skin	12	300
Canned, liquid pack, solids and liquid, regular packed in syrup	48	(120)
Dehydrated flakes, prepared with water	45	140
Tangerine, raw (Dancy variety)	2	126
Tapioca, dry	3	18
Tapioca desserts, tapioca cream pudding	156	135
Tartar sauce, regular	707	78
Tea, instant (water-soluble solids), carbohydrate added		
Dry powder	—	4350
Beverage	—	25
Tomato catsup, bottled	1042[§§§]	363
Tomato juice, canned or bottled		
Regular pack	200	227
Special dietary pack (low sodium)	3	227
Tomato juice cocktail, canned or bottled	200	221
Tomato puree, canned		
Regular pack	399	426
Special dietary pack (low sodium)	6	426
Tomatoes, ripe		
Raw	3	244
Canned, solids and liquid, regular pack	130	217
Tuna, canned		
In oil, solids and liquid	800	301
In water, solids and liquid	41[||||]	279[||||]
Turkey, all classes		
Light meat, cooked, roasted	82	411
Dark meat, cooked, roasted	99	398
Turkey potpie, commercial, frozen, unheated	369	114
Turnips, cooked, boiled, drained	34	188
Turnip greens, leaves, including stems		
Canned, solids and liquid	236*	243
Frozen, cooked, boiled, drained	17	149
Veal, retail cuts, untrimmed	80	500
Vinegar, cider	1	100
Waffles, frozen, made with enriched flour	644	158
Walnuts		
Black	3	460
Persian or English	2	450
Watercress, leaves including stems, raw	52	282
Watermelon, raw	1	100

FOOD AND DESCRIPTION	SODIUM (mg)	POTASSIUM (mg)
Yogurt, made from whole milk	47	132
Zwieback	250	150

Numbers in parentheses denote valued input, usually from another form of the food or from a similar food. Dashes (—) denote a lack of reliable data for a constituent that is believed to be present in measurable amount. Values are selected from Watt BK, Merril AL: *Composition of foods—raw, processed, prepared,* Agriculture Handbook No. 8, Washington, DC, 1963, U.S. Department of Agriculture.

*Estimated average based on the addition of salt in the amount of 0.6% of the finished product.

†Processed, partially debranned, whole-kernel wheat with salt added.

‡Processed, partially debranned, whole-kernel wheat with chicken fat, chicken stock base, dehydrated onion flakes, salt, monosodium glutamate, and herbs.

§Values apply to unsalted butter. Unsalted butter contains less than 10 mg of either sodium or potassium per 100 g. The value for vitamin A is the year-round average.

||Applies to unsalted nuts. For salted nuts, the value is approximately 200 mg per 100 g.

¶Values for phosphorus and sodium are based on the use of 1.5% anhydrous disodium phosphate as the emulsifying agent. If the emulsifying agent does not contain either phosphorus or sodium, the content of these two nutrients in milligrams per 100 g is as follows:

FOOD	SODIUM	PHOSPHORUS
American processed cheese	650	444
Swiss processed cheese	681	540
American cheese food	—	427
American cheese spread	1139	548

**Value for product without added salt.

††Values apply to salted margarine. Unsalted margarine contains less than 10 mg/100 g of either sodium or potassium. The vitamin A value is based on the minimum required to meet federal specifications for margarine with vitamin A added (i.e., 15,000 IU/lb).

‡‡Applies to product without added salt. If salt is added, an estimated average value for sodium is 236 mg/100 g.

§§Sodium content is variable. For example, very thick pretzel sticks contain approximately twice the amount listed.

||||Prepared with butter or margarine, lemon juice, or vinegar.

¶¶Values apply to products that contain salt. For those without salt, the sodium content is low, and it ranges from less than 10 to 50 mg/100 g; the amount is usually indicated on the label.

***A sample dipped in brine contained 215 mg sodium/100 g.

†††For product that is canned without added salt, the value is approximately the same as that of raw salmon.

‡‡‡Values for sauerkraut and sauerkraut juice are based on a salt content of 1.9% and 2.0%, respectively, in the finished products. The amounts in some samples may vary significantly from these estimates.

§§§Applies to regular pack. For special dietary pack (low sodium), values range from 5 to 35 mg/100 g.

|||||One sample with salt added contained 875 mg of sodium/100 g and 275 mg of potassium.

****Value of 90 mg potassium/100 g contributed by flour. Small quantities of additional potassium may be provided by other ingredients.

Index

Page numbers followed by "*f*" indicate figures, "*b*" indicate boxes, and "*t*" indicate tables.

A

ABCDEFs of nutrition assessment, 430*b*
Abdomen, signs of nutrient imbalance in, 296*t*-297*t*
Abdominal thrusts, 306
Absorption, 56, 60-66
  of carbohydrates, 60-63
  competitive, and micronutrient bioavailability, 63*b*
  of fats, 35-37, 37*f*, 60-63
  in gastrointestinal tract, 67*f*
  in intestinal wall surface, 63-64
  in large intestine, 65
  of macronutrients and micronutrients, 65, 65*t*
  in microvilli, 64
  mineral, 111
  in mucosal folds, 64
  nutrient, sodium in, 116
  process of, 64-65
  of proteins, 60-63
  in small intestine, 63-65, 63*f*
  structures in, 63-64
  in villi, 64
  of water, 65
Academy of Nutrition and Dietetics
  on breastfeeding, 164
  on eating disorders, 268
  on nutrition care process model, 291
  on registered dietitian qualifications, 290*b*
  on vegetarian diets, 46
  on weight management, 258
Acetone, 355
α-Acetyl-CoA carboxylase, 103
β-Acetyl-CoA carboxylase, 103
Achalasia, 307
Acid-base balance
  in body fluids, 144-145
  ketosis upsetting, 21
  phosphate in, 114
Acid-base buffer system, 146
Acidity
  for nutrient absorption, 59*b*
  and proteins, 44
Acidosis, 21, 145
Acids, 145, 145*b*
  and digestion, 59
Acquired immunodeficiency syndrome (AIDS)
  HIV evolution, 422-423
  types and incidence of, in American populations, 423*b*
Acrodermatitis enteropathica, 126-127, 127*f*
Active lifestyle, 79*b*
Active transport
  in absorption, 65
  and water balance, 141
Activities of daily living (ADLs), and exercise, 278
Activity level, and water requirement, 134-135
Acute cardiovascular disease, 334-336. *see also* Myocardial infarction (MI)
Acute glomerulonephritis, 375, 375*t*
Acute kidney injury, 376-378
Acute renal failure, 376
Adaptive thermogenesis, 76
Additives, food, 210, 211*t*-212*t*
Adenosine triphosphate (ATP), 67, 71
Adequate intake, 7. *see also* individual micronutrients/macronutrients
Adipocytes, 256
Adipose tissue, 32
  as energy storage, 73
  as storage site, 68

Administration on Aging, of the U.S. Department of Health and Human Services, 198
Adolescence
  elevated basal energy expenditure in, 75-76
  life cycle growth pattern, 166
  mineral supplements during, 131
  nutrition requirements during, 183-184
    eating disorders, 184
    eating patterns, 184
    physical growth, 183-184
  positive nitrogen balance in, 43
  zinc intake in, 126
Adolescents
  benefits of exercise for, 272, 275*b*
  obesity and, 245, 246*f*
  vitamin supplementation for, 107
Adulthood
  dietary energy intake in, 80
  life cycle growth pattern, 166
  mineral supplements during, 131
Adult-onset diabetes, 348-349
Adults. *see also* Middle adults (45 to 64 years old); Older adults
  benefits of exercise for, 272-273, 275*b*
  diet modifications for, 197
  energy needs, estimation of, 263*b*
  growth and development
    continuing, 186-190
    shaping influences in, 187-190
  impact on health care, 186-187
  life expectancy, 186
  nutrition needs of, 190-193
    aging process and, 190-193
    macronutrients and fluids, 191-192
    micronutrients and health concerns, 192-193
    nutrient supplementation, 193
  overweight and obesity in, prevalence of, 196*f*
  physical growth of, 188-189
  population and age distribution of, 186, 187*f*
  psychosocial development of, 189
  quality of life, 186
  socioeconomic status of, 189-190, 190*f*
Advance directives, 404*b*
Advanced care planning, 404*b*
Advocates, 290
Aerobic capacity, 279
Aerobic exercise
  benefits of, 272
  for children and adolescents, 272
  weight management benefits of, 262*b*
Aflatoxin, 222
African American
  calcium retention and peak bone mass of, 172*b*
  cancer percentages in, 412*b*, 412*f*
  food habits, 233, 233*t*
  food insecurity, 6*b*
  heart disease death rate, 344*f*-345*f*
  HIV incidence in, 423*b*, 423*f*
  kidney transplant failures in, 384*b*
  lipid metabolism in, 38*b*
  prevalence of type 2 diabetes mellitus, 349*b*
Age
  as pregnancy risk factor, 154
  and water intake needs, 134*t*, 135
Aging. *see also* Older adults
  Dietary Guidelines for Americans and, 7, 9*f*
  polypharmacy increases with, 197-198, 198*b*
  process
    individuality of, 191
    nutrition needs and, 190-193
Agricultural pesticides, 207-210

Agricultural Research Service, 202-203
Air displacement plethysmography, 248
Albumin, 139
Alcohol
  absorption of, 68, 69*b*
  as pregnancy risk factor, 154-156
Alcohol abuse/alcoholism
  and cancer, 422
  and cirrhosis, 322
  and fatty liver disease, 321
  and fetal alcohol syndrome, 154, 156*f*
  and hepatitis, 321-322
  and hypertension, 339
  iron deficiency and, 131
  and pancreatitis, 325
  thiamin deficiency due to, 95-96
  Wernicke's encephalopathy and, 95-96
  zinc deficiency and, 132
Alcohol use
  Dietary Guidelines for Americans on, 9*f*
  limitations in diabetics, 363*b*, 366-368
  Muslim prohibition of, 240
  and peptic ulcer, 311*b*
  and vitamin supplementation, 107
Aldosterone, 144, 372
Aldosteronoma, 351
Algal polysaccharides, 16, 16*t*
Alkaline, and water balance, 145
Alkaline diet, 389
Alkalinity, and proteins, 44
Alkalizing agents, 286*b*
Alkalosis, 145
Allergens, 177
  common food, 319
Allergies
  definition of, 319
  and digestion, 70
Alpha-linolenic acid, 28*f*, 29-30, 48*t*
  DRIs for, 39
Alternative agriculture, 207-210
Alternative living arrangements, 200-201
Alzheimer's disease, protein-folding mistakes and, 41
Amenorrhea, 281
  in female athletes, 283*b*
American Academy of Pediatrics
  on breastfeeding, 164
  on milk content for premature infants, 173
  on solid food additions, 176
American Cancer Society, guidelines for cancer prevention, 420-422
American diet, 106*b*
  acculturation to, 230, 230*b*
American Dietetic Association. *see* Academy of Nutrition and Dietetics
American food pattern, changing, 241-244, 243*b*
  frequency, 243
  household dynamics, 241-243
American Geriatrics Society, 199-200
American Heart Association (AHA)
  on benefits of exercise, 275
  dietary guidelines, 332-333, 333*b*
  on trans fat avoidance, 30
American Institute for Cancer Research, guidelines for cancer prevention, 420-422
American Psychiatric Association, diagnostic criteria for eating disorders, 269*b*
Amino acids, 4, 41, 393. *see also* Proteins
  branched-chain, 286
  as building blocks, 4, 41, 42*f*
  classes of, 41-42, 42*b*

Amino acids *(Continued)*
  conditionally indispensable, 41-42, 42*b*
  dietary importance of, 41
  dispensable, 41-42, 42*b*
  indispensable, 41-42, 42*b*
  supplements, 286*b*
  tissue building function of, 4
Aminopeptidase, 49
Amniotic fluid, protein in, 148
Amphiphilic molecule, 30
Amylase, 44, 58
Anabolism, 42-43, 66-67
Anaerobic microorganism, 219
Anaphylactic shock, 319
Androgens, 286-287
Anemia, 120
  with B vitamin deficiencies, 104*t*
  during childhood, 182
  global prevalence of, 123*f*
  iron-deficiency
    causes of, 120
    following surgery, 394
    mineral supplementation for, 131
  with kidney disease, 379
  milk, 182
  in pregnancy, 157
Anencephaly, 150-151
  with folate deficiency, 100
Angina pectoris, 327
Angiotensin I, 143-144
Angiotensin II, 144
Angiotensin-converting enzyme (ACE), 144
Angiotensinogen, 143-144
Animal fats, 32-33
Anions, 139, 139*t*
Anorexia
  with cancer, 414
  cannabis to treat, 415-416, 416*b*
  and hepatitis, 321-322
  with nephron diseases, 375
  nutritional management of, 418-419, 418*t*-419*t*
Anorexia nervosa
  description and clinical signs of, 268-270, 269*b*
  and female athlete triad, 283*b*
  nutrition-related clinical signs commonly associated with, 270*t*
Antacids, affecting mineral depletion, 131*b*
Anthropometrics
  for enteral feeding monitoring, 401*b*
  measurements, 167, 293-295
  during nutrition care, 293-295, 299
Antibiotics, vitamin K and, 92*b*
Antibody, 413
Anticoagulants, vitamin K and, 92*b*
Anticonvulsants, and nutrient metabolism, 182*b*
Antidepressants, drug-nutrient interaction of, 198*b*
Antidiuretic hormone (ADH)
  mechanism, and water balance, 143, 143*f*
  role in kidney, 372-373
Antiestrogens, and breast cancer, 417*b*
Antigen, 412-413
Antihistamines, drug-nutrient interaction of, 198*b*
Antihyperlipidemics, drug-nutrient interaction of, 198*b*
Antihypertensives, drug-nutrient interaction of, 198*b*
Antiketogenic effect, 21
Antineoplastic drugs, drug-nutrient interactions with, 414, 414*t*
Antioxidants
  ascorbic acid as, 94
  for cancer patients, 417
  and chemotherapy interactions, 417*b*
  vitamin A as, 85-86
  vitamin E as, 90
  vitamins as, 84
Antiretroviral drugs
  nucleoside reverse transcriptase inhibitors, 426, 427*t*-429*t*
  side effects of, 426, 427*t*-429*t*
Anuria, 375
Appetite
  loss with cancer, 414
  nutritional management of loss of, 418-419, 418*t*-419*t*

Appetite *(Continued)*
  radiation therapy affecting, 414
  suppressants, 256
Appetite-regulating network, 250
Appropriate for gestational age (AGA), 173
Arginine, 417
Ariboflavinosis, 96, 104*t*
Arteriole, definition of, 373
Artificial loop graft, 381*f*
Artificial sweeteners, 20, 21*t*
Ascites, 323
  with nephrotic syndrome, 375-376
Ascorbic acid. *see* Vitamin C
Asian food patterns, 234-235, 237*t*
Aspartame, and phenylketonuria, 43*b*
Aspiration, risk for, 177-178
Aspirin
  and iron absorption, 394*b*
  in peptic ulcer disease, 309
Assisted living facilities, 200
Atherosclerosis, 327-334, 328*f*
  dietary recommendations to reduce risk of, 331-334
  disease process, 327-328, 328*f*
  drug therapy in, 334
  fat metabolism and, 328-330
    cholesterol, 328-329, 330*t*
    lipoproteins, 329-330, 330*t*
    triglycerides, 330, 330*t*
  and lipoprotein density, 30
  risk factors, 330-331, 331*b*
Athletics, 282-287
  and body mass index (BMI), 247
  carbohydrate loading, 284*t*
  competition, 284-285
  fitness levels and body fat percentages, 249*f*
  general training diet, 282-284
  kilocalories (kcal) burned in various, 280
  pregame meals, 284-285, 285*b*
Atonic, 405
Atrophy, and immunity, 413
Auscultation, 399
Autoimmune thyroid disorders, 76*b*
Azotemia, 378

B
Baby bottle tooth decay, 175, 175*f*
Baby-Friendly Hospital Initiative, 159
Bacillus cereus, 220*t*
Bacterial food infections, 215-217
Bacterial food poisoning, 217-219
Bacterial urinary tract infection, 373-374, 374*b*
Balance, 42-44
  nitrogen balance, 43-44
    negative, 43-44
    positive, 43
  protein balance, 42-43, 43*f*
Balanced diet, importance of, 2-3
Bariatric surgery, 257, 405-407, 406*b*
Barrett's esophagus, 307
Basal energy expenditure (BEE), 73-76
  factors that influence, 74-76
  magnesium in, 119
  measurement of, 73-74
  median values according to age and gender, 81*t*
  prediction of, 74
  total energy expenditure and, 78*f*
Basal metabolic rate (BMR), 73, 252
  following surgery, 393
Bases, 145, 145*b*
Base-to-acid ratio, 145
B-complex vitamins, 104*t*. *see also* Vitamin B
  postoperative needs for, 394
Behavior modification
  Therapeutic Lifestyle Changes (TLC) diet, 333
  for weight management, 258, 259*b*
Beriberi, 95-96, 104*t*
Beta-alanine, 286*b*
Bile
  during digestion, 58, 60
  in fat digestion, 34-36, 35*f*
  and Questran, 36*b*
Biliary system, 60
  organs of, 60*f*
Binge eating disorder, 262*b*, 268, 269*b*, 270
Bioelectrical impedance analysis (BIA), 247-248

Biologic age, definition of, 166
Biologic changes, aging and, 190-191
Biotechnology, 208-209, 209*f*
  genetically modified (GM) foods and, 209
Biotin, 102-103, 104*t*
Biotinidase deficiency, 103
Birth defects, congenital hypothyroidism and, 77*b*
Blindness, with vitamin A deficiency, 86, 86*f*
Blood cholesterol profile, 330-331
Blood clotting
  calcium in, 112
  function of vitamin K in, 91-92, 91*f*, 92*b*
  and liver function, 61*b*
Blood glucose
  in diabetes mellitus
    energy supply and, 352-355, 353*f*
    laboratory tests, 352
    monitoring, 361
    sources of, 353, 353*f*
    uses of, 353, 354*f*
  gluconeogenesis, 68
  glycemic index, 22*b*
  storage in liver, 67-68
Blood lipids. *see* Lipids
Blood pressure
  benefits of exercise for managing, 275
  levels of, hypertensive, 339-340, 339*t*
  potassium in, 117
Blood urea nitrogen (BUN)
  and nephron function, 376
  tests, during nutrition care process, 295
Blood volume, protein needs and, 148
BOD POD, for body composition, 248, 248*f*
Body composition, 279
  during adolescence, 183-184
  assessment during nutrition care process, 295
  and weight management, 245-248, 247*f*
Body defense system. *see* Immune system
Body dysmorphic disorder, 268
Body fat
  assessment tools, 247*f*
  benefits of aerobic exercise, 262*b*
  menopause and, 190-191
  necessity of, 249-250
  weight *versus*, 245-246
Body fat calipers, 247, 247*f*
Body fluids
  ionic composition of, 116*f*
  phosphate in homeostasis of, 114
  sodium and, 116*f*
Body frame, 249, 249*t*
Body mass index (BMI), 80, 245
  assessment during nutrition care process, 294-295
  body fat percentage, 247*f*
  calculations, 170*b*, 249
  classifications of, 245, 246*b*
  -for-age charts, 167
  and growth charts, 245, 246*f*
  and height/weight tables, 248-249
  median values according to age and gender, 81*t*
  and obesity, overweight, 245
Body temperature
  influencing basal energy expenditure, 76
  and water requirement, 134
Body weight. *see* Weight
Body work, involuntary, 71
Body wraps, clothing and, 256
BodyGem device, 74, 74*f*
Bolus feeding, 401
Bone density
  calcium retention and peak bone mass, 172*b*
  in women, 283
Bone diseases
  benefits of exercise for, 275*b*, 277
  osteodystrophy, 378, 386
  osteopenia, 283
  osteoporosis
    and calcitriol, 88
    in female athletes, 283*b*
Bone marrow
  complications with chemotherapy, 414
  and immune system, 412-413, 413*f*
Bone mass
  and female athlete triad, 283*b*
  in women, 283*b*

Bone mineral density (BMD)
    during adolescence, 184
    calcium retention and peak bone mass, 172b
    in female athletes, 283b
    osteoporosis levels of, 113b
    in women, 283b
Bones
    building, vitamins in, 84
    development of
        function of vitamin K in, 92
        role of vitamins in, 4
    formation of
        calcium in, 111-112
        phosphorus in, 114
    health, of adults, 192, 192f
    mineralization, vitamin D in, 88
    protein needs for healing of, 393
    strengthening of, in children and adolescents,
        272
Bottle caries. see Baby bottle tooth decay
Bottle mouth. see Baby bottle tooth decay
Bottles, cleaning, 175
Botulism, food-borne, 218-219
Bovine colostrum, 286b
Bowels
    and fiber, 20b
    large intestine
        constipation, 318
        diverticular disease, 317-318, 317f
        irritable bowel syndrome, 318
    small intestine
        absorption in, 63-65, 63f
        in digestion, 59-60
        role in carbohydrate digestion, 23, 24f
        role in fat digestion, 34-37, 35f
        role in protein digestion, 48-49, 50f
Bowman's capsule, 371-372, 372f
Bran layers, in wheat kernel, 15f
Branched-chain amino acids, 286
Bread
    calcium in, 114t
    folate in, 100t
    iron in, 124t
    niacin in, 98t
    pantothenic acid in, 103t
    potassium in, 118t
    pyridoxine in, 99t
    riboflavin in, 97t
    thiamin in, 96t
    vitamin E in, 91t
    zinc in, 127t
Breast, anatomy of, 161f
Breast cancer
    antiestrogens and, 417b
    benefits of exercise for prevention of, 275b
    recent research findings regarding, 422
Breast milk, 174
    substitute, 174-175
        versus human milk, 184b
        nutritional values of, 175t
        risk of using, 163
Breastfeeding, 158. see also Lactation
    advantages of, 163-164, 164b, 164t
    complications in, 162-163
    composition of, 162, 162t
    Healthy People 2020, 159
    of newborn infant, 174f
    summary guidelines for, 177
    ten steps to successful, 161b
    trends, in United States, 159f-160f, 160b-161b,
        160t-161t
Bronchodilators, 301
Brush border, 64
    of intestinal tract, 23
Buddhists, vegetarian diets of, 45
Buffer ions, in digestion, 57
Buffer systems
    for acid-base balance, 145
    and water balance, 145
Bulimia nervosa
    description and clinical signs of, 268, 269b, 270
    and female athlete triad, 283b
    nutrition-related clinical signs commonly
        associated with, 270t
Burns
    acute or flow phase of, 409
    follow-up reconstruction for, 410

Burns (Continued)
    increased need for proteins for, 50-51
    medical nutrition therapy for, 409-410
    shock or ebb phase, 408-409
    stages of nutrition care, 408-410
    total body surface area in, 408
    type and extent of, 408, 408f
Butter, 32

C
Cachexia, 415
Caffeine, 286b
    as pregnancy risk factor, 156
    and water requirement, 135
Cajun, 233
Calciferol. see Vitamin D
Calcitriol, 87
Calcium, 111-114, 121t
    concerns for vegetarians, 46-47, 48t
    deficiency, 112-113, 112f
    food sources of, 113-114, 114t, 115b, 115f
    functions of, 111-112
    homeostasis, vitamin D in, 88
    and kidney disease, 377, 379, 381-382, 385t, 388,
        388t
    in lacto-ovo-vegetarian diet pyramid, 46, 47f
    needs
        for growth, 171-172
        during pregnancy, 149-150
    requirements, 112
    retention, racial differences in, 172b
    toxicity of, 113
Calcium stones, 386f, 387-389
Calories, 71. see also Kilocalories
    intake for different calorie levels, 260t-261t
Campylobacter jejuni, 220t
Canada's Food Guide, 235f
Cancer
    cultural considerations of, 412b
    development process of
        and body's defense system, 412-413, 413f
        carcinogenesis, 411
        causes of, 411-412
        metastasis, 411
        mutation, 411
        nature of, 411
    FDA on health claims and, 421
    Kaposi's sarcoma and, 425
    medical nutrition therapy for
        dietary modifications for side effects,
            418t-419t
        energy needs, 416
        enteral nutrition support, 420
        fluid needs, 418
        objectives of nutrition plan, 415-416
        oral diet with nutrient supplementation,
            418-420
        parenteral nutrition support, 420
        prevention guidelines of, 420-422
        protein, 416
        and symptom relief, 416
        vitamins and minerals, 417
    nutritional complications with treatment for,
        413-414
        chemotherapy, 414
        drug-nutrient interactions, 414, 414t
        radiation, 413-414, 413f
        surgery, 413
    research in, 421-422
    systemic effects of, 414-415
"Cancer cures", 422
Candida albicans
    with HIV, 424-425
    in mouth ulcers, 305
Candidiasis, 305
Canker sores, 305
Cannabis, for anorexia, 415-416, 416b
Capillary fluid shift mechanism, 141
Capillary membranes, water movement between,
    139-140
Carbamazepine, 182b
Carbohydrate loading, 284t
    for endurance performance, 284b
Carbohydrates, 12-26, 18t-19t, 281, 283-284
    absorption of, 60-63
    as basic fuel source, 12
    case study for identifying dietary, 17b

Carbohydrates (Continued)
    classes of, 13-20, 13t
        disaccharides, 13f, 13t, 14
        monosaccharides, 13-14, 13f, 13t
        polysaccharides, 13f, 13t, 15-20
    complications, 22b
    for diabetes mellitus
        counting, 365-366
        in nutrient balance, 362-364
    Dietary Guidelines for Americans, 24
    dietary importance of, 12-13
    Dietary Reference Intakes (DRIs) for, 23-24, 25b
    digestion of, 22-23, 24f, 60, 66b
    energy provided by, 4, 71, 283-284
    and energy-production system, 12
    food sources of, 21, 37
    functions of, 20-21
        as basic fuel supply, 20
        as reserve fuel supply, 20-21
    gram content and calories of, 18t-19t
    MyPlate food guidance system, 25
    nature of, 12-20
    needs, of adults, 191
    nutrient balance, 263
    recommended percentage intake of, 4, 4f, 256
    special tissue functions of, 21
        in central nervous system, 21
        in liver, 21
        in protein and fat sparing, 21
Carboxylase enzymes, 102-103
Carboxypeptidase, 49, 60
Carcinogenesis, 411
Cardiovascular disease (CVD), 327, 328f, 331b
    acute, 334-336
Cardiovascular fitness, 279
β-carotene, 86
Carotenes, 86-87, 86b
Carotenoids, 85-86, 86b, 422
Catabolism, 42-48, 66-67
    prevention in cancer patients, 415-416
    protein balance and, 42-43
Catheter, placement for parenteral nutrition, 403f
Cations, 139, 139t
Caucasian, calcium retention and peak bone mass
    of, 172b
CCR5 antagonist, 427t-429t
CD4+ T-lymphocyte, 424
Celiac disease (CD), 76b, 319-320, 320f, 321t
Cell membranes, 140
    fatty structure, 32
Cellulitis, 356
Cellulose, 16t
Center for Food Safety and Applied Nutrition,
    202
Centers for Disease Control and Prevention
    (CDC)
    on cancer, 422
    on food safety regulations, 203t
    growth charts, 167, 168f-169f
    on HIV classification, 423b, 424-425, 424t
    on neural tube defects (NTDs), 150
    on osteoporosis, 192f
Cereal
    calcium in, 114t
    folate in, 100t
    iron in, 124t
    lacto-ovo-vegetarian diet pyramid and, 47f
    niacin in, 98t
    pantothenic acid in, 103t
    potassium in, 118t
    pyridoxine in, 99t
    riboflavin in, 97t
    thiamin in, 96t
    vitamin E in, 91t
    zinc in, 127t
Cerebrovascular accident, 328
Challah, 240
Cheilosis, 305, 305f
Chelating agents, affecting mineral depletion,
    131b
Chelator, definition of, 16
Chemical buffer system, and water balance, 145
Chemical digestion, 56-58
    gastrointestinal secretions, 57-58
    intestinal enzymes, 60
    in mouth and esophagus, 58
    pancreatic enzymes, 60

Chemical digestion *(Continued)*
  in small intestine, 59-60
  in stomach, 58-59
Chemical processes, for energy and building
    tissue, 4
Chemical score, of proteins, 49, 51*t*
Chemotherapy
  and antioxidant interactions, 417*b*
  nutritional complications with, 414
Chewing, 22-23
Childhood
  elevated basal energy expenditure in, 75-76
  growth, measuring, 166-167
  life cycle growth pattern, 166
  nutrition problems during, 180-183
    anemia, 182
    failure to thrive, 181-182
    lead poisoning, 183
    obesity, 182-183, 183*b*, 183*f*
  nutrition requirements during, 178-183
    preschool-aged children (3 to 5 years old),
      178
    school-aged children (5 to 12 years old),
      178-180
    toddlers (1 to 3 years old), 178
  PA coefficient in, 75*b*
  positive nitrogen balance in, 43
  zinc intake in, 126
Children
  benefits of exercise for, 275*b*
  caloric allowance for, 80*t*
  early-onset obesity, 250
  obesity statistics and trends, weight
    management and, 245, 246*f*
  vitamin supplementation for, 107
Chinese
  food guides, 236*f*
  food habits/traditions, 234, 237*t*
Chloride, 118-119, 121*t*
  shift, 118
Choking, risk for, 177-178
Cholecalciferol, 87-88
Cholecystectomy, 407
Cholecystitis, 324-325, 407
Cholecystokinin, 60
Cholelithiasis, 324-325, 407, 407*f*
Cholesterol
  definition of, 29-31
  and *Dietary Guidelines for Americans*, 31
  excess in, 37
  in fat metabolism, 328-329, 330*t*
  foods high in, 32
  National Cholesterol Education Program
    (NCEP), 333
  niacin as treatment for high, 98*b*
Cholesterol esterase, 34-35
Choline, 103-105
Chromium, 129, 130*t*
Chronic dieting syndrome, 256
Chronic diseases
  of aging, 197-198
  in elderly, reducing risk for, 193
Chronic hypertension, 157
  pre-eclampsia superimposed on, 157
Chronic kidney disease (CKD), 378-379
  case study of, 380*b*
  manifestations of, 375*t*
  medical nutrition therapy for, 379, 385*t*
  prevalence of, 374*f*
  risk factors for, 374, 374*b*
  signs and symptoms of, 379
  stages of, 378, 378*t*, 385*t*
Chronic kidney disease-mineral and bone
    disorder, 378
Chronologic age, 166
Chylomicrons, 36-37, 36*f*, 329, 329*f*
Chyme, 58
Chymotrypsin, 49, 60
Cirrhosis, 322-324, 323*f*
Cis form, 30, 30*f*
Citrate, 387
Citric acid cycle, 67
Clinical nutrition specialist, 1
Clinically severe obesity, 257, 257*f*
Clostridial food poisoning, 218-219
Clostridium botulinum, 218-219, 220*t*
Clostridium perfringens, 218, 220*t*

Cobalamin, 101-102, 101*f*, 102*t*, 104*t*
Coenzyme A (CoA), 102
Coenzymes, from vitamins, 84
Cognitive function, benefits of exercise for, 275*b*
Cold sores, 305
Cold storage, of foods, 214*t*-215*t*
Collagen
  structure of, sulfur in, 120
  vitamin C in synthesis of, 84, 93
Collecting duct, of kidney, 373*t*
Colloidal osmotic pressure (COP), 139
Colloids, 139
Colon cancer, benefits of exercise for prevention
    of, 275*b*
Colorectal cancer, recent research findings
    regarding, 422
Colostomy, 407-408, 407*f*
Colostrum, 162
Commodity Supplemental Food Program, 199,
    224
Common bile duct, 23
Community resources, government program,
    198-199
  Commodity Supplemental Food Program, 199
  congregate nutrition services, 198-199
  extension services, 199
  home-delivered meals, 199
  Older Americans Act, 198-199
  research centers, 199
  Senior Farmers' Market Nutrition Program, 199
  Supplemental Nutrition Assistance Program
    (SNAP), 199
  United States Department of Agriculture, 199
Competitive absorption, and micronutrient
    bioavailability, 63*b*
Competitive foods, 225
Complementary and alternative medicine (CAM),
    antioxidants and chemotherapy, 417*b*
Complementary foods, commercial or
    homemade, 176-177
Complementary proteins, 45
Complete blood count, tests during nutrition care
    process, 295
Complete proteins, 45
Complex carbohydrates, 13, 15*f*, 281
Conditionally indispensable amino acids, 41-42,
    42*b*
Congenital hypothyroidism, 77*b*
Congestive heart failure, 336-338
Congregate care arrangements, 200
Congregate nutrition services, 198-199
Connective tissue, ascorbic acid in, 93
Constipation, 318
  nutritional management of, 418*t*-419*t*, 420
  during pregnancy, 153
Consumer Education and Research, 202-203
Contamination
  fecal, 216-217
  food, 215-223, 216*f*
Continuing care retirement communities, 200
Continuous ambulatory peritoneal dialysis, 382,
    383*f*
Continuous cyclic peritoneal dialysis, 382, 383*f*
Continuous feeding, 401
Continuous renal replacement therapy (CRRT),
    377
Copper, 128-129, 130*t*
Coronary arteries, 327
Coronary heart disease, 274-275, 275*b*, 327-338
  acute cardiovascular disease, 334-336
  atherosclerosis, 327-334, 328*f*
    dietary recommendations to reduce risk of,
      331-334
    disease process, 327-328, 328*f*
    drug therapy in, 334
    fat metabolism and, 328-330
    risk factors, 330-331, 331*b*
  congestive heart failure, 336-338
  hypertension, 338-343
  Therapeutic Lifestyle Changes (TLC) diet and,
    333
Corticosteroids, 301
Costs
  of dangers, in food fads, 265
  economical buying, 244
  and socioeconomic nutrition disparities. *see*
    Socioeconomics

Cow's milk, 14, 175-176
  human milk *versus*, 162, 162*t*
  summary guidelines for, 177
Crawfish boil, 234
Creatine, as performance enhancer, 286*b*
Creatinine, 377
Creatinine height index, 295
Cretinism, 125
Crohn's disease, 315-316, 315*t*, 316*f*
Cryptosporidium, 220*t*
Cultural considerations
  and acculturation to American diet, 230*b*
  aging composition of the U.S. population, 187*b*,
    188*f*
  American diet, 106*b*
  in bone health, 113*b*
  breastfeeding trends in the United States,
    160*b*-161*b*, 160*f*, 160*t*-161*t*
  cancer, types and incidence, in American
    populations, 412*b*
  continued burden of lead poisoning, 222*b*,
    222*f*
  ethnic differences in lipid metabolism, 38*b*
  ethnicity and sociodemographics, for heart
    disease, 344*b*-345*b*
  food insecurity, 6*b*
  genetics and predisposition for obesity, 252*b*
  growth charts for children, 184*b*
  HIV populations and, 423*b*
  hypermetabolism and hypometabolism, 77*b*
  Id al-Fitr festival, 241, 241*b*
  indispensable amino acids, and complementary
    food proteins, 46*b*
  and kidney transplants, 384*b*
  lactose intolerance, 23*b*
  prescription medications and dietary
    supplement use, 302*b*
  racial differences in calcium retention and peak
    bone mass, 172*b*
  regarding advanced care planning, 404*b*
  social disparities and dental status, 305*b*
  type 2 diabetes, prevalence of, 349*b*
Cultures
  food habits in different, 229-241
    African American, 233, 233*t*
    Asians, 234-235, 237*t*
    Chinese, 234
    French American and Cajun, 233-234, 233*t*
    Greek, 238, 240*t*
    Italian, 236-238, 240*t*
    Japanese, 234
    Mediterranean, 235-238, 240*t*
    Mexican, 230, 231*t*
    Native American, 231-233, 231*t*
    Puerto Rican, 230-231, 231*t*
    Southeast Asian, 234-235, 237*t*
    Spanish, 230-233, 231*t*
  and religious dietary laws, 238-241, 242*t*
  strength of personal, 229
  traditional food patterns, 229-238
Cunningham equation, 284*b*
Cushing's syndrome, 351
Cyanocobalamin, 101
Cyclospora cayetanensis, 220*t*
Cysteine, 119
Cystic fibrosis (CF), 312-314, 314*b*
Cystine stones, 387, 389

D
Daily food plan, for pregnant women, 149*t*
Daily Food Plan for Moms, 163
Daily reference value, 205*b*
Daily values, 205*b*
Dairy. *see also* Milk
  intake for different calorie levels, 260*t*-261*t*
  MyPlate food guidance system
    recommendations and, 8*f*
  as saturated fat, 27-28, 29*f*, 32
DASH diet, 341, 342*t*, 343*b*
Deamination, 42-43
Death rates
  in cancer, 411
  disparities in kidney transplant, 384*b*
  from eating disorders, 268
Deficiency diseases, prevention of, vitamins in,
    84-85
Dehiscence, 393

Dehydration
adverse effects of progressive, 136f
definition of, 135-136
in elderly, 194
nutritional management of, 418t-419t
oral rehydration therapy for, 142b
prevention during exercise, 280
Density, 72
Dental health
in elderly, 194
problems, 304, 305b
Deoxyadenosylcobalamin, 101
Deoxyribonucleic acid (DNA), 411
Depression
in adults, 189-190
benefits of physical activity for, 275b
Designer foods, 108
Dextrins, 22-23
Diabetes mellitus, 347-370
classification of, 347-352
gestational, 349-351, 350b
juvenile-onset, 348
type 1, 347-348, 350t
type 2, 348-349, 349b, 350t
defining factor, 347
diagnosis of, criteria for, 352b
glucose intolerance and, 347-352
insulin, history and discovery of, 348b
kidney disease with, 374, 374b, 374f
long-term complications of, 355-357
dyslipidemia, 356, 357t
heart disease, 356-357
hypertension, 357
nephropathy, 356
neuropathy, 356
retinopathy, 355-356
management of, 357-361
diet management, 365-369, 365t
early detection and monitoring, 357
food distribution, 364-365
goals of care in, 357-361
medical nutrition therapy (MNT), 361-362
nutrient balance, 362-364, 363b
total energy balance, 362
metabolic pattern of, 352-357
blood glucose control in, 353, 353f-354f
energy supply in, 352
pancreatic hormonal control in, 353-355, 354f
nature of, 347-352
self-management education and support, 359-361, 360b
diet and lifestyle management in, 360-361
medications in, 361
monitoring in, 361
problem solving in, 361
reducing risk in, 361
resource awareness in, 361
symptoms of, 352, 352t
uncontrolled, abnormal metabolism in, 355
Dialysate, 377
Dialysis, process, 371
Diarrhea, 316-317
oral rehydration therapy for, 142b
strategies to treat cancer-related, 418, 418t-419t
Diastolic blood pressure, 275, 339
Diet history questionnaire, 293t
Dietary energy intake
estimating, 72
recommendations for, 80
Dietary fiber. see Fiber
Dietary folate equivalencies (DFEs), 99-100
Dietary Guidelines for Americans, 7-10, 9f, 80, 193, 225, 332-333, 333b, 343
on benefits of physical activity, 194-196
for carbohydrates, 24
for fats, 39
meals for children, 180
on physical fitness, 272, 273b
on potassium, 117
for pregnant and lactating women, 147, 148b
for proteins, 52-54
on trans fat avoidance, 30
on weight management, 259
Dietary Reference Intakes (DRIs), 6-7, 80, 147
for adults, 190
for calcium, 112

Dietary Reference Intakes (DRIs) (Continued)
for carbohydrates, 15, 23-24, 25b
energy calculation, 75b
for fats, 39
for iodine, 124
for iron, 120
panels of, 6-7, 7b
for phosphorus, 114
for proteins, 52, 53b
for sodium, 116
for vitamins, 85
for water, 134, 134t
water-soluble. see Water-soluble vitamins
for zinc, 126
Dietary Supplement Health and Education Act (DSHEA), 106
Dietary supplements, 106. see also Minerals; Vitamins
iron for athletes, 282b
during life cycle periods, 107, 131
minerals, 131-132
use of, 292b, 302b
vitamins, 106-108, 172
Diet-drug interactions, 301b
resources for, 301b
Dietetics, 1
Diets
alkaline, 389
chronic dieting syndrome, 256
Dietary Guidelines for Americans, 9f
fad, 107, 252-256
gluten-free, for celiac disease, 320, 321f, 321f
high-protein, 53b, 54t
importance of balanced, 2-3
during lactation, 163
low-fat, for gallbladder disease, 324t
management of, for diabetes mellitus, 360-361, 365-369, 365t
carbohydrate counting in, 365-366
food exchange system in, 366, 366t-367t
sample menu prescription, 2200 kilocalories, 368b
modification, 258-264
during pregnancy, 152
routine house, 396-397, 398t
types of, weight-loss program comparison, 253t-255t
vegetarian, 45-47
types of, 45-46
Diffusion, 64-65, 64f, 140, 140f
Digestion, 56, 57f, 62f
and allergies, 70
basic principles of, 56, 57f
of carbohydrates, 22-23, 60, 66b
chemical, 56-58
gastrointestinal secretions, 57-58
intestinal enzymes, 60
in mouth and esophagus, 58
pancreatic enzymes, 60
in small intestine, 59-60
in stomach, 58-59
chloride in, 118
errors in, 68-70
galactosemia, 68-69
glycogen storage disease, 69
phenylketonuria, 68
of fats, 34-37, 35f, 60
and lactose intolerance, 69
and liver function, 60, 61b
mechanical, 56-58
in mouth and esophagus, 58
in small intestine, 59
in stomach, 58
mineral, 111
muscles in, 56-57
nerves in, 57
of proteins, 47-49, 50f, 60
Digestive secretions
concentration of, 143t
volume of, 142t
Dipeptidase, 49
Dipeptide, 41
Disaccharides, 13f, 13t, 14, 60
lactose, 14
maltose, 14
sucrose, 14

Diseases
increased need for proteins during, 50-51
influencing basal energy expenditure, 76
prevention and health promotion, 1
vitamin supplementation and, 107
Disordered eating, 268-271
Dispensable amino acids, 41-42, 42b
Disproportionately small for gestational age (dSGA), 173
Distal tubule, 372, 372f, 373t
Diuresis, 394
Diuretics
affecting mineral depletion, 131b
and water requirement, 135
Diverticular disease, 317-318, 317f
Diverticulitis, 317
Do-not-resuscitate order, 404b
Doubly labeled water method, 291
Down syndrome, growth charts and, 167
Drug abuse, HIV due to injection, 423b
Drug-nutrient interactions, 311
affecting mineral depletion, 131b
anticonvulsants and nutrient metabolism, 182b
antiestrogens and breast cancer, 417b
antioxidants and chemotherapy, 417b
aspartame and phenylketonuria, 43b
aspirin and iron absorption, 394b
classification of, 300t
drug-resistant Escherichia coli, 217b
exenatide and glucose control, 359b
grapefruit juice and drug metabolism, 341b
herbs, 301
hyperemesis gravidarum, 153b
immunosuppressive therapies after kidney transplantation, 383b-384b
introduction to, 3b
iron supplementation, 282b
medication use in the adult, 198b
Orlistat and, 256-257, 257b
phytic acid and mineral absorption, 17b
polypharmacy by older adults, 300
propofol and lipids, 403b
proton pump inhibitors and micronutrient absorption, 311b
Questran and bile, 36b
tetracycline and mineral absorption, 311b
on water and electrolyte balance, 135b
Drugs
for diabetes mellitus, 365
for peptic ulcer disease, 310-311
as pregnancy risk factor, 156
weight loss, 256-257
Dry beans. see Legumes
Dry mouth, 138
Dual-energy x-ray absorptiometry (DEXA), 248, 248f
Dumping syndrome, 257, 405
Dynamic equilibrium, 133
Dysbiosis, 318
Dyslipidemia, 330, 356, 357t
Dysphagia, 306-307

E
Early-onset obesity, 250
Eating disorders
during adolescence, 184
anorexia nervosa, 268-270, 269b
APA diagnostic criteria and, 269b
binge eating disorder, 262b, 268, 269b, 270
bulimia nervosa, 268, 269b, 270
and female athlete triad, 283b
not otherwise specified, 268, 269b
Eating habits. see also Food habits
behavior modification, 258
in different cultures. see Cultures
Eating patterns. see also Food patterns
of adolescents, 184
changing behaviors, 259, 259b, 262b
and Dietary Guidelines for Americans, 9f
Eclampsia, 157
Edema
with low protein levels, 393
with nephron diseases, 375, 375t
from water intoxication, 136, 136f
Eggs
calcium in, 114t
cobalamin in, 102t

Eggs (Continued)
   folate in, 100t
   iron in, 124t
   niacin in, 98t
   pantothenic acid in, 103t
   potassium in, 118t
   pyridoxine in, 99t
   riboflavin in, 97t
   as saturated fat, 27-28, 29f, 32
   thiamin in, 96t
   vitamin A in, 87t
   vitamin D in, 90t
   vitamin E in, 91t
   zinc in, 127t
Eicosanoids, 31
Eicosapentaenoic acid, 417
Elderly. see Older adults
Electrolytes, 138-139
   balance, 133-146
     drug effects on, 135b
     with kidney disease, 378
   in digestion, 58
   in digestive fluids, 143t
   needed for burn patients, 409
   and postoperative wound healing, 394-395
   tests during nutrition care process, 295
Elemental formula, 316, 392
Emotional needs, food and, 265
Empty calories, 21, 72
Emulsifier, 34
Endocrine system, functions of kidneys, 373
Endorphins, 277
End-stage renal disease (ESRD), 371
   disease process of, 380
   hemodialysis for, 380-381, 380f-381f
   kidney transplantation for, 382-385, 384b, 384f
   medical nutrition therapy for, 380-385
   peritoneal dialysis for, 382, 383f
Energy
   balance, 71-82, 263
     basal energy expenditure in, 73-76
     case study on, 78b
     components, 259-262
     energy intake and, 72-73
     equations for estimating resting energy
       needs, 75b
     estimated energy requirement in, 79b
     output in, 73-79
     physical activity in, 76-77
     resting energy expenditure in, 73-74, 73f-74f
     thermic effect of food in, 77
     total energy expenditure in, 77-79, 78f
   and blood glucose control, 352-355, 353f
   catabolism and anabolism, 66-67
   Dietary Guidelines for Americans
     recommendations, 80
   dietary reference intake recommendations for,
     80, 81t
   for exercise needs, 280-281
   extra, storage of, 67-68
   fat as fuel for, 31
   food sources of, 71-72
   imbalance over time, 78b
   interwoven influence among, 251f
   and kilocalorie, 12
   measurement of, 71
   MyPlate and, 80
   needs, 71
     in burn patients, 409, 409t
     for cancer patients, 416
     for growth, 167-171
     with kidney disease, 377, 379, 381, 385t
     during lactation, 163
     postoperative, 393
     during pregnancy, 147-148
     preoperative reserves, 391
   and nutrient stores, 280-281
   and obesity, 250
   protein as fuel for, 44
   sources of, 3-4
   stored, 72-73
   total, 282-283
   vitamins and minerals needs, 281
   and weight management, 250
Energy density, 72
Energy metabolism, phosphorus in, 114
Enriched grain, 15

Enteral feeding
   advantages following surgery, 399-401
   definition of, 390
   determining during nutrition care process,
     298-299
   formula, 400
   monitoring patient for, 401b
   with mouth, throat, and neck surgery, 404-405
   problem-solving tips for, 402t
   routes of, 399, 399f
   types of, 399f
Enteral nutrition support, for cancer patients, 420
Enterohepatic circulation, 35-36
Enterokinase, 49, 60
Environment, and water requirement, 134
Environmental food contaminants, 219-223
Environmental Protection Agency, on food safety
     regulations, 203t
Enzymes
   in digestion, 57
   intestinal, 60
   metabolic functions of, 44
   from pancreas, role in fat digestion, 34-35,
     35f-36f
   pancreatic, 60
   pepsin, 59
   role of
     in carbohydrate digestion, 22-23
     in protein digestion, 47, 50f
   from small intestine, role in fat digestion, 35
   from stomach, in digestion, 59
   from vitamins, 84
   zinc and, 126
Epilepsy, 182b
Ergocalciferol, 87
Ergogenic, 285, 286b
Erroneous claims, of food misinformation and
    fads, 264-265
   dangers and, 264-265
Erythropoietin, 373
Escherich, Theodor, 216-217
Escherichia coli, 216-217, 220t
   drug-resistant, 217b
Esophageal varices, 322
Esophagitis, 307
Esophagostomy, 399
Esophagus
   in digestion, 58
   diseases/disorders of, 307-308
     central tube disorders, 307
     esophageal varices, 322
     esophagitis, 307
     gastroesophageal reflux disease, 307-308,
       308f, 308t
     hiatal hernia, 308, 309f
     lower esophageal sphincter defects, 307
Essential fatty acids, 29-30
   deficiency in, 38
Essential hypertension, 338-343
Estimated Average Requirement, 7
Estimated energy requirements (EER), 79b
Estrogen, 111
   antiestrogens and breast cancer, 417b
Ethnicity. see also Cultural considerations
   and abnormal thyroid function, 344b-345b
   growth charts for children, 184b
   and lipid metabolism, 38b
   and sociodemographics, for heart disease,
     344b-345b
Etiology, definition of, 297-298
Euvolemia, 393
Evaluation, in nutrition care process model,
    299-300
Excess supplementation, of adults, 193
Exclusively breastfed, 158
Excretion, 373
Exenatide, glucose control and, 359b
Exercise
   behaviors, 259-262
   dietary needs during, 279-281
   energy and, 76, 285
   expenditure per hour, 278t
   health benefits of, 273
     for blood lipid levels, 274, 275b
     for bone disease, 275b, 277
     for depression, 275b
     for diabetes mellitus, 275, 275b, 364, 364t

Exercise (Continued)
     for heart muscle function, 274
     for hypertension, 275, 275b
     for mental health, 275b, 277
     for oxygen-carrying capacity (VO$_2$ max), 275,
       275b
     for weight management, 275, 275b
   intensity, frequency and duration components,
     272
   PA coefficient and, 75b
   during pregnancy, 152
   preparation and care, 279
   source of energy for, 277t
   treadmill stress test, 334, 334f
   voluntary, 71
Exogenous insulin, 348
Expanded-criteria donors, 382
Extension services, for older Americans, 199
External energy cycle, 72
Extracellular fluid (ECF), and water balance, 137,
    137f, 137t
Extremely low birth weight (ELBW) infant, 173
Extrusion reflex, 177
Exudate, 393
Eyes, signs of nutrient imbalance in, 296t-297t

F
Facilitated diffusion, 64f, 65, 140
Fad diets, 107, 252-256
Failure to thrive, 181-182
   in adults, 189-190
Familial hypercholesterolemia, 330
Familial hypertriglyceridemia, 330
Family history
   and cardiovascular disease, 330
   and chronic kidney disease, 374b
Family reinforcement, as genetic and
    environmental factors, 251
Fast food, 30
Fasting, 256
Fasting glucose, tests during nutrition care
    process, 295
Fat substitutes, 32
Fats, 27-40, 281
   absorption of, 35-37, 37f, 60-63
   American diet consumption of, 106b
   animal, 32-33
   average intake of, 38b
   in the body, 32
   and cancer, 421
   and chylomicrons, 36-37, 36f
   dietary, recommendations for, 37-39
   Dietary Guidelines for Americans on, 9f, 24, 39
   dietary importance of, 27
   Dietary Reference Intakes for, 39
   digestion of, 34-37, 35f, 60
   energy provided by, 4, 284
   food label information for, 33-34, 33t, 34f
   food sources of, 32-33
     characteristics of, 33
     digestibility of, 37
     variety in, 32-33
   functions of, 31-32
     as energy source, 31
     as essential nutrient, 31
     flavor and satisfaction as, 32
   and health problems, 37-38
     amount of fats in, 37
     type of, 37
   and kidney stones, 387
   in lacto-ovo-vegetarian diet pyramid, 47f
   lipogenesis, 68
   metabolism of, 328-330
     cholesterol in, 328-329, 330t
     lipoproteins, 329-330, 329f, 330t
     role of carbohydrates in, 21
     triglycerides, 330, 330t
   micelle formation, 35-36
   nature of, 27-31
   needs, of adults, 191
   in nutrient balance, 263
     for diabetes mellitus, 364
   plant, 33
   and post-surgery healing, 393
   recommended intake of, 4, 4f
   structure and classes of, 27
   in uncontrolled diabetes, 355

Fats (Continued)
  vitamin A in, 87t
  vitamin D in, 90t
  vitamin E in, 91t
Fat-soluble vitamins, 85, 93t
  vitamin A (retinol), 85-87, 86b, 86f, 87t
  vitamin D (calciferol), 87-89, 88f-89f, 90t
  vitamin E (tocopherol), 89-91, 91f, 91t, 92b
  vitamin K, 91-92, 92t
Fatty acids, 27
  classification of, 27-31, 28f
  Dietary Guidelines for Americans, 9f
  tissue-building function of, 4
Fatty liver disease, 321
  from choline deficiency, 103
FDA. see Food and Drug Administration (FDA)
Fecal contamination, 216-217
Federal Food Safety Regulations, enforcement of, 202, 203t
Federal Trade Commission, on food safety regulations, 203t
Feeding
  commercial formula, 174-175
  determining method of, 298-299
  older adults with sensitivity, 194b
  physiologic delays relevant to, 173
  for premature infants, 173-174
Feeding America, 6
Feeding Infant and Toddlers Study (FITS), 179b
Feeding Made Simple, 179b, 182-183
Female athlete triad, 281, 283b
Females. see Women
Ferritin, 120, 122f
Fetal alcohol spectrum disorders, 154-156
Fetal alcohol syndrome (FAS), 154, 156f
Fetus, growth of, protein needs, 148
Fever blisters, 305
Fiber, 16, 65
  and cancer, 421
  case study for identifying, 17b
  classes of, 16, 16t
  health benefits of, 20b
  in nutrient balance, for diabetes mellitus, 363-364
  recommended daily intake of, 19
  regulation and control functions of, 5
  soluble and insoluble, 16t
Fiber-restricted diet, 392t
Fibrin, 112
Fight-or-flight reflexes, metabolic rate and, 76
Filé powder, 234
Filipino, food habits/traditions, 237t
Filippo, Pacini, 217
Filtration
  function of kidney, 373
  and water balance, 141
Fish
  calcium in, 114t
  and cancer, 421
  cobalamin in, 102t
  Dietary Guidelines for Americans on, 9f
  folate in, 100t
  iron in, 124t
  niacin in, 98t
  pantothenic acid in, 103t
  potassium in, 118t
  pyridoxine in, 99t
  riboflavin in, 97t
  thiamin in, 96t
  as unsaturated dietary fat, 28, 29f
  vitamin A in, 87t
  vitamin D in, 90t
  vitamin E in, 91t
  zinc in, 127t
Fish oil, 420
Fistulas, 414
Flatulence, 66b
Flavor
  additives to improve, 211t-212t
  from fats, 32
Flexibility, 274f, 277
Fluids
  cancer-related dehydration, 418t-419t
  during lactation, 163
  needs
    of adults, 192
    for burn patients, 408-409

Fluids (Continued)
  for cancer patients, 418
  during hemodialysis, 382
  for hydration when exercising, 280
  for kidney disease patients, 280, 377-379, 382, 385t, 388
  and postoperative wound healing, 394
Fluoride, 128, 128f, 130t
  supplementation, 178
Fluorosis, 128, 128f
Folacin, 104t
Folate, 99-101, 100f, 100t, 104t
  needs
    during hemodialysis, 382
    during pregnancy, 150-151
    postoperative needs for, 394
Folic acid, 104t
Food, 3
  buying and handling practices, 225-226
  definition of, 228
  functional, 108, 108b
  functions of nutrients in, 3-5
  guides and recommendations for, 7-10
  misinformation and fads, 264-266
  needs and costs, 223-226
  water content of, 138t
Food additives, 210, 211t-212t
Food allergies, 319-320. see also Allergens
Food and Drug Administration (FDA), 202-203, 266
  on cancer-related health claims, 421
  enforcement duties of, 202
  food label information
    on cancer risk, 421
    on fats, 33, 33t, 34f
  on food safety regulations, 203t
  health claim approval by, 205b, 207
  on weight loss drugs, 256
Food and Nutrition Science Alliance, 266, 266b
Food assistance programs, 224-225
Food choices, factors that influence personal, 228-229, 229b
  economic, 229
  food and psychosocial, 228
  marketing and environmental, 229
  psychologic, 228
Food combinations, 264
Food contamination, 215-223, 216f
Food costs. see Costs
Food diaries, 259
Food environment, changing, 10
Food exchange system, for diabetes mellitus, 366, 367t
Food fads, 264-265
  claims, types of, 264
Food frequency questionnaires, 293t
Food guides, 264
  Canada, 235f
  China, Japan, and Korea, 236f
  for health promotion, 5-10
  for hypertension, 343-344
  for Mexico and Puerto Rico, 232f
  Southern Arizona American Indian Food Guide, 232f
Food habits, 228-244. see also Eating habits
  cultural development of, 229-241
  economic influences on, 228-229
  psychologic influences on, 228-229
  social influences on, 228-229, 229b
Food insecurity, 6b, 182, 223
Food intolerances, 319
Food jag, 178
Food label information
  on cancer risk, 421
  on fats, 33-34, 33t, 34f
Food labels, 203-207
  current format of, 204-207
    front-of-package labeling, 205-207, 206f
    health claims, 205b, 207
    nutrition facts label, 204-205, 204f, 205b
  food standards and, 203
  nutrition information, 203
  regulations
    early development of, 203
    U.S. Food and Drug Administration on, 203-204

Food market, distrust of, in food fads, 265
Food neophobia, 228
Food patterns. see also Eating patterns
  aging effect on, 191
  alternative, during pregnancy, 152
Food poisoning, bacterial, 217-219
  clostridial, 218-219
  staphylococcal, 217-218
Food safety
  actions for, 212, 213f
  for adults, 192-193
  buying and storing food, 212, 214t-215t
  "Fight BAC!", 213f
  health promotion and, 202-207
  preparing and serving food, 213
Food Safety and Inspection Service, on food safety regulations, 203t
Food sources
  of calcium, 113-114, 114t, 115b, 115f
  of carbohydrates, 21, 37
  of chloride, 119
  of energy, 3-4, 71-72
  of fats, 32-33
    digestibility of, 37
    variety in, 32-33
  of folate, 100t
  of iodine, 125
  of iron, 123f, 123t-124t
  of magnesium, 119
  of niacin, 98t
  of pantothenic acid, 103t
  of phosphorus, 116
  of potassium, 118t
  of proteins, 44-47, 45f, 46b, 47f, 48t, 149
  of pyridoxine, 99t
  of riboflavin, 97t
  of selenium, 128
  of sodium, 117
  of sulfur, 120
  of thiamin, 96t
  of vitamin A, 87, 87t
  of vitamin B_{12} (cobalamin), 102t
  of vitamin C, 95t
  of vitamin D, 89, 90t
  of vitamin E, 91t
  of vitamin K, 92t
  of zinc, 127, 127t
Food standards, 203
  organic, 208b
Food supply
  community, 202-227
  food assistance programs, 224-225
  hunger and malnutrition, 223-224
  Nutrition Services Incentive Program, 225
  school meals program, 225
Food technology, 207-210
  agricultural pesticides, 207-210
  biotechnology, 208-209, 209f
  food additives, 210, 211t-212t
  irradiation, 209-210, 210f
  organic farming, 207-208
Food-borne disease, 210-223, 220t
  bacterial food infections, 215-217
  bacterial food poisoning, 217-219
  environmental food contaminants, 219-223
  food contamination and, 215-223, 216f
  food safety and, 212-213
    buying and storing food, 212, 214t-215t
    preparing and serving food, 213
  parasites, 219
  prevalence of, 210, 213f
  viruses, 219
Food-drug interactions, 301b
Football players, body mass index versus overweight, 245-246
Forearm arteriovenous fistula, 381f
Formulas
  elemental, 316, 392
  enteral feeding, 400
  general food supplement, 395-396
  high-protein, high-kilocalorie liquid formulas, 305t
  infant
    versus breastfeeding, 163
    choosing, 174
    feeding, 174-175

Formulas *(Continued)*
    iron-fortified, 177
    preparing, 174
    polymeric, 316
Fortified foods, 15
Free radicals, 84, 95*b*
French American and Cajun, food habits, 233-234, 233*t*
Front-of-package labeling, 205-207, 206*f*
Fructose, 14, 14*f*
Fruits
    American diet deficiency in, 106*b*
    calcium in, 114*t*
    and cancer, 421
    Dietary Guidelines for Americans on, 9*f*
    folate in, 100*t*
    intake for different calorie levels, 260*t*-261*t*
    iron in, 124*t*
    in lacto-ovo-vegetarian diet pyramid, 47*f*
    pantothenic acid in, 103*t*
    potassium in, 118*t*
    pyridoxine in, 99*t*
    recommended servings, 19
    vitamin A in, 87*t*
    vitamin C in, 95*t*
    vitamin E in, 91*t*
Fuel factors, 72
Fuel sources, 279-280
Functional food categories, 108, 108*b*
Functional losses, and water requirement, 135
Fusion inhibitor, 427*t*-429*t*

G
Galactose, 14
Galactosemia, 68-69
Gallbladder
    disease in, 324-325
    role in fat digestion, 34, 35*f*
    surgery of, 407, 407*f*
Gallstones, 324
Gastrectomy, 405, 406*b*
Gastric cancer, recent research findings regarding, 422
Gastric glands, 61*f*
Gastric ulcer, peptic ulcer and, 308-309, 309*f*, 310*b*
Gastrin, 59
Gastroesophageal reflux disease (GERD), 307-308, 308*f*, 308*t*
Gastrointestinal accessory organs, 320-325
    gallbladder disease, 324-325
        cholecystitis and cholelithiasis, 324-325, 324*t*
    liver disease, 321-324
        cirrhosis, 322-324, 323*f*
        fatty, 321
        hepatitis, 321-322, 322*b*
    pancreatic disease, 325
    pancreatitis, 325
Gastrointestinal circulation, in water balance, 141-143
Gastrointestinal system
    function of, tests during nutrition care process, 295
    motility, 56-57
    problems
        in elderly, 193-194
        during pregnancy, 152-153
    surgery for, 404-408
        bariatric surgery, 405-407, 406*b*
        dumping syndrome, 405
        gallbladder surgery, 407, 407*f*
        gastrectomy, 405, 406*b*
        gastric surgery, 405
        intestinal surgery, 407-408, 407*f*
        mouth, throat, and neck surgery, 404-405
        rectal surgery, 408
Gastrointestinal tract
    complications with chemotherapy, 414
    diseases/disorders of
        lower. *see* Lower gastrointestinal (GI) tract
        upper. *see* Upper gastrointestinal (GI) tract
Gastroscopy, 310
Gender
    bone health and, 113*b*
    predisposition for obesity and, 252*b*
General food supplement formula, 395-396

Genetic defects, 374
    in digestion and metabolism, 68-69
        galactosemia, 68-69
        glycogen storage disease, 69
        phenylketonuria, 68
Genetically modified (GM) foods, 209, 209*f*
Genetics
    and environmental factors, 250-252
    and predisposition for obesity, 250-251, 252*b*
Gerontological Society of America, 199
Gestational age, 173
Gestational diabetes mellitus (GDM), 158, 349-351, 350*b*
Gestational hypertension, 157
Ghrelin, 250
Giardiasis, 219
Gingivitis, 304, 305*f*
Globulin, 139
Glomerular filtration rate (GFR), 372, 378*t*
Glomerulus, 371-372, 372*f*
    definition of, 371
Glossitis, 305, 305*f*
Glucagon, 44, 354
β-Glucans, 16*t*
Gluconeogenesis, 68
Glucose, 14. *see also* Blood glucose
    control, exenatide and, 359*b*
    metabolism of, 120
    tolerance in, impaired, 351-352
    in uncontrolled diabetes, 355, 355*f*
Glucose intolerance, diabetes mellitus and, 347-352
GLUT4, 355
Glutamine, 417
Gluten, 320
Gluten-free diet, for celiac disease, 320, 321*f*, 321*t*
Glycemic control, in diabetes mellitus, 347, 364, 364*t*
    medication and, 357-358
Glycemic index, in nutrient balance, for diabetes mellitus, 363
Glycerides, 27
Glycogen, 13-20
    in blood glucose, 353
    as energy storage, 73
    liver storage of, 67-68
    as quick energy storage, 4
    stores of, in liver, 21
Glycogen loading, 284
Glycogen storage disease, 69
Glycogenesis, 67-68
Glycolipid, 30-32
Goiter, 124-125, 125*f*
Gout, 387
Grains
    intake for different calorie levels, 260*t*-261*t*
    in lacto-ovo-vegetarian diet pyramid, 47*f*
Greek, food habits/traditions, 238, 240*t*
Growth and development, 166-167
    adolescence, 166
    adulthood, 166
        continuing, 186-190
        physical growth during, 188-189
        shaping influences in, 187-190
    and basal energy expenditure, 75-76
    childhood, 166
        growth measurement, 166-167
        preschool-aged children, 178
        psychosocial development, 167
        school-aged children, 178
        toddlers, 178
    dietary energy intake during, 80, 80*t*
    infancy, 166
    life cycle growth pattern, 166
    nutritional requirements for, 167-172
        energy needs, 167-171
        mineral and vitamin needs, 171-172
        protein needs, 171
        water requirements, 171, 171*t*
    positive nitrogen balance in, 43
Growth charts, 167, 168*f*-169*f*
    for children, 184*b*
    with special health care needs, 167
    use and interpretation of, 170*b*
Growth hormone, 76, 286*b*
Gums, 16*t*

Gustatory distress, 402*t*
Gynecomastia, 287

H
Hair
    signs of nutrient imbalance in, 296*t*-297*t*
    sulfur and, 119
Hair follicle, 414
Hamwi method, 249
Harmful foods, 264
Harris-Benedict equation, 74, 75*b*, 282-283
Hazard Analysis & Critical Control Point (HACCP), 213
Healing
    balance nutrition and, 413
    increased need for proteins during, 50-51, 392-393
Health, 1-2
    and balanced diet, 3
    danger to, 265
    defined, 1-4
    traditional and preventive approaches to, 2
Health care, impact on, 186-187
Health care team, in nutrition care process, 288-290
Health promotion, 1-3
    basic definitions regarding, 1-2
    and decreasing dietary fats, 38-39
    and disease prevention, 193-197
    food safety and, 202-207
    and goals of *Healthy People 2020*, 2*f*
    importance in nutrition science, 1
    nutrient and food guides for, 5-10
Healthy People 2020
    on breastfeeding, 159
    goal regarding cancer, 412*b*
    goals for physical fitness, 272, 273*b*
    goals of, 2, 2*f*
    health promotion goals of, 186
Heart, signs of nutrient imbalance in, 296*t*-297*t*
Heart disease. *see also* Coronary heart disease
    and diabetes, 356-357
    and fats, 38-39
    and Mediterranean diet, 239*b*
    modifiable risk factors for, 332*b*
Heartburn, 58
    during pregnancy, 153
Height
    assessment during nutrition care process, 294
    median values according to age and gender, 81*t*
Height/weight tables, standard, 248-249
Heimlich maneuver, 306
Helicobacter pylori, in peptic ulcer disease, 309, 309*f*, 310*b*
Hematuria, with nephron diseases, 375, 375*t*
Heme iron, 123, 123*t*
Hemicellulose, 16*t*, 17
Hemochromatosis, 122-123
Hemodialysis, 380-381, 380*f*-381*f*
Hemoglobin, 110
    synthesis of, iron in, 120
Hemolytic uremic syndrome, 217
Hemorrhoids, 153
Hepatic encephalopathy, 322
Hepatitis, 219, 321-322, 322*b*
Hepatitis A, 220*t*
Herbs, and drug interactions, 301
Herpes simplex virus, in mouth ulcers, 305
Hiatal hernia, 58, 308, 309*f*
Hiatus, 308
High blood pressure, benefits of exercise for prevention of, 275*b*
High-density lipoproteins (HDLs), 30, 329-330, 329*f*
    composition of, 31*f*
    reduction in, 38
High-fructose sugars, U.S. consumption of, 14, 14*f*, 21
Highly active antiretroviral therapy (HAART), 426, 431*b*
High-oxalate foods and drinks, 387*b*
High-protein diets, 53*b*, 54*t*
Hindus, vegetarian diets of, 45
Hispanics. *see* Cultural considerations; Cultures
Histamine H2-receptor antagonists, for peptic ulcer disease, 310

Home-delivered meals, 199
Homeostasis, and water balance, 133
Honey, for infants, 177
Hormones
    changes with aging, 190-191
    controls, and water balance, 143-144
    mammary glands, 159-161
    secretions during digestion, 59-60, 61f
    status, influencing basal energy expenditure, 76
24-hour food recall, 293t
Human immunodeficiency virus (HIV)
    evolution of, 422-423
    medical management of, 425-430
        drug therapy, 426-430, 427t-429t
        initial evaluation and goals, 425-426, 426b
        vaccine development, 426-430
    medical nutrition therapy for, 430-432
        ABCDEFs of nutrition assessment, 430b
        assessment of, 430
        intervention of, 430
        lipodystrophy, 431, 431b
        nutrition counseling, education, and
            supportive care, 431-432
    opportunistic infections and, 425b
    parasitic nature of, 423-425
    population and, 423b
    progression of, 422-425
    transmission and stages of, 423-424, 424f
    types and incidence of, in American
        populations, 423b
Human milk, 174
    versus breast milk substitutes, 184b
    versus cow's milk, 162, 162t
    fortifiers, 173
    lactose in, 14
    nutritional values of, 175t
Hunger, malnutrition and, 223-224
Hydration, of athletes, 280b, 285
Hydrochloric acid
    in digestion, 57
    in protein digestion, 47-48, 50f
Hydrogenation, 30
Hydrophilic molecules, 30
Hydrophobic molecules, 30
Hydrostatic pressure, 141
Hydrostatic weighing, 247
1α-hydroxylase, 88, 88f
Hydroxylysine, 93
β-Hydroxymethylbutyrate (HMB), 286b
Hydroxyproline, 93
Hypercalcemia, 113, 387
Hypercalciuria, 387
Hypercholesterolemia, 328
Hyperemesis gravidarum, 153, 157
    drug-nutrient interaction, 153b
Hyperglycemia, 347
    symptoms of, 369t
Hyperhomocysteinemia, 99
Hyperkalemia, 118
Hyperlipidemia, 27
Hypermetabolism, 77b
Hypernatremia, 117
Hyperoxaluria, 387
Hyperphosphatemia, 116
Hypertension
    benefits of physical activity for, 275, 275b
    blood pressure levels, 339-340, 339t
    as coronary heart disease, 338-343
    diabetes and, 357
    education and prevention for, 343-344
        education principles, 344, 344b-345b,
            344f-345f
        practical food guides, 343-344
    with kidney disease, 379
    medical nutrition therapy for, 340-343
        DASH diet, 341, 342t, 343b
        physical activity, 340-341
        sodium control, 343
        weight management, 340
    prehypertension, 339-340, 340t
    resistant, 343
    stage 1, 340
    stage 2, 340, 341b
Hypertensive disorders of pregnancy, 157-158
Hyperthyroidism, 77b, 125
    and underweight, 266
Hypertriglyceridemia, 330

Hyperuricosuria, 387
Hypervitaminosis A, 86-87
Hypocalcemia, 112
Hypocitraturia, 387
Hypogeusia, 126
Hypoglycemia, 354, 366
    avoiding during exercise, 281
    symptoms of, 369t
Hypoglycemic agents, 301, 358, 360t
Hypokalemia, 117
Hypomagnesemia, 119
Hypometabolism, 77b
Hyponatremia, 116
Hypophosphatemia, 114
Hyposmia, 126
Hypotension, 376
Hypothyroidism, 77b
    and iodine, 125
    and levothyroxine absorption, 76b
Hypovolemia, 143

I
Ibuprofen, in peptic ulcer disease, 309
Id al-Fitr festival, 241, 241b
Idiopathic diseases, 315
Ileostomy, 407-408, 407f
Illness
    and blood glucose control, 368
    increased need for proteins during, 50-51
Immune cells, vitamin A in, 85-86
Immune system
    balanced nutrition supporting, 413
    and cancer, 412-413, 413f
    protein functions in, 44
    T cells and B cells, 412-413
    zinc in, 126
Immunocompetence, 413
Immunosuppressive therapies, after kidney
    transplantation, 383b-384b
Incomplete proteins, 45
Indispensable amino acids, 41-42, 42b
Individual variation, of weight, 249
"Infant and Young Child Feeding", 164
Infants
    caloric allowance for, 80t
    classifications of, 173
        maturity, 173
        size for gestational age, 173
        weight, 173
    height measurement of, 294f
    learning how to eat, 177b, 177f
    life cycle growth pattern of, 166
    mature, feeding, 174-178
    nutrition requirements of, 173-178
    positive nitrogen balance in, 43
    vitamin supplementation for, 107
    weaning, 175
Infarct, 327-328
Infarction, 334
Infection, protein needs for resisting, 393
Inflammatory bowel disease (IBD), 315-316
Inhalation toxicity, 129
Insulin, 44
    control in, 353-354
    definition of, 347
    exogenous, 348
    history and discovery of, 348b
    pen, 358f
    pump, 358f
    release of, potassium in, 117
    types of, 357-358, 358t, 359b, 359f
Integrase inhibitor, 427t-429t
Intensity, component of exercise, 272
Intermediate-density lipoproteins (IDLs), 329,
    329f
Internal energy cycle, 72
Intervention, nutrition, in nutrition care process
    model, 298-299
Intestinal enzymes, in digestion, 60
Intestinal glands, 60, 61f
Intestinal surgery, 407-408, 407f
Intestinal wall, 49
    surface, absorption in, 63-64
Intracellular fluid (ICF), and water balance, 137,
    137f, 137t
Intramural nerve plexus, 57
Intrauterine growth restriction (IUGR), 157

Invisible fat, 33
Iodine, 77b, 123-125, 124f-125f, 130t
Iodine uptake levels, 74
Ionic composition, of body fluid compartment,
    116f
Ions, 138-139
Iron, 120-123, 130t
    absorption and aspirin, 394b
    concerns for vegetarians, 46-47, 48t
    deficiency, 120
    food sources of, 123, 123f, 123t-124t
    functions of, 120
    needs
        for growth, 172
        during pregnancy, 150
    requirements, 120
    supplementation in athletes, 282b
    toxicity of, 122-123
Iron-deficiency anemia
    in athletes, 282b
    causes of, 120
    following surgery, 394
    mineral supplementation for, 131
Irradiation, 209-210, 210f
Irritable bowel syndrome (IBS), 318
Islets of Langerhans, 353, 354f
Italian, food habits/traditions, 236-238, 240t

J
Japanese
    food guides, 236f
    food habits/traditions, 234, 237t
Jaw, fractured, surgical procedures in, 304, 305t
Jejunostomy tube, 399
Jewish, dietary laws, 238-240
Joule (J), 71
"Junk foods", 263-264
Juvenile-onset diabetes, 348

K
Kashin-Bek disease, 127
Keratin, 119
Keshan disease, 127
Ketoacidosis, 352
Ketones, 355
Ketosis, 21, 376
Kidney
    anatomy and structures of, 371-373, 372f
        Bowman's capsule, 371-372, 372f
        collecting duct, 373t
        collecting tubule, 372-373
        distal tubule, 372, 372f, 373t
        glomerulus, 371-372, 372f
        loop of Henle, 372, 372f, 373t
        nephron, 371, 372f, 373t
        proximal tubule, 372, 372f, 373t
    disease. see Kidney disease
    failure. see Kidney disease
    functions of
        endocrine, 373
        excretory and regulatory, 373
    and water balance, 143
Kidney disease, 371-389
    acute kidney injury, 376-378
    chronic kidney disease, 378-379
        case study of, 380b
        medical nutrition therapy, 379, 385t
        signs and symptoms of, 379
        stages of, 378, 378t, 385t
    end-stage renal disease, 371
        disease process, 380
        hemodialysis for, 380-381, 380f-381f
        medical nutrition therapy for, 380-385
        peritoneal dialysis, 382, 383f
        transplantation for, 382-385, 384b, 384f
    kidney stone disease. see Kidney stones
    nephron diseases
        acute glomerulonephritis, 375, 375t
        nephritic syndrome, 375, 375t
        nephrotic syndrome, 375-376, 375t
    process and dietary considerations
        bacterial urinary tract infection, 373-374, 374b
        causes of, 373-374, 374b
        diabetes mellitus, 374, 374b, 374f
        genetic or congenital defects, 374
        infection and obstruction, 373-374
        kidney stone obstruction, 373-374, 374b

Kidney disease (Continued)
  medical nutrition therapy, 375
    risk factors for, 374, 374b
    urinary tract infection, 373-374, 374b
  renal calculi, 386f
Kidney stones
  calcium stones, 386f, 387-389
  cystine stones, 387, 389
  medical nutrition therapy for, 388-389, 388t
  obstruction from, 373-374, 374b
  risk factors for developing, 386b
  struvite stones, 386f, 387
  uric acid stones, 386f, 387, 389
Kidney transplantation, 382-385, 384b, 384f
Kilocalories (kcal)
  adjustment necessary for weight loss, 263b
  allowances from birth to 18 years, 80t
  balance, Dietary Guidelines for Americans, 9f
  changing food behaviors, 262b
  definitions of, 3
    and energy, 12
  and energy, 71
  energy expenditure during various activities, 78t
  and nutrient density, 72
Kilojoules, conversion of, 71
Kinesiotherapist, 289
Korean food guides, 236f
Kosher rules, 238
Krebs cycle, 67
Kwashiorkor, 44, 51, 52f

L
Laboratory tests
  blood glucose test, 352
  complete blood count, 295
  liver enzymes, 295
Lactated Ringer's solution, 408
Lactation, 158-164. see also Breastfeeding
  mineral supplements during, 131
  nutrition and lifestyle needs of, 163
  physiologic process of, 159-163
  positive nitrogen balance in, 43
  recommended energy intake during, 81t
  supply and demand in, 161-162
  trends in, 158-159, 159f
  vitamin supplementation during, 107
Lactation specialist, 163
Lacto-ovo-vegetarian diet pyramid, 46, 47f
Lactose intolerance, 23b, 69
  drug absorption and, 76b
Lacto-vegetarians, 45
Laparoscopic cholecystectomy, 407
Laparoscopic fundoplication, 308
Large for gestational age (LGA), 173
Large intestine
  absorption in, 65
  disease in, 317-318
    constipation, 318
    diverticular disease, 317-318, 317f
    irritable bowel syndrome, 318
Latinos. see Cultural considerations; Cultures
Law of isotonicity, 142
Lead poisoning, 219, 222b
  in childhood, 183
Lean body mass, influencing basal energy
  expenditure, 75
Lecithin, 30-31
Lecithinase, 35
Legumes
  calcium in, 114t
  and cancer, 421
  cobalamin in, 102t
  and daily fiber recommendations, 19
  folate in, 100t
  iron in, 124t
  in lacto-ovo-vegetarian diet pyramid, 47f
  niacin in, 98t
  pantothenic acid in, 103t
  potassium in, 118t
  pyridoxine in, 99t
  riboflavin in, 97t
  thiamin in, 96t
  vitamin A in, 87t
  vitamin D in, 90t
  vitamin E in, 91t
  zinc in, 127t
Leptin, 250

Let-down reflex, 162f
Levothyroxine, absorption of, 76b
Life cycle. see also Growth and development
  dietary energy intake in, 80
  energy expenditure in, 81t
  mineral supplements in, 131
  vitamin supplementation in, 107
Life expectancy, 186
  and good nutrition, 2-3
Lifestyle
  and cancer risk, 420-421
  and hypertension, 339-340, 340t, 343
  and lactation, 163
  management of, for diabetes mellitus, 360-361
  physical activity pyramid, 274f
Lignin, 16-17, 16t
Limeys, 83
Linoleic acid, 28f, 29-30
  DRI for, 39
Lipase, 34, 44, 58, 60
  pancreatic, 60
Lipectomy, 258
Lipids, 27
  and cancer, 421
  classification of, 27-31, 28f
    cholesterol, 29-30
    lipoproteins, 30, 30f
    monounsaturated fats, 28, 28f-29f
    phospholipids, 30-31, 31f
      eicosanoids, 31
      lecithin, 30-31
    polyunsaturated fats, 28, 28f-29f
    saturated fatty acid, 27-28, 28f-29f
    sterols, 31
    unsaturated fatty acid, 28-30, 29f
      essential fatty acids, 29-30
      nomenclature of, 28-29
      omega-3 and omega-6 fatty acids, 30
      trans-fatty acids, 30
  metabolism of, ethnic differences in, 38b
  and post-surgery healing, 393
Lipiduria, 376
Lipodystrophy, 431, 431b
Lipogenesis, 68
Lipoproteins, 30, 30f
  in fat metabolism, 329-330, 329f, 330t
  and post-surgery healing, 393
Liquid feedings, high-protein, high-kilocalorie
  formula for, 305t
Lister, Baron Joseph, 216
Listeria monocytogenes, 216, 220t
Listeriosis, 216
Liver
  bile production, 58, 60
  function of, 60, 61b
  portal circulation, 66
  storage of glycogen by, 13-14, 16, 21
Liver disease, 321-324
  cirrhosis, 322-324, 323f
  fatty, 321
  hepatitis, 321-322, 322b
Liver enzymes, tests during nutrition care
  process, 295
Living wills, 404b
Lobectomy, 321
Loop of Henle, 372, 372f, 373t
Low active lifestyle, 79b
Low birth weight infant, 156b, 173
Low blood sugar, 21
Low energy availability, causes of underweight,
  266
Low-density lipoproteins (LDLs), 30, 329, 329f
  increase in, 38
  niacin as treatment for high, 98b
Lower esophageal sphincter (LES), defects in, 307
Lower gastrointestinal (GI) tract, 312-318
  large intestine disease, 317-318
    constipation, 318
    diverticular disease, 317-318, 317f
    irritable bowel syndrome, 318
  small intestine diseases, 312-317
    cystic fibrosis, 312-314, 314b
    diarrhea, 316-317
    inflammatory bowel disease, 315-316, 315t,
      316f
    malabsorption, 312, 313t
    steatorrhea, 312

Lubricant, water as, 134
Lymphatic system, in transport, 66
Lymphocytes
  immune system functions of, 412-413, 413f
  post-surgery roles of, 393

M
Macronutrients
  absorption of, 65, 65t
  chemical and mechanical actions on, 56
  digestion of. see Digestion
  needs of older adults, 191-192
  restrictions, specific, 256
Macrosomia, 158, 349
Macular degeneration, vitamin A in prevention
  of, 85
Magnesium, 119, 121t
Major minerals, 110, 111b, 121t
  calcium, 111-114, 112f, 113b, 114t, 115b, 115f
  chloride, 118-119
  magnesium, 119
  phosphorus, 114-116
  potassium, 117-118, 118t
  sodium, 116-117, 116f
  sulfur, 119-120
Malabsorption, 312, 313t
  causes of, 266
  radiation therapy causing, 414
Males. see Men
Malnutrition, 5
  in America, 223-224
  causes of, 223f, 266
  characteristics of, 391t
  cycle of, 223, 224f
  defined, 5
  in elderly women, individual approach for,
    197b
  HIV-related, 430
  in hospitalized patients, 390
  hunger and, 223-224
  in older adults, in long-term care facilities, 267b
  in oral tissue inflammation, 304-305
  treatments for, 266
  worldwide, 223
Mammary glands, 159-161
Manganese, 129, 130t
Marasmus, 51-52
Margarine, 30, 33
Masculinization, 287
Mastication, 22-23
Maternal blood volume, protein needs for, 148
Maternal tissues, growth of, protein needs, 148
Meal patterns, changing food behaviors, 262b
Meal planning, 264
Meat
  calcium in, 114t
  and cancer, 421
  cobalamin in, 102t
  folate in, 100t
  intake for different calorie levels, 260t-261t
  invisible fat in, 33
  iron in, 124t
  niacin in, 98t
  pantothenic acid in, 103t
  potassium in, 118t
  pyridoxine in, 99t
  riboflavin in, 97t
  as saturated fat, 27-28, 29f
  thiamin in, 96t
  visible fat in, 33
  vitamin A in, 87t
  vitamin D in, 90t
  vitamin E in, 91t
  zinc in, 127t
Mechanical digestion, 56-58
  in mouth and esophagus, 58
  in small intestine, 59
  in stomach, 58
Mechanical soft diet, 304
MedGem device, 74, 74f
Medical marijuana, 416b
Medical nutrition therapy (MNT), 289
  for acute kidney injury, 377-378
  for burn patients, 409-410
  for cancer patient, 414-420
  for chronic kidney disease, 379, 385t
  for coronary heart disease, 334-335, 335b

Medical nutrition therapy (MNT) (Continued)
  defining in therapeutic process model, 289
  for diabetes mellitus, 361-362
  for end-stage renal disease, 380-385
  for hemodialysis, 381-382
  for HIV patient, 430-432
  for hypertension, 340-343, 342t, 343b
  for kidney disease, 375
  for kidney stones, 388-389, 388t
  for pulmonary edema, 336-338
Medications
  polypharmacy by older adults, 300
  and water requirement, 135
Mediterranean diet, 37, 335-336, 338f, 422
  heart disease and, 239b
Mediterranean Diet Pyramid, 238f
Mediterranean food habits, 235-238
Megaloblastic anemia, 104t
  macrocytic, 100
Melatonin, 190
Membranes
  capillary, 139-140
  cell, 140
Men
  healthy weight range of, 249
  PA coefficient in, 75b, 79b
  recommended energy intake for, 81t
Menaquinone, 92b
Menkes' disease, 128-129
Menopause, 190
Mental health, benefits of physical activity for,
  275b, 277
Mercury, 222
Metabolic needs, and water requirement, 135
Metabolic syndrome, 331, 331t, 351-352
  benefits of exercise for prevention of, 275b
Metabolism, 3, 56, 66-68, 68f, 73
  changes with aging, 190
  errors in, 68-70
    galactosemia, 68-69
    glycogen storage disease, 69
    phenylketonuria, 68
  mineral, 111
    absorption, 111
    calcium in, 112
    digestion, 111
    iron in, 120
    magnesium in, 119
    occurrence in body, 111
    phosphorus in, 114
    potassium in, 117
    sulfur in, 119
    tissue uptake, 111
    transport, 111
  role of ascorbic acid in, 94
  role of proteins in, 44
  role of vitamins in, 84
Metalloenzymes, zinc and, 126
Metastasis, 411
Methionine, 119
Methyl mercury, 222
Methylcobalamin, 101
Methylcrotonyl-CoA carboxylase, 103
Mexican, 230, 231t
Micelle formation, 35-36
Microalbuminuria, 356
Microbiome, 317
Micronutrients
  absorption of, 65, 65t
  bioavailability of, and competitive absorption,
    63b
  and mechanical and chemical digestion, 56
Microvilli
  in absorption, 64
  brush border, 64
Middle adults (45 to 64 years old), psychosocial
  development of, 189
Mifflin-St. Jeor equation, 74, 75b, 263b
Milk
  American diet of, 106b
  anemia, 182
  calcium in, 113-114, 114t
  content, for premature infants, 173
  delivery, methods of, 173-174
  and Dietary Guidelines for Americans, 9f
  lactose in, 14
  pantothenic acid in, 103t

Milk (Continued)
  potassium in, 118t
  production, physiology of, 162f
  and rennin, 48
  riboflavin in, 97t
  versus supplements, calcium from, 115b
  vitamin A in, 87t
  vitamin D in, 90t
  whole, invisible fat in, 33
  zinc in, 127t
Minerals, 110-132
  absorption of, 17b
  classes of, 110
  as coenzyme factors, 5
  depletion of, medications in, 131b
  digestion of, 56
  functions of, 110
  in human nutrition, 110-111
  major, 110, 111b, 121t
    calcium, 111-114, 112f, 113b, 114t, 115b, 115f
    chloride, 118-119
    magnesium, 119
    phosphorus, 114-116
    potassium, 117-118, 118t
    sodium, 116-117, 116f
    sulfur, 119-120
  metabolism of, 111
    absorption, 111
    digestion, 111
    occurrence in body, 111
    tissue uptake, 111
    transport, 111
  needs
    for growth, 171-172
    during pregnancy, 149-150
  and postoperative wound healing, 394
  regulation and control functions of, 5
  supplementation of, 131-132
  trace, 110, 111b, 130t
    chromium, 129
    copper, 128-129
    fluoride, 128, 128f
    iodine, 123-125, 124f-125f
    iron, 120-123, 122f-123f, 123t-124t
    manganese, 129
    molybdenum, 129
    other essential, 129
    selenium, 127-128
    zinc, 126-127, 126b, 127f, 127t
Mini Nutritional Assessment, 194, 195f-196f
Moderately active lifestyle, physical activity (PA)
  coefficient, 263b
Molybdenum, 129, 130t
MONA protocol, 334
Monitoring and evaluation, in nutrition care
  process model, 299-300
Monosaccharides, 13-14, 13f, 13t
  disaccharides converted into, 60
  fructose, 14, 14f
  galactose, 14
  glucose, 14
Monounsaturated fats, 28, 28f-29f
  cardio-protective, 37
"Morning sickness", 152
Mouth
  problems in, 304-307
  role in digestion, 22-23, 24f, 58
    fat, 34, 35f
    protein, 47, 50f
  signs of nutrient imbalance in, 296t-297t
  surgery of, 404-405
  xerostomia, 138, 270
Mucilages, 16t
Mucosal folds, and absorption, 64
Mucosal protectors, for peptic ulcer disease, 311
Mucositis, 414, 418t-419t
Mucus, secretions of, and digestion, 58-59
Multiple-day food record, 293t
Muscle mass, as energy storage, 73
Muscle strengthening
  for children and adolescents, 272
  for physical fitness, 272, 273b
Muscles
  actions
    calcium in, 112
    energy needed for, 279-280
    magnesium in, 119

Muscles (Continued)
    potassium in, 117
    sodium in, 116
  in digestion, 56-57
Musculoskeletal extremities, signs of nutrient
  imbalance in, 296t-297t
Muslim, dietary laws, 240-241
  influence of festivals, 241
Mutation, 411
Myelomeningocele, 100f
Myocardial infarction (MI), 327-328
  cardiac rest, as objective, 334
  long-term dietary modifications, 335-336
  medical nutrition therapy in, 334-335, 335b
MyPlate, 7, 8f, 80
  on carbohydrates, 25
  on fats, 39
  on proteins, 54
  on weight management, 264
  on young children, 178, 180f-181f
Myxedema, 125

N
Nails
  signs of nutrient imbalance in, 296t-297t
  sulfur and, 119
National Health and Nutrition Examination
  Survey (NHANES)
  on adequate water intake, 134
  on social disparities and dental status, 305b
  on sodium consumption, 116-117
  on US fruit and vegetable consumption, 19
National Organic Program, 208b
National School Lunch program, 225
Native American, food habits, 231-233, 231t
Natural foods, 208, 264
Natural toxins, as food contaminants, 222-223
Nausea
  with cancer, 414
  cannabis to treat, 415-416, 416b
  "morning sickness", 152-153
  nutrition management of, 418t-419t
Neck surgery, 404-405
Negative energy balance, 256, 258
Neonatal abstinence syndrome (NAS), 156
Neoplasm, definition of, 411
Nephritic syndrome, 375, 375t
Nephrolithiasis, 386
Nephron
  description and illustration of, 371, 372f, 373t
  diseases of
    acute glomerulonephritis, 375, 375t
    nephritic syndrome, 375, 375t
    nephrotic syndrome, 375-376, 375t
Nephropathy, 356
Nephrosis, 375
Nephrotic syndrome, 375-376, 375t
Nephrotoxic drugs, 374, 374b
Nerves
  and calcium, 112
  and digestion, 57
Net protein utilization, 49, 51t
Neural tube defects (NTDs), 100
  folate and, 150
Neuropathy, 356
  with dialysis, 386
Niacin, 97-98, 97f, 98b, 98t, 104t
Nicotinamide, 104t
Nicotine, as pregnancy risk factor, 156
Nicotinic acid, 104t
Nipples, cleaning, 175
Nitrate (beet juice), 286b
Nitrogen
  balance with cancer, 414
  protein as primary source of, 41
  retention with kidney disease, 378
Nonambulatory patients, alternative measures
  for, 294b
Noncellulose polysaccharides, 17-20
Nonheme iron, 123, 123t
Non-nucleoside reverse transcriptase inhibitors,
  427t-429t
Nonnutritive sweeteners, 20
Nonresidue elemental formulas, 392
Nonsteroidal antiinflammatory drugs (NSAIDs)
  drug-nutrient interaction of, 198b
  for peptic ulcer disease, 309

Noroviruses, 220*t*
Nucleoside reverse transcriptase inhibitors, 426, 427*t*-429*t*
Nurses, role in nutrition care process, 288-289
Nursing bottle caries. *see* Baby bottle tooth decay
Nursing diagnosis, 288
Nursing homes, 200-201
Nursing process, 290
Nutraceuticals, 108
Nutrient
  absorption of
    acidity for, 59*b*
    sodium in, 116
  balance, 263
  density, 72
  drug-nutrient interactions, 301, 301*b*
  energy-yielding, 3
  essential, 3
  functions in food, 3-5
  needs, during lactation, 163
  nonessential, 3
  recommended intake of, 4, 4*f*
  signs indicating imbalances, 296*t*-297*t*
  standards for, 5-7
    Dietary Reference Intakes, 6-7
  and tissue building, 4
Nutrition, 1, 272-287
  across the life cycles. *see* Growth and development
  for adults, 186-201
  definition of, 1
  diagnosis, 297-298
  drug-nutrient interactions, 301
  and immune system, 413
  during infancy, childhood, and adolescence, 166-185
  during lactation, 147-165
  during pregnancy, 147-165
  signs of good, 2-3
  signs of nutrient imbalance in, 296*t*-297*t*
  six essential nutrients in human, 3
  study of, importance of, 1
  support and nursing process. *see* Nutrition care process model
  ten red flags for junk foods, 266*b*
  Therapeutic Process, 288-290
Nutrition care process model, 288, 289*f*. *see also* Nutrition care
  anthropometric measurements of, 293-295
  client history, 295-297
  coordination of nutrition care, 299
  diet-drug interactions, 300-301, 300*t*
  drug-food interactions, 300-301
  drug-herb interactions, 301
  drug-nutrient interactions, 301, 301*b*
  food and/or nutrient delivery, 298-299
  health care team and, 288-290
  history, 292*b*
  nutrition education and counseling, 299
  nutrition-focused physical findings and, 295
  person-centered care and, 291-293
  phases of, 291-300
    food- and nutrition-related history, 291-293
    monitoring and evaluation, 299-300
    nutrition diagnosis, 297-298
    nutrition intervention categories, 298-299
  physician and support staff, 289
  problem, 297
  registered dietitians (RDs)
    qualifications of, 290*b*
  roles of nurse and clinical dietitian, 289-290
  signs and symptoms of, 298
  signs of nutrient imbalance in, 296*t*-297*t*
  strengths and limitations of techniques, 293*t*
  Therapeutic Process, 288-290
Nutrition facts label, 204-205, 204*f*, 205*b*
Nutrition information, FDA food label information, 203
Nutrition science, definition of, 1
Nutrition Services Incentive Program, 198, 225
Nutrition support
  conditions require, 395*t*-396*t*
  process of. *see* Nutrition care process model
  route of administration for, 397*f*
  with surgery, 390-410
Nutritional states, 5
Nutritive sweeteners, 20

Nuts
  calcium in, 114*t*
  cobalamin in, 102*t*
  and daily fiber recommendations, 19
  folate in, 100*t*
  iron in, 124*t*
  niacin in, 98*t*
  pantothenic acid in, 103*t*
  potassium in, 118*t*
  pyridoxine in, 99*t*
  riboflavin in, 97*t*
  thiamin in, 96*t*
  as unsaturated dietary fat, 28, 29*f*
  vitamin A in, 87*t*
  vitamin D in, 90*t*
  vitamin E in, 91*t*
  zinc in, 127*t*

O
Obesity. *see also* Weight loss; Weight management
  adolescents, 245, 246*f*
  in adults, 196*f*
  benefits of exercise for prevention of, 275*b*
  cancer risks with, 421
  causes of, 250-252
    genetic and environmental factors, 250-252
    hormonal control, 250
  in childhood, 182-183, 183*b*, 183*f*
  clinically severe, 250
  and *Dietary Guidelines for Americans*, 9*f*
  and health, 250
  high-protein diets, 53*b*, 54*t*
  and overnutrition, 5
  predisposition for, genetics and, 251, 252*b*
  as pregnancy risk factor, 154
  surgery and, 257
  trends in, 246*f*
  and weight control, 245-258
Oils
  American diet consumption of, 106*b*
  intake for different calorie levels, 260*t*-261*t*
  vitamin A in, 87*t*
  vitamin D in, 90*t*
  vitamin E in, 91*t*
Older adults
  alternative living arrangements for, 200-201
  benefits of exercise for, 273, 275*b*
  chronic disease in, reducing risk for, 193
  clinical needs of, 193-198
  community resources for, 198-200
  dehydration in, 138
  feeding, with sensitivity, 194*b*
  individual approach for, 197
  medications for, 197-198, 198*b*
  nutritional status, 193-194
  physical activities
    benefits of, 197*b*
    physical fitness goals, 273
  psychosocial development of, 189
  quality of life of, 189*f*
  vitamin supplementation for, 107
  weight loss problems in long-term care facilities, 267*b*
  weight management and physical activity in, 194-197
Older Americans Act, 198-199
Oleic acid, 28*f*, 30
Oliguria, 375, 375*t*
Olive oil, 29*f*, 32
Omega-3 fatty acids, 30, 38
  supplements, for pancreatic cancer patients, 417
  and vegetarians, 46-47, 48*t*
Omega-6 fatty acids, 30
"One-Step" method, 158
Opportunistic infections, 425*b*
Optimal nutrition, 5, 358
Oral feedings
  following surgery, 395-397, 398*b*
  with mouth, throat, and neck surgery, 404
Oral glucose tolerance test, 158
Oral rehydration therapy, principles of, 142*b*
Oral tissue inflammation, 304-305, 305*f*
Organic compounds, small, and water balance, 139
Organic farming, 207-208
Organic food standards, 208*b*

Organic seal, 207-208, 207*f*
Orlistat, 256-257, 257*b*
Osmosis, 140, 140*f*
Osmotic pressure, 44, 140
Osteoblasts, 277
Osteodystrophy, 378, 386
Osteopenia, 192
Osteoporosis, 112, 112*f*, 192
  calcitriol for, 88
  in gender and racial groups, 113*b*
Outcomes, in nutrition care process model, 299
Overnutrition, 5
Overweight
  in adults, 196*f*
  in childhood, 183*b*, 183*f*
  defining *versus* obesity, 245
  and health problems, 250
Ovo-vegetarians, 45
Oxalate foods, and drinks, 387*b*, 388
Oxidation, 84
Oxygen, dietary needs during exercise, 279
Oxygen-carrying capacity (VO$_2$ max), 275
Oxytocin, 161

P
Pacific Islanders. *see* Cultural considerations
Pain, 416, 420
Palmitic acid, 28*f*
Pancreas
  in carbohydrate digestion, 23
  and diabetes, 351
  disease in, 325
  enzymes from
    in digestion, 60
    role in fat digestion, 34-35, 35*f*-36*f*
  and intestinal enzymes in digestion, 59
  in protein digestion, 48-49, 50*f*
Pancreatic amylase, 60
Pancreatic hormonal control, diabetes and, 353-355, 354*f*
Pancreatic lipase, 60
Pancreatitis, 325
Pandemic, 423
Pantothenic acid, 102, 103*t*-104*t*
Parasites, 423
  food-borne disease, 219
Parenteral feeding, 401-402
  definition of, 390
  determining during nutrition care process, 299
Parenteral nutrition support, for cancer patients, 420
Parity, as pregnancy risk factor, 154
Parotid glands, 306
Pasta
  calcium in, 114*t*
  folate in, 100*t*
  iron in, 124*t*
  niacin in, 98*t*
  pantothenic acid in, 103*t*
  potassium in, 118*t*
  pyridoxine in, 99*t*
  riboflavin in, 97*t*
  thiamin in, 96*t*
  vitamin E in, 91*t*
  zinc in, 127*t*
Patient Self-Determination Act of 1991, 404*b*
Pectins, 16*t*
Pellagra, 97, 97*f*, 104*t*
Pepsin, 48, 59
Peptic ulcer disease (PUD), 308-312, 309*f*, 310*b*-311*b*
Peptide hormones, 44
Percent daily value (% DV), 205
Percutaneous endoscopic gastrostomy, 399
Percutaneous endoscopic jejunostomy, 399
Peripheral parenteral nutrition, 401-402, 402*f*
Peristalsis, 23, 56-57
Peritoneal cavity, 382
Peritoneal dialysis, 382, 383*f*
Pernicious anemia, and vitamin B$_{12}$, 102, 104*t*
Personal adaptation, 298
Personal needs, meeting, 278-279
Person-centered care, 10
  in nutrition care process model, 291-293
Pesticides, agricultural, 207-210

pH levels
  and proteins, 44
  respiratory control of, 145
  and uric acid stones, 389
  urinary control of, 145
  and water balance, 144-145
Pharynx, 306
Phenylketonuria (PKU), 42, 68
  and aspartame, 43b
Pheochromocytoma, 351
Phosphate, 377
Phospholipids, 30-31, 31f
  eicosanoids, 31
  lecithin, 30-31
Phosphorus, 114-116, 121t
  homeostasis, vitamin D in, 88
Photosynthesis, 12
Phylloquinone, 91
Physical activity. *see also* Exercise; Physical fitness
  activities of daily living (ADLs), 278
  cancer risks with, 421
  for diabetes, 358-359
  energy expenditure in, 76-77
  fitness levels and body fat percentages, 249f
  health benefits and, 273-277, 273b, 275b
    for blood lipid levels, 274, 275b
    for bone disease, 275b, 277
    for diabetes, 275, 275b
    for heart muscle function, 274
    for hypertension, 275, 275b
    for mental health, 275b, 277
    for oxygen-carrying capacity (VO₂ max), 275, 275b
    for weight management, 275, 275b
  for hypertension, 340-341
  for older adults, 194-197
    benefits of, 197b
  Physical Activity Guidelines for Americans, 190, 272
  recommendations and benefits of, 272-279
  total energy expenditure and, 78f
  and water requirement, 134
Physical activity (PA) coefficient
  estimating resting energy needs, 75b
  on weight management, 263b
Physical Activity Guidelines for Americans, 190, 272
Physical activity pyramid, 274f
Physical Activity Readiness Questionnaire, 273, 276f
Physical fitness, 272-287. *see also* Physical activity
  aerobic benefits, achieving and, 278-279, 279t
  and athletic performance, 282-287
    carbohydrate loading, 284
    competition, 284-285
    general training diet, 282-284
    hydration, 285
    pregame meal, 284-285, 285b
  defining, 272
  goals and guidelines for achieving, 272
  macronutrient and micronutrient recommendations, 281
  muscle strengthening, 272
  types of activities
    activities of daily living, 278
    aerobic exercises for, 277, 277t
    resistance training, 277
    weight-bearing exercise, 277-278
  vitamins and minerals needed, 281
Physiologic buffer systems, and water balance, 145
Physiologic changes, in aging process, 190-191
Phytic acid, and mineral absorption, 17b
Phytochemicals, 105-106
Phytosterols, 31
Pica, as pregnancy risk factor, 156-157
Pinocytosis, 64f, 65, 141
Placenta, development of, protein needs, 148
Plant fats, 33
Plaque, 327
Plasma proteins
  tests during nutrition care process, 295
  and water balance, 139
Plateaus, in weight management, 262b
Polarity, of water, 133
Polydipsia, 136
Polymeric formula, 316
Polypeptides, 48

Polypharmacy, 197
Polysaccharides, 15-20
  cellulose, 16
  dietary fibers, 16
  glycogen, 4, 16
  lignin, 16-17
  noncellulose, 17-20
  starch, 15
Polyunsaturated fats, 28, 28f-29f
Polyuria, 139
Poor living situation, causes of underweight, 266
Portal circulation, 23, 66
Portal hypertension, 322
Portion sizes, in eating, 243
Potassium, 117-118, 121t, 377, 379, 381, 385t
Poultry
  calcium in, 114t
  cobalamin in, 102t
  folate in, 100t
  intake for different calorie levels, 260t-261t
  iron in, 124t
  niacin in, 98t
  pantothenic acid in, 103t
  potassium in, 118t
  pyridoxine in, 99t
  riboflavin in, 97t
  thiamin in, 96t
  vitamin A in, 87t
  vitamin D in, 90t
  vitamin E in, 91t
  zinc in, 127t
Poverty
  and cancer percentage, 412b
  and food insecurity, 6b
  and undernutrition, 5
  and underweight individuals, 266
Prebiotic, 316
Prediabetes, 351, 361-362
  syndrome, 196-197
Pre-eclampsia, 157
  superimposed on chronic hypertension, 157
Preexisting diseases, pregnancy and, 158
Pregame meal, 284-285, 285b
Pregnancy
  complications of, 157-158
  daily food plan for, 149t, 152
  folate requirements during, 99-100
  gastrointestinal problems during, 152-153
  hypertensive disorders of, 157-158
  increased basal energy expenditure in, 75-76
  mineral supplements during, 131
  nutritional demands of, 147-152
    energy needs, 147-148
    key mineral and vitamin needs, 149-151
    protein needs, 148-149
  nutrition-related risk factors in, 153, 154b
  positive nitrogen balance in, 43
  recommended energy intake during, 81t
  risk factors for, 153-154
  special counseling needs in, 154-157
    age and parity, 154
    alcohol, 154-156
    caffeine, 156
    drugs, 156
    nicotine, 156
    obesity, 154
    pica, 156-157
    socioeconomic difficulties, 157
  teenage, 154, 155b, 155f
  vitamin supplementation during, 107
  weight gain during, 151-152, 151f, 151t-152t
Prehypertension, 339-340, 340t
Premature infants, 173
  feeding considerations for, 173-174
  milk content for, 173
Preschool-aged children (3 to 5 years old), nutrition requirements of, 178
Prescription medications, 302b
Pressure sores, increased need for proteins for, 50-51
Prevention, goals of *Healthy People 2020*, 2
Primary hypertension, 338-339
Probiotic, 316
Processed foods
  and cancer, 421
  high-fructose sugars in, 14, 14f
Proenzymes, 47

Professional organizations and resources, for older adults, 199-200
  community groups, 199-200
  national groups, 199
  volunteer organizations, 200
Prohormone, 87
Prolactin, 161
  inhibitors, 163
Propionyl-CoA carboxylase, 103
Propofol, and lipids, 403b
Proportionately small for gestational age (pSGA), 173
Prostate cancer, recent research findings regarding, 422
Protease inhibitors, 427t-429t
Proteases, 44
Protein efficiency ratio, 50, 51t
Protein-energy malnutrition (PEM), 390-391, 391b
Proteins, 41-55, 281, 286b
  absorption of, 60-63
  American diet consumption of, 106b
  amino acids
    as building blocks of, 41
    classes of, 41-42, 42b
    conditionally indispensable, 41-42, 42b
    dispensable, 41-42, 42b
    indispensable, 41-42, 42b
  balance, 42-43, 43f
  biologic value of, 49, 51t
  complementary, 45
  complete, 45
  concerns for vegetarians, 48t
  dietary guides, 52-54
    Dietary Guidelines for Americans, 52-54
    Dietary Reference Intakes (DRIs) for, 52, 53b
    MyPlate, 54
  dietary quality of, 49-50, 51t
  digestion of, 47-49, 50f, 60
  energy provided by, 4, 71, 284
  excess dietary intake of, 52
  food sources of, 44-47, 45f, 46b, 47f, 48t, 149
    types of, 44-45
  functions of, 44, 44b
    as body defense system, 44
    as energy system, 44
    in metabolism and transportation, 44
    tissue building as, 44
    and water and pH balance, 44
  and high-protein diets, 53b, 54t
  incomplete, 45
  intake for different calorie levels, 260t-261t
  and kidney disease, 377, 379, 382, 385t, 388
  metabolism of, role of carbohydrates in, 21
  nature of, 41-44
  needs
    of adults, 191, 192t
    for burn patients, 409
    for cancer patients, 416
    for growth, 171
    during lactation, 163
    during pregnancy, 148-149
    for wound healing, 392-393
  nutrient balance, 263
    for diabetes mellitus, 364
  preoperative reserves, 390-391
  protein-energy malnutrition, 51-52
  recommended intake of, 4, 4f
  synthesis, magnesium in, 119
  tissue building function of, 4
  in uncontrolled diabetes, 355
  vegetarian diets and, 45-47
    types of, 45-46
Proteinuria, with nephron diseases, 375, 375t
Proton pump inhibitors, for peptic ulcer disease, 310-311, 311b
Provitamin A, 86
Proximal tubules, 372, 372f, 373t
Psychologic influences, on food habits, 228, 229b
Psychosocial development
  adults, 189
  childhood, 167
Psychosocial support, for HIV, 432
Ptyalin, 58
Public health departments, 199

Public health nutritionist, 1
Puerto Rican, 230-231, 231t
Pulmonary edema, 336
Purging, 270
Pyloric valve, 58
Pyridine ring, 98
Pyridoxine, 98, 99t, 104t
Pyruvate carboxylase, 103

Q

Quality of life, goals for cancer patients, 416
Questran, and bile, 36b

R

Radiation therapy, nutritional complications with, 413-414, 413f
Radura symbol for irradiation, 209-210, 210f
Ramadan, 241
RDAs. see Recommended Dietary Allowances (RDAs)
Reabsorption, function of kidneys, 373
Realistic goals, diet and, 258
Recommended Dietary Allowances (RDAs), 6, 52, 84b, 225
Recovery after exercise, 285
Rectal surgery, 408
Refeeding syndrome, 317
Registered dietitians (RDs)
    definition of, 1
    qualifications of, 290b
    role of, 289-290
Religious dietary laws, 238-241, 242t
Renal calculi. see Kidney stones
Renal circulation, in water balance, 143
Renin, 143-144, 373
Renin-angiotensin-aldosterone system, 143-144, 144f, 373
Rennin, 48-49
Research centers, for older Americans, 199
Resistance training, 277
Resistant hypertension, 343
Resorption, bone, 112-113
    vitamin D and, 88
Respiration, chloride in, 118
Resting energy expenditure (REE), 73
    equations for estimating, 75b
    measurement of, 73-74, 73f-74f
    prediction of, 74
Resting metabolic rates, tests during nutrition care process, 295
Retinoic acid, 85
Retinol. see Vitamin A
Retinopathy, 355-356
Rhodopsin, 85
Riboflavin, 96, 97t, 104t
Rice
    calcium in, 114t
    folate in, 100t
    iron in, 124t
    niacin in, 98t
    pantothenic acid in, 103t
    potassium in, 118t
    pyridoxine in, 99t
    riboflavin in, 97t
    thiamin in, 96t
    vitamin E in, 91t
    zinc in, 127t
Rickets, 89, 89f, 112
Risk factors, and health promotion, 2
Rooting reflex, 174, 174f
Routine house diets, 396-397, 398t
Rules of Kashrut, 238

S

Saccharides, definition of, 13
Salivary amylase, 22-23, 58-59
Salivary glands
    in digestion, 58
    disorders of, 306
    location of, 306f
Salmon, Daniel, 215
Salmonella, 215, 220t
Salmonellosis, 215-216
Salt, 117, 125
Sarcopenia, 190
Satiety, from fats, 32
Satisfaction, from fats, 32

Saturated fat, excess in, 37
Saturated fatty acids, 27-28, 28f-29f
    foods high in, 32-33
"Sauna suits", 256
School Breakfast and Lunch Programs, 180, 225
School meals program, 225
School-aged children (5 to 12 years old), nutrition requirements of, 178-180
Scientifically, thinking, 265-266
Screen time, 178
Scurvy, 83, 94f, 104t
Secondary hypertension, 338-339
Secretin, 60
Sedentary lifestyle, 79b
    avoidance of, 272
    PA coefficient and, 75b
Selenium, 127-128, 130t
    metabolism of, vitamin E in, 90
Selenoproteins, 127
Self-care
    for diabetes mellitus management, 359-361
    and lifestyle. see Lifestyle
Senescence, 191
Senior farmers' market nutrition program, 199
Sepsis, 394
Serum protein-bound iodine, 124
Seventh-Day Adventists, vegetarian diets of, 45
Shiga, Kiyoshi, 216
Shigella, 220t
Shigella dysenteriae, 216
Shigellosis, 216
Shock, 393, 408-409
Significant obesity, 250
Simple carbohydrates, 13
Simple diffusion, 64f, 65
Skeletal system integrity, tests during nutrition care process, 295
Skin
    signs of nutrient imbalance in, 296t-297t
    sulfur and, 119
    vitamin D and, 88f
Small for gestational age (SGA), 152, 173
Small intestine
    absorption in, 63-65, 63f
    in digestion, 59-60
    diseases in, 312-317
        cystic fibrosis of, 312-314, 314b
        diarrhea of, 316-317
        inflammatory bowel disease of, 315-316, 315t, 316f
        malabsorption in, 312, 313t
        steatorrhea in, 312
    enzymes in role in fat digestion, 35
    roles of
        in carbohydrate digestion, 23, 24f
        in fat digestion, 34-37, 35f
        in protein digestion, 48-49, 50f
Smoking
    ascorbic acid needs and, 95b
    cancer and, 421
    vitamin supplementation and, 107
Social influences, on food habits, 228-229, 229b
Sociodemographics
    and heart disease, 344b-345b
    and kidney disease, 374b
Socioeconomics
    difficulties, as pregnancy risk factor, 157
    and health of older adults, 189-190, 267b
    poverty. see Poverty
Sodium, 116-117, 116f, 121t
    Dietary Guidelines for Americans, 9f
    food sources of, 117
    in hypertension, 343
    recommendation with kidney disease, 377, 379, 381, 385t, 388
    restriction, for myocardial infarction, 336, 336b-337b
Sodium phosphate, 286b
Soft diets, with mouth, throat, and neck surgery, 404
Solid foods
    additions, 176-177, 176t
        summary guidelines for, 177
    iron-fortified, 176
Solute particles, in solution, 138-139

Solvent, water as, 133, 136-138
Somatostatin, 354-355
Sorbitol, 20
Sound knowledge, lack of, in food fads, 265
Southeast Asian, food habits, 234-235, 237t
Spanish, food habits, 230-233, 231t
Special Milk Program, 225
Special Supplemental Food Program for Women, Infants, and Children, 225
Speech-language pathologist, 306
Spina bifida, 150-151
    with folate deficiency, 100, 100f
Sports. see Athletics; Physical fitness
Sports drinks, 280b, 285
Staphylococcal food poisoning, 217-218, 218b
Staphylococcus aureus, 220t
Starch, 15
    as carbohydrate food source, 21
    and carbohydrate loading, 281
    in nutrient balance, for diabetes mellitus, 362-363
State land grant universities, 199
Steatohepatitis, 321
Steatorrhea, 312
Steatosis, 321
Steroids, 31, 286-287
Sterols, 31
Stillbirth, 158
Stoma, 393, 407-408, 407f
Stomach
    in digestion, 58-59, 58f
    and duodenum, problems in, 308-312, 309f, 310b-311b
    roles of
        in carbohydrate digestion, 23, 24f
        in fat digestion, 34, 35f
        in protein digestion, 47-48, 50f
Stomatitis, 305, 305f, 418t-419t
Streptococcus, hemolytic, in mouth ulcers, 305
Stress
    in cancer patients, 416
    in glycemic control, 369
    of surgery, 394
Stress eating, 262b
Stroke. see Cerebrovascular accident
Struvite stones, 386f, 387
Sugar
    American diet consumption of, 106b
    as carbohydrate food source, 21
    classification of, 13
    Dietary Guidelines for Americans, 9f
    fructose, 14, 14f
    galactose, 14
    glucose, 14
    lactose, 14
    maltose, 14
    in nutrient balance, for diabetes mellitus, 362-363
    substitutes and sweeteners, 364
    sucrose, 14
    sweetness of, 21t
    U.S. consumption of, 14, 14f, 21
    vitamin A in, 87t
    vitamin D in, 90t
    vitamin E in, 91t
Sugar alcohols, 20
Sulfur, 119-120, 121t
Supersaturation, 386
Supplemental Nutrition Assistance Program (SNAP), 199, 224-225
Supplementation. see Dietary supplements
Surgery, 390-410
    advanced planning care and, 404b
    bariatric, 257, 405-407, 406b
    burn patient nutritional needs, 408-410
    for cancer, nutritional complications with treatments, 413
    emergency, 392
    gastrointestinal, 404-408
        bariatric surgery, 405-407, 406b
        dumping syndrome, 405
        gallbladder surgery, 407, 407f
        gastrectomy, 405, 406b
        gastric surgery, 405
        intestinal surgery, 407-408, 407f
        mouth, throat, and neck surgery, 404-405
        rectal surgery, 408

Surgery (Continued)
    methods of feeding
        enteral, 390, 391b, 395, 395t-396t, 396b,
            399-401
        oral, 395, 397, 398b
        parenteral, 390, 395, 395t-396t, 396b, 401-402,
            403b
    nonresidue elemental formulas, 392
    nutrition needs
        postoperative, 392-394
        preoperative, 390-392
    nutrition support following, 395-402, 395t-396t
    weight loss and, 257-258, 405, 406b
Swallowing disorders, 306-307
Sweeteners, 364
    nonnutritive, 20
    nutritive, 20
    sweetness of, 21t
Systolic blood pressure, 275, 339

T
Tanita bioelectrical impedance analysis, 247f
Taste
    nutrition management and, 418t-419t, 419-420
    radiation therapy affecting, 414
T cells, and cancer, 412-413, 413f
Teaching opportunities, remaining alert to, 265
Technology, food, 207-210
    agricultural pesticides, 207-210
    biotechnology, 208-209, 209f
    food additives, 210, 211t-212t
    irradiation, 209-210, 210f
    organic farming, 207-208
Teenage pregnancy, 154, 155b, 155f
Temperatures, for cooking various foods, 213,
    213f
Teratogen, 156
    vitamin A as, 86-87
Teratogenic effect, 149
Term infants, 173
Terminal sterilization method, 175
Tetracycline, and mineral absorption, 311b
Tetrahydrofolic acid (TH₄), 99, 150
Therapeutic Lifestyle Changes (TLC) diet, 333
Thermic effect, of food, 73, 77, 251f
    total energy expenditure and, 78f
Thermoregulation, water for, 134
Thiamin (vitamin B₁), 95-96, 96t, 104t
Throat, 404-405
Thrush, 305, 424-425
Thyroid function tests, for basal energy
    expenditure, 74
Thyroid-stimulating hormone (TSH), 111
Thyrotropin, 111
Thyrotropin-releasing hormone (TRH), 124
Thyroxine (T₄), 74-76, 123-124, 124f
Tissues
    building of, 4
        role of fatty acids in, 4
        role of proteins, 4, 44
        role of vitamins and minerals in, 4
    and protein balance, 42-43
    structure and protection, vitamins in, 84
    turnover, 43
    uptake, of mineral, 111
Tocopherol. see Vitamin E
α-Tocopherol, 90
Toddlers (1 to 3 years old), nutrition
    requirements of, 178
Tolerable upper intake level, 7
    antioxidants in cancer patients, 417
    for calcium, 113
    for major minerals, 121t
    for trace minerals, 130t
Tooth, formation of
    calcium in, 111-112
    phosphorus in, 114
Total Diet Study, 202
Total energy balance, for diabetes mellitus,
    362
Total energy expenditure (TEE), 77-79, 78f, 78t
    equations for estimating, 75b
    median values according to age and gender,
        81t
Total lymphocyte count, tests during nutrition
    care process, 295
Toxins, and nephrotoxic drugs, 374

Trace minerals, 110, 111b, 130t
    chromium, 129
    copper, 128-129
    fluoride, 128, 128f
    iodine, 123-125, 124f-125f
    iron, 120-123, 122f-123f, 123t-124t
    manganese, 129
    molybdenum, 129
    other essential, 129
    selenium, 127-128
    zinc, 126-127, 126b, 127f, 127t
Trans-fatty acids, 30
    Dietary Guidelines for Americans, 9f
    and health, 38
Transferrin, 120, 122f
Transport
    mineral, 111
    nutrients, 56, 64f, 65-66
    water for, 134
Travel, in diet management, 368-369
Traveler's diarrhea, 316-317
Treadmill stress test, 334, 334f
Tributyrinase, 34, 59
Triglycerides, 27, 28f
    and absorption of fats, 35-36, 37f
    in fat metabolism, 330, 330t
    niacin as treatment for high, 98b
Triiodothyronine (T₃), 124, 124f
Tripeptide, 41
Trypsin, 49, 60
Tube feeding, calculating, 400, 400b
Tumors
    HIV related, 425
    malignant cancer, 411
"Two-Step" method, 158
Type 1 diabetes mellitus, 347-348
    dietary strategies for, 365t
    versus type 2, 350t
Type 2 diabetes mellitus, 348-349
    benefits of exercise for prevention of, 275, 275b
    dietary strategies for, 365t
    prevalence of, 349b, 349f
    risk factors for, 349b
    versus type 1, 350t
Tyramine diet, 414t

U
Ulcerative colitis (UC), 315t, 316, 316f
Ulcers
    in mouth, 305
    peptic, 308-312, 309f, 310b-311b
Ultraviolet (UV) light, and vitamin D, 87, 88f
Undernutrition, 5
Underweight, 266-271
    causes of, 266
    dietary treatment of, 266-268
    eating disorders. see Eating disorders
    extremes in, 266
    general causes and treatment, 266-268
    treatment of, 271
Unintentional weight loss, 189
United Nations Committee on World Food
    Security, 223
United States Department of Agriculture, 199
Unsaturated fatty acids, 28-30, 29f
    essential fatty acids, 29-30
    nomenclature of, 28-29
    omega-3 and omega-6 fatty acids, 30
    trans-fatty acids, 30
Upper gastrointestinal (GI) tract, 304-312
    dental problems, 304, 305b
        surgical procedures in, 304, 305t
    esophageal problems, 307-308
    gastroesophageal reflux disease, 307-308, 308f,
        308t
    hiatal hernia, 308, 309f
    lower esophageal sphincter defects, 307
    mouth problems, 304-307
    oral tissue inflammation, 304-305, 305f
    salivary glands disorders, 306, 306f
    stomach and duodenum disorders, 308-312,
        309f, 310b-311b
    swallowing disorders in, 306-307
Urea, 378
Uric acid, hyperuricosuria, 387
Uric acid stones, 386f, 387, 389
Urinary tract infection, 373-374, 374b

Urinary urea nitrogen excretion, tests during
    nutrition care process, 295
U.S. Department of Agriculture
    on food safety regulations, 203t
    intake for different calorie levels, 260t-261t
    and MyPlate, 7
    on protein intake in US, 52

V
Vaccine, for HIV, 426-430
Vagotomy, 405
Vascular system, in transport, 65-66
Vasculitis, 313
Vasopressin, 143
Vegans, 46
Vegetables
    American diet of, 106b
    calcium in, 114t
    and cancer, 421
    and daily fiber recommendations, 19
    Dietary Guidelines for Americans, 9f
    folate in, 100t
    intake for different calorie levels, 260t-261t
    iron in, 124t
    in lacto-ovo-vegetarian diet pyramid, 47f
    pantothenic acid in, 103t
    potassium in, 118t
    pyridoxine in, 99t
    vitamin A in, 87t
    vitamin C in, 95t
    vitamin E in, 91t
    vitamin K in, 92t
Vegetarian diets, 45-47
    nutrient considerations for, 48t
    types of, 45-46
Venous catheter, 381f
Very active lifestyle, 79b
Very low birth weight (VLBW) infant, 173
Very low-density lipoproteins (VLDLs), 329, 329f
Viandas, 230-231
Vibrio, 217
Vibrio parahaemolyticus, 220t
Vibrio vulnificus, 220t
Villi
    and absorption, 64
    loss with radiation therapy, 414
Viruses, food-borne disease, 219
Visible fat, 33
Vision, vitamin A in, 85
Visual purple, 85
Vitamin A, 85-87, 93t
    and cancer, 421
    deficiency, 86
    food sources of, 87, 87t
    functions of, 85-86
        for growth, 85
        for tissue strength and immunity, 85-86
        for vision, 85
    requirements, 86
        and body storage, 86
        food forms and units of measure in, 86
    stability of, 87
    toxicity, 86-87
Vitamin B₁, 95-96, 96t, 104t
Vitamin B₂, 96, 97t
Vitamin B₃, 97-98, 97f, 98b, 98t, 104t
Vitamin B₆, 98-99, 99t, 104t
    needs during hemodialysis, 382
Vitamin B₁₂, 101-102, 101f, 102t, 104t
    concerns for vegetarians, 46-47, 48t
    needs
        for adults, 193
        during hemodialysis, 382
Vitamin C, 93-95, 104t
    and cancer, 421
    in collagen synthesis, 84
    deficiency, 94, 94f
    and Dietary Reference Intakes, 6
    food sources of, 94-95, 95t
    functions of, 93-94
    importance of, during hemodialysis, 382
    importance of, postoperative, 394
    requirements, 94
    for scurvy, 83
    stability of, 94-95
    tissue building function of, 4
    toxicity, 94

Vitamin D, 87-89, 93t
  activation by kidneys, 373
  and cancer, 422
  concerns for vegetarians, 46-47, 48t
  deficiency, 89, 89f
  food sources of, 89, 90t
  functions of, 88
  needs
    for adults, 193
    for growth, 172
    during pregnancy, 151
  requirements, 88-89
  and rickets, 112
  stability of, 89
  toxicity, 89
Vitamin E, 89-91, 93t, 382, 417
  deficiency, 90
  food sources of, 90-91, 91t
  functions of, 90
  requirements, 90
  stability of, 90-91
  toxicity of, 90
Vitamin K, 91-92, 93t, 394
  deficiency, 92
  food sources of, 92, 92t
  functions of, 91-92
  needs, for growth, 172
  requirements, 92
  stability of, 92
  toxicity, 92
Vitamins, 83-109
  as coenzyme factor, 5
  definition of, 84
  Dietary Reference Intakes for, 85
  digestion of, 56
  discovery of, 83-84
  fat-soluble, 85, 93t
    vitamin A (retinol), 85-87, 86b, 86f, 87t
    vitamin D (calciferol), 87-89, 88f-89f, 90t
    vitamin E, 91-92, 91f, 92b
    vitamin E (tocopherol), 89-91, 91t
  functions of, 84-85
    as antioxidants, 84
    coenzymes and enzymes, 84
    in metabolism, 84
    in prevention of deficiency diseases, 84-85
    in tissue structure and protection, 84
  megadoses of, 108
  metabolism of, 85
  milligram and microgram measurements of, 84b
  and mineral needs
    in cancer patients, 417
    for exercise, 281
    for kidney disease, 377, 379, 382, 388
  and mineral needs, in burn patients, 409
  nature of, 83-85
  needs
    for growth, 171-172
    during pregnancy, 150-151
  phytochemicals, 105-106
  postoperative needs for, 394
  preoperative reserves, 392
  regulation and control functions of, 5
  structure, sulfur in, 119
  supplementation of, 106-108
    based on life cycle, 107
    based on lifestyle and health status, 107
    principles of, 107-108
  supplements, 172
  tissue building function of, 4
  water-soluble. see Water-soluble vitamins
Vomiting, 418t-419t
  during pregnancy, 152-153

W

Waist circumference, measuring during nutrition
    care process, 295
Walking
  benefits, 273
  intensity levels, 278f
Wasting
  cachexia, 415
  causes of, 266
  HIV related, 430-431

Water. see also Water balance
  absorption of, 65
  compartments of, 133
  functions of, 133-134
  as fundamental nutrient, 133
  intake of, 137-138, 138f
  intoxication from, 136, 136f
  needs
    adequate intake per day, 134-135, 134t
    age and, 135
    for growth, 171, 171t
    hydration of athletes, 280, 280b
    postoperative, 394
  output of, 138, 138f
  particles in, 133
  and pH balance, 44
  polarity of, 133
  regulation and control functions of, 5
  role in digestion, 58
  as solvent, 133, 136-138
  as unified whole, 133
Water balance, 133-146
  acids and bases on, 144-145, 145b
  active transport in, 141
  buffer systems for, 145
  capillary fluid shift mechanism in, 141
  compartments and, 137f, 137t
  and dehydration, 135-136, 136f
  diffusion in, 140, 140f
  distribution and, 136-137, 137f
  drug effects on, 135b
  electrolytes and, 138-139
  extracellular fluid and, 137, 137f, 137t
  facilitated diffusion in, 140
  filtration in, 141
  and gastrointestinal circulation, 141-143
  homeostasis and, 133
  hormonal controls in, 143-144
  intracellular fluid and, 137, 137f, 137t
  and kidney disease, 378
  and law of isotonicity, 142
  organ system circulation in, 141-143
  osmosis in, 140, 140f
  and pH, 145
  pinocytosis in, 141
  plasma proteins and, 139
  potassium and, 117
  and renal circulation, 143
  small organic compounds and, 139
  sodium and, 116, 116f
  solute particles in solution and, 138-139
  water intake and, 137-138, 138f, 139t
  water output and, 138, 138f, 139t
Water-soluble vitamins, 85, 93-105, 104t
  biotin, 102-103
  choline, 103-105
  cobalamin (vitamin B_{12}), 101-102, 101f, 102t
  folate, 99-101, 100f, 100t
  niacin (vitamin B_3), 97-98, 97f, 98b, 98t
  pantothenic acid, 102, 103t
  riboflavin (vitamin B_2), 96, 97t
  thiamin (vitamin B_1), 95-96, 96t
  vitamin B_6, 98-99, 99t
  vitamin C (ascorbic acid), 93-95, 94f, 95b, 95t
Weaning, 175
Weight. see also Weight management
  assessment during nutrition care process,
    294-295
  control, obesity and, 245-258
  extreme practices, 252-258
  extremes and health problems, 250
  healthy range of, 249-250
  individual energy balance levels, 252
  measurement and maintenance goals, 248-250
  median values according to age and gender, 81t
  obesity. see Obesity
Weight gain
  energy imbalance and, 77-78, 78b
  with hypothyroidism, 77b
  obesity. see Obesity
  during pregnancy, 151-152, 151f, 151t-152t
Weight loss
  bariatric surgery and, 257, 405, 406b
  comparison of select weight-loss programs,
    253t-255t

Weight loss (Continued)
  with dehydration, 136f
  eating disorders, 268
  energy imbalance and, 77-78
  and high-protein diets, 53b, 54t
  HIV related, 430
  overweight and health problems and,
    250
  problems in, in older adults, 267b
  protein-energy malnutrition, 390, 391b
  wasting. see Wasting
Weight management, 245-271
  benefits of physical activity for, 275, 275b
  case study of, 263b
  energy balance, 250
  for hypertension, 340
  obesity. see Obesity
  in older adults, 194-197
  preventive approach of, 264
  sound program, 258-264
    basic principles, 258
    basic strategies and actions, 258
    behavior modification, 258
    distribution balance, 263-264
    energy balance, 263
    food plan, 262-264
    portion control, 263-264
  underweight of, 266-271
    causes and treatment, 266-268
Weight-bearing exercise, benefits of, 277-278
Weir equation, 74
Wellness, 1-2
  definition of, 1-2
Wernicke's encephalopathy, 95-96
White blood cells, immune system functions of,
    412-413
Whole grains
  and cancer, 421
  and daily fiber recommendations, 19
  definition of, 15, 15f
  Dietary Guidelines for Americans, 9f, 24
  intake for different calorie levels, 260t-261t
Wilson's disease, 128-129
Women
  female athlete triad, 281, 283b
  healthy weight range of, 249
  PA coefficient in, 75b, 79b
  recommended energy intake for, 81t
Women, Infants, and Children (WIC) Food and
    Nutrition Services program, 155
Work, voluntary, 71
World Cancer Research Fund, guidelines for
    cancer prevention, 420-422
World Health Organization (WHO)
  on breastfeeding, 164
  growth charts, 167, 168f-169f
  on HIV clinical staging and classification,
    424
  in iodine-deficiency disorders, 124
  in osteoporosis, 113b
Worldwide malnutrition, 223
Wound healing, 393
  increased need for proteins for, 50-51

X

Xanthophylls, 86b
Xerophthalmia, 86
Xerosis, 86
Xerostomia, 138, 270, 418t-419t

Y

Young adults (20 to 44 years old), psychosocial
    development of, 189

Z

Zinc, 126-127, 127f, 127t, 130t
  barriers, 126b
  concerns for vegetarians, 46-47, 48t
  deficiency, 132
  food sources of, 127, 127t
  functions of, 126
  needs during hemodialysis, 382
  and postoperative wound healing, 394
Zoosterols, 31
Zymogen, 47